# Heptinstall's Pathology of the Kidney

Sixth Edition

# Heptinstall's Pathology of the Kidney

## Sixth Edition

## Volume Two

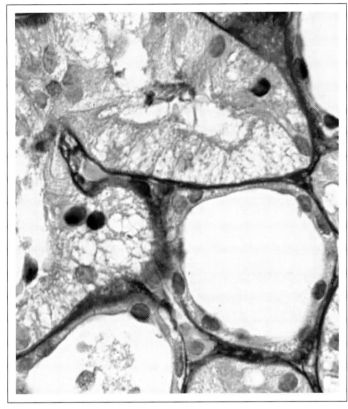

**EDITORS**

### J. CHARLES JENNETTE, MD

Department of Pathology and Laboratory Medicine
University of North Carolina at Chapel Hill
Chapel Hill, North Carolina

### JEAN L. OLSON, MD

Department of Pathology
University of California, San Francisco
San Francisco, California

### MELVIN M. SCHWARTZ, MD

Department of Pathology
Rush University Medical Center
Chicago, Illinois

### FRED G. SILVA, MD

US and Canadian Academy of Pathology
Adjunct Professor of Pathology
Emory University and The Medical College of Georgia
Augusta, Georgia

Lippincott Williams & Wilkins
a Wolters Kluwer business
Philadelphia • Baltimore • New York • London
Buenos Aires • Hong Kong • Sydney • Tokyo

*Acquisitions Editor:* Jonathan Pine
*Managing Editor:* Jean McGough
*Developmental Editor:* Dovetail Content Solutions
*Project Manager:* Bridgett Dougherty
*Senior Manufacturing Manager:* Benjamin Rivera
*Marketing Manager:* Angela Panetta
*Design Coordinator:* Steve Druding
*Production Service:* TechBooks
*Printer:* Walsworth Publishing Co.

© 2007 by LIPPINCOTT WILLIAMS & WILKINS
530 Walnut Street
Philadelphia, PA 19106 USA
LWW.com

**Library of Congress Cataloging-in-Publication Data**

Heptinstall's pathology of the kidney.—6th ed. / editors, J. Charles
    Jennette . . . [et al.].
      p. ; cm.
    Includes bibliographical references and index.
    ISBN-13: 978-0-7817-4750-9
    ISBN-10: 0-7817-4750-3
    1. Kidneys—Diseases.  2. Kidneys—Pathophysiology.    I. Jennette,
J. Charles.  II. Heptinstall, Robert H., 1920-   .  III. Title: Pathology
of the kidney.
    [DNLM: 1. Kidney Diseases—pathology.   WJ 300 H5295 2007]
RC903.9.H47 2007
616.6'2207—dc22
                                       2006023033

10 9 8 7 6 5 4 3 2 1

To my loving wife, Yvonne, my wonderful daughters, Jennifer and Caroline, and my amazing granddaughters, Olivia and Augusta.

J.C.J.

In loving memory of my parents, Caroline and Arthur Olson.

J.L.O.

To my wife, Lisa, for the hours taken from her.

M.M.S.

To my lovely wife, Jean, and our wonderful daughter, Lindsay.

F.G.S.

# Contents

# Contributors

**CORINNE ANTIGNAC, M.D.**
Institut National de la Santé et de la
Recherche Scientifique
Hôpital Necker–Enfants Malades
Paris, France

**LOIS J. AREND, M.D.**
Associate Professor and Director, Renal
Pathology and Electron Microscopy
Pathology and Laboratory Medicine
Department
University of Cincinnati Medical Center
Cincinnati, Ohio

**JAY BERNSTEIN, M.D,**
Past-Director and Chairman
Research Institute and Department
of Pathology
William Beaumont Hospital
Royal Oak, Michigan

**STEPHEN M. BONSIB, M.D.**
Director, Surgical Pathology
Pathology and Laboratory Medicine
Department
Indiana University School of Medicine
Indianapolis, Indiana

**ARTHUR H. COHEN, M.D.**
Professor
Pathology and Medicine Department
University of California,
Los Angeles School of Medicine
Director, Anatomic Pathology
Pathology Department
Cedars-Sinai Medical Center
Los Angeles, California

**ROBERT B. COLVIN, M.D.**
Benjamin Castleman Professor
of Pathology
Harvard Medical School
Chief of Pathology
Massachusetts General Hospital
Boston, Massachusetts

**VIVETTE D. D'AGATI, M.D.**
Professor
Pathology Department
Columbia University College of
Physicians and Surgeons
Director
Renal Pathology Laboratory
Columbia University Medical Center
New York, New York

**JOHN N. EBLE, M.D.**
Department of Pathology
Indiana University Medical Center
Indianapolis, Indiana

**LAURA S. FINN, M.D.**
Associate Professor
Pathology Department
University of Washington
Medical Center
Staff Pathologist
Department of Laboratories
Children's Hospital and Regional
Medical Center
Seattle, Washington

**AGNES B. FOGO, M.D.**
Professor of Pathology, Medicine,
and Pediatrics
Director, Renal/EM Laboratory
Pathology Department
Vanderbilt University Medical Center
Nashville, Tennessee

**DAVID J. GRIGNON, M.D.**
Professor and Chairman
Pathology Department
Wayne State University
Specialist-in-Chief
Pathology and Laboratory
Medicine Department
Detroit Medical Center
Detroit, Michigan

**MARIE-CLAIRE GUBLER, M.D.**
Institut National de la Santé et de la
Recherche Scientifique
Hôpital Necker–Enfants Malades
Paris, France

**MARK HAAS, M.D., Ph.D.**
Professor
Director, Renal Pathology and
Electron Microscopy
Pathology Department
Johns Hopkins Medical Institutions
Baltimore, Maryland

**LAURENCE HEIDET**
Institut National de la Santé et de la
Recherche Scientifique
Hôpital Necker–Enfants Malades
Paris, France

**GUILLERMO HERRARA, M.D.**
Chairman and Professor
Pathology Department
St. Louis University School of Medicine
Chief
Pathology Department
St. Louis University Health Center
St. Louis, Missouri

**MICHAEL HUGHSON, M.D.**
Professor
Pathology Department
Former Chair and Chief of Service
Pathology Department
University of Mississippi Medical Center
Jackson, Mississippi

**DAGAN JENKINS, B.Sc.**
PhD Student
Nephro-Urology Unit
Institute of Child Health
University College
London, United Kingdom

**J. CHARLES JENNETTE, M.D.**
Brinkhous Distinguished Professor
and Chair
Pathology and Laboratory
Medicine Department
University of North Carolina
at Chapel Hill
Chapel Hill, North Carolina

**MICHAEL KASHGARIAN, M.D.**
Professor
Pathology, Molecular, Cellular, and
Developmental Biology
Yale University
Director
Diagnostic Electron Microscopy
and Renal Pathology
Yale–New Haven Hospital
new Haven, Connecticut

**ZOLTAN G. LASZIK, M.D., Ph.D.**
Associate Professor
Pathology Department
University of California/San Francisco
San Francisco, California

**HELEN LIAPIS, M.D.**
Associate Professor of Pathology
and Immunology
Asssociate Professor of Internal
Medicine (Renal Division)
Washington University School
of Medicine
St. Louis, Missouri

**TIBOR NADASDY, M.D., Ph.D.**
Professor
Pathology Department
Ohio State University
Director of Renal Pathology
Pathology Department
Ohio State University Medical Center
Columbus, Ohio

**CYNTHIA C. NAST, M.D.**
Professor
Pathology Department
University of California, Los Angeles
Pathology Department
Cedars-Sinai Medical Center
Los Angeles, California

**VOLKER NICKELEIT, M.D.**
Associate Professor
Pathology Department
(Nephropathology Laboratory)
University of North Carolina
Medical School
Chapel Hill, North Carolina

**JEAN L. OLSON, M.D.**
Professor
Pathology Department
University of California,
San Francisco
San Francisco, California

**MARIA M. PICKEN, M.D., Ph.D**
Professor
Pathology Department
Director
Renal Pathology and Electron
Microscopy Laboratory
Loyola University Medical Center
Maywood, Illinois

**LORRAINE C. RACUSEN, M.D.**
Professor
Active Staff
Pathology Department
Johns Hopkins University School of
Medicine and Hospital
Baltimore, Maryland

**MELVIN M. SCHWARTZ, M.D.**
Otho S.A. Sprague
Professor of Pathology
Pathology Department
Rush University Medical Center
Chicago, Illinois

**DANIEL D. SEDMAK, M.D.**
Professor
Executive Vice-Dean, COM
Pathology Department
The Ohio State University
Columbus, Ohio

**FRED G. SILVA, M.D.**
Adjunct Professor
Pathology Department
Emory University and The Medical
College of Georgia
Atlanta, Georgia
Secretary-Treasurer and Executive
Vice President
U.S. and Canadian Academy of
Pathology
Augusta, Georgia

**HARSHARAN K. SINGH, M.D.**
Associate Professor
Director, Electron Microscopy Services
Pathology and Laboratory
Medicine Department
University of North Carolina School of
Medicine and Hospital
Chapel Hill, North Carolina

**DAVID B. THOMAS, M.D.**
Assistant Professor
Assistant Director, Nephropathology
Laboratory
Pathology and Laboratory
Medicine Department
University of North Carolina School
of Medicine and Hospital
Chapel Hill, North Carolina

**JOHN E. TOMASZEWSKI, M.D.**
Vice Chair for Anatomic Pathology–
Hospital Services
Professor of Pathology and
Laboratory Medicine
Hospital of the University
of Pennsylvania
Philadelphia, Pennsylvania

**MARK A. WEISS, M.D.**
Medical Director, Pathology Services
The Urology Group
Cincinnati, Ohio

**PAUL WINYARD, B.M., B.Ch., M.A.,
F.R.C.P.C.H., Ph.D.**
Senior Lecturer
Nephro-Urology Unit
Institute of Child Health
University College, London
Honorary Consultant
Renal Unit
Great Ormond Street Hospital for
Children NHS Trust
London, United Kingdom

**ADRIAN S. WOOLF, M.D.**
Professor
Nephro-Urology Unit
Institute of Child Health
University College, London
London, United Kingdom

**XIN J. ZHOU, M.D.**
Professor
Pathology and Internal
Medicine Department
Director, Division of Renal Pathology
University of Texas Southwestern
Medical Center
Dallas, Texas

# Preface

This sixth edition of *Heptinstall's Pathology of the Kidney* has the most dramatic and substantive changes in content of any new edition of this preeminent book on kidney diseases. Yet, still at the core of this edition is the bedrock foundation established by Robert H. Heptinstall, who edited and to a substantial degree authored the first four editions of this classic text. The sixth edition is in essence the 40th anniversary edition of this monumental and comprehensive work, which was first published in 1966.

Since the fifth edition, published in 1998, there have been extraordinary advances in the understanding of the molecular and cellular basis for many kidney diseases, in the knowledge of pathologic and clinical manifestations of kidney diseases, and in the utilization of pathologic findings for directing new and better treatment of kidney diseases. The text of the sixth edition has been extensively modified to include authoritative, thoroughly referenced discussions of these remarkable new advances. Another striking and extremely valuable change in this edition is the transition to color photomicrographs that are even more informative than the traditionally excellent images that have been a hallmark of previous editions.

In his preface to the third edition, Dr. Heptinstall wisely noted that the "two main ingredients for writing a successful medical book are personal experience and an ability to discern what is important in the writing of others." The 36 authors who contributed to the sixth edition fulfill these criteria admirably. They are among the most capable and accomplished renal pathologists in the world. All of these authors have extensive hands-on experience with diagnostic renal pathology, teaching renal pathology at major medical centers, and advancing the field through clinical and translational research. They have contributed thousands of articles to the literature on renal pathology. In fact, many of the major advances in our current understanding of renal pathology have been made by authors of chapters in this book. The editors thank all of them for their truly outstanding contributions. We are convinced that the sixth edition of *Heptinstall's Pathology of the Kidney* is the most comprehensive, most authoritative, most thoroughly referenced, and best illustrated book on renal pathology ever produced.

All the editors are honored by the opportunity and challenge afforded us by Dr. Heptinstall to sustain his book on renal pathology. We and all others who are interested in the study of kidney diseases are forever indebted to him for establishing this classic text.

J.C.J.

# Robert H. Heptinstall
## A Tribute

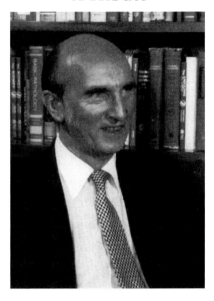

The first edition of *Pathology of the Kidney* by Robert H. Heptinstall marked the watershed between autopsy- and biopsy-based studies of renal disease in human beings. Before The Pathology of the Kidney renal pathology textbooks related the clinical evolution of "renal syndromes" and the associated autopsy findings. The percutaneous renal biopsy initially described by Iversen and Brun only 15 years prior to the publication of *Pathology of the Kidney* allowed a more dynamic view of kidney disease, and the text drew heavily on renal biopsy studies and immunofluorescence and electron microscopic findings in renal tissue. This new information had to be integrated with the autopsy-based renal literature for, as "Heppy" wrote in the preface to the first edition, "we are almost completely ignorant of the sequence of events that takes place during the evolution of a given disease, and ... the nomenclature in use at the moment is most unsatisfactory. Most of our concepts and nomenclature of renal disease have been based on kidneys studied at autopsy, which except in rare instances represent the end stage of a process that has been going on for years. The renal biopsy has presented us with histological pictures that in the light of our present concepts are not only difficult to interpret but defy satisfactory labeling." The enduring contribution of *Pathology of the Kidney* is that it brought order out of chaos and in doing so defined the central issues of modern renal pathology. Over the years, this classic textbook and its subsequent editions have provided guidance and insight not only to nephropathologists but to nephrologists, renal physiologists, and the entire renal community.

The first edition of *Pathology of the Kidney* is also an outstanding example of medical authorship. The book was written with wit and style, and it is scholarly, authoritative, and comprehensive. This monumental achievement is even more remarkable when one considers that the first four editions were essentially monographs.

How Heppy accomplished his goals of presenting biopsy-based pathology, relating it to the existing classifications, and identifying a pathogenetic sequence deserves exposition. Much of the text is written in the first person because it was based on his extensive experience with renal pathology in biopsy and autopsy material. When writing on disputed topics, however, he was careful to quote "widely the opinions of others." A complete and critical reading of the literature allowed him to correlate biopsy studies of acute and evolving renal diseases with the end-stage findings and nomenclature from autopsy studies. In the few areas where he did not have personal experience, he was exact in quoting published material, and whenever possible he reviewed the pathology material obtained by others. The superb illustrations complemented the text by demonstrating the pathologic lesions in all their phases allowing a pathogenetic connection between acute and end-stage lesions. Finally, his experience as an experimental pathologist aided him in critically evaluating and identifying relevant experimental studies.

The late Ramzi S. Cotran, no mean scholar himself, acknowledged the comprehensive and scholarly nature of the *Pathology of the Kidney* by insisting that it was the place to begin not only the work-up of a difficult case but also an experimental study. Thus, Heppy has provided a fair template for those who would write chapters in pathology textbooks. In so far as we succeed, the credit is his, and if we fail, the responsibility is ours.

# Preface to the First Edition (1966)

The task of presenting a comprehensible account of the pathology of the kidney is surprisingly difficult, as I have found to my cost over the past three years. The main difficulties are twofold: first, we are almost completely ignorant of the sequence of events that takes place during the evolution of a given disease and, second, the nomenclature in use at the moment is most unsatisfactory. Most of our concepts and nomenclature of renal disease have been based on kidneys studied at autopsy, which except in rare instances represent the end stage of a process that has been going on for years. The renal biopsy has presented us with histological pictures that in light of our present concepts are not only difficult to interpret but defy satisfactory labeling. Many of these pictures are doubtless early stages of a process whose end stage we already recognize, but others very likely represent processes with which we are quite unfamiliar. Only by conducting intelligently planned studies with repeat biopsies over a long period of time can we hope to resolve these problems, and a greater degree of cooperation between the various groups of investigators will be required than has been the case up to now.

Accepting the imperfect state of our knowledge, I have attempted to present an account of the more common diseases that affect the kidney. The book is mainly for the pathologist and the internist specializing in renal problems, but it is hoped that it will be of use to others, such as the urologist and the obstetrician.

The pathology of the various diseases has been presented in the light of both autopsy and biopsy experience, and although many of the views expressed are my own, this being an author's privilege, a balanced presentation has been attempted by quoting widely the opinions of others. The clinical sections are of necessity brief, for these aspects have been authoritatively dealt with on numerous occasions by people better qualified than I am. Experimental contributions have been quoted when appropriate, and in most chapters the role of the newer techniques such as electron and fluorescence microscopy has been described. The traditional chapter on renal physiology has been omitted, and for this I offer no apology. This is a highly complex subject that can hardly be compressed into one chapter; it is also one that I am not competent to discuss. Renal tumors are not discussed because they are adequately considered in existing texts on surgical pathology.

I have been fortunate in persuading Dr. J.M. Kissane to write chapters on the development and congenital defects of the kidney, and Dr. K.A. Porter to write on renal transplantation. These two former colleagues of mine are experts in their fields, and their respective chapters amply reflect their competence.

I am very grateful to all those who supplied us with illustrations and material from which illustrations were made. Professor Paul Beeson was asked to read the two chapters on pyelonephritis and promptly replied with four single-spaced pages of comments and suggestions; I was chastened but grateful. Dr. Abou Pollack has been a constant source of pearls of wisdom and exotic material; I am much indebted to this fine pathologist. Most of the photomicrographs for my own chapters were prepare by Mr. Chester Reather, and these, as always, were of matchless quality. The wearisome job of checking the references was bravely carried out by Miss Virginia Shriver, and her efforts, and those of the staff of the William H. Welch Medical Library at Johns Hopkins, are much appreciated. The most difficult job of all was done by Miss Mary Lakin, my secretary, who, starting out with scraps of paper adorned by nearly undecipherable handwriting, restored order out of chaos and produced the final manuscript. It is impossible to thank her enough.

Lastly, it is a great pleasure to acknowledge the help and stimulus over the years of Dr. A.M. Joekes. The biopsies we saw together provided a nucleus for many of the thoughts that have been expressed in this book, and to him belongs much of the credit (or blame) for the finished product.

R.H.H.

# Acknowledgments

Dr. Jennette thanks his wife, Yvonne, daughters, Jennifer and Caroline, and granddaughters, Olivia and Augusta, for forgiving the time spent away from them pursuing his passion for renal pathology. He thanks Dr. Fred Dalldorf for sparking his interest in renal pathology, Dr. Ron Falk for his decades of stimulating professional collaboration, and the many nephropathologists and nephrologists who have shared their insights on kidney disease with him. He also thanks his long-term associate, Alice "Sandy" Wilkman, for her assistance with this and innumerable other projects over the past 40 years.

Dr. Olson thanks Drs. Glenn Chertow, Chi-Yuan Hsu, and Timothy Meyer for their discussions regarding nephrology and providing many helpful comments. For their help during the formative part of her career, Dr. Olson thanks Drs. Manjeri Venkatachalam, Helmut Rennke, and Ramzi Cotran. She also gives special thanks to Dr. Robert H. Heptinstall, her mentor and friend, for steering her toward renal pathology and for nurturing her early career.

Dr. Schwartz thanks his wife Lisa for understanding his commitment to this book. He thanks his teachers, Dr. Manjeri Venkatachalam and the late Dr. Ramzi S. Cotran, for introducing him to the mysteries of the kidney and leading him into nephropathology. He also thanks his clinical colleagues, Dr. Edmund J. Lewis and Dr. Stephen M. Korbet, for keeping his focus on the clinical relevance of the renal biopsy, for helpful discussions leading to evolving concepts of disease, and for career-long collaborative efforts that have found their way into the text. Dr. Silva thanks all of the members of the Southwest Pediatric Nephrology Group (under the able direction of Dr. Ron Hogg) for the renal biopsy material used in the preparation of his chapters. He also thanks Dr. Conrad L. Pirani for all his years of mentoring.

# Renal Diseases Associated With Plasma Cell Dyscrasias, Amyloidoses, Waldenström Macroglobulinemia, and Cryoglobulinemic Nephropathies

**19**

*Guillermo A. Herrera    Maria M. Picken*

## HISTORICAL PERSPECTIVE

The historical events that occurred more than 150 years ago and brought attention to an association between plasma cell dyscrasias and renal disease that were most remarkable and deserve recollection. Review of these historical events serves the purpose to follow chronologically how our understanding of renal damage associated with dysproteinemias has advanced throughout the years.

Thomas Alexander McBean, a tradesman from London, sought medical attention in September 1844 because while vaulting out of an underground cavern he felt as if something had snapped or given away within his chest, producing persistent intense pain (1). Dr. William MacIntire, McBean's attending physician, removed a pint of blood, applied a strengthening plaster to the chest, and recommended abstention from all bodily exertion, resulting in temporary relief and return to his "ordinary avocations." The improvement did not last long, and further treatment with steel and quinine was performed, with favorable results. However, in the following months, Mr. McBean eventually developed severe weakness, wasting, pallor, hepatic enlargement, pleuritic chest pain, and edema of the face and ankles. These new clinical developments forced a surgeon, whom he consulted, to "take blood from the arm to the amount of one pound, and to apply leeches and blisters topically."

Dr. MacIntire observed peculiar abnormalities in his patient's urine, which was noted to be "opaque, acid and of high density with a specific gravity of 1.035" (1). Fifteen months after the incident, on October 30, 1845, Dr. Thomas Watson, a leading clinician in London at the time, evaluated Dr. MacIntire's patient and examined Mr. McBean's urine, corroborating the previous findings. Seeking help from a well-recognized chemical pathologist, Dr. Henry Bence-Jones, was the logical way to proceed. The letter that Dr. Watson sent to Dr. Bence-Jones remains an exact description of the urinary abnormalities that are en-countered in many patients with renal disease and dysproteinemias. This was the beginning of a saga that deciphered the relationship between a totally unknown blood disorder and the kidney. Dr. Watson stated in this letter:

> The tube contains urine of very high specific gravity. When boiled it becomes slightly opaque. On the addition of nitric acid, it effervesces, assumes a reddish hue, and becomes quite clear; but as soon as it cools assumes the consistency and appearance which you see. Heat reliquifies it. What is it? (2).

Dr. Bence-Jones took special interest in this specimen, analyzed the urine, and reported his findings. He deduced that the substance responsible for the urine abnormalities was not albumin because it was soluble in acid, and after performing a number of tests, he concluded that it was of a proteinaceous nature and referred to it as an "oxide of albumin, the hydrated deutoxide" (3). He calculated that the patient excreted 67 grams/day of this substance. Today, we know this material as Bence-Jones (BJ) protein, in recognition of his contribution to our understanding of its nature, in spite of the fact that it was really MacIntire who first discovered the abnormalities in McBean's urine. Bence-Jones was the first to provide a detailed account of McBean's disease, referring to it as ". . . a hitherto undescribed disease, essentially malignant in nature . . . (affecting the) osseous system;" indeed this is an accurate characterization of a previously unknown disease (3).

Mr. McBean's condition did not improve. He continued to have excruciating bone pain and developed intractable diarrhea, progressive generalized weakness, and emaciation. He died January 1, 1846, at 46 years of age.

An autopsy performed on Mr. McBean by Alexander Shaw revealed soft, friable ribs, sternum, and vertebrae, and they contained a "gelatiniform substance of blood-red color and unctuous feel." The ribs were "brittle, soft, and easily cut with a knife," and as described by Dr. MacIntire they "crumbled under the heel of the scalpel" (4). A diagnosis of *mollities et fragilitas ossium*, also known at the time as *mollities ossium*, quite descriptive terms for the disease in question (1,4–6), was made. Microscopic sections of the bones were examined by Dr. John Dalrymple, a surgeon at the Royal Ophthalmic Hospital in Moorfields, England, who documented the presence of abnormal cells in detailed drawings he made to illustrate his findings. These cells showed characteristics typical of malignant plasma cells (5), but plasma cells had not even been described at the time. Both Dalrymple and MacIntire believed that the disorder responsible for McBean's death was essentially a malignant disease of bone. On his death certificate, the cause of death was "atrophy from albuminuria" (4), once again alluding to the renal component of this disorder as an essential manifestation of the disease process. The kidneys at autopsy were essentially normal on gross examination. It would take many years of clinicopathologic analysis and research to comprehend the scope of this patient's disease and to explain the different clinical manifestations.

Although the term *multiple myeloma* was introduced by von Rustizky in 1873 (7), the disease was rarely recognized until 1889, when Kahler published a case report (8). Kahler recognized that his patient had a similar substance in the urine to that described in McBean's urine. In 1900, Wright determined that multiple myeloma was a disease of plasma cells (9) when he recognized the similarity of the malignant cellular proliferation in this disease to cells initially described in 1875 by Waldeyer and fully characterized by Ramón y Cajal 15 years later in syphilitic condylomata (10). The association between plasma cells, their secretory products, and nephrotoxicity was not recognized until more than 50 years after McBean's death, in 1899 (11). Dr. James Ewing, lecturing to medical students in 1932, summarized the available knowledge by stating: "A very peculiar protein (BJ protein), specific of the disease and supposed to be derived from the adsorption of bone" (12). A definitive relationship between BJ proteinuria and the abnormal proteins seen in the serum of patients with myeloma was not demonstrated until 1956 in a study performed by Korngold and Lipari (13). These investigators determined that there were two types of pathologic light chains: κ and λ. Edelman and Gally demonstrated in 1962 that the light chains from the serum and BJ proteins of a myeloma patient were the same (14).

## CLARIFICATIONS IN TERMINOLOGY: MULTIPLE MYELOMA AND OTHER MANIFESTATIONS OF DYSPROTEINEMIAS (PLASMA CELL DYSCRASIAS)

There are three clinical entities related to a diagnosis of dysproteinemia: multiple myeloma (often referred to as myeloma), plasma cell dyscrasia (dysproteinemia), and monoclonal gammopathy of unknown significance (MGUS). It should be noted that *plasma cell dyscrasia* and *dysproteinemia* are frequently used as generic terms for all of these disorders. Criteria for differentiating these three conditions have been clearly delineated by Durie (15). An understanding of the kinetics associated with plasma cell disorders is important for management of these patients and therapeutic purposes (16,17).

Myeloma represents the most striking and advanced manifestation of a plasma cell dyscrasia. It is typically associated with lytic ("punched out") bone lesions, which are often multiple. There is a monoclonal spike in the serum and/or BJ proteinuria resulting from the production of either complete immunoglobulins or fragments of immunoglobulins by the neoplastic plasma cells. Finally, a significant increase in the number of bone marrow plasma cells (usually in the 15% to 20% range), often arranged in sheets with atypical cellular forms, is present.

Myeloma accounts for approximately 1% of all malignancies and 10% of all hematologic neoplasms (18). It is the second most common hematologic malignancy in the United States, with approximately 40,000 individuals suffering from myeloma at any time, and approximately 16,000 new cases will have been diagnosed in 2005 (19). The incidence of myeloma is approximately 4 in 100,000 individuals; it is higher among Blacks than in the general population and more common in males than in females (20–22). The disease is most common with advancing age (mean age 65), but it is seen in individuals in the fourth and fifth decades of life. It is rare to find it in patients younger than 40 years of age (18), but there are reports of cases in the second decade of life. Renal insufficiency is a frequent complication of myeloma and the second most common cause of death after infection in these patients (18,21). Elevated serum creatinine was found in more than 50% of patients with myeloma, at initial examination, in a series of 869 cases described by Kyle (18).

The term *plasma cell dyscrasia* or *dysproteinemia* denotes a less than full-blown neoplastic plasma cell disorder. The affected patients often have circulating light chains in the serum or urine detected as a monoclonal (M) spike; they may have clinical manifestations, including renal findings, but the bone marrow is not diagnostic of myeloma. Although there may be a small increase in the number of plasma cells, they are not significantly atypical and are not clustered in sheets. In our experience, in approximately 5% of patients with dysproteinemia, the percentage of plasma cells is within the normal range (<5%). Lytic bone lesions are absent, and clinical manifestations are subtle or nondetectable. Routine bone marrow studies may be incorrectly considered as normal. When ancillary testing is performed (flow cytometry or immunomorphologic evaluations), a clone of plasma cells responsible for the production of the abnormal immunoglobulins is usually found (23). To establish monoclonality in these cases, immunophenotyping can also be performed on cytospin preparations using antibodies that recognize the major Vκ or Vλ subgroups or gene families and those that preferably identify free light chains (24).

The third group of patients with dysproteinemia have an isolated monoclonal M protein peak or gammopathy in the serum, and this condition is diagnosed as an MGUS. The amount of M protein must be lower than 3 g/dL and there must be fewer than 5% plasma cells in the bone marrow (25–29). Other criteria include the absence or only small amounts of light chains in the urine, absence of lytic bone lesions, and no related anemia, hypercalcemia, or renal failure (25). The individual with an MGUS is otherwise normal. In patients with a diagnosis of MGUS, significant BJ proteinuria, even in the absence of recognizable renal disease, usually precedes clinical and laboratory manifestations of either myeloma or AL amyloidosis, but it may take more than 20 years for clinical disease to develop (27). Monoclonal gammopathy of unknown significance (MGUS) is found in approximately 3% of persons older than 70 years of age in Sweden (28). The prevalence of MGUS is higher in older patients, and only 4% of MGUS patients were younger than 40 years in a study by the Mayo Clinic group (25). Some of these patients essentially have "smoldering or indolent myeloma" and, with time, develop full-blown disease. In the Mayo Clinic study, 26% of the patients with MGUS developed either multiple myeloma, Waldenström's macroglobulinemia, or AL amyloidosis (25). Once a patient with a diagnosis of MGUS develops evidence of organ damage as a consequence of the circulating M protein, the diagnosis of MGUS is no longer tenable. A significant number of MGUS patients eventually develop renal disease. In fact, renal dysfunction is often the first systemic manifestation of progression.

The distinction between myeloma and MGUS based on bone marrow morphology is not reproducible, and it is virtually impossible to unequivocally separate one entity from the other (30). While the percentage of plasma cells is the most predictive feature of myeloma, the cytologic differences are not sharply defined. Interobserver variability is high in the assessment of morphologic atypia of plasma cells, and atypical plasma cells can be seen in patients with MGUS. This emphasizes the importance of identifying renal or other organ involvement in a given patient, because this finding objectively negates a diagnosis of MGUS.

The fundamental reason for making a distinction between plasma cell dyscrasia and multiple myeloma is because there is far greater consensus regarding the management of myeloma and renal disease compared to patients with renal disease who do not meet criteria for myeloma. The reality is that the pathogenesis for all these disorders is directly related to the overproduction of monoclonal light or heavy chains by a neoplastic plasma cell clone. The most recent literature stresses the indication for aggressive chemotherapy to eradicate the existing plasma cell clone. In fact, waiting to fulfill the criteria for myeloma before initiating treatment may deny the patient the early intervention that is needed to achieve optimum results.

## Synthesis of Immunoglobulin Components by Plasma Cells and Abnormalities in Plasma Cell Dyscrasias

Plasma cells synthesize and secrete specific immunoglobulin molecules with a minor excess of κ or λ light chains. The plasma cells synthesize a variety of immunoglobulins, including IgG, IgM, IgD, IgE, and IgA, which can be detected using serum protein electrophoresis (SPEP). Each immunoglobulin molecule is composed of two identical heavy chains (with molecular weight of approximately 50,000 daltons each) and two light chains (molecular weight of approximately 25,000 daltons each) linked by variable numbers of disulfide bonds. Both types of light chains consist of a common basic structure composed of a 107- to 111-residue amino-terminal variable ($V_L$) region and a 107-residue carboxyl-terminal constant ($C_L$) domain. The $V_L$ is the product of two genes, V (variable) and J (joining), that encode the first 95 to 99 amino acids and the remaining 12 amino acids, respectively. The light chain variable region of the germ line DNA includes multiple V and J sequences. There are approximately 30 Vκ and Vλ germline genes that specify proteins on the basis of homology into Vκ 1, 2, 3, and 4 and Vλ 1, 2, 3, 6, and 8 subgroups (31–37). Variations in the V sequence result from the presence of approximately 30 Vκ and Vλ germ-line genes, with somatic mutations and differences resulting from recombinations of the V and J gene encoded segments. These variations account for the variability in light chain pathogenicity and the site of pathologic action within the nephron. The carboxyl terminal of each light chain does not vary and is known as the constant C region. Each heavy chain has constant domains $C_H1$, $C_H2$, and $C_H3$ and a variable domain ($V_H$). There are five types of heavy chains, named γ (IgG), α (IgA), μ (IgM), δ (IgD), and ε (IgE). Immunoglobulin G and IgA have variable numbers of disulfide bonds linking the heavy chains and the heavy chains to the light chains. These characterize different isotypes of these Ig molecules, known as IgG1, IgG2, IgG3, and IgG4, as well as IgA1 and IgA2. Immunoglobulin A and IgG2 tend to exist in pairs of units known as "dimers" or may even polymerize to produce larger molecules. Immunoglobulin M exists primarily as a pentamer molecule composed of five Ig units.

Normal light chains synthesized by the plasma cells maintain a ratio of κ to λ of 2 to 1 in the serum. κ molecules occur predominantly as monomers or noncovalent dimers, with molecular weights of 22,000 and 44,000 daltons, respectively, whereas λ molecules typically exist as covalent dimers. The $V_H$ and $V_L$ comprise the antigen binding site. The $C_H2$ and $C_H3$ components are involved in effector functions such as binding to immune cells and host tissues and fixing complement. The synthesis of light chains occurs independently from heavy chains, and they combine in the rough endoplasmic reticulum to form the complete immunoglobulin molecule. The fact that light and heavy chains are synthesized independently is the pathogenetic basis for the existence of light chain- and heavy chain-related disorders as specific entities, as well as occasional overlap entities (36,37).

In neoplastic plasma cell disorders, there is proliferation of a clone of plasma cells secreting a single type of Ig molecule or subunit that may be identified as a monoclonal peak on SPEP or urine protein electrophoresis (UPEP) and characterized by immunoelectrophoresis or immunofixation (38). In some cases, only light chains are produced by the neoplastic plasma cells, and they are not generally detectable on SPEP but can be identified in the urine. The demonstration of a monoclonal protein in the serum or urine is important to corroborate a diagnosis of dysproteinemia. In a series of patients with myeloma reported by Kyle (18), a monoclonal protein was demonstrated in 90% of the patients using SPEP. The urine contains light chains in 60% to 80% of myeloma patients as detected by means of UPEP. Urinary light chains (BJ proteins) can also be found in the urine of patients with other B-cell neoplasms. While free light chains readily circulate in the body, for heavy chains to be found in the circulation they need to be released from the endoplasmic reticulum by binding with light chains. This is the reason why heavy chains do not circulate freely in normal individuals. Quantitation of serum free light chains can be used in the diagnosis and follow-up of patients with plasma cell dyscrasias/myeloma (39).

During the process of cellular replication and differentiation in the bone marrow, mutations typically take place when mature B lymphocytes are transforming into plasmablasts. The mutated plasmablasts produce a colony of identical mutated plasma cells or what is referred to as a *plasma cell clone* in a particular bone marrow site. The abnormal plasma cells eventually travel to additional bone marrow locations and other organs, disseminating the pathologic process and producing the various lesions seen in cases of advanced myeloma. Most malignant plasma cell disorders actively produce immunoglobulins, and these are generally composed of one type of light and one type of heavy chain.

In dysproteinemias, the normally controlled production of antibodies is replaced by an inappropriate production of larger amounts of immunoglobulin molecules by the bone marrow. The normally equal production of light and heavy chains may be imbalanced, resulting in free light or heavy chains. Imbalance of immunoglobulin production most commonly results in an excess of abnormal light chains (35).

Furthermore, in dysproteinemic patients, biosynthesis of abnormal light chains, either large, polymeric, or fragmented, has been documented in bone marrow cell cultures from patients with monoclonal immunoglobulin deposition diseases (MIDDs) and amyloidosis (36,37). It has become clear that mutations resulting in amino acid substitutions in the light or heavy chain molecules are crucial in determining their pathogenicity or absence thereof, along with the type of renal involvement. In some cases, certain physicochemical characteristics of these immunoglobulin components make them nephrotoxic, and even in cases where the production of these immunoglobulins by plasma cells is small, significant renal damage may occur.

Fewer than 1% of myelomas produce no immunoglobulin molecules (nonsecretory), and approximately 5% to 10% produce only light chains, which may only be detectable in the urine (40). The SPEP in these patients could be normal or show nonspecific alterations.

The light chains in patients with plasma cell dyscrasia may be larger or smaller than normal, with molecular weights ranging from 12,000 to 30,000 daltons. Glycosylation of light chains contributes to an increase in their molecular weight. In a small number of myeloma cases (<5%) two different abnormal immunoglobulin molecules or fragments of these molecules are produced, indicating the presence of two distinct clones of neoplastic plasma cells (37). Immunoglobulin G is the most common immunoglobulin produced in myeloma cases (52%), followed by IgA (25%). Myelomas producing IgD, IgE, and IgM together account for fewer than 1% of all cases.

The primary structure of light and heavy chains is responsible for whether a given molecule is pathogenic to the kidney or not, as has been clearly shown in studies with recombinant variable portions of light chains. Not all light chains from patients with plasma cell dyscrasias result in renal damage. Particular amino acid alterations will result in changes in the tertiary conformation of the proteins, leading to either partial or complete unfolding and changes in stability, potentiating aggregation. The three-dimensional configuration of a given light or heavy chain molecule can be predicted using computer modeling techniques; taking this information into account, the effects of a particular protein can be anticipated (41–56). It is known that λ light chains are preferentially associated with amyloidosis, while κ light chains are most common in light chain deposition disease (LCDD) (50,57–59). λ proteins of two Vλ gene families, 6a and 3r, are typically associated with amyloidosis (50), and patients with λ VI are the most common ones with renal amyloidosis. In LCDD, the majority of patients are κ Vκ I or IV related. Changes in the stability and glycosylation of these light chains also affect their ability to produce renal damage (60). Fanconi syndrome–related acute tubulopathy is almost invariably κ light chain related. In these patients, a specific amino acid substitution in position 30 of the variable portion of the light chain molecule accounts for the failure of complete processing and catabolism of the involved light chain in the proximal tubular lysosomal compartment (61,62). Biosynthetic data from studies of bone marrow plasma cells from patients with myeloma indicate that those light chains, which are heavier than normal, are usually glycosylated, and this alteration can make the light chains more nephrotoxic or change their pattern of nephrotoxicity (63).

## Metabolism of Light and Heavy Chains in Normal Individuals and Pathologic Behavior in Patients with Plasma Cell Dyscrasia

Because light chains are low–molecular-weight proteins, they are freely filtered through the glomeruli and delivered to the proximal tubules. Glomerular clearance of light chains may be affected by a number of factors, including their physicochemical characteristics, size, isoelectric point, hydrophobicity, and state of aggregation. For example, light chain polymers and heavy chains do not cross the filtration barrier. Once the light chains are filtered by the glomerulus, 90% are reabsorbed by the proximal tubules, endocytosed, and catabolized through a lysosomal process, with their amino acids eventually returning to the circulation (64,65). This process is very efficient in normal individuals, with only a small amount of free light chains found in the urine. The cubilin-megalin receptor located on the brush border of proximal tubular cells working in tandem controls the endocytosis of the light chains (66–68). Light chain endocytosis occurs by a very specific, saturable, receptor-mediated process. There are a number of ligands that compete with light chains for brush border binding. The internalized light chains are then transported into vesicles, where the endosomal system catabolizes them. Hydrolytic enzymes present in the endosomes digest the light chains. Some of the process of light chain digestion appears to take place at the brush border itself, before endocytosis. The κ and λ light chain susceptibility to catabolism varies and accounts for the fact that the ratio of κ to λ light chains is reversed in the urine (2:1, λ to κ) (69).

In the setting of a plasma cell dyscrasia, the quantity of light chains in the filtrate may exceed the maximal reabsorptive capacity of the proximal tubular cells. When this occurs, the light chains pass into the distal nephron, where they may precipitate or remain in the tubular filtrate, resulting in light chain (BJ) proteinuria. Light chains precipitate out of solution when the urine is heated to approximately 56°C and redissolve as the temperature rises. As the urine is allowed to cool again, a precipitate forms, followed by dissolution as further cooling occurs. These are the characteristics documented by Dr. Bence-Jones in Mr. McBean's urine (2). The monoclonal light chains in the urine may be detected by UPEP or by testing for BJ proteins. Sensitive techniques such as immunoelectrophoresis or immunofixation may be required to detect small amounts of monoclonal proteins in the urine of these patients.

The usual synthesis rate of monoclonal light chains in normal patients is less than 0.9 g/day, whereas in patients with myeloma it increases to approximately 3 to 85 g/day (70,71). Normal patients may excrete small amounts of light chains (up to 50 mg/day). There is no apparent specific relationship between some of the characteristics of the monoclonal light chains excreted by individuals (i.e., chemical properties, subtype κ v λ, monomer versus dimer, anionic versus cationic) and the presence of pathologic findings demonstrated clinically or experimentally.

Normal light chains are not attracted to the mesangium and do not interact with mesangial cells. In contrast, some physicochemically abnormal light chains from patients with plasma cell dyscrasias interact with purported mesangial receptors and alter mesangial homeostasis.

Also, in patients with myeloma, the concentration of light chains reaching the kidneys is usually much higher,

and the inability of the proximal tubules to properly catabolize the abnormal light chains leads to pathologic alterations. In patients with myeloma, the light chains commonly circulate as polymers that cannot be properly broken down by the endosomal/lysosomal system in the proximal tubules, enhancing their propensity to produce pathologic alterations. After the glomerular filtration barrier is compromised, as a result of monotypic light chains interacting with the glomerular basement membranes, such polymers can freely go through.

While there is a mechanism to deal with the small amounts of light chains that circulate in normal individuals, that is not the case concerning heavy chains, because they cannot be filtered though the glomerulus owing to their high molecular weight. If free heavy chains are released to the circulation, they interact with the capillary endothelium and mesangium, where they engage in pathologic processes. Presumably, the physicochemical characteristics of the particular heavy chains will dictate how they produce pathology. There is no information currently available on how heavy chains are processed by the kidneys, and the knowledge available regarding pathogenesis of heavy chain–related diseases is rather limited at this time. In Waldenström's macroglobulinemia, the circulating IgM molecules become entrapped in subendothelial zones and generally do not significantly alter mesangial homeostasis or produce tubular lesions.

## LABORATORY DIAGNOSIS

The identification of a monoclonal protein in the serum and/or urine is important to confirm a diagnosis of dysproteinemia. Immunoelectrophoresis is routinely used to characterize the monoclonal protein that is detected in serum or urine. Serum protein electrophoresis is a good screening test for plasma cell dyscrasia, even though light chain secreting and nonsecreting plasma cell disorders lack a monoclonal spike. In these cases examination of the urine for BJ proteins is important to make or solidify a diagnosis. The urine must be properly concentrated to detect small amounts of the monoclonal light chains. Immunoelectrophoresis or immunofixation may be necessary to confirm a diagnosis in some instances.

Immunofixation electrophoresis, a faster technique than immunoelectrophoresis, is the most sensitive and commonly used method available for the detection of monoclonal proteins. It is very helpful in identifying a monoclonal protein associated with a polyclonal increase of light chains, subtle bands associated with faint monoclonal or biclonal proteins, and monoclonal heavy chain fragments in the urine. Clarification of banding patterns noted on electrophoresis gels is possible by direct comparison of results. The superior resolution, simplicity, and enhanced sensitivity of immunofixation make it the diagnostic modality of choice to detect monoclonal gammopathies. One caution with immunofixation is that it requires precise dilution of the antibodies to avoid a prozone effect (38).

High-resolution electrophoresis (thin-layer agarose gels) may be combined with transfer onto nitrocellulose, followed by resolution of bands with monospecific enzyme-tagged antisera or monoclonal antibodies (Western blotting). This procedure is extremely sensitive, more discriminating than immunofixation, and allows detection of minute amounts of monoclonal light chains (72). The technique can be utilized in selected instances when the monoclonal protein is in very small amounts.

## RENAL INVOLVEMENT IN PLASMA CELL DYSCRASIAS

Renal involvement in dysproteinemia/plasma cell dyscrasias/myeloma is heterogeneous. Approximately 85% of all light chains with plasma cell dyscrasias are nephrotoxic. The morphologic manifestations vary, depending on the renal compartments targeted by the nephrotoxic light or heavy chains. In some instances, more than one renal compartment is affected, and combinations of different patterns of renal damage can be seen in the same patient. The majority of the nephrotoxic light chains (approximately 70%) affect the tubular interstitial compartment and are referred to as *tubulopathic*. The other 30% of nephrotoxic light chains preferentially involve the glomerular compartment, producing glomerulopathies (*glomerulopathic* light chains). The physicochemical characteristics of the involved immunoglobulin molecule appear to be the primary pathologic determinant. There are also some uncharacterized host factors that may influence the pathologic alterations and the degree of damage. In this chapter, the light chain- and heavy chain-associated disorders will be discussed separately, but the reader must understand that on occasions they may be found acting in concert. Each of the diseases has specific clinical manifestations, pathologic findings, pathogenesis, prognosis, and management, and these specific features support viewing them as separate diseases. These diseases include:

- Light chain (myeloma) cast nephropathy
- Acute tubulopathy (acute tubular damage or necrosis)
- Inflammatory tubulointerstitial nephritis
- Amyloidosis (light chain- [AL] or heavy chain- [AH] related) (AL/AH amyloidosis)
- Deposition diseases (light chain- [L] or heavy chain- [H] related]) (LCDD/HCDD)

Light chain cast nephropathy, acute tubulopathy, and inflammatory tubulointerstitial nephritis are part of the spectrum of renal damage produced by tubulopathic light chains. The glomerular and vascular compartments are not typically affected by the tubulopathic light chains. Amyloidosis and the deposition diseases generally exhibit glomerular manifestations, but they are also commonly associated with tubular interstitial and vascular pathology. In very rare circumstances, alterations in the vasculature (i.e., in AL amyloidosis) may be the predominant (73) or the first morphologic manifestation of renal involvement, preceding pathologic damage to other renal compartments. Combined patterns such as AL amyloidosis and LCDD, LCDD and light chain cast nephropathy, and LCDD and HCDD are uncommon (74–76).

Infiltration of the renal parenchyma by neoplastic plasma cells is rare and usually occurs in terminal patients with myeloma (77). Renal insufficiency or failure because of renal parenchymal infiltration is very unusual. Neoplastic aggregates of plasma cells seen in autopsies from these patients (77) may be associated with malignant plasma cells in the urinary sediment (78).

### Light Chain (Myeloma) Cast Nephropathy

#### Historical Perspective

Cast nephropathy was the first renal lesion to be recognized in patients with myeloma. It was well documented by Decastello in 1909 (79), but the first cases had been recorded in the literature a few years earlier by Ellinger (11). In the early 1920s, Krauss (80) championed the concept of nephrotoxic light chains, but others noted that, at least in some patients, large amounts of BJ proteinuria were not associated with renal insufficiency. Thennhauser and Krauss hypothesized in 1920 that the tubular casts were concretions of serum proteins and BJ "albumose" (81). In a comprehensive study by Bell in 1933 addressing renal lesions in myeloma, which included a complete review of the literature, he concluded that "it seems highly probable that casts are the chief cause of renal insufficiency resulting from multiple myeloma" (82). Other series of patients with myeloma have shown that light chain cast nephropathy is the most common lesion seen in these patients (77,82–85). This has not changed through the years (77,85).

#### Clinical Presentation and Laboratory Findings

The most typical presentation of cast nephropathy is acute renal deterioration or frank renal failure (86,87). It remains the most common cause of acute renal failure in patients with myeloma. In some cases, there are identifiable precipitating factors, such as dehydration, hypercalcemia, contrast media, nonsteroidal anti-inflammatory drugs, hyperuricemia, infections, nephrotoxins, or loop diuretics, such as furosemide. Renal biopsy may establish the diagnosis of underlying myeloma, or the patients may already have an established diagnosis of myeloma and are biopsied because of renal insufficiency to determine the renal lesion. After the diagnosis of light chain cast nephropathy, approximately 90% of patients are found to have overt myeloma (84). These patients frequently also have nephrotic range proteinuria, predominantly composed of light chains. Routine urinalysis using a dipstick, which primarily detects albuminuria, commonly fails to pick up light chain proteinuria.

## Gross Pathology

There are no specific gross features in kidneys with light chain cast nephropathy (77,82,83,85). The kidneys may have subcapsular pathology, including granularity and occasional petechiae, but these are likely related to vascular disease (85). The mean weight of the kidneys from patients with myeloma cast nephropathy was 166 g in one autopsy series (85).

## Light Microscopy

The glomerular and vascular compartments are normal in appearance or show changes related to other existing conditions, i.e., benign nephrosclerosis. The most striking changes are in the tubular interstitial compartment when casts are present in the distal nephron (Fig. 19.1A) (86–89). In fact, most casts are located in the collecting ducts, and if medulla is not included in the specimen, the diagnosis may be missed. The typical casts exhibit irregular, angulated, and geometric shapes; fracture planes; and occasionally a lamellated internal appearance, attesting to their protein-rich composition, which imparts to them a firm and often brittle consistency. In some casts, the fragments come together in a jigsaw puzzle–type of arrangement, which is quite peculiar and characteristic (Fig. 19.1A). Casts in the proximal tubules and even in the urinary space are the result of retrograde filling. An interstitial inflammatory reaction, predominantly with mononu-

clear inflammatory cells and sometimes eosinophils, often accompanies the tubular casts. Tubulopathic light chains associated with nephron obstruction can elicit an interstitial inflammatory reaction by stimulating cytokines (90).

The casts contain predominantly light chains and Tamm-Horsfall protein, but they may also include cell debris from proximal tubular damage (91–95). The epithelial cells in the tubules with casts often appear reactive and, at times, enlarged. Multinucleated cells of macrophage origin may also be seen inside tubules surrounding the casts (Fig. 19.1B), and it has been postulated that these cells migrate from the interstitium through the tubular basement membranes into the tubules (96–98). If the casts break through the tubular basement membranes, then a multinucleated giant cell reaction may be elicited in the adjacent interstitium surrounding the expelled material. These giant cells have also been shown to exhibit a macrophage phenotype. Interestingly, some of the casts are congophilic and upon polarization elicit apple green birefringence; they also exhibit thioflavin T and S positivity (99,100). Certain histochemical and staining properties of renal tubular casts in human multiple myeloma and in "mouse myeloma" are similar to those of amyloid (100). The casts are generally eosinophilic and weakly periodic acid-Schiff (PAS) positive; however, there is significant variability in the tinctorial characteristics, as the composition of these casts may be quite variable. In rare cases, the casts are composed exclusively of, or contain, crystals (Fig. 19.2). Whereas the morphology of casts is quite characteristic, there are cases in which the morphology is not pathognomonic. In some of these atypical cases, immunofluorescence may be helpful. However, some cases require careful clinicopathologic correlation for accurate interpretation. The extent of cast formation correlates with the degree of interstitial fibrosis, tubular atrophy, and dropout (101), and there is also a correlation with renal function in many but not all cases (101).

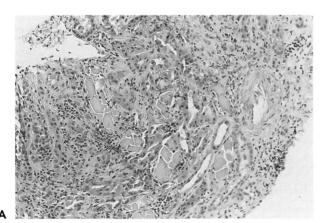
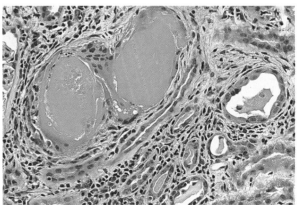

**Figure 19.1.** Light chain cast nephropathy. **A:** Typical distal nephron casts with brittle consistency, resulting in fracture planes. (H&E; ×350.) **B:** Multinucleated cell reaction around cast. (H&E; ×500.)

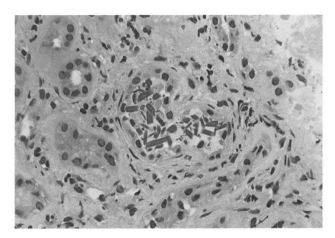

**Figure 19.2.** Light chain cast nephropathy. Distal nephron cast containing crystals. (H&E; ×500.)

## Immunofluorescence

The glomeruli and vasculature reveal no specific findings. Tamm-Horsfall protein can be demonstrated in the casts, because they form as a result of interactions between this protein and light chains (91–95). Albumin can also be found in the casts. Monotypic (restricted) light chain staining (either κ or λ) of the casts is only seen when the casts have been formed acutely and not when they have remained in place for a prolonged period of time. In most cases, there is trapping of the other light chain, and as a consequence, fluorescence staining of similar intensity is noted for both light chains. When there is fluorescence for both light chains, the light chain involved in the plasma cell dyscrasia may predominate. Silva et al (99) found that the tubular casts contained the light chain identified in the urine in more than 50% of 40 patients with multiple myeloma.

## Electron Microscopy

The glomeruli and the vasculature are unremarkable. In most cases, the casts contain abundant fibrillary material admixed with cellular debris. Granular, electron-dense material is seen in many casts, and their specific light chain identity can be substantiated by employing ultrastructural labeling techniques (102,103).

In selected cases, the casts are composed of variably sized and shaped crystalline-like structures. Such casts are fairly specific for light chain cast nephropathy (102–104), and the diagnosis can be confirmed by using ultrastructural immunogold labeling to demonstrate monoclonality when immunofluorescence studies fail to make the diagnosis.

## Etiology and Pathogenesis

Casts, in general, form in the distal nephron, and light chain casts are not an exception (86). Local factors combine to optimize cast formation. At this site, Tamm-Horsfall protein, produced by the thick ascending limb of the loop of Henle, is most abundant and provides a perfect nidus for cast formation. The casts form as a result of co-aggregation of Tamm-Horsfall protein and light chains (90). The light chains are delivered to the distal portion of the nephron after they exceed the proximal tubule threshold for light chain reabsorption and/or after damage to the proximal tubules impairs reabsorption (88).

It was proposed that a high isoelectric point in the monoclonal light chain predisposed to cast formation (105–111), but this theory has not found universal acceptance. Another determinant of cast formation is pH (112). It has been shown that cast-forming monoclonal light chains bind to a common portion of the peptide backbone of Tamm-Horsfall protein, with the carbohydrate moiety in this protein being responsible for facilitating co-aggregation. The binding site for Tamm-Horsfall protein on monoclonal light chains is located within the CDR-3 (complementarity determining region 3) (113). These findings lend support to the current view that the structure of the pathogenic light chain must be such that certain interactions occur. The slower fluid flow in the distal nephron is a contributing factor to effective cast formation.

In 1976, Koss et al produced an obstructive renal lesion in mice by the intraperitoneal injection of a light chain from a patient with light chain cast nephropathy (105), and Solomon et al published similar findings in 1991 (106). Clyne et al proposed in the late 1970s that electrostatic interactions between various proteins involved resulted in precipitation and cast formation (104,107). Microperfusion of rat tubules with light chains purified from the urine of patients with light chain cast nephropathy has reproduced the distal nephron obstructive lesion in the research laboratory, further attesting to the importance of the physicochemical characteristics of a given light chain in the pathogenesis of the distal nephron lesion (114,115).

Myeloma casts have been found to be resistant to urinary and macrophage metalloproteinases, making their destruction difficult in some cases (116). The destructive interstitial nephritis that accompanies this lesion has been attributed to rupture of the basement membranes of tubules with spillage of the cast contents, including Tamm-Horsfall protein, into the interstitium, leading to the release of potent cytokines and other mediators and resulting in irreversible interstitial damage (95).

## Differential Diagnosis

The light microscopic appearance of the tubular casts in light chain cast nephropathy is often times pathognomonic, and there are no other conditions that show similar findings (103). Crystals in casts should create a strong suspicion for a diagnosis of light chain cast nephropathy

(102,103). However, when the casts are not classic in appearance, the nephropathologist must carefully evaluate all immunomorphologic data available to make a final determination. When monoclonality cannot be demonstrated by immunofluorescence, the diagnosis of cast nephropathy may be suspected but not confirmed. The clinician must then conduct the necessary studies to confirm the suspicion or rule out this possibility. The differential diagnosis should include nephropathies with cast formation. In rare circumstances, light chain protein excretion is increased in unrelated conditions (117). In rifampin-associated light chain proteinuria, a pathologic picture similar to that of myeloma cast nephropathy may occur (118).

## Treatment, Course of the Disease Process, and Prognosis

The great majority of patients with light chain cast nephropathy have a clearly identifiable plasma cell dyscrasia and meet the criteria for myeloma (approximately 90% of these patients) (84). This is responsible for the alternative diagnosis for this condition: myeloma cast nephropathy. The main therapy of myeloma cast nephropathy is aimed at avoiding the formation of additional casts by reducing the amount of circulating light chains, which is most efficaciously accomplished by treating the plasma cell dyscrasia, and facilitating the clearance of existing casts (119). Plasmapheresis, especially in younger patients, has been used to acutely decrease the concentration of circulating light chains while the chemotherapy decreases plasma cell mass and diminishes light chain secretion (120). This therapeutic strategy is particularly useful in patients with acute renal failure. To facilitate the clearance of existing tubular casts, proper hydration is of utmost importance. Maintenance of a high urine output (aiming at about 3 L/day) is the goal (121). Loop diuretics must not be used, and other agents that promote cast formation or produce renal damage should be avoided. These include radiocontrast agents, nonsteroidal anti-inflammatory drugs, and any nephrotoxic agents. Infections, hypercalcemia, and electrolyte imbalances should be promptly treated. Alkalinization of the urine may facilitate solubility of BJ proteins, but by itself it is of virtually no value.

Colchicine was promoted as an agent that would prevent the formation of new casts as a consequence of its effect on Tamm-Horsfall protein removing its carbohydrate component (89,101), but the clinical benefit of colchicine treatment remains doubtful. Cysteamine, a reducing agent, may be used to aid in dissolving the existing casts, and vincristine can disrupt casts already in place. Dimethyl sulfoxide has also been used to dissolve casts (122).

While renal function is compromised, many of these patients require dialysis (123,124). Dialysis is also recommended for those with acute-onset renal failure (122,125).

Aggressive chemotherapy should be considered seriously and administered to all newly diagnosed patients and already diagnosed patients who are in otherwise relatively good shape (119). Alkylating agents and prednisone not only directly act on the proliferating plasma cells but also result in a decrease of proteinuria, ameliorate nephrotic syndrome if present, and directly impact favorably on renal function (119,121,123,126). The treatment of those patients who do not meet minimal criteria for a diagnosis of myeloma is more controversial. Melphalan and prednisone have been used with good initial results in 50% to 60% of these patients (119,123). However, the trend is to be even more aggressive with patients with low tumor burden to effect a cure of the underlying plasma cell dyscrasia.

Renal function improves in about 54% of the patients who present in acute renal failure when the plasma light chain concentration is decreased (124). However, progressive loss of renal function occurs in the majority with time, especially if the myeloma can not be adequately controlled. The prognosis has not changed in the last 30 years. The overall median survival for patients with myeloma cast nephropathy and renal failure has been reported to range from 13 months (124) to 20 to 30 months, with a 5-year survival rate of 18% to 27% (18,127). Renal transplantation is generally not considered a viable therapeutic avenue because of the poor prognosis.

## Acute Tubular Damage (Acute Tubulopathy)

### Historical Perspective

Most of the initial publications linking renal damage to myeloma concentrated on cast nephropathy. However, early reports indicated that direct tubular damage by nephrotoxic light chains was an important pathologic mechanism. In 1921, Löhlein first reported crystalline inclusions in proximal tubules in a patient with multiple myeloma (128). The inclusions were also seen in Fanconi syndrome associated with acute tubulopathy in patients with plasma cell dyscrasias (129). In 1963, Costanza and Smoller (130) and in 1975, Maldonado et al (131) suggested that proximal tubular damage was an important pathogenetic mechanism in a subset of patients with myeloma and renal damage. Clyne et al (104) injected BJ proteins intraperitoneally in rats and produced intracytoplasmic inclusions in proximal tubules. However, the glomerular filtration rate did not decline, leading the authors to conclude that although tubular alterations could occur, there was no direct association with renal failure. When these experiments were repeated 5 years later using intravenous infusion of BJ proteins, the same investigators demonstrated that severe reduction in glomerular filtration rate occurred, but in these animals a significant component of distal tubule cast formation was also noted (107). DeFronzo et al (132) indicated that the degree of renal failure correlated best with tubular atrophy rather than obstruction and that some patients developed defects in urine-concentrating ability and acidification. Damage to proximal tubules by some nephrotoxic light chains was clearly demonstrated in experimental nephron microperfusion studies by Smolens et al (114) and Sanders et al (115). Some light chains were capable of producing both distal nephron obstruction and proximal tubule damage (115). In a clinical study, renal biopsies from patients with myeloma were found to have evidence of proximal tubular damage (133). Pote et al have further emphasized the role of nephrotoxic light chains in proximal tubular damage and demonstrated experimentally the direct toxic effect of some tubulopathic light chains on proximal tubules (134).

## Clinical Presentation and Laboratory Findings

It is not difficult to conceptualize proximal tubular damage in patients with plasma cell dyscrasias, because light chains are usually metabolized in proximal tubules. The delivery of excessive amounts of physiochemically abnormal light chains to the proximal tubules may lead to overload of the lysosomal system, followed by release of lysosomal enzymes and tubular cell damage. This type of tubular damage may be seen in combination with other renal manifestations in patients with plasma cell dyscrasias, and the clinical manifestations that predominate in those cases may be those related to the other conditions (i.e., those associated with AL amyloidosis or LCDD). When this lesion is found by itself, the usual clinical presentation is acute renal deterioration or acute renal failure. Some patients with this pattern of renal damage present with tubular dysfunction, including aminoaciduria, phosphaturia, and glucosuria. Other clinical manifestations include subnephrotic range proteinuria, uricosuria, and at times, renal tubular acidosis

type II (of proximal tubular origin) (130,135). This is the typical constellation of findings of acquired Fanconi syndrome. Virtually all cases that have been described with this type of renal pathology have been κ light chain-related, indicating that the composition of the light chains is a crucial determinant of this specific pathologic manifestation. An abnormal clone of plasma cells is detected in approximately 50% of these patients at first presentation (136), and there may be a prolonged interval between the diagnosis of Fanconi syndrome and clinical evidence of myeloma. In one case, the renal abnormalities preceded the demonstration of an underlying plasma cell disorder by 16 years (131). While some degree of clinically insignificant proximal tubular damage is present in most patients with plasma cell dyscrasias and nephrotoxicity (133), this lesion can be responsible for rapid renal deterioration (103). Acute tubular damage associated with light chain-related Fanconi syndrome occurs in fewer than 5% of patients with renal involvement in plasma cell dyscrasias (88,103).

## Gross Pathology

Macroscopic features of kidneys from patients with Fanconi syndrome associated with proximal tubular damage have been documented only rarely. The kidneys have been noted to be enlarged with pale cortical areas (129), findings similar to those seen in association with acute tubular necrosis, regardless of etiology.

## Light Microscopy

Proximal tubular damage by nephrotoxic light chains results in acute tubular necrosis (102,103). The early changes include vacuolization of the tubular cells followed by apical blebbing with loss of surface microvillous borders, desquamation, and fragmentation (Fig. 19.3A). In some

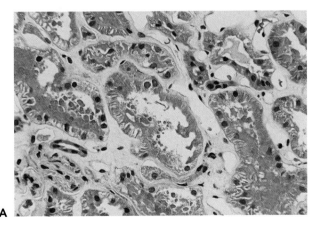
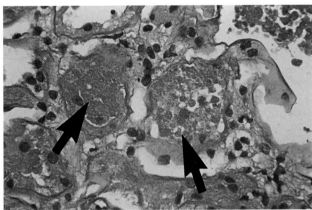

**Figure 19.3.**   Acute tubulopathy, light chain related. **A:** Early mild changes in proximal tubules, with fragmentation and desquamation of tubular cells. (H&E; ×500.) **B:** Severe tubulopathy with loss of tubular integrity resulting from cell necrosis (*arrows*) with loss of nuclei. (H&E; ×750.)

cases, tubular integrity is compromised to the point where only tubular outlines remain (arrows in Fig. 19.3B). Evidence of tubular regeneration with mitotic figures can be seen. In cases associated with clinical Fanconi syndrome, needle-like intracytoplasmic tubular inclusions may be identified with PAS and trichrome (137–139). There are a few reported cases with Fanconi syndrome containing typical intracytoplasmic crystals in tubular cells coexisting with myeloma cast nephropathy (140).

## Immunofluorescence

Monoclonal light chains may be detected in the cytoplasm of the tubular cells corresponding to the localization of the light chain in lysosomes. In other cases, even though staining for both light chains is noted, there is obvious predominance of the pertinent light chain (103,140,141). This is explained by filtration of the non-pertinent light chain and uptake by the proximal tubules. The preferential or monotypic staining for a type of light chain should be taken as a clue that the acute tubulopathy is related to an underlying plasma cell dyscrasia. However, the absence of detectable staining for either of the light chains does not rule out this condition. Sometimes, the abnormal light chains, partially digested in the lysosomes, are not detected by the available antisera. In the Fanconi syndrome-associated cases, the needle-shaped prox-imal tubular inclusions may fluoresce intensely for κ (extremely rarely for λ) light chains and be very easy to detect (87,140). However, in the majority of the cases, fluorescence evaluation does not aid in identifying the cytoplasmic inclusions.

## Electron Microscopy

Proximal tubular damage can be confirmed ultrastructurally. In experimental work and in clinical material, lysosomal proliferation, tubular cell vacuolization and fragmentation, apical cytoplasmic blebs, and segmental loss of microvillous borders are generally present, although with variable degrees of severity. The lysosomal system appears overactive, and large and atypical lysosomes are often found (Fig. 19.4) (102,103). With ultrastructural immunogold labeling, the lysosomes are seen to be packed with monotypic light chains (102). In cases associated with Fanconi syndrome, there are needle-shaped, round or rectangular to rodlike, electron-dense structures in the cytoplasm of the proximal tubular cells. The needle-like inclusion bodies can appear crystalline (Fig. 19.5) or fibrillary. At high magnification, the crystalline-appearing inclusions sometimes exhibit parallel linear arrays. These structures can also be labeled for the specific light chain using ultrastructural immunogold techniques (Fig. 19.5B) (102,142,143).

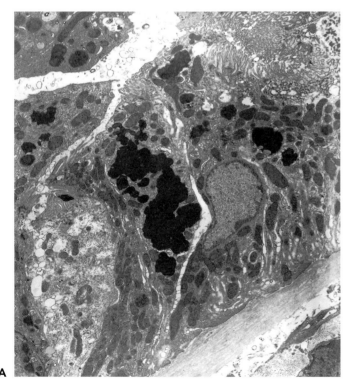
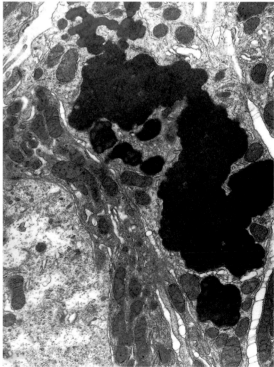

**A**    **B**

**Figure 19.4.** Acute tubulopathy, light chain related. Atypical lysosomes in proximal tubular cells exposed to tubulopathic light chains with segmental loss of microvillous border. Transmission electron microscopy. (Uranyl acetate and lead citrate; **A:** ×11,000; **B:** ×17,500.)

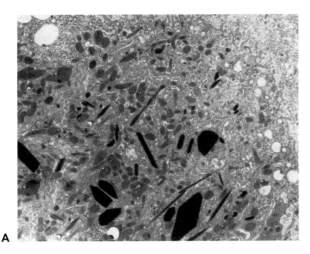 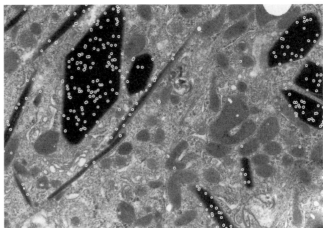

**Figure 19.5.**   Acquired light chain–related Fanconi syndrome. **A,B:** Crystalline cytoplasmic inclusions labeled for κ light chains in proximal tubular cells. **B:** Intense gold labeling for κ light chains in cytoplasmic inclusions. Ten-nanometer gold particles have been traced with computer-assisted technology to highlight the labeling. Transmission electron microscopy. (Uranyl acetate and lead citrate; **A:** ×8500; **B:** ×12,500.)

## Etiology and Pathogenesis

The pathogenesis of this type of renal damage is directly related to the inability of the lysosomal system to degrade the nephrotoxic light chain, resulting in "clogging" of the lysosomes in the proximal tubules (115,144). When immunogold labeling is performed, the lysosomes are found to be overfilled with the monotypic light chain that they are unable to properly degrade. Lysosomal overload causes release of their proteolytic enzymes into the cytosol, leading to cytoplasmic vacuolization, simplification, and even frank necrosis. As a consequence, fragmentation, desquamation, and apical blebbing of the proximal tubular cells occur with accompanying segmental or total loss of microvillous borders. Most cases of Fanconi syndrome are associated with the κ 1 subgroup, most originating from two germ lines: LCO2 and LCO12 (136). In the case of Fanconi syndrome-associated proximal tubular damage, the partially digested light chains form the fibrillary or crystalline inclusions in the cytoplasm of the proximal tubules. The crystalloid structures have been shown to contain a complete monoclonal κ light chain and a truncated NH-terminal fragment corresponding to the variable domain that is necessary for crystallization to occur (61,62). These partially digested fragments result from degradation by cathepsin B, and they do not bind Tamm-Horsfall protein except in very exceptional cases. This observation explains why cast nephropathy is so rarely associated with Fanconi syndrome.

## Differential Diagnosis

The main differential diagnosis is acute tubular necrosis from other causes. The best way to make an unequivocal diagnosis of light chain-related acute tubulopathy or acute tubular necrosis is by demonstrating monoclonal light chains in association with the lesion in question using immunofluorescence, electron microscopy, or immuno-electron microscopy, or a combination of these techniques (102,103). Unfortunately, the commercially available antibodies to κ and λ light chains do not always detect the abnormal light chain deposited in the kidneys. Good clinicopathologic correlation may be helpful in solidifying this diagnosis. In the case of light chain-associated Fanconi syndrome, the presence of the characteristic tubular cytoplasmic inclusions and the demonstration that these contain monotypic light chains suffices to make a solid diagnosis (84,140,142,143).

## Treatment, Course of the Disease Process, and Prognosis

This lesion is often seen in conjunction with other patterns, and the clinical course and prognosis of light chain-associated acute tubular necrosis or tubulopathy as a specific entity have not been carefully analyzed. The disease course and prognosis of the concomitant process tend to prevail in these combined patterns of disease. However, anecdotal cases indicate that, by itself, this lesion is fully reversible if the circulating light chains can be controlled. Therefore, aggressive treatment of the underlying plasma cell dyscrasia, together with clinical support while the tubules are regenerating, is the standard of care. Some patients may require temporary dialysis during the acute renal failure episode. It is also important to realize that when combined lesions are present (i.e., LCDD and light chain-associated acute tubular necrosis), the acute tubulopathy may be the main culprit responsible for the renal failure

(103). If tubular function can be reinstated, renal failure can improve dramatically.

There are degrees of acute tubulopathy, and the mild forms are probably of no significant clinical importance. The long-term effects of recurring acute tubular necrosis in the setting of an underlying plasma cell dyscrasia are not known. More careful clinicopathologic studies are needed to clarify the overall importance of this lesion on patients' prognosis and renal survival.

Because this may be the only renal pathology, a definitive diagnosis in a patient with a circulating paraprotein represents objective morphologic evidence of organ damage and should be taken as an indicator that treatment of the plasma cell dyscrasia is warranted.

## Inflammatory Tubular Interstitial Nephritis

This is perhaps the least recognized of the patterns of renal damage associated with plasma cell dyscrasias. It mimics acute tubular interstitial nephritis. It is important to recognize it so that its association with an undiagnosed underlying plasma cell dyscrasia can be established and to rule out other forms of tubular interstitial nephritis.

### Historical Perspective

Two patients were reported in the 1980s with inflammatory tubular interstitial changes and/or isolated tubular basement membrane monotypic κ light chain deposits. The patients had myeloma with no associated glomerular or vascular light chain deposition, and they were considered atypical LCDD cases (36,145). For many years, it has been recognized that in patients with cast nephropathy, interstitial inflammation may be a significant finding. Some patients with known myeloma and renal insufficiency show no evidence of cast nephropathy or any other forms of plasma cell dyscrasia-associated pathology, but the biopsy shows a patchy interstitial inflammatory infiltrate associated with tubulitis, providing a clue that such a lesion could be part of the spectrum of plasma cell-associated renal pathology. A series of eight such patients has been compiled recently (146) to emphasize this rather unusual pattern of light chain-related renal disease, which could be confused with an acute tubular interstitial nephritis unrelated to the plasma cell dyscrasia because of the similarity in histologic findings (147). All but one of these patients and the two previously published cases have been κ light chain related.

### Clinical Presentation and Laboratory Findings

Among patients with plasma cell dyscrasias and related renal disease, this morphologic pattern accounts for approximately 10% of cases (146). All the patients with this disease process have presented in acute renal failure, and the cause is either unknown or is related to a plasma cell dyscrasia, most often overt myeloma. The patients are usually older than 50. Serum and urine electrophoresis showed seven patients with κ light chains and one with λ light chains. Nonnephrotic range proteinuria may be found. Serum creatinine is quite variable, but it is generally more than 3 mg/dL at presentation (146).

### Gross Pathology

The kidneys from two patients exhibiting this lesion in a recent autopsy series showed normal weight and no specific gross findings (77).

### Light Microscopy

The glomerular and vascular compartments are unremarkable. The tubular interstitial compartment shows an inflammatory process composed predominantly of lymphocytes and plasma cells associated with tubulitis (Fig. 19.6).

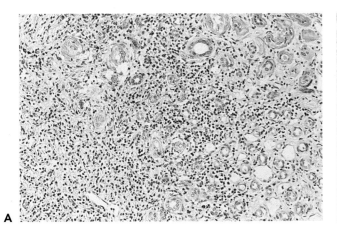
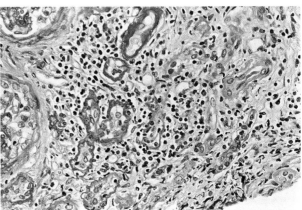

**Figure 19.6.** Inflammatory light chain–related tubular interstitial nephritis. **A:** Intense interstitial inflammation associated with lymphocytes extending through tubular basement membranes into tubules. (H&E, ×350.) **B:** This is better seen on PAS stain. (×500.)

The inflammatory process can be intense. Tubular damage can be variable but is frequently marked. There is no tubular cast formation. The absence of casts in multiple sections taken from autopsy kidneys represents substantial evidence that this lesion is clearly separable from light chain cast nephropathy and that it represents a specific pattern of renal damage in patients with plasma cell dyscrasias (77). Because the diagnosis requires the demonstration of monotypic light chains along the tubular basement membranes, it cannot be established by light microscopy alone.

## Immunofluorescence

Linear monotypic light chain staining may be demonstrated outlining the tubular basement membranes in association with the most intense interstitial inflammation. There may also be intracytoplasmic staining in proximal tubular cells for the monotypic light chain (145,146). As with acute tubulopathy, there are cases in which staining for both light chains is present, but if the pertinent light chain is more prominently stained, this finding supports the diagnosis.

## Immunohistochemistry

In some of these cases, monotypic light chain staining deposition along tubular basement membranes in areas with interstitial inflammation and tubulitis can be clearly demonstrated using immunohistochemistry (146). In these cases monotypic staining for the pertinent light chain can be striking, whereas there is no staining for the other light chain (Fig. 19.7).

## Electron Microscopy

No specific glomerular or vascular changes are identified. Specifically, there are neither light chain deposits nor evidence of amyloid deposition. In some cases there may be focal deposition of light chains, represented by punctate to powdery, electron-dense material along the outer aspect of the tubular basement membranes (146), but in most cases such is not the case. The lysosomal system may be prominent in the proximal tubules. By ultrastructural immunogold technique, distinct labeling for monotypic light chains can be demonstrated along the tubular basement membranes in areas with prominent interstitial inflammation and in tubules exhibiting tubulitis. Both proximal and distal tubules may be labeled, but the findings are usually more striking along distal tubules (143). Highly concentrated monotypic light chains are also noted in proteinaceous material in tubular lumina, which does not organize into well-formed casts (146).

## Etiology and Pathogenesis

The inflammatory interstitial reaction that may occur in these cases is probably induced by the binding of pathogenic light chains to the tubular basement membranes, which alters intrinsic tissue antigens and promotes the release of cytokines, resulting in chemoattraction and activation of interstitial mononuclear inflammatory components. Light chains may reach the tubular basement membranes by transcytosis after reabsorption or by passive tissue diffusion from peritubular capillaries (146). Conceptually speaking, this pattern of renal disease could be considered as a type of LCDD with pathologic manifestations restricted to the tubular interstitial compartment.

## Differential Diagnosis

An important differential diagnosis is acute tubular interstitial nephritis (147). When eosinophils are present, a hypersensitivity reaction is an important consideration in the

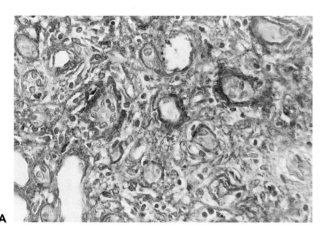
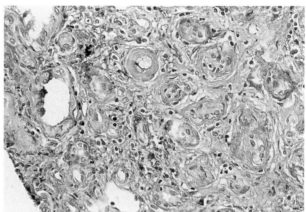

**Figure 19.7.** Inflammatory light chain-related tubular interstitial nephritis. Note labeling of tubular basement membranes for κ (**A**) but not λ (**B**) light chains in an area with prominent interstitial inflammatory activity. Immunohistochemistry for κ (**A**) and λ (**B**) light chains. (Peroxidase anti-peroxidase stain, diaminobenzidine as marker; ×500.)

differential diagnosis. It is imperative for an accurate diagnosis to demonstrate that monotypic light chains are associated with the tubular interstitial compartment using ancillary diagnostic techniques. There are no light microscopic findings that allow separation of the light chain-related type of inflammatory tubular interstitial nephritis from the other types of acute tubular interstitial nephritis.

## Treatment, Course of the Disease Process, and Prognosis

This disease is a relatively recently recognized entity, and there are no studies addressing kidney survival or the clinical course of this disease.

## MONOCLONAL IMMUNOGLOBULIN DEPOSITION DISEASES

Monoclonal immunoglobulin deposition diseases are systemic disorders characterized by deposition of monoclonal immunoglobulins in many organs, but the kidneys are the most commonly involved. In most cases, light chains are the immunoglobulin components that deposit in tissues, giving rise to LCDD, but recently, heavy chain-associated monoclonal deposition disease, also referred to as *heavy chain deposition disease* (HCDD), has been recognized. Interestingly, the pathologic findings in both light chain and heavy chain deposition diseases are quite similar (84,103,140,148,149). Our understanding of the pathogenesis of light chain-related deposition diseases is more complete than that of heavy chain-related diseases. This is mainly because light chain-associated diseases were described long before their counterparts, and they are more prevalent. A few cases of combined light and heavy chain deposition disease have been reported (140). The morphologic spectrum of these conditions is extensive, so routine staining of renal biopsies for κ and λ light chains is imperative to identify unusual and early manifestations of these disorders.

## Historical Perspective

In 1957, Kobernick and Whiteside showed nonamyloid glomerular abnormalities in patients with myeloma and recognized the similarity of these lesions with diabetic nephropathy (150). About 10 years later, Abrahams et al reported a myeloma patient with renal disease and deposition of subendothelial material in glomeruli described as "coarse and more granular than the glomerular basement membrane" (151). The next year Rosen et al (152) reported a similar case, with what he described as glomerular "osmiophilic subendothelial densities." It was Antonovych et al (153) in 1974 who first recognized the association of

the ultrastructural findings noted above with the deposition of κ light chains. Randall et al (154) in 1976 published two autopsies from patients with plasma cell dyscrasias and documented the widespread pathologic findings of a disease that he referred to as "systemic LCDD." Heavy chain deposition disease was first described 17 years later by Aucouturier et al (155), who emphasized that in this disorder, instead of deposition of light chain immunoglobulin components, there were deposits composed of monotypic heavy chains. In 1985 Jacquot et al (74) were the first to describe three cases of LCDD associated with light chain (AL) amyloidosis.

## Light Chain Deposition Disease

### Clinical Presentation and Laboratory Findings

There is no significant sex predilection for this disease, but males predominate slightly in most series (7:5). The average age of patients with LCDD with renal manifestations is 55 to 60 years. At the time of diagnosis, acute renal failure is present in 30%, and a similar percentage is dialysis-dependent. Most (more than 90%) present with proteinuria, and the average protein excretion per 24 hours is in the nephrotic range (generally 4 to 5 g/day) in 53% of LCDD patients. Interestingly, full-blown nephrotic syndrome is noted in a minority of these cases (140). Seventy-eight percent of LCDD patients present with hypertension, 52% have hematuria, and varying degrees of renal insufficiency are detected in 95% of these patients (140). In selected LCDD cases, tubular dysfunction is the predominant clinical manifestation (156,157). As the clinicopathologic heterogenicity of this disease is better appreciated, patients are diagnosed earlier, and the manifestations of renal insufficiency tend to be less pronounced (158–163).

Rapid deterioration of renal function occurs as the disease advances, if not treated aggressively. Renal biopsy preceded any other clinical signs or evidence of dysproteinemia in 70% of the cases with pure LCDD (140,149). Classic features of underlying myeloma are present in more than half of these patients, but there is a significant number of patients with LCDD that have either a normal bone marrow biopsy and aspirate or rather unimpressive plasmacytosis at presentation that is often incorrectly considered reactive (103,149). Careful evaluation of the plasma cells in the latter case using either immunohistochemical techniques or flow cytometry can identify a monoclonal population of plasma cells, albeit a small clone in many cases. Biosynthetic studies of the plasma cells often demonstrate paraprotein production, even when serum and urine electrophoresis fail to show any abnormalities (36). In autopsy of patients who died with a clinical diagnosis of myeloma, approximately 3% to 5% exhibited LCDD (77,83). This figure is conservative, as the less characteristic cases of LCDD are not diagnosed because immunofluorescence and electron microscopy of the kidneys was not part of the evaluation of these autopsies. The most commonly involved light chains in these cases are κ, and subtypes IV and I predominate (164). The ratio of κ to λ is 9:1 in LCDD (140).

Bone marrow biopsy and aspirate revealed sufficient criteria to diagnose myeloma in 35% of LCDD cases, osteolytic lesions in 13%, and hypogammaglobulinemia in 33%. Of the patients with LCDD at the time of clinical presentation and diagnosis, 39% carried a diagnosis of MGUS (165). Up to 30% of patients with MIDD have no detectable monoclonal proteins in urine or serum, and even using the most sensitive techniques available, the percentage of patients falling in this category remained at 15% to 20% (165).

When LCDD coexisted with light chain cast nephropathy, 82% of these patients presented with acute renal failure, and 64% required dialysis (84). Renal biopsy preceded any clinical evidence of dysproteinemia in 64% of the patients with combined LCDD and cast nephropathy. Cases of combined cast nephropathy and LCDD are mainly associated with κ light chains. Light chain deposition disease can also occur in combination with light chain-associated (AL) amyloidosis (74–76) and HCDD (140). The paraprotein composition of LHCDD is typically IgG-κ or IgG-λ (140).

## Gross Pathology

There are only two autopsy studies in patients with myeloma performed after LCDD was described in 1976. Three patients with LCDD were noted in the series by Ivanyi et al, and the mean weight of the kidneys was 271 g (83,166). Herrera et al (77) reported the autopsy findings in 77 patients with myeloma. These cases comprised approximately 10% of all cases with myeloma that died during the period of time this study covered at the institution. There were two cases with LCDD, both with small kidneys with

average weight of 130 g and evidence of surface scarring attributed to coexistent vascular disease.

## Light Microscopy

The most characteristic finding in patients with LCDD is nodular glomerulopathy (Fig. 19.8) that mimics the nodular glomerulosclerosis pattern of diabetic nephropathy (167–173). Capsular drops, hyaline caps, and capillary microaneurysms are not present in LCDD, and the absence of these features helps in the differential diagnosis from diabetic nephropathy. In addition, the mesangial nodules in LCDD are more evenly distributed, although there is significant variation depending on the stage of the disease process (57,58,163,168,169), whereas the nodules in diabetic nephropathy tend to be asymmetric. The mesangial nodules are argyrophilic and composed of extracellular matrix proteins admixed with monotypic light chains (174,175), and the principal matrix protein deposited is tenascin (175). In silver methenamine-stained sections, there may be lamellation of the peripheral portions of the mesangial nodules. Mesangial hypercellularity accompanies the increase in extracellular matrix in some of the cases. The peripheral capillary walls are variably thickened, and the capillary wall alterations are uneven from one glomerulus to the other and even within the same glomerulus. The thickened walls are a consequence of the subendothelial deposition of light chains (103,143). There are a number of glomerular morphologic patterns, including mesangial, membranoproliferative, and crescentic (176–179), that precede the nodular glomerulopathy. Progression from one of these "early" patterns to a classic nodular glomerulosclerosis has been shown to occur when repeat kidney biopsies are performed. A recently recognized "atypical" variant of LCDD shows peculiar light microscopic features and ultrastructural findings (180) simulating an immune complex–mediated disease. The light chain deposits, regardless of

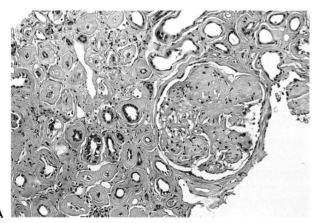
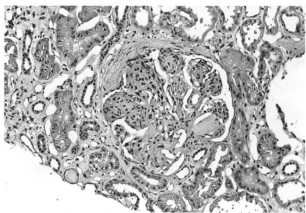

**Figure 19.8.** Light chain deposition disease. Nodular glomerulopathy characteristic of LCDD is evident. Note variation in cellularity, with hypercellular nodules present in **(B)**. (H&E; ×500.)

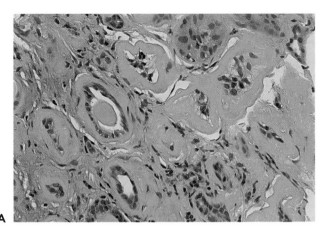 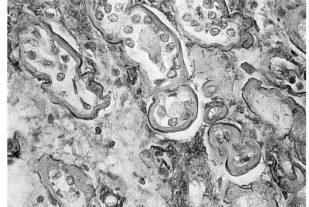

A    B

**Figure 19.9.** Light chain deposition disease. **A:** Thickened tubular basement membranes. (H&E; ×500.) **B:** κ Light chain deposition on the outer aspect of the tubular basement membranes. (Immunohistochemistry for κ light chain, peroxidase anti-peroxidase stain, diaminobenzidine as marker; ×500.)

whether they are in renal or extrarenal sites, are always Congo red negative.

In patients with early LCDD, the glomeruli at times appear essentially unremarkable, and these cases may be incorrectly diagnosed as minimal change glomerulopathy if immunofluorescence staining for light chains is not performed (102,103,143,149). Recognition of this LCDD pattern is very challenging (103,149) and requires careful immunomorphologic evaluation and/or immunoelectron microscopy (143) to confirm the association of monoclonal light chain deposits with the capillary walls.

The extraglomerular changes may also be quite impressive. The tubular basement membranes may be thickened and tortuous, as a result of deposition of light chains, generally on the outer aspect of the tubular basement membranes (Figs. 19.8A and 19.9). In our experience, thickening of vessel walls by light chain deposits is seen in ap-

proximately 40% of LCDD cases. In half of LCDD patients with vascular changes, concentric thickening of the small and medium arteries accompanied by focal light chain deposits (149) creates a striking hyperplastic vasculopathy. Light chain deposits can be found in many organs, including lung, liver, small and large intestine, thyroid, prostate, pancreas, rectum, skin, spleen, and choroid plexus, among others (154).

## Immunofluorescence

Deposition of monoclonal light chains can be seen along peripheral capillary walls in glomeruli, alongside tubular basement membranes, and in vessel walls (Fig. 19.10); the staining can be interrupted and in some cases is subtle (103,143,162). The pattern and intensity of staining depend on the amount and distribution of light chain

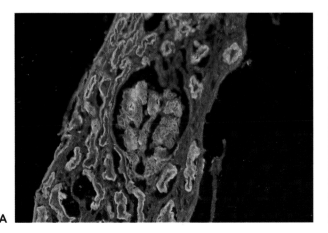 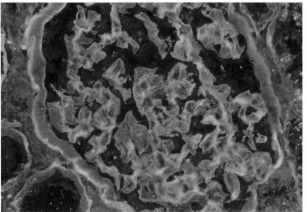

A    B

**Figure 19.10.** Light chain deposition disease. **A:** Low-power view showing linear staining along tubular basement membranes and mesangial staining in glomeruli for κ light chains. (Fluorescein; ×150.) **B:** Linear peripheral glomerular capillary wall staining and staining along tubular basement membranes and Bowman's capsule. Direct immunofluorescence for κ light chain. (Fluorescein; ×500.)

deposits. No staining is noted for the other light chain, defining the monotypic nature of the labeling pattern. In most cases, there is also granular monotypic light chain mesangial staining in glomeruli, but mesangial staining is rare without accompanying capillary wall staining. In a subset of these patients, there is also focal granular staining in the interstitium proper. In some cases, there is a discrepancy between the fluorescence staining and the demonstration of light chains by electron microscopy. In fact, there are a few reported cases of combined LCDD and light chain cast nephropathy, in which the monotypic light chain deposition has been demonstrated by immunofluorescence and no corresponding deposits were found ultrastructurally (84,140).

Generic antibodies to κ and λ light chains cannot detect all pathologic light chains deposited in the kidney in patients with LCDD. Only when a specific antibody is raised against the pathologic light chain can it be guaranteed that the light chain will be detected. Also, in patients with concomitant diabetes mellitus and LCDD, the abnormal light chains are frequently glycosylated to a degree that impairs their detection. Immunogold electron microscopy is successful in labeling the abnormal light chains even when generic antibodies are used, attesting to the increased sensitivity of this technique (143). Immunofluorescence techniques have detected deposits in virtually every organ (154).

## Electron Microscopy

Light chain deposition manifested by flocculent to granular to powdery electron-dense material can be seen in all renal compartments (Figs. 19.11 and 19.12), especially in cases with nodular glomerulosclerosis (advanced lesion). Visualization of light chain deposits may be challenging because the deposits may blend with the mesangial matrix and glomerular/tubular basement membranes. In rare cases, the electron-dense light chain material is noted superimposed upon the glomerular basement membrane, mimicking dense deposit disease (102,181). At low magnification, the light chain deposits may simulate immune complexes (180). Light chain material is generally also present along the tubular basement membranes, Bowman's capsule, and in the interstitium (Fig. 19.12A) (182,183). There may also be distinct deposition of light chains in the vasculature (Fig. 19.12B) (149). The light chain deposits may be subtle when the amount of light chain deposits is limited (102), and they may blend with surrounding structures. In combined MIDD and cast nephropathy cases, the light microscopic alterations in glomeruli and other compartments may be subtle and easily missed, but combining the data obtained from immunofluorescence and electron microscopic evaluation should suffice to make the correct diagnosis (Fig. 19.13) (87,140).

## Etiology and Pathogenesis

Conclusive evidence that the abnormal light chain protein is primarily responsible for light chain-associated disease has been provided from an in vivo model using mice injected with human BJ proteins from patients with LCDD. Solomon et al (59) demonstrated nodular and diffuse light chain precipitates in the tubular basement membranes, mesangium, and vessel walls, recapitulating the key findings in the kidneys of these patients. Khamlichi et al (45) confirmed these results.

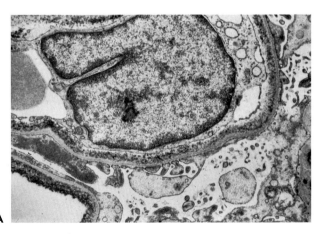 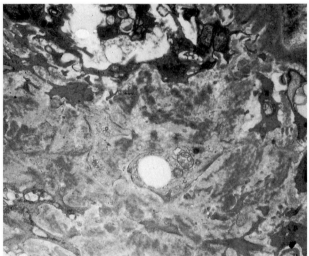

**Figure 19.11.** Light chain deposition disease. **A:** Continuous, punctate, subendothelial, electron-dense material (light chains) outlines the peripheral glomerular capillary wall. (Uranyl acetate and lead citrate; ×8500.) **B:** Mesangial light chain deposition. Transmission electron microscopy. (Uranyl acetate and lead citrate; ×9500.)

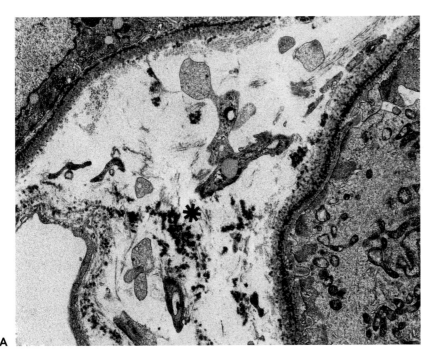
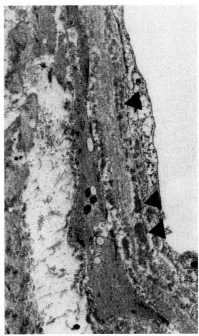

A                                                                                          B

**Figure 19.12.** Light chain deposition disease. Punctate, electron-dense material along tubular basement membranes and in the interstitium proper (*asterisk* in **A**) and along vessel wall (*arrowheads* in **B**). Transmission electron microscopy. (Uranyl acetate and lead citrate; **A:** ×7500; **B:** ×9500.)

Since then, the pathogenesis of LCDD has been scrutinized using renal biopsy material and an in vitro mesangial cell culture model. Studies on renal biopsies demonstrating platelet-derived growth factor-β (PDGF-β) and transforming growth factor-β (TGF-β) in the mesangium of patients with LCDD in various morphologic stages suggested a role for these two growth factors in the pathogenesis of this disorder (184). The in vitro model confirmed the findings in the renal specimens and showed that interactions between mesangial cells and light chains from these patients were crucial in the pathogenesis. Rat and human mesangial cells grown on coverslips and in a matrix with composition similar to that of an altered mesangial "milieu" and incubated with light chains purified from the urine of patients with LCDD recapitulated the biopsy findings (184–186). Human mesangial cells incubated with light chains purified from the urine of patients with LCDD transform from their usual smooth muscle to a myofibroblastic phenotype (187), endowing them with the necessary machinery to engage in active synthesis of extracellular matrix proteins. The initial events were activation of PDGF-β, leading to cellular proliferation through c-fos activation, and later TGF-β activation, resulting in matrix deposition (187,188). The in vitro model clearly demonstrated the crucial role of TGF-β in the production of extracellular matrix proteins by mesangial cells in LCDD (188). Tenascin is the main extracellular matrix protein in the nodules formed in the in vitro model, as well as in the mesangial nodules in nodular glomerulosclerosis in LCDD (175,185,186) by transformed

mesangial cells with a myofibroblastic phenotype (189). Tenascin is mainly degraded by matrix metalloproteinase 7 (MMP-7), with minor contributions by MMP-1 and MMP-3 (190). Matrix metalloproteinase 7 secretion by mesangial cells is impaired in LCDD, making tenascin degradation virtually impossible (191). The specific mechanism responsible for this has not yet been elucidated. The interactions between the light chains responsible for LCDD and mesangial cells occur through a receptor-mediated mechanism (192).

Although κ light chains are preferentially associated with LCDD, amino acid substitutions introducing hydrophobic residues in the exposed portions of the variable region of the light chains, usually in the CDR 1 and CDR 3 and less often CDR 2 and FR regions, are associated with LCDD, regardless of light chain subtype (193,194). Some light chains with posttranslational glycosylation have also been associated with LCDD (195).

## Treatment, Course of the Disease Process, and Prognosis

The outcome in LCDD remains uncertain and depends on how early in its course the disease is detected. Overall, patient survival at 1 and 5 years (89% versus 70%), respectively is better than renal survival (67% at 1 year versus 17% at 5 years) (140). Approximately one third of the LCDD patients without diagnostic features of myeloma develop overt myeloma during the course of the disease, affecting

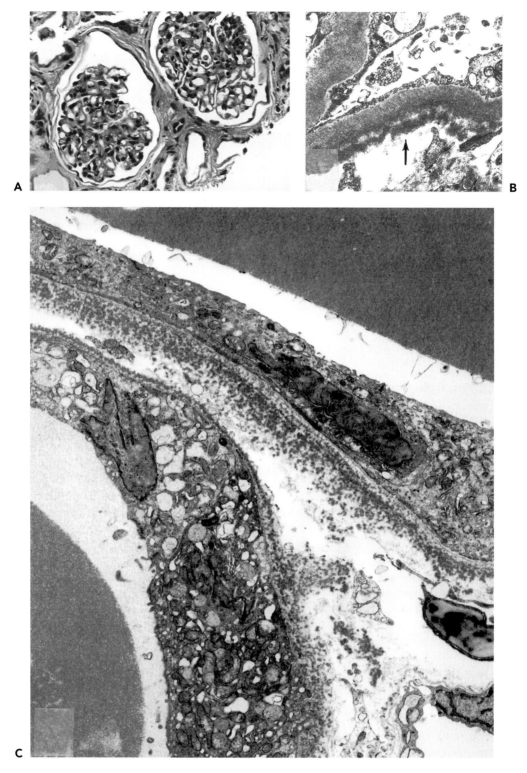

**Figure 19.13.** Light chain deposition disease and light chain cast nephropathy, combined. **A:** Glomeruli are unremarkable by light microscopy. (H&E; ×500.) **B:** However, ultrastructurally, deposition of light chain material is noted along peripheral glomerular capillary walls (*arrow*) and (**C**) along tubular basement membranes, associated with abundant distal tubular casts. **B, C:** Transmission electron microscopy. (Uranyl acetate and lead citrate; **B:** ×9500, **C:** ×7500.)

survival adversely. Extrarenal deposits can be asymptomatic or associated with organ damage (161).

Treatment is aimed at controlling and reducing the abnormal light chain production by the clone of plasma cells. Chemotherapy with melphalan and prednisone has been employed with success in patients with LCDD and myeloma (196), but the benefit of chemotherapy has been debated when the bone marrow findings are inconclusive, especially if a monoclonal protein cannot be demonstrated in serum or urine (195). Chemotherapy is most effective in cases with a serum creatinine lower than 2 mg/dL. The severity of the underlying plasma cell dyscrasia and the degree of renal failure at presentation, as expected, significantly affect prognosis (88). Bone marrow transplantation has been used, especially in cases detected early, before compromise of other organs has occurred (195–198). Those patients with overt myeloma do much worse than those with no detectable paraprotein/proliferation of plasma cells and systemic manifestations. However, even in those cases with poor response, renal progression to end-stage disease may take several years.

Early diagnosis and aggressive therapy appear to offer the best hope for these patients in terms of preservation of renal function and overall survival (198). High-intensity chemotherapy followed by stem cell rescue and bone marrow transplantation have been used in several trials, resulting in increased patients' survival and improvement in renal function (198,199), but this is not yet standard therapy.

There are a few reports of resolution or disappearance of nodular glomerulosclerosis after therapy in patients with LCDD, suggesting that early intervention can reverse renal damage in these patients (200,201).

## Transplantation in Light Chain Deposition Disease

Renal transplantation has been successful in patients with disease confined to the kidneys (202,203). If the production of the precursor protein is not controlled or eliminated before transplantation, the disease will recur in the transplanted kidney. Because complete control of the plasma cell dyscrasia is virtually impossible, recurrence is inevitable, and recurrence occurs in more than 50% of the patients 8 to 48 months after transplantation and may eventually lead to graft loss (202–206). In a series of patients documenting the outcome of seven LCDD patients that were transplanted, recurrence occurred in five of the allografts (202). Recurrence is not always associated with rapid loss of the transplanted kidney; the median time to reach end-stage renal failure was 33.3 months. One of these transplanted patients was alive with no evidence of recurrence 13 years after transplantation (202). Therefore, renal trans-

plantation can be used to improve quality of life in certain patients but not as a long-term solution in the majority. Unfortunately, even when it is believed that control of the plasma cell clone has been achieved, it can re-emerge, followed by light chain deposition. Light chain deposition disease can recur without clinical evidence of underlying myeloma (206). There is a case report of de novo LCDD arising in a transplanted cadaver kidney 16 years after transplantation (207).

## Heavy Chain Deposition Disease

### Clinical Presentation and Laboratory Findings

Heavy chain disease (HCD) is a disorder characterized by the production of monoclonal immunoglobulins with truncated heavy chains and no associated light chains. Abnormal heavy chains circulate in the blood of patients with this disorder, and these paraproteins must be identified in the serum and characterized to make a definitive diagnosis. Heavy chain disease involving three immunoglobulin classes has been described: α-HCD is the most common of the three, followed by γ-HCD and then μ-HCD. Patients with α-HCD present with malabsorption and protein-losing enteropathy; renal disease is not a significant clinical manifestation of this condition and only occurs sporadically. Approximately 150 cases of γ-HCD have been reported, and it is a heterogeneous disorder, which some believe does not justify its diagnosis as a single entity (208). This disease usually manifests with lymphadenopathy, splenomegaly, and constitutional symptoms. Palatal edema and uvula swelling, initially thought to be characteristic of the disease, are only noted in approximately 10% to 15% of all patients with γ-HCD (208). Skeletal involvement occurs in approximately 30% of these patients, and differentiation from myeloma and Waldenström macroglobulinemia may be difficult on clinical grounds (208). γ–heavy chain disease is the most common type of HCD associated with renal manifestations (208).

The majority of patients with HCD do not develop HCDD. Bence-Jones proteinuria is common. Heavy chain disease and cast nephropathy have been documented to coexist (140). There is not much experience with μ-HCD and renal disease (148,208). Heavy chain deposition disease is mainly associated with γ (γ 1 and γ 3 subtypes) and rarely with α-heavy chains.

Only approximately 75 to 100 patients with HCDD have been described in the literature (87,140,208). There is no sex predilection for HCDD. Patients with HCDD and renal disease tend to be younger than those with LCDD by a few years (average age 53 to 55 years of age); but some patients in the third decade have also been reported (140,148). The clinical presentation is similar to that of LCDD patients. Hypertension, nephrotic syndrome, microhematuria, and renal insufficiency are usually present at the time of the renal biopsy (148). Hypocomplementemia is not uncommon in HCDD and correlates with the presence of γ 1 or 3 subtypes of γ heavy chain (148). Signs of complement activation with C3 deposition in the kidney represent an additional feature of this condition (140,148). Hypertension and hematuria are more common in HCDD than in LCDD (148). In some patients with HCDD, a monoclonal component is not detectable in serum and or urine. Whereas most patients with HCDD have a monoclonal gammopathy, only a few meet the minimal criteria for myeloma (84).

It is likely that HCDD is underdiagnosed in renal biopsies, and the incidence of this condition is very likely underestimated. For example, two recent autopsy series of patients with myeloma (77,83) failed to identify any patients with HCDD, suggesting that the overall knowledge about this disease and methods available to diagnose it remain suboptimal. Patients with findings in their renal biopsies that are suggestive of deposition disease with negative stains for κ and λ by immunofluorescence should be worked up for HCDD.

Some cases are combined LCDD and HCDD (142), and γ is the most frequent heavy chain component in these cases. Both κ and λ light chains have been found in the LCDD component of these cases (140). The combined variety occurs in older patients—by approximately 10 years—than patients with LCDD or HCDD alone (140). Overall renal function is more significantly impaired at presentation when the two deposition disorders coexist, with an average serum creatinine in the neighborhood of 5 mg/dL. However, proteinuria is usually in the range of 3 g/24 h. The diagnosis of combined LHCDD requires careful pathologic evaluation of the renal biopsies and a high index of suspicion (140). The diagnosis cannot be reached by light microscopy alone; immunofluorescence with the use of specific antisera is required.

## Gross Pathology

There are no studies describing specific gross findings in patients with HCDD.

## Light Microscopy

In the great majority of the reported cases of HCDD, nodular glomerulosclerosis with features identical to those seen in association with LCDD has been identified (Fig. 19.14) (140,209–212). Crescents were described in four of nine cases, involving 11% to 75% of the glomeruli in one series (140,213). The broad spectrum of glomerular lesions described in LCDD has not been documented in HCDD, with the exception of a single case of intracapillary proliferative glomerulonephritis (214). Tubular basement membrane deposits with no glomerular or vascular heavy chain deposition have been reported (140). Congo red stain is always negative.

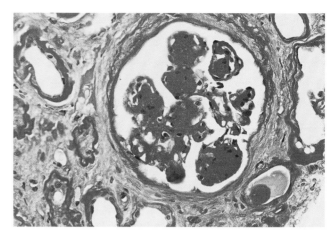

**Figure 19.14.**   Heavy chain deposition disease. Morphological findings in HCDD are identical to those in LCDD, with nodular glomerulopathy as the typical pattern. (H&E; ×500.)

## Immunofluorescence

Only heavy chain components are positive, and staining for light chains is negative. Cases with γ 1, γ 3, γ 4, α, and μ chain deposits have been reported, and γ chain deposits are the most common (140). The distribution of staining is similar as that for LCDD (Fig. 19.15), but the degree of staining along tubular basement membranes is generally less than in LCDD. The staining for the heavy chain components varies from a predominantly linear to a much less common granular pattern (84,140). The heavy chain deposits usually display a uniform, continuous pattern of deposition at the various sites responsible for the linear fluorescence staining pattern noted in the great majority of the cases. Specific antibodies for portions of the heavy chain molecule that are missing in this condition (anti-$C_H$1 and anti-$C_H$2) can be used to confirm the absence of these

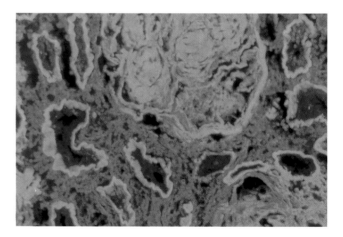

**Figure 19.15.**   Heavy chain deposition disease. Intense peripheral capillary wall and mesangial staining, associated with linear tubular basement membrane staining. Direct immunofluorescence staining for μ heavy chain. (Fluorescein; ×350.)

components and confirm the diagnosis (80,142,204,213). Extrarenal deposits of heavy chain components have been reported in pancreas, thyroid, striated muscle, and liver but are less frequent than in LCDD (84,140).

## Electron Microscopy

The ultrastructural findings in HCDD are similar to those in LCDD in most instances. The heavy chain deposits can be subtle or massive. Overall, heavy chain deposits are variable in quantity and distribution in the various renal compartments. In one case the deposits were described as fibrillary, consisting of 13- to 18-nm-diameter fibrils without periodicity, judged ultrastructurally to be different from those found in fibrillary glomerulopathy. The fibrils exhibited various lengths, with the shorter ones having smooth walls and the longer fibrils exhibiting a "barbed-wire" appearance (215). This case appears to represent an unusual morphologic manifestation of μ-chain HCDD. The patient had no clinical manifestations of Waldenström's macroglobulinemia. Another μ-HCDD had massive fibrillary deposits in the mesangium that varied from 16 to 18 nm in diameter and were determined not to be compatible with the material seen in fibrillary glomerulopathy by electron microscopic criteria (210). These two cases suggest that there may be a variant of HCDD with peculiar fibrillary ultrastructural appearance, but this deserves further consideration.

## Etiology and Pathogenesis

The deletions in the domains of heavy chain portion of the immunoglobulin molecule (i.e., $C_H1$, $C_H2$, and very rarely, hinge region) result in premature secretion of the heavy chain into the circulation, and these structurally abnormal heavy chains are deposited in target organs, including the kidneys (216). The γ-heavy chain protein normally is retained in the endoplasmic reticulum during IgG assembly by binding of the $C_H1$ domain (and to some extent $C_H2$ and hinge region) to heavy chain binding protein. The specific mechanisms involved in the pathogenesis of the renal alterations that occur in this disorder have not been elucidated.

## Treatment, Course of the Disease Process, and Prognosis

The therapy employed is similar to that of LCDD, and the results appear to be comparable (198). However, there are no controlled trials addressing the therapy and management of patients with HCDD. Nevertheless, it appears that, based on anecdotal experience, the overall outcome is poor in terms of renal and patient survival. One patient had γ-HCDD for 10 years and subsequently developed γ AL amyloidosis (217).

## Transplantation in Heavy Chain Deposition Disease

The experience with transplantation in this disease is extremely limited. One transplanted HCDD patient developed recurrent disease approximately 1.5 years after transplantation, so the fate of renal transplants in this condition may be similar to the more extensive experience in LCDD (218).

## Differential Diagnosis for LHCDD (Light and Heavy Chain Deposition Disease)

Because the light microscopic appearance of LHCDD is so variable, the differential diagnosis includes many diseases, and it must be differentiated from minimal change disease in those cases where the glomeruli appear essentially normal, from mesangial proliferative glomerulonephritis when mesangial proliferation is present, and from membranoproliferative glomerulonephritis, including dense deposit disease; also, crescentic glomerulonephritis must be distinguished from the proliferative variants of LCDD (103). When considering the most characteristic expression of LCDD and HCDD—nodular glomerulosclerosis—the main differential diagnosis is diabetic nephropathy or "idiopathic" nodular glomerulosclerosis (219). In most instances, demonstration of monoclonal light or heavy chain determinants in the proper histopathologic setting is the essential diagnostic finding. Careful attention to the tubular interstitial and vascular compartments for light chain deposits is also imperative, as there is a subset of LCDD patients with no glomerular light chain deposition and only interstitial manifestations of this disease (103,140). It is also important to identify heavy chain deletions using specific antisera to the mutated components of the heavy chain molecule in HCDD to confirm that diagnosis. Rarely, amyloidosis needs to be ruled out, especially in cases with nodular glomerulopathy. In the great majority of these situations, immunofluorescence and electron microscopy suffice, and a solid, unequivocal diagnosis can be obtained. Selective use of immunoelectron microscopy is indicated when the usual diagnostic techniques do not provide enough data to establish an unequivocal diagnosis (143). In the experience of one of the authors (GAH), approximately 5% of the cases require an extended workup beyond routine light, immunofluorescence, and ultrastructural evaluation.

## AMYLOIDOSES

AL and AH amyloidosis (formerly "primary" and "associated with multiple myeloma") are included in this chapter because these forms of disease are associated with a paraprotein, and the amyloid fibrils are derived from

**TABLE 19.1**

**SYSTEMIC AMYLOIDOSES IN HUMANS: AMYLOID FIBRIL PROTEINS AND THEIR PRECURSORS**

| Amyloid Protein | Precursor | Systemic (S) or Localized (L) | Syndrome |
|---|---|---|---|
| AL/AH | Immunoglobulin light/heavy chain | S, L | Primary, myeloma associated |
| AA | Serum AA protein | S, ?L | Sporadic: secondary, reactive, familial |
| ATTR | Transthyretin | S, ?L | Familial, senile, systemic |
| AFib | Fibrinogen A α chain | S | Familial |
| AApoAI, II, IV | Apolipoprotein AI, AII, AIV | S, L | Familial, sporadic (aging) |
| AGel | Gelsolin | S | Familial |
| ALys | Lysozyme | S | Familial |
| ACys | Cystatin C | S | Familial |
| $A\beta_2M$ | $\beta_2$ microglobulin | S, ?L | Dialysis associated |

immunoglobulin light (AL) or heavy (AH) chains. AA amyloidosis (formerly "secondary") and familial, dialysis-related, and localized types of amyloidoses, which are not related to myeloma or paraproteinemia, are also discussed in this chapter because they have pathologic and pathogenetic similarities to AL amyloidosis and for historical reasons.

## Definition

Amyloidosis comprises a group of protein-folding disorders of diverse etiology in which deposits of abnormally folded proteins share unique staining properties and fibrillar ultrastructural appearance (220). These deposits ultimately lead to destruction of tissues and progressive disease. Despite the biochemical diversity, all types of amyloid have a β-pleated sheet secondary structure that confers their diagnostic staining characteristics and stability under physiologic conditions (220–222). The term *amyloid* was first coined by Schleiden in 1838 to describe a normal constituent of plants. He used the iodine/sulfuric acid reaction to produce a blue or violet color, first described in 1814, to identify starch and related compounds (223,224). In 1839, botanists started using this reaction to identify cellulose, a compound related to starch that, like starch, is made up of glucose repeat units (225). In 1853, Virchow demonstrated that amyloid behaved similarly to cellulose when tested and applied the term *amyloid*, meaning "starch-like" (224,225). Freidrich and Kekule were the first to recognize that the material found by Virchow in a waxy spleen, and believed to be amyloid, was probably proteinaceous rather than cellulose-like (226,227). More than a century later, biochemical studies of the isolated amyloid fibrils demonstrated that amyloid is indeed derived from protein.

## Classification

A biochemical approach is the basis for the current classification of amyloid, and the World Health Organization classification is based upon the type of amyloid fibril protein, also referred to as the *precursor protein* (Table 19.1) (228,229). By convention, the amyloid fibril type is designated A for amyloid, followed by an abbreviated form of the name of the fibril protein. In primary amyloidosis, multiple myeloma-associated amyloidosis, and in many cases of tumor-forming amyloidosis, the amyloid is designated AL (light chain related) or AH (heavy chain related). The second major form of systemic amyloid, seen in amyloidosis secondary to chronic inflammatory conditions and familial Mediterranean fever, is derived from an acute phase reactant—serum amyloid A protein (SAA)—and the amyloid type is designated AA. There are more than 20 types of precursor proteins associated with various clinical forms of amyloidosis and many more variants. While some amyloidoses are localized, others are systemic, or systemic and localized (229).

Amyloidosis is a rare disease, with an estimated prevalence of 1 per 60,000 (230). The prevalence of amyloidosis increases with age. Among adult patients with nephrotic syndrome, approximately 1% to 5% have amyloidosis (231). It is extremely rare in children (232). The autopsy incidence of systemic amyloidosis is 0.8% (230).

The most common type of amyloidosis depends on the population studied. In the United States and the Western world, amyloidosis associated with an underlying plasma cell dyscrasia (AL amyloidosis) is by far the most prevalent, followed by AA amyloidosis. A large series from the Mayo Clinic examining data from 1977 to 1986 demonstrated that 74% of patients with amyloidosis were AL type, 4% were AA type, and among the remaining patients 20%

had localized and 2% had familial amyloidoses (233). In the developed countries the prevalence of AA amyloidosis varies, with lower numbers in the United States than in Europe (234,235; see also the section "AA Amyloidosis"). Recent data from the United Kingdom (National Amyloidosis Centre) show that AA amyloidosis was diagnosed in 18% of systemic amyloidoses. This is in contrast to developing countries, where secondary (AA) amyloidosis is far more common than AL amyloidosis (236). In fact, worldwide, an estimated 45% of all generalized amyloidoses are of the AA type, which makes it the second most frequent type of systemic amyloidosis (recently reviewed by Röcken and Shakespeare [237]). Familial amyloidoses are diagnosed with increasing frequency as awareness increases. While older series (233,238) showed that, among amyloid patients, only 2% had the familial form, more recent series (during the 2000–2004 period) show that 10% of new patients (239) have genetic abnormalities.

The following sections describe the pathology of renal amyloidosis in general, followed by specific features of the various types of amyloidosis presented in the different sections that follow.

## Gross Pathology

Postmortem examination of patients with amyloidosis have generally revealed enlarged kidneys with pale, waxy-appearing cut surfaces. The first study of amyloidosis by Bell clearly demonstrated an increase in the weight of kidneys, with only 5 of 65 cases showing either normal or small kidneys (82). In the study by Dikman et al (240), which included 33 autopsies and 1 nephrectomy from patients with different types of amyloidosis, the kidneys weighed more than 200 g in 9 patients and between 100 and 200 g in 16 patients. By intravenous pyelogram, the kidneys were shown to be increased in size in 36 cases and smaller than normal in 5 cases. Interestingly, the weight

of the kidneys did not correlate with renal function or the site of renal amyloid deposition and was generally inversely proportional to the amount of renal amyloid (240). This indicates that, in advanced cases, parenchymal atrophy is the determining factor accounting for kidney size. The average kidney weight of four patients with AL amyloidosis in a recent autopsy study was 200 g (77).

## Light Microscopy

The light microscopic features of amyloidosis are the same regardless of the type of amyloid. Amyloid deposits can be found in any of the renal compartments. In hematoxylin and eosin–stained sections, amyloid appears as eosinophilic, amorphous, "hyaline" material (Fig. 19.16). Glomerular amyloid formation begins in the mesangium (Fig. 19.16A), eventually replacing the normal mesangial matrix (Fig. 19.16B) and extending into peripheral capillary walls. Amyloid can also be seen in the interstitium, beginning its deposition generally in areas adjacent to blood vessels. Another site of significant amyloid deposition is in the renal vasculature. Amyloid is defined by its tinctorial characteristics, which include Congo red positivity (salmon pink or pale rose staining) (Fig. 19.17A,B) and fluorescence with thioflavin T or S (103,241) (Fig. 19.17C). Congo red–positive (congophilic) material must polarize and produce apple green birefringence to be considered diagnostic of amyloid (Fig. 19.17B). To demonstrate small amounts of amyloid in tissue sections, it is recommended that the sections be cut to a thickness of 9 or 10 μm, instead of the customary 4 μm (241). Alternatively, examination of additional sections of regular thickness (typically two or more) may yield similar results. Adequate polarization equipment is a must (reviewed by Röcken and Sletten [242]). Thioflavin fluorescence is much more sensitive than congophilia in the detection of small amounts of amyloid (103,163). It is very difficult to demonstrate

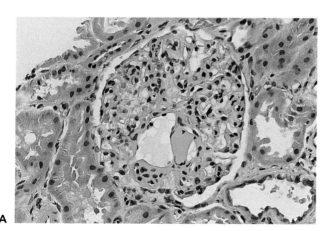
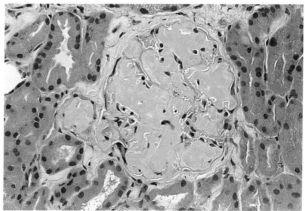

**Figure 19.16.** AL amyloidosis. **A:** Early segmental mesangial amyloid deposition. **B:** Complete obliteration of the glomerular architecture by amyloid deposits in an advanced case. (H&E; ×500.)

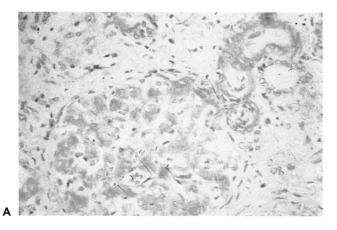

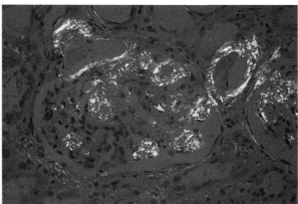

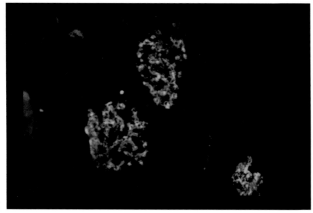

**Figure 19.17.** AL amyloidosis. **A:** Salmon pink staining of amyloid with Congo red. (×500.) **B:** Apple green birefringence is elicited on polarization of sample shown in (**A**). (×500.) **C:** Thioflavin-T stain depicts mesangial amyloid deposits. (×350.)

Congo red staining in small amyloid deposits, and even if the typical staining appearance is noted in small foci, it is extremely challenging to demonstrate the expected polarization. Proper detection of birefringence depends on the intensity of the transmitted light and, therefore, a strong light source is highly recommended to maximize results. All color filters should be removed. Examination of sections in the dark is also strongly recommended. If excessive Congo red dye is retained by the tissue, it can lead to false birefringence (243). Even when the technique is optimized, amyloid may only exhibit a weak affinity for Congo red and not show birefringence. "Pre-amyloidotic" deposits, i.e., deposits with immunohistochemistry that is positive for the amyloid precursor protein but negative by Congo red staining, have been detected in some hereditary amyloidoses such as those derived from transthyretin (ATTR) and associated with dialysis (244). In these cases, electron microscopy becomes essential to establish an unequivocal diagnosis. Another way to demonstrate small amyloid deposits is to perform a Congo red stain and place the stained section under fluorescence light; amyloid then becomes bright red (245). This peculiar appearance of Congo red–stained specimens was described many years ago. The Eastwood Congo red method enhances staining of amyloid when viewed by light microscopy and quenches background fluorescence when viewed by fluorescence mi-

croscopy (246). Other stains, such as crystal violet, methyl violet, Sirius red, and sulfated Alcian blue, are less sensitive and specific. Moreover, some of these stains also fade. Thioflavin T stain may also yield false-positive results (247).

Amyloid deposition in glomeruli may occur in segmental, diffuse mesangial, nodular, and pure basement membrane patterns (231,240,248). Early segmental amyloid deposits are small, discrete, and confined to the mesangium without creating easily detectable nodularity. It is very easy to miss this early form of amyloidosis, and detection may require careful evaluation of the special stains, immunofluorescence, and electron microscopy. In the diffuse form, the mesangium is uniformly expanded by weakly PAS-positive acellular deposits. Nearly complete glomerular obliteration by amyloid is typically seen in amyloid derived from fibrinogen (AFib) (249,250). In the nodular form, the mesangium is asymmetrically expanded by large masses of amyloid that compress and compromise capillary spaces (103,248). The nodular form should be distinguished from diabetic nephropathy and other forms of nodular glomerulosclerosis. The glomerular lesions may be uniform among the lobules within a glomerulus. The basement membrane may remain normal, even when massive mesangial amyloidosis is present. However, fraying, loss of argyrophilia, and discontinuities are seen along the glomerular capillary walls with the Jones methenamine silver stain as amyloid deposits increase in this location. A multinucleated giant cell reaction may accompany glomerular amyloid deposition (251). Rarely, crescents can be seen, highlighting the fact that capillary wall rupture has occurred (252). Subepithelial amyloid deposition may be associated with spikes that project into the urinary space or can be seen at the periphery of mesangial areas (82,240,253).

The tubular interstitial compartment may be variably affected. The tubules may show nonspecific findings or vacuolization and damage. Interstitial and peritubular deposits of amyloid are seen in approximately 50% of cases (251). Medullary amyloid deposits are more frequent and more extensive, with a predilection for deposition around vasa recta, loops of Henle, and collecting ducts (240,251). Watanabe and Saniter reported interstitial involvement in 57 of 122 cases of amyloidosis, and in 12 cases the involvement was characterized as massive (251). Occasionally, patients with AA amyloidosis and amyloidosis derived from certain mutants of transthyretin and apolipoprotein AI may show amyloid deposition limited to the interstitium and medulla. Such patients present with renal failure not associated with proteinuria (249,254–256). Inflammation is not a typical feature of amyloidosis, but scattered aggregates of lymphoplasmacytic cells may be present, particularly in AL (240). Aggregates of foam cells can also be seen in the interstitium, primarily in cases with large amounts of proteinuria (240). Tubular atrophy is seen most often in advanced cases with interstitial amyloid deposition.

Renal vessels are often involved, with arteriolar deposits being most frequent, followed by deposits in arteries, peritubular capillaries, and veins (73,240). The amyloid deposits in the vessel walls may be subtle or completely replace the vessel walls and be associated with occlusion of the lumina. Vascular amyloid may be mimicked by hyalinosis and even fibrinoid necrosis, and special stains may be necessary to establish a distinction. Vascular deposits frequently coexist with glomerular amyloid, but the extent of vascular amyloid deposition is unrelated to the pattern of glomerular involvement. Watanabe and Saniter found amyloid in interlobular arteries or arterioles in 97 of 122 renal biopsies (251). In rare cases, the vessels are the only site in the kidney where amyloid can be demonstrated. In some familial amyloidoses, for example, AApoAI (A amyloid derived from apolipoprotein AI), amyloid deposits may involve the blood vessels and spare the glomeruli (249). In certain cases of AA amyloidosis, only vascular deposits were detectable in the kidney (73,257,258).

In making the diagnosis of amyloidosis, abdominal fat aspiration is as sensitive as rectal biopsy and more sensitive than bone marrow biopsy. The sensitivity (52% to 100%) and the specificity (99%) suggest that although a positive result is good evidence for the disease, a negative result does not exclude it (234,242).

## Immunopathology

In view of the expanding spectrum of systemic amyloidoses and the emergence of amyloid type-specific therapies, the typing of deposits is currently the standard of care. A variety of techniques have been used to identify the amyloid fibril protein type in amyloidosis. Gallo et al (259) applied immunofluorescence techniques to frozen tissues, and this approach remains the preferred option. Since then, immunoperoxidase stains have been applied to paraffin sections, and immuno-electron microscopic labeling has been pioneered by Herrera et al (102,141). The biochemical typing of amyloid protein in formalin-fixed, paraffin-embedded specimens has also been reported (260–262). The most recent approach involves the use of proteomic techniques to detect and type amyloid deposits (263). These newer techniques are available only in specialized laboratories; thus, immunofluorescence and immunoperoxidase are the most widely used. However, the two latter stains are not always straightforward, because amyloid deposits are associated with a high background stain (particularly in paraffin sections), which may result in false-positive results. Therefore, the use of a panel of antibodies and the inclusion of a stain for amyloid P component is strongly recommended (242,264). Clinicopathologic correlation is required in all cases, not simply in those with equivocal results.

Despite the biochemical diversity of amyloid fibril proteins, all types of amyloid have been shown to contain amyloid P component by biochemical and immunohistochemical methods. In contrast, deposits of MIDD lack the amyloid P component (265,266). However, the amyloid P component is not specific for amyloid, because it may also be seen in the organized deposits of fibrillary glomerulopathy (265), as well as in normal glomerular basement membranes and blood vessels, but in significantly lesser amounts than in amyloid deposits (265).

The rationale behind the use of a panel of antibodies is that it permits the selection of antiserum, which provides the strongest staining, comparable to that of the amyloid P component, and this then serves as a built-in positive control. The use of immunohistochemistry for the detection of κ and λ light or heavy chains in paraffin-embedded tissues generally results in very high background staining, which often makes interpretation challenging or even impossible. However, immunofluorescence typing performed on unfixed samples (frozen tissue, air-dried fat aspirates, bone marrow smears) gives much better results (please see also the next section on "Immunofluorescence"). In contrast, AA amyloidosis is relatively easy to demonstrate immunohistochemically (237,267,268) (Fig. 19.18). While many deposits of ATTR give good results in both unfixed samples and paraffin sections, in some cases the results may be difficult to interpret (250,268). The same situation may apply to certain cases of ApoAI and other

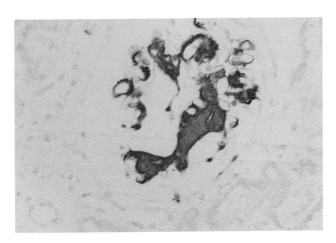

**Figure 19.18.** Immunohistochemical immunofluorescence typing of amyloid in AA amyloidosis. Intense staining of amyloid deposits for AA protein. Immunohistochemistry for AA protein. (Peroxidase auto-peroxidase stain for AA protein, diaminobenzidine as marker; ×500.)

hereditary amyloidoses (249,268). In particular, evaluation of paraffin sections may require pretreatment of sections with formic acid or guanidine for antigen retrieval (250,269).

It is recommended that a limited panel of antibodies be used for amyloid typing routinely, with the recognition that some cases may require an additional workup, which should be done in specialized centers. The typical antibody panel should include human amyloid P component, κ and λ immunoglobulin light chains, amyloid A protein, transthyretin, and fibrinogen. The stain for $\beta_2$-microglobulin should be added in the setting of dialysis. In the present author's experience (MP) this antibody panel allowed definitive typing of amyloid deposits in 90% of kidney biopsies. The author has used the same antibody

panel for the typing of amyloid deposits in other tissues, with 90% and 85% success rates in frozen and paraffin sections, respectively. Stains for Apolipoprotein AI and AII and lysozyme may also be included, depending on the differential diagnosis. However, these latter stains are best performed at laboratories that are specialized in the typing of amyloid (please also see previous and following sections). When stains for κ and λ light chains and fibrinogen are included in the immunofluorescence antibody panel used for native kidney biopsies, the amyloid typing panel would require only the addition of stains for amyloid P component, AA, transthyretin, and $\beta_2$ microglobulin.

## Immunofluorescence

Immunofluorescence is the technique of choice for detection of amyloid derived from immunoglobulin light and heavy chains. Restriction for the light chain (for either κ or λ) or for heavy chain determinants (γ, μ) must be demonstrated, in association with Congo red–positive deposits, for a diagnosis of AL amyloidosis (Fig. 19.19). Most AL amyloidosis cases are λ light chain related (Fig. 19.19A), and most cases of renal AL amyloidosis are λ VI (269). The few cases of AH amyloidosis that have been reported have been either γ or μ related (270–274). Specific antibodies to the heavy chains should be used in the diagnosis of this condition. In AH amyloidosis, the amyloidogenic protein is composed of fragments of heavy chains and not of intact, complete heavy chains. The $C_H1$ constant domain has not been detected in any of the cases reported (274).

Unfortunately, not all AL amyloid deposits are immunoreactive with commercial antibodies for κ or λ light chain (275). AL amyloid fibril proteins are very heterogeneous as a consequence of the antigenic diversity of their variable regions. The outcome of the

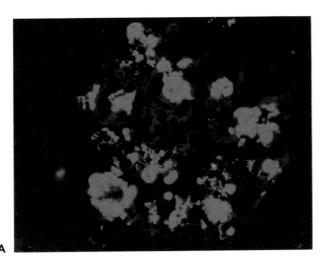

A

B

**Figure 19.19.** Immunohistochemical direct immunofluorescence typing of amyloid. AL amyloidosis. Mesangial λ light chain amyloid deposits are clearly depicted **(A)**, with completely essentially negative stain for λ light chains **(B)**. (Fluorescein; ×500.)

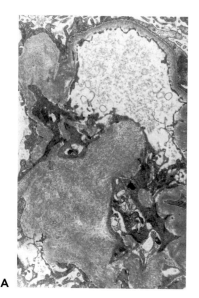 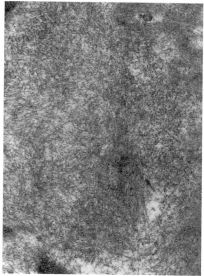 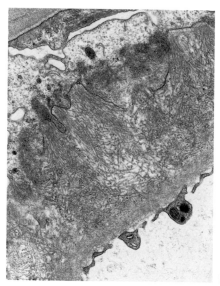

A                                                                                                                                                    B,C

**Figure 19.20.**   AL amyloidosis. Typical ultrastructural appearance of amyloid fibrils in mesangium, extending into peripheral capillary walls and occupying a subepithelial location, as shown in **(C)**. Transmission electron microscopy. (Uranyl acetate and lead citrate; **A:** ×7500; **B:** ×12,500; **C:** ×13,500.)

immunohistochemical stain depends largely on the extent to which the C region is present. Therefore, in cases where the amyloid fibril protein is derived from the variable region alone, typing will be inconclusive or frankly negative with commercial antibodies. The proportion of renal biopsies with subsequently proven AL, where the amyloid deposits were not reactive in frozen sections with antibodies against κ or λ light chain, varies between 13.6% (MP, author unpublished data) and 35.3% (275). Keeping in mind this limitation of the method, it is strongly recommended that all equivocal or frankly negative cases be studied further. Lachmann et al (276) studied 350 patients with systemic amyloidosis, in whom the diagnosis of AL amyloidosis was suggested by clinical and laboratory findings and by the absence of a family history. This study showed that 9.7% of patients actually had familial amyloidosis. Interestingly, a low-grade monoclonal gammopathy was detected in 24% of these patients. Thus, confirmation of the amyloid type by careful clinicopathologic correlation, as well as exclusion of other types, is important. Additional studies may include screening for transthyretin (TTR) variants by isoelectric focusing and mass spectrometric characterization and analyses for genetic mutation by direct DNA sequencing and restriction fragment-length polymorphism. Variants of apolipoprotein AI, apolipoprotein AII, fibrinogen α-chain, lysozyme, and gelsolin should be excluded, and referral to an amyloid center should be considered.

A single patient may suffer from different amyloid diseases simultaneously. Examples include renal glomerular AL and vascular AA deposits in a patient with ankylosing spondylitis (257) and cardiac deposits derived from wild type ATTR and AApoAIV (277).

It is also becoming evident that immunohistochemical stains can detect deposits of amyloid protein that are Congo red–negative and are considered pre-amyloidotic. This has been documented in occasional patients with hereditary amyloidosis (ATTR) and dialysis-related amyloidosis (244).

## Electron Microscopy

Regardless of the type of amyloid, the ultrastructural findings are essentially similar. Amyloid is characterized by randomly disposed, rigid, nonbranching, variably long (up to 14,000 A), 7- to 10-nm-diameter fibrils (102,278–280) (Fig. 19.20). Amyloid can be found in any of the renal compartments. Ultrastructural immunogold labeling can depict the precursor protein in amyloid fibrils in any of the renal compartments (Fig. 19.20A,B). In glomeruli, fibrils are invariably found in mesangial areas replacing the normal mesangial matrix. They are also seen in Bowman's capsule and space, and they may extend into the peripheral capillary walls occupying the subendothelial or subepithelial spaces (280). Amyloid can also infiltrate and replace the basal lamina, possibly contributing to the loss of argyrophilia and fraying seen by light microscopy. Epithelial cells may be destroyed, the entire lamina densa of the glomerular basement membrane is replaced by amyloid, and amyloid may be found in the urinary space in end-stage amyloidosis. New layers of basement membrane may be seen surrounding amyloid deposits. Extremely rare cases of amyloidosis exhibit massive aggregates of amyloid fibrils in subendothelial and mesangial areas arranged in tightly packed, electron-dense structures, which can be easily confused with a number of entities, including membranoproliferative glomerulonephritis, cryoglobulinemic glomerulopathy, and even diffuse proliferative lupus nephritis (281). These cases show the expected tinctorial characteristic of amyloid and are usually associated with monoclonal κ light chains. In the few documented cases of regression of amyloidosis, the glomerular basement membrane remains a complicated lattice of basal lamina, and there may be a few remaining fibrils or amorphous debris in between the lacunae left behind by the lamellated lamina densa (280). The overall resultant appearance mimics that of stage IV membranous nephropathy.

There are reports suggesting that $\beta_2$ microglobulin-associated amyloidosis has some unique ultrastructural characteristics (282–284). The authors noted that the amyloid fibrils in this condition exhibited a peculiar arrangement in short curvilinear bundles (283,284).

## AL/AH Amyloidosis

### Historical Perspective

The first case of amyloidosis associated with myeloma (discovered retrospectively, since myeloma was not recognized as a pathologic entity then) was reported in 1867 (285). In 1872, Adams documented an association between renal amyloidosis and myeloma (285). The first case of amyloidosis in a patient with myeloma was published in 1902 by Jochmann and Schumm (286), and 15 years later Glaus reported a second case of amyloidosis associated with myeloma (287). Approximately 50 years later, Schmiedeberg described the amino acid composition of amyloid and noted that it resembled that of serum globulin (225). The Congo red stain was introduced in 1933 by Bennhold as a diagnostic clinical test and later used as a histologic stain (288,289). Six years later, Divry and Florkin reported green birefringence when amyloid was stained with Congo red and then viewed under polarized light (290). In 1931, Magnus-Levy first suggested a relationship between amyloid and light chain proteinuria (291). Two years later, Bell studied 90 autopsies from patients with multiple myeloma (including a literature review), and discovered 3 patients with amyloidosis, further substantiating a possible association (82).

In 1949 Sikl, in another literature review, compiled information from 40 cases with amyloidosis and myeloma and clearly demonstrated that the two diseases were not merely coincidental (292). It took almost another 30 years (in 1959) for Cohen and Calkins (293) to demonstrate the fibrillary nature of amyloid using the transmission electron microscope. In 1961, Osserman recognized that abnormal light chains were directly involved in the pathogenesis of amyloidosis (294). Four years later, Eanes and Glenner reported for the first time the fact that amyloid was composed of β-pleated sheets (295), and in the early 1970s, Glenner

et al further demonstrated the amino acid composition of an amyloid protein, which matched the N terminus of an immunoglobulin light chain (296). In 1972, Levin et al described the amino acid composition and sequence of amyloid from a patient with secondary amyloidosis and labeled it *amyloid A protein* (297). In the late 1960s and early 1970s, Shirahama and Cohen emphasized the essential role that mesangial cells played in the pathogenesis of glomerular AA amyloidosis (298,299). Their studies with splenic macrophages engaged in amyloid formation also strongly suggested a crucial role for lysosomes in the process of amyloidogenesis. Linke et al in 1973 (300) and Epstein the following year (301) digested BJ proteins with proteolytic enzymes, forming amyloid fibrils.

The study of renal amyloidosis was then essentially ignored until the early 1990s, when the work of Solomon et al, who injected light chain proteins intraperitoneally, demonstrated the formation of vascular amyloidosis in the kidney (59). This seminal work was followed by elegant studies on the molecular modeling of amyloid and analysis of the amino acid sequence and conformation of amyloidogenic light chains. In 1996, Tagouri et al (302) demonstrated amyloid formation by mesangial cells incubated with amyloidogenic light chains purified from the urine of patients with AL amyloidosis, thus establishing an in vitro model to study renal amyloidogenesis. This was followed by the use of an isolated kidney perfusion model, whereby amyloidogenic light chains were delivered to the kidney via the renal artery (303). Additional studies by Comenzo et al (304) convincingly showed that λ VI light chains display a striking renal tropism and, as a consequence, are the most common light chains involved in renal amyloidosis, as had been previously proposed by Solomon et al (50). The first case of heavy chain-related amyloidosis was reported by Eulitz et al in 1990 (270), and since then, only a handful of similar patients have been documented (271–274).

## Clinical Presentation and Laboratory Findings

The clinical manifestations of AL/AH amyloidosis in general are frequently rather nonspecific and virtually always include fatigue and weight loss. Other findings may include edema, orthostatic hypotension, hepatomegaly without filling defects, peripheral neuropathy, cardiac arrhythmias, carpal tunnel syndrome, and congestive heart failure resulting from restrictive cardiomyopathy (268). Gastrointestinal symptoms (motility abnormalities, atony, pseudoobstruction, malabsorption, diarrhea, bleeding) may also be seen in fewer than 10% of patients. In 4% of patients with AL, gastrointestinal symptoms are the dominant syndrome (268). Hepatic involvement is much more common, involving some 70% of patients with AL amyloidosis. The most common clinical presentation is proteinuria with or without renal insufficiency. The amount of proteinuria is very variable and depends on the extent of renal involvement. Renal failure may ensue in the advanced stages.

The kidneys may be involved in all types of amyloidosis. Glomerular involvement by amyloidosis is frequent and explains the proteinuria that these patients exhibit. Amyloidosis is often diagnosed by renal biopsy. Only a minority of patients have an established diagnosis of amyloidosis prior to renal biopsy.

Amyloidosis related to plasma cell dyscrasia is also called *primary amyloidosis*. In most cases of immunoglobulin-associated amyloidosis, the precursor protein is an immunoglobulin light chain or fragment (AL amyloidosis). In a minority of the cases, amyloidosis originates from truncated immunoglobulin heavy chains (AH amyloidosis) (270–274). In these cases there is an underlying plasma cell dyscrasia responsible for the amyloidosis.

AL/AH amyloidosis primarily affects older individuals; it is unusual to find a patient with this condition younger than 40 years of age. Early studies of renal amyloidosis by Bell clearly documented that all renal compartments may be involved and that it was a systemic disease; in only 2 of the 65 cases reported amyloid was amyloid found only in the kidney (82). However, renal involvement may be the first manifestation of systemic disease, with subsequent studies demonstrating the systemic nature of the amyloidosis. Extrarenal localized AL amyloid deposits are frequently seen in the genitourinary tract (see under "Localized Amyloidoses").

## Etiology and Pathogenesis of Renal AL Amyloidosis

Shirahama and Cohen studied AA amyloidogenesis and demonstrated the importance of mesangial cells and lysosomes in the process (298,299) of renal amyloidogenesis. Studies in the early 1980s focusing on amyloidogenesis revealed that the mesangium was the first site where amyloid is formed in the glomerulus (305). More recent studies have elucidated the precise mechanisms at play in renal AL amyloidogenesis. When rat or human mesangial cells were incubated with light chains purified from the urine of patients with AL amyloidosis, the light chains were endocytosed into phenotypically changed mesangial cells with a macrophage phenotype (189) and delivered to the mature lysosomal system, where amyloid formation took place (192). The internalization process is clathrin mediated (192). Amyloid formation can be influenced by altering lysosomal function or the mesangial milieu (186,192,306). Once amyloid is produced and delivered to the extracellular mesangial matrix, activation of metalloproteinases occurs, with eventual destruction of the mesangial matrix and replacement by amyloid (191).

Certain amino acid sequences, as well as posttranslational modifications of the light chains such as glycosylation, dipole moment formation, and charge–charge interactions, are responsible for the amyloidogenic potential of a given light chain. Some of these alterations include mutations of Arg61 leading to loss of a critical buried salt-bridge, mutations of Pro residues in B turns, or replacement of isoleucine (Ile) at position 27b, which enhances fibrillogenesis by destabilizing the variable portion of the light chains. Replacement of lysine (Lys) 31 is also highly destabilizing and strongly associated with amyloidosis. Replacement mutations in positions 61 (arginine [Arg] -aspartate [Asp]), 31 (Asp-Lys), 36 (tyrosine [Tyr] -phenylalanine [Phe]), and 27 (threonine [Thr] -Ile), among others, may be responsible for the above-mentioned alterations. Other changes in the light chains are also associated with propensity for development of AL amyloidosis (35,63,307–308). Such alterations in the physicochemical composition of a light chain may govern specific interactions with mesangial receptors, potentiating endocytosis into the mesangial cells and eventual amyloid formation (192). The mechanisms involved in AH amyloidosis remain unclear (294).

## AA Amyloidosis (Formerly Secondary Amyloidosis)

### Historical Perspective

AA amyloidosis usually arises in the context of an acute-phase response such as is seen in inflammatory arthritides, periodic fevers, chronic infections, and malignancies (234–238,309–313). For this reason, this form of amyloidosis was formerly referred to as "secondary" amyloidosis. However, it is now designated *AA amyloidosis* to reflect its origin from amyloid A protein. Amyloid A fibril protein is derived from a larger precursor protein, an acute-phase reactant, termed *serum amyloid A* or SAA (297,314–316). An association between familial Mediterranean fever (FMF) and the development of AA amyloidosis has been known for decades (317,318). In recent years, a number of other hereditary autoinflammatory diseases have been discovered and linked with the development of AA amyloidosis as their major complication (319–322). However, the majority of cases of AA amyloidosis have no apparent familial component. Therefore, AA amyloidosis should be considered in the context of sporadic systemic amyloidosis as well as familial amyloidosis associated with hereditary autoinflammatory diseases.

### Clinical Presentation and Laboratory Findings

AA amyloidosis affects patients of various ages; three series found an age range of 11 to 87 years, with a median of 50 (238,309,311). However, in younger patients affected by AA amyloidosis, a hereditary component must be considered (322) (see "Familial Mediterranean Fever").

There are many conditions that have been associated with AA amyloidosis. Often the underlying disease has been longstanding and is severe in nature, and this underlying process dominates the clinical picture (235,238, 309,323).

These associated conditions include inflammatory arthritides, chronic inflammatory states, chronic infections, and malignancies. Rheumatoid arthritis is the most frequent followed by ankylosing spondylitis and other arthritides (323–326). Among chronic inflammatory states are inflammatory bowel disorders (Crohn's disease), sarcoidosis, and an ever-expanding group of familial periodic fevers, of which FMF is the prototype (235,309, 323,327). Tuberculosis, osteomyelitis, bronchiectasis, leprosy, pyelonephritis, decubitus ulcers, Whipple's disease and acne conglobata (323), hypogammaglobulinemia, agammaglobulinemia, paraplegia, cystic fibrosis, and "skin poppers" may be associated with AA amyloidosis (310,328). Several malignancies, namely hepatoma, renal cell carcinoma, Castleman's disease, Hodgkin's disease, and Waldenström macroglobulinemia (WM), have been associated with AA amyloidosis (323,329). Interestingly, between 6% and 13% of patients with AA amyloidosis have no evidence of an underlying inflammatory process (235,267,309,311,330). In the Western world, inflammatory arthritides and inflammatory bowel disorders have replaced infectious diseases as the underlying process most commonly associated with AA amyloidosis (235,309,311). In two recent large Western series, rheumatoid arthritides accounted for 39% and 64% of AA amyloid cases, while chronic infections contributed only 13% and 14% of patients (235,309). However, outside the Western world, infectious diseases (tuberculosis in particular) are more common.

The incidence and prevalence of AA amyloidosis in the general population are largely unknown. For unknown reasons, the incidence varies worldwide and by geographical area, with a higher incidence in Europe than in the United States, even in the setting of the same underlying disease (234). Familial Mediterranean fever remains an important cause of AA amyloid in regions around the Mediterranean (317,318,322) and in immigrant populations of Mediterranean origin.

Proteinuria and nephrotic syndrome are the most common presenting symptoms. In one recent large series (309) 97% of patients had significant proteinuria. Occasionally, patients may present with renal failure without significant proteinuria (254,331). AA amyloidosis usually takes many years to develop. In rheumatoid arthritis, it is at least 2 years, with a mean of 15 years (309,332). Some patients have a preclinical phase of amyloidosis during which AA deposits can be detected in tissues without clinical manifestations (332). The overall 5-year survival rate in patients with overt renal disease in AA amyloidosis has been reported to be 40% (238,311). The prognosis can be markedly improved with control of the underlying inflammatory process (309).

## Gross and Microscopic Pathology

Autopsy studies have shown amyloid in nearly every organ. The kidneys are almost always involved (238,309, 311,313,333,334). However, the gastrointestinal tract, spleen, liver, thyroid, and adrenal gland are common sites of amyloid deposition (335,336). Myocardial involvement is rare (309,337). Renal deposits of amyloid are mostly glomerular. However, in patients without proteinuria, amyloid deposits may be limited to the interstitium and affect predominantly the medulla (254) or tubules (331). Less common patterns of renal amyloidosis are heavy tubular deposits with tubular dysfunction or crescentic glomerulonephritis (254,310). It is generally agreed that AA amyloidosis can be reliably diagnosed by immunohistochemical methods in virtually all cases in both frozen and paraffin-embedded sections (237,267,313) (Fig. 19.18A). There are several case reports of co-deposition of AA and AL. Pettersson et al (257) reported a patient with ankylosing spondylitis with renal glomerular AL and vascular AA amyloidosis. Similar consideration must also be given to patients with WM, who typically develop AL. However, in some patients, WM may be associated with AA amyloidosis (329). A large study of patients with rheumatoid arthritis from Japan (334) demonstrated amyloid in 19% of patients. In one recent study from Japan, gastrointestinal amyloid correlated better with renal involvement than abdominal fat aspirate (336).

## Familial AA Amyloidoses

Familial AA amyloidoses develop in the context of mutations in genes for nonamyloid fibril proteins that play a permissive role in the development of amyloid (322). In contrast, other familial amyloidoses are associated with heritable abnormalities in the amyloid fibril precursor proteins (see "Hereditary Amyloidoses Resulting from Amyloid Fibril Protein Precursor Mutations").

Although the role of genetic factors in the development of AA amyloidosis in FMF has long been suspected, the underlying mechanisms have only recently been discovered (318,322,338–340). At the same time, several other chronic inflammatory diseases, which may be complicated by the development of AA amyloidosis, have also been shown to have genetic components (319,321,322). Most patients with hereditary periodic fevers, including familial Mediterranean fever, have mutations in the pyrin, cryopyrin, or tumor necrosis factor (TNF) receptor genes (321,322). Their products modulate the activity of apoptotic proteins and signal transduction pathways, playing a crucial role in the inflammatory response of the innate immune system. Thus, collectively, these diseases can be considered to be a consequence of an inborn error of inflammation. Apart from FMF, there are several other periodic fevers that have recently been clinically as well as genetically characterized: TNF receptor-1 associated periodic syndrome (TRAPS), cryopyrin-associated periodic syndrome (CAPS), and others (321,322,341). As a group, these disorders are referred to as *infevers*. Their database was recently established (321). Familial Mediterranean fever is autosomal recessive; all others are autosomal dominant and rare. A thorough diagnosis is warranted, because clinical and therapeutic management is specific for each of these diseases (340).

## Familial Mediterranean Fever

Familial Mediterranean fever is by far the most common form of the nephropathic familial amyloidoses, and it occurs in ethnic groups from around the Mediterranean basin and in their descendants: non-Ashkenazi (Sephardic) Jews of North African or Middle Eastern descent, Armenians, Middle Eastern Arabs, and Turks (reviewed by Padeh [322]). However, clinical cases in individuals of non-Mediterranean ancestry are increasingly reported as genetic testing becomes available (340). It is speculated that heterozygotes carrying mutant alleles have a selective survival advantage owing to their heightened inflammatory state, which helps them clear a putative endemic Mediterranean pathogen(s). The gene responsible for this febrile disorder, *MEFV* (mapped to the short arm of chromosome 16), codes for pyrin (reviewed in 322,338,339,342).

### Clinical Presentation and Laboratory Findings

Familial Mediterranean fever is characterized by regular, unpredictable, and painful febrile episodes lasting 1 to 4 days accompanied by sterile peritonitis, pleuritis, synovitis, or an erysipelas-like erythema involving the lower extremities. The symptoms related to synovitis may be prolonged. No specific factor inciting the attacks has been identified (317). The symptoms resolve without treatment and with no apparent ill effects until amyloidosis supervenes. AA amyloidosis is the main and potentially lethal complication of the disease. It affects most patients before 40 years of age, but has been reported in children as young as 5 years old (322).

Renal involvement is the principal clinical manifestation of AA amyloidosis in patients with FMF (317,343). Proteinuria is typically followed by nephrotic syndrome and uremia. Proteinuria during the nephrotic stage may be massive, and the course may be complicated by renal vein thrombosis, with abrupt deterioration of renal function (344). The uremic stage supervenes as glomerular amyloid occludes the tufts, and hypertension is found in up to 50% of patients at this stage. The duration of clinical renal disease, from the onset of proteinuria to terminal renal failure, varies from 2 to 13 years (317). Development of amyloid nephropathy may follow a period of active disease (phenotype I) or, on rare occasions, may be the presenting manifestation (phenotype II) (318,322).

Amyloidosis appears to be the inevitable consequence of untreated disease, but the prevalence of AA in inadequately treated FMF patients varies with population group. In untreated patients, amyloidosis occurred in 60% of Turkish patients and in 27% of non-Ashkenazi Jews (317). Amyloidosis was the cause of death in virtually all autopsied patients with FMF who were not treated with colchicine (317).

### Gross and Microscopic Pathology

Amyloid deposits in FMF are distributed throughout the body in small vessels. In autopsy kidneys, the glomeruli are always extensively involved, with gross replacement of the tufts. Amyloid deposits are also seen in dense rings around the tubules. Interstitial deposits are inconstant, but when present, they appear to preferentially accumulate in the medulla (317,345,346). Glomerular amyloid deposits begin in the mesangium and spread via the subendothelial space to involve the tuft in the same fashion as other forms of systemic amyloidosis. Whereas in a patient with FMF, proteinuria is presumptive evidence of amyloidosis, other renal pathologies should be considered, particularly in patients treated with colchicine. Said et al (346) performed biopsies on 15 patients with FMF, principally to elucidate the cause of proteinuria, and only 7 patients had amyloidosis. Also, increased incidence of vasculitides and Henoch-Schönlein disease has been reported in patients suffering from FMF (347,348).

### Etiology and Pathogenesis of AA Amyloidosis

The amyloid fibril protein in sporadic AA amyloidosis, FMF, and other periodic fevers is derived from proteolytically cleaved SAA (314,315,349). Serum amyloid A protein is a major acute-phase reactant produced primarily by the liver (350), although extrahepatic expression of SAA has also been documented. The normal physiologic function of SAA is unknown. Serum amyloid A protein has been linked to functions related to inflammation, pathogen defense, high-density lipoprotein metabolism, and cholesterol transport. It is best known for its response to inflammatory stimuli such as infection and tissue injury, in which SAA levels are markedly increased.

The human SAA genes are located on chromosome 11. (For details, see Uhlar and Whitehead [316].) Amyloid A forms by proteolysis of SAA1 and SAA2. Evidence is emerging that certain *SAA* polymorphisms may be associated with an increased risk for the development of AA amyloidosis. Thus, among Europeans, the incidence of AA amyloidosis appears to be increased in persons homozygous for the 1.1 allele (351). However, in Japan, homozygosity for the 1.3 allele appears to correlate positively with renal AA (352). AA amyloidosis is a result of the interplay of three major mechanisms (237,353–355): increased production of SAA, its proteolysis, and participation of the extracellular matrix. A permanent acute-phase response, with overproduction of SAA induced by proinflammatory cytokines (237), appears to be a prerequisite for the development of AA amyloidosis. In patients with FMF, serum levels of SAA are elevated two to three times above normal under basal conditions and may rise by 50 times above normal during febrile episodes (356).

The *FMF* gene (MEFV) encodes pyrin. Pyrin belongs to the pyrin gene family, which encompasses several related genes involved in autoinflammatory diseases by affecting apoptotic and inflammatory signaling pathways. Data derived from an animal model of AA amyloidosis show that amyloidogenesis is preceded by changes in the composition of the extracellular matrix. There is increased deposition of glycosaminoglycans and amyloid P component accompanying amyloid fibril protein deposition (354,355,357). Interestingly, extracellular matrix, in particular glucosaminoglycans and the amyloid P component, appear to be involved in fibril formation in all types of amyloidosis thus far studied (265,266). The role of these ancillary components is not clear. Several functions have been proposed, including facilitating aggregation and protein misfolding, leading to fibril formation, substrate adhesion, and protection from degradation (237,354,355). Protein aggregation has recently developed into an area of intensive research, because inhibition of aggregation has been targeted as a potentially useful approach to decreasing the amyloid burden during disease (358–362). Amyloid P component, a glycoprotein related to C-reactive protein, can be detected in amyloid deposits by scintigraphy. This feature has been successfully used by some amyloid centers in Europe to assess the kinetics of amyloid deposition following treatment (363).

It is postulated that proteolytic processing of SAA to AA protein takes place within macrophages (237,298, 299,349). Experimental studies have shown that, in the kidney, mesangial cells are involved in the processing of AA protein (as well as AL protein) (298,299). It is as yet unknown why some patients with inflammatory disease and high levels of SAA develop amyloidosis whereas others do not (364). It is postulated that other factors must also be implicated, such as genetic SAA subtypes (see previous) (351,352) and factors affecting the degradation of SAA to AA protein (237,349,365).

## Hereditary Amyloidoses Resulting from Amyloid Fibril Protein Precursor Mutations

### Historical Perspective

The hereditary systemic amyloidoses are a diverse group of autosomal dominant diseases that occur much less frequently than AL or AA amyloidoses. In these amyloidoses, the variant structure of the amyloid precursor protein is the pivotal factor in amyloidogenesis (249,268,311). Diagno-

sis can be challenging, since the phenotype can be similar to AL or AA and a family history may not be present (276). Until the amyloid fibril proteins and their precursors were identified, familial amyloidosis was classified by clinical and pathologic phenotype (366). While certain hereditary amyloidoses are concentrated in particular geographic locations or affect defined ethnic groups, many patients from throughout the world have been diagnosed with these various phenotypes. Thus, hereditary amyloidosis should not be excluded in a given patient based on ethnicity alone. Currently, in keeping with the present-day classification of amyloidoses, these disorders are named after the amyloid fibril protein. Among these diseases are amyloidoses derived from the fibrinogen A α-chain (AFib), transthyretin (ATTR), apolipoprotein AI (AApoAI), apolipoprotein AII (AApoAII), gelsolin (AGel), lysozyme (ALys), and cystatin (ACys) (249,276,367). Whereas several of the familial disorders are distinctly neuropathic or cardiopathic, virtually all of them can affect kidneys, although in some of these amyloidoses, renal deposits may be clinically silent. At Boston University, 10% of patients were diagnosed with familial amyloidosis, with 85% of the familial amyloidosis attributed to ATTR and 5% caused by AFib (239). In contrast, in the United Kingdom, AFib is the most frequent hereditary amyloidosis (276). The low incidence of these disorders may be a consequence of underdiagnosis. Testing for familial amyloidosis should be considered in all inconclusive cases, and DNA analysis is mandatory to support the diagnosis. Serum screening for variants of transthyretin by isoelectric focusing and mass spectrometric characterization of variants are also performed. Although rare, these forms need to be properly recognized because of the implications for patient management.

## Amyloid Derived from Fibrinogen

### Clinical Presentation and Laboratory Findings

Amyloid derived from a mutant fibrinogen A α chain (AFib) causes isolated renal amyloidosis not associated with peripheral neuropathy or cardiac involvement. The protein was characterized in 1993 by Benson et al (reviewed in 249). Kindreds have been identified in the United Kingdom, Mexico, United States, France, and Asia (368,369). Typically, age at presentation ranges from the third to the eighth decade (median 57 years). There is variable penetrance, and de novo mutation has been documented (368). Clinically, there is rapid kidney failure from initial presentation (proteinuria, hypertension, mild renal impairment) to end-stage renal failure and dialysis dependence within 1 to 5 years (249,368,369).

### Gross and Microscopic Pathology

AFib shows a remarkable tropism for the kidney. Histology is virtually pathognomonic, showing near replacement of the glomeruli by amyloid, without any interstitial or vascular involvement. Deposits stain specifically with antibodies to fibrinogen (249,276).

## Amyloid Derived from Transthyretin

Transthyretin is a carrier protein for thyroid hormone and retinol binding protein (311,370). More than 100 different TTR mutations have been reported (239). The most frequent worldwide is the mutation leading to the valine 30 methionine substitution (Met30). There are well-established foci of familial ATTR in Portugal, Sweden, and Japan. However, the disease has been documented in many countries. A recent study showed that almost 4% of African Americans carry an abnormal TTR, with substitution of Ile for valine at position 122 (V122I) (371).

### Clinical Presentation and Laboratory Findings

The age at onset and the phenotype may vary between different kinships. In general, males are more often affected than females. There are also geographic differences. The same variant (Met30) produces an earlier age of onset in Portuguese and a later onset in Swedish endemic foci. A low penetrance in carriers of the mutation has been observed; therefore, the family history may be absent (276), and occasional reports of apparently sporadic ATTR cases have been noted (250). In elderly patients, wild-type TTR may form amyloid, which shows cardiac tropism. This senile ATTR (termed *senile systemic amyloidosis*) affects an estimated 20% to 25% of people over the age of 80 (311,372,373).

Despite being inherited, the disease is generally not clinically apparent until middle or later life. Although polyneuropathy and cardiomyopathy are the major clinical manifestations, nephropathic and ocular forms have also been reported. Microalbuminuria may be the first stage of clinical ATTR nephropathy and is premonitory of neuropathy (374). The most frequent form of presentation of ATTR nephropathy is nephrotic proteinuria with renal dysfunction (374). Some mutations appear to be associated with renal impairment without proteinuria (255).

### Gross and Microscopic Pathology

Amyloid deposits are systemic but typically affect peripheral nerves and myocardium, depending on the phenotype. Varying degrees of renal involvement have been reported with primarily glomerular deposits, but in some patients, amyloid may be limited to interstitium in the medulla (256). End-stage renal disease may develop (256). Pre-amyloidotic deposits can be detected in nerves of some carriers without clinical evidence of the disease (244). Mixed deposits of amyloid, i.e., derived from two different proteins (TTR and ApoAIV), have also been reported (277).

## Miscellaneous Types of Familial Amyloidosis

Other types of familial systemic amyloidoses, which include amyloid derived from apolipoprotein I (AApoAI), apolipoprotein II (AApoAII), lysozyme (ALys), gelsolin (AGel), and cystatin (ACys), are relatively rare and are associated with amino acid substitutions in the corresponding native protein (250,367). It is quite possible that additional types will be discovered in the future. All of these amyloidoses can involve the kidney. In AApoAI, renal disease with progression to hypertension without nephrotic syndrome is frequent, and renal insufficiency is common (249,375–377). In the kidney, amyloid deposits are small and limited to large arteries and interstitium, whereas the glomeruli are generally spared. Apolipoprotein II-derived amyloidosis is characterized by slowly progressing renal disease with glomerular, interstitial, and vascular involvement by amyloid (249,377,378). Lysozyme-derived amyloidosis is characterized by nephropathy, dermal petechiae, gastrointestinal involvement with bleeding, hepatic involvement, and ocular or oral sicca syndrome. In the kidney, there are glomerular and vascular deposits of amyloid (249,379). Gelsolin-derived amyloidosis is characterized by cranial neuropathy, corneal dystrophy, and cutis laxa (380,381). Involvement of the kidneys has also been documented in homozygous patients (380) with marked glomerular amyloid deposits. Cystatin-derived amyloidosis is typified by involvement of the cerebral vessels in the form of familial cerebral congophilic angiopathy. However, there are also systemic deposits of amyloid, including the kidneys, where the deposits are clinically silent (382).

### Etiology and Pathogenesis

It is believed that the presence of a mutant form of the amyloid protein precursor is pivotal in the development of amyloidosis. However, there is considerable variation in affected gene penetration and phenotype (249,250,311). For example, in ATTR, the same variant (Met30) produces an earlier age of onset in Portuguese, and a later onset in Swedish, endemic foci (311). Similar variations in phenotype have been observed in other hereditary amyloidoses (377). Several modifiers (genetic and/or environmental factors) of precursor protein gene mutation effects have been hypothesized.

## Dialysis-Related Amyloidosis: Amyloid Derived from $\beta_2$-Microglobulin

### Historical Perspective

$\beta_2$-Microglobulin amyloidosis (A$\beta_2$M) is a type of systemic amyloidosis that commonly develops in patients with chronic renal failure who are undergoing long-term hemodialysis (383–385) and is referred to as *dialysis-related amyloidosis*. Although clinical symptoms of dialysis-related amyloidosis were observed in the mid-1970s, the amyloid fibril protein was not identified until 1985 (282,283). The amyloid fibril precursor protein is $\beta_2$-microglobulin, which is a small, 11,800-dalton protein with a predominantly $\beta$-pleated sheet secondary structure. $\beta_2$-Microglobulin is a subunit of the class I histocompatibility antigens. It circulates unbound as a monomer, and 95% is eliminated by glomerular filtration, tubular resorption, and metabolism. Thus, the serum level is inversely related to the glomerular filtration rate. Normal serum concentration (1 to 3 mg/L) increases by up to 60 times in patients receiving maintenance hemodialysis, because this protein is not effectively removed during dialysis (385).

## Clinical Presentation and Laboratory Findings

There is peripheral osteoarthropathy, with symptoms ranging from acute arthritis to progressive joint destruction (386); spondyloarthropathy, predominantly involving the cervical spine, and carpal tunnel syndrome are frequently present. Extra-articular symptoms may include ischemic colitis with perforation, macroglossia, and heart failure (387–389).

Clinical manifestations of the disease are zero at 5 years but increase to 50% at 12 years (386). Most patients with visceral amyloid had been on dialysis for 15 years or more. The incidence of amyloid in peritoneal dialysis is less well known, since very few patients remain for prolonged periods of time on this type of dialysis. However, since peritoneal dialysis is unable to remove $\beta_2$M, the risk may be similar. By serum amyloid P component scintigraphy, among 13 patients on peritoneal dialysis for more than 5 years, the prevalence of dialysis-related amyloidosis was similar to that seen in hemodialysis patients (390). However, the development of bone cysts required much longer periods of dialysis (17 years), and many patients were asymptomatic (391).

## Gross and Microscopic Pathology

$\beta_2$-Microglobulin amyloidosis has a predilection for bones, joints, and synovium. Radiologic and pathologic studies demonstrate juxta-articular cysts at insertion sites of capsule or tendons, which are filled with collagen and A$\beta_2$M. These cysts may become large enough to cause pathologic fractures (386,388,391–393).

$\beta_2$-Microglobulin amyloid is deposited in end-stage kidneys, but this has no clinical significance. $\beta_2$-Microglobulin amyloidosis has also been shown to have a systemic distribution and to involve other organs, with deposits of amyloid in the subcutis, gastrointestinal tract, liver, spleen, myocardium, lungs, skin, thyroid, ears, and perineural space. Although many of these deposits may be seen predominantly in the vessel wall, bulky visceral deposits have also been reported (387–389). Electron microscopic studies suggest that in some cases the A$\beta_2$M fibrils are arranged in short curvilinear bundles (284,393).

Tissue deposition occurs much earlier than any clinical or radiographic manifestations of the disease. At autopsy, amyloid was found in joints in 21% of patients on hemodialysis for less than 2 years, 50% for 4 to 7 years, and 100% for more than 13 years (392).

## Etiology and Pathogenesis

Although there is no direct correlation between the absolute concentration of $\beta_2$M and amyloidosis-related symptoms, high serum levels of this protein are believed to be the basis of amyloid deposition in tissues (385). Moreover, no significant accumulation of $\beta_2$M is observed in the synovial fluid, even though periarticular tissues are preferentially involved in this type of amyloidosis. Therefore, the involvement of factors modifying $\beta_2$M has been postulated. To this end, it has been proposed, but not as yet conclusively proven, that modification of $\beta_2$M by advanced glycation end products may facilitate amyloid formation (394). It has also been hypothesized that chronic inflammatory stress, induced by repeated stimuli from dialysis systems, may be involved in the pathogenesis of A$\beta_2$M. Interestingly, in recent years, there has been a decrease in the prevalence of A$\beta_2$M (395). This decrease has been observed in the absence of any major modification in serum levels of $\beta_2$M. However, it has been noted that this decline coincides with improvements in dialysis techniques, such as the use of endotoxin-free dialysates, which leads to better control of the inflammatory reaction associated with dialysis (385).

## Treatment, Course of the Disease Process, and Prognosis

The relative efficiency of different forms of dialysis in removing $\beta_2$M from the circulation and the bioreactivity of certain dialysis membranes have been intensively studied in an effort to prevent A$\beta_2$M (383,384,395). However, so far, renal transplantation remains the only effective method of preventing and treating dialysis-related amyloidosis (384,385). Renal transplantation generally arrests the disease process and leads to rapid relief of osteoarticular pain. Scintigraphy studies also suggest that there may be some regression of the amyloid deposits (396).

### Localized Amyloidoses

Localized amyloid may form a single amyloid mass referred to as an *amyloid tumor* or *amyloidoma*, which clinically may mimic neoplasia (268,311). Localized amyloid may be seen in the respiratory, gastrointestinal, and genitourinary tracts; skin; soft tissues; conjunctiva; lymph nodes; and elsewhere in individuals who do not have systemic amyloidosis

(397,398). In the urinary tract, the most common localized deposits of amyloid are in the urinary bladder, but the ureter, urethra, renal pelvis, glans penis, prostate gland, and seminal vesicles may also be involved (399–401).

While localized genitourinary amyloid is most often of the AL type, other types of amyloid have also been detected: ATTR, AA and, in patients on hemodialysis, $A\beta_2M$ (400,401). In localized AL deposits, there is frequently infiltration of plasma cells in the vicinity of the deposits. Immunohistochemical and molecular studies have shown that the plasma cell populations associated with local amyloid deposits are clonal (402), which suggests local production of the amyloid precursor protein. It is postulated that in other types of localized deposits, local tissue factors may create a milieu favorable for fibrillogenesis (268). Treatment is local and involves excision of the lesion or radiation; some patients receive no treatment (397,400). The most critical aspect is the correct determination of the localized nature of the deposits.

## Systemic Amyloidoses

### Treatment, Course of the Disease Process, and Prognosis

This section will discuss the systemic amyloidoses. The localized and dialysis-related amyloidoses were discussed earlier in their respective sections. Although the overall prognosis in amyloidosis is poor, it varies with the type of amyloidosis and extent of clinical organ involvement.

AL amyloidosis has the worst prognosis. Although long-term survival of patients with AL amyloidosis (more than 20 years) has been documented (403), such indolent progression of the disease is very uncommon (fewer than 5% of AL amyloidosis patients). The median survival of patients with AL amyloidosis is 9 to 20 months, depending on the series (231,233,240).

In general, in other amyloidoses, survival rates have been shown to improve with early treatment. However, the prognosis also depends on the extent of systemic involvement, with progressive neuropathy and/or cardiac involvement dominating the clinical picture in several hereditary amyloidoses (366,367,370,372,373). The involvement of kidney, liver, and gastrointestinal tract may also be seen (367–370,374–382). Thus, once a diagnosis of the type of amyloidosis is confirmed, it is important to assess the extent of systemic involvement and the prognosis.

Cardiac involvement is the most important negative predictor of survival in AL amyloidosis (233). Congestive heart failure resulting from cardiac infiltration by amyloid, or sudden death as a result of an arrhythmia, are the most common immediate causes of death. In one large study, the median survival was 13.2 months, and death resulted predominantly from cardiac involvement and heart failure. Exertional dyspnea usually precedes death, and, once

it occurs, most patients with AL amyloidosis die within 3 months. In AA amyloidosis, cardiac involvement is relatively rare, but when it occurs, it is an unfavorable predictive factor (337,404). In one recent study, estimated survival at 5 years was 30% in patients with cardiac involvement, versus 60% in patients without evidence of cardiac involvement at the time of diagnosis (404). However, survival may be longer with other types of cardiac amyloidosis; 5-year survival has been reported in some patients with ATTR, in particular in the senile form where the amyloid fibril is derived from a wild-type protein (373).

The kidney is one of the most important and common sites for amyloid deposition, with evidence of clinical renal disease in 48% to 97% of patients, depending on the series (240,309). Renal involvement also affects prognosis adversely, but not to the same extent as cardiac involvement. In AL amyloidosis, eradication or suppression of the underlying plasma cell dyscrasia is the focus of treatment for these patients; this, in turn, improves renal function. Treatment with oral melphalan and prednisone can prolong the life of patients with AL amyloidosis (405). Unfortunately, the overall response of AL amyloidosis to chemotherapy is limited (405). Nephrotic range, frequently massive proteinuria, and refractory peripheral edema are the predominant clinical manifestations in these patients. Skinner et al reported a decrease in proteinuria in approximately 10% of patients treated with melphalan and prednisone (406), and Kyle and Gertz (233) found a decrease in proteinuria of more than 50% in 18% of similarly treated patients.

As the disease progresses, proteinuria usually becomes more marked, and a progressive decrease in renal function typically occurs. Long-term dialysis is the usual outcome if the patients live long enough. Dialysis usually begins at approximately 13.8 months after diagnosis. After patients are placed on dialysis, median survival is 8.2 months (407).

In AA amyloidosis, the clinical picture is frequently determined by renal involvement (309). In a recent large study from a single referral center in the United Kingdom, among patients not on dialysis, 97% had significant proteinuria and 58% were nephrotic. In older series (234), nephrotic AA amyloidosis patients had a life expectancy similar to that of AL amyloidosis. However, recent studies show that effective control of the underlying inflammatory activity, as assessed by median SAA concentration, is associated with improved survival (309). However, renal insufficiency at the time of diagnosis adversely influences the clinical outcome. Thus, early diagnosis is critical.

Although most of the hereditary amyloidoses affect the kidney, there is significant variability in the degree of renal damage. Fibrinogen A $\alpha$-chain-derived amyloidosis leads to rapid renal failure (367), whereas renal failure in AApoAI, AApoII, and ALys is slower. There is also considerable variability in the renal damage incurred in various forms of ATTR, with some mutations being associated with renal failure (250,256). Clinically silent renal deposits can be seen in several systemic amyloidoses, including ATTR (some mutations), ACys, and AGel (250).

From a patient management point of view, the diagnosis of renal amyloid should be considered to comprise three broad categories: AL, AA, and hereditary types. The clinical management of patients with systemic AL amyloidosis targets the control of the underlying plasma cell dyscrasia. In patients with AA amyloidosis, control of the acute-phase response is currently the standard of care. In hereditary amyloidoses, liver transplantation is used to eliminate the source of abnormal protein. Moreover, because of the genetic component, perinatal screening and counseling need to be considered in patients with hereditary amyloidoses.

Treatment of AL amyloidosis with high-dose melphalan and autologous blood stem cell transplantation has led to an improvement in overall survival rates (408–412). At least four randomized studies using high-dose chemotherapy and autologous stem cell transplantation have demonstrated clinical benefit in patients with AL amyloidosis, including improvement of renal function (410). Seventy-seven percent of patients with proteinuria above 1 g/day who were treated using this regimen survived more than 1 year, and 80% of patients with nephrotic syndrome showed significant improvement (409,410). Only four became dialysis dependent at 12 to 30 months after treatment (411). The overall benefit of this aggressive therapy is largely restricted to patients who achieve complete eradication of the plasma cell dyscrasia (408). In another large study comprising more than 200 patients with AL amyloidosis, 60% of the patients were alive 4 years after follow-up, with the percentage increasing to 85% if no cardiac involvement was detected at the beginning of therapy (409).

Hematopoietic cell transplantation can reverse amyloid deposition and reduce or eliminate the clonal plasma cell disorder (409,410). Performance status and quality of life of patients with AL amyloidosis can be improved considerably (408). The main drawback is that early mortality of hematopoietic cell transplantation is approximately 26% (range, 13% to 44%), making it a risky therapeutic modality (408–412).

In AA amyloidosis, control of the acute-phase response is currently the standard of care (309). Disease-modifying antirheumatic drugs, alkylating agents, anti-TNF therapies, and other biologic agents have been used to treat inflammatory arthritides. Antibiotics and surgery have been used in the control of chronic sepsis, whereas corticosteroids, anti-TNF therapies, and surgery have been recommended for the control of Crohn's disease. In Castleman's disease, surgery and anti-interleukin-6 therapies showed success. Among familial periodic fevers, treatment regimens vary. Familial Mediterranean fever has been successfully treated with colchicine (413). Anti-TNF therapies and corticosteroids have been used in the treatment of TRAPS, while in Muckle-Wells syndrome (a CAPS), anti-interleukin-1 therapies have been tried (413–415).

In patients with FMF, treatment with colchicine prevents the attacks and may even cause a remission of amyloidosis. However, this treatment is not effective in halting the progression of renal disease in patients with initial serum creatinine above 1.5 mg/dL (413).

Nonetheless, the above regimens are not successful for, or applicable to, patients diagnosed at advanced stages of the disease, with refractory underlying disease, or with undetermined or ubiquitously produced circulating precursors. Thus, new therapies have been explored (235,358–362,415–417). The first of a new class of anti-amyloid agents is designed to block the formation of amyloid fibrils by inhibition of glycosaminoglycan binding (362) (see also "AA Amyloidoses," subsection "Etiology and Pathogenesis").

In hereditary amyloidoses, most of the abnormal precursor proteins are produced by the liver. Hence, liver transplantation is currently offered to many of the affected patients in an attempt to eliminate the input of an abnormal amyloid precursor protein (369,378,418–421). In several patients, liver transplantation was combined with cardiac and/or kidney transplantation (419–421). While the long-term effects of liver transplantation on disease progression remain to be determined, the initial results are encouraging.

## Renal Transplantation in Amyloidoses

Renal transplantation for systemic AL amyloidosis has a relatively good outcome, with 5-year patient and graft survival rates of 63% and 65%, respectively, despite a significant increase in early posttransplantation complication rates (mainly sepsis) (422,423). Still better outcomes have been observed in systemic AA amyloidosis, with 92% and 89% 5-year patient and graft survival rates, respectively (National Amyloid Centre Database, United Kingdom). In AL amyloidosis, renal transplantation is most clearly indicated for patients without systemic manifestations of myeloma or systemic deposition of amyloid, while in AA amyloidosis, successful control of the acute phase response is essential.

Renal transplantation in patients with hereditary neuropathic amyloidoses has typically been performed in combination with orthotopic liver transplant (419,420). However, in patients with hereditary amyloidoses predominantly affecting the kidneys, solitary kidney transplantation has been tried (369,378), with mixed results. In patients with AFib treated with a solitary renal transplant, there was a high recurrence rate of amyloid in the allograft (four of five). Thus, currently, hepatorenal transplantation is offered to these patients, with excellent outcomes (369). In contrast, in AApoAII, in which renal failure develops slowly, solitary kidney transplantation has been successful in at least one case (378), where a 9-year follow-up showed no allograft dysfunction.

Cardiac amyloidosis is a contraindication for renal transplant in AL and AA amyloidoses, because survival is markedly compromised (233,337,405). However, combined cardiac and renal transplantations have been offered to selected patients with hereditary amyloidoses targeting those organs (419). Data from several studies show that 65% of transplanted patients with systemic amyloidosis were alive 5 years after renal transplantation (422–424). Systemic complications are responsible for a significant percentage of posttransplant morbidity and mortality. Overall, amyloidosis recurrence rates are approximately 15% to 25%, and graft failure from recurrent amyloidosis is unusual (422–424). The great majority of transplants have been performed in patients with AA amyloidosis, which has a slower and more indolent clinical course in patients in whom the acute-phase response has been successfully controlled. Because long-term survival in AL/AH amyloidosis has been relatively low until recently and the clinical course has been generally stormy, opportunities for considering renal transplantation have been limited. Data pertaining to renal transplants in patients with AL amyloidosis is incomplete and the numbers are small, making it impossible to draw conclusions regarding graft survival and the development of amyloidosis in transplants and extrarenal tissues. However, it has been estimated that recurrence in the transplanted kidney occurs in approximately 20% of patients with AL amyloidosis (422–424). Therefore, renal transplantation may be appropriate in some AL amyloidosis cases, i.e., where the underlying plasma cell dyscrasia has been controlled, heart involvement is absent, and the patient is in relatively good shape. Renal transplantation continues to be offered to patients with other amyloidoses who have severe kidney amyloid deposition. In contrast to AL and AA amyloidoses, in hereditary amyloidoses, cardiac involvement is not an absolute contraindication to renal transplantation (419).

De novo amyloidosis in transplanted kidneys in patients with AL and non-AL amyloidoses has also been reported (425,426). As more experience is accumulated, a better definition of the role of renal transplantation in these diseases will emerge.

### Differential Diagnosis for Amyloidosis

The diagnosis of amyloid can be made with certainty in the great majority of cases by using a combined approach, including light microscopic, histochemical, and ultrastructural analysis (279). It is as important to identify the precursor protein using ancillary diagnostic techniques, with immunofluorescence and immunohistochemistry playing crucial roles in this process, so that the amyloid can be properly classified for patients' management and therapeutic purposes (220,242,264,268,313).

To diagnose early amyloidosis, a high level of suspicion is needed to avoid missing the correct diagnosis. Congo red and thioflavin T or S stains may not clearly identify small foci of amyloid deposition, and an incorrect diagnosis may be made. Ultrastructural evaluation, if representative material is available, is often the best way to substantiate the diagnosis of amyloidosis in these cases. Segmental glomerular and vascular hyalinosis may be confused at times with amyloidosis because of the similar eosinophilic ("hyaline") light microscopic appearance.

Other infiltrative glomerular processes must be ruled out. Fibrillary and immunotactoid glomerulopathies may be associated with expanded mesangium and loss of argyrophilia, features that can also be seen in amyloidosis. The negative Congo red stain in the above conditions and ultrastructural findings should readily differentiate these diseases (278,279). The reader is referred to Chapter 20 on these entities for a full description of the differential diagnostic points. Nodular glomerular amyloidosis can be confused with other nodular glomerulopathies, such as diabetic nephropathy and light and heavy chain deposition disease; the tinctorial characteristics of amyloid, as described in the light microscopy section of this chapter, and ultrastructural features should provide enough evidence to make the right diagnosis.

Although the ultrastructural appearance of amyloid is unique, a source of confusion with amyloid fibrils may be mesangial matrix with an accentuated fibrillary appearance (i.e., mesangiolysis and diabetic fibrillosis) (278,279,306). The random distribution and rather constant diameter of amyloid fibrils should provide the necessary criteria for making a distinction in these situations.

## RENAL INVOLVEMENT IN WALDENSTRÖM MACROGLOBULINEMIA

### Historical Perspective

Waldenström macroglobulinemia was originally described by Jan Waldenström in 1944. He reported two elderly patients with "signs of severe derangement of protein metabolism with very high globulin and low albumin values." These patients also had a severe normochromic anemia, high serum viscosity, and a very large molecule with a molecular weight of 1,000,000 in the serum, which migrated next to β-globulin (427). Dutcher and Fahey detailed the histopathologic and clinical features of WM in 1959 and described perivascular infiltrates of neoplastic lymphoplasmacytic cells in the kidneys in one of three autopsies that they reported (428).

Several case reports in the 1940s and 1950s noted an association between WM and amyloidosis. It was Lamm in 1961 who called attention to peculiar renal alterations in patients with WM. He described hyaline thrombi in glomerular capillaries and in an interlobar band of the renal artery in one of two autopsies of patients with WM

(429). In 1966, Forget et al (430) reported one case and summarized the literature. Although the pathogenesis was unclear at the time, their paper served to affirm that a small percentage of patients with WM during their clinical course develop amyloidosis. Argani and Kipkie coined the term *macroglobulinemic nephropathy* in 1969 (431). A comprehensive publication in 1970 by Morel-Maroger et al reviewed findings of 5 renal biopsies and 13 autopsies of patients with WM (432).

## Clinical Presentation and Laboratory Findings

Waldenström macroglobulinemia is a rare disease; it is much less common than myeloma. It is far more common in whites than in blacks, and it is more frequent in female whites, with an incidence of 6.1 cases per million individuals (433). It is a lymphoproliferative disorder characterized by a monoclonal proliferation of lymphoplasmacytic cells producing IgM, which can be detected as an M spike in serum protein electrophoresis. It generally occurs in older patients (median age of 63 to 70 years), and 99% of the patients are older than 40 years (434). IgM is the paraprotein found in 16% of all myeloma patients, but only 17% to 26% of these patients develop WM (433). IgM monoclonal gammopathy may exist for years before WM develops (435). A consensus panel has made recommendations regarding the clinicopathologic definition of WM (436), as the definition of this syndrome has been controversial (437).

The diagnosis of WM is sometimes made in the course of workup for anemia, elevated sedimentation rate, or increased serum proteins (434,437–439). Patients may also present with a variety of clinical signs and manifestations, including fatigue, weakness, recurring bleeding, lymphadenopathy, splenomegaly, anemia, elevated erythrocyte sedimentation rate, high serum viscosity, and decreased fibrinogen (429,437–439). The serum level of IgM is variable, but symptomatology generally occurs when the serum IgM levels exceed 3 g/dL, and hyperviscosity occurs as a consequence of the high molecular weight of IgM. Monoclonal IgM proteins have very high molecular weights, and when they accumulate, increased plasma osmotic pressure and plasma volume follow. In about one third of patients with WM, a hyperviscosity syndrome occurs (439), characterized by chronic nasal, gum, and gastrointestinal bleeding; headaches; tinnitus; vertigo; impaired hearing; ataxia; mental confusion; blurring and loss of vision with sausage-shaped retinal veins; flame-shaped hemorrhages in the optic fundus; and papilledema (439). Finally, high-output heart failure, stupor, and coma may occur. Osteolytic lesions are rare in this condition (440). Cryoglobulinemia may be an associated condition (434). Unusual manifestations occur in rare cases, such as multifocal osteolytic lesions, bone fractures, and those related to infiltration by neoplastic plasma cells of multiple sites, pro-

ducing such clinical manifestations as cardiac tamponade, obstruction of bile ducts, and severe headache, lethargy, and stupor (441).

In contrast with classic plasma cell dyscrasia and myeloma, renal abnormalities occur rather infrequently in WM. Glomerular abnormalities predominate (432). Renal function is mildly or moderately impaired in about 15% of patients with this condition (431). Patients may present uremic and dehydrated and exhibit nonselective proteinuria (442). Rarely, a patient with WM presents in acute renal failure (431). Patients with WM are typically not hypercalcemic. The degree of BJ proteinuria is low, explaining why cast nephropathy is so rare in this condition. While Krajny and Pruzanski found that BJ proteinuria was identified in 71% of 45 patients, the light chain excretion was very low (less than 200 mg/24 h in all but 9 patients) (443). Kyle and Garton reported a monoclonal spike in the urine in 25 of 57 patients with a median excretion of 1 g/24 h (434). Occasional patients develop nephrotic or nephritic syndrome. Eleven of these patients also had albuminuria (434,444). Infiltration of the renal parenchyma by neoplastic cells can also occur (445,446). Amyloidosis develops in 20% of patients with WM; when this happens the kidneys are often affected. Amyloidosis is the most common cause of nephrotic syndrome in these patients. Significant albuminuria is usually related to amyloidosis (447,448).

Acute renal failure in patients with WM is usually a result of extensive vascular occlusion by circulating IgM, dehydration (432,442), massive renal infiltration by neoplastic lymphoplasmacytic cells (445), and distal nephron obstruction, as seen in myeloma (449).

## Gross Pathology

Not much is known about the gross appearance of kidneys in patients with WM. There is one report of giant kidneys found in this condition in a patient with massive infiltration of the renal parenchyma by neoplastic cells (445).

## Light Microscopy

The most typical glomerular lesions are variably sized, sometimes massive, amorphous, PAS-positive subendothelial deposits (Fig. 19.21A), which may result in compromise of the capillary spaces. In some cases, well-defined thrombi occlude the capillary spaces. Either a few thrombi or massive thrombosis can be seen (431,432). Glomerular necrosis, which may be segmental, is rare and is a result of complete occlusion of glomerular capillaries or arterioles. Cryoglobulins may be identified in 7% to 20% of these patients, and the thrombi may contain cryoglobulins (432,450,451). Therefore, there is significant morphologic overlap between patients with WM and those with cryoglobulinemia associated with other disorders.

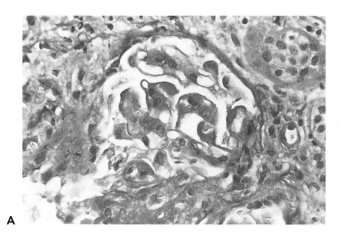

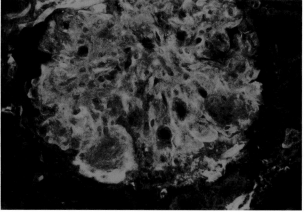

**Figure 19.21.** Waldenström macroglobulinemia. **A:** Typical massive subendothelial deposits, which are PAS-positive. **B:** Corresponding fluorescence staining for IgM depicts peripheral capillary wall staining in areas where subendothelial deposits are present. (×500.)

Waldenström macroglobulinemia was identified in 7 of 21 patients with type I cryoglobulinemia and 8 of 22 patients with type II cryoglobulinemia, attesting to the close association between these two diseases and the morphologic overlap that may occur (450). Amyloid deposition can be seen in any of the renal compartments.

Other renal lesions have been reported in patients with WM, including minimal change disease (452), membranous nephropathy (453), and MIDD (454). Cast nephropathy is unusual but has also been documented (449).

Infiltration of the renal parenchyma by neoplastic cells represents an additional pathologic manifestation of WM. These infiltrating neoplastic cells are seen in both cortical and medullary areas and may play a crucial role in the majority of WM patients who develop significant renal insufficiency. In some cases the neoplastic cellular infiltration results in the formation of renal or perirenal masses (455).

### Immunofluorescence

The glomerular deposits vary in their distribution, stain for IgM and often concomitantly for IgG, and appear as granular to massive peripheral capillary wall deposits (Fig. 19.21B). In some cases, the deposits are accompanied by C3 or C4 staining along the peripheral capillary walls. Light chain monotypicality (restriction) may be identified along with the Ig deposits (432). If thrombi are present, they also frequently stain for IgM, with their peripheral zones generally staining more intensely than their centers (432,442–445). Even in normal-appearing glomeruli, there may be deposition of IgM. Arterioles and small arteries may also reveal IgM staining in their walls. Some of the staining may be related to the fact that these patients have large amounts of circulating IgM, which adheres to various structures in the kidney.

### Electron Microscopy

The deposits are usually electron dense and are located either subendothelially, in capillary spaces in glomeruli, or in the extraglomerular vasculature. Most of the capillary thrombi are electron dense and amorphous (454), but they may contain cryoglobulins with their typical ultrastructural appearance (298,299). Cryoglobulins may also be seen in thrombi located anywhere in the renal vasculature.

### Treatment, Course of the Disease Process, and Prognosis

There are a number of features in this condition at presentation that adversely affect survival: male sex, age greater than 60 years, anemia, and neutropenia. A number of patients with monoclonal IgM in their serum evolve over years to develop WM (434,435). Treatment may not be needed until years after the diagnosis of WM is established; treatment is usually required because of hematologic complications such as severe anemia, hyperviscosity, or visceral involvement.

Renal insufficiency is common in patients who are biopsied. Renal manifestations rarely require dialysis (431,442). In the small percentage of patients with hyperviscosity and renal failure characterized by vascular occlusion on renal biopsy by circulating IgM, plasma exchange may be very useful. In some patients, repeated plasmapheresis is employed to delay the use of cytotoxic drugs. However, in most patients, plasmapheresis alone is not enough to reverse the renal insufficiency, and the concomitant use of chemotherapy to suppress the underlying neoplastic process is indicated. Oral alkylating agents are employed most often, with chlorambucil administration on a daily basis at low dose or intermittently at higher doses (456). Approximately 50% of the patients achieve a sustained partial response. Steroids may be added to the treatment, especially if there is associated cryoglobulinemia or autoimmune hemolytic anemia.

In essence, the treatment of patients with WM and renal compromise consists of systemic chemotherapy to reduce tumor load and the use of plasmapheresis to remove pathologic circulating IgM. When cryoglobulinemia accompanies WM, proteinuria and renal function may improve with primary therapy of the condition, such as is seen when interferon α therapy is used for the treatment of patients with hepatitis C and WM (451,453,457). The median survival for all patients is 5 years and, as expected, is better with responders to the therapy (438). When amyloidosis complicates WM, the overall survival is 28 months; this is even shorter for those patients with cardiac involvement at presentation (447). The most common cause of death in WM is gastrointestinal hemorrhage (434). A small percentage (3.8% to 7.4%) of these patients die of renal failure (434,445,458).

### Transplantation in Waldenström Macroglobulinemia

There is minimal experience with renal transplantation in patients with WM. A renal transplant was performed in a patient, who died 7 months later of a pulmonary embolus. Postmortem examination established a diagnosis of WM with renal involvement and served to retrospectively confirm a diagnosis of WM in a previous renal biopsy performed on this patient, diagnosed initially as chronic pyelonephritis (459).

### Differential Diagnosis for Waldenström Macroglobulinemia–Associated Nephropathy

The histopathologic findings in WM-associated glomerulopathy overlap significantly with those seen in cryoglobulinemic nephropathy (see "Cryoglobulinemic Nephropathy," which follows this section). Hyaline thrombi are characteristic of both conditions, and proliferative and exudative glomerular activity can be seen in selected WM-associated glomerulopathy, although it is more frequently seen in cryoglobulinemic nephropathy. Cryoglobulins can be identified in WM-associated nephropathy, further complicating the differential diagnosis between these two conditions (451). Therefore, the clinical history and laboratory data become very important when this differential diagnosis is considered. Fortunately, in the great majority of the cases the renal biopsy is performed after a diagnosis of WM has been established, and the role of the renal pathologist is to determine the type of lesion present and the extent of the abnormalities encountered.

However, it should be noted that in a significant number of cases, the light microscopic and immunofluorescence findings clearly point to a diagnosis of WM-associated glomerulopathy. Identifying by immunofluorescence glomerular deposits or capillary thrombi that stain dominantly or codominantly for IgM with associated light chain restriction in the proper clinical setting should immediately suggest a diagnosis of WM-associated nephropathy (432).

## CRYOGLOBULINEMIC NEPHROPATHY

Cryoglobulins are serum proteins (immunoglobulins) that are soluble at 37°C (i.e., monoclonal cryoglobulins), precipitate in the cold, and redissolve when heated. Cryoglobulins may precipitate in the vasculature, forming thrombi in virtually every organ in the body, and may also elicit an inflammatory reaction (vasculitis) in the vessel walls. A cryoglobulin may be of a single class of immunoglobulins or complexes in which one component, usually IgM, exhibits antibody activity against IgG (i.e., mixed cryoglobulins). Although the precipitation of cryoglobulins is generally most striking at 4°C, some precipitation occurs at temperatures around 20°C (450,460). Precipitation of cryoglobulins depends on temperature, pH, cryoglobulin concentration, and weak noncovalent factors (461). The discussion regarding cryoglobulinemia in this chapter will address the subject in general; details of cryoglobulinemia associated with certain disorders (i.e., systemic lupus erythematosus) will be covered in detail in the corresponding chapters.

### Historical Perspective

Wintrobe and Buell in 1933 were the first to describe a patient with myeloma who had cryoprecipitable serum, presumably containing cryoglobulins (461), but it was not until 1947 that Lerner and Watson coined the term *cryoglobulins* (462). A syndrome associated with cryoglobulinemia was described in the 1960s by Meltzer and others (463,464), which included purpura, arthralgias, asthenia, and renal disease. Brouet et al (450) classified cryoglobulins into three different types. Type I cryoglobulins are associated with monoclonal gammopathies, usually IgM, and with underlying B-cell neoplasms and plasma cell dyscrasias. Type II cryoglobulins are associated with a monoclonal component, usually IgM, which exhibits activity against the Fc portion of polyclonal IgG. Type III cryoglobulins are polyclonal immunoglobulins of more than one isotype (mixed composition) and are not associated with underlying plasma cell dyscrasias. Mixed cryoglobulins, containing two or more classes of immunoglobulins and encompassing types II and III, constitute 60% to 65% of all cryoglobulins. Brouet's original series (450) included approximately 30% of all cryoglobulinemia cases that could not be related to any underlying disorder (essential or primary cryoglobuline-mia). In the last 20 years cryoglobulinemia has been found in association with an increasing variety of diseases, predominantly hepatitis C, and the number of cases within the essential category has become very small (464–466).

## Clinical Presentation and Laboratory Findings

Significant overlap exists in the clinical features of the different types of cryoglobulinemia. Cryoglobulinemia is more common in females. Patients with circulating cryo-globulins may have a variety of clinical conditions, includ-ing lymphoproliferative disorders, infections, chronic liver disease, systemic lupus erythematosus, other connective tissue diseases, and other conditions, which will exhibit their characteristic symptoms and clinical findings (464–476). Hepatitis C is the most common disease associated with cryoglobulinemia. Extrarenal manifestations are not uncommon, including Raynaud's phenomenon and pur-pura. Cases of cryoglobulinemic glomerulonephritis asso-ciated with an underlying plasma cell dyscrasia are rela-tively uncommon (477).

The prevalence of cryoglobulinemia depends on the population studied. Cryoglobulins are present in approx-imately 5.5% to 49% of patients with renal disease, pri-marily membranoproliferative glomerulonephritis type I and lupus nephritis (469). Approximately 21% to 29% of patients with cryoglobulinemia have renal involvement (450,478). Renal disease is most common with type II cryo-globulinemia (474). Cryoglobulinemic nephropathy oc-curs almost exclusively in connection with type II cryoglob-ulinemia where a circulating IgM κ is present (464). Renal disease generally follows purpuric manifestations by ap-proximately 4 years (465,470). Proteinuria greater than 0.5 g/day and hematuria are the most common renal manifes-tations (459,465,470). Nephrotic and nephritic syndromes are found in 20% to 25% of these patients, respectively (479,480). Hypertension is usually present, and manifes-tations of vasculitis can be observed (459,465,470,477). Hypocomplementemia and splenomegaly are identified in the most aggressive cases (481). All cryoglobulinemias are characterized by exacerbations and remissions. Clini-cal and histologic activity does not always correlate directly with detection of circulating cryoglobulins (470), but there are cases documented in the literature with clinical remis-sion associated with the disappearance of the circulating cryoglobulinemia (470,472–478,482).

To detect cryoglobulins in the serum, a blood specimen is drawn and maintained at 37°C until clotting is com-pleted, during transport to the laboratory. After that, the serum, separated at 37°C is incubated at 4°C to identify ag-glutination or gelation, which would be indicative of cryo-globulins, for at least 72 hours. The inadvertent storage of clotted blood in a refrigerator remains an important rea-son for failing to identify cryoglobulins. A gross screening method has been referred to as the "cryocrit" determina-tion, in which the serum is cold-incubated in a hematocrit tube, which is then centrifuged in the cold after maximal cryoprecipitation has occurred. The relative volume occu-pied by the cryoprecipitate is then expressed on a percent-age basis (483).

## Gross Pathology

There are no documented gross pathologic findings in the kidneys of patients with cryoglobulinemic nephropathy in the literature.

## Light Microscopy

Membranoproliferative glomerulonephritis (MPGN) type I is the renal pattern most commonly identified in pa-tients with cryoglobulinemia (Fig. 19.22A) (484,485).

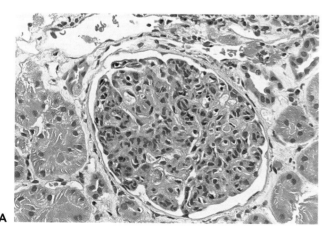
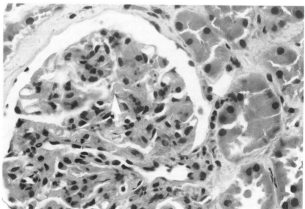

**Figure 19.22.** Essential cryoglobulinemic glomerulopathy. **A:** Membranoproliferative pattern is shown, with accentuation of glomerular lobules and segmentally thickened peripheral capillary walls. (H&E; ×350.) **B:** Hyalin thrombi may be found in only a few capillaries (*arrow*). (H&E; ×500.)

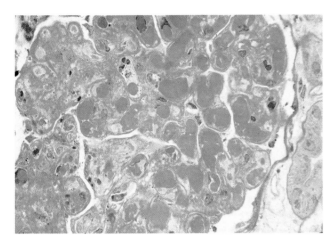

**Figure 19.23.** Type II cryoglobulinemic glomerulopathy. Glomerular capillaries completely filled with thrombi containing cryoglobulins. (PAS; ×750.)

Membranoproliferative glomerulonephritis is responsible for approximately 80% of all renal lesions in type II cryoglobulinemic nephropathy (465). The glomeruli have hypercellular mesangia, resulting in accentuation of glomerular lobulation. The capillary spaces are variably obliterated, and reduplication of the peripheral capillary walls may be appreciated on silver-stained sections. However, the marked hypercellularity seen in classic MPGN type I is sometimes absent or the proliferative activity is segmental (279). Infiltration of capillary spaces by monocytes is frequently seen and polymorphonuclear cells may also be seen in segmental glomerular areas. Intracapillary thrombi are often focal, but when extensive (Fig. 19.22B), or when thrombi are identified in larger renal vessels, the typical clinical presentation is rapid deterioration of renal function or renal failure. The capillary thrombi are eosinophilic on hematoxylin and eosin stain, are PAS-positive (Fig. 19.21B), and may occlude most of the capillary spaces (Fig. 19.23) (471). Thrombi are seen in approximately half of these cases (480,486). When massive intracapillary thrombi are present, the patient usually has either type I or II cryoglobulins (464).

Vasculitis with a prominent inflammatory cell component is seen in approximately 25% to 33% of cases with cryoglobulinemic nephropathy and is almost always accompanied by intraluminal hyaline thrombi (486). The combination of vasculitis and glomerular thrombi should suggest cryoglobulinemic nephropathy, but proliferative lupus nephritis with associated vasculitis (not related to cryoglobulins) is also in the differential diagnosis.

### Immunofluorescence

Three distinct patterns of immunofluorescence staining are described. Strong staining of the intraluminal thrombi associated with spotty granular to pseudolinear staining along peripheral capillary walls is perhaps the most characteristic pattern, and it should immediately suggest the diagnosis of cryoglobulinemia (465,486,487). Thrombi sometimes only show peripheral staining, with their centers remaining negative (465,468). The circulating cryoglobulin and the type deposited in the kidneys are obviously of the same type, indicating that the cryoglobulins become trapped or precipitate in the kidney (450,465,488,489). However, only a minority of patients with cryoglobulinemia exhibit this typical appearance. Subtle, discontinuous granular staining along peripheral glomerular capillary loops represents the second staining pattern, which is much less specific. The third pattern is that of intense, granular, diffuse, finely to coarsely granular to pseudolinear subendothelial staining, similar to what is seen in classic MPGN type I. The immunoreactants that can be detected vary from case to case and depend on the type of circulating cryoglobulins (490). Occasionally only one of the immunoglobulins present in the cryoglobulins can be demonstrated in the kidneys. Because IgG is the most common type of cryoglobulin, deposits with IgG staining predominate. There are also a significant number of cases with IgM as well as C3 deposits (92% of all cases); the latter follow in intensity and distribution the immunoglobulin deposits in most instances, but it is rare to find it in thrombi even when the immunoglobulins are detected (465). C4 is detectable in approximately one third of cases but is uncommon in capillary thrombi (465). Frequently, fibrinogen is detected in the glomeruli and vasculature, especially in cases with overt vasculitis. In rare cases, isolated mesangial or peripheral capillary wall deposits are detected by immunofluorescence (465). Because of the cyclical nature of this disorder, deposits can be abundant or scanty in a given patient during the course of the disease. There is also some correlation between the clinical disease activity and the findings in the renal biopsy, but this is not always the case (465,487).

### Electron Microscopy

Discrete, electron-dense deposits of the immune complex type can be seen in subepithelial, subendothelial, intramembranous, or mesangial areas. Some of the subepithelial deposits mimic "humps" (490). The appearance of the deposits is frequently similar to that of the cryoprecipitate of the same patient (488–490). Varying degrees of intraglomerular cellular proliferation and duplication of peripheral capillary walls by mesangial cell interposition (491–494) can be present. Inflammatory cells, including polymorphonuclear cells and most characteristically monocytes, may be found in glomerular capillaries (495).

The most classic deposits seen in cryoglobulinemia are characterized by thick-walled microtubular or annular, frequently curved structures that measure 10 to 25 nm in width (Fig. 19.24) (278,279,486). The microtubules may be paired, randomly arranged, or in groups in what has

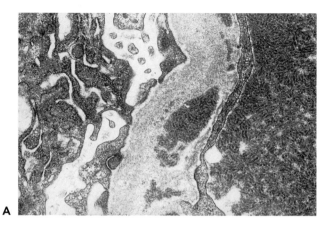

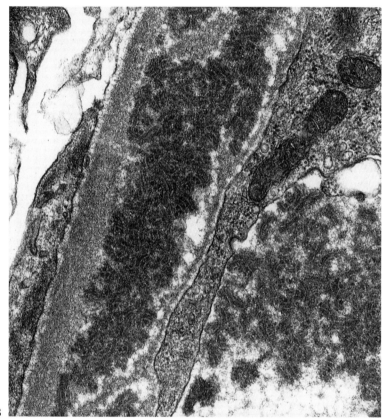

**Figure 19.24.** Cryoglobulinemic glomerulopathy associated with hepatitis C. Classic curved microtubular aggregates typical of cryoglobulin deposits are seen in the subendothelial zone and in intracapillary thrombi. Transmission electron microscopy. (Uranyl acetate and lead citrate; **A:** ×12,500; **B:** ×25,000.)

been described as "paracrystalline arrays" (480,490). On cross section, they appear as hollow, ringlike structures approximately 300 A in diameter or annular structures with spokes. Both the tubular and annular patterns may be present in the same case. This appearance is most commonly seen in the IgG–IgM type of mixed cryoglobulinemia, but sometimes similarly well organized deposits can be found in type I cryoglobulinemia and other conditions (472,490). The number of capillary thrombi containing cryoglobulins can be variable, and at times, careful evaluation of the material submitted for ultrastructural examination is required to identify the few thrombi with diagnostic features.

Although the microtubular/annular pattern predominates overall, the deposits may exhibit fingerprints (495) or a fibrillary or crystalloid substructure (465,467). For example, the cryoglobulin deposits associated with type I cryoglobulinemia may be composed of either straight fibrils forming bundles 80 nm wide, which in cross section appear cross-hatched, or tubular structures in a fingerprint-like array (467).

Rhomboid, variably shaped, membrane-bound osmiophilic structures in the cytoplasm of mesangial and glomerular epithelial cells in patients with cryoglobulinemic nephropathy are documented in a few publications (488,494). The structures resemble the crystalloid structures seen in the Fanconi lesion associated with plasma cell dyscrasias and detected also rarely in patients with myeloma in resident glomerular cells (primarily mesangial cells) but differ in that they are PAS-negative (489,494,495).

Even when cryoglobulinemic nephropathy is suspected on the basis of the light and immunofluorescence findings, ultrastructural confirmation is crucial for a definitive diagnosis. Cryoglobulins most notably coexist with classic immune complexes in lupus nephritis cases. In rare instances, immune complexes without internal substructure are the only ultrastructural findings in a case with typical clinicopathologic features of cryoglobulinemic nephropathy (488).

## Treatment, Course of the Disease Process, and Prognosis

In many cases cryoglobulinemia is an indolent disorder, especially cases associated with hepatitis C and glomerular involvement (485). Often, the renal biopsy establishes the diagnosis of cryoglobulinemia.

The disease process is generally characterized by periods of disease inactivity, recurrences, and exacerbations. Remissions are generally associated with the disappearance of the circulating cryoglobulins and resolution of the clinical renal manifestations. Patients with cryoglobulinemia only infrequently (10% of the cases) progress to end-stage renal disease requiring dialysis within 5 to 10 years (465,479,480).

Difficult-to-control cryoglobulinemia is treated with immunosuppressive therapy, steroids, and plasmapheresis. In these cases skin manifestations and arthralgias respond quickly, but renal disease is more unpredictable (496). It depends primarily on the chronicity of renal involvement. Acute nephropathy responds well to this aggressive treatment (496,497).

## Transplantation in Cryoglobulinemia

Renal transplantation is extremely uncommon in patients with cryoglobulinemic nephropathy because of the characteristic good renal prognosis of this condition. Renal transplant patients with active hepatitis may develop either de novo or recurrent cryoglobulinemic nephropathy in renal allografts (498).

## Differential Diagnosis for Cryoglobulinemic Glomerulopathy

A definitive diagnosis of cryoglobulinemic nephropathy requires ultrastructural demonstration of cryoglobulins (278,279) or strong clinicopathologic evidence of this condition with an associated immune complex-mediated glomerulonephritis, which characteristically shows features of MPGN type I (498). Familiarization with the various morphologic appearances of cryoglobulins is essential to avoid missing this diagnosis. Ultrastructural confirmation of cryoglobulin deposition is crucial in establishing a solid diagnosis. On light microscopic evaluation, the finding of hyaline thrombi elicits a rather interesting differential diagnosis that includes lupus nephritis and thrombotic microangiopathy (499). Electron microscopy is very important in characterizing the composition of the capillary thrombi. The fact that cryoglobulins can be seen in otherwise typical lupus nephritis further complicates the differential diagnosis. However, proper and careful evaluation of the immunofluorescence and ultrastructural findings should provide crucial data (499). Clinical and serologic findings should also be considered in the final evaluation of each case.

## REFERENCES

1. MacIntire W. Case of mollities and fragilitas ossium accompanied by urine strongly charged with animal matter. Med Chir Tr 1850;33:211.
2. Bence-Jones H. On a new substance occurring in the urine of a patient with "mollities ossium." Philos Trans R Soc Lond 1848;138:55.
3. Bence-Jones H. Papers on chemical pathology; Prefaced by the Gulstonian lectures, at the Royal College of Physicians. Lancet 1847;2:88.
4. Clamp JR. Some aspects of the first recorded case of multiple myeloma. Lancet 1967;2:1354.
5. Dalrymple J. On the microscopic character of mollities ossium. Dublin J Med Sci 1846;2:85.
6. Kyle RA. Multiple myeloma: How did it begin? Mayo Clin Proc 1994;69:680.
7. von Rustizky J. Multiples myelom. Dtsch Z Chir 1873;3:162.
8. Kahler O. Zur Symptomatologie des multiplen Myeloms: Beobachtung von Albumosurie. Prag Med Wochenschr 1889;14:33.
9. Wright JH. A case of multiple myeloma. Johns Hopkins Hosp Rev 1900;9:359.
10. Ramón y Cajal S. Estudios histológicos sobre los tumores epiteliales. Rev Trimest Microgr 1896;1:83.
11. Ellinger A. Das Vorkommen des Bence-Jones'schen Korpers im Harn bei Tumoren des Knochenmarks und seine diagnostische Bedeutung. Dtsch Arch Klin Med 1899;62:255.
12. Ewing J. Lectures on tumor pathology. In: Cornell University Medical School, Class of 1934, 2nd ed. New York City: Robert C. Gall and Associates, 1977:54.
13. Korngold L, Lipari R. Multiple-myeloma proteins. III. The antigenic relationship of Bence Jones proteins to normal gamma-globulin and multiple-myeloma serum proteins. Cancer 1956;9:262.
14. Edelman GM, Gally J. The nature of amyloid proteins. Chemical similarities to polypeptide chains of myeloma globulins and normal gamma globulins. J Exp Med 1962;116:207.
15. Durie BGM. Staging and kinetics of multiple myeloma. Semin Oncol 1986;13:300.
16. Sullivan PW, Salmon SE. Kinetics of tumor growth and regression in IgG multiple myeloma. J Clin Invest 1972;51:1697.
17. Drewinko B, Alexanian R. Growth kinetics of plasma cell myeloma. J Natl Cancer Inst 1977;58:1247.
18. Kyle RA. Multiple myeloma: Review of 869 cases. Mayo Clin Proc 1975;50:29.

19. Multiple Myeloma Research Foundation website (www.multiple myeloma.org).
20. MacLennan IC, Drayson M, Dunn J. Multiple myeloma. Br Med J 1994;308:1033.
21. Niesvizky R, Siegel D, Michaeli J. Biology and treatment of multiple myeloma. Blood Rev 1993;7:24.
22. Bataille R, Harousseau JL. Multiple myeloma. N Engl J Med 1997;336:1657.
23. Abe M, Goto T, Kennel SJ. Production and immunodiagnostic applications of antihuman light chain monoclonal antibodies. Am J Clin Pathol 1993;100:67.
24. Perfetti V, Bellotti V, Garini P, et al. AL amyloidosis. Characterization of amyloidogenic cells by anti-idiotypic monoclonal antibodies. Lab Invest 1994;71:853.
25. Kyle RA. Monoclonal gammopathy of undetermined significance. Natural history in 241 cases. Am J Med 1978;64:814.
26. Kyle RA. Monoclonal gammopathy of undetermined significance. Blood Rev 1994;8:135.
27. Vastni PS, Erickson DG, Williams RC Jr, et al. Benign monoclonal gammaglobulinemia and glomerulonephritis. Am J Med 1977;62:324.
28. Axelsson U. An eleven-year follow-up on 64 subjects with M-components. Acta Med Scand 1977;201:173.
29. Kyle RA. "Benign" monoclonal gammopathy—after 20 to 35 years of follow-up. Mayo Clin Proc 1993;68:26.
30. Milla F, Oriol A, Aguilar J, et al. Usefulness and reproducibility of cytomorphologic evaluations to differentiate myeloma from monoclonal gammopathies of unknown significance. Am J Clin Pathol 2001;115:127.
31. Klein R, Jaenichen R, Zachau HG. Expressed human immunoglobulin kappa genes and their hypermutation. Eur J Immunol 1993;23:3248.
32. Kawasaki K, Minoshima S, Nakato E, et al. One-megabase sequence analysis of the human immunoglobulin lambda gene locus. Genome Res 1997;7:250.
33. Solomon A, Weiss DT. Protein and host factors implicated in the pathogenesis of light chain amyloidosis (AL amyloidosis). Amyloid. Int J Exp Clin Invest 1995;2:269.
34. Putnam FW. From the first to the last of the immunoglobulins: Perspectives and prospects. Clin Physiol Biochem 1983;1:63.
35. Buxbaum J. Aberrant immunoglobulin synthesis in light chain amyloidosis: Free light chains and light chain fragment production by human bone marrow cells in short-term tissue culture. J Clin Invest 1986;78:798.
36. Preud'homme JL, Morel-Maroger L, Brouet JC, et al. Synthesis of abnormal immunoglobulins in lymphoplasmacytic disorders with visceral light chain deposition. Am J Med 1980;69:703.
37. Preud'homme JL, Morel-Maroger L, Brouet JC, et al. Synthesis of abnormal heavy and light chains in multiple myeloma with visceral deposition of monoclonal immunoglobulin. Clin Exp Immunol 1980;42:545.
38. Ritchie RF, Smith R. Immunofixation: III. Applications to the study of monoclonal proteins. Clin Chem 1976;22:1982.
39. Abraham RS, Katzmann JA, Clark RJ, et al. Quantitative analysis of serum free light chains: A new marker for the diagnostic evaluation of primary systemic amyloidosis. Am J Clin Pathol 2003;119:274.
40. Bladé J, Kyle RA. Nonsecretory myeloma, immunoglobulin D myeloma, and plasma cell leukemia. Hematol Oncol Clin North Am 1999;13:1259.
41. Wetzel R. Domain stability in immunoglobulin light chain deposition disorders. Adv Protein Chem 1997;50:183.
42. Hurle MR, Helms LR, Li L, et al. A role for destabilizing amino acid replacements in light-chain amyloids. Proc Natl Acad Sci U S A 1994;94:5446.
43. Stevens FJ, Myatt EA, Chang CH, et al. A molecular model for self-assembly of amyloid fibrils: Immunoglobulin light chains. Biochem 1995;34:10697.
44. Cogne M, Preud'homme J-L, Bauwens M, et al. Structure of a monoclonal kappa chain of the V kappa IV subgroup in the kidney and plasma cells in light chain deposition disease. J Clin Invest 1991;42:545.
45. Khamlichi AA, Aucouturier P, Silvain C, et al. Primary structure of a monoclonal kappa chain (FRA) in myeloma with light chain deposition disease. Clin Exp Immunol 1992;87:122.
46. Stevens FJ, Myatt EA, Chang CH, et al. A molecular model for self-assembly of amyloid fibrils: Immunoglobulin light chains. Biochemistry 1995;34:10697.
47. Wally J, Kica G, Zhang Y, et al. Identification of a novel substitution in the constant region of a gene coding for an amyloidogenic kappa 1 light chain. Biochim Biophys Acta 1999;1454:49.
48. Wall JS, Gupta V, Wilkerson M, et al. Structural basis of light chain amyloidogenicity: Comparison of the thermodynamic properties, fibrillogenic potential and tertiary structural features of four λ 6 proteins. J Mol Recognit 2004;17:323.
49. Decourt C, Cogne M, Rocca A. Structural peculiarities of a truncated V kappa III immunoglobulin light chain in myeloma with light chain deposition disease. Clin Exp Immunol 1996;106:357.
50. Solomon A, Frangione B, Franklin EC. Bence Jones proteins and light chains of immunoglobulins. Preferential association of the lambda VI subgroup of human light chains with amyloidosis (AL) lambda. J Clin Invest 1982;70:453.
51. Gallo G, Goni F, Boctor F, et al. Light chain cardiomyopathy. Structural analysis of the light chain tissue deposits. Am J Pathol 1996;148:1397.
52. Preud'homme JL, Aucouturier P, Striker L, et al. Monoclonal immunoglobulin deposition disease (Randall type). Relationship with structural abnormalities of immunoglobulin chains. Kidney Int 1994;46:965.
53. Picken MM, Frangione B, Barlogie B, et al. Light chain deposition disease derived from the V kappa light chain subgroup: Biochemical characterization. Am J Pathol 1989;134:749.
54. Cogne M, Preud'homme JL, Bauwens M, et al. Structure of a monoclonal kappa chain of the V kappa IV subgroup in the kidney and plasma cells in light chain deposition disease. J Clin Invest 1991;87:2186.
55. Rocca A, Khamlichi AA, Aucouturier P, et al. Primary structure of a variable region of the V kappa I subgroup (ISE) in light chain deposition disease. Clin Exp Immunol 1993;91:506.
56. Stevens FJ. Four structural risk factors identify most fibril-forming kappa light chains. Amyloid 2000;7:200.
57. Solomon A, Weiss, DT, Herrera GA. Renal diseases associated with multiple myeloma and related plasma cell dyscrasias. In: Berenson J, ed. Biology and Management of Multiple Myeloma. Totowa, NJ: Humana Press, 2004:281.
58. Solomon A, Weiss DT, Herrera GA. Light chain deposition disease features. In: Mehta J, Singhal S, eds. Myeloma. Oxford, UK: Martin Dunitz, 2002:507.
59. Solomon A. Bence-Jones proteins and light chains of immunoglobulins. N Engl J Med 1976;294:17.
60. Abraham RS, Geyer SM, Price-Troska TL, et al. Immunoglobulin light chain variable (V) region genes influence clinical presentation and outcome in light chain–associated amyloidosis (AL). Blood 2003;101:3801.
61. Deret S, Denoroy L, Lamarine M, et al. Kappa light chain–associated Fanconi's syndrome: Molecular analysis of monoclonal immunoglobulin light chains from patients with and without intracellular crystals. Protein Eng 1999;12:363.
62. Aucouturier P, Bauwens M, Khamlichi AA, et al. Monoclonal Ig L chain and L chain V domain fragment crystallization in myeloma-associated Fanconi's syndrome. J Immunol 1993;150:3561.
63. Omtvedt LA, Bailey D, Renouf DV, et al. Glycosylation of immunoglobulin light chains associated with amyloidosis. Amyloid 2000;7:227.
64. Herrera GA. Low molecular weight proteins and the kidney. Physiological and pathological considerations. Ultrastruct Pathol 1994;18:89.
65. Maack T. Renal handling of low molecular weight proteins. Am J Med 1975;58:57.
66. Batuman V, Guan S. Receptor-mediated endocytosis of immunoglobulin light chains by renal proximal cells. Am J Physiol 1997;272:F521.
67. Batuman V, Verroust PJ, Navar GL, et al. Myeloma light chains are ligands for cubilin (gp280). Renal Physiol 1998;F246.

68. Verroust PJ, Birn H, Nielsen R, et al. The tandem endocytic receptors megalin and cubilin are important proteins in renal pathology. Kidney Int 2002;62:745.

69. Abe M, Goto T, Kosaka M, et al. Differences in kappa to lambda (kappa:lambda) ratios of serum and urinary free light chains. Clin Exp Immunol 1998;111:457.

70. Solomon A, Waldmann TA, Fahey JL, et al. Metabolism of Bence Jones proteins. J Clin Invest 1964;43:103.

71. Jensen K. Metabolism of Bence Jones proteins in multiple myeloma patients and in patients with renal disease. Scand J Clin Lab Invest 1970;26:13.

72. Briault S, Courtois-Capella M, Duarte F, et al. Isotype of serum monoclonal immunoglobulins in human immunodeficiency virus–infected adults. Clin Exp Immunol 1988;74: 182.

73. Falck HM, Tornroth T, Wegelius O. Predominantly vascular amyloid deposition in the kidney in patients with minimal or no proteinuria. Clin Nephrol 1983;19:137.

74. Jacquot C, Saint-Andre JP, Touchard G, et al. Association of systemic light-chain deposition disease and amyloidosis: A report of three patients with renal involvement. Clin Nephrol 1985;24: 93.

75. Ganeval D, Noel LH, Preud'homme JL, et al. Light chain deposition disease: Its relation to AL-type amyloidosis. Kidney Int 1984;26:1.

76. Buxbaum JN, Chuba JV, Hellman GC, et al. Monoclonal immunoglobulin deposition disease: Light chain and light and heavy chain deposition diseases and their relationship to light chain amyloidosis. Ann Int Med 1990;112:455.

77. Herrera GA, Joseph L, Gu X, et al. Renal pathologic spectrum in an autopsy series of patients with plasma cell dyscrasias. Arch Pathol Lab Med 2004;128:875.

78. Pringle JP, Graham RC, Bernier GM. Detection of myeloma cells in the urine sediment. Blood 1974;43:137.

79. Decastello A. Beitrage zur Kenntnis der Bence-Jonesschen Albuminurie. Zeitschr Klin Med 1909;67:319.

80. Krauss E. Studien zur Bence-Jones'schen Albuminurie. Dtsch Arch Klin Med 1921–1922;137:257.

81. Thannhauser SJ, Krauss E. Über eine degerative Erkrankung der Harnkanälchen (Nephrose) bei Bence-Jones'scher Albuminurie mit Nierenschwund (kleine, glatte, weisse Niere). Dtsch Arch Klin Med 1920;133:183.

82. Bell ET. Renal lesions associated with multiple myeloma. Am J Pathol 1933;9:393.

83. Ivanyi B. Frequency of light chain deposition nephropathy relative to renal amyloidosis and Bence Jones cast nephropathy in a necropsy study of patients with myeloma. Arch Pathol Lab Med 1990;114:986.

84. Lin J, Markowitz GS, Valeri AM, et al. Renal monoclonal immunoglobulin deposition disease: The disease spectrum. J Am Soc Nephrol 2001;12:1482.

85. Kapadia SB. Multiple myeloma: A clinicopathologic study of 62 consecutively autopsied cases. Medicine 1980;39:380.

86. Start DA, Silva FG, Davis LD, et al. Myeloma cast nephropathy: Immunohistochemical and lectin studies. Mod Pathol 1988;1:336.

87. Cohen AH. The kidney in plasma cell dyscrasias: Bence-Jones cast nephropathy and light chain deposit disease. Am J Kidney Dis 1998;32:529.

88. Sanders PW, Herrera GA. Monoclonal immunoglobulin light chain–related renal diseases. Sem Nephrol 1993;13:324.

89. Smolens P. The kidney in dysproteinemic states. AKF Nephrol Lett 1987;4:27.

90. Huang ZQ, Sanders PW. Biochemical interaction between Tamm-Horsfall glycoprotein and Ig light chains in the pathogenesis of cast nephropathy. Lab Invest 1995;73:810.

91. Hoyer JR, Seiler MW. Pathophysiology of Tamm-Horsfall protein. Kidney Int 1979;16:279.

92. Sanders PW, Booker BB. Pathobiology of cast nephropathy from human Bence Jones proteins. J Clin Invest 1992;89:630.

93. Sanders PW, Booker B, Bishop JB, et al. Mechanisms of intranephronal cast formation by low molecular weight proteins. J Clin Invest 1990;85:570.

94. Rhodes DCJ, Hinsman EJ, Rhodes JA. Tamm-Horsfall glycoprotein binds IgG with high affinity. Kidney Int 1993;44:1014.

95. Thomas DB, Davies M, Peters JR, et al. Tamm Horsfall protein binds to a single class of carbohydrate specific receptors on human neutrophils. Kidney Int 1993;44:423.

96. Sedmak DD, Tubbs RR. The macrophagic origin of multinucleated giant cells in myeloma kidney: An immunohistologic study. Hum Pathol 1987;18:304.

97. Alpers CE, Magil AB, Gown AM. Macrophage origin of the multinucleated cells of myeloma cast nephropathy. Am J Clin Pathol 1989;92:662.

98. Sessa A, Torri Tarelli L, Meroni M, et al. Multinucleated giant cells in myeloma kidney: An ultrastructural study. Appl Pathol 1984;2:185.

99. Silva FG, Pirani CL, Mesa-Tejada R, et al. The kidney in plasma cell dyscrasias: A review and a clinicopathologic study of 50 patients. In: Fenoglio C, Wolff M, eds. Progress in Surgical Pathology. New York: Masson, 1983:131.

100. Coleman RF, Mowry RW. Certain histochemical and staining properties of renal tubular casts in human multiple myeloma and in "mouse myeloma" compared to those of amyloid [Abstract]. Fed Proc 1964;23:446.

101. DeFronzo RA, Humphrey RL, Wright JR, et al. Acute renal failure in multiple myeloma. Medicine 1975;54:209.

102. Herrera GA. The contributions of electron microscopy to the understanding and diagnosis of plasma cell dyscrasia-related renal lesions. Med Electron Microsc 2001;34:1.

103. Herrera GA. Renal manifestations in plasma cell dyscrasias: An appraisal from the patients' bedside to the research laboratory. Ann Diagn Pathol 2000;4:174.

104. Clyne DH, Brendstrup L, First MR, et al. Renal effects of intraperitoneal kappa chain injection: Induction of crystals in renal tubular cells. Lab Invest 1974;31:131.

105. Koss MN, Parani CL, Osserman EF. Experimental Bence-Jones cast nephropathy. Lab Invest 1976;34:579.

106. Solomon A, Weiss DT, Kattine AA. Nephrotoxic potential of Bence Jones proteins. N Engl J Med 1991;324:1845.

107. Clyne DH, Pesce AJ, Thompson RE. Nephrotoxicity of Bence Jones proteins in the rat: Importance of isoelectric point. Kidney Int 1979;16:345.

108. Hill GS, Morel-Moreger L, Mery JP, et al. Correlations between relative electrophoretic mobilities of light chains and renal lesions in multiple myeloma [Abstract]. Kidney Int 1978;14: 712.

109. Coward RA, Delamore IW, Mallick NP, et al. The importance of urinary immunoglobulin light chain isoelectric point (pI) in nephrotoxicity in multiple myeloma. Clin Sci 1984;66:229.

110. Johns EA, Turner R, Cooper EH, et al. Isoelectric points of urinary light chains in myelomatosis: Analysis in relation to nephrotoxicity. J Clin Pathol 1986;39:833.

111. Melcion C, Mougenot B, Baudouin B, et al. Renal failure in myeloma: Relationship with isoelectric point of immunoglobulin light chains. Clin Nephrol 1984;22:138.

112. Holland MD, Galla JH, Sanders PW, et al. Effect of urinary pH and diatrizoate on Bence Jones protein nephrotoxicity in the rat. Kidney Int 1985;27:46.

113. Ying WZ, Sanders PW. Mapping the binding domain of immunoglobulin light chains for Tamm-Horsfall protein. Am J Pathol 2001;158:1859.

114. Smolens P, Venkatachalam M, Stein JH. Myeloma kidney cast nephropathy in a rat model of multiple myeloma. Kidney Int 1983;24:192.

115. Sanders PW, Herrera GA, Chen A, et al. Differential nephrotoxicity of low molecular weight proteins including Bence Jones proteins in the perfused rat nephron in vivo. J Clin Invest 1988;82:2086.

116. Ronco PM, Mougenot B, Touchard G, et al. Renal involvement in hematological disorders: Monoclonal immunoglobulins and nephropathy. Curr Opin Nephrol Hypertens 1995;4:130.

117. Groop L, Mäkipernaa A, Svante S, et al. Urinary excretion of kappa light chains in patients with diabetes mellitus. Kidney Int 1988;37:1120.

118. Soffer O, Nassar VH, Campbell WG, Bourke E. Light chain

nephropathy and acute renal failure associated with rifampin therapy. Am J Med 1987;82:1052.

119. Misiani R, Tiraboschi G, Mingardi G, et al. Management of myeloma kidney: An anti-light chain approach. Am J Kidney Dis 1987;10:28.

120. Zucchelli P, Pasquali S, Cagnoli L, et al. Controlled plasma exchange trial in acute renal failure due to multiple myeloma. Kidney Int 1988;33:1175.

121. Anderson KC, Kyle RA, Dalton WS, et al. Multiple myeloma: New insights and therapeutic approaches. Hematology (Am Soc Hematol Educ Program) 2000;147

122. Rayner HC, Haynes AP, Thompson JR, et al. Perspectives in multiple myeloma: Survival, prognostic factors and disease complications in a single center between 1975 and 1988. Q J Med 1991;79:517.

123. Bear RA, Cole EH, Lang A, et al. Treatment of acute renal failure due to myeloma kidney. Can Med Assoc J 1980;123:750.

124. Winearls CG. Acute myeloma kidney. Kidney Int 1995;48:1347.

125. Port FK, Nissenson AR. Outcome of end-stage renal disease in patients with rare causes of renal failure. II: Renal or systemic neoplasms. Q J Med 1989;73:1161.

126. Sanders PW. Pathogenesis and treatment of myeloma kidney. J Lab Clin Med 1994;124:484.

127. Kyle RA, Elveback LR. Management and prognosis of multiple myeloma. Mayo Clin Proc 1976;51:751.

128. Löhlein M. Euweisskrystalle in den harnkanälchen bei multiplen myelom. beitr zi Path Anat Vz Allg Path 1921;69:295.

129. Engle RL Jr, Wallis LA. Multiple myeloma and the adult Fanconi syndrome. I. Report of a case with crystal-like deposits in the tumor cells and in the epithelial cells of the kidney. Am J Med 1957;22:5.

130. Costanza DJ, Smoller M. Multiple myeloma with the Fanconi syndrome: Study of a case, with electron microscopy of the kidney. Am J Med 1963;34:125.

131. Maldonado JE, Velosa JA, Kyle RA, et al. Fanconi syndrome in adults. A manifestation of a latent form of myeloma. Am J Med 1975;58:354.

132. DeFronzo RA, Cooke CR, Wright JR, et al. Renal function in patients with multiple myeloma. Med 1978;57:151.

133. Sanders PW, Herrera GA, Lott RL, et al. Morphologic alterations of the proximal tubules in light chain—related renal disease. Kidney Int 1988;33:881.

134. Pote A, Zwizinski C, Simon EE, et al. Cytotoxicity of myeloma light chains in cultured human kidney proximal tubule cells. Am J Kidney Dis 2000;36:735.

135. Maldonado JE, Velosa JA, Kyle RA, et al. Fanconi syndrome in adults: A manifestation of a latent form of myeloma. Am J Med 1975;58:354.

136. Messiaen T, Deret S, Mougenot B, et al. Adult Fanconi syndrome secondary to light chain gammopathy: Clinicopathologic heterogeneity and unusual features in 11 patients. Medicine (Baltimore) 2000;79:135.

137. Raman SBK, Van Slyck EJ. Nature of intracytoplasmic crystalline inclusions in myeloma cells (morphologic, cytochemical, ultrastructural and immunofluorescent studies). Am J Clin Pathol 1983;80:224.

138. Mullen B, Chalvardjian A. Crystalline tissue deposits in a case of multiple myeloma. Arch Pathol Lab Med 1981;105:94.

139. Gu X, Barrios R, Cartwright J, et al. Light chain crystal deposition as a manifestation of plasma cell dyscrasia: The role of immunoelectron microscopy. Hum Pathol 2003;34:270.

140. Markowitz GS. Dysproteinemia and the kidney. Adv Anat Pathol 2004;11:49.

141. Herrera GA, Paul R, Turbat-Herrera EA, et al. Ultrastructural immunolabeling in the diagnosis of light chain—related renal disease. Pathol Immunopathol Res 1986;5:170.

142. Truong LD, Mawad J, Cagle P, et al. Cytoplasmic crystals in multiple myeloma-associated Fanconi's syndrome. Arch Pathol Lab Med 1989;113:781.

143. Herrera GA, Sanders PW, Reddy BV, et al. Ultrastructural immunolabeling: A unique diagnostic tool in monoclonal light chain related renal diseases. Ultrastruct Pathol 1994;18:401.

144. Sanders PW, Herrera GA, Galla JH. Human Bence Jones protein toxicity in rat proximal tubule epithelium in vivo. Kidney Int 1987;32:851.

145. Venkataseshan VS, Faraggiana T, Hughson MD, et al. Morphologic variants of light-chain deposition disease in the kidney. Am J Nephrol 1988;8:272.

146. Gu X, Herrera GA. Light chain—mediated acute tubular interstitial nephritis: A poorly recognized pattern of renal disease in patients with plasma cell dyscrasia. Arch Pathol Lab Med 2006;130:165.

147. Rastegar A, Kashgarian M. The clinical spectrum of tubulointerstitial nephritis. Kidney Int 1998;54:313.

148. Kambham N, Markowitz GS, Appel GB, et al. Heavy chain deposition disease: The disease spectrum. Am J Kidney Dis 1999;33:954.

149. Sanders PW, Herrera GA, Kirk KA, et al. Spectrum of glomerular and tubulointerstitial renal lesions associated with monotypical immunoglobulin light chain deposition. Lab Invest 1991; 64:527.

150. Kobernick SD, Whiteside JH. Renal glomerulus in multiple myeloma. Lab Invest 1957;6:478.

151. Abrahams C, Pirani CL, Pollar VE. Ultrastructure of the kidney in a patient with multiple myeloma. J Pathol Bacteriol 1966;92: 220.

152. Rosen S, Cortell S, Adner MM, et al. Multiple myeloma and the nephrotic syndrome. Am J Clin Pathol 1967;47:567.

153. Antonovych TT, Lin RC, Mostofi FK. Light chain deposits in multiple myeloma. Ultrastructural and immunofluorescence findings in the kidney [Abstract]. Lab Invest 1974;30:370A.

154. Randall RE, Williamson WC Jr, Mullinax F, et al. Manifestations of systemic light chain deposition. Am J Med 1976;60:293.

155. Aucouturier P, Khamlichi AA, Touchard G, et al. Heavy-chain deposition disease. N Engl J Med 1993;329:1389.

156. Smithline N, Kassirer JP, Cohen JJ. Light-chain nephropathy: Renal tubular dysfunction associated with light-chain proteinuria. N Engl J Med 1976;294:71.

157. Pirani CL, Silva FG, Appel GB. Tubulointerstitial disease in multiple myeloma and other nonrenal neoplasias. In: Cotran RS, ed. Contemporary Issues in Nephrology, Vol 10. New York: Churchill Livingstone, 1983:287.

158. Gallo GR, Feiner HD, Katz LA, et al. Nodular glomerulopathy associated with nonamyloidotic kappa light chain deposits and excess immunoglobulin light chain synthesis. Am J Pathol 1980;99:621.

159. Feiner HD. Pathology of dysproteinemia: Light chain amyloidosis, non-amyloid immunoglobulin deposition disease, cryoglobulinemia syndromes, and macroglobulinemia of Waldenström. Hum Pathol 1988;19:1255.

160. Ronco PM, Alyanakian MA, Mougenot B, et al. Light chain deposition disease: A model of glomerulosclerosis defined at the molecular level. J Am Soc Nephrol 2001;12:1558.

161. Ganeval D, Mignon F, Preud'homme JL, et al. Visceral deposition of monoclonal light chains and immunoglobulins: A study of renal and immunopathologic abnormalities. In Grunfeld JP, Maxwell MH (eds): Advances in Nephrology, pp. 25–63, Chicago, Year Book Medical Pub Inc., 1982.

162. Herrera GA. Light chain deposition disease (nodular glomerulopathy, kappa light chain deposition disease): A case report. Ultrastruct Pathol 1994;18:119.

163. Isaac J, Herrera GA. Renal biopsy as a primary diagnostic tool in plasma cell dyscrasias. Pathol Case Rev 1998;3:183.

164. Denoroy L, Deret S, Aucouturier P. Overrepresentation of the V kappa IV subgroup in light chain deposition disease. Immunol Lett 1994;42:63.

165. Verroust P, Mery JP, Morel-Maroger L, et al. Glomerular lesions in monoclonal gammopathies and mixed essential cryoglobulinemias IgG-IgM. Adv Nephrol Necker Hosp 1971;1:161.

166. Ivanyi B, Varga G, Nagy J, et al. Light chain deposition nephropathy in necropsy material. Zentralbl Pathol 1991;137:366.

167. Tubbs RR, Gephardt GN, McMahon JT, et al. Light chain nephropathy. Am J Med 1981;71:263.

168. Gallo GR, Lazowski P, Kumar A, et al. Renal and cardiac manifestations of B-cell dyscrasias with nonamyloidotic monoclonal

light chain and light and heavy chain deposition diseases. Adv Nephrol Necker Hosp 1998;28:355.

169. Morel-Maroger L, Verroust P. Glomerular lesions in dysproteinemias. Kidney Int 1974;5:249.

170. Bangerter AR, Murphy WM. Kappa light chain nephropathy: A pathologic study. Virchows Arch A Pathol Anat Histopathol 1987;410:531.

171. Hill GS, Morel-Maroger L, Mery JP, et al. Renal lesions in multiple myeloma: Their relationship to associated protein abnormalities. Am J Kidney Dis 1983;2:423.

172. Kaplan NG, Kaplan KC. Monoclonal gammopathy, glomerulonephritis and the nephrotic syndrome. Arch Intern Med 1970;125:696.

173. Sanders PW, Herrera GA. Monoclonal immunoglobulin light chain–related renal diseases. Semin Nephrol 1993;13:324.

174. Bruneval P, Foidart JM, Nochy D, et al. Glomerular matrix proteins in nodular glomerulosclerosis in association with light chain deposition disease and diabetes mellitus. Hum Pathol 1985;16:477.

175. Turbat-Herrera EA, Isaac J, Sanders PW, et al. Integrated expression of glomerular extracellular matrix proteins and B1 integrins in monoclonal light chain related renal diseases. Mod Pathol 1997;10:485.

176. Silva FG, Meyrier A, Morel-Maroger L, et al. Proliferative glomerulonephropathy in multiple myeloma. J Pathol 1980;130:229.

177. Lapenas DJ, Drewry SJ, Luke RL III, et al. Crescentic lightchain glomerulopathy: Report of a case. Arch Pathol Lab Med 1983;107:319.

178. Dhar SK, Smith EC, Fresco R. Proliferative glomerulonephritis in monoclonal gammopathy. Nephron 1977;19:288.

179. Meyrier A, Simon P, Mignon F, et al. Rapidly progressive ("crescentic") glomerulonephritis and monoclonal gammopathies. Nephron 1984;38:156.

180. Chang A, Peutz-Kootstra CJ, Richardson CA, et al. Expanding the pathologic spectrum of light chain deposition disease: A rare variant with clinical follow-up of 7 years. Mod Pathol 2005;18:998.

181. Knobler H, Kopolovic J, Kleinman Y, et al. Multiple myeloma presenting as dense deposit disease: Light chain nephropathy. Nephron 1983;34:58.

182. Linder J, Croker BP, Vollmer RT, et al. Systemic kappa light-chain deposition: An ultrastructural and immunohistochemical study. Am J Surg Pathol 1983;7:85.

183. Kirkpatrick CJ, Curry A, Galle J, et al. Systemic kappa light chain deposition and amyloidosis in multiple myeloma: Novel morphological observations. Histopathology 1986;10: 1065.

184. Herrera GA, Shultz JJ, Soong SJ, et al. Growth factors in monoclonal light chain related renal diseases. Hum Pathol 1994;25: 883.

185. Herrera GA, Russell WJ, Isaac J, et al. Glomerulopathic light chain-mesangial interactions modulate in vitro extracellular matrix remodeling and reproduce mesangiopathic findings documented in vivo. Ultrastruct Pathol 1999;23:107.

186. Teng J, Zhang PL, Russell WJ, et al. Insights into mechanisms responsible for mesangial alterations associated with fibrogenic glomerulopathic light chains. Nephron Physiol 2003;94: 28.

187. Russell WJ, Cardelli J, Harris E, et al. Monoclonal light chainmesangial cell interactions: Early signaling events and subsequent pathologic effects. Lab Invest 2001;81:689.

188. Zhu L, Herrera GA, Murphy-Ullrich JE, et al. Pathogenesis of glomerulosclerosis in light chain deposition disease: Role for transforming growth factor. Am J Pathol 1995;147:375.

189. Keeling J, Teng J, Herrera GA. AL-amyloidosis and light chain deposition disease light chains induce divergent phenotypic transformations of human mesangial cells. Lab Invest 2004;84: 1322.

190. Imai K, Kusakabe M, Sakakura T, et al. Susceptibility of tenascin to degradation by matrix metalloproteinases and serine proteinases. FEBS Lett 1994;352:216.

191. Keeling J, Herrera GA. The role of matrix metalloproteinases and tissue inhibitors of metalloproteinases in mesangial remodeling in light chain-related glomerular damage. Kidney Int 2005;68:1590.

192. Teng J, Russell WJ, Gu X, et al. Different types of glomerulopathic light chains interact with mesangial cells using a common receptor but exhibit different intracellular trafficking patterns. Lab Invest 2004;84:440.

193. Decourt C, Touchard G, Preud'homme JL, et al. Complete primary sequences of two lambda immunoglobulin light chains in myelomas with nonamyloid (Randall-type) light chain deposition disease. Am J Pathol 1998;153:313.

194. Preud'homme JL, Aucouturier P, Tonchard G, et al. Monoclonal immunoglobulin deposition disease: A review of immunoglobulin chain alterations. Int J Immunopharmacol 1994;16:425.

195. Sanders PW. Management of paraproteinemic renal disease. Curr Opin Nephrol Hypertens 2005;14:97.

196. Heilman RL, Velosa JA, Holley KE, et al. Long term follow-up and response to chemotherapy in patients with light chain deposition disease. Am J Kidney Dis 1992;20:34.

197. Munshi NC, Barlogie B, Desikan KR, et al. Novel approaches in myeloma therapy. Semin Oncol 1999;26:28.

198. Royer B, Arnulf B, Martinez F, et al. High dose chemotherapy in light chain or light and heavy chain deposition disease. Kidney Int 2004;65:642.

199. Barlogie B, Shaughnessy J, Tricot G, et al. Treatment of multiple myeloma. Blood 2004;103:20.

200. Komatsuda A, Wakui H, Ohtani H, et al. Disappearance of nodular mesangial lesions in a patient with light chain nephropathy after long-term chemotherapy. Am J Kidney Dis 2000;35:E9.

201. Hotta O, Taguma Y. Resolution of nodular glomerular lesions in a patient with light-chain nephropathy. Nephron 2002;91:504.

202. Leung N, Lager DJ, Gertz MA, et al. Long-term outcome of renal transplantation in light-chain deposition disease. Am J Kidney Dis 2004;43:147.

203. Gerlag PG, Koene AK, Berden JHM. Renal transplantation in light chain nephropathy: Case report and review of the literature. Clin Nephrol 1986;25:101.

204. Alchi B, Nishi S, Iguchi S, et al. Recurrent light and heavy chain deposition disease after renal transplantation. Nephrol Dial Transplant 2005;20:1487.

205. Howard AD, Moore J Jr, Tomaszewski MM. Occurrence of multiple myeloma three years after successful renal transplantation. Am J Kidney Dis 1987;10:147.

206. Alpers CE, Marchioro TL, Johnson RJ. Monoclonal immunoglobulin deposition disease in a renal allograft: Probable recurrent disease in a patient without myeloma. Am J Kidney Dis 1989;13:418.

207. Ecder T, Tbakhi A, Braun WE, et al. De novo light-chain deposition disease in a cadaver renal allograft. Am J Kidney Dis 1996;28:461.

208. Fermand JP, Brouet JC. Heavy-chain diseases. Hematol Oncol Clin North Am 1999;13:1281.

209. Moulin B, Deret S, Mariette X, et al. Nodular glomerulosclerosis with deposition of monoclonal immunoglobulin heavy chains lacking $C_H1$. J Am Soc Nephrol 1999;10:519.

210. Liapis H, Papadakis I, Nakopoulou L. Nodular glomerulosclerosis secondary to μ heavy chain deposits. Hum Pathol 2000; 31:122.

211. Yasuda T, Fujita K, Imai H, et al. Gamma-heavy chain deposition disease showing nodular glomerulosclerosis. Clin Nephrol 1995;44:394.

212. Soma J, Sato K, Sakuma T, et al. Immunoglobulin $\gamma_3$-heavy chain deposition disease: Report of a case and relationship with hypocomplementemia. Am J Kidney Dis 2004;43:E2.

213. Cheng IK, Ho SK, Chan DT, et al. Crescentic nodular glomerulosclerosis secondary to truncated immunoglobulin alpha heavy chain deposition. Am J Kidney Dis 1996;28:283.

214. Vedder AC, Weening JJ, Krediet RT. Intracapillary proliferative glomerulonephritis due to heavy chain deposition disease. Nephrol Dial Transplant 2004;19:1302.

215. Nabarra B, Larquet E, Diemert MC, et al. Unusual IgM fibrillar deposits in glomerulonephritis: Ultrastructural and diffraction studies in a case report. Hum Pathol 2003;34:1350.

216. Hendershot L, Bole D, Kohler G, et al. Assembly and

secretion of heavy chains that do not associate posttranslationally with immunoglobulin heavy chain-binding protein. J Cell Biol 1987;104:761.

217. Komatsuda A, Maki N, Wakui H, et al. Development of systemic lambda-light chain amyloidosis in a patient with gamma-heavy chain deposition disease during long-term follow-up. Nephrol Dial Transplant 2005;20:434.

218. Buxbaum J, Gallo G. Nonamyloidotic monoclonal immunoglobulin deposition disease. Light-chain, heavy-chain, and light- and heavy-chain deposition diseases. Hematol Oncol Clin North Am 1999;13:1235.

219. Markowitz GS, Lin J, Valeri AM, et al. Idiopathic nodular glomerulosclerosis is a distinct clinicopathologic entity linked to hypertension and smoking. Hum Pathol 2002;33:826.

220. Kisilevsky R. Amyloid and amyloidoses: Differences, common themes, and practical considerations. Mod Pathol 1991;4:514.

221. Gertz MA, Lacy MQ, Dispenzieri A. Immunoglobulin light chain amyloidosis and the kidney. Kidney Int 2002;61:1.

222. Harada M, Isersky C, Cuatrecasas P, et al. Human amyloid protein: Chemical variability and homogeneity. J Histochem Cytochem 1971;19:1.

223. Aterman K. A historical note on the iodine-sulphuric acid reaction of amyloid. Histochemistry 1976;49:131.

224. Haas LF. Rudolph Ludwig Carl Virchow (1821–1902). J Neurol Neurosurg Psychiatry 1996;61:578.

225. Gertz MA, Lacy MQ, Dispenzieri A. Amyloidosis. Hematol Oncol Clin North Am 1999;13:1211.

226. Ruske W. August Kekule and the development of the theory of chemical structure [in German]. Naturwissenschaften 1965;52:485.

227. Puchtler H, Sweat F. A review of early concepts of amyloid in context with contemporary chemical literature from 1839–1859. J Histochem Cytochem 1966;14:123.

228. WHO-IUS Nomenclature subcommittee: Nomenclature of amyloid and amyloidosis. Bull World Health Organ 1993;71:105.

229. Westermark P, Benson MD, Buxbaum JN, et al. Amyloid: Toward terminology clarification. Amyloid 2005;12:1.

230. Thornton C. Amyloid disease: An autopsy review of the decades 1937–1946 and 1961–1970. Ulster Med J 1983;52:31.

231. Ogg CS, Cameron JS, Williams DG, et al. Presentation and course of primary amyloidosis of the kidney. Clin Nephrol 1981;15:9.

232. Woo P. Amyloidosis in children. Baillieres Clin Rheumatol 1994;8:691.

233. Kyle RA, Gertz MA. Systemic amyloidosis. Crit Rev Oncol Hematol 1990;10:49.

234. Hazenberg BPC. The changing face of AA amyloidosis. In: Grateau G, Kyle RA, Skinner M, eds. Amyloid and Amyloidosis. Boca Raton, FL: CRC Press, 2005:517.

235. Skinner MD. Therapeutic management of AA amyloidosis: From bench to bedside. In: Grateau G, Kyle RA, Skinner M, eds. Amyloid and Amyloidosis. Boca Raton, FL: CRC Press, 2005:524.

236. Tuglular S, Yalcinkaya F, Paydas S, et al. A retrospective analysis for aetiology and clinical findings of 287 secondary amyloidosis cases in Turkey. Nephrol Dial Transplant 2002;17:2003.

237. Röcken C, Shakespeare A. Pathology, diagnosis and pathogenesis of AA amyloidosis. Virchows Arch 2002;440:111.

238. Gertz MA, Kyle RA. Secondary systemic amyloidosis: Response and survival in 64 patients. Medicine 1991;70:246.

239. Connors LH, Prokayeva T, Akar H, et al. Familial amyloidosis: Recent novel and rare mutations in a clinical population. In: Grateau G, Kyle RA, Skinner M, eds. Amyloid and Amyloidosis. Boca Raton, FL: CRC Press, 2005:360.

240. Dikman SH, Churg J, Kahn T. Morphologic and clinical correlates in renal amyloidosis. Hum Pathol 1981;12:160.

241. Elghetany MT, Saleem A, Barr K. The Congo red stain revisited. Ann Clin Lab Sci 1989;19:190.

242. Röcken C, Sletten K. Amyloid in surgical pathology. Virchows Arch 2003;443:3.

243. Carson FL, Kingsley WB. Non-amyloid green birefringence following Congo red staining. Arch Pathol Lab Med 1980;104:333.

244. Koike H, Misu K, Sugiura M, et al. Pathology of early- vs late-onset TTR Met30 familial amyloid polyneuropathy. Neurology 2004;63:129.

245. Puchtler H, Sweat F. Congo red as a stain for fluorescence microscopy of amyloid. J Histochem Cytochem 1965;13:693.

246. Churukian CJ, Schenk EA. Eastwood Congo red method for demonstrating amyloid. J Histotechnol 1988;11:105.

247. Hobbs JR, Morgan AD. Fluorescence microscopy with Thioflavine-T in the diagnosis of amyloid. J Pathol Bacteriol 1963;86:437.

248. Nakamoto Y, Hamanaka S, Akihama T, et al. Renal involvement patterns of amyloid nephropathy: A comparison with diabetic nephropathy. Clin Nephrol 1984;22:188.

249. Benson MD. Ostertag revisited: The inherited systemic amyloidoses without neuropathy. Amyloid 2005;12:75.

250. Hawkins PN. Hereditary systemic amyloidosis with renal involvement. J Nephrol 2003;16:443.

251. Watanabe T, Saniter T. Morphological and clinical features of renal amyloidosis. Virchows Arch 1975;366:125.

252. Moroni G, Banfi G, Maccario M, et al. Extracapillary glomerulonephritis and renal amyloidosis. Am J Kidney Dis 1996;28:695.

253. Triger DR, Joekes AM. Renal amyloidosis: A fourteen-year follow-up. Q J Med 1973;165:15.

254. Westermark P, Sletten K, Eriksson M. Morphologic and chemical variation of the kidney lesions in amyloidosis secondary to rheumatoid arthritis. Lab Invest 1979;41:427.

255. Haagsma EB, Hawkins PN, Benson MD, et al. Familial amyloidotic polyneuropathy with severe renal involvement in association with transthyretin Gly47Glu in Dutch, British and American families. Amyloid 2004;11:44.

256. Lobato L. Portuguese-type amyloidosis (transthyretin amyloidosis, ATTR V30M). J Nephrol 2003;16:438.

257. Pettersson T, Antilla P, Tornroth T. Renal glomerular AL and vascular AA amyloidosis in a patient with ankylosing spondylitis. In: Grateau G, Kyle RA, Skinner M, eds. Amyloid and Amyloidosis. Boca Raton, FL, CRC Press: 2005:284.

258. Rivera F, Gil CM, Gil MT, et al. Vascular renal AA amyloidosis in adult Still's disease. Nephrol Dial Transplant 1997;12:1714.

259. Gallo GR, Feiner HD, Chuba JV, et al. Characterization of tissue amyloid by immunofluorescence microscopy. Clin Immunol Immunopathol 1986;39:479.

260. Kaplan B, Hrncic R, Murphy CL, et al. Microextraction and purification techniques applicable to chemical characterization of amyloid proteins in minute amounts of tissue. Methods Enzymol 1999;309:67.

261. Kaplan B, Martin BM, Livneh A, et al. Biochemical subtyping of amyloid in formalin-fixed tissue samples confirms and supplements immunohistologic data. Am J Clin Pathol 2004;121:794.

262. Murphy CL, Eulitz M, Hrncic R, et al. Chemical typing of amyloid protein contained in formalin-fixed paraffin-embedded biopsy specimens. Am J Clin Pathol 2001;116:135.

263. Picken MM, Thulasiraman V, Picken RN, et al. Tissue detection and characterization of amyloid: Is proteomics the answer? In: Grateau G, Kyle RA, Skinner M, eds. Amyloid and Amyloidosis. Boca Raton, FL: CRC Press, 2005:27.

264. Picken MM. The changing concepts of amyloid. Arch Pathol Lab Med 2001;25:38.

265. Yang GCH, Nieto R, Stachura I et al. Ultrastructural immunohistochemical localization of polyclonal IgG, C3, and amyloid P component on the Congo red negative amyloid-like fibrils of fibrillary glomerulopathy. Am J Pathol 1992;141:409.

266. Gallo G, Picken MM, Buxbaum J, Frangione B. Deposits in monoclonal immunoglobulin deposition disease lack amyloid P component. Mod Pathol 1988;1:453.

267. Picken MM, Pelton K, Frangione B, et al. Primary amyloidosis A: Immunohistochemical and biochemical characterization. Am J Pathol 1987;129:536.

268. Merlini G, Westermark P. The systemic amyloidoses: Clearer understanding of the molecular mechanisms offers hope for more effective therapies. J Intern Med 2004;255:159.

269. Picken MM, Larrondo-Lillo M, Coria F, et al. Distribution of the protease inhibitor alpha 1-antichymotrypsin in cerebral and systemic amyloid. J Neuropathol Exp Neurol 1990;49:41.

270. Eulitz M, Weiss DT, Solomon A. Immunoglobulin heavy-chain-associated amyloidosis. Proc Natl Acad Sci U S A 1990;87:6542.

271. Solomon A, Weiss DT, Murphy C. Primary amyloidosis associated with a novel heavy-chain fragment (AH amyloidosis). Am J Hematol 1994;45:171.

272. Tan SY, Murdoch IE, Sullivan TJ, et al. Primary localized orbital amyloidosis composed of the immunoglobulin gamma heavy chain CH3 domain. Clin Sci (Lond) 1994;87:487.

273. Mai HL, Sheikh-Hamad D, Herrera GA, et al. Immunoglobulin heavy chain can be amyloidogenic: Morphologic characterization, including immunoelectron microscopy. Am J Surg Pathol 2003;27:541.

274. Yazaki M, Fushimi T, Tokuda T, et al. A patient with severe renal amyloidosis associated with an immunoglobulin γ-heavy chain fragment. Am J Kidney Dis 2004;43:e23.

275. Novak L, Cook WJ, Herrera GA, Sanders PW. AL-amyloidosis is underdiagnosed in renal biopsies. Nephrol Dial Transplant 2004;19:3050.

276. Lachmann HJ, Booth DR, Booth SE, et al. Misdiagnosis of hereditary amyloidosis as AL (primary) amyloidosis. N Engl J Med 2002;346:1786.

277. Bergström J, Murphy CL, Weiss DT, et al. Two different types of amyloid deposits—apolipoprotein A-IV and transthyretin—in a patient with systemic amyloidosis. Lab Invest 2004;84:981.

278. Howell D, Gu X, Herrera GA. Organized deposits and look-alikes. Ultrastruct Pathol 2003;27:295.

279. Iskandar SS, Herrera GA. Glomerulopathies with organized deposits. Semin Diag Pathol 2002;19:116.

280. Jao W, Pirani CL. Renal amyloidosis: Electron microscopic observations. Acta Pathol Microbiol Scand [A] 1972;233:217.

281. Veeramachaneni R, Gu X, Herrera GA. Atypical amyloidosis: Diagnostic challenges and the role of immunoelectron microscopy in diagnosis. Ultrastruct Pathol 2004;28:75.

282. Gejyo F, Odani S, Yamada T, et al. Beta 2-microglobulin: A new form of amyloid protein associated with chronic hemodialysis. Kidney Int 1986;30:385.

283. Gorevic PD, Casey TT, Stone WJ, et al. Beta-2 microglobulin is an amyloidogenic protein in man. J Clin Invest 1985;76:2425.

284. Nishi S, Ogino S, Maruyama Y, et al. Electron-microscopic and immunohistochemical study of beta-2-microglobulin-related amyloidosis. Nephron 1990;56:357.

285. Adams W. Mollitis ossium. Trans Pathol Soc London 1872;23:186.

286. Jochmann G, Schumm O. Zur kenntniss des myeloms und der sogenannten Kahler'schen Krankheit (multiple myeloma, einhergehend mit Bence-Jones'scher albumosurie. Ztschr Klin Med 1902;14:445.

287. Glaus A. Ueber multiples myelozytom mit eigenartigen, zum teil kristallahnlichen zelleinlagerungen, kombiniert mit elastolyse und ausgedehneter amyloidose und verkalkung [Basel]. Virchows Arch 1916–1917;223:301.

288. Bock HE. 80th anniversary of Prof. Dr. Hans Hermann Bennhold on Sept. 11, 1973 [in German]. Med Welt 1973;24:1341.

289. Kallee E. The 100th birthday of Hans Hermann Bennhold [in German]. Dtsch Med Wochenschr 1993;118:1336.

290. Reznik M. Paul Divry. The discovery of cerebral amyloidosis [in French]. Acta Neurol Belg 1989;89:168.

291. Magnus-Levy A. Bence-Jones-Eiweiss und Amyloid. Zirschr Klin Med 1931;116:510.

292. Sikl H. A case of diffuse plasmacytosis with deposition of protein crystals in the kidneys. J Pathol Bacteriol 1949;61:149.

293. Cohen AS, Calkins E. Electron microscopic observations on a fibrous component in amyloid of diverse origins. Nature 1959;183:1202.

294. Osserman EF. Amyloidosis. Tissue proteinosis: Gammaloidosis. Ann Intern Med 1961;55:1033.

295. Eanes ED, Glenner GG. X-ray diffraction studies on amyloid filaments. J Histochem Cytochem 1968;16:673.

296. Glenner GG, Harbaugh J, Ohma JI, et al. An amyloid protein: The amino-terminal variable fragment of an immunoglobulin light chain. Biochem Biophys Res Commun 1970;41:1287.

297. Levin M, Franklin EC, Frangione B, et al. The amino acid sequence of a major nonimmunoglobulin component of some amyloid fibrils. J Clin Invest 1972;51:2773.

298. Shirahama T, Cohen AS. An analysis of the close relationship of lysosomes to early deposits of amyloid: Ultrastructural evidence in experimental mouse amyloidosis. Am J Pathol 1973;73:97.

299. Shirahama T, Cohen AS. Intralysosomal formation of amyloid fibrils. Am J Pathol 1975;81:101.

300. Linke RP, Zucker-Franklin D, Franklin EC. Morphologic, chemical and immunologic studies of amyloid-like fibrils formed from Bence Jones proteins proteolysis. J Immunol 1973;111:10.

301. Epstein WV, Tan M, Wood IS. Formation of "amyloid" fibrils in vitro by action of human kidney lysosomal enzymes on Bence Jones proteins. J Lab Clin Med 1974;84:107.

302. Tagouri YM, Sanders PW, Picken MM, et al. In vitro AL-amyloid formation by rat and human mesangial cells. Lab Invest 1996;74:290.

303. Herrera GA, Welbourne TC, Russell WJ. Isolated perfused rat kidney: A new model to evaluate light chain nephrotoxicity [Abstract]. Lab Invest 2001;81:188A, Mod Pathol 2001;14:188A.

304. Comenzo RL, Zhang Y, Martinez C, et al. The tropism of organ involvement in primary systemic amyloidosis: Contributions of IgVL germline gene use and clonal plasma cell burden. Blood 2004;98:714.

305. von Gise HV, Christ H, Bohle A. Early glomerular lesions in amyloidosis. Virchows Arch 1981;390:259.

306. Isaac J, Kerby JD, Russell WJ, et al. In vitro modulation of AL-amyloid formation by human mesangial cells exposed to amyloidogenic light chains. Amyloid 1998;5:238.

307. Harada M, Isersky C, Cuatrecasas P, et al. Human amyloid protein: Chemical variability and homogeneity. J Histochem Cytochem 1971;19:1.

308. Bellotti V, Merlini G. Current concepts on the pathogenesis of systemic amyloidosis. Nephrol Dial Transplant 1996;11:53.

309. Lachmann HJ, Goodman HJB, Gallimore J, et al. Characteristics and clinical outcome of 340 patients with systemic AA amyloidosis. In: Grateau G, Kyle RA, Skinner M, eds. Amyloid and Amyloidosis. Boca Raton, FL: CRC Press, 2005:173.

310. Neugarten J, Gallo GR, Buxbaum J, et al. Amyloidosis in subcutaneous heroin abusers ("skin poppers' amyloidosis"). Am J Med 1986;81:635.

311. Buxbaum JN. The systemic amyloidoses. Curr Opin Rheumatol 2004;16:67.

312. Joss N, McLaughlin K, Simpson K, et al. Presentation, survival and prognostic markers in AA amyloidosis. Q J Med 2000;93:535.

313. Hazenberg BP, van Gameren II, Bijzet J, et al. Diagnostic and therapeutic approach of systemic amyloidosis. Neth J Med 2004;62:121.

314. Benditt EP, Hoffman JS, Eriksen N, et al. SAA, an apoprotein of HDL: Its structure and function. Ann N Y Acad Sci 1982;389:183.

315. Husby G, Marhung, Dowton B. Serum amyloid A (SAA): Biochemistry, genetics, and the pathogenesis of AA amyloidosis. Int J Exp Invest 1994;1:119.

316. Uhlar CM, Whitehead AS. Serum amyloid A: The major vertebrate acute phase reactant. Eur J Biochem 1999;265:501.

317. Sohar E, Gafni J, Pras M, et al. Familial Mediterranean fever: A survey of 470 cases and review of the literature. Am J Med 1967;43:227.

318. Bakkaloglu A. Familial Mediterranean fever. Pediatr Nephrol 2003;18:853.

319. McDermott MF, Aksentijevich I. The autoinflammatory syndromes. Curr Opin Allergy Clin Immunol 2002;2:511.

320. Stjernberg-Salmela S, Ranki A, Karenko L, et al. The genetic background of tumour necrosis factor receptor-associated periodic syndrome and other systemic autoinflammatory disorders. Scand J Rheumatol 2004;33:133.

321. Touitou I, Lesage S, McDermott M, et al. Infevers: An evolving mutation database for auto-inflammatory syndromes. Hum Mutat 2004;24:194.

322. Padeh S. Periodic fever syndromes. Pediatr Clin North Am 2005;52:577.

323. Merlini G. Uncommon conditions underlying AA amyloidosis. In: Grateau G, Kyle RA, Skinner M, eds. Amyloid and Amyloidosis. Boca Raton, FL: CRC Press, 2005:521.

324. Berglund K, Thysell H, Keller C. Results, principles and pitfalls in the management of renal AA amyloidosis: A 10–21 year follow-up of 16 patients with rheumatic disease treated with alkylating cytostatics. J Rheumatol 1993;20:2051.

325. Chevrel G, Jenvrin C, McGregor B, et al. Renal type AA amyloidosis associated with rheumatoid arthritis: A cohort study showing improved survival on treatment with pulse cyclophosphamide. Rheumatology 2001;40:821.

326. Anderson CJ, Gregory MC, Groggel GC, et al. Amyloidosis and Reiter's syndrome: Report of a case and review of the literature. Am J Kidney Dis 1989;14:319.

327. Levasseur R, Le Goff C, Richer C, et al. AA amyloidosis complicating sarcoidosis. Rev Med Interne 1999;20:168.

328. Tan AU Jr, Cohen, AH, Levine, BS. Renal amyloidosis in a drug abuser. J Am Soc Nephrol 1995;5:1653.

329. Gardyn J, Schwartz A, Gal R, et al. Waldenström's macroglobulinemia associated with AA amyloidosis. Int J Hematol 2001;74:76.

330. Knutar O, Pettersson T, Tornroth T, et al. AA amyloidosis without definable underlying disease. In: Bely M, Apathy A, eds. Amyloid and Amyloidosis. Hungary, 2001:168

331. Hiki Y, Horii A, Kokubo T, et al. A case of rheumatoid arthritis with renal tubular amyloidosis. Nephron 1994;68:394.

332. Hazenberg BPC, van Rijswijk MH. Where has secondary amyloid gone? Ann Rheum Dis 2000;59:577.

333. Boers M, Croonen AM, Dijkmans BAC. Renal findings in rheumatoid arthritis: Clinical aspects of 132 necropsies. Ann Rheum Dis 1987;46:658.

334. Nakano M, Ueno M, Nishi S, et al. Analysis of renal pathology and drug history in 158 Japanese patients with rheumatoid arthritis. Clin Nephrol 1998;50:154.

335. Kobayashi H, Tada S, Fuchigami T, et al. Secondary amyloidosis in patients with rheumatoid arthritis: Diagnostic and prognostic value of gastroduodenal biopsy. Br J Rheumatol 1996;35:44.

336. Kuroda T, Tanabe N, Sakatsume M, et al. Comparison of gastroduodenal, renal and abdominal fat biopsies for diagnosing amyloidosis in rheumatoid arthritis. Clin Rheumatol 2002;21:123.

337. Reyners AK, Hazenberg BP, Reitsma WD, et al. Heart rate variability as a predictor of mortality in patients with AA and AL amyloidosis. Eur Heart J 2002;23:157.

338. Pras E, Aksentijevich I, Gruberg L, et al. Mapping of a gene causing familial Mediterranean fever to the short arm of chromosome 16. N Engl J Med 1992;326:1509.

339. The International FMF Consortium (1997). Ancient missense mutations in a new member of the RoRet gene family are likely to cause familial Mediterranean fever. Cell 1997;90:797.

340. Touitou I, Notarnicola C, Grandemange S. Identifying mutations in autoinflammatory diseases: Towards novel genetic tests and therapies? Am J Pharmacogenomics 2004;4:109.

341. Dode C, Cuisset L, Delpech M, et al. TNFRSF1A-associated periodic syndrome (TRAPS), Muckle-Wells syndrome (MWS) and renal amyloidosis. J Nephrology 2003;16:435.

342. Bakkaloglu A, Duzova A, Ozen S, et al. Influence of serum amyloid A (SAA1) and SAA2 gene polymorphisms on renal amyloidosis, and on SAA/C-reactive protein values in patients with familial Mediterranean fever in the Turkish population. J Rheumatol 2004;31:1139.

343. Zemer D, Livneh A, Pras M, et al. The kidney in familial Mediterranean fever. Contrib Nephrol 1993;102:187.

344. Reuben A, Hirsch M, Berlyne GM. Renal vein thrombosis as the major cause of renal failure in familial Mediterranean fever. Q J Med 1977;182:243.

345. Ben-Chetrit E. Familial Mediterranean fever (FMF) and renal AA amyloidosis: Phenotype–genotype correlation, treatment and prognosis. J Nephrol 2003;16:431.

346. Said R, Hamzeh Y, Said S, et al. Spectrum of renal involvement in familial Mediterranean fever. Kidney Int 1992;41:414.

347. Tekin M, Yalcinkaya F, Tumer N, et al. Familial Mediterranean fever: Renal involvement by diseases other than amyloid. Nephrol Dial Transplant 1999;14:475.

348. Akpolat T, Akpolat I, Karagoz F, et al. Familial Mediterranean fever and glomerulonephritis and review of the literature. Rheumatol Int 2004;24:43.

349. Kluve-Beckerman B, Liepnieks JJ, Wang L, et al. A cell culture system for the study of amyloid pathogenesis: Amyloid formation by peritoneal macrophages cultured with recombinant serum amyloid A. Am J Pathol 1999;155:123.

350. Kluve-Beckerman B, Dwulet FE, Benson MD. Human serum amyloid A. J Clin Invest 1988;82:1670.

351. Booth DR, Booth SE, Gillmore JD, et al. SAA1 alleles as risk factors in reactive systemic AA amyloidosis. Amyloid 1998;5:262.

352. Moriguchi M, Terai C, Koseki Y, et al. Influence of genotypes at SAA1 and SAA2 loci on the development and the length of latent period of secondary AA-amyloidosis in patients with rheumatoid arthritis. Hum Genet 1999;105:360.

353. Yakar L, Kaplan P. The molecular basis of reactive amyloidosis. Semin Arthritis Rheum 1995;24:255.

354. Kisilevsky R. The relation of proteoglycans, serum amyloid P and apo E to amyloidosis: Current status, 2000. Amyloid 2000;7:23.

355. Ancsin JB. Amyloidogenesis: Historical and modern observations point to heparan sulfate proteoglycans as a major culprit. J Protein Folding Disord 2003;10:67.

356. Knecht A, de Beer FC, Pras M. Serum amyloid A protein in familial Mediterranean fever. Ann Intern Med 1985;102:71.

357. Moss J, Shore I, Woodrow D. AA glomerular amyloid. An ultrastructural immunogold study of the colocalization of heparan sulphate proteoglycan and P component with amyloid fibrils together with changes in distribution of type IV collagen and fibronectin. Histopathology 1994;24:427.

358. Kisilevsky R, Szarek WA. Novel glycosaminoglycan precursors as anti-amyloid agents part II. J Mol Neurosci 2002;19:45.

359. Snow AD, Castillo GM. Specific proteoglycans as potential causative agents and relevant targets for therapeutic intervention in Alzheimer's disease and other amyloidoses. Amyloid. Int J Exp Clin Invest 1997;4:133.

360. Pepys MB, Herbert J, Hutchinson WL, et al. Targeted pharmacological depletion of serum amyloid P component for treatment of human amyloidosis. Nature 2002;417:254.

361. Lachmann HJ, Hawkins PN. Novel pharmacological strategies in amyloidosis. Nephron Clin Pract 2003;94:c85.

362. Hauk W, Dember LM, Hawkins PN, et al. A prospective analysis of demography, etiology, and clinical findings of AA amyloidosis patients enrolled in the international clinical phase II/III Fibrillex study. In: Grateau G, Kyle RA, Skinner M, eds. Amyloid and Amyloidosis. Boca Raton, FL: CRC Press, 2005:179.

363. Hawkins PN. Serum amyloid P component scintigraphy for diagnosis and monitoring amyloidosis. Curr Opin Nephrol Hypertens 2002;11:649.

364. DeBeer FC, Mallya RK, Faga EA. Serum amyloid A protein concentration in inflammatory diseases and its relationship to the incidence of reactive systemic amyloidosis. Lancet 1982;2:231.

365. Prelli F, Pras M, Frangione B. Degradation and deposition of amyloid AA fibrils are tissue specific. Biochemistry 1987;26:8251.

366. Varga J, Wohlgethan JR. The clinical and biochemical spectrum of hereditary amyloidosis. Semin Arthritis Rheum 1988;18:14.

367. Benson MD. Non-transthyretin hereditary amyloidoses. In: Grateau G, Kyle RA, Skinner M, eds. Amyloid and Amyloidosis. Boca Raton, FL: CRC Press, 2005:309.

368. Bybee A, Kang HG, Ha IS, et al. A novel complex indel mutation in the fibrinogen Aα chain in an Asian child with systemic amyloidosis. Familial Amyloidosis: Recent novel and rare mutations in a clinical population. In: Grateau G, Kyle RA, Skinner M, eds. Amyloid and Amyloidosis. Boca Raton, FL: CRC Press, 2005:315.

369. Stangou AJ, Lachmann HJ, Goodman HJB, et al. Fibrinogen A α-chain amyloidosis: Clinical features and outcome after hepatorenal or solitary kidney transplantation. In: Grateau G, Kyle RA, Skinner M, eds. Amyloid and Amyloidosis. Boca Raton, FL: CRC Press, 2005:312.

370. Benson M, Uemichi T. Transthyretin amyloidosis. Amyloid 1996;3:44.

371. Jacobson DR, Pastore RD, Yaghoubian E, et al. Variant-sequence transthyretin (isoleucine 122) in late onset cardiac amyloidosis in black Americans. N Engl J Med 1997;336:466.

372. Westermark P, Bergström J, Solomon A, et al. Transthyretin-derived senile systemic amyloidosis: Clinico-pathologic and structural considerations. Amyloid 2003;10(suppl 1):48.

373. Picken MM, Leya F, Picken RN. Wild type transthyretin-derived senile systemic amyloidosis with limited proteolytic digestion of the monomer: Clinico-pathologic studies with DNA and amyloid protein characterization. In: Grateau G, Kyle RA, Skinner M, eds. Amyloid and Amyloidosis. Boca Raton, FL: CRC Press, 2005:466.

374. Lobato L, Beirao I, Silva M, et al. Familial ATTR amyloidosis: Microalbuminuria as a predictor of symptomatic disease and clinical nephropathy. Nephrol Dial Transplant 2003;18: 532.

375. Booth DR, Tan SY, Booth SE. et al. Hereditary hepatic and systemic amyloidosis caused by a new deletion/insertion mutation in the apolipoprotein A1 gene. J Clin Invest 1996;97:2714.

376. Murphy CL, Wang S, Weaver K, et al. Renal apolipoprotein A-I amyloidosis (AApo-A-I) associated with a novel mutant Leu64Pro. In: Grateau G, Kyle RA, Skinner M, eds. Amyloid and Amyloidosis. Boca Raton, FL: CRC Press, 2005:363.

377. Hawkins PN, Bybee A, Goodman HJB, et al. Phenotype, genotype and outcome in hereditary ApoAI amyloidosis. In: Grateau G, Kyle RA, Skinner M, eds. Amyloid and Amyloidosis. Boca Raton, FL: CRC Press, 2005:316.

378. Magy N, Liepnieks JJ, Yazaki M, et al. Renal transplantation for apolipoprotein AII amyloidosis. Amyloid 2003;10:224.

379. Valleix S, Drunat S, Philit JB, et al. Hereditary renal amyloidosis caused by a new variant lysozyme W64R in a French family. Kidney Int 2002;61:907.

380. Maury CP. Homozygous familial amyloidosis, Finnish type: Demonstration of glomerular gelsolin-derived amyloid and non-amyloid tubular gelsolin. Clin Nephrol 1993;40:53.

381. Kiuru S. Gelsolin-related familial amyloidosis, Finnish type (FAF), and its variants found worldwide. Amyloid 1998;5:55.

382. Olafsson I, Grubb A. Hereditary cystatin C amyloid angiopathy. Amyloid 2000;7:70.

383. Floege J, Ketteler M. Beta2-microglobulin-derived amyloidosis: An update. Kidney Int Suppl 2001;78:S164.

384. Gejyo F, Narita I. Current clinical and pathogenetic understanding of β₂-m amyloidosis in long term dialysis patients. Nephrology 2003;8:S45.

385. Argiles A, Charnet A, Schmitt-Bernard CF, et al. β2 Microglobulin amyloidosis. In: Grateau G, Kyle RA, Skinner M, eds. Amyloid and Amyloidosis. Boca Raton, FL: CRC Press, 2005:415.

386. Schaffer J, Floege J, Koch KM. Clinical aspects of dialysis-related amyloidosis. Contrib Nephrol 1995;112:90.

387. Choi HS, Heller D, Picken MM, et al. Infarction of intestine with massive amyloid deposition in two patients on long-term hemodialysis. Gastroenterology 1989;96:230.

388. Campistol JM, Argiles A. Dialysis-related amyloidosis: Visceral involvement and protein constituents. Nephrol Dial Transplant 1996;11(suppl 3):142.

389. Takahashi S, Morita T, Koda T, et al. Gastrointestinal involvement of dialysis-related amyloidosis. Clin Nephrol 1988;30:168.

390. Tan S-Y, Baillod R, Brown E, et al. Clinical, radiological and serum amyloid P component scintigraphic features of β2-microglobulin amyloidosis associated with continuous ambulatory peritoneal dialysis. Nephrol Dial Transplant 1999;14:1467.

391. Jadoul M, Garbar C, Vanholder R, et al. Prevalence of histological β2-microglobulin amyloidosis in CAPD patients compared with hemodialysis patients. Kidney Int 1998;54:956.

392. Jadoul M, Garbar C, Noel H, et al. Histologic prevalence of beta2-microglobulin amyloidosis in hemodialysis: A prospective post-mortem study. Kidney Int 1997;51:1928.

393. Picken MM, Shen S. Beta2-microglobulin amyloidosis: Illustrative cases. Ultrastruct Pathol 1994;18:135.

394. Miyata T, Ueda Y, Saito A, et al. "Carbonyl stress" and dialysis-related amyloidosis. Nephrol Dial Transplant 2000;15(suppl 1):25.

395. Schwalbe S, Holzhauer M, Schaeffer J, et al. Beta 2-microglobulin associated amyloidosis: A vanishing complication of long-term dialysis? Kidney Int 1997;52:1077.

396. Floege J, Schaffer J, Koch KM. Scintigraphic methods to detect beta2-microglobulin associated amyloidosis (Abeta2-microglobulin amyloidosis). Nephrol Dial Transplant 2001;16 (suppl 4):12.

397. Biewend ML, Menke DM, Calamia KT. The spectrum of localized amyloidosis: A case series of twenty patients. In: Grateau G, Kyle RA, Skinner M, eds. Amyloid and Amyloidosis. Boca Raton, FL: CRC Press, 2005:421.

398. Paccalin M, Rubi M, Hachulla E, et al. Localized amyloidosis: About 36 cases. In: Grateau G, Kyle RA, Skinner M, eds. Amyloid and Amyloidosis. Boca Raton, FL: CRC Press, 2005:424.

399. Fushimi T, Takei Y, Touma T, et al. Bilateral localized amyloidosis of the ureters: Clinicopathology and therapeutic approaches in two cases. Amyloid 2004;11:260.

400. Tirzman O, Wahner-Roedler DL, Malek RS, et al. Primary localized amyloidosis of the urinary bladder: A case series of 31 patients. Mayo Clin Proc 2000;75:1264.

401. Boorjian S, Choi BB, Loo MH, et al. A rare case of painless gross hematuria: Primary localized AA-type amyloidosis of the urinary bladder. Urology 2002;59:137.

402. Setoguchi M, Hoshii Y, Kawano H, et al. Analysis of plasma cell clonality in localized AL amyloidosis. Amyloid 2000;7:41.

403. Goldsmith DJA, Sandooran D, Short CD, et al. Twenty-one years survival with systemic AL-amyloidosis. Am J Kidney Dis 1996;278.

404. Tanaka F, Migita K, Honda S, et al. Clinical outcome and survival of secondary (AA) amyloidosis. Clin Exp Rheumatol 2003;21:343.

405. Sanchorawala V, Wright DG, Seldin DC, et al. An overview of the use of high-dose melphalan with autologous stem cell transplantation for the treatment of AL-amyloidosis. Bone Marrow Transplant 2001;28:637.

406. Skinner M, Sanchorawala V, Seldin DC, et al. High-dose melphalan and autologous stem-cell transplantation in patients with AL-amyloidosis: An 8-year study. Ann Intern Med 2004;140:85.

407. Gertz MA, Kyle RA, O'Fallon WM. Dialysis support of patients with primary amyloidosis: A study of 211 patients. Arch Intern Med 1992;152:2245.

408. Seldin DC, Anderson JJ, Sanchorawala V, et al. Improvement in quality of life of patients with AL amyloidosis treated with high-dose melphalan and autologous stem cell transplantation. Blood 2004;104:1888.

409. Sanchorawala V, Wright DG, Seldin DC, et al. High-dose intravenous melphalan and autologous stem cell transplantation as initial therapy or following two cycles of oral chemotherapy for the treatment of AL amyloidosis: Results of a prospective randomized trial. Bone Marrow Transplant 2004;33:381.

410. Skinner M, Sanchorawala V, Seldin DC, et al. High-dose melphalan and autologous stem-cell transplantation in patients with AL amyloidosis: An 8-year study. Ann Intern Med 2004;140:85.

411. Dember LM, Sanchorawala V, Seldin DC, et al. Effect of dose-intensive intravenous melphalan and autologous blood stem-cell transplantation on AL-amyloidosis-associated renal disease. Ann Intern Med 2001;134:746.

412. Comenzo RL, Vosburgh E, Falk RH, et al. Dose-intensive melphalan with blood-cell support for the treatment of AL (amyloid light chain) amyloidosis: Survival and responses in 25 patients. Blood 1998;10:3662.

413. Livneh A, Zemer D, Langevitz P, et al. Colchicine treatment of AA amyloidosis of familial Mediterranean fever: An analysis of factors affecting outcome. Arthritis Rheum 1994;37:1804.

414. Hawkins PN, Lachmann HJ, Aganna E, et al. Spectrum of clinical features in Muckle-Wells syndrome and response to anakinra. Arthritis Rheum 2004;50:607.

415. Hawkins PN, Lachmann HJ, McDermott MF. Interleukin-1-receptor antagonist in the Muckle-Wells syndrome. N Engl J Med 2003;348:2583.

416. Hoffman HM, Rosengren S, Boyle DL, et al. Prevention of cold-associated acute inflammation in familial cold autoinflammatory syndrome by interleukin-1 receptor antagonist. Lancet 2004;364:1779.

417. Adamski-Werner SL, Palaninathan SK, Sacchettini JC, et al. Diflunisal analogues stabilize the native state of transthyretin. Potent inhibition of amyloidogenesis. J Med Chem 2004;47:355.

418. Nowak G, Suhr OB, Wikstrom L, et al. The long-term impact of liver transplantation on kidney function in familial amyloidotic polyneuropathy patients. Transpl Int 2005;18:111.

419. Stangou AJ, Hawkins PN. Liver transplantation in transthyretin-related familial amyloid polyneuropathy. Curr Opin Neurol 2004;17:615.

420. Gillmore JD, Stangou AJ, Tennent GA, et al. Clinical and biochemical outcome of hepatorenal transplantation for hereditary systemic amyloidosis associated with apolipoprotein AI Gly26Arg. Transplantation 2001;71:986.

421. Lobato I, Ventura A, Beirao I, et al. End-stage renal disease in familial amyloidosis ATTR Val30Met: A definitive indication to combined liver-kidney transplantation. Transplant Proc 2003;35:1116.

422. Hartmann A, Holdaas H, Fauchaud P, et al. Fifteen years experience with renal transplantation in systemic amyloidosis. Transplant Int 1992;5:15.

423. Pasternak A, Ahonen H, Kulback B, et al. Renal transplantation in 45 patients with amyloidosis. Transplant 1986;42:598.

424. Tan SY, Pepys MB, Hawkins PN. Treatment of amyloidosis. Am J Kidney Dis 1995;26:267.

425. Harrison KL, Alpers CE, Davis CL. De-novo amyloidosis in a renal allograft: A case report and review of the literature. Am J Kidney Dis 1993;22:468.

426. Le QC, Wood TC, Alpers CE. De-novo AL amyloid in a renal allograft. Am J Nephrol 1998;18:67.

427. Waldenström J. Incipient myelomatosis or "essential" hyperglobulinemia with fibrinogenopenia: A new syndrome? Acta Med Scand 1944;117:216.

428. Dutcher TF, Fahey JL. The histopathology of the macroglobulinemia of Waldenström. J Natl Cancer Inst 1959;22:887.

429. Lamm ME. Macroglobulinemia: report of two cases. Am J Clin Pathol 1961;35:53.

430. Forget BG, Squires JW, Sheldon H. Waldenström's macroglobulinemia with generalized amyloidosis. Arch Intern Med 1966;118:363.

431. Argani I, Kipkie GF. Macroglobulinemic nephropathy. Acute renal failure in macroglobulinemia of Waldenström. Am J Med 1964;36:151.

432. Morel-Maroger L, Basch A, Danon F, et al. Pathology of the kidney in Waldenström's macroglobulinemia: Study of sixteen cases. N Engl J Med 1970;283:123.

433. Herrinton LJ, Weiss NS. Incidence of Waldenström's macroglobulinemia. Blood 1993;82:3148.

434. Kyle RA, Garton JP. The spectrum of IgM monoclonal gammopathy in 430 cases. Mayo Clin Proc 1987;62:719.

435. Montoto S, Rozman M, Rosinol L, et al. Malignant transformation in IgM monoclonal gammopathy of undetermined significance. Semin Oncol 2003;30:178.

436. Owen RG, Treon SP, Al-Katib A, et al. Clinicopathological definition of Waldenström's macroglobulinemia: Consensus panel recommendations from the Second International Workshop on Waldenström's Macroglobulinemia. Semin Oncol 2003;30:110.

437. Treon SP, Dimopoulos M, Kyle RA. Defining Waldenström's macroglobulinemia. Semin Oncol 2003;30:107.

438. Dimopoulos MA, Alexanian R. Waldenström's macroglobulinemia. Blood 1994;83:1452.

439. Crawford J, Cox EB, Cohen HJ. Evaluation of hyperviscosity in monoclonal gammopathies. Am J Med 1985;79:13.

440. Moulopoulos LA, Dimopoulos MA, Varma DG, et al. Waldenström macroglobulinemia: MR imaging of the spine and CT of the abdomen and pelvis. Radiology 1993;188:669.

441. Fudenberg HH, Virella G. Multiple myeloma and Waldenström macroglobulinemia: Unusual presentations. Semin Hematol 1980;17:63.

442. Veltman GA, van Veen S, Kluin-Nelemans JC, et al. Renal disease in Waldenström's macroglobulinaemia. Nephrol Dial Transplant 1997;12:1256.

443. Krajny M, Pruzanski W. Waldenstrom's macroglobulinemia: Review of 45 cases. Can Med Assoc J 1976;114:899.

444. Soetekouw R, Bruijn JA, Hogewind BL, et al. A 66-year-old woman with nephrotic syndrome and an IgM monoclonal gammopathy. Ann Hematol 1998;76:227.

445. Grossman ME, Bia MJ, Goldwein MI, et al. Giant kidneys in Waldenström's macroglobulinemia. Arch Intern Med 1977;137:1613.

446. Berkel J, Granillo-Bodansky C, v d Borne AE. Acute renal failure associated with a malignant lymphoproliferative disorder with monoclonal light chain immunoglobulin production: Report of a case. Scand J Haematol 1978;20:377.

447. Gertz MA, Kyle RA, Noel P. Primary systemic amyloidosis: A rare complication of immunoglobulin M monoclonal gammopathies and Waldenström's macroglobulinemia. J Clin Oncol 1993;11:914.

448. Muso E, Tamura I, Yashiro M, et al. Waldenström's macroglobulinemia associated with amyloidosis and membranous nephropathy. Jpn J Nephrol 1993;35:1265.

449. Isaac J, Herrera GA. Cast nephropathy in a case of Waldenström's macroglobulinemia. Nephron 2002;91:512.

450. Brouet JC, Clauvel JP, Danon F, et al. Biologic and clinical significance of cryoglobulins: A report of 86 cases. Am J Med 1974;57:775.

451. Keshgegian AA, Sevin P. Waldenström macroglobulinemia associated with mixed cryoglobulins: Report of a case with partial precipitation in vitro at 37 degrees C. Arch Pathol Lab Med 1979;103:270.

452. Hory B, Saunier F, Wolff R, et al. Waldenström macroglobulinemia and nephrotic syndrome with minimal change lesion. Nephron 1987;45:68.

453. Martelo OJ, Schultz DR, Pardo V, et al. Immunologically-mediated renal disease in Waldenström's macroglobulinemia. Am J Med 1975;58:567.

454. Gallo GR, Feiner HD, Buxbaum JN. The kidney in lymphoplasmacytic disorders. Pathol Ann 1982;17:291.

455. Moore DF, Moulopoulos LA, Dimopoulos MA. Waldenström's macroglobulinemia presenting as renal or perirenal mass: Clinical and radiographic features. Leuk Lymphoma 1995;14:331.

456. Facon T, Brouillard M, Duhamel A, et al. Prognostic factors in Waldenström's macroglobulinemia: A report of 167 cases. J Clin Oncol 1993;11:1553.

457. Tsuji M, Ochiai S, Taka T, et al. Nonamyloidotic nephrotic syndrome in Waldenström's macroglobulinemia. Nephron 1990;54:176.

458. Debre P, Zittoun R, Cadiou M, et al. Waldenström's macroglobulinemia: Developmental and prognostic study. Semin Hop 1975;51:2921.

459. Bradley JR, Thiru S, Bajallan N, et al. Renal transplantation in Waldenström macroglobulinemia. Nephrol Dial Transplant 1988;3:214.

460. Grey HM, Kohler PF. Cryoimmunoglobulins. Semin Hematol 1973;10:87.

461. Wintrobe MM, Buell MV. Hyperproteinemia associated with multiple myeloma: With report of a case in which an extraordinary hyperproteinemia was associated with thrombosis of the retinal veins and symptoms suggesting Raynaud's disease. Bull Johns Hopkins Hosp 1933;52:156.

462. Lerner AB, Watson CJ. Studies of cryoglobulins: Unusual purpura associated with the presence of a high concentration of cryoglobulin (cold precipitable serum globulin). Am J Med Sci 1947;214:410.

463. Meltzer M, Franklin EC. Cryoglobulinemia: A study of twenty-nine patients. I. IgG and IgM cryoglobulins and factors affecting cryoprecipitability. Am J Med 1966;40:828.

464. Meltzer M, Franklin EC, Elias K, et al. Cryoglobulinemia: A clinical and laboratory study. II. Cryoglobulins with rheumatoid factor activity. Am J Med 1966;40:837.

465. D'Amico G, Colasanti G, Ferrario F, et al. Renal involvement in essential mixed cryoglobulinemia. Kidney Int 1989;35:1004.

466. Schifferli JA, French LE, Tissot JD. Hepatitis C virus infection, cryoglobulinemia, and glomerulonephritis. Adv Nephrol Necker Hosp 1995;24:107.

467. Cordonnier D, Vialtel P, Renversez JC, et al. Renal diseases in 18 patients with mixed type II IgM—IgG cryoglobulinemia:

Monoclonal lymphoid infiltration (2 cases) and membranoproliferative glomerulonephritis (14 cases). Adv Nephrol Necker Hosp 1983;12:177.

468. Karras A, Noel LH, Droz D, et al. Renal involvement in monoclonal (type I) cryoglobulinemia: Two cases associated with IgG3 kappa cryoglobulin. Am J Kidney Dis 2002;40:1091.

469. Druet P, Letonturier P, Contet A, et al. Cryoglobulinaemia in human renal diseases: A study of seventy-six cases. Clin Exp Immunol 1973;15:483.

470. Gorevic PD, Kassab HJ, Levo Y, et al. Mixed cryoglobulinemia: Clinical aspects and long-term follow-up of 40 patients. Am J Med 1980;69:287.

471. Monti G, Galli M, Invernizzi F, et al. Cryoglobulinaemias: A multi-centre study of the early clinical and laboratory manifestations of primary and secondary disease. GISC. Italian Group for the Study of Cryoglobulinaemias. Q J Med 1995;88:115.

472. Bengtsson U, Larsson O, Lindstedt G, et al. Monoclonal IgG cryoglobulinemia with secondary development of glomerulonephritis and nephrotic syndrome. Q J Med 1975;44:491.

473. Florin-Christensen A, Roux ME, Arana RM. Cryoglobulins in acute and chronic liver diseases. Clin Exp Immunol 1974;16:599.

474. Agnello V, Chung RT, Kaplan LM. A role for hepatitis C virus infection in type II cryoglobulinemia. N Engl J Med 1992;327:1490.

475. Hurwitz D, Quismorio FP, Friou GJ. Cryoglobulinaemia in patients with infectious endocarditis. Clin Exp Immunol 1975;19:131.

476. Weisman M, Zvaifler N. Cryoglobulins in rheumatoid arthritis. Rheumatology 1975;6:60.

477. Ferri C, La Civita L, Longombardo G, et al. Mixed cryoglobulinaemia: A cross-road between autoimmune and lymphoproliferative disorders. Lupus 1998;7:275.

478. Burstein DM, Rodby RA. Membranoproliferative glomerulonephritis associated with hepatitis C virus infection. J Am Soc Nephrol 1993;4:1288.

479. D'Amico G. Renal involvement in hepatitis C infection: Cryoglobulinemic glomerulonephritis. Kidney Int 1998;54:650.

480. Tarantino A, Campise M, Banfi G, et al. Long-term predictors of survival in essential mixed cryoglobulinemic glomerulonephritis. Kidney Int 1995;47:618.

481. Linscott WD, Kane JP. The complement system in cryoglobulinaemia: Interaction with immunoglobulins and lipoproteins. Clin Exp Immunol 1975;21:510.

482. Adam C, Morel-Maroger L, Richet G. Cryoglobulins in glomerulonephritis not related to systemic disease. Kidney Int 1973;3:334.

483. Grey H, Kohler P. Cryoimmunoglobulins. Sem Hematol 1973;2:87.

484. Faraggiana T, Parolini C, Previato G, et al. Light and electron microscopic findings in five cases of cryoglobulinemic glomerulonephritis. Virchows Arch 1979;384:29.

485. Ferrario F, Colasanti G, Barbiano Di Belgioioso G, et al. Histological and immunohistological features in essential mixed cryoglobulinemia glomerulonephritis. In: Ponticelli C, Minetti L, D'Amico G, eds. Antiglobulins, Cryoglobulins and Glomerulonephritis. Boston: Martinus Nijhoff, 1986:193.

486. D'Amico G, Fornasieri A. Cryoglobulinemic glomerulonephritis: A membranoproliferative glomerulonephritis induced by hepatitis C virus. Am J Kidney Dis 1995;25:361.

487. Cordonnier D, Martin H, Groslambert P, et al. Mixed IgG-IgM cryoglobulinemia with glomerulonephritis: Immunochemical, fluorescent and ultrastructural study of kidney and in vitro cryoprecipitate. Am J Med 1975;59:867.

488. Porush JG, Grishman E, Alter AA, et al. Paraproteinemia and cryoglobulinemia associated with atypical glomerulonephritis and the nephrotic syndrome. Am J Med 1969;47:957.

489. Pais B, Panades MJ, Ramos J, et al. Glomerular involvement in type I monoclonal cryoglobulinaemia. Nephrol Dial Transplant 1995;10:130.

490. Feiner H, Gallo G. Ultrastructure in glomerulonephritis associated with cryoglobulinemia: A report of six cases and review of the literature. Am J Pathol 1977;88:145.

491. Bartlow BG, Oyama JH, Ing TS, et al. Glomerular ultrastructural abnormalities in a patient with mixed IgG–IgM essential cryoglobulinemic glomerulonephritis. Nephron 1975;14:309.

492. Mazzucco G, Monga G, Casanova S, et al. Cell interposition in glomerular capillary walls in cryoglobulinemic glomerulonephritis (CRYGN): Ultrastructural investigation of 23 cases. Ultrastruct Pathol 1986;10:355.

493. Monga G, Mazzuco G, Casanova S, et al. Ultrastructural glomerular findings in cryoglobulinemic glomerulonephritis. Appl Pathol 1987;5:108.

494. Verroust P, Mery JP, Morel-Maroger L, et al. Glomerular lesions in monoclonal gammopathies and mixed essential cryoglobulinemias IgG–IgM. Adv Nephrol Necker Hosp 1971;1:161.

495. Ogihara T, Saruta T, Saito I, et al. Finger print deposits of the kidney in pure monoclonal IgG kappa cryoglobulinemia. Clin Nephrol 1979;12:186.

496. Ben-Bassat M, Boner G, Rosenfeld J, et al. The clinicopathologic features of cryoglobulinemic nephropathy. Am J Clin Pathol 1983;79:147.

497. Valbonesi M, Montani F, Mosconi L, et al. Plasmapheresis and cytotoxic drugs for mixed cryoglobulinemia. Haematologia (Budap) 1984;17:341.

498. Dussol B, Tsimaratos M, Lerda D, et al. Viral hepatitis C and membranoproliferative glomerulonephritis in a renal transplant patient [in French]. Nephrologie 1995;16:223.

499. Herrera GA. The value of electron microscopy in the diagnosis and clinical management of lupus nephritis. Ultrastruct Pathol 1999;23:63.

# Glomerular Diseases With Organized Deposits

20

*Melvin M. Schwartz*

Organized glomerular deposits, seen by electron microscopy, are among the most dramatic findings in renal pathology. Most frequently, the deposits are organized into elongated, nonbranching fibrils or larger tubules. They also take the form of short curved microtubules (1), spheres (2), crystals (3), "fingerprints" (4), or fibrils with lateral spines (barbed wire) (5). The deposits are usually extracellular in the mesangium, the basal laminae, and the capillary lumens. Rarely, the glomerular cells contain crystals. The pathologist must distinguish organized deposits from the small and intermediate-sized fibrils that are normal features of the extracellular matrix in the immature and adult kidney (6) and the cytoskeletal microtubules and microfilaments of glomerular cells. Glomerular organized deposits occur in various diseases of known and unknown pathogenesis (Table 20.1), and morphologically identical deposits may occur in different diseases.

| TABLE 20.1 |
| --- |
| **CLASSIFICATION OF THE FIBRILLARY GLOMERULOPATHIES** |

Amyloid (Congo red–positive)
  AL amyloid
    Primary
    Multiple myeloma
  AA amyloid
    Chronic inflammation
    Granulomatous infections
    Tumors
  Other types of amyloid

Nonamyloid (Congo red–negative)
  Immunoglobulin-derived fibrils
    Cryoglobulinemia
      Mixed essential cryoglobulinemia
      Multiple myeloma
      Chronic lymphocytic leukemia
    Monoclonal gammopathies
      "Benign"
      Multiple myeloma
    Light chain deposition disease
    Chronic lymphocytic leukemia
    Systemic lupus erythematosus
    Immunotactoid glomerulopathy

  Non–immunoglobulin-derived fibrils
    Nail-patella syndrome
    Collagenofibrotic glomerulopathy
    Diabetes mellitus
    Fibrin
    Fibronectin glomerulopathy
    Others

From Korbet SM, Schwartz MM, Lewis EJ. The fibrillary glomerulopathies. Am J Kidney Dis 1994;23:751.

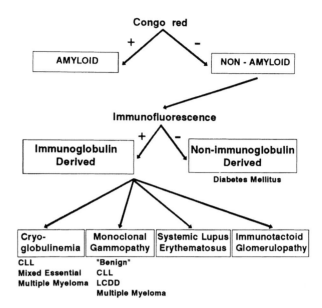

**Figure 20.1** Algorithm for the evaluation of a patient with organized glomerular electron-dense deposits. CLL, chronic lymphocytic leukemia; LCDD, light chain deposition disease. (From Korbet SM, Schwartz MM, Lewis EJ. The fibrillary glomerulopathies. Am J Kidney Dis 1994;23:751.)

clinically useful diagnostic approach than either strictly clinical or morphologic classification. The differential diagnosis of organized glomerular electron-dense deposits may be represented as a diagnostic algorithm based on the Congo red stain and the immunochemical composition of the deposits (Fig. 20.1), and this is the approach that will be followed in this chapter.

## DIAGNOSTIC ALGORITHM FOR ORGANIZED GLOMERULAR DEPOSITS

Determining whether patients with organized glomerular deposits have an underlying disease is a primary concern because a specific diagnosis often has therapeutic and prognostic implications. Although the pathologist working without a complete history and laboratory examination may be tempted to render a descriptive diagnosis based solely on the morphology of the organized deposits, this is inadvisable because despite their striking appearance, the morphology of the deposits is usually not pathognomonic. Also, the renal presentations of diseases with organized glomerular deposits are often similar with proteinuria, the nephrotic syndrome, and variable renal insufficiency, and complete clinical, hematologic, and laboratory studies may be necessary to distinguish among them. Therefore, the composition of the deposits, defined by immunohistologic and histochemical analysis, provides a more

## CONGO RED–POSITIVE ORGANIZED DEPOSITS

### Amyloidosis

The Congo red stain dichotomizes organized deposits into those that are Congo red–positive (green birefringence under polarized light with the quality of dichromism) (Fig. 20.2) and –negative, and a positive stain is pathognomonic for amyloid. Amyloidosis is the prototypical disease with organized deposits (Fig. 20.3) (see Chapter 19) that appear as 8- to 10-nm-diameter, nonbranching, extracellular fibrils. The principal amyloid fibril proteins seen in renal disease are AA (derived from serum amyloid A protein [SAA], an acute phase reactant) and AL (derived from immunoglobulin light chains). Because the reaction of amyloid fibrils with Congo red dye is a function of the tertiary structure of the amyloid molecule rather than the nature of its precursor proteins, this reaction, which is shared by all forms of amyloid, is the gold standard for the diagnosis (7). However, the current standard of practice

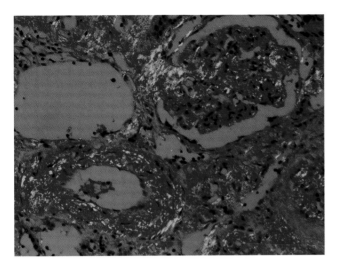

**Figure 20.2** Congo red–positive stain from a biopsy with AL amyloidosis. There is positive staining in the glomerulus, the interstitium, and an interlobular artery. Amyloid fibrils were seen in the same distribution by electron microscopy. (×85.)

for the diagnosis of amyloidosis requires identification of the amyloid fibril protein, and the pathologist should use immunohistochemistry including specific antisera to kappa and lambda light chains, SAA, and other precursor proteins (see Chapter 19). The next step in the evaluation of organized glomerular deposits is an immunohistochemi-

cal evaluation to separate the diseases into those with and without immunoglobulin molecules or fragments in the deposits.

## CONGO RED–NEGATIVE IMMUNOGLOBULIN-DERIVED ORGANIZED DEPOSITS

Normal or neoplastic plasma cells or B lymphocytes produce immunoglobulin molecules and fragments that can form organized glomerular deposits when deposited in the kidney as aggregates or immune complexes. Diseases that may have glomerular organized immunoglobulin deposits include cryoglobulinemia (primary and secondary), benign monoclonal gammopathy (monoclonal gammopathy of unknown significance [MGUS]), multiple myeloma, light chain deposition disease. and chronic lymphocytic leukemia (Chapter 19), systemic lupus erythematosus (Chapter 12), and hepatitis C (8). The presence of organized glomerular deposits is not pathognomonic for any of these diseases. In each instance, the diagnosis requires clinicopathologic correlation and adherence to established criteria. Discussion of these diseases will be limited to the ultrastructural appearance of the deposits and differential diagnostic features. This section concludes with an in-depth discussion of immunotactoid glomerulopathy.

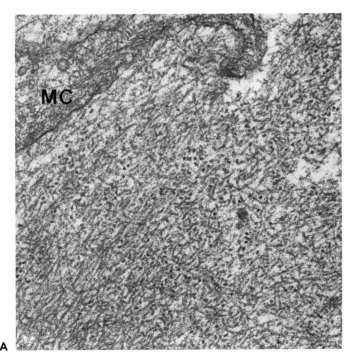
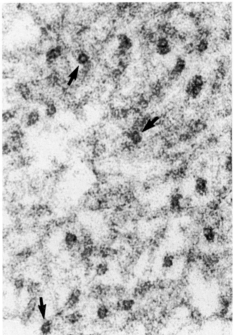

**Figure 20.3** Electron micrographs showing glomerular amyloidosis. **A:** Mesangial deposits of randomly arranged, 12-nm fibrils. MC-mesangial cell process. (Uranyl acetate and lead citrate, ×70,000.) **B:** Electron-lucent core in amyloid fibrils (*arrows*). (Uranyl acetate and lead citrate, ×250,000.) (From Korbet SM, Schwartz MM, Lewis EJ. The fibrillary glomerulopathies. Am J Kidney Dis 1994;23: 751.)

## Cryoglobulinemia

Cryoglobulins are usually immunoglobulins that precipitate from cooled serum and redissolve on heating. Their immunoglobulin composition is the basis for classification: *type I cryoglobulins* are monoclonal immunoglobulins usually seen with hematolymphoid neoplasms. *Type II cryoglobulins* contain a monoclonal immunoglobulin with antiglobulin activity (rheumatoid factor) against a polyclonal immunoglobulin, and they are seen with infections, autoimmune diseases, chronic liver disease (especially hepatitis C), and various forms of proliferative glomerulonephritis. *Type III cryoglobulins*, composed of a polyclonal immunoglobulin with antiglobulin activity against a polyclonal immunoglobulin, are seen in systemic lupus erythematosus, infections, and various other conditions (9,10). Although type I and II cryoglobulins have both been associated with hematolymphoid neoplasms, it is important to note that glomerular deposits of a monoclonal immunoglobulin are not synonymous with an underlying malignancy (11,12). Ultrastructural study of cryoprecipitates have shown organization into rods, annuli, filaments, cylindrical and annular bodies, globular condensations, and fingerprintlike periodic condensations, and the morphology varies with the class and quality (1) of the immunoglobulin components. Patients with cryoglobulinemia may have similar organized deposits in the glomeruli, usually in the form of tubules measuring up to 1 micron long and from 20 to 30 nm wide. They may be arranged in pairs, bundles, pseudocrystalline arrays, or randomly, or tightly packed (1,13–16). The tubules often have a thick wall, a definite electron-lucent core, an ill-defined surface coat, and a substructure seen as globular units in the annuli and striations in the tubules. Organized deposits are most frequently seen in type II cryoglobulinemia (Fig. 20.4), but similar structures have also been described with type I cryoglobulinemia (15,17). Although cryoglobulins composed of polyclonal IgG (type III) or monoclonal IgG and small amounts of IgM (type II) form 6-nm-diameter, randomly arranged filaments in vitro, the renal electron-dense deposits seen in the associated diseases are usually amorphous.

## Paraproteinemias

The presence of a serum or urine monoclonal immunoglobulin (paraprotein) is part of the definition of plasma cell dyscrasias and dysproteinemias. The clonal proliferation producing the monoclonal immunoglobulin may be subtle (benign monoclonal gammopathy/MGUS) or there may be local and systemic signs and symptoms related to a neoplasm or its paraprotein product. The renal

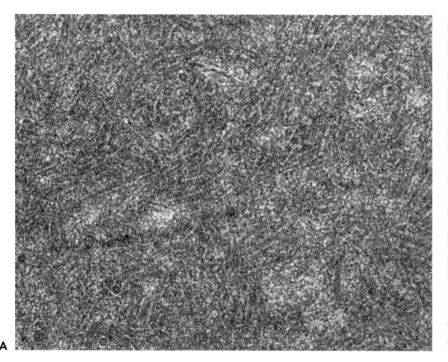
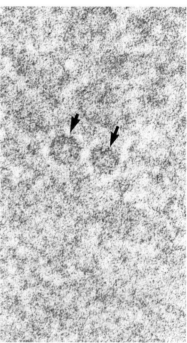

A                                                                                                    B

**Figure 20.4**   Mixed essential cryoglobulinemia. Subendothelial electron-dense deposit from a patient with hematuria, proteinuria, hypocomplementemia, and 760 μg/mL mixed IgG-IgM cryoglobulin. **A:** The deposits contain randomly arranged, closely packed tubules seen as annuli in cross section. (Uranyl acetate and lead citrate, ×70,000.) **B:** The tubules are thick walled, with cross-sectional diameter of 30 nm and an electron-lucent core (*arrows*). (Uranyl acetate and lead citrate, ×250,000.) (From Korbet SM, Schwartz MM, Lewis EJ. The fibrillary glomerulopathies. Am J Kidney Dis 1994;23: 751.)

pathology seen with the dysproteinemias includes amyloidosis (AL), myeloma kidney, cryoglobulinemic glomerulonephritis, monoclonal immunoglobulin deposition disease (MIDD) (see Chapter 19), and glomerulopathy with organized immune deposits. In *multiple myeloma*, the principal pathology is immunoglobulin light chain casts in the tubules, but there are reports of crystals in the renal tubules and tubular epithelium, associated with Fanconi's syndrome (see Chapter 19). Glomerular crystals are rare (18,19). Two thirds of the cases of *monoclonal immunoglobulin deposition disease* (MIDD) have a monoclonal protein in the serum or urine that may be related to multiple myeloma (20,21), and the remainder have no evidence of a plasma cell dyscrasia. The electron-dense deposits in MIDD are usually punctate and finely granular and are located in the lamina rara interna of the glomerular basal lamina and on the interstitial side of the tubular basal lamina. A few reports (22–25) describe 10- to 15-nm-diameter, randomly arranged or irregularly clustered microfilaments in the tubular basal lamina and in the characteristic glomerular nodules. The fibril size in these cases of MIDD overlaps that of amyloid fibrils, but the deposits are Congo red–negative. It is possible that the fibrils occasionally seen in MIDD are a secondary phenomenon and do not represent an aggregated or polymerized form of the monoclonal immunoglobulin. Because light chains stimulate the production of matrix proteins by mesangial cells in vivo (26), the fibrils may represent matrix proteins rather than organized immunoglobulin molecules (23,24).

The definition of benign monoclonal gammopathy or monoclonal gammopathy of unknown significance (MGUS) includes a circulating paraprotein and the absence of signs of malignant B-cell neoplasm or multiple myeloma. An associated systemic or renal disease related to the paraprotein should exclude patients from this diagnosis. MGUS is an important clinical diagnosis because of its unpredictable long-term outcome. Approximately one third of the patients with this condition develop multiple myeloma, macroglobulinemia, or B-cell lymphoma after 20 years of follow-up (27). On the other hand, many patients with renal diseases that are associated with plasma cell dyscrasias have a serum or urine paraprotein. These include 30% of patients with monoclonal immunoglobulin deposition disease (28), 64% of patients with primary amyloidosis (29), occasional patients with Waldenström's macroglobulinemia (30), and many patients with types I and II cryoglobulinemia (9,10). All these patients could be classified as MGUS, but I consider the glomerular deposits, with or without organization, as complications of the underlying diseases. This allows the clinician to treat the patients with disease-specific therapy. When patients with MGUS and Congo red–negative glomerular immunoglobulin deposits are studied by electron microscopy (31–39), 13- to 25-nm-diameter microfilaments or 19- to 51-nm-diameter microtubules are described in

subepithelial, subendothelial, and luminal deposits. When such cases are reported as fibrillary glomerulonephritis or immunotactoid glomerulopathy (see below, Immunotactoid Glomerulopathy), it should come as no surprise that some of them develop a long-term complication of MGUS. Bridoux et al (36) reported on a patient (no. 6) in whom AL amyloidosis ($\lambda$ type) developed 3 years after the diagnosis of immunotactoid glomerulopathy and an IgG$\lambda$ monoclonal gammopathy.

In patients found by screening of serum and urine for monoclonal immunoglobulins using immunoelectropheresis or the more sensitive immunoblotting technique, renal diseases unrelated to the monoclonal protein are found in 46% of the cases (36,40). In my experience, biopsies performed for isolated monoclonal immunoglobulins in the absence of renal functional abnormalities often show no or nonspecific glomerular pathology.

## Chronic Lymphocytic Leukemia/Lymphoma and Lymphoproliferative Disorders

Patients with *chronic lymphocytic leukemia/lymphoma* and other lymphoproliferative disorders may have an associated cryoglobulinemia or paraproteinemia, and some develop glomerulonephritis and the nephrotic syndrome (see Chapter 19). The glomeruli may contain electron-dense deposits, organized as microfibrils or microtubules ranging from 10 to 48 nm in diameter. They are either randomly distributed or focally packed in parallel arrays (Fig. 20.5) (41–48). In most instances, the microfibrils/microtubules have an electron-lucent core. Organized deposits in patients with cryoglobulins or a paraprotein are an indication for a hematologic evaluation because neither the organized glomerular deposits nor the serum protein abnormalities are diagnostic of an underlying hematologic neoplasm. This is a critical diagnostic point with therapeutic implications because treatment with remission of the malignancy is frequently associated with resolution of proteinuria and improvement of renal function (36,43).

## Systemic Lupus Erythematosus

*Systemic lupus erythematosus* (SLE) is an autoimmune disease, and approximately one half the cases have an immune complex–mediated glomerulonephritis. Although the pathology is characteristic, the diagnosis of SLE glomerulonephritis requires clinical evidence of systemic involvement (49). Electron-dense deposits, corresponding to immune aggregates seen by immunofluorescence microscopy, are usually amorphous, but in some cases, there are vague small, short, curved microtubules that fail to resolve into definite structures at high magnification. Occasionally, organized deposits occur in subepithelial, subendothelial, transmembranous, and mesangial locations, and similar deposits occur in extraglomerular sites including

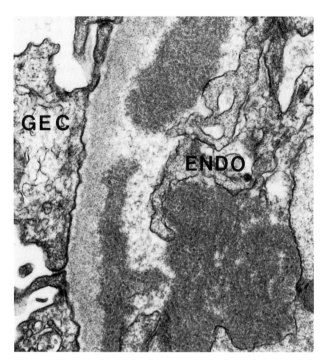

**Figure 20.5** Lymphoproliferative disorder with lymphocytosis, hypocomplementemia, cryoglobulinemia and rapidly progressive glomerulonephritis. Subendothelial electron-dense deposits composed of randomly arranged short tubules, with an electron-lucent core in cross section. GEC, glomerular epithelial cell. ENDO, endothelial cell. (Uranyl acetate and lead citrate, ×25,000.)

the interstitium, the tubular basement membrane, the peritubular capillary basement membrane, and in the juxtaglomerular apparatus (50). "Fingerprints" are the most characteristic and frequent form of organized deposits, consisting of two to six regularly stacked curved or straight electron-dense bands, 8 to 15 nm in diameter with a center-to-center distance of 19 to 29 nm (Fig.20.6A) (4,51). At high magnification, the substructure is more complex with cross-striations produced by small lateral projections seen at regular intervals with a center-to-center distance of 10 to 15 nm (4). There are reports of similar deposits in cryoglobulins consisting of polyclonal IgG with traces of IgM (1). Even more rarely, there are distinct tubules or fibrils in association with the fingerprints or in isolation. The tubules have an electron-lucent core and measure 25 to 40 nm in diameter with variable length (52,53) (Fig. 20.6B), and the fibrils measure 8 to 27 nm. Hvala et al (50) found organized glomerular deposits in 37 of 185 biopsies (20%) from patients with SLE: The deposits were organized as fingerprints in 32 biopsies (86%), 20- to 100-nm tubules in 3 biopsies (8%), and 18-nm fibrils in 2 biopsies (5%). The fingerprint form of the deposits is quite specific for SLE. In 626 kidney biopsies from patients with primary renal and systemic diseases other than SLE, there were no fingerprint deposits. Finally, organized extracellular deposits are different from the intracellular tubuloreticular structures that are often present within dilated cisterna of the endoplasmic reticulum of glomerular endothelial cells in SLE.

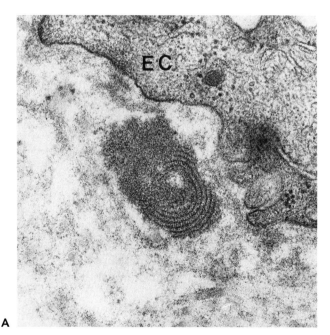

A

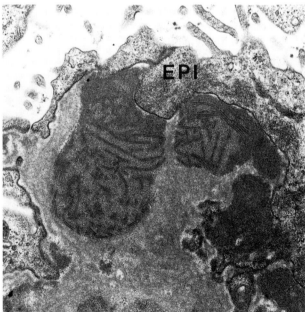

B

**Figure 20.6** Systemic lupus erythematosus. **A:** "Fingerprint" electron-dense deposit in the perivascular interstitium, composed of five parallel, sharply curved lines with lateral projections. There were similar structures throughout the glomeruli, which showed diffuse glomerulonephritis. EC, endothelial cell. (Uranyl acetate and lead citrate, ×25,000.) **B:** Subepithelial electron-dense deposits contain elongated, straight, randomly arranged tubules. Note that the organized deposits are within a larger amorphous deposit. The glomeruli also showed subendothelial electron-dense deposits and diffuse glomerulonephritis. EPI, glomerular epithelial cell. (Uranyl acetate and lead citrate, ×15,000.)

## Immunotactoid Glomerulopathy (Fibrillary Glomerulonephritis)

There are established clinicopathologic and serologic criteria to diagnose systemic diseases and hematologic neoplasms with glomerular involvement, and in the presence of organized glomerular deposits, chronic lymphocytic leukemia/lymphoma, lymphoproliferative disorders, SLE, and cryoglobulinemia are appropriate diagnoses. Regardless of the morphology of the deposits, these diagnoses are preferred over a diagnosis that focuses on the appearance of the deposits because the diseases have specific prognostic and therapeutic implications, and so far, the ultrastructural character of the electron-dense deposits does not add diagnostic specificity, prognostic information, or therapeutic guidance to the pathology of these diseases. By exclusion, there remains a group of patients with Congo red–negative, organized glomerular immunoglobulin deposits with no associated systemic disease.

Rosenmann and Eliakim (54) were the first to report glomerular Congo red–negative, "amyloidlike" fibrillary deposits that contained IgG and C3. Similar cases have been reported as nonamyloidotic fibrillary glomerulopathy (55,56), fibrillary nephritis (6), Congo red–negative amyloidosislike glomerulopathy (57), amyloid stain–negative microfibrillary glomerulopathy (58), and Congo red–negative idiopathic fibrillary glomerulopathy (without detectable cryoglobulins or monoclonal gammopathy) (59). These diagnoses take their descriptive names from the ultrastructure of the deposits that are similar in their morphology and random organization to amyloid fibrils and from the negative Congo red reaction. Other cases have been reported as fibrillary glomerulonephritis (FGN) (37,60–63). However, this diagnosis confuses the lesion specified by the presence of organized immunoglobulin deposits with the general category of fibrillary glomerulopathies (6,64,65) and the β-fibrilloses (7), diseases with biochemically diverse organized deposits (66). Most of these names are long and cumbersome, and none specifies the immunoglobulin content of the fibrils.

In 1980, Schwartz and Lewis (67) reported the clinical and pathologic findings of a 49-year-old man who had an 11-year history of proteinuria and the nephrotic syndrome. His renal biopsy was Congo red– and thioflavin T–negative, and the glomeruli contained immunoglobulin and complement (C3) deposits. By electron microscopy, the deposits comprised thick-walled tubules, measuring 35 nm in diameter, organized in parallel arrays. Despite repeated evaluation over a 17-year course of nephrotic syndrome and progressive renal insufficiency that terminated in end-stage renal disease, the patient never developed any of the diseases that previously had been associated with organized immunoglobulin deposits. By analogy to the linear crystallization of hemoglobin S that forms elongated tactoids in red blood cells during sickle cell crisis, the term *immunotactoid glomerulopathy* (ITG) was coined to emphasize the morphology and the composition of the glomerular deposits.

Korbet et al (68) proposed that biopsies showing either of the ultrastructural forms of the organized immunoglobulin deposits should be included under the single diagnostic rubric of ITG, when patients with diseases associated with organized glomerular immune deposits were excluded from the analysis. It was the author's intention that the diagnosis of ITG, defined as a primary glomerular disease, would accumulate data concerning clinical features, response to therapy, cause, and pathogenesis independent of well-defined diseases that may have similar glomerular deposits. However, not all accept this definition of ITG with its exclusions, and some pathologists, seeing a biopsy with organized glomerular immunoglobulin deposits, especially when the clinical information is too limited to make all the exclusions, may feel justified in diagnosing the smaller diameter fibrils as fibrillary glomerulopathy and the larger tubules with a hollow center as immunotactoid glomerulopathy. Consequently, the diagnoses of ITG and FGN will both contain a mixture of primary and secondary glomerular diseases, and by including patients with systemic diseases and lymphoproliferative disorders, the clinical characteristics of both groups will become a function of the underlying diseases (36,37). The validity and utility of this approach depends on the demonstration that the different ultrastructural appearances define discrete and mutually exclusive morphologic categories of glomerular disease and that the fibrillar and tubular forms of Congo red–negative organized glomerular immune deposits have specific and different clinical associations (41). Unless these differences are clearly apparent, the clinician, confronted by two entities that are similar clinically, pathologically, and biochemically and are differentiated only by the ultrastructural appearance of the deposits, may find this distinction unnecessary and confusing.

## Clinical Implications of Fibril Size, Appearance, and Organization

When organized glomerular deposits are grouped by their ultrastructural appearance, the diagnosis of ITG is reserved for cases with larger, parallel tubules, and cases with smaller, randomly arranged fibrils are called *fibrillary glomerulonephropathy/glomerulonephritis* (FGN). The rationale for this distinction is that it allegedly provides a reproducible division with important and unique clinical implications (37,41,61,63,69). However, Korbet et al (68) used ITG to describe patients with both types of deposits, and FGN more properly denotes glomerular diseases with fibrils seen by electron microscopy without regard to their biochemical composition (64,66,70). In spite of these problems, I will use these terms to consider the validity and utility of separating biopsies containing

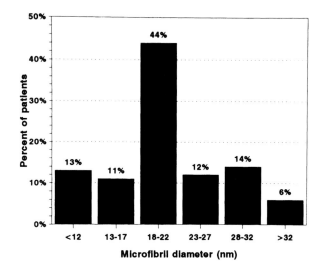

**Figure 20.7**   Fibril diameter in 88 patients diagnosed with immunotactoid (fibrillary) glomerulopathy. (From Korbet SM, Schwartz MM, Lewis EJ. The fibrillary glomerulopathies. Am J Kidney Dis 1994;23:751.)

glomerular nonamyloid, organized immune deposits into two categories on the sole basis of the appearance of the deposits.

The morphologic features that reportedly discriminate between the tubules in ITG and the fibrils in FGN include cross-sectional diameter, lumens, and random versus parallel arrangements. Although fibril/tubule diameter is consistent within a biopsy and among biopsies from the same patient, there is a range of diameters from 10 to 49 nm (71) (Fig. 20.7). Generally, the fibrils of FGN have an average diameter from 18 to 22 nm, approximately twice the diameter of amyloid fibrils, and virtually all cases measure less than 30 nm (37,60,61,63,69). When Pronovost et al (59) defined ITG by fibril size larger than 30 nm, it composed only 6.5% of the 186 cases they reviewed. In contrast, when they defined ITG by focal parallel arrangement of the fibrils, it almost doubled its prevalence (12%). Some have argued that the morphologic definition of ITG also includes a "hollow," electron-lucent tubular lumen, but the fibrils in many if not all cases of what has been called FGN also have an electron-lucent lumen (64,68). Bridoux et al (36) reported on 14 ITG patients with hollow-core microtubules in (focal) parallel arrays. In the four patients who did not have a disease that has been associated with organized glomerular immunoglobulin deposits including lymphoma, leukemia, or a MGUS, the microtubules measured 15 ± 6 nm in diameter. Using an arbitrary definition of the fibril morphology, one can separate some cases (FGN) from a much smaller number of cases (ITG), but there is considerable overlap between the two diagnostic categories. Using fibril size of 30 nm as the cutoff, Rosenstock et al (37) reported that 61 cases of FGN had a mean diameter of 20.1 nm ± 0.4 (range 13 to 29 nm) and 6

cases of ITG had a mean diameter of 38.2 nm ± 5.7 (range, 20 to 55 nm). Even if it were possible to separate ITG and FGN into mutually exclusive morphologic groups, there is no compelling reason to do so unless the ultrastructural features have significant clinical implications.

Korbet et al (68,71) reported their experience with ITG and reviewed the literature, and they found no significant differences between patients with the fibrillar and the tubular forms of deposits. The clinical presentation, the immunopathology, the prognosis, and the response to therapy were the same. Two recent series comparing ITG and FGN that included patients with either monoclonal proteins in the urine or serum (37) or lymphomas, leukemia, or MGUS (36) found no significant difference in the clinical features or demographics at presentation. In addition, the clinical outcome and response to therapy was either not different or the number of patients with ITG was too small to analyze. Pronovost et al (59) compared the demographics and clinical features of 186 patients with ITG and FGN. There was a slight female predominance, but there were no age differences. They found no difference in the prevalence of hypertension, hematuria, nephrotic syndrome, and renal insufficiency at presentation whether the diagnosis was established by fibril size (FGN up to 30 nm and ITG larger than 30 nm) or fibril arrangement (FGN random and ITG focally parallel). They also evaluated the association between FGN and ITG and lymphoproliferative disease. As might be predicted, patients with a serum or urine paraprotein and a lymphoproliferative disorder frequently (44%) had organized glomerular deposits of a tubular nature, as is seen in ITG. However, when patients with a paraprotein were excluded, the prevalence of neoplasia in both ITG and FGN was similar and low. The authors concluded that it was premature to subclassify ITG/FGN because of their similar clinical presentations, the similar prevalence of lymphoproliferative malignancy when patients with a paraprotein were excluded, and the insufficiency of biochemical and pathogenetic information to justify subclassification on the basis of fibril composition or mechanisms of fibrillogenesis (70).

These considerations lead to the conclusion that there is too much overlap in fibril morphology to dichotomize the biopsies in a nonarbitrary manner, and the morphologic differences, which some believe to support a distinction between ITG and FGN, are of unknown significance. The clinical utility of this distinction is also in question because there are no consistent differences in clinical presentation, demographics, prognosis, or response to therapy related to fibril size, morphology, or organization, and when secondary causes of organized glomerular immunoglobulin deposits are excluded (including patients with a paraprotein), the prevalence of hematologic malignancy is low and similar. In my opinion, if it is to be clinically useful, pathologists should diagnosis ITG only after excluding diseases known to be associated with organized glomerular immunoglobulin deposits. Therefore, I consider ITG to be a primary glomerular disease characterized by deposits of immunoglobulin and complement that have variable electron microscopic appearances, and the diagnosis requires exclusion of diseases known to be associated with organized glomerular immune deposits. In the following discussion of the clinical findings, pathologic features, and outcome, I will refer to the entity as ITG regardless of the ultrastructural appearance of the deposits. However, when an author distinguishes between ITG and FGN, I will follow the article's convention in presenting the data.

## Clinical Findings

ITG is an uncommon condition, but more than 200 cases have been reported as ITG or one of its synonyms since it was first described in 1977 (54). The clinical features have been the subject of several reviews and large series that summarize the data and give the primary references (59,60,63,64,68–71). Additionally, case reports and series have accumulated since the 5th edition of *Heptinstall's Pathology of the Kidney* (36,37,53,72–79). In a study restricted to biopsies with fibrils less than 30 nm in diameter, the prevalence was 0.8% of 3785 consecutive nontransplant renal biopsies (63). Another large biopsy series reported 60 biopsies with fibrils smaller than 30 nm (0.6%) and 6 biopsies with fibrils 30 nm or larger (0.06%) among 10,108 native kidney biopsies (37). The prevalence of ITG is similar to that of amyloidosis (63). Fogo et al (69) reported 32 cases of FGN (1.2%) and 52 cases of amyloidosis (2%) in 2649 biopsies over an 11-year period. In our series of adult patients with the nephrotic syndrome, ITG constituted 4% of the biopsies (13 of 340), and the prevalence of amyloidosis was similar (11 cases) (80).

The clinical presentation of ITG does not distinguish it from the other primary causes of proteinuria and the nephrotic syndrome (71), and this point was confirmed in a review of 186 patients with ITG and FGN (59). The disease presents in the fifth decade with an equal distribution between men and women (63,71), and a disproportionate number of the patients are White (37,59,63). All patients with ITG have proteinuria, and at the time of presentation, more than half have nephrotic syndrome. Despite the prominence of proteinuria and symptoms related to the nephrotic syndrome, some patients are frankly nephritic at presentation or develop rapidly progressive glomerulonephritis. Hypertension, hematuria, and renal insufficiency frequently accompany proteinuria (37,59,71). ITG is rare in children (78,81,82). By definition, there is no evidence of cryoglobulinemia, paraproteinemia, lymphoproliferative disorder, or plasma cell dyscrasia. Even though up to 19% of ITG patients have a positive antinuclear antibody, it is usually in low titer or in a speckled pattern (63,68), and those patients fulfilling the clinical criteria for systemic lupus erythematosus are excluded. With rare exceptions, clinical involvement is limited to the kidney.

Nonglomerular renal deposits and systemic involvement with organ dysfunction are very unusual. There are two reports of ITG in patients with pulmonary hemorrhage, and in one, pulmonary involvement was associated with rapidly progressive glomerulonephritis (83). Fibrillar deposits in the lung were identical to those in the kidneys in both cases (83,84): The deposits stained for IgA in one case (83) and IgG in the other (84). Ozawa et al (85) reported on a 56-year-old Japanese man who died of liver failure. Postmortem examination of the liver and kidney demonstrated identical Congo red–negative fibrillar deposits. Sabatine et al (86) reported a patient with glomerular and myocardial deposits of 8- to 12.4-nm fibrils that were positive for IgG and complement (C3) by fluorescence microscopy and were Congo red–negative.

## Pathologic Findings

### Light Microscopy

In the 43 cases of ITG that I have studied, the *glomerular* pathology generally reflects the distribution of the deposits (personal observation, 2005). Every case showed some degree of mesangial expansion by eosinophilic, PAS-positive material from a slight increase to massive deposits with glomerular distortion (Fig. 20.8). More than half (25 of 43) had glomerular basement membrane (GBM) abnormalities, but they were variable in extent and character. There were focal thickening of the GBM (63,68,71) and other abnormalities, including irregularities, subepithelial projections (spikes), silver-negative defects (holes), and splitting (Fig. 20.9). These pathologic changes reflect the subepithelial and subendothelial location of the deposits and widespread infiltration of the GBM by deposits (see Electron Microscopy). Cases with diffuse spikes and holes or splitting were rare, and only three cases seriously suggested the diagnosis of membranous glomerulonephritis (Fig. 20.10). Mild mesangial hypercellularity (two to four cells per mesangial area) often accompanied mesangial expansion and GBM abnormalities (Fig. 20.11A), but mesangial hypercellularity was moderate to severe in only 5 of 43 cases (Fig. 20.11B). Two cases had prominent glomerular capillary thrombi (Fig. 20.12). Hyalinized and obsolescent glomeruli were a nonspecific but common finding in ITG: on average, one third of the glomeruli were hyalinized, and more than half of the glomeruli were hyalinized in 12 of 43 cases. The deposits in the mesangium and the GBM are periodic acid-Schiff (PAS)–positive and blue with the trichrome stain, and they are negative with the Congo red and thioflavin T stains for amyloid. There are no specific lesions of the tubules, interstitium, or blood vessels, but interstitial fibrosis and tubular atrophy are commensurate with the degree of glomerular obsolescence.

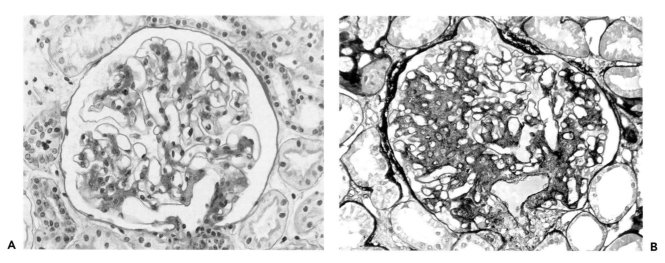

**Figure 20.8** Immunotactoid glomerulopathy. **A:** Glomerulus showing mild expansion of the mesangium by PAS-positive material and a slight increase in mesangial cells. The GBM appears normal. (PAS, ×170.) **B:** Glomerulus with severe mesangial expansion. The capillaries are patent, and the GBM appears normal. (Methenamine silver–PAS, ×170.)

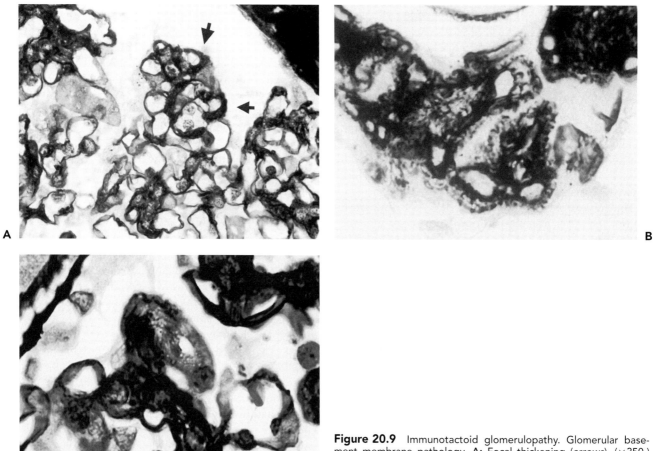

**Figure 20.9** Immunotactoid glomerulopathy. Glomerular basement membrane pathology. **A:** Focal thickening (*arrows*). (×350.) **B:** Diffuse spikes. (×550.) **C:** Basement membrane staining is irregular with mottling and well-defined holes. (×550.) (**A–C,** Methenamine silver–PAS [Jones].)

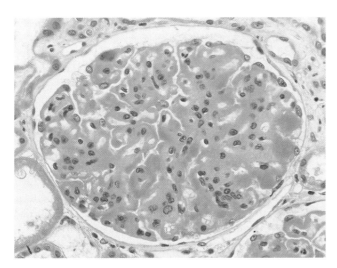

**Figure 20.10** Immunotactoid glomerulopathy. The basement membranes are diffusely thickened and have focal intense eosinophilia, reflecting widespread subepithelial, intramembranous, and subendothelial organized deposits. Also, the mesangium is expanded and shows segmental mild hypercellularity. (H&E, ×170.)

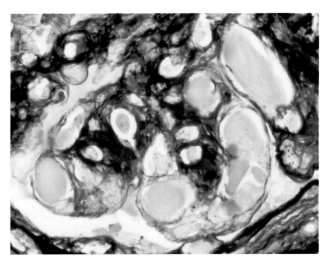

**Figure 20.12** Immunotactoid glomerulopathy. Glomerular thrombi. The capillaries contain hyalin thrombi that stained for IgG, but the thrombi were fibrin-negative by fluorescence microscopy. By electron microscopy the capillaries contained organized immune deposits. Note that the glomerular basement membranes are split. (Methenamine silver–PAS; ×550.)

Biopsies diagnosed as ITG or FGN are sometimes associated with significant glomerular inflammation including crescents, endocapillary proliferation, membranoproliferative glomerulonephritis, and segmental necrosis with neutrophil infiltration. Iskandar et al (63) reported crescents in 19% of 31 renal biopsies showing FGN, and crescentic involvement ranged from 10% to 80%. Fogo et al (69) found crescents in seven cases that involved from 13% to 75% of the glomeruli in 32 patients with FGN. Most were fibrous crescents, but in one case, there were active cellular crescents. In addition, there was a diffuse proliferative or lobular pattern of glomerulonephritis in 25 of 32 biopsies. In 60 patients with FGN (fibril diameter <30 nm), Rosenstock et al (37) found MPGN in 44% (27 cases) and diffuse endocapillary proliferative glomerulonephritis (DPGN) with leukocytic infiltration in 15% (9 cases). Thirty-one percent of 60 FGN cases had cellular or fibrocellular crescents, and they were most frequent in the DPGN group involving a mean of 25% of the glomeruli (range 0% to 57%). In the six patients with fibril diameter of 30 nm or more, three had MPGN and three had DPGN. None had crescents. In addition, there are isolated reports of ITG with a rapidly progressive course and crescents or necrosis in more than half of the glomeruli (76,83,87–89).

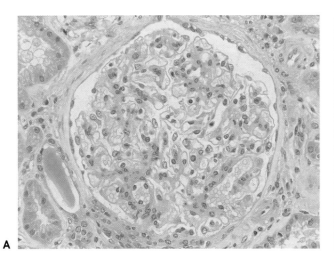

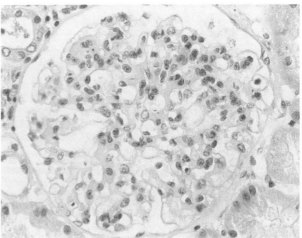

**Figure 20.11** Immunotactoid glomerulopathy. **A:** Mild mesangial proliferation with three to six cells per mesangial area. **B:** Moderate proliferation with five to nine cells per mesangial area. The capillaries are patent and the GBM appear normal in both photographs. (**A** and **B**, H&E, ×170.)

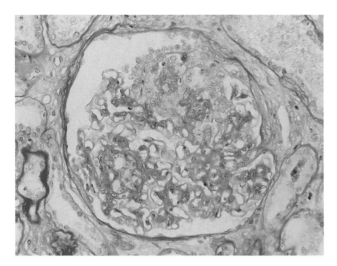

**Figure 20.13**  Immunotactoid glomerulopathy. There is a segmental area of glomerular necrosis with destruction of capillaries, proliferation of the overlying epithelial cells, and adhesion to Bowman's capsule. The uninvolved glomerular tuft shows mesangial expansion with minimal hypercellularity, patent capillaries, and normal basement membranes. (PAS, ×170.)

When cryoglobulinemia, paraproteinemia, and systemic diseases were excluded, the 43 cases of ITG that I studied had less diffuse inflammation, and when necrosis was present, it was segmental and focal. Four biopsies had focal segmental glomerular necrosis superimposed on mesangial expansion and focal GBM thickening (Fig. 20.13). In two cases, one glomerulus was involved, and in two cases, two glomeruli showed necrosis. A crescent was associated with an area of necrosis in one case (Fig. 20.14), and crescents were seen in the surviving glomeruli in an end-stage

kidney showing extensive glomerular sclerosis. None of the remaining 38 biopsies had active, cellular crescents or glomerular necrosis.

## Immunohistopathology

The pattern of glomerular immunoglobulin and complement deposition in ITG is variable, and it reflects the mesangial and GBM locations of deposits seen by electron microscopy (60,63,69,71). Most commonly, both mesangial and GBM deposits are present, but in a few cases, the deposits are isolated to the GBM or the mesangium. The mesangial deposits are either discrete and granular (Fig. 20.15A) or diffusely expand the mesangium and focally extend into the basement membrane (Fig. 20.15B). The GBM deposits are usually irregular, discontinuous linear, and granular (Fig. 20.16A), or ribbonlike, but a few cases show diffuse granular staining (Fig. 20.16B). Until recently, there were no reports of tubular basement membrane, interstitial, or vascular deposits. Adeyi et al (75) reported on two patients with polyclonal deposits of IgG in the glomeruli and along the tubular basement membranes. The histochemical stains for amyloid were negative. The fibrils measured 28 nm in one case, and the second had 30-nm fibrils in the glomeruli and 15-nm fibrils in the tubular basement membranes.

In a review of the cases of ITG reported up to 1994, IgG was the most frequent immunoglobulin seen in the deposits (103 of 110 reported cases, 94%). IgA was found in 29 of 101 (29%), IgM in 62 of 102 (60%), and C3 in 99 of 103 (96%). The IgG usually contained both κ and λ light chains (62 of 86 cases, 72%) (64,71). Two large series (37,63) confirmed this composition of the deposits, and

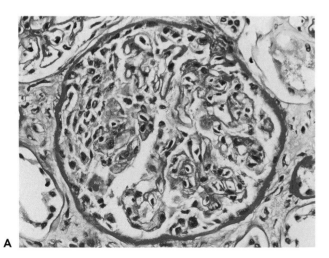
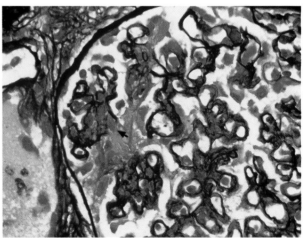

**Figure 20.14**  Immunotactoid glomerulopathy. **A:** A small crescent in Bowman's space overlies a damaged glomerular segment. The uninvolved portion of the glomerulus shows mesangial expansion and normal basement membranes. (PAS, ×170.) **B:** The basement membrane is disrupted (*arrow*) in the necrotic glomerular segment in the same glomerulus seen in (**A**). (Methenamine silver–PAS [Jones], ×350.)

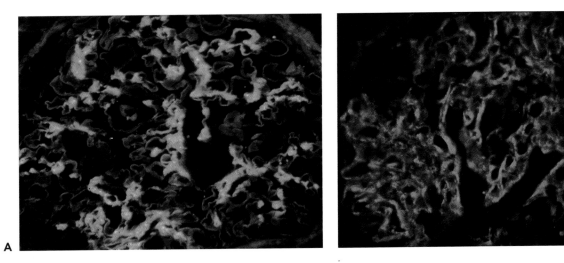

**Figure 20.15** Immunotactoid glomerulopathy. Mesangial deposits. **A:** Immunoglobulin G (IgG) is deposited in a pure mesangial pattern. Note the total sparring of the glomerular capillary walls. Light microscopic changes were also confined to the mesangium and consisted of PAS-positive expansion. **B:** There is massive mesangium expansion by irregularly staining deposits of immunoglobulin G (IgG). The deposits also focally involve the glomerular basement membranes.

they both demonstrated that IgG and C3 had the strongest staining intensity. Monoclonal immunoglobulin deposits were present in 16 of 86 cases (19%) of ITG studied with light chain antisera, and κ light chain restriction was in all reported cases, usually in combination with γ heavy chain (32,34,35,46,60,68,90–95). Rosenstock et al (37) reported a case of FGN with λ light chain restriction. I have seen a similar case, but it was complicated by the presence of an IgGκ paraprotein (see above, Paraproteinemia). There are case reports in which the glomerular deposits contained IgAλ (73) and IgMκ (5). In two studies that dichotomized the biopsies on the basis of fibril size (<30 nm versus 30 nm or larger) (37) or appearance (fibrillary versus tubular) (69), the immunoglobulin distribution was similar in both groups with IgG dominance. Iskandar et al (63) studied the IgG subgroups in 28 patients with fibril diameters less than 30 nm (mean 22.2 nm ± (7.4). The deposits were restricted to IgG subgroup 4 (IgG4). This was in contrast to the predominance of IgG1 and IgG3 in the glomerular deposits of control patients with diffuse lupus glomerulonephritis and was similar to that seen in control patients with idiopathic membranous glomerulonephritis. Monoclonal IgG3κ was reported in a case with 35-nm microtubular deposits (67).

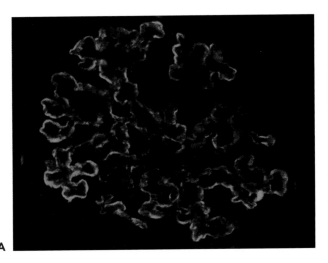
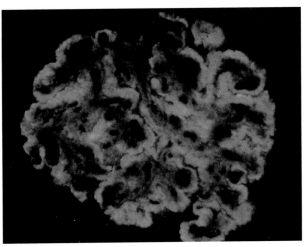

**Figure 20.16** Immunotactoid glomerulopathy. Glomerular basement membrane deposits. **A:** Immunoglobulin G (IgG) is seen as discontinuous linear and focal granular staining. The mesangium is largely uninvolved. **B:** There are massive granular deposits of immunoglobulin G along the basement membranes and in the mesangium. (**A** and **B**, fluorescein isothiocyanate conjugated rabbit anti-human IgG, ×170.)

The relationship between monoclonal glomerular deposits and fibril morphology and size is inconstant. Most of the reported cases with monoclonal glomerular deposits do not have large-diameter microtubular deposits. At presentation, 13 of the 65 biopsies studied with immunoglobulin light chain antisera showed light chain restriction. This was usually IgGκ although other heavy and light chain specificities are described. On the one hand, 12 of the 13 cases with monoclonal deposits were associated with smaller diameter (<30 nm), randomly arranged microfibrils/microtubules, and in only one case were the associated microtubules 30 nm or larger and closely packed (68). An additional ten biopsies with organized microtubules 30 nm or larger were not studied for light chains (9 biopsies) or had no restriction (1 biopsy).

## Electron Microscopy

The extracellular deposits in ITG are elongated, nonbranching fibrils or tubules (6,37,59,60,64,68,70,71). They do not show periodicity or substructure, and their localization at the same sites as immune deposits seen by fluorescence microscopy implies that they contain immunoglobulins and complement as principal components. Additional ultrastructural findings include mesangial expansion and hypercellularity, basal lamina splitting, mesangial circumferential extension, and diffuse glomerular epithelial cell (GEC) foot process effacement.

Organized deposits are found throughout the glomerulus, but the mesangium is nearly always involved (6,60,61,63,64,71) (Fig. 20.17). In approximately 25% of the cases, only the mesangium is involved, but usually mesangial and basal lamina deposits are found together. The basal lamina deposits have a predilection for the lamina densa and the lamina rara externa (32,60,93–96). In some cases subepithelial deposits are discrete, isolated, and extensive (Fig. 20.18). In a few instances the subepithelial fibrils are oriented perpendicular to the basal lamina and resemble spicular amyloid (6,54,68,92). In other cases there are prominent subendothelial deposits that encroach on the lumen as pseudothrombi (58,63,68,93–96) (Fig. 20.19). New layers of basal lamina form over both

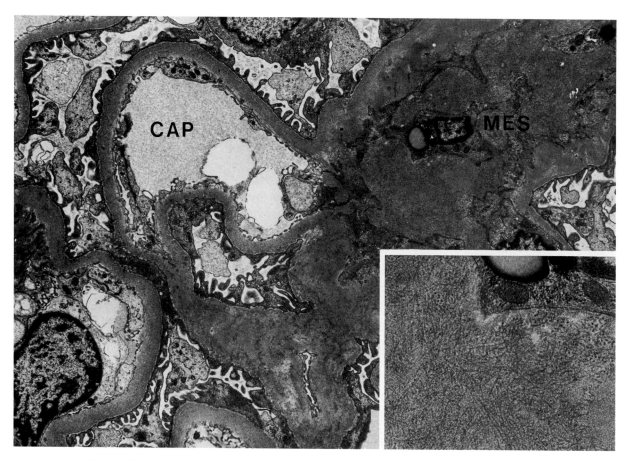

**Figure 20.17**  Immunotactoid glomerulopathy. The mesangium (MES) is expanded by vague electron-dense deposits, which spare the GBM. (Uranyl acetate and lead citrate, ×8600.) CAP, capillary lumen. **Inset:** At higher magnification, the mesangial deposits comprise randomly arranged fibrils that measure 21.3 ± 4 nm in diameter. (Uranyl acetate and lead citrate, ×28,800.) (From Korbet SM, Schwartz MM, Rosenberg BF, et al. Immunotactoid glomerulopathy. Medicine 1985;64:228.)

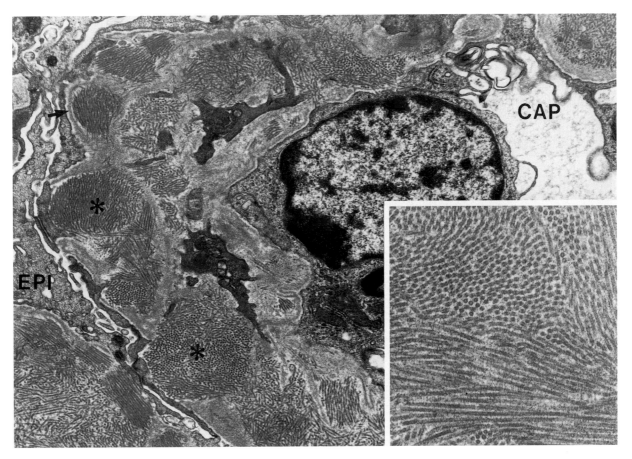

**Figure 20.18** Immunotactoid glomerulopathy. Deposits of 35.4 ± 2 nm in diameter tubules occur as discrete subepithelial masses (*asterisks*) and as masses incorporated into the capillary wall and covered by newly formed GBM (*arrow*). CAP, glomerular capillary lumen. EPI, glomerular epithelial cell. (Uranyl acetate and lead citrate, ×12,500.) **Inset:** The immunotactoids are seen as closely packed tubules in longitudinal and cross-sectional arrays demonstrating their regular diameter, thick walls, and electron-lucent core. (Uranyl acetate and lead citrate, ×35,000.) (From Korbet SM, Schwartz MM, Rosenberg BF, et al. Immunotactoid glomerulopathy. Medicine 1985;64:228.)

the subendothelial and subepithelial deposits. In other instances, the GBM appears diffusely infiltrated and replaced by fibrils (Fig. 20.20).

The appearance of the fibrils and their state of organization varies from case to case, but within a biopsy and between biopsies performed in the same patient at different times, the deposits are similar. The reported microfibril/microtubule diameter varies from the size of amyloid (9 to 11 nm) to greater than 50 nm, and the estimated length ranges from 1000 to 1500 nm (Fig. 20.7). The cross-sectional appearance varies from a solid dot to tubules with either a thin or a thick wall (Fig. 20.21). A lucent center or a lumen is easily seen in tubules with a diameter of 30 nm or more, but careful examination often reveals a lumen in fibrils with a diameter smaller than 30 nm (68). High-resolution studies have failed to demonstrate either periodicity or substructural organization in the deposits (6). In most cases the fibrils/tubules are randomly arranged in the mesangium and in the GBM, but in some cases with larger diameter tubules, the deposits are seen in a tightly

packed, parallel arrangement (61,67,69,94,97). Granular unorganized deposits have been seen separately from the organized deposits or intermixed with them in the GBM and the mesangium (6,54,60–62,69,90,92,93,98), suggesting that they are only partially organized. However, Yang et al (98) studied seven patients with glomerular Congo red–negative, 15- to 20-nm microfibril deposits by protein A gold immunoelectron microscopy, and although they noted nonfibrillar electron-dense areas in the biopsies, positive staining for IgG, both light chains, and C3 were confined to the fibrils. In contrast to organized deposits in immune complex diseases such as SLE, the immune reactants were confined to the microfibrils in the cases studied, and the nature of nonfibrillar electron-dense deposits remained unelucidated.

Extraglomerular deposits are rare in ITG. In a few cases, deposits are described in the tubular basement membranes or the interstitium (6,60,67,68,75) (Fig. 20.22). In association with typical glomerular pathology, organized immunoglobulin deposits have been described in the liver

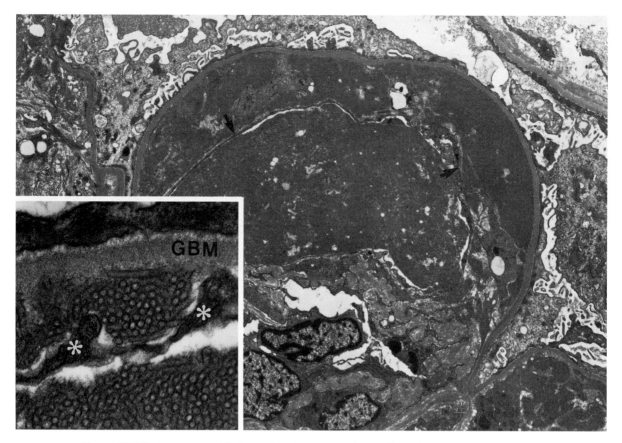

**Figure 20.19** Immunotactoid glomerulopathy. Glomerular capillary almost occluded by a large subendothelial deposit and a luminal thrombus separated by the preserved endothelium (*arrows*). (Uranyl acetate and lead citrate, ×5300.) **Inset:** At higher magnification, deposits comprise tightly packed tubules with an external diameter of 48.9 nm beneath the glomerular basement membrane (GBM), and they are separated from similar deposits in the capillary lumen by the endothelial cell (*asterisks*). (Uranyl acetate and lead citrate, ×45,000.) (Korbet SM, Schwartz MM, Rosenberg BF, et al. Immunotactoid glomerulopathy. Medicine 1985;64:228.)

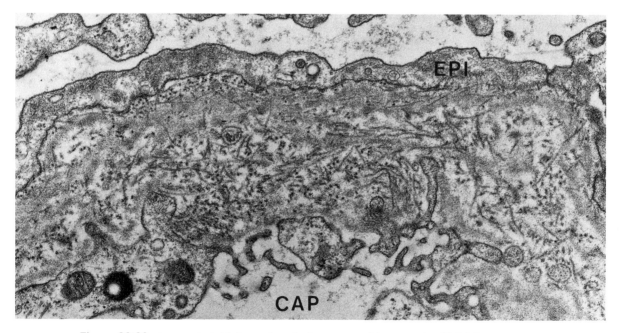

**Figure 20.20** Immunotactoid glomerulopathy. Immunotactoids, measuring 22.8 ± 3 nm, are seen as solid dots in cross section and elongated fibrils in the subepithelial and subendothelial regions of the capillary wall, penetrating and displacing the substance of the basal lamina. EPI, glomerular epithelial cell; CAP, capillary lumen. (Uranyl acetate and lead citrate, ×30,000.) (From Korbet SM, Schwartz MM, Rosenberg BF, et al. Immunotactoid glomerulopathy. Medicine 1985;64:228.)

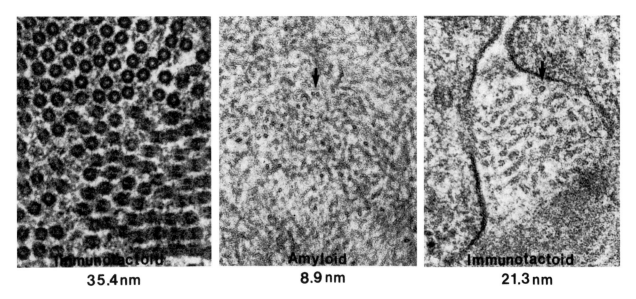

**Figure 20.21** The spectrum of immunotactoid fibril diameter. Immunotactoids of large (35.4 nm) and small (21.3 nm) diameter shown with amyloid **(center)** at the same magnification for comparison. On the **left** are the thick-walled tubules seen on four successive biopsies of one patient. Illustrated on the **right** are the 21.3-nm microtubules characteristic of most cases of ITG. Arrowheads indicate an electron-lucent core in amyloid **(center)** and immunotactoid fibrils **(right)**. Uranyl acetate and lead citrate, ×118,000. (From Korbet SM, Schwartz MM, Rosenberg BF, et al. Immunotactoid glomerulopathy. Medicine 1985;64:228.)

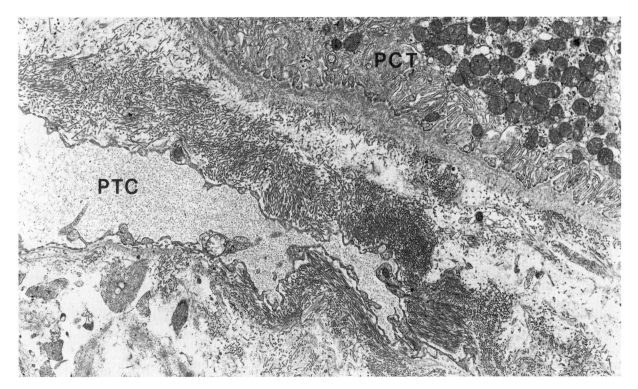

**Figure 20.22** Immunotactoid glomerulopathy. Extraglomerular immunotactoids are present in the interstitium, concentrated around a peritubular capillary (PTC). This feature was seen in only one of four biopsies from this patient. PCT, proximal convoluted tubules. (Uranyl acetate and lead citrate, ×19,000.) (From Korbet SM, Schwartz MM, Rosenberg BF, et al. Immunotactoid glomerulopathy. Medicine 1985;64:228.)

(85) and the lung (83,84). In these cases there was clinical evidence of extrarenal disease, but when clinically uninvolved organs were studied, deposits were not present (92). In an autopsy study of a patient with ITG, random sections of liver, spleen, heart, and skin did not contain organized deposits and the sections were Congo red–negative. Furthermore, there was no evidence of plasma cell dyscrasia or lymphoproliferative disease (68).

## Etiology and Pathogenesis

The etiology and pathogenesis of ITG are unknown, and there are no clinical or experimental data to suggest that deposits with different-sized and organized fibrils/tubules have separate causes or pathogenetic mechanisms. Any proposed pathogenic mechanism must account for three general features of ITG, however: lymphocytes or plasma cells produce the immunoglobulins found in the deposits; the precursors reach the kidney via the circulation; and the deposits are predominant in the glomeruli. The first two features suggest that the pathogenesis of ITG is similar to that of cryoglobulinemia or monoclonal gammopathy. Because cryoglobulins and paraproteins constitute exclusions from the diagnosis of ITG, the immunoglobulin must circulate in quantities that escape routine testing. It is also possible that non–cold precipitable immunoglobulins or immune complexes that are able to form organized deposits in the glomerulus explain this phenomenon. Additionally, B-cell or plasma cell neoplasia is not a necessary condition because the glomerular deposits are polyclonal in most cases. The third feature implies a role for local factors in fibrillogenesis. For example, plasma concentration produced by glomerular ultrafiltration may be a prerequisite for fibril formation.

The ultrastructural similarities between ITG and amyloidosis suggest that the pathogenesis of the two conditions is similar, and the morphologic and immunologic heterogeneity of the glomerular deposits in ITG may be the result of several mechanisms and precursors analogous to amyloid fibril formation. Yang et al (98) studied the relationship between amyloid and ITG and showed that in their patients the fibrils contained amyloid P component in addition to γ heavy chain and both κ and λ light chains and C3. GBM matrix proteins (type IV collagen, heparan sulfate proteoglycan, fibronectin, and fibrillin) were not present. The presence of amyloid P component suggests that the fibrils in ITG form in an analogous fashion to amyloid, but the final product does not form a beta pleated sheet and thus, is Congo red–negative. Casanova et al (92) stained the fibrils for IgG, both light chains, and C3, but they did not contain amyloid fibril proteins. In both studies (92,98), protein A gold immunoelectron microscopy demonstrated that the positive elements were localized to the fibrils, leading to the conclusion that all the pathologic immunoglobulins were present in an organized state. Neither group

studied examples of ITG with tubules 30 nm or more in diameter.

It cannot be assumed that deposits with different appearances have different compositions. Rastagno et al (88) reported a unique case in which biochemically identical fibrils were seen in the glomeruli and in a serum precipitate that formed after four months at 4°C. The fibronectin content of the fibrils, seen in the glomeruli and in the serum precipitate, suggested that fibronectin plays a role in fibrillogenesis. Although that remains a possibility in their unique case, the authors failed to find fibronectin in the glomerular deposits in other patients with FGN (98). The extreme conditions required to form the cryoprecipitate (4 months at 4°C) and its failure to dissolve on rewarming suggest that it is not a classic cryoglobulin. Furthermore, the fibrils appeared quite different in the glomeruli and the cryoprecipitate: The serum fibrils were large (diameter 90 nm) and showed periodicity in contrast to those in the glomeruli that were 15 to 20 nm without periodicity. The role of physical conditions and the glomerular environment illustrated in this case supports our original conjecture that the filtration somehow favors fibrillogenesis and precipitation (67,68,71).

Pathogenic speculation concerning ITG has focused on systemic factors such as the characteristics of normal or pathologic immunoglobulins whose properties favor glomerular precipitation and fibrillogenesis. Recurrent disease following renal transplantation supports a role for systemic factors (37,55,59,60,99). However, the absence of a demonstrable paraprotein and a population of neoplastic plasma cells or lymphocytes suggest that local glomerular factors are involved. The CD2-associated protein (CD2ap) knock-out mouse provides support for defective glomerular function in ITG and localizes the defect to the podocyte (100,101). CD2ap is an 80-kD protein found in the specialized junction between T lymphocytes and antigen-presenting cells (100,102), and it is also found throughout the developing and mature kidney (100). In the glomerulus, CD2ap binds to the cytoplasmic domain of nephrin, a key component of the podocyte slit diaphragm (100), where it contributes to the filtration barrier. CD2ap knock-out mice have congenital nephrotic syndrome and compromised immune function, and they die of renal failure 6 to 7 weeks after birth. The podocytes show pathologic changes (103), and the glomeruli have mesangial and subendothelial deposits of parallel arrays of tubules seen by electron microscopy (103). Although the composition of the tubules is unknown, the ultrastructural pathology is similar to that seen in ITG in human beings. Thus, it may be that glomerular deposits in ITG are secondary to acquired defects in critical podocyte cellular functions involved in the clearance of filtered and retained immunoglobulins. In addition, the organized nature of the deposits suggests that physicochemical homogeneity of the precursor molecules remains an important distinguishing pathogenetic feature between ITG and other primary immunoglobulin-mediated glomerular diseases in which the deposits are not organized.

## Clinical Course, Prognosis, Therapy, and Clinicopathologic Correlations

### Clinical Course and Prognosis

Renal insufficiency is a presenting feature in 50% of patients with ITG, and the disease progresses to end-stage renal disease in almost half the cases within 2 to 4 years of follow-up (37,59,63,64,69). Because systemic diseases or hematologic disorders associated with organized glomerular ultrastructural deposits are exclusions, the patients do not develop signs or symptoms related to these conditions. The renal course with persistent proteinuria, frequently in the nephrotic range, and the progressive loss of renal function is similar to that seen in other primary forms of glomerular disease.

### Therapy

There are case reports that suggest that treatment with prednisone and various immunosuppressive agents induces a reduction of protein excretion (74,77), but no statistically supported clinical trial has been published. The reports of therapeutic responses emphasize the critical importance of the definition of ITG. In one case, a patient with a malignant lymphoma reduced the level of proteinuria while being treated with alternate-day prednisone (46). In a small series, treatment with prednisone and various chemotherapeutic reagents led to a complete or partial remission of the nephrotic syndrome in five of seven patients with organized glomerular immunoglobulin deposits and malignant lymphoproliferative disease. However, there was a relapse of the nephrotic syndrome often accompanied by hematologic relapse in six of seven patients following treatment withdrawal (36). In these cases, reversal of renal disease is a known result of therapy of chronic lymphocytic lymphoma and leukemia (44). A patient with de novo ITG and hypocomplementemia following renal transplantation completely reversed massive subendothelial and focal mesangial immunotactoid deposits while on antirejection therapy (104). Although there were organized glomerular deposits in this case, the clinical setting and the presence of hypocomplementemia disqualify this case for the diagnosis of typical ITG. Therefore, treatment with steroids alone, steroids with plasma exchange, and steroids with cyclophosphamide have not been effective or offer limited benefit in the treatment of patients with ITG when underlying diseases that may respond to such treatment (cryoglobulinemia, lymphoproliferative malignancy, and systemic lupus erythematosus) are excluded (37,70,71).

Patients with ITG frequently present with renal insufficiency, and they have a progressive course that does not respond to current therapy. Because they generally do not have systemic involvement, their prognosis, independent of renal survival, is quite good. A limited number of patients with ITG have received renal transplants, and the disease recurred with identical immunopathology and ultrastructural pathology in the grafts and the native kidneys in approximately half of the cases (37,55,59,60,99). Although recurrent disease in one patient occurred 21 months after transplantation and led to graft loss 3 years later (100), graft function remained adequate after 5 to 11 years of follow-up in the others (37,55,59,60,99). There are three reports of de novo ITG following renal transplantation (37,83,104). Therefore, renal transplantation is appropriate therapy for patients with ITG that has reached end stage, and this good result is in contrast with the poor patient survival in primary amyloidosis (64).

### Clinicopathologic Correlations

The clinicopathologic correlation with the most potential is also the most controversial. It has been suggested that the tubular deposits with a lucent core and at least focal organization into parallel arrays (usually >30 nm) are associated with hematologic malignancy (37,41,46,69) and dysproteinemia (31,35,41,69), and smaller (<30 nm) randomly arranged fibrils are not. As Korbet et al (68,71) and others (59) have shown, this association is dependent on including patients with paraproteinemias in the diagnosis of ITG. When paraproteinemias are excluded, the prevalence of hematologic malignancy is equally low in patients with deposits smaller than 30 nm and in those with deposits 30 nm in diameter and larger. Nevertheless, the literature contains at least 47 cases reported with the diagnosis of ITG or one of its synonyms and an antecedent hematologic malignancy or monoclonal serum immunoglobulin (32,34,36,41,46,52,68,69,91,105). Twenty-five of these cases, including one reported by Korbet et al (68), had fibrils that were less than 30 nm in diameter and randomly oriented, demonstrating that the association with hematologic neoplasia is not limited to cases with larger microtubular deposits (106). In contrast, the glomeruli in the index case of ITG (67) contained monoclonal deposits of IgG that appeared as large-diameter (35.4 nm), closely packed tubules by electron microscopy. Repeated evaluations of the patient and his serum and bone marrow never had clinical or serologic evidence of dysproteinemia, cryoglobulinemia, lymphoproliferative disorder, or systemic disease. He progressed to end-stage kidney disease and died of unrelated causes after a clinical course that covered almost 18 years. There is a known association between hematologic malignancies and monoclonal gammopathy and organized glomerular deposits (see above), and the diagnosis of ITG should not include these patients.

More than 50% of patients with ITG progress to end-stage renal disease, and identification of those who will develop progressive renal disease has been a focus of clinical study. Korbet et al (68) followed 11 patients with ITG (mean fibril diameter <30 nm in 8 and 30 nm or more in 3) for a mean of 52.6 months (range 22 to 94 months), and 6 progressed to a serum creatinine greater than 5.0 mg/dL. Male gender, poorly controlled blood pressure, and nephrotic-range proteinuria were more prevalent in the patients who progressed compared with those who did not progress. The authors noted that the two patients with strictly mesangial involvement were in the nonprogressive group. Pronovost et al (59) stratified 25 patients with ITG/FGN (defined by fibril diameter and arrangement) into three groups according to the slope of 1/serum creatinine (1/Cr). Ten patients had no or slow progression (1/Cr = −0.103); nine had intermediate progression (1/Cr = 0.121); and six had rapid progression (1/Cr = 0.466). The three groups did not differ in age, the prevalence of hematuria and proteinuria, or the serum creatinine at presentation. Although patients with more rapid progression of renal dysfunction had a greater prevalence of nephrotic syndrome and worse hypertension, the differences were not statistically significant. Rosenstock et al (37) analyzed outcome in 56 patients with FGN (fiber diameter <30 nm), and after a mean of 23 months (range 0 to 128 months), 25 progressed to end-stage renal disease. The authors reported diverse patterns of glomerular pathology in FGN, and patients with pure mesangial and membranous patterns (times to end-stage renal disease 80 and 87 months, respectively) had longer renal survival than patients with membranoproliferative, diffuse proliferative, and diffuse sclerosing glomerulonephritis (times to end-stage renal disease 44, 20, and 7 months, respectively). In a univariate analysis of presenting clinical and pathologic findings, the histologic subtype, nephrotic syndrome, severity of interstitial disease, presence of crescents, percent crescents, hematocrit, level of protein excretion, serum creatinine, and the percentage of sclerotic glomeruli correlated with outcome. However, multivariate analysis showed that the initial serum creatinine and the severity of interstitial disease were the only clinical and pathologic features that independently predicted progression to end-stage renal disease.

## DISEASES WITH CONGO RED–NEGATIVE (NONAMYLOID) NON–IMMUNOGLOBULIN-DERIVED ORGANIZED DEPOSITS

Diseases with Congo red–negative deposits of diverse biochemical composition constitute a third group with organized glomerular deposits. There are collagen fibers in the thickened glomerular basal lamina in the *nail-*

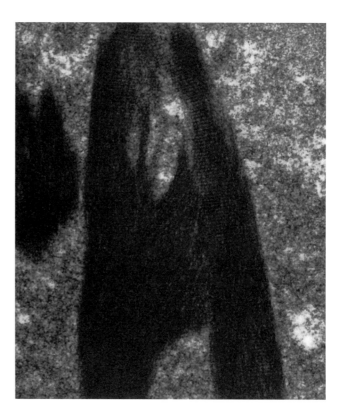

**Figure 20.23** Fibrin tactoids from a patient with chronic glomerulonephritis. Polymerized fibrin forms electron-dense, elongated masses with characteristic periodicity. (Uranyl acetate and lead citrate, ×30,000.)

*patella syndrome* and in the expanded subendothelium and mesangium in *collagenofibrotic nephropathy (type III collagen nephropathy)* (see Chapter 11). There may be deposits of fibrin in inflammatory glomerular diseases, and the polymerized fibrin usually forms amorphous electron-dense masses. Rarely, there are *fibrin tactoids* with typical periodicity (Fig. 20.23). The mesangium in diabetic glomerulosclerosis may contain 10- to 20-nm-diameter fibrils (Fig. 20.24). They are the postulated result of advanced glycosylation end product–related cross linking of normal matrix proteins (23,107) (see Chapter 18). *Fibronectin glomerulopathy* is a rare hereditary disease with glomerular fibronectin deposits that sometimes form organized deposits (see below).

Churg and Venkataseshan (66) reported three cases of glomerulopathy with Congo red–negative deposits that did not contain immunoglobulin, complement, or fibronectin. Electron microscopy demonstrated mesangial and tubular basement membrane fibrils measuring from 13 to 20 nm in diameter. The authors reported the cases to warn physicians of the possibility that a biochemical spectrum of organized deposits, including presently unidentified substances, may cause fibrillary glomerulonephritis. They used the term *fibrillary glomerulonephritis* to indicate the class of diseases with fibrillary deposits rather than a specific disease.

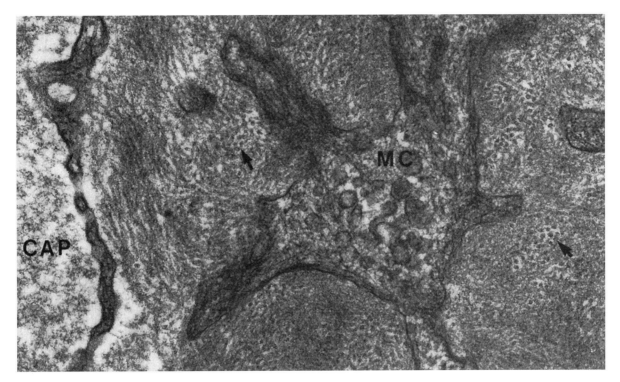

**Figure 20.24** Diabetes mellitus. The patient was a 25-year-old man with insulin-dependent diabetes mellitus for 9 years and proteinuria for 2 years. The mesangium was diffusely expanded by PAS-positive matrix, and there was diffuse linear staining of the GBM for IgG. The mesangium, underlying the capillary lumen (CAP), contains randomly arranged, 16-nm tubules that have an electron-lucent center in cross section (*arrows*). MC, mesangial cell. (Uranyl acetate and lead citrate, ×70,000.) (From Korbet SM, Schwartz MM, Lewis EJ. The fibrillary glomerulopathies. Am J Kidney Dis 1994;23: 751.)

Ferluga et al (108) reported a case of advanced diabetic nodular glomerular sclerosis that also had prominent subendothelial deposits of microtubules, 67 nm in diameter, with similar localization of IgG, IgM, κ, λ, C3, and fibrin. The patient had an IgG-IgM cryoglobulinemia (200 mg/L) that provides an alternative explanation for the organized deposits. However, as our experience with glomerular disease with organized deposits accumulates, it is predictable that further biochemically specific forms of fibrillary glomerulonephritis will be recognized (109,110), further clinical associations will be recognized (8,78), and cases with more than one population of organized deposits will be reported (39).

## Fibronectin Nephropathy

Fibronectin nephropathy (FN), a disease with an autosomal dominant mode of inheritance, presents with proteinuria and slowly progressive loss of renal function. It was first reported as an atypical form of lobular glomerulonephritis with massive subendothelial and mesangial, focally fibrillar, electron-dense deposits that did not stain for immunoglobulins and complement (41,111–113). Once fibronectin was identified as a major component of

the deposits (66,114,115), the initially identified families were restudied, and the deposits were shown to contain fibronectin (116). Since the last edition of *Heptinstall's Pathology of the Kidney*, further cases have accumulated (117,118).

Twenty-eight patients with FN (66,114,116) were 29.4 ± 15 years old at the time of diagnosis. All but two of the patients (66) had an affected first-degree relative, and the disease presented in parents and children of either sex and in multiple siblings. Proteinuria was the most common presentation (26 of 28), and in 12 patients it was in the nephrotic range (at least 3 g/24 hours). Twelve of 19 patients had microscopic hematuria, and mild hypertension was present in 11 of 19 patients. There were no consistent serologic abnormalities, and fibronectin levels were normal. Renal function was initially abnormal (elevated serum creatinine) in 5 of 21 patients. Despite persistent high-grade proteinuria, after 6.6 ± 4.2 years of follow-up, only 5 patients reached end-stage renal disease and required dialysis. However, 13 affected family members in one large kindred progressed to end-stage renal disease (119). Four patients received renal transplants, and 1 had a recurrence 27 months posttransplantation that progressed to graft failure.

The principal *light microscopic change* is glomerular enlargement and lobulation resulting from PAS and trichrome-positive mesangial deposits and mild mesangial proliferation (Fig. 20.25). This process displaces the glomerular capillaries to the periphery of the lobule and decreases their luminal diameters. With the Jones stain, the preserved GBM is usually at the periphery of the thickened capillary wall, and focal areas of duplication and subepithelial spikes are inconstant (112). There are no specific changes in the renal tubules, interstitium, and blood vessels. Special stains for amyloid are negative. By *immunofluorescence microscopy*, the glomeruli do not consistently stain for immunoglobulin or complement components. However, one case (111) did have intense mesangial and parietal staining for IgG and C3, and two patients (116) had positive staining for IgG, IgM, C3, and fibrinogen. In contrast, immunohistologic stains for fibronectin are strongly positive in all cases in the same mesangial and subendothelial location as the PAS-positive deposits. The most consistent *ultrastructural finding* is large (giant), mesangial and subendothelial electron-dense deposits that mirror the location

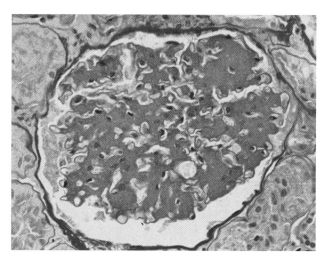

**Figure 20.25** Hereditary glomerulopathy with fibronectin deposits. The glomerulus shows massive mesangial expansion by intensely PAS positive deposits that were silver- and Congo red–negative. Note the capillaries remain patent although reduced in size at the periphery of the expanded lobules. Kidney biopsy from a 22-year-old man with a strong family history of renal disease and proteinuria of 604 mg/24 hours and normal renal function. (PAS, ×235.) (Photomicrograph prepared from material supplied by Dr. Daniel D. Sedmak.)

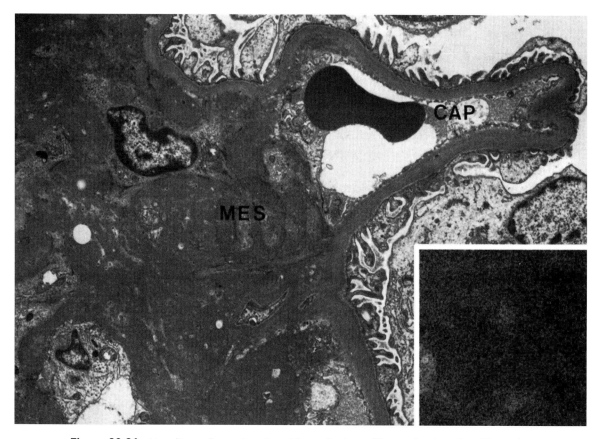

**Figure 20.26** Hereditary glomerulopathy with predominant fibronectin deposits. Glomerulus showing massive mesangial (MES) electron-dense deposits. Although there were focal subendothelial electron-dense deposits, the capillary (CAP) illustrated is free of deposits. (Uranyl acetate and lead citrate, ×6250.) **Inset:** High magnification of the deposits shows poorly formed, short microtubules with the suggestion of a hollow core. (Uranyl acetate and lead citrate, ×75,000.) (Electron micrographs prepared from material supplied by Dr. Daniel D. Sedmak).

of the PAS-positive, fibronectin deposits (Fig. 20.26). The GBM is usually normal and not directly involved (114,116), but subepithelial and intramembranous deposits were seen in one family (112). Extraglomerular deposits are infrequent, but they have been described in the basement membrane of Bowman's capsule (112) and the tubular basement membrane (113). The electron-dense deposits are predominantly amorphous and granular, but they may contain electron-lucent areas and scattered, focal fine filaments 10 to 14 nm in diameter (112,114–116). The morphology of the deposits falls between the highly organized fibrils derived from mutant protein precursors seen in hereditary amyloidosis and the amorphous, infrequently fibrillar deposits of abnormal light chains in MIDD (see Chapter 28).

Fibronectin is a multifunctional, extracellular matrix glycoprotein that is active in cellular adhesion and migration. Fibronectin is produced locally in the glomerulus by mesangial cells (cellular fibronectin), and the liver synthesizes fibronectin isoforms that circulate (plasma fibronectin). Upregulation of fibronectin production occurs in diverse glomerular diseases (120). Massive glomerular accumulation of plasma fibronectin, the central pathogenetic event in FN, implies that the precursor is derived from the circulation (114,116), but plasma levels of fibronectin are not elevated (115). Therefore, plasma fibronectin accumulates because either the clearance mechanism is faulty or the fibronectin is in a form that frustrates normal clearance mechanisms. Because other extracellular matrix proteins and immunoglobulins are inconstantly present in the deposits (114,116), a general defect of mesangial clearance is unlikely. Haplotype analysis in a 197-member pedigree with 13 relatives developing end-stage renal failure from the disease excluded mutations in fibronectin as the cause of the glomerulopathy (121). Although the gene has not been identified, Vollmer et al (122) postulated a genetic defect in a circulating factor that binds to fibronectin and leads to its glomerular retention. This is the apparent mechanism of glomerular localization of fibronectin in the uteroglobin knock-out mouse (123), but uteroglobin has been excluded from the pathogenesis of fibronectin glomerulopathy (124) in human beings. Vollmer et al (124) mapped the gene to a 4.1-cM interval on chromosome 1q32, and they propose a candidate gene from the regulation of complement activation cluster that is localized to this region. Interestingly, amyloid P component has been demonstrated in the deposits of one patient with FN (114), an observation that may explain the fibrillar organization seen in some cases.

## REFERENCES

1. Stoebner P, Renversez J, Groulade J, et al. Ultrastructural study of human IgG and IgG-IgM crystal cryoglobulins. Am J Clin Pathol 1979;71:404.
2. Dales S, Wallace AC. Nuclear pore complexes deposited in the glomerular basement membrane are associated with autoantibodies in a case of membranous nephritis. J Immunol 1985;134:1588.
3. Matsuyama N, Joh K, Yamaguchi Y, et al. Crystalline inclusions in the glomerular podocytes in a patient with benign monoclonal gammopathy and focal segmental glomerulosclerosis. Am J Kidney Dis 1994;23:859.
4. Grishman E, Porush JC, Rosen SM, Churg J. Lupus nephritis with organized deposits in the kidneys. Lab Invest 1967;16:717.
5. Nabarra B, Larquet E, Diemert MC, et al. Unusual IgM fibrillar deposits in glomerulonephritis: Ultrastructural and diffraction studies in a case report. Hum Pathol 2003;34:1350.
6. Duffy JL, Khurana E, Susin M, et al. Fibrillary renal deposits and nephritis. Am J Pathol 1983;113:279.
7. Glenner GG. Amyloid deposits and amyloidosis. The beta-fibrilloses (first of two parts). N Engl J Med 1980;302:1283.
8. Markowitz GS, Cheng JT, Colvin RB, et al. Hepatitis C viral infection is associated with fibrillary glomerulonephritis and immunotactoid glomerulopathy. J Am Soc Nephrol 1998;9:2244.
9. Brouet J, Clauvel J, Danon F, et al. Biologic and clinical significance of cryoglobulins: A report of 86 cases. Am J Med 1974;57:775.
10. Gorevic PD, Kassab HJ, Levo Y, et al. Mixed cryoglobulinemia: Clinical aspects and long-term follow-up of 40 patients. Am J Med 1980;69:287.
11. Gorevic PD, Frangione B. Mixed cryoglobulinemia cross-reactive idiotypes: Implications for the relationship of MC to rheumatic and lymphoproliferative diseases. Semin Hematol 1991;28:79.
12. Monteverde A, Rivano MT, Allegra GC, et al. Essential mixed cryoglobulinemia, type II: A manifestation of a low-grade malignant lymphoma? Clinical-morphological study of 12 cases with special reference to immunohistochemical findings in liver frozen sections. Acta Haematol 1988;79:20.
13. D'Amico G, Colasanti G, Ferrario F, Sinico RA. Renal involvement in essential mixed cryoglobulinemia. Kidney Int 1989;35:1004.
14. Faraggiana T, Parolini C, Previato G, Lupo A. Light and electron microscopic findings in five cases of cryoglobulinemic glomerulonephritis. Virchows Arch A Pathol Anat Histol 1979;384:29.
15. Feiner H, Gallo G. Ultrastructure in glomerulonephritis associated with cryoglobulinemia: A report of six cases and a review of the literature. Am J Pathol 1977;88:145.
16. Tarantino A, De Vecchi A, Montagnino G, et al. Renal disease in essential mixed cryoglobulinemia. Q J Med 1981;197:1.
17. Ogihara T, Saruta T, Saito I, et al. Finger print deposits of the kidney in pure monoclonal IgG kappa cryoglobulinemia. Clin Nephrol 1979;12:186.
18. Kowalewska J, Tomford RC, Alpers CE. Crystals in podocytes: An unusual manifestation of systemic disease. Am J Kidney Dis 2003;42:605.
19. Verroust P, Mery J-P, Morel-Maroger L, et al. Glomerular lesions in monoclonal gammopathies and mixed essential cryoglobulinemias IgG-IgM. Adv Nephrol 1971;1:161.
20. Buxbaum JN, Chuba JV, Hellman GC, et al. Monoclonal immunoglobulin deposition disease: Light chain and light and heavy chain deposition diseases and their relation to light chain amyloidosis: Clinical features, immunopathology, and molecular analysis. Ann Intern Med 1990;112:455.
21. Preud'homme J-L, Aucouturier P, Touchard G, et al. Monoclonal immunoglobulin deposition disease (Randall type): Relationship with structural abnormalities of immunoglobulin chains. Kidney Int 1994;46:965.
22. Alpers CE, Hopper J, Biava CG. Light-chain glomerulopathy with amyloid-like deposits. Hum Pathol 1984;15:444.
23. Bruneval P, Foidart JM, Nochy D, et al. Glomerular matrix proteins in nodular glomerulosclerosis in association with light chain deposition disease and diabetes mellitus. Hum Pathol 1985;16:477.
24. Gallo GR, Feiner HD, Katz LA, et al. Nodular glomerulopathy associated with nonamyloidotic kappa light chain deposits

and excess immunoglobulin light chain synthesis. Am J Pathol 1980;99:621.

25. Gipstein R, Cohen A, Adams D, et al. Kappa light chain nephropathy without evidence of myeloma cells: Response to chemotherapy with cessation of maintenance hemodialysis. Am J Nephrol 1982;2:276.

26. Zhu L, Herrera GA, Murphy-Ullrich JE, et al. Pathogenesis of glomerulosclerosis in light chain deposition disease: Role for transforming growth factor-beta. Am J Pathol 1995;147:375.

27. Kyle RA. Monoclonal gammopathy of undetermined significance. Blood Rev 1994;8:135.

28. Ganeval D, Noel LH, Preud'homme JL, et al. Light-chain deposition disease: Its relation with AL-type amyloidosis. Kidney Int 1984;26:1.

29. Kyle RA, Greipp PR. Amyloidosis (AL): Clinical and laboratory features in 229 cases. Mayo Clin Proc 1983;58:665.

30. Kyle RA, Garton JP. The spectrum of IgM monoclonal gammopathy in 430 cases. Mayo Clin Proc 1987;62:719.

31. Cadnapaphornchai P, Sillix D. Recurrence of monoclonal gammopathy-related glomerulonephritis in renal allograft. Clin Nephrol 1989;31:156.

32. Esparza AR, Chazan JA, Nayak RN, Cavallo T. Fibrillary (immunotactoid) glomerulopathy: A possible role for kappa light chain in its etiology and/or pathogenesis. Am J Surg Pathol 1991;15:632.

33. Kebler R, Kithier K, McDonald F, Cadnapaphornchai P. Rapidly progressive glomerulonephritis and monoclonal gammopathy. Am J Med 1985;78:133.

34. Orfila C, Meeus F, Bernadet P, et al. Immunotactoid glomerulopathy and cutaneous vasculitis. Am J Nephrol 1991;11:67.

35. Rollino C, Coppo R, Mazzucco G, et al. Monoclonal gammopathy and glomerulonephritis with organized microtubular deposits. Am J Kid Dis 1990;15:276.

36. Bridoux F, Hugue V, Coldefy O, et al. Fibrillary glomerulonephritis and immunotactoid (microtubular) glomerulopathy are associated with distinct immunologic features. Kidney Int 2002;62:1764.

37. Rosenstock JL, Markowitz GS, Valeri AM, et al. Fibrillary and immunotactoid glomerulonephritis: Distinct entities with different clinical and pathologic features. Kidney Int 2003;63:1450.

38. Da'as N, Kleinman Y, Polliack A, et al. Immunotactoid glomerulopathy with massive bone marrow deposits in a patient with IgM kappa monoclonal gammopathy and hypocomplementemia. Am J Kidney Dis 2001;38:395.

39. Mukai K, Kitazawa K, Totsuka D, et al. A case of immunotactoid glomerulopathy with unusual microtubular deposits. Clin Nephrol 1998;49:321.

40. Pauecksakon P, Revelo MP, Horn RG, et al. Monoclonal gammopathy: Significance and possible causality in renal disease. Am J Kidney Dis 2003;42:87.

41. Alpers CE. Immunotactoid (microtubular) glomerulopathy: An entity distinct from fibrillary glomerulonephritis? Am J Kidney Dis 1992;19:185.

42. Duwaji MS, Shemin DG, Medeiros LJ, Esparza AR. Proliferative glomerulonephritis with unusual, organized, cylindrical deposits associated with angioimmunoblastic lymphadenopathy-like T-cell lymphoma. Arch Pathol Lab Med 1995;119:377.

43. Moulin B, Ronco PM, Mougenot B, et al. Glomerulonephritis in chronic lymphocytic leukemia and related B-cell lymphomas. Kidney Int 1992;42:127.

44. Touchard G, Preud'homme JL, Aucouturier P, et al. Nephrotic syndrome associated with chronic lymphocytic leukemia: An immunological and pathological study. Clin Nephrol 1989;31:107.

45. Galea HR, Bridoux F, Aldigier JC, et al. Molecular study of an IgG1kappa cryoglobulin yielding organized microtubular deposits and glomerulonephritis in the course of chronic lymphocytic leukaemia. Clin Exp Immunol 2002;129:113.

46. Rosenmann E, Brisson M, Bercovitch D, Rosenberg A. Atypical membranous glomerulonephritis with fibrillar subepithelial deposits in a patient with malignant lymphoma. Nephron 1988;48:226.

47. Garibaldi DC, Gottsch J, de la Cruz Z, et al. Immunotactoid keratopathy: A clinicopathologic case report and a review of reports of corneal involvement in systemic paraproteinemias. Surv Ophthalmol 2005;50:61.

48. Jacobson E, Sharp G, Rimmer J, MacPherson B. A 59-year-old woman with immunotactoid glomerulopathy, heavy-chain disease, and non-Hodgkin lymphoma. Arch Pathol Lab Med 2004;128:689.

49. Tan EM, Cohen AS, Fries JF, et al. The 1982 revised criteria for the classification of systemic lupus erythematosus. Arthritis Rheum 1982;25:1271.

50. Hvala A, Kobenter T, Ferluga D. Fingerprint and other organised deposits in lupus nephritis. Wiener Klinische Wochenschrift 2000;112:711.

51. Kim YH, Choi YJ, Reiner L. Ultrastructural "fingerprint" in cryoprecipitate and glomerular deposits: A case report of systemic lupus erythematosus. Hum Pathol 1981;12:86.

52. Lai FM, Lai KN, Li EK, et al. Immunotactoid glomerulopathy with fingerprint immune deposits: A variant of lupus nephritis? Virchows Arch A Pathol Anat Histopathol 1989;415:181.

53. Hvala A, Ferluga D, Vizjak A, Koselj-Kajtna M. Fibrillary noncongophilic renal and extrarenal deposits: A report on 10 cases. Ultrastruct Pathol 2003;27:341.

54. Rosenmann E, Eliakim M. Nephrotic syndrome associated with amyloid-like glomerular deposits. Nephron 1977;18:301.

55. Sturgill BC, Bolton WK. Non-amyloidotic fibrillary glomerulopathy. Kidney Int 1989;35:233.

56. Neill J, Rubin J. Nonamyloidotic fibrillary glomerulopathy. Arch Pathol Lab Med 1989;113:553.

57. Sturgill BC, Bolton WK, Griffith KM. Congo red–negative amyloidosis-like glomerulopathy. Hum Pathol 1985;16:220.

58. Kobayashi Y, Fujii K, Kurokawa A, et al. Glomerulonephropathy with amyloid-stain–negative microfibrillar glomerular deposits. Nephron 1988;48:33.

59. Pronovost PH, Brady HR, Gunning ME, et al. Clinical features, predictors of disease progression and results of renal transplantation in fibrillary/immunotactoid glomerulopathy. Nephrol Dial Transplant 1996;11:837.

60. Alpers CE, Rennke HG, Hopper J, Biava CG. Fibrillary glomerulonephritis: An entity with unusual immunofluorescence features. Kidney Int 1987;31:781.

61. D'Agati V, Sacchi G, Truong L, et al. Fibrillary glomerulopathy: Defining the disease spectrum. J Am Soc Nephrol 1991;2:591.

62. Perry GJ, Lin BP, Wyndham RN, Kalowski S. Fibrillary glomerulonephritis: A report of two cases. Aust NZ J Med 1989;19:250.

63. Iskandar SS, Falk RJ, Jennette JC. Clinical and pathologic features of fibrillary glomerulonephritis. Kidney Int 1992;42:1401.

64. Korbet SM, Schwartz MM, Lewis EJ. The fibrillary glomerulopathies. Am J Kidney Dis 1994;23:751.

65. Schwartz MM. Renal amyloidosis and other fibrillar glomerular diseases. Curr Opin Nephrol Hypertens 1993;2:238.

66. Churg J, Venkataseshan VS. Fibrillary glomerulonephritis without immunoglobulin deposits in the kidney. Kidney Int 1993;44:837.

67. Schwartz MM, Lewis EJ. The quarterly case: Nephrotic syndrome in a middle-aged man. Ultrastruct Pathol 1980;1:575.

68. Korbet SM, Schwartz MM, Rosenberg BF, et al. Immunotactoid glomerulopathy. Medicine 1985;64:228.

69. Fogo A, Qureshi N, Horn RG. Morphologic and clinical features of fibrillary glomerulonephritis versus immunotactoid glomerulopathy. Am J Kidney Dis 1993;22:367.

70. Brady HR. Fibrillary glomerulopathy. Kidney Int 1998;53:1421.

71. Korbet SM, Schwartz MM, Lewis EJ. Immunotactoid glomerulopathy. Am J Kidney Dis 1991;17:247.

72. Kawashima M, Horita S, Nakayama H, et al. Immunoelectron microscopic analysis of intraglomerular deposits in IgA-dominant immunotactoid glomerulopathy [in Japanese]. Rinsho Byori Jpn J Clinl Pathol 2002;50:1085.

73. van Ginneken EE, Assmann KJ, Koolen MI, et al. Fibrillary-immunotactoid glomerulopathy with renal deposits of

IgAlambda: A rare cause of glomerulonephritis. Clin Nephrol 1999;52:383.

74. Dickenmann M, Schaub S, Nickeleit V, et al. Fibrillary glomerulonephritis: Early diagnosis associated with steroid responsiveness. Am J Kidney Dis 2002;40:E9.

75. Adeyi OA, Sethi S, Rennke HG. Fibrillary glomerulonephritis: A report of 2 cases with extensive glomerular and tubular deposits. Hum Pathol 2001;32:660.

76. Sethi S, Adeyi OA, Rennke HG. A case of fibrillary glomerulonephritis with linear immunoglobulin G staining of the glomerular capillary walls. Arch Pathol Lab Med 2001;125:534.

77. Kurosu M, Ando Y, Takeda S, et al. Immunotactoid glomerulopathy characterized by steroid-responsive massive subendothelial deposition. Am J Kidney Dis 2001;7:E21.

78. Aviles DH, Craver R, Warrier RP. Immunotactoid glomerulopathy in sickle cell anemia. Pediatr Nephrol 2001;16:82.

79. Cheah PL, Looi LM, Ghazalli R, Chua CT. Immunotactoid glomerulopathy: An unusual deposition disease: Report of the first Malaysian case. Malay J Pathol 1999;21:59.

80. Korbet SM, Genchi RM, Borok RZ, Schwartz MM. The racial prevalence of glomerular lesions in nephrotic adults. Am J Kidney Dis 1996;27:647.

81. Chung WY, Lee SY, Joo JE. Fibrillary glomerulonephritis in a 9-year-old girl. Nephron 1995;69:79.

82. Takemura T, Yoshioka K, Akano N, et al. Immunotactoid glomerulopathy in a child with Down syndrome. Pediatr Nephrol 1993;7:86.

83. Calls GJ, Torras A, Ricart MJ, et al. Fibrillary glomerulonephritis and pulmonary hemorrhage in a patient with renal transplantation. Clin Nephrol 1995;43:180.

84. Masson RG, Rennke HG, Gottlieb MN. Pulmonary hemorrhage in a patient with fibrillary glomerulonephritis. N Engl J Med 1992;326:36.

85. Ozawa K, Yamabe H, Fukushi K, et al. Case report of amyloid-like glomerulopathy with hepatic involvement. Nephron 1991;58:347.

86. Sabatine MS, Aretz HT, Fang LS, Dec GW. Images in cardiovascular medicine: Fibrillary/immunotactoid glomerulopathy with cardiac involvement. Circulation 2002;105:e120.

87. Adey DB, MacPherson BR, Groggel GC. Glomerulonephritis with associated hypocomplementemia and crescents: An unusual case of fibrillary glomerulonephritis. J Am Soc Nephrol 1995;6:171.

88. Rostagno A, Vidal R, Kumar A, et al. Fibrillary glomerulonephritis related to serum fibrillar immunoglobulin-fibronectin complexes. Am J Kidney Dis 1996;28:676.

89. Rovin BH, Bou-Khalil P, Sedmak D. Pulmonary-renal syndrome in a patient with fibrillary glomerulonephritis. Am J Kidney Dis 1993;22:713.

90. Devaney K, Sabnis S, Antonovych T. Nonamyloidotic fibrillary glomerulonephritis, immunotactoid glomerulopathy, and the differential diagnosis of filamentous glomerulopathies. Mod Pathol 1991;4:36.

91. Yeun JY, Whitaker WR, Garcia-Kennedy R, et al. Fibrillary glomerulonephritis: A case report. Am J Kidney Dis 1991;18:131.

92. Casanova S, Donini U, Zucchelli P, et al. Immunohistochemical distinction between amyloidosis and fibrillary glomerulopathy. Am J Clin Pathol 1992;97:787.

93. Mazzucco G, Casanova S, Donini U, et al. Glomerulonephritis with organized deposits: A new clinicopathologic entity? Light-electron-microscopic and immunofluorescence study of 12 cases. Am J Nephrol 1990;10:21.

94. Olesnicky L, Doty SB, Bertani T, Pirani CL. Tubular microfibrils in the glomeruli of membranous nephropathy. Arch Pathol Lab Med 1984;108:902.

95. Sadjadi SA, Sobel HJ. Congo red-negative amyloidosis-like glomerulopathy: Report of a case. Am J Kidney Dis 1987;9:231.

96. Schifferli JA, Merot Y, Chatelanat F. Immunotactoid glomerulopathy with leukocytoclastic skin vasculitis and hypocomplementemia: A case report. Clin Nephrol 1987;27:151.

97. Griffel B, Bernheim J. Glomerular deposits in idiopathic membranous glomerulopathy. Arch Pathol Lab Med 1980;104:56.

98. Yang GCH, Nieto R, Stachura I, Gallo GR. Ultrastructural immunohistochemical localization of polyclonal IgG, C3, and amyloid P component on the congo red-negative amyloid-like fibrils of fibrillary glomerulopathy. Am J Pathol 1992;141:409.

99. Korbet SM, Rosenberg BF, Schwartz MM, Lewis EJ. Course of renal transplantation in immunotactoid glomerulopathy. Am J Med 1990;89:91.

100. Li C, Ruotsalainen V, Tryggvason K, et al. CD2AP is expressed with nephrin in developing podocytes and is found widely in mature kidney and elsewhere. Am J Physiol Renal Physiol 2000;279:F785.

101. Take H, Watanabe S, Takeda K, et al. Cloning and characterization of a novel adaptor protein, CIN85, that interacts with c-Cbl. Biochem Biophys Res Commun 2000;268:321.

102. Dustin ML, Olszowy MW, Holdorf AD, et al. A novel adaptor protein orchestrates receptor patterning and cytoskeletal polarity in T-cell contacts. Cell 1998;94:667.

103. Shih NY, Li J, Karpitskii V, Nguyen A, et al. Congenital nephrotic syndrome in mice lacking CD2-associated protein. Science 1999;286:312.

104. Rao KV, Hafner GP, Crary GS, et al. De novo immunotactoid glomerulopathy of the renal allograft: Possible association with cytomegalovirus infection. Am J Kidney Dis 1994;24:97.

105. Abraham G, Bargman JM, Blake PG, et al. Fibrillary glomerulonephritis in a patient with metastatic carcinoma of the liver. Am J Nephrol 1990;10:251.

106. Verani RR. Fibrillary glomerulonephritis. Kidney 1993;2:63.

107. Sohar E, Ravid M, Ben Shaul Y, et al. Diabetic fibrillosis: A report of three cases. Am J Med 1970;49:64.

108. Ferluga D, Hvala A, Vizjak A, et al. Immunotactoid glomerulopathy with unusually thick extracellular microtubules and nodular glomerulosclerosis in a diabetic patient. Pathol Res Pract 1995;191:585.

109. Hill P, Dwyer K, Kay T, Murphy B. Severe chronic renal failure in association with oxycodone addiction: A new form of fibrillary glomerulopathy. Hum Pathol 2002;33:783.

110. Akimoto H, Shirai M, Usutani S, et al. Membranoproliferative glomerulonephritis-like lesion with fibrillary deposition associated with multicentric Castleman's disease. Nippon Jinzo Gakkai Shi 1998;40:301.

111. Abt AB, Wassner SJ, Moran JJ. Familial lobular glomerulopathy. Hum Pathol 1991;22:825.

112. Burgin M, Hofmann E, Reutter FW, et al. Familial glomerulopathy with giant fibrillar deposits. Virchows Arch A Pathol Anat Histol 1980;388:313.

113. Tuttle SE, Sharma HM, Bay W, Hebert L. A unique familial lobular glomerulopathy. Arch Pathol Lab Med 1987;111:726.

114. Assmann KJ, Koene RA, Wetzels JF. Familial glomerulonephritis characterized by massive deposits of fibronectin. Am J Kidney Dis 1995;25:781.

115. Mazzucco G, Maran E, Rollino C, Monga G. Glomerulonephritis with organized deposits: A mesangiopathic, not immune complex-mediated disease? A pathologic study of two cases in the same family. Hum Pathol 1992;23:63.

116. Strom EH, Banfi G, Krapf R, et al. Glomerulopathy associated with predominant fibronectin deposits: A newly recognized hereditary disease. Kidney Int 1995;48:163.

117. Niimi K, Tsuru N, Uesugi N, Takebayashi S. Fibronectin glomerulopathy with nephrotic syndrome in a 3-year-old male. Pediatr Nephrol 2002;17:363.

118. Uesugi N, Katafuchi R, Taguchi H, et al. Clinicopathological and morphometrical analysis of 5 cases from 4 families of fibronectin glomerulopathy. Nippon Jinzo Gakkai Shi Jpn J Nephrol 1999;41:49.

119. Vollmer M, Jung M, Ruschendorf F, et al. The gene for human fibronectin glomerulopathy maps to 1q32, in the region of the regulation of complement activation gene cluster. Am J Hum Genet 1998;63:1724.

120. Assad L, Schwartz MM, Virtanen I, Gould VE. Immunolocalization of tenascin and cellular fibronectins in diverse glomerulopathies. Virchows Arch B Cell Pathol Incl Mol Pathol 1993;63:307.

121. Hildebrandt F, Strahm B, Prochoroff A, et al. Glomerulopathy associated with predominant fibronectin deposits: Exclusion of the genes for fibronectin, villin and desmin as causative genes. Am J Med Genet 1996;63:323.

122. Vollmer M, Kremer M, Ruf R, et al. Molecular cloning of the critical region for glomerulopathy with fibronectin deposits (GFND) and evaluation of candidate genes. Genomics 2000;68:127.

123. Zhang Z, Kundu GC, Yuan CJ, et al. Severe fibronectin-deposit renal glomerular disease in mice lacking uteroglobin. Science 1997;276:1408.

124. Vollmer M, Krapf R, Hildebrandt F. Exclusion of the uteroglobin gene as a candidate for fibronectin glomerulopathy (GFND). Nephrol Dial Transplant 1998;13:2417.

# Renal Disease Caused by Hypertension

*Jean L. Olson*

## DEFINITION

Hypertension, or increased blood pressure, is a worldwide problem with a prevalence of greater than 1 billion people (1). The Joint National Committee on Prevention, Detection, Evaluation, and Treatment of High Blood Pressure (JNC-7) has published guidelines for the classification of different levels of blood pressure (1), as follows: normal pressure is considered to be less than 120/80 mm Hg, prehypertension is 120 to 139/80 to 89 mm Hg, stage 1 hypertension is 140 to 159/90 to 99 mm Hg, stage 2 hypertension is greater than 160/100 mm Hg. Awareness of the importance of hypertension has increased in the general population as well as among medical professionals, and more people receive antihypertensive medications. This greater awareness accompanied by more effective treatment has led to reductions in the rates of both cardiovascular disease and stroke, well-known complications of hypertension over the past 20 years (1). However, the prevalence of hypertension has increased to 31.3% of adult Americans parallel to an increase in obesity and decrease in physical activity (2). Using data from the NHANES III study and the new definitions of hypertension from the JNC-7 report, Qureshi et al (3) found an estimated 80 million Americans with prehypertension, 25 million with stage 1 hypertension, and 11 million with stage 2 hypertension.

Hypertension can have a known cause, such as renal artery stenosis, but in most cases, the etiologic factors are unknown, and the condition is deemed "essential" hypertension. The prevalence of the secondary forms of hypertension, in which the cause can be determined, is generally thought to be 5% (4). This chapter covers all forms of hypertension but focuses mainly on essential hypertension.

## ESSENTIAL HYPERTENSION

### Clinical Presentation

### Prevalence, Age, and Gender

The prevalence of hypertension is estimated to be 31.3% in the adult population of the United States for the years 1999 to 2000 when one includes patients using antihypertensive agents (2). Each year, an additional 3 million adult residents of the United States are diagnosed with hypertension (2). Furthermore, 140,000 patients with hypertension show signs of increased serum creatinine levels, and 5300 hypertensive patients with a history of renal insufficiency (generally with a glomerular filtration rate [GFR] <50 mL/min) progress to end-stage renal disease (ESRD) each year. ESRD may be defined as a requirement for renal replacement therapy and is usually associated with a GFR less than 10 to 15 mL/min. The interval between the development of renal insufficiency in hypertensive patients and ESRD is about 6 years (5).

Although essential hypertension first becomes manifest in middle life, evidence suggests that factors such as low birth weight owing to maternal malnutrition may contribute to its development later in life (6–9). Small placental size correlates to higher blood pressure even in early childhood (9). Others have related low birth weight and diminished nephron numbers to a higher risk of hypertension in adolescence or adulthood (7,8). In rats maternal protein restriction during nephrogenesis resulted in hypertension in the offspring (10). Systolic blood pressure rises throughout life with a difference of 20 to 30 mm Hg from early to late adulthood (11). Diastolic blood pressure also rises but to a lesser degree and only until the sixth decade (1). In general, cardiovascular risk is related to levels of diastolic pressure in patients younger than 60 years of age. However, pulse pressure (the difference between systolic and diastolic pressure) is the best predictor of cardiovascular risk in patients older than 60 years as it is a marker of central vascular stiffness (12). The prevalence of hypertension in children is estimated at 1% to 2% with most of the cases owing to secondary forms, but a few represent early onset of essential hypertension. More than half of all individuals aged 60 to 69 are hypertensive, and this proportion increases to 75% of those 70 years and older (1). Secondary forms of hypertension should be considered in patients younger than 30 years of age and in those older than 60 years with sudden onset of hypertension (13). A careful family history should also be obtained, because many of these forms have a genetic basis. Although hypertension has no gender preference, at younger ages through middle age, men predominate; however, this trend reverses with increasing age (2).

## Genetic Factors

Essential hypertension is now thought to be a polygenic quantitative trait with only a small contribution from each gene and with modulation by sex, race, age, and environmental factors. The evidence of a genetic effect has been gathered from several sources, including family studies, twin studies, an examination of single gene traits that appear to increase susceptibility to hypertension, and more recently, evaluation of genetic polymorphisms and their relation to the presence of essential hypertension on different genetic backgrounds. The first evidence of genetic factors was accomplished in family and twin studies. In one such study, Mo et al (14) studied 520 offspring with two hypertensive parents, two normotensive parents, or one of each. Those offspring who had two normotensive parents had a mean blood pressure of 121 mm Hg, and 1.3% of them were taking antihypertensive drugs. The intermediate group with one parent of each type showed an average blood pressure of 125 mm Hg, and 2.4% of them used antihypertensive drugs. The group with two hypertensive parents had an average blood pressure of 135 mm Hg, and 11.7% had been prescribed antihypertensive medications. These differences were significant among all three groups. Twin studies are even more powerful because it can be assumed that any differences are due to environmental influences in the case of monozygotic twins but that dizygotic twins represent both genetic and environmental differences (15,16). Greater concordance for hypertension is found between monozygotic than dizygotic twins (16). Carmelli et al (15) found that hypertension accompanied obesity in 31.2% of monozygotic twins but in only 14.9% of dizygotic twins. Furthermore, these investigators found that hypertension occurred in the context of diabetes in 34% of monozygotic twins but in only 8.1% of dizygotic twins.

In the last few years the hope that investigators would be able to discover several candidate genes that might be responsible for essential hypertension was expressed (17). In fact, seven genes have been discovered that are responsible for monogenic types of hypertension (18). Many of these will be discussed later in the section on secondary forms of hypertension. However, it has become equally clear that despite an enormous proliferation of papers on various associations between polymorphisms and hypertension (e.g., more than 1000 hits in a literature search for angiotensin-converting enzyme I/D polymorphism alone), we do not yet understand the role of various mutations and the pathophysiology of hypertension (19). Nevertheless, I will briefly discuss several strategies and summarize the results to date.

The strategies used in recent investigations include association studies examining polymorphisms of candidate genes, linkage analysis including genome-wide screening, and animal models. These will be discussed in turn. Several candidate genes have been definitely linked to hypertension (20,21). The first such demonstration was a study by Jeunemaitre et al (22) of the angiotensinogen gene. They found that hypertensive members of sib-pairs in two large populations inherited a variant of angiotensinogen with threonine rather than methionine at position 235 in higher frequency than normotensive members of the pair. Furthermore, these hypertensive patients had greater concentration of angiotensinogen in their sera. They concluded that this polymorphism might contribute to the hypertension. Studies attempting to confirm this finding were supportive in some populations but contrary in others (20). The next step was to determine how the polymorphism affects the function of the protein. Hopkins et al (23) found that homozygous patients with the 235T genotype had a blunted renal vascular response to the infusion of angiotensin II. Many other investigators have examined polymorphisms in a number of genes thought to be involved in regulation of blood pressure. Most of these studies have shown only small effects in limited populations including gender or ethnic group or race specificity. Table 21.1 lists several of the genes with polymorphisms that show increased susceptibility to essential hypertension. This table lists only a few examples, many of which have not been tested in larger populations. It should also be noted that other studies failed to show any association between the polymorphisms listed and hypertension. For example, several investigators have not found an association between the deletion-insertion allele of angiotensin-converting enzyme and hypertension (24–26).

Genome-wide screens for genes controlling blood pressure are now being performed by linkage analysis using various genotypic markers usually at 10-cM intervals in hypertensive populations (27–29). The screens published up to the end of 2003 were reviewed by Mein et al (30), who found that all chromosomes except 13 and 20 have hyper-

## TABLE 21.1

### GENES WITH POLYMORPHISMS ASSOCIATED WITH ESSENTIAL HYPERTENSION[a]

Adducin (409,410)
Aldosterone synthase (24,411)
Angiotensin-converting enzyme
   Insertion allele (412)
   Deletion allele (413)
Angiotensinogen (24,414)
Angiotensin II types 1 and 2 receptors (24,415)
Apolipoprotein E (416)
Bradykinin receptors (417)
Catalase (418)
Dopamine β-hydroxylase (419)
Endothelial nitric oxide (NO) synthase (420)
Epithelial sodium channel (421)
Hepatocyte growth factor (422)
Sodium-calcium exchanger (423)
WNK1 (424)

[a]These and additional candidate genes are also listed in Staessen JA, Wang J, Bianchi G, et al. Essential hypertension. Lancet 2003; 361:1629.

tension, blood pressure, or pre-eclampsia loci. Chromosome 2 is particularly promising as several studies found linkages to overlapping areas on it. A more recent study has shown replication of some of the sites found in earlier studies including chromosome 16 at 65 cM, chromosome 17 at 70 cM, and chromosome 22 at 35 cM (29). They suggested that future studies should do fine mapping of these regions that likely contain candidate genes. Benjafield et al (27) have done that, combining a genome-wide scan that found suggestive loci on chromosomes 1 and 4 followed by fine mapping using sib-pairs. The locus on chromosome 4 overlapped with a quantitative trait locus for blood pressure in an earlier study as well as a syntenic locus in the spontaneously hypertensive rat. The area of interest on chromosome 1 contains genes for chloride channels, natriuretic peptides, and tumor necrosis factor receptor 2. Mitochondrial DNA is also being subjected to genome-wide screen, particularly in families with maternal transmission of hypertension (31).

Experimental models of hypertension, chiefly in mice and rats, have been used extensively to help in the determination of candidate genes as well as to understand the pathophysiology of hypertension. It is beyond the scope of this chapter to review all of this work, but a few representative examples are given. Cvetkovic and Sigmund (32) reviewed the use of knock-out and transgenic mice in this endeavor. Friese et al (33) studied the spontaneously hypertensive rat (SHR) and the blood pressure–high mouse at a stage before the onset of hypertension in an attempt to understand the mechanisms for its development. Graham et al (34) applied genome-wide screening to the stroke-prone SHR and then applied congenic/consomic breeding models to confirm the quantitative trait loci and dissect the genes further.

Genetic background may also be used in the future to determine the best therapy for individuals. For example, Matayoshi et al (35) examined polymorphisms in 17 genes and found 2 (one each in thiazide-sensitive cotransporter gene and adrenergic receptor-beta 3 gene) which were associated with good therapeutic response to thiazide diuretics that was not seen in those patients without the polymorphisms. Other investigators have begun to study other polymorphisms with an eye to tailoring therapy to the individual patient. This is described further in the section on therapy (see later) (36,37).

Thus it is evident that hypertension does not rely on a single gene but is a polygenic complex trait as first predicted by Hamilton et al in 1954 (38). In summary, it is apparent that although a few single genes may cause hypertension by themselves, most genetic effects act by increasing susceptibility to develop hypertension under certain conditions. In other words, most of these traits are permissive and require other environmental or racial factors to cause blood pressure to rise. These additional factors are discussed next.

## Environmental Factors

Several studies have shown clearly that environmental factors are important in the control of blood pressure (1,15). Individual factors that have been examined include body weight, salt intake, physical activity, smoking, alcohol consumption, cocaine abuse, use of oral contraceptives, socioeconomic class, and psychological stress. The effects of many of these risk factors depend on an interaction between genes and the environment. Tyroler et al (39) noted that obesity led to an increase in both incidence and prevalence of hypertension. Change in weight led to alteration of blood pressure, lending further credence to the importance of this relationship. The role of salt intake in the etiology of hypertension is becoming accepted with the understanding that it may be modified owing to different sensitivities to salt within different populations. The role of dietary intake of both sodium and potassium was reviewed by He and Whelton (40). They put particular emphasis on meta-analysis of randomized controlled trials, which showed a 4.8-mm Hg reduction in systolic pressure and a 2.5-mm Hg reduction in diastolic pressure in hypertensive patients when placed on a sodium-restricted diet.

Physical inactivity may also increase the risk of hypertension. In a study by Miall and Oldham (41), people with light occupations had higher blood pressure than those who engaged in heavy physical labor. Smoking, alcohol consumption, and cocaine abuse are all known to increase blood pressure (1). Oral contraceptives are also associated with high blood pressure, and this risk is even greater with advancing age, duration of use, and increased body mass (1). Socioeconomic class and psychological stress may act in concert to raise blood pressure, or they may be independent factors. One of the explanations for the importance of class is in the area of access to health care (42). Stress may increase blood pressure mediated by any of several stress response genes including heat shock protein (hsp) 27 and hsp 70 or tumor necrosis factor-α (43).

## Racial Factors

The prevalence of hypertension in non-Hispanic black men and women is 38.8% compared with 27.2% for non-Hispanic whites (2). Furthermore, the number of non-Hispanic black adults as a percentage of hypertensive patients in the United States is 21.2% higher than would be expected based on the percentage of non-Hispanic adults in the general population (2). Hypertension begins at an earlier age, is more severe, and is more difficult to control in blacks (44). Blacks also progress to ESRD owing to hypertension 17.7 times more frequently than do whites (45).

It is likely that environmental and genetic factors just outlined above may account for most of the racial differences in susceptibility to hypertension. Parmer et al (45) examined the effects of high- and low-salt diets on a group of white and black men matched for blood pressure and found an impaired ability to excrete a salt load in the black group. Proposed causes for this altered salt handling in blacks include failure to respond appropriately to angiotensin II (AngII), reduction in kallikrein–kinin excretion, and hyperinsulinemia (16). Suthanthiran et al (46) found hyperexpression of transforming growth factor-beta (TGF-β) in hypertensive patients independent of renal disease and that such hyperexpression was more severe in African American hypertensives than in whites. They suggested that these findings preceded the development of the complications of hypertension but might contribute to the vascular and fibrosing lesion seen in patients with hypertension. Differences in the pathology of hypertension-associated renal disease have been described by others (47). As noted earlier, low nephron number has also been associated with the development of hypertension, and blacks as a group do have lower birth weights and likely lower nephron number (7,8,44,48,49).

## Clinical Features

### Initial Presentation

In the earliest stages, most patients are asymptomatic, and the condition is recognized only at routine examination, when injury to the vessels may already be present. Symptoms that may be recognized include headache, epistaxis, tinnitus, and dizziness, but symptoms are unusual.

Excessive weight, smoking, abnormal serum lipid patterns, and diabetes mellitus are common. When there is a family history of hypertension, the patient may be lean. Repeated blood pressure readings may be necessary to establish the diagnosis and to determine the appropriate therapy (50).

As the duration of hypertension becomes protracted, symptoms of the complications may appear. The target organs of hypertension include the heart, brain, kidney, peripheral arteries, and the eye (51–53). Hypertension accelerates atherosclerosis in the systemic circulation, whereas the lower-pressure pulmonary circulation rarely develops atherosclerotic plaques even in the face of elevated serum lipids (52). It has also been hypothesized that hypertension produces a hypercoagulable state (53), which would also accelerate atherosclerosis. The chief manifestations of hypertension in the heart include concentric left ventricular hypertrophy, congestive heart failure, and coronary artery atherosclerosis leading to increased risk of myocardial infarction (52,54). Additional cardiovascular risk is seen in hypertensive patients with the metabolic syndrome (55), defined as three or more of the following conditions: abdominal obesity, triglycerides greater than 150 mg/dL, high-density lipoprotein cholesterol less than 40 mg/dL in men or 50 mg/dL in women, blood pressure greater than 130/85 mm Hg or being treated for hypertension, and a fasting glucose greater than 110 mg/dL. Hypertension is associated with cerebral hemorrhage owing to lesions in the penetrating vessels in the midbrain or to rupture of berry aneurysms. The effects of hypertension in the kidney will be discussed below. Aortic aneurysms as well as claudication are well-known peripheral artery manifestations of hypertension. Hypertension may cause retinal arteriolar thickening, hemorrhage, exudates, or papilledema (50).

Proteinuria is present in 10% to 18% of patients with essential hypertension (56). The prevalence of microalbuminuria, defined as 20 to 200 mg/dL, in patients with newly detected hypertension was 23% to 37% (56). This albuminuria correlated with the level of arterial pressure because 11% of patients with borderline levels of hypertension had microalbuminuria, whereas 37% of those with mild hypertension had albuminuria. Furthermore, only 26% of lean hypertensive patients had microalbuminuria, whereas 35% of overweight patients showed this urinary finding (56). In those patients who progress to significant renal disease with renal insufficiency, a few may manifest nephrotic-range proteinuria (57). Furthermore, it is now recognized that microalbuminuria is an excellent predictor of cardiovascular risk (58,59). These issues are discussed more completely in the section Proteinuria and Hypertension (see p. 940).

## Accelerated Hypertension (Malignant Hypertension)

The current classification of hypertension no longer uses the term *malignant hypertension* (1). However, this term remains in the literature. The terms malignant hypertension and *accelerated hypertension* may be used interchangeably. In the past, malignant hypertension was defined as severe elevation of mean arterial pressure (>140 mm Hg) in combination with funduscopic changes including retinal hemorrhages, exudates, and papilledema (60). It is often accompanied by target organ damage. The clinical symptoms may include visual disturbances, headache, headache with visual disturbance, heart failure, stroke or transient ischemic attack, or dyspnea (61). Hematuria is present in as many as 21% of patients, and some patients have gross hematuria. Significant proteinuria is present in at least 67% of patients (61). The presence of significant proteinuria was also associated with higher serum creatinine levels (61). The causes of proteinuria in this context are discussed at greater length later.

Malignant hypertension may occur without any history of hypertension, or it may be preceded by a period of essential hypertension (62). It may also complicate secondary forms of hypertension such as cocaine abuse (63), renal artery stenosis, or various endocrinologic causes of hypertension (64). Lip et al (61) studied 242 patients with malignant hypertension in England. Of these patients, 136 had primary malignant hypertension, but only 11 had a known history of hypertension. The remaining 44% of patients had secondary hypertension caused by renal artery stenosis, renal parenchymal diseases, or other such conditions (Table 21.2). They found an incidence of 1 to 2 cases of malignant hypertension per 100,000 per year and believe that there is no apparent decline in this disease. An excess of black and Asian patients was noted relative to the number expected for the population studied (61). A definite association of cigarette smoking with the development of the malignant phase of essential hypertension has been established by these authors as well as by others (61,65). This form of hypertension is also more prevalent in men (61,65). Survival has increased with the introduction of more effective antihypertensive drugs (64).

The cause of the switch from benign to malignant hypertension is not yet understood. Many authors have suggested that the renin–angiotensin axis is important. This theory has been supported by a transgenic model of malignant hypertension that has been developed by the insertion of the mouse *ren-2* renin gene into Sprague-Dawley rats (66). The affected rats had increased blood pressure and typical renal changes of malignant hypertension and died at 50 to 90 days of age. Further examination of this model suggested overexpression of the renin gene in the adrenal cortex, leading to activation of the adrenal renin–aldosterone system, which then increased circulating prorenin (67). Heterozygotes showed target organ damage in the heart and kidney but no other characteristics of malignant hypertension. Treatment of these rats with angiotensin-converting enzyme (ACE) inhibitors prevented the transition to a malignant phase of hypertension in these rats (68). The

## TABLE 21.2

### SECONDARY FORMS OF HYPERTENSION

Renal parenchymal disease
  Glomerulonephritis, acute or chronic
  Chronic pyelonephritis
  Polycystic disease
  Diabetes mellitus
  Renal artery stenosis
  Urinary tract obstruction
  Scleroderma
  Hemolytic uremic syndrome
  Polyarteritis
  Irradiation injury
  Tumors, including those secreting rennin
  Analgesic nephropathy
  End-stage renal disease (multiple causes)

Endocrine abnormalities
  Adrenal gland
    Pheochromocytoma
    Cortical alterations
      Cushing's syndrome
      Primary aldosteronism
      Congenital hyperplasia
  Hyperparathyroidism
  Hyperthyroidism
  Paragangliomas

Pregnancy related
  Preeclampsia
  Eclampsia
  Postpartum acute renal failure

Neurologic disorders
  Tumor
  Cerebrovascular disease
  Encephalitis
  Acute porphyria
  Neurofibromatosis

Miscellaneous
  Oral contraceptives
  Licorice ingestion
  Various medications
  Carcinoid syndrome
  Obstructive sleep apnea

expression of this disease varied depending on the strain used as a background. Genome-wide screening of these different transgenic strains showed that those with more severe expression of disease had loci associated with higher plasma ACE activity (68). Additional studies of these transgenic rat models have been reviewed by Fleming (68).

## Laboratory Findings Including Proteinuria

Hemolytic anemia is frequently seen in malignant hypertension, with schistocytes on the peripheral blood smear. Thrombocytopenia and negative results on Coombs test are also part of this hematologic picture, which is also known as microangiopathic hemolytic anemia or thrombotic microangiopathy. Other conditions associated with this condition include hemolytic uremic syndrome, thrombotic thrombocytopenic purpura, scleroderma renal crisis, and various drug-related injuries. These conditions are described in Chapters 16 and 23.

The occurrence of low levels of proteinuria in hypertension has long been recognized (69). When microalbuminuria is defined as 20 to 200 μg/min (30 to 300 mg/24 hours), the prevalence of microalbuminuria ranges between 5% and 37% in hypertensive patients (70). The degree of either proteinuria (69) or albuminuria (56) correlates to the level of arterial pressure. In addition, high-density lipoprotein cholesterol is lower in patients with microalbuminuria (71). Insulin resistance and serum levels of cholesterol, triglycerides, and uric acid are higher in hypertensive patients with microalbuminuria (58). Microalbuminuria is associated with left ventricular hypertrophy, increased carotid intima-media thickness, increased risk of myocardial infarcts, and peripheral vascular disease (70,72,73). Furthermore, microalbuminuria is predictive of increased cardiovascular disease and death in hypertensive patients (56,59,72). Bianchi et al (58) during 7 years of follow-up saw 12 cardiovascular events in 54 hypertensive patients (22%) with microalbuminuria as compared with 2 out of 87 hypertensive patients (2.3%) with normal urinary albumin excretion. Wang et al (74) went one step further and examined urinary albumin to creatinine ratio in 1499 nonhypertensive individuals. During a mean follow-up period of 2.9 years, 15% of these persons developed hypertension and another 33% progressed to a higher level of hypertension. The authors found that urinary albumin excretion predicted these changes in blood pressure even at levels lower than the conventional threshold for microalbuminuria. Genome-wide linkage analysis has shown a possible linkage to urinary microalbumin in hypertensive individuals to chromosomes 12 and 19 (75) and in the general population to chromosome 8 with a possible candidate gene, hyaluronan synthase (76).

Although the mechanism underlying the relationship between microalbuminuria and increased risk for both hypertension and cardiovascular risk is not completely understood, it is believed that endothelial damage is one common factor. Some evidence for this belief comes from a study by Cottone et al (77) in which microalbuminuric essential hypertensive patients had higher serum levels of circulating endothelin-1 and basic fibroblast growth factor. Furthermore, there was a correlation between these factors and the level of microalbuminuria. Glomerular alterations are also considered to be important. Hypertensive patients with proteinuria, particularly when it is in the nephrotic range, frequently have enlarged glomeruli (78,79). In some patients, focal segmental glomerulosclerosis was seen. These changes will be discussed later in the section on glomerular pathology. The pathogenesis of both the glomerular lesion and proteinuria in the setting of hypertension is interesting. Ten percent of patients at the onset of their hypertension are found to have hyperfiltration (56). Hyperfiltration is one of the proposed factors in the causation of glomerular injury in general, and it may play a role in glomerular injury in hypertension as well. Another important factor that may contribute to the pathogenesis of glomerular injury and thus, proteinuria in hypertension, is endothelial injury (80). Pedrinelli et al (80) examined levels of von Willebrand factor (vWF) in 10 hypertensive patients with microalbuminuria and compared them with 10 hypertensive patients without microalbuminuria and 10 controls without microalbuminuria for endothelial injury. These investigators found that vWF was increased in the serum of patients with microalbuminuria. Furthermore, serum levels of vWF correlated with urinary albumin excretion (UAE), mean blood pressure, and age. Mean blood pressure and vWF both contributed to the rise in UAE when multiple regression analysis with UAE as the dependent variable was performed. Patients with microalbuminuria had higher serum creatinine levels and lower creatinine clearance than did hypertensive patients without microalbuminuria. An inverse correlation was found between vWF and creatinine clearance. The authors concluded that blood pressure may contribute to endothelial damage and thereby may promote microalbuminuria. They also suggested that smoking may predispose to microalbuminuria, perhaps by causing endothelial damage. Kario et al (81) also compared hypertensive patients with microalbuminuria with patients with normoalbuminuria. They found that patients with microalbuminuria had higher serum levels of creatinine, factor VIIa, vWF, and thrombomodulin. Furthermore, they found a significant correlation between factor VIIa and both thrombomodulin and vWF. Levels of factor VIIa also correlated well with 24-hour systolic and diastolic blood pressures. This study differed from that of Pedrinelli in that vWF did not correlate with UAE.

## Pathologic Findings

## Gross Pathology

The kidneys in benign nephrosclerosis are typically reduced in size, with a total weight ranging between 120 g and 250 g. The two kidneys are usually affected equally. The capsular surface is most commonly finely granular, reflecting disease in small arteries and arterioles. The granules are formed by zones of relatively preserved or even hypertrophied renal parenchyma alternating with neighboring nephrons with diseased arterioles, which are scarred and depressed. When larger renal arteries show intimal thickening and damage larger clusters of nephrons, however, coarser granularity may be superimposed against a background of fine granularity with scattered V-shaped pits. Such larger scars will take the form of pits, which, on

cut surface, extend only through the cortex and not the medulla, indicating their relationship to the interlobular or arcuate vessels. This feature differentiates them from pyelonephritic scars, which are larger, U-shaped, and extend through a fibrotic medulla to end in a dilated, distorted and inflamed calyx. The capsule may strip with difficulty over such pitted scars. The kidney may be difficult to cut because of the interstitial fibrosis. The cut surface also reveals cortical thinning. Glomeruli may be difficult to identify. Atherosclerosis may be evident in the main renal artery or in any of its branches. Cortical cysts or small adenomas may also be present. If the patient has a short history of hypertension or only mild elevations, there may not be any gross alterations.

The gross appearance of the kidney from an untreated patient with accelerated hypertension differs from that of a patient who has been treated or who has had a period of less severe hypertension preceding the onset of malignant hypertension. In the untreated patient, the combined kidney weights can range from 130 g to 410 g (82). The capsular surface may be smooth in those patients without preceding hypertension but may show a granular surface for those with long-standing hypertension. Petechial hemorrhages, frequently representing congested glomeruli sometimes with hemorrhage into local tissue, are prominent and may also be seen on the cut surface. Small infarcts may also be noted (Fig. 21.1). In patients who have been treated, the petechial hemorrhages and infarcts are less prominent or not visible at all.

## Light Microscopy

### Glomeruli

The glomeruli may be normal or may simply show age-related changes (83). A few obsolete glomeruli are seen in all adults despite the absence of increased blood pressure. Even when some glomeruli show alterations related to hypertension, many glomeruli may not show significant changes. The earliest change is that of collapse of the capillary loops with apparent thickening of their walls on hematoxylin and eosin (H&E)–stained sections. Periodic acid–Schiff (PAS) reaction, however, shows that the apparent thickening is chiefly owing to wrinkling of the capillary basement membrane (Fig. 21.2). With time, the entire glomerular tuft shrinks and retracts to the vascular pole. This is accompanied by the filling in of Bowman's space by a faintly eosinophilic material. H&E-stained sections of such glomeruli reveal only pink, nondescript balls (Fig. 21.3). However, PAS staining demonstrates the shrunken tuft as well as mild thickening of Bowman's capsule (Fig. 21.4). Furthermore, the material filling Bowman's space is PAS negative, a characteristic staining pattern for collagen. This change may begin in the hilar portion of the tuft, but it soon fills the entire space emptied by the shrinking glomerulus (84).

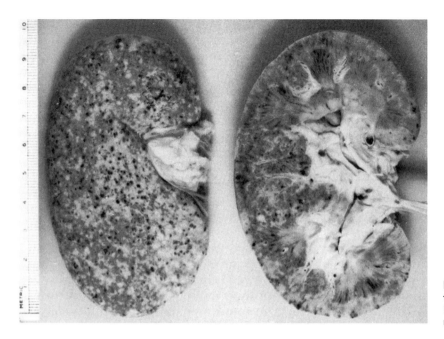

**Figure 21.1**  Kidney from a patient who had the malignant phase of essential hypertension. Kidney weights: left, 150 g; right 130 g. Note numerous petechial hemorrhages.

Another type of glomerular change can be seen in certain cases. It consists of an increase in the mesangial matrix, which results in either segmental or global solidification (sclerosis) of the glomerular tuft (Fig. 21.5), without collagenization of Bowman's space. This change was sometimes accompanied by the hyalinosis lesion and has been particularly emphasized in what has been described as "decompensated benign nephrosclerosis" (DBN) (85,86). This term is used by Bohle et al (85,86) to describe those cases of benign nephrosclerosis in which many glomeruli show prominent hyalinosis accompanied by mesangial widen-

ing. In a study of hypertensive patients, these authors found that 775 kidneys showed the ischemic glomeruli described above accompanied by hyaline arteriolosclerosis. An additional 251 patients had the solidified glomeruli of DBN (86). These patients developed chronic renal failure within a few years and had higher levels of blood pressure, proteinuria, and higher serum creatinine than patients with solely ischemic lesions. This form of glomerular solidification is readily distinguished from that described in the previous paragraph by use of the PAS staining technique, which reveals that the solidification is taking place in the tuft itself. Marcantoni et al (47) recognized these solidified glomeruli of DBN in a higher proportion of African

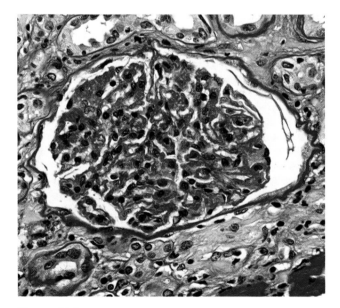

**Figure 21.2**  Glomerulus with wrinkling of glomerular basement membrane accompanied by reduction of capillary lumen diameter. (PAS, ×390.)

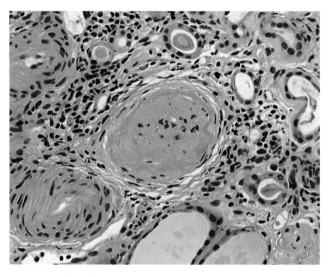

**Figure 21.3**  Sclerotic glomerulus with obliterated capillary loops. (H&E, ×260.)

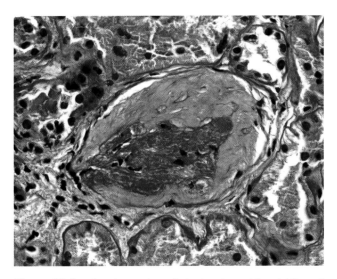

**Figure 21.4** The glomerular tuft is shrunken with wrinkling of the capillary walls. The capsular space contains pale-staining material. The PAS technique clearly distinguishes between the collapsed tuft and the collagenous material occupying the capsular space. (PAS, ×340.)

American hypertensive patients than in Caucasians. They also reported a higher frequency of segmental sclerosis in the patients with DBN. It is also possible to consider this alteration a secondary form of focal segmental glomerulosclerosis (FSGS). Kincaid-Smith (87) has suggested that the increase in segmental glomerular lesions may be related to the increase in the association between the metabolic syndrome (chiefly obesity and insulin resistance) and hypertension. She posits that these factors are producing the segmental glomerular sclerosis rather than the hypertension. Hughson et al (88), in a careful morphometric anal-

ysis in a racially mixed population, did not find any solidified glomeruli in the 13 hypertensive patients they studied. This is most likely owing to the small sample size. Considerable confusion has arisen in the literature owing to the failure to distinguish between these two lesions—the collapsed glomerulus and the solidified glomerulus. The juxtaglomerular apparatus (JGA) is slightly enlarged with respect to numbers of cells in patients with benign hypertension compared with normotensive controls (89).

The glomerular changes in accelerated (malignant) hypertension may be acute or chronic (90–92). These changes are also present in the secondary forms of malignant hypertension in association with some pre-existing renal parenchymal disease; the alterations described here are superimposed on the changes of the respective condition. The acute changes are focal; most glomeruli appear unchanged. The most obvious change is that of fibrinoid necrosis, which is usually segmental (Fig. 21.6). This lesion is eosinophilic but it is most easily seen with a silver stain, which demonstrates interruption of the glomerular basement membrane (GBM). Furthermore, the intense eosinophilia of the area of necrosis stands in sharp contrast to the black staining of the GBM and mesangial matrix (Fig. 21.7). The mesangial matrix may also show loosening, so-called mesangiolysis. The fibrinoid necrosis may extend from a similar lesion in the afferent arteriole, or it may be associated with a crescent. Fibrin, which accounts for the eosinophilia of the lesion, may also be seen in other capillary lumina within the glomerular tuft or may accumulate under endothelial cells. Endothelial cells of arterioles and capillaries may become swollen and obscure the lumen. Fibrin platelet thrombi with red blood cell

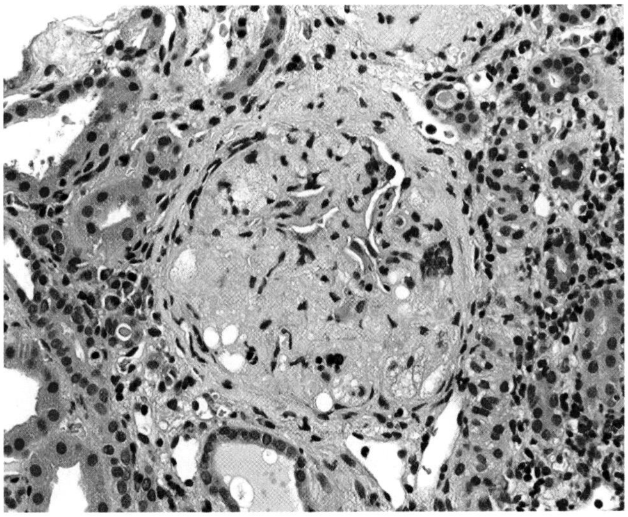

**Figure 21.5** Solidified glomerulus extending to Bowman's capsule without collagenization of Bowman's space. Foam cells may be seen within the glomerulus (H&E, ×260).

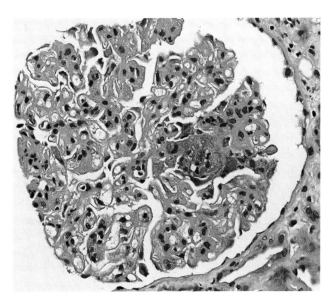

**Figure 21.6** Glomerulus with segmental necrotizing lesion (fibrinoid necrosis) characterized by eosinophilia, karyorrhexis, and apparent disruption of glomerular architecture (H&E, ×260).

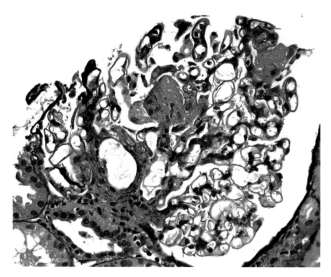

**Figure 21.7** Fibrinoid necrosis involving several lobules in the center and upper right of the tuft, with segmental disruption of basement membrane at the central portion (periodic acid–methenamine silver, ×260).

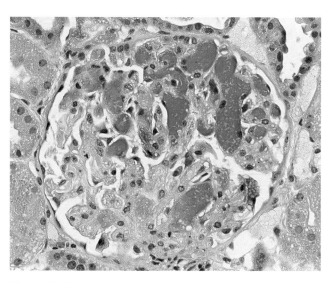

**Figure 21.9** Glomerulus with congested capillary loops (H&E, ×260).

fragments may also be seen (Fig. 21.8). In other glomeruli, the predominant alteration is one of intense congestion with dilatation of the capillary lumina (Fig. 21.9). Such glomeruli may be seen under the dissecting microscope as bright red dots. The final acute alteration is that of thickening of capillary walls in open capillary lumina. Silver stain demonstrates double contours indicative of subendothelial widening (Fig. 21.10). (See also Chapter 16.)

The chronic changes are of two different types. The first is similar to that seen in benign hypertension, in that there

is collapse of the tuft with wrinkling of the GBM accompanied by collagenization of Bowman's space. This change may occur with or without a preceding period of benign hypertension, although it is much more prominent in patients with a history of hypertension. In the second type, glomeruli are also collapsed but seem almost acellular and, on silver stain, show the subendothelial widening described earlier in this paragraph. Thus, the collapsed glomeruli have evolved from those that showed subendothelial widening.

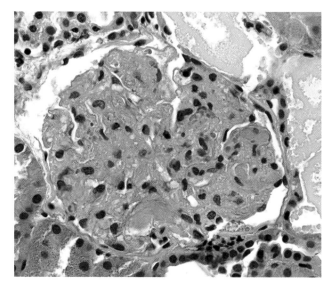

**Figure 21.8** Glomerulus with dilated capillaries filled with red cells, red-cell fragments, and amorphous material probably representing platelets and fibrin. An identical picture is seen in other conditions with thrombotic microangiopathy such as hemolytic uremic syndrome and scleroderma (H&E, ×520).

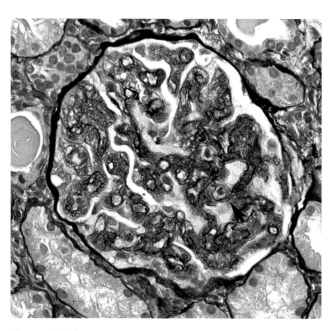

**Figure 21.10** Glomerulus with double contours (*arrow*) representing duplication of the glomerular basement membrane and subendothelial widening (periodic acid–methenamine silver, ×370).

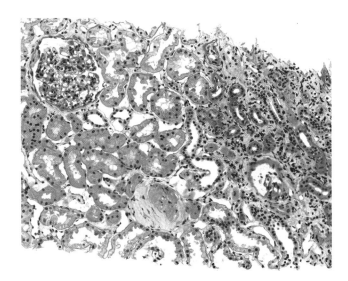

**Figure 21.11** Renal biopsy showing zone of atrophic tubules and interstitial fibrosis to right with normal tubules and interstitium to left. Some of the normal tubules show mild dilatation. (PAS, ×125.)

### Tubules

The tubules in either benign or malignant hypertension may be atrophic and sometimes contain hyaline casts. The epithelial cells are flattened and surrounded by thickened tubular basement membrane, which may be wrinkled. If the biopsy is performed soon after the onset of malignant hypertension, however, the basement membranes are not likely to be thickened. Many tubules will not be affected. Actual loss of tubules may also occur. Such atrophic areas often alternate with zones of tubules with dilated lumina (Fig. 21.11). Such zones form the granularity seen on the capsular surface of gross specimens owing to the fact that the renal vessels do not have collaterals and the capsular surface is therefore the most ischemic. The size of the scars, or fields of atrophic tubules, depends on the diameter of the narrowed vessel supplying the area, thus determining the number of nephrons affected. Although such atrophic tubules are frequently near an obsolete glomerulus, this is not always the case, a finding that may reflect the greater susceptibility of tubules to ischemia. If the patient has proteinuria, protein reabsorption droplets may be present in the tubular epithelial cells. In patients with sudden onset of malignant hypertension, patchy necrosis of tubules may be evident, and there may be cortical infarcts. Such areas are more common in scleroderma-associated thrombotic microangiopathy than in that associated with malignant hypertension. (See also Chapter 16.)

### Interstitium

The interstitium is widened in areas with atrophic tubules. Increased collagen is noted. Chronic inflammatory cells, usually small lymphocytes, may be widely dispersed in the areas of scarring; however, larger aggregates of lymphocytes

may be present in the scars in subcapsular zones. Morphometric studies by Grund et al (93) have shown a correlation between the amount of interstitium and the serum creatinine level. These authors hypothesized that the renal intertubular capillaries had diminished cross-sectional area resulting from interstitial fibrosis and that this change may have contributed to the decrease in the GFR. They did not determine whether the fibrosis preceded the loss of capillaries or vice versa. The changes in accelerated hypertension are similar to those seen in benign nephrosclerosis.

### Blood Vessels

The changes vary with the size of the vessel involved and also differ among individual patients. Arcuate and larger arteries show the alterations typical of atherosclerosis, as manifested by fibrous intimal thickening that results in reduction of the vessel lumen. The internal elastic lamina may show splitting, which is best seen with either a silver or elastic stain. This change is different from the abrupt breaks seen in vasculitis. Lipid-containing macrophages are not usually evident except in the intima of the main renal artery or its branches. In cases in which malignant hypertension is primary and not secondary to a period of lower levels of hypertension, the larger arteries may not show any alteration. Otherwise, the arteries are similar in appearance to those seen with any level of hypertension.

Interlobular arteries show fibroelastic intimal thickening with reduplication of the internal elastic lamina (Fig. 21.12). The degree of intimal thickening in arteries is closely linked to this change in arterioles (94). The media may be thickened in small arteries and/or arterioles (Fig. 21.13), reflecting hypertrophy, hyperplasia, or remodeling. In any case lumen size is decreased, and this decrease may be the result of remodeling, alterations in stiffness

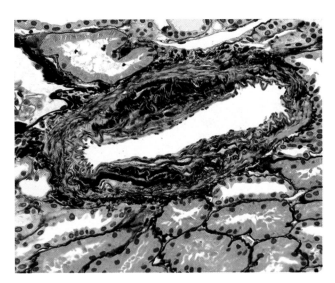

**Figure 21.12** Interlobular artery with reduplication of internal elastic lamina. (Periodic acid–methenamine silver, ×260.)

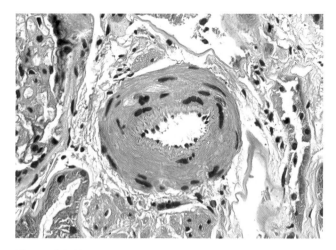

**Figure 21.13** Small artery showing medial thickening with multiple layers of smooth muscle cells and wrinkling of internal elastic lamina. (H&E, ×325.)

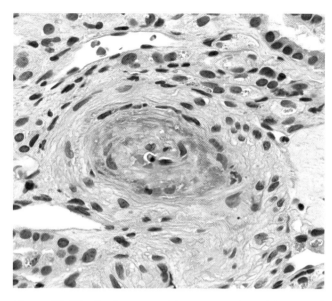

**Figure 21.15** Small artery with mucinous basophilic intimal thickening. (H&E, ×470.)

or compliance, and functional abnormalities. Remodeling and functional changes will be discussed below. Stiffness may be dependent on alterations in the amount and type of collagen, the collagen-elastin ratio and the presence of proteoglycans (95). The latter has been described in humans. An abnormal interaction among these elements may also lead to increased stiffness (95). In patients with accelerated hypertension, the smaller of the interlobular arteries may also show fibrinoid necrosis, which is a segmental change causing localized destruction of a vessel (Fig. 21.14). However, thickening of the intima with mucoid matrix and widely spaced, concentrically arranged cells are more typical changes (Fig. 21.15). The matrix has

sparse collagen in a basophilic edematous-appearing matrix. This thickened intima may also show lipid-containing macrophages as well as marked reduplication of the elastic lamina (Fig. 21.16). Elastic reduplication is particularly prominent in those patients who had a prolonged period of benign hypertension before the onset of malignant hypertension. In these cases, the intimal thickening is luminal to the elastic reduplication. The intimal thickening extends along most of the length of the vessels and causes marked narrowing of the lumen that results in the

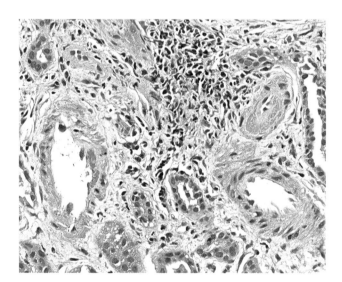

**Figure 21.14** Small artery to left showing segmental fibrinoid necrosis characterized by intense eosinophilia and granular texture. Arteriole at upper right shows fibrinoid necrosis with near occlusion of the lumen. (H&E, ×260.)

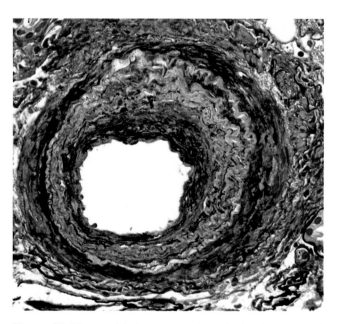

**Figure 21.16** Interlobular artery with marked reduplication of the internal elastic lamina. (Periodic acid–methenamine silver, ×170.)

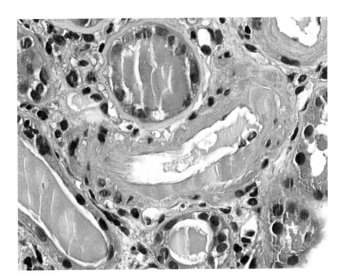

**Figure 21.17** Arteriole with circumferential intimal hyalin deposition. Note glassy appearance. (H&E, ×520.)

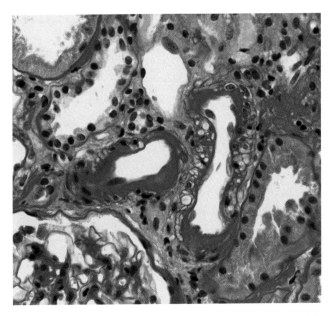

**Figure 21.18** Small artery with intimal hyalin and arteriole to left with intimal deposition of hyalin extending toward the media and compressing smooth muscle cells. (PAS, ×400.)

devastating ischemic alterations that can cause renal failure. The most common terms used to describe this lesion are *onion skin thickening, endarteritis fibrosa,* and *musculomucoid intimal thickening.* These alterations in the kidney in malignant hypertension, including the findings of fibrinoid necrosis of the afferent arteriole, glomerulitis, and onion skin thickening of small arteries, were first described by Volhard and Fahr (96).

Arterioles are commonly affected by hyaline arteriolosclerosis, although this change is by no means universal (89). Burchfiel et al (97) found that the risk of arteriolar hyalinization increased with increases in diastolic blood pressure. The severity of arteriolar hyalinization also correlates with the degree of larger artery intimal thickening (98). This lesion is characterized by the presence of homogeneous eosinophilic material, sometimes with lipid in the subendothelium of the arterioles (Fig. 21.17). It may extend into the media and is more easily seen using the PAS stain (Fig. 21.18). Use of the term *hyaline* suggests that it appears glassy, to distinguish it from the more granular texture of fibrinoid necrosis, a lesion typical of the malignant phase of hypertension discussed below. Sommers and Melamed (89), in a study of 2300 renal biopsies performed at the time of sympathectomy for benign hypertension, found evidence of arteriolar nephrosclerosis in 82% of the specimens. They proposed the following sequence for the evolution of these renal lesions: arteriolar intramural hydropic swelling followed by cellular degeneration, with pooling of ground substance and partial replacement of smooth muscle cells by fibrosis. They found that arterioles were thickened by fibrous replacement of the smooth muscle with or without hyalin. The arterioles lengthened and became tortuous. They also found that the ratio of the wall thickness to the lumen diameter increased with higher di-

astolic blood pressure (89). The nature and pathogenesis of hyalin accumulation is discussed in the section Pathogenesis of Small-Vessel Changes.

The characteristic lesion of severe (malignant) hypertension is fibrinoid necrosis. Eosinophilic material with a granular texture supplants the medial smooth muscle cells with loss of cell nuclei (Fig. 21.14). This granular material must be differentiated from the glassy appearance of hyaline arteriolosclerosis, the more typical lesion of benign hypertension (Fig. 21.17). Of course, hyaline arteriolosclerosis may also be present in patients with malignant hypertension, but the identification of true fibrinoid necrosis suggests the diagnosis of the accelerated phase. Fibrinoid necrosis also impinges on the vascular lumen. Areas of fibrinoid necrosis can be distinguished easily with the use of the PAS/Jones (silver) and the recognition of the granular texture rather than the glassy appearance of hyalin. The elastic lamina of the vessel wall as well as the interstitium between smooth muscle cells stains black from the silver. This finding is in sharp contrast to the bright pink staining of the fibrinoid material. Masson trichrome stain also delineates fibrinoid necrosis well as the fibrin stains bright red (Fig. 21.19). Thrombus formation is often superimposed on the area of necrosis, resulting in complete occlusion of the vessel. Fragmented red blood cells are frequently seen within either the thickened intima or the vessel wall, evidence of thrombotic microangiopathy (Fig. 21.20). Mixed inflammatory cells are occasionally present, but their presence is not necessary to make the diagnosis.

Hughson et al (99), in a study of patients with malignant nephrosclerosis, identified nodules in small arteries

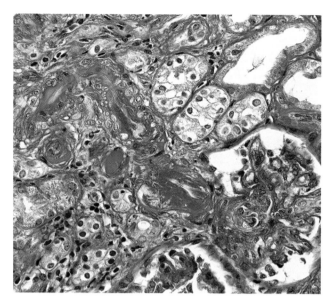

**Figure 21.19** Afferent arteriole with fibrinoid necrosis staining bright red. The lumen is nearly totally occluded, resulting in collapse of glomerulus being fed by the vessel. (Masson trichrome, ×310.)

and arterioles. These nodules were composed of spindled cells with a vascular network similar to the plexiform lesion seen in pulmonary hypertension. He hypothesized that the pathogenesis was owing either to arterial necrosis or organization of thrombi or to a combination of the two, with the necrosis occurring first followed by the thrombus. Hughson also suggested that the intimal hyperplasia was caused by turbulent blood flow. These changes were seen most commonly in the kidneys, followed by periadrenal fat, pancreas, intestines, gallbladder, and heart.

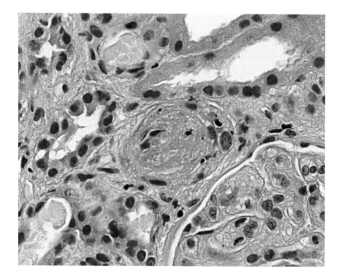

**Figure 21.20** Arteriole showing thrombotic microangiopathy with platelet-fibrin thrombus occluding lumen. Also note fragmented red blood cells within vessel wall. (H&E, ×520.)

## Thrombotic Microangiopathy and Malignant Nephrosclerosis

The term *malignant nephrosclerosis* was first used by Fahr (100) in a description of the renal pathologic characteristics of a patient who had an accelerated or malignant form of hypertension. Bohle et al (101) examined the issue of malignant nephrosclerosis in great detail. They divided their patients into two groups: one with the changes of fibrinoid necrosis in glomeruli and arterioles and the other with onion skin alterations in the intima of arteries. They designated the first group with either normal blood pressure or recent onset of hypertension as primary malignant hypertension. Bohle et al believed that in these cases the renal vascular morphologic changes preceded the hypertension. The other group had long-standing accelerated hypertension that was considered secondary malignant hypertension. The authors believed that the vascular changes in these cases were caused by the hypertension. Patients in the primary malignant hypertension group were younger than those in the secondary group. Furthermore, women outnumbered men, and the primary group had more severe hemolytic anemia and often presented in acute renal failure. Hence, many of these patients could be classified into the hemolytic uremic syndrome. Investigators now recognize that several diseases show morphologic changes identical to those seen in malignant nephrosclerosis. These include the following, which are discussed in Chapter 16, hemolytic uremic syndrome, thrombotic thrombocytopenic purpura, renal involvement in systemic sclerosis (scleroderma), toxicity of certain drugs such as cyclosporine and mitomycin C, complications of radiation and bone marrow transplantation, and postpartum acute renal failure (see Chapter 17). The term used to encompass these various clinical entities is *thrombotic microangiopathy*. It is characterized by fibrinoid changes in both glomeruli and renal arterioles accompanied by fragmented erythrocytes (Fig. 21.20). The glomeruli may also show collapse and wrinkling of the tuft. The renal arterioles and small arteries show intimal thickening, often with a mucoid appearance resulting in marked narrowing of their lumina. As suggested in the name, thrombotic occlusion of the lumen is often superimposed on this narrowing. Thus, malignant nephrosclerosis may be considered a form of thrombotic microangiopathy. A fuller description of these alterations is given in Chapter 16.

The question of the primacy of malignant levels of hypertension in the pathogenesis of these microangiopathic lesions is still controversial. Most of the cases I see now that have the changes I consider representative of malignant nephrosclerosis are superimposed on kidneys with primary glomerular disease. In these patients, severe renal parenchymal disease is present, and the history is consistent with pre-existence of the glomerular disease before the onset of the malignant levels of hypertension. Thus, they can be considered as cases of secondary malignant hypertension. However, I have also seen a patient with IgA nephropathy and the changes of malignant nephrosclerosis in whom glomerular disease was not severe and the tubules and interstitium showed only focal fibrosis and atrophy. Nevertheless, the arteries showed changes consistent with the malignant hypertension, which was present clinically. In that case, I believe that the malignant hypertension was separable from the renal parenchymal disease and was thus primary or essential malignant hypertension. In most cases with microangiopathic changes, malignant hypertension is prominent clinically. However, I have seen the alterations of thrombotic microangiopathy without documentation of malignant levels of hypertension. In one particularly memorable case of scleroderma renal crisis, the patient never had a recorded blood pressure exceeding 120/80 mm Hg yet had spectacular fibrinoid necrosis of both glomeruli and arterioles.

## Immunofluorescence Findings

Arterioles with hyaline accumulation have been shown to contain IgM and C3 most commonly, but IgG, IgA, IgE, and fibrinogen have also been recorded (57,102) (Fig. 21.21). C3 may also be observed without accompanying immunoglobulins. The most common reactant seen in immunofluorescence studies of malignant hypertension is fibrinogen (101,103). It may be seen in areas of fibrinoid necrosis, as would be expected, but it is also seen in glomerular capillary loops and in larger vessels without obvious fibrinoid necrosis. These changes are more prominent in the more active cases. On occasion, other immunoglobulins can be identified, presumably accumulating nonspecifically in areas of injury.

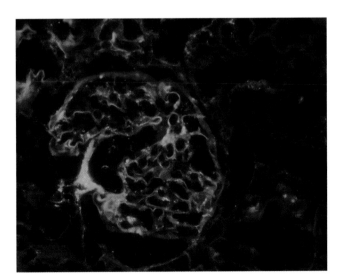

**Figure 21.21** Immunofluorescence micrograph of afferent arteriole staining with C3 antiserum. (C3 antiserum, ×260.)

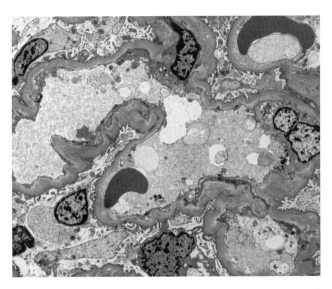

**Figure 21.22** Electron micrograph showing wrinkling of glomerular basement membrane with variability in its thickness. Foot processes are coarsened but frank effacement is not seen. (Uranyl acetate and lead citrate, ×3600.)

## Electron Microscopy

Ultrastructural studies (91,104,105) of glomeruli from patients with hypertension have shown wrinkling and thickening of the GBM, which also becomes more dense (Fig. 21.22). Electron microscopy also confirms the presence of collagen fibrils with scattered cells within the capsular space and reduplication of the basement membrane material of Bowman's capsule (Fig. 21.23). The presumption has always been that the shrinkage of the tuft results from ischemia (104,105) but little evidence indicates that ischemia is responsible for the accumulation of collagenous material in Bowman's space, and at the moment, no good explanation exists for its presence. In open glomeruli one may see mild but widespread subendothelial widening (Fig. 21.24).

Ultrastructural studies of intimal thickening of larger arteries in hypertension show that the intimal cells are myofibroblasts as characterized by both abundant rough endoplasmic reticulum and myofibrils distributed along the periphery of the cell. Immunohistochemistry confirms the smooth muscle differentiation of these cells as well. Electron microscopy also demonstrates the presence of extracellular proteoglycans (small granules), which are responsible for imparting the mucoid appearance to the thickening (91,106).

Ultrastructural studies (91,103) of glomeruli from patients with accelerated hypertension demonstrate dense amorphous material in the areas of fibrinoid necrosis, sometimes with fibrin tactoids. The mesangium may be intact or show areas of loosening of the matrix, sometimes with finely granular material. Loss of attachment of the GBM to the matrix denotes areas of mesangiolysis

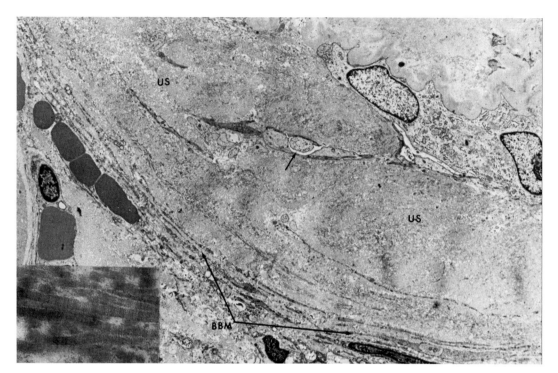

**Figure 21.23** Electron micrograph from an obsolescent glomerulus. Remains of the capillary tuft with wrinkled GBM and epithelial cell are seen in the top right corner. The urinary space (US) is filled with collagen as confirmed at higher magnification in the lower left **inset** (×10,000; **inset**, ×36,000). (From Nagle R, et al. Lab Invest 1969;21:419. Copyright © 1969 by the U.S. Canadian Division of the International Academy of Pathology.)

(103), which results in capillary dilatation and even microaneurysm formation, an alteration that can also be seen in the other conditions associated with thrombotic microangiopathy (see Chapter 16). Red blood cell fragments, platelets, and fibrin thrombi may be found in arterioles and

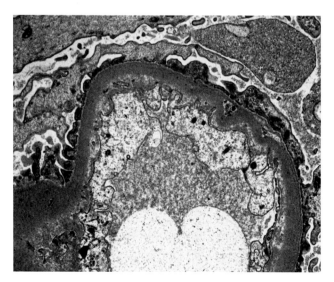

**Figure 21.24** Electron micrograph showing mild subendothelial widening with new basement membrane formation. (Uranyl acetate and lead citrate, ×13,100.)

capillaries. Endothelial cells may be swollen or, in more severely affected areas, they may become necrotic and disappear. The widened subendothelial space contains flocculent material of variable density, sometimes with fibrin tactoids. The glomeruli with long-term changes show wrinkling of the GBM, which becomes both thicker and denser. Areas with subendothelial widening have more flocculent material, which becomes more lucent, and new basement membrane material is laid down immediately below the endothelial cell (Fig. 21.25). Ultrastructural studies have suggested that the smooth muscle cells of the media are hypertrophied (91). Furthermore, such studies have also shown the presence of cells with smooth muscle features in the intima (91).

Ultrastructural studies of vessels in severe hypertension confirm the presence of fibrin within fibrinoid necrosis, with frequent tactoids noted (91). Smooth muscle cells are necrotic or show various degenerative changes, including loss of microfibrils, vacuole formation, and increased numbers of autophagosomes. In those areas where the endothelium remains intact, one may see swelling of these cells or increased microfilaments, so-called stress fibers, at either the luminal surface or near its attachment to the basal lamina (107,108). An increase in the number of cellular organelles and myofilaments has been shown to occur in vascular endothelium when exposed to shear stress in vitro (109,110).

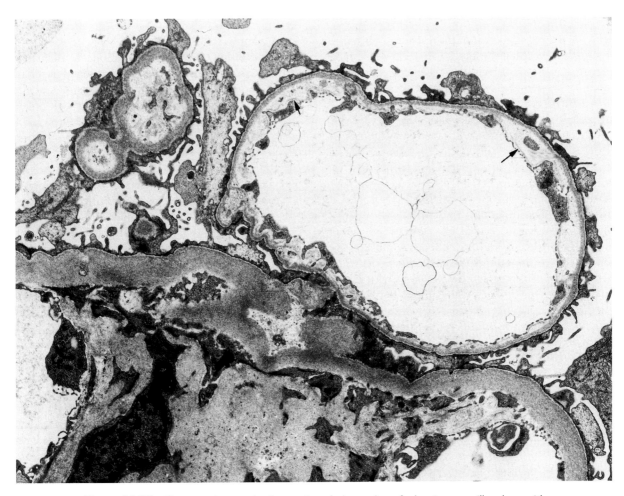

**Figure 21.25** Electron micrograph of a portion of glomerular tuft showing a capillary loop with subendothelial widening and new basement membrane (*arrows*) immediately subjacent to endothelial cell. The electron-lucent area between the two basement membranes contains flocculent material, most notably to the left. Occasional denser material may represent degraded fibrin-related material. (Uranyl acetate and lead citrate, ×5,650.)

## Etiology and Pathogenesis

### Pathophysiology of Hypertension

The pathogenetic mechanisms of essential hypertension are complex, but it is recognized that sodium and fluid balance and vasomotor tone are the major determinants of blood pressure. Blood pressure regulation depends on both cardiac output (CO) and vascular resistance. One cause of increased CO is augmented renal salt reabsorption. The resulting increased tissue perfusion is not needed, producing autoregulation mediated by vasoconstriction, which leads to increased blood pressure (111). Resistance is determined by Hagen-Poiseuille's law and is directly related to the length of the vessels and the blood viscosity, as represented by the hematocrit level. Resistance is inversely related to the fourth power of the diameter of the blood vessels (112). Thus, it is clear that arteriolar diameter is the most powerful determinant of resistance in the short term.

In the long term, other factors, such as increased wall-to-lumen ratio, which affects lumen diameter, and rarefaction, which results in a decrease in the number of arterioles and capillaries, also become important. Many factors contribute to the vascular changes including the sympathetic nervous system, the renin-angiotensin system, and endothelial dysfunction. These will be discussed briefly in turn. Then I will discuss an interesting new hypothesis put forward by Johnson et al (113) trying to unify these systems and other new concepts that have appeared in the literature such as the effect of reduced number of nephrons and the roles of uric acid and aldosterone.

The sympathetic nervous system (SNS) is clearly involved in blood pressure regulation. The role of the SNS in chronic hypertension has been difficult to dissect owing to the complex nature of the SNS. Several studies (114) suggest that increased SNS activity as measured by heart rate, high levels of norepinephrine, or increased urinary catecholamine is present in subjects prior to the onset of hypertension. The SNS plays a role in chronic hypertension chiefly by increasing tubular sodium reabsorption, renin release, and renal vascular resistance (115). These changes shift the pressure–natriuresis curve to the right so that there is a resetting of arterial pressure upward to re-establish sodium balance (115,116). SNS activity is also increased in hypertensive patients (115). However, it is not yet clear whether this increase is primary or represents an epiphenomenon. The link between obesity and hypertension may be owing to the possibility that leptin may activate the SNS (117). The role of stress and the SNS in acute hypertension is well accepted (114). Mental stress has been shown to cause a larger increase in GFR in hypertensive patients than in normotensive subjects (115), perhaps indicating greater reactivity in vessels to SNS changes. Increases in SNS activity are also important in secondary hypertension.

The renin-angiotensin system (RAS) plays a central role in blood pressure regulation; and a review of all of the actions and interactions is beyond the scope of this chapter. Angiotensin II (AII) is the most potent of the peptides in the system with the AT1 receptor activating the most hypertensive effects (116). AII causes renal vasoconstriction, increases the sensitivity of the tubuloglomerular feedback, and increases tubular reabsorption of sodium. AII may also have direct toxic effects on vessels and/or may be a stimulus to remodeling (see below). Intrarenal AII levels are also increased in hypertension, resulting in the resetting of the pressure–natriuresis relationship. Obesity may also be involved in this resetting of the pressure–natriuresis curve as there is increased sodium reabsorption and activation of the RAS in obesity (118). When this relationship cannot be counterbalanced by other physiologic mechanisms, hypertension is the result (119).

The normal basal state of salt repletion is one of vasodilatation controlled by the production of nitric oxide (NO) by the endothelial cells (120). Endothelial dysfunction was initially defined as impaired vasodilation in response to such substances as acetylcholine or bradykinin. However, it is now thought to encompass not only reduced vasodilation but also a proinflammatory and prothrombotic state related to loss of function of the endothelium (121). The endothelium produces many vasodilatory substances including NO, prostacyclin, endothelium-derived hyperpolarizing factors, and C-type natriuretic peptide. It also produces vasoconstrictors such as endothelin-1 (ET-1), AII, thromboxane A2, and reactive oxygen species (ROS). Endothelial dysfunction has been described in humans with hypertension and in families prior to the onset of hypertension (122).

NO is one of the most important vasodilators, but it is also an anti-inflammatory substance, is antiproliferative, and inhibits platelet aggregation. It is synthesized from L-arginine by a family of NO synthases and exists in two constitutive forms: endothelial and neuronal. The constitutive forms of NO are both calcium- and calmodulin-dependent. Release of the constitutive forms of NO produces various effects, including smooth muscle relaxation, inhibition of platelet aggregation and adhesion, and increased neurotransmission in peripheral sympathetic nerves. Larger, local doses affect both afferent and efferent arterioles. NO may also modify mesangial cell tone mediated by antagonism of AII-induced contraction (123,124). Loss or decrease in NO is almost always one of the signs of endothelial dysfunction (121). Diminished NO can result from a decrease in endothelial NO synthase (eNOS) owing to inhibitors or reduction in its substrate, arginine. NO synthase is inhibited by L-nitro ethyl arginine as well as by certain other substances that are normally produced endogenously (125). Long-term blockade of NO synthase brings about sustained hypertension and end organ damage (123). Providing arginine may overcome the blockade and result in lowered blood pressure, further supporting the role of NO in controlling blood pressure (126). ROS have been associated with decreased NO mediated by an uncoupling of eNOS to a reductase function by which it produces more ROS and less NO. In an in vitro model of vessels from skeletal muscle, Huang et al (127) showed that elevated shear stress could induce ROS that then diminished NO. Similarly in humans, markers of oxidative stress have been associated with lower levels of NO in hypertension and in chronic renal disease (121).

Hyperhomocysteinemia is now recognized as a cardiovascular risk factor with more recent demonstration of a link to essential hypertension (128). Homocysteine has been shown to decrease NO bioavailability by enhancing lipid peroxidation evidenced by increased plasma levels of $F_2$-isoprostanes (128). These isoprostanes stimulate production of ET-1, the most powerful vasoconstrictor known. ET-1 is produced by endothelial and vascular smooth muscle cells in response to such stimuli as shear stress, hypoxia, AII, and vasopressin. ET-1 interacts with $ET_A$ receptors to cause vascular smooth muscle contraction. Homocysteine and ET-1 have also been shown to have structural effects on vessels (128,129). These changes will be discussed below.

Hyperuricemia is also associated with increased blood pressure. Certain families with hyperuricemia have recently been found to have hypertension and progressive renal disease (130). In a community-based study, serum uric acid has also been shown to be an independent predictor of hypertension incidence and of progression to hypertension (131). Mazzali et al (132) developed an animal model of hyperuricemia in the rat in which the hyperuricemia induced reduction in endothelial NO and stimulated renin production. Furthermore, they showed that the arteriolar lesions that developed were followed by development of salt sensitivity that was independent of the level of serum uric acid (133).

Johnson et al (113) have put forth an interesting hypothesis that weaves many of these strands into a common pathway to understand the pathogenesis of essential hypertension. It is briefly summarized here, but the reader is advised to refer to the review cited for a fuller explanation. These authors believe that in the prehypertensive state repeated but intermittent episodes of vasoconstriction are initiated by a hyperactive sympathetic nervous system (SNS), by genetic alterations in the RAS, or by hyperuricemia. At first the hypertension is salt resistant and pressure natriuresis is intact. However, as arteriolar lesions develop (by mechanisms that will be described below), ischemia results as well as defective autoregulation. Tubulointerstitial disease results, leading to increased sodium reabsorption. Another contributing factor to the impairment of autoregulation may be a reduction in nephron number (49,134). This structural alteration then reduces blood flow to glomeruli, shifting the pressure–natriuresis curve and resulting in increased salt sensitivity and increased blood pressure.

The preceding discussion has introduced endothelial dysfunction and its attendant decreased NO induced by hyperuricemia, hyperhomocysteinemia, and stimulated RAS as potential factors involved in the pathogenesis of hypertension. Advances in our knowledge of molecular biology have led to the uncovering of these substances and enhanced our understanding of their differing functions and interactions. Possible links to the structural abnormalities seen are discussed below. Other hormones such as aldosterone may also be involved in essential hypertension (135,136). Its role in the pathogenesis of hypertension will also be discussed in the secondary forms associated with hyperaldosteronism. In summary, the pathogenesis of hypertension remains a complex issue. Although we now can list some of the substances that play an important part in its genesis, we still understand little of the interrelationships among them. Just as blood pressure is controlled by many genes and numerous factors, it is virtually certain that pathogenetic mechanisms of action are multiple.

## Pathogenesis of Glomerular Lesions

### Experimental Studies

The observations of Wilson and Byrom (137) using the 2K1C rat model, in which a renal artery from one kidney is clipped to reduce blood flow to induce hypertension, form the basis of much of our understanding of the pathologic manifestations of hypertension in the kidney. In this model, the clipped kidney is protected in the short term from hypertension while the nonclipped kidney is exposed to the elevated systemic pressure and, as a result, manifests both glomerular and vascular injury. Changes in the nonprotected glomeruli include segmental or global necrosis with adhesions and eventual total sclerosis of the tuft. Fibrinoid necrosis is present in afferent arterioles and small renal arteries. These alterations are those seen in human malignant hypertension. Studies in various other ex-

perimental models of hypertension have confirmed these findings (138–140).

Many different experimental models of hypertension have been developed. A comparison of four different models showed a relationship between preglomerular resistance and the occurrence of glomerular injury (140). Another experimental model used inhibition of NO synthase through inhibition of its synthesis by nitro arginine methyl ester (NAME) producing vasoconstriction (123). When NO synthesis was inhibited for 2 months, blood pressure was elevated, the GFR decreased, proteinuria occurred, and glomerular injury appeared. Addition of sodium chloride to the diet exacerbated the hypertension and the glomerular injury (141). The glomerular lesions included glomerular collapse, segmental necrosis, and segmental glomerulosclerosis. Those glomeruli that showed collapse had decreased perfusion, whereas those glomeruli with either sclerosis or necrosis had been exposed to increased pressures.

Although ischemia owing to vasoconstriction or luminal narrowing seems likely to be important in the collapsing form of glomerular injury in hypertension, it does not adequately explain all the alterations seen. Increased glomerular pressure may occur because of increased postglomerular pressure leading to increased pressure within the glomerulus itself. Early evidence that the direct transmission of increased pressure to the glomerulus could induce injury came from the studies of Byrom (142), in which removal of the clip from animals with 2K1C hypertension produced acute glomerular injury. More studies have supported the concept that increased glomerular pressure, whatever its pathogenesis, can be crucially important as a mechanism for direct glomerular injury, which, in its obsolete form, would be the solidified type.

It is now well known that hypertension accelerates most forms of glomerular injury. In most cases, the common finding is increased glomerular capillary pressure resulting from the loss of effective afferent arteriolar constriction in the face of increased systemic pressure (i.e., loss of autoregulation) confirmed by micropuncture studies in various experimental models of hypertension (143–145). Autoregulation refers to the ability of the kidney to maintain renal blood flow and GFR in a narrow range despite wider variation in systemic blood pressure. This is accomplished chiefly through two mechanisms, namely, a myogenic reflex in the afferent arteriole and tubuloglomerular feedback (TGF) (146). During impaired autoregulation the sensitivity of TGF is reset owing to changes in NO and AII. This is the same idea as the resetting of the pressure–natriuresis curve discussed above. When there is sustained delivery of NaCl to the macula densa, the neuronal type of NO synthase is increased, offsetting the usual vasoconstrictive effect of TGF on the afferent arteriole. These changes are found early in the course of the development of hypertension in the spontaneously hypertensive rat, the Milan hypertensive strain, and the Dahl salt-sensitive rat (146). It is thought that this mechanism may be particularly important in salt-sensitive hypertension. Loss of autoregulation is seen in many models characterized by progressive renal injury, and many of these show up-regulation of transforming growth factor-beta. Sharma et al (147) found that transforming growth factor-beta impaired the autoregulatory response owing to both the myogenic and TGF-sensitive components whereas other growth factors such as platelet-derived GF did not. This effect of transforming growth factor-beta seems to involve the ROS system.

The loss of autoregulation also plays an important role in subsequent glomerular injury. The vasodilation resulting from the loss of autoregulation allows the transmission of higher pressure to the glomerulus, in effect an increase in glomerular capillary pressure ($P_{gc}$). The role of loss of autoregulation as one mechanism for the hemodynamic alterations has been studied by Griffin et al first in the renal ablation model (148) and more recently in the normotensive renal ablation model as well as in the stroke-prone spontaneously hypertensive rat using high-salt diets (149,150). In the normotensive renal ablation model, the systemic pressure is slightly higher than in controls but does not attain hypertensive levels. Nevertheless, when followed for 14 to 15 weeks, these animals develop glomerular lesions that correlate to the level of their systolic pressure as well as their pulse pressure (150). The authors believe that it is the transmission of this elevated pressure to the glomerulus that results in the glomerular injury. This supposition was also supported by the comparison of changes in autoregulation in the stroke-prone spontaneously hypertensive rat (SHRsp) and their progenitors, the stroke-resistant SHR (149). In this study the SHRsp had higher blood pressure and renal blood flow (RBF) than the SHR, and the RBF increased more with added salt. The authors concluded that these increased pressures were transmitted to the glomeruli leading to the increased glomerular injury documented by others in this model (151).

The glomeruli in experimental models characterized by loss of autoregulation show severe injury. The alterations include endothelial injury with loss of attachment from the GBM, accumulation of plasma proteins in the subendothelial space (the hyalinosis lesion), epithelial injury manifested by variable foot process effacement, protein reabsorption droplets and vacuoles, and mesangial injury with mesangiolysis. This last form of extreme glomerular injury is associated with capillary microaneurysms and, in later stages, with mesangial sclerosis. The capillary loops may also contain fibrin thrombi (138,140,144). Chander et al (152) have shown that aldosterone may play an important role in the thrombotic microangiopathy seen as part of the glomerular injury in SHRsp. Glomeruli throughout the cortex may be affected, with juxtamedullary glomeruli affected slightly more frequently (140). In models with vasoconstriction, the glomerular injury is much less severe

and is almost restricted to juxtamedullary glomeruli (140). This finding is thought to be related to a greater loss of autoregulation in juxtamedullary as compared with superficial glomeruli in these two models.

Endothelial injury is caused by shear stress and direct mechanical injury. Endothelial dysfunction may precede hypertension and is associated with decreased NO levels and an increase in AII. There has been a long-standing controversy regarding the role of the increased pressure (induced by AII) as the mediator of injury versus the nonpressor actions of AII itself. Mori and Cowley (153) inserted a servo-controlled device in the aorta of Sprague-Dawley rats between the two renal arteries to control renal perfusion pressure. The rats were then fed a 4% salt diet and received a continuous infusion of AII for 2 weeks. The juxtamedullary glomeruli of the kidney that were exposed to uncontrolled pressure showed more injury than those glomeruli in the kidney in which the perfusion pressure was controlled. The superficial glomeruli were similar between the two sides. The authors concluded that both AII and the increased pressure were factors, but that the nonpressor actions of AII contributed only 25% of the injury. An editorial comment on this paper agreed with the study, but cautioned that subtle changes that may have been induced by AII were not assessed (154). Mechanisms of glomerulosclerosis have been reviewed (155–157). Several recent papers have examined some of these mechanisms in the setting of hypertensive injury. Camp et al (158) examined the role of matrix metalloproteinases (MMPs) in interstitial fibrosis and glomerular changes such as increased mesangial matrix accumulation in SHR. Previous studies had shown that these MMPs were increased in vessels in response to increased shear stress (159). They found that MMP-2 and MMP-7 were increased at the onset of hypertension, but that there was no increase in tissue inhibitor of metalloproteinase (TIMP)-4. This suggested an imbalance with increased degradation of elastin relative to collagen, possibly resulting in increased stiffness and dysfunction (158). The forces that bring about visceral epithelial cell injury have been studied by Kretzler et al (160) and involve capillary loop distension with epithelial cell hypertrophy and eventual loss of attachment of the epithelial cell from the GBM. In addition, epithelial cells may show blebs and vacuoles. A possible link between mechanical strain and podocyte injury has been studied in vitro by Durvasula et al (161). They found that increased mechanical strain was followed by increased AII production, a fivefold increase in $AII_1$ receptor mRNA expression, and an increase in transforming growth factor-beta mRNA expression. This was also accompanied by an increase in apoptosis of the epithelial cells (161).

### Clinical Studies

Obsolete glomeruli show two different forms. In the first of these forms, the glomeruli are solidified or hyalinized; thus, an increase in matrix is often accompanied by

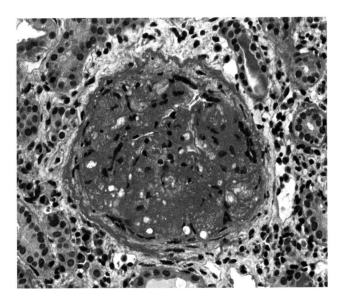

**Figure 21.26**   Solidified glomerulus extending to Bowman's capsule with increased mesangium, sclerosis of capillary loops, and occasional foam cells. (PAS, ×400.)

remnants of hyalinosis lesions (Fig. 21.26). The other lesion is characterized by wrinkling of the GBM with retraction of the tuft to one side of Bowman's capsule and collagenization of Bowman's space (see Fig. 21.4). This may be viewed as a form of collapse of the glomerular tuft. This latter lesion is predominant in essential hypertension. The wrinkled glomerulus is likely the result of chronic ischemia. Kasiske (162) compared autopsy kidneys from patients with moderate to severe systemic atherosclerosis to those from patients of similar age with mild atherosclerosis with respect to the number of sclerotic glomeruli, the degree of vascular narrowing of arcuate and interlobular arteries, and the presence or absence of hypertension. He found that the extent of glomerular obsolescence depended on both the age of the patient and the degree of intrarenal vascular disease. Although hypertension correlated with the degree of glomerulosclerosis, it was not independent of the other two factors. The degree of narrowing of the renal artery correlated strongly with the extent of glomerular obsolescence, a finding supporting the idea that the sclerosis was caused by ischemia, as represented by the vascular narrowing. It is well known that glomeruli may become sclerotic with increasing age, independent of increased blood pressure (83,163). Kaplan et al (83) stated that 95% of the population up to 40 years of age should have fewer than 10% globally sclerotic glomeruli. Kappel and Olsen (163) countered that no more than 1% of glomeruli should be obsolete by age 40 years, but that as many 30% of glomeruli may become globally sclerotic by age 80 years. Smith et al (164) developed a formula that provides a rough approximation of the upper limit of the expected number of sclerotic glomeruli as the age of the patient divided by 2 minus 10.

The solidified glomerulus is the alteration that Bohle (85,86) described in decompensated benign nephrosclerosis, a form associated with a more rapid course to end-stage renal disease. Marcantoni et al (47) studied 62 hypertensive patients (19 African Americans and 43 Caucasians) with regard to the types of glomerular injury present in their renal biopsies. They found that 25% of glomeruli in the African American patients were of the solidified form as compared with 8% in Caucasians. A subgroup of patients also had segmental sclerosis, also seen more frequently in African Americans. In addition to the segmental lesions, the African Americans in this subgroup had 38% solidified glomeruli. The authors suggested that this lesion may be related to vasospasm/functional vasoconstriction in African American patients. Another possible explanation is the hypothesis that African Americans are subject to glomerular hyperfiltration (165,166). Aviv et al (165) hypothesize that a high-salt diet (or other mechanism for increased sodium delivery to the distal tubule) causes tubular hyperperfusion at the macula densa with consequent resetting of the tubuloglomerular feedback mechanism and change in the balance between afferent and efferent vascular tone, ending in glomerular hyperfiltration. Because glomerular hyperfiltration is one of the factors thought to play a role in the pathogenesis of segmental sclerosis, it may be important in the prevalence of segmental lesions perhaps progressing to the solidified glomeruli in these patients. In aging kidneys, Hill et al (167) describe two types of hyaline arteriolosclerosis, one with occlusion of the lumen and one without such occlusion. They found that the arterioles with nonocclusive hyalin had dilated lumens and the glomeruli were hypertrophied. Furthermore, they believe that these findings support a loss of autoregulation at such sites. Another factor in the pathogenesis of these lesions may be the presence of reduced numbers of glomeruli in some patients with hypertension (49,134).

Brenner and Chertow (134) suggested that early gestational age or fetal growth retardation might affect nephronogenesis so that a reduced number of nephrons occurs with consequent hyperfiltration of those that are present. Keller et al (49) found a reduced number of nephrons at autopsy in patients with hypertension. Rostand (168) in a review cautioned that relationships between low birth weight and later hypertension have only been weak in studies to date but cited other studies that suggest that it is worthwhile to look for reduced renal reserve, microalbuminuria, and other evidence for end organ damage in such patients.

## Pathogenesis of Small-Vessel Changes

Considerable examination of the pathogenesis of the different vascular changes seen in human hypertension has been undertaken over the years. These changes include hyaline arteriolosclerosis, intimal thickening, and medial thickening. Each of the major alterations is discussed in turn.

## Hyaline Arteriolosclerosis

Hyaline arteriolosclerosis is an alteration seen in patients with benign hypertension, in the aged, in patients with diabetes mellitus, and in patients with various glomerular diseases. Thus, it is not specific for hypertension. Moritz and Oldt (169) examined small arteries and arterioles defined by an external diameter of less than 500 µm at autopsy from 100 patients with hypertension and compared them with 100 control cases. These researchers found that hyaline arteriolosclerosis increased with age in various organs. A clear relationship between hyaline arteriolosclerosis and hypertension was seen only in the kidney. Tracy et al (170) confirmed that renal hyaline arteriolosclerosis correlated with blood pressure. In addition, these investigators found a direct relationship between the degree of plaques in the coronary arteries and the severity of hyaline arteriolosclerosis in the kidney.

Electron microscopic studies of arteriolar hyalin have suggested that the material represents an accumulation of plasma-derived materials (171). Many investigators have used immunofluorescence techniques to identify the various materials within the hyaline lesions (102,170). In such studies, the usual substances used included the various immunoglobulins, complement components, and fibrinogen. C3 has always been identified, often in the company of IgM. Gamble (102) studied splenic arteries with hyaline arteriolosclerosis and found C3 and its fragments only without other complement components or immunoglobulins. In particular, he identified C3b, C3c, and C3d, with C3b in its inactive form. When IgM or C1q was present, it was always bound to C3 and not to the arteriolar wall. Tracy et al (170) also found inactive C3b in hyaline lesions. In addition, these investigators found cholesterol, phospholipid, triglycerides, tryptophan, tyrosine, and cysteine, sometimes accompanied by small amounts of fibrin. This accumulation was thought to be a natural consequence of aging, but it could be accelerated by either hypertension or diabetes mellitus. In such cases, increased vascular permeability could account for the acceleration of lesion formation. Williams et al (172) examined the question of increased vascular permeability in hypertension. They showed that AII can increase vascular permeability independent of its pressor activity. Hill and Bariety (167) suggested that hyaline often accumulates in areas of smooth muscle thinning, but they did not demonstrate a cause and effect.

## Intimal Arterial Thickening

The observation of intimal thickening in hypertension is well established. Hypertensive nephrosclerosis is often defined by the presence of intimal thickening or fibroplasia. Tracy et al (173) related nephrosclerosis to arterial fibroplasia, blood pressure, and age and compared populations

in New Orleans, Japan, and Guatemala. They found that all patients had at least some arterial fibroplasia. Kloczko et al (174) examined 84 patients with newly diagnosed essential hypertension and grouped them by retinal findings. They found significantly higher levels of von Willebrand factor (vWF) antigen in the serum of hypertensive patients compared with nonhypertensive controls. In addition, vWF antigen was higher in those patients with worse eye ground changes and with higher grades of hypertension, although no direct correlation was seen with either systolic or diastolic blood pressure. This study documented the presence of endothelial injury in patients with hypertension.

Although the presence of intimal thickening in hypertension is well described, its pathogenesis has not been defined. The relationship between hypertension and atherosclerosis is well accepted (175). Thus one possible explanation is the accumulation of platelets in areas of acute endothelial injury followed by secretion of growth factors and subsequent proliferation of smooth muscle cells into the intima (176). Endothelial dysfunction is now recognized to play a central role in the pathophysiology of both atherosclerosis and hypertension (121,177,178). Shear stress can be sensed by mechanosensors, such as the vascular endothelial growth factor receptor, ion channels, G proteins, intercellular junction proteins, and membrane lipids (179,180). Both shear stress and increased pulse pressure may induce release of endothelium-derived NO (178,181,182), which would then produce vasodilation and lowered blood pressure. Shear stress can be thought of as tangential friction, whereas increased pulse pressure acts in a perpendicular fashion to the wall of the vessel (181). In an in vitro experiment, continuous shear stress resulted in transient release of NO with an unresponsive interval of 15 minutes followed by a second transient release with a similar unresponsive interval. Increase in the amount of stress resulted in the release of a greater amount of NO (181). Another in vitro study of endothelial cells under cyclic strain confirmed the up-regulation of endothelial-derived NO synthase (183). This strain resulted in altered production of vasoactive substances, increased endothelial cell proliferation, changes in endothelial cell morphology, and increased protein synthesis (183).

In hypertension NO is decreased, and this decrease is an indicator of endothelial dysfunction. The decrease may be the result of either a decrease in synthesis or an increase in degradation. Some of the possible mechanisms for decreased synthesis include deficiency in the precursor, L-arginine, changes in the L-arginine transporter, production of endogenous NO synthase inhibitors such as asymmetric dimethyl arginine (ADMA), cofactor deficiency, decreased eNOS gene, decreased half-life of eNOS mRNA, changes in Gi proteins, changes in calcium-independent pathways of eNOS activation, and changes in the interactions between eNOS and caveolin-90 (178). Shear stress has been shown to increase gene expression of protein arginine methyltransferase (PRMT-1), ADMA synthase, resulting in increased levels of ADMA (184). This is accomplished via the NF-κB pathway. Increased NO degradation or inactivation occurs secondary to oxidative stress through interactions with superoxide ions mediated chiefly through increased NADPH and xanthine oxidase (178). Another mechanism of increased oxidative stress may be hyperhomocysteinemia (128). Endothelial cell superoxide generation is reviewed by Li and Shah (185). Endothelial dysfunction also plays a role in vascular remodeling and will be further discussed in the next section. However, we still do not understand the reasons for the increased intimal thickness, which is most pronounced where shear stress varies over time and is of lower magnitude.

## Medial Thickening

The presence of increased wall thickening is also an old observation in arteries from patients with hypertension. The reduced diameter of the lumen was thought to be the structural equivalent of increased peripheral resistance. An important measurement used to document this alteration is an increase in the wall-to-lumen ratio. Short (186) dilated and fixed by perfusion the mesenteric arteries of patients with hypertension and controls at autopsy. He then compared the wall-to-lumen ratio of arterioles in deciles by size and found that this ratio was higher for hypertensive patients for all but the smallest 20% of arterioles. Short also found that the cross-sectional area was not increased. Studies in humans using accessible tissue from the gluteal region showed an increase in the wall-to-lumen ratio in hypertensive patients as compared with nonhypertensive controls (187,188). Christensen (189) compared the mesenteric vessels of SHR and WKY rats. Multiple regression analysis showed that pulse pressure was the main factor responsible for change in wall-to-lumen ratio, with heart rate a minor factor and mean blood pressure not an independent predictor. Pulse pressure also correlated with vessel wall thickness.

The changes in the vessel wall now called remodeling were first recognized by Baumbach and Heistad (190) in the cerebral arterioles of stroke-prone SHRs. These authors noted that both external and internal diameters of these vessels were reduced at a time of maximal dilation. As the concept developed, remodeling became defined as a rearrangement of the existing cells around a smaller lumen (190). Two forms of remodeling are now recognized. Eutrophic remodeling is characterized by reduction in the outer diameter and lumen, but the media cross-section does not increase because of the rearrangement of the cells themselves (191,192). This form of remodeling is found most frequently in renin-associated forms of hypertension (192). Simon (193) considers angiotensin II to be central to the pathogenesis of these lesions in the kidney. Studies of vessels from subcutaneous gluteal tissues have shown that eutrophic remodeling may be present in humans with mild

to moderate levels of hypertension (194). In contrast, in hypertrophic remodeling, the external diameter remains the same, and the increased size of the muscle cells causes direct reduction of the lumen by encroachment (191,192). Hypertrophic remodeling has been demonstrated by Rizzoni et al (195) without evidence of hyperplasia. AII is also critical in the induction of smooth muscle hypertrophy (196). Investigators transfected ACE into both the medial smooth muscle cells and intimal endothelial cells of rat carotid arteries. The increase in ACE was accompanied by a parallel increase in DNA synthesis, which was abrogated with the administration of AII receptor antagonist. Two weeks after the transfection, the wall-to-lumen ratio was increased without an increment in cell number. No systemic effects of ACE were detected, suggesting the presence of a paracrine effect and supporting the idea that AII can directly cause smooth muscle cell hypertrophy. Sventek et al (197) examined the role of ET-1 in several different experimental models of hypertension and found that in the non–renin-dependent models, ET-1 was associated with smooth muscle hypertrophy. Endothelins are known to have both mitogenic and hypertrophic effects. It is also now clear that both forms of remodeling may occur in the same patient or experimental animal at the same time and that these changes may increase with longer exposures to hypertension (95). The presence of these changes in the resistance vessels is also predictive along with increased pulse pressure of increased risk for cardiovascular events (198). The importance of changes in the renal afferent arterioles in the pathogenesis of hypertension has been reviewed by Skov and Mulvany (199) and is unquestioned. It is likely that several different factors contribute to the pathogenesis of these changes.

Remodeling of the smooth muscle cells of the vessels is also accompanied by an increase in the intercellular matrix in vessels of all sizes. O'Callaghan and Williams (200) showed a link between chronic cyclical strain and increased production of extracellular matrix by vascular smooth muscle cells grown in culture. This was mediated by increased transforming growth factor-β. Other investigators have shown an increase in matrix metalloproteinase-2 (MMP-2) (201), but MMP-3 and MMP-9 have also been implicated (202). Others have suggested that AII or aldosterone may be important in increased stiffness (203). Such changes result in increased stiffening and decreased compliance in all vessels and are associated with increased cardiovascular morbidity and mortality (202). Yasmin et al (204) studied arterial stiffness using an augmentation index and pulse wave velocity in the young adult offspring of hypertensive and nonhypertensive families. They found that the augmentation index was increased in the offspring of hypertensive families, suggesting that patients likely to develop hypertension might have changes in arterial compliance prior to the onset of increased blood pressure. In the resistance vessels, these changes in the extracellular matrix further increase the thickness of the media in hypertrophic remodeling and contribute to the reorganization of the vessel wall in eutrophic remodeling (95,192). Another possible mechanism for changes in compliance is alteration in elastin. Known mutations in the elastin gene in supravalvular aortic stenosis and in Williams syndrome are associated with hypertension (205).

Remodeling can be reversed with therapy, as shown in both experimental models and in human beings (192,194,206–211). Notoya et al (209) administered an angiotensin-converting enzyme (ACE) inhibitor to SHR and found a reversal of vascular remodeling. Ledingham and Laverty (206,208) performed a series of studies in the New Zealand genetically hypertensive rat. They found that an ACE inhibitor prevented remodeling as did two different angiotensin receptor antagonists. Furthermore, they found that fluvastatin also prevented remodeling in this model despite the fact that it did not lower blood pressure (207). Pu et al (210) studied the deoxycorticosterone acetate (DOCA)–salt hypertensive rat, a model with low renin and vasodilation rather than vasoconstriction in micropuncture studies (143). They used omapatrilat, which inhibits both ACE and neutral endopeptidase (NEP). They also administered an ACE inhibitor in a second group and a NEP inhibitor in a third group. They found that omapatrilat and the NEP inhibitor decreased vascular remodeling, but that the ACE inhibitor alone had no effect. They concluded that NEP inhibition was necessary in the DOCA–salt model to prevent remodeling. Schiffrin et al (194) contrasted the ability of losartan, an angiotensin type receptor-1 antagonist (AT1RA), to that of atenolol, a beta-blocker, to reverse remodeling in human beings. They found that the AT1RA reduced the ratio of media width to lumen diameter following 1 year of treatment but that atenolol did not have such an effect. Schiffrin (192) has reviewed the various studies of the effect of different antihypertensive agents on the structure of small arteries in patients. This review showed that the ACE inhibitors, AT1RAs, and calcium channel blockers reversed remodeling. However, the beta-blockers did not. This failure has been attributed to the vasoconstricting effect of beta-blockers as well as their lack of effect on oxidative stress (192).

As discussed above in the pathophysiology of hypertension section, increased levels of uric acid in the serum may also play a primary role in essential hypertension (113). In a rat model of hyperuricemia, Mazzali et al (132) showed that the elevated serum uric acid produced hypertension that was associated with arteriolopathy of the afferent arteriole. Ablation of the hypertension by treatment with hydrochlorothiazide did not affect development of the vascular lesion (132). Micropuncture studies of these rats showed that the hyperuricemia was associated with vasoconstriction and a decrease in renal plasma flow (212). It has been posited that the uric acid may enter the smooth muscle cell by an organic anion transporter and is then able to ac-

tivate mitogen-activated protein kinases and transcription factors to result in increased cellular proliferation, increased inflammatory mediators such as cyclo-oxygenase 2, and up-regulation of the AT1R (113,213).

Aldosterone is also emerging as an important player in the pathogenesis of hypertension and in the structural changes in vessel walls (135,136,152,214). Rocha et al (214), using the stroke-prone spontaneously hypertensive rat, showed that administration of an ACEI could prevent glomerular and vascular lesions and reduce the plasma aldosterone levels. However, when aldosterone was given with the ACEI, the beneficial effects were eliminated with greater injury than in animals that received no therapy (214). These effects were independent of changes in blood pressure, suggesting a direct tissue effect. Aldosterone induces both hypertrophy and pericellular fibrosis in vascular smooth muscle cells (135). Aldosterone is also important in the regulation of plasminogen activator inhibitor-1 (PAI-1) and may act together with AII to alter the vascular fibrinolysis system (135). This idea is further supported by Chander et al (152) in their study of the role of aldosterone in the pathogenesis of thrombotic microangiopathy in rats with severe hypertension. Other potential mechanisms for aldosterone in potentiating vascular injury include stimulation of ROS, increased sodium influx into vascular smooth muscle cells, and inhibition of nitric oxide (135).

### Summary

The mechanism for the remodeling is uncertain although some aspects are understood. It seems likely that different factors are important depending on the type of hypertension and the underlying genetic abnormalities. However, a broad outline may be seen as drawn by a simpleminded pathologist (Fig. 21.27). Several different inciting factors may be involved in the vascular injury including prolonged shear stress, AII, aldosterone, homocysteine, and uric acid. Shear stress is transduced to cause release of several factors that may promote remodeling. AII, aldosterone, and homocysteine increase ROS, resulting in decreased NO. AII also increases ET-1. Decreased NO with an additional effect from aldosterone and probably AII has a prothrombotic effect. The decreased NO, increased ET-1, and uric acid lead to increased vasoconstriction, cellular migration, and cellular proliferation, leading to remodeling. The various signaling pathways within the cells for these various processes are reviewed by Touyz and Schiffrin (215,216) but are beyond the scope of this chapter.

## Pathogenesis of Interstitial Disease

Considerable interest exists in the relationship between changes in the interstitium and in the remainder of the kidney in hypertension as well as in other renal disease. Mai et al (217) studied the 2K1C model at 1-week intervals after clipping for 4 weeks. The rats developed hypertension

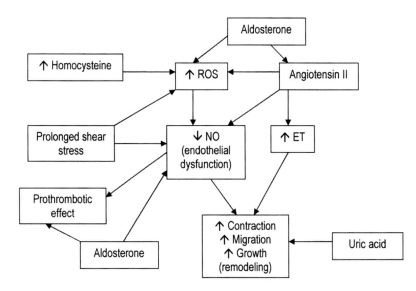

**Figure 21.27** Flow chart showing inciting factors for vascular injury and mechanisms that possibly result in remodeling of the vessel wall. ROS, reactive oxygen species; NO, nitric oxide; E-1, endothelin.

by day 7, accompanied by an early 37% expansion of interstitial volume in the unclipped kidney. This change preceded the occurrence of glomerular or vascular changes. Immunofluorescence studies showed the accumulation of collagen types I, III, IV, V, and VI and fibronectin. Other interstitial alterations included increased proliferating cell nuclear antigen in tubular epithelial cells, as well as an increase in infiltrating macrophages and T lymphocytes, all occurring by day 7. Renal arteries showed significantly increased wall thickness, but this increase also followed the interstitial changes. In general, extracellular matrix deposition depended on the enhanced growth of fibroblasts with prolonged mitotic life span and a more active production of matrix proteins.

Other investigators have also observed the early occurrence of interstitial disease in the setting of experimental hypertensive injury (158,218). Johnson et al (218) noted the parallel development of tubulointerstitial disease and hypertension. The tubulointerstitial injury was characterized by a "striped" pattern suggesting vascular origin that was most severe in the outer medulla and juxtamedullary cortex accompanied by increased osteopontin and macrophages, capillary rarefaction, and increased collagen deposition. *Capillary rarefaction* refers to the ablation of the peripheral microvessels and has been recognized in the setting of hypertension for many years. Some have attributed a portion of the increased peripheral resistance to this reduction in capillaries (219). The exact mechanism of rarefaction is unknown but apoptosis in capillary endothelial cells has been shown to be increased (220,221). Ischemia secondary to arteriolar vasoconstriction is thought to be important (153,222). Mori and Cowley (153) also believe that increased perfusion pressure transmitted to the vasa recta leads to endothelial dysfunction in those microvessels with increased ROS and the consequences described above. Another possible factor is reduction in vascular en-

dothelial growth factor (222). Johnson et al (113) believe that early often subtle tubulointerstitial injury may be critical in the development of salt-sensitive hypertension.

## Differential Diagnosis

Several conditions resemble the pathologic changes seen in hypertension. These include aging, thrombotic microangiopathy, and antiphospholipid antibody syndrome (APS). Hypertension may be a complication of other renal diseases as renal parenchyma becomes scarred during the progression of renal disease. These will be discussed in turn. The secondary forms of hypertension may produce changes that are indistinguishable from essential hypertension. The pathology of these forms is discussed later in the chapter.

Aging produces many of the same changes seen with hypertension in both experimental models and in humans (83,167,173,201,222,223). These include glomerular obsolescence of the wrinkled capillary wall type, interstitial fibrosis, tubular atrophy, intimal thickening, and hyaline arteriolosclerosis (83,98,167,223). However, the solidified form of obsolescence is not expected because of aging. In addition, although some remodeling of vessel walls may occur with increased age, widespread medial thickening is unusual. Finally, reduplication of elastic lamina is not usually seen in older individuals in the absence of hypertension. At least some of these changes are caused by alterations in the phenotype of individual cells (224). The similarities are likely owing to the common mechanism of ischemia (223).

Thrombotic microangiopathy is characterized by the presence of fibrin platelet thrombi with schistocytes contained within arterioles and glomerular capillaries. Subendothelial widening with double contours on silver stain is frequently seen. TMA is a common pathologic finding in several disorders including malignant hypertension, hemolytic uremic syndrome, thrombotic thrombocytopenic purpura, and scleroderma and with the administration of several drugs such as calcineurin inhibitors and various chemotherapeutic agents. It is not possible to distinguish among these diagnoses without clinical information. These disorders are discussed in Chapter 18.

Antiphospholipid antibody syndrome is defined by the presence of antiphospholipid antibodies and/or lupus anticoagulant-associated arterial or venous thrombosis and spontaneous miscarriages (225,226). The patients frequently have severe hypertension as well. It may occur as a primary lesion or may complicate autoimmune disease, in particular systemic lupus erythematosus (227). Nochy et al (225) examined the changes in the kidney of 16 patients with primary APS. They found TMA in 31%, fibrous intimal hyperplasia in 75%, fibrous and fibrocellular vascular occlusions in 68%, and focal cortical atrophy in 61% of the biopsies. The fibrous intimal hyperplasia frequently showed a cellular proliferation with actin positive cells. They found the involvement of larger vessels, the increased cellularity of the intimal hyperplasia, and the focal cortical atrophy to be useful features allowing differentiation from TMA in general. In addition, the medial walls did not show the changes typically associated with essential hypertension.

Chronic kidney disease is commonly accompanied by hypertension (157,228). Fifteen to 80% of patients with chronic glomerular disease without renal failure had hypertension (157). In a study of patients with end-stage renal disease, the prevalence of hypertension was 90% (228). The lesions are identical to those described above for essential hypertension. The differentiation between primary hypertension and hypertension complicating a parenchymal renal disease is made by the presence of a primary glomerular or tubulointerstitial disease preceding the onset of hypertension. In addition, if collapsed and wrinkled glomeruli predominate, then the likelihood increases that hypertensive vascular injury has contributed to the changes seen, whereas if the glomeruli show the solidified form, then an end-stage kidney disorder is more likely to have resulted from some other glomerular disease such as chronic glomerulonephritis in which enlargement or expansion of the glomerulus may precede the sclerosing process (see Chapter 27).

## Clinical Course, Prognosis, Therapy, and Clinicopathologic Correlation

### Clinical Course

The natural history of hypertension has changed and continues to evolve as new antihypertensive drugs are developed. Review of older studies, before effective therapy protocols were developed, provides an interesting backdrop to a consideration of the current progression of the disease. One of the best of these studies is that of Perera (229), who studied 500 untreated hypertensive patients with diastolic pressures greater than 90 mm Hg. He found that 50% of patients suffered from congestive heart failure, 16% had angina, and 12% had strokes. These complications led to shortening of life by 15 to 20 years. Seven percent of patients, mostly men, progressed to the malignant phase of hypertension. Effective therapy has resulted in a lower mortality rate from the hypertension itself and has reduced the incidence of complications. However, in the age group between 35 and 64 years, hypertension continues to increase risk for coronary disease, 2.0 and 2.2 times for men and women respectively, for stroke 3.8 and 2.6 times, for peripheral artery disease, 2.0 and 3.7 times, and for heart failure 4.0 and 3.0 times (52). Risk is also increased in patients older than 64 years with relative risks ranging between 1.6 and 2.3 for the various cardiovascular complications (52).

Before antihypertensive therapy was available, nearly 70% of patients died of renal failure within months of the onset of the malignant phase of hypertension (90). Lip et al (61) in their study in Birmingham, England, showed no decline in the incidence of malignant hypertension over a 20-year period ending in 1994. Scarpelli et al (230) studied 121 consecutive cases of accelerated hypertension between 1974 and 1996. They divided them into two groups by date of presentation (1974 to 1980 and 1981 to 1996) using 1980 as the breakpoint because of the introduction of newer effective drugs. They found a decrease in the prevalence of the disease as well as a reduction in the severity of the presentation. In particular, they found fewer cases with papilledema. The overall survival rate was 69.8% at 12 years. However, analysis of the patients who presented in 1986 or later showed no morbidity in the 10 years since development of the disease. The reasons for improvement were thought to be related to less severe blood pressure elevations than in years past, detection of the disease before severe cardiac disease had supervened, as well as the improvement of therapeutic regimens (230). Effective therapy returns the patient to the typical course for hypertension, but the severe levels of hypertension can recur and put the patient at risk for cerebral hemorrhage or myocardial infarction (231). Other complications include chronic renal failure (31.7%), heart failure, hypertensive cardiomyopathy, and angina (61).

Hypertension is the second most common cause of ESRD in the United States, accounting for 23% of the incidence of ESRD (232). This percentage is a decrease from that reported in the previous edition of this text (30.1%) owing to an increase in the total number of patients with ESRD mainly because of a parallel increase in diabetic nephropathy. However, the absolute number of patients with ESRD owing to hypertension has remained largely unchanged. Factors that increase the risk of progression to ESRD for a hypertensive patient include lack of treatment, diastolic blood pressure (greater than 87 mm Hg), male sex, and Black race (233). However, the true incidence of primary hypertension resulting in ESRD is difficult to determine. A recent study by Hsu et al (234) showed that the adjusted relative risk of developing ESRD is 1.62 (CI 1.27 to 2.07) for patients with blood pressures of 120 to 129/80 mm Hg compared with patients with blood pressure less than 120/80 mm Hg. As levels of blood pressure become more elevated, the adjusted relative risk of ESRD also increases to 2.59 at blood pressures of 140 to 159/90 to 99 mm Hg and to 3.88 for blood pressures of 180 to 209/110 to 119 mm Hg. At times, a clinician evaluates a patient, discovers high blood pressure, and then finds ESRD. Renal biopsy is usually unrewarding in these late circumstances, although in a few cases, a primary glomerular disease may be found. The characteristic pathologic manifestations of hypertensive nephrosclerosis, however, are nonspecific, especially in the context of ESRD. Furthermore, it is not always possible to distinguish between primary and secondary hypertension on a renal biopsy.

## Prognosis

The factors that determine prognosis are those that affect the development of the complications of hypertension. The risks for cardiovascular disease have been outlined above. I will limit this discussion to the factors that determine the likelihood of developing renal disease in association with hypertension. Many of these have been suggested in the section Pathogenesis of Hypertension above. Walker (235) showed that a subset of patients with diastolic pressures that did not exceed 115 mm Hg would be predicted to progress to ESRD using the slope of the plot of the reciprocal of the serum creatinine against time. This author also showed that the progression could be halted by maintaining diastolic pressures lower than 95 mm Hg. Data suggest that 140,000 patients with hypertension in the United States develop increased serum creatinine levels each year, whereas 5300 hypertensive patients with previous renal insufficiency develop ESRD (235). An intriguing case report suggests that optimal blood pressure control is capable of reversing hypertensive nephrosclerosis (GFR from 20 mL/min to 80 mL/min) as well as improvement in retinal findings and in left ventricular wall thickness (from 19 to 12 mm) over a 3-year period (236). Some factors that predispose the hypertensive patient to renal failure are increasing age, poor serum glucose control in diabetic patients, level of systolic blood pressure, male gender, black race, and elevated uric acid and triglycerides (237,238). Diastolic blood pressure is a good predictor of progression to ESRD (235). On the other hand, effective therapy reduces the likelihood of progression to renal insufficiency (64,230).

Large epidemiologic studies are plagued by several problems such as lack of renal biopsy in diagnosis, differences in criteria for entry into the study or dialysis program, differing therapies, questions concerning inclusion of secondary forms of hypertension, and lack of distinction between benign and malignant hypertension. However, biopsy studies are limited by the smaller numbers of patients who can be studied. In one biopsy study, Pillay et al (239) confirmed the presence of hypertensive nephrosclerosis without evidence of other renal disease on biopsy or autopsy study in seven black patients with grade 2 retinal changes who either died of uremia or who were undergoing dialysis.

Genetic studies are also being undertaken for an examination of the relationship between genetic polymorphisms and the presence of renal insufficiency in hypertensive patients. Mallamaci et al (240) showed an association between the presence of the D allele in the *ACE* gene with biopsy-proven hypertensive renal disease. Another group found albuminuria and a mild increase in left ventricular size in hypertensive patients with the D allele of *ACE* (241). In a more elaborate study, Fabris et al (242) examined polymorphisms in the renin-angiotensin-aldosterone system owing to its central role in the pathogenesis of hypertension in hypertensive patients with and without renal failure. They examined the insertion/deletion of angiotensin-converting enzyme (*ACE* I/D), angiotensinogen (*AGT*) M235T, angiotensin II type 1 receptor (*AT1R*) A1166C and aldosterone synthase (*CYP11B2*)-344C/T polymorphisms. They found that each of the genetic polymorphisms examined was associated with renal failure. The associations *AGT* TT-*AT1R* AC and *CYP11B2* CC-*ACE* DD were present more frequently in hypertensive patients with renal insufficiency. On the other hand, patients with *AGT* MM-*AT1R* AA and *AGT* MM-*AT1R* AA-*CYP11B2* TT or TC combinations showed a reduced risk for renal failure (242).

Thus, it seems that even benign hypertension can result in renal failure, particularly in patients with higher levels of diastolic blood pressure. However, the frequency of this occurrence has not been determined because of the aforementioned problems of case acquisition in the large epidemiologic studies and the lack of documentation by renal biopsy studies. A likely course of events in those cases of hypertension that proceed to renal insufficiency is that vasoconstriction causes renal ischemia and tubulointerstitial injury with functional early renal failure (113). Vasoconstriction may maintain hypertension by interfering with sodium handling, and established hypertension then leads ultimately to decreased GFR because of progressive luminal narrowing of afferent arterioles, glomerular obsolescence, and tubular atrophy. Alternatively, transmission of elevated pressures to the glomerulus through damaged and dilated afferent arterioles may induce glomerular capillary hypertension and hyperperfusion and may cause glomerular injury and progressive renal insufficiency (47,86,140).

## Therapy

Numerous drugs are available to treat hypertension. They fall into different classes of action. Those currently in use include diuretics, β-adrenergic blockers, α-adrenoceptor blockers, ACE inhibitors, calcium antagonists, AII receptor antagonists, adrenergic inhibitors, and direct smooth muscle vasodilators. New drugs and classes are also under development or in clinical trials including endothelin antagonists, mineralocorticoid receptor antagonists, vasopeptidase inhibitors, and renin inhibitors. It is critically important to control the blood pressure to 120/80 mm Hg or less (1). It has been shown that lowering the blood pressure to these optimal levels can slow the progression of hypertensive nephropathy (243,244).

Depending on the severity of the hypertension, patients are started on one of the first-line drugs and additional agents are added as needed. The drug therapy is tailored to the individual patient's needs (18). It has been known for some time that ACE inhibitors are renoprotective and it is now apparent that the angiotensin II subtype 1 receptor antagonists (AT[1]RA) protect the kidneys as well (245). Some drugs have been shown to reverse pathophysiologic alterations in vessels (194). Studies of the various polymorphisms in the renin–angiotensin–aldosterone system are leading to clinical studies to examine whether these polymorphisms can predict efficacy of one agent over another in particular patients (36,37). Williams et al (37) noted that a loss-of-function mutation in the gene encoding renal 11beta-hydroxysteroid dehydrogenase type 2 (*HSD11B2*) enzyme resulted in overstimulation of the mineralocorticoid receptor leading to salt-sensitive hypertension. Cytosine-adenine (CA) repeat microsatellite in intron 1 of *HSD11B2* was determined, and the CA repeat length was strongly associated with the response to hydrochlorothiazide, a diuretic. Likewise Spiering et al (36) showed that AII sensitivity is associated with the A1166C polymorphism of the AII type 1 receptor (*AT1R*) gene. They investigated the hormonal as well as systemic and renal hemodynamic responses to acute AT1R blockade with an active metabolite of losartan in 15 AA and 14 CC essential hypertensive patients. They found that lowering of blood pressure during high salt was significantly blunted in CC patients compared with AA patients. During low salt, decrease in renal vascular resistance was less in CC patients compared with AA patients.

## Clinicopathologic Correlation

Many clinical factors have been found to correlate with progression of renal as well as cardiovascular complications of hypertension. The one factor that links all of these complications is the acceleration of atherosclerosis by hypertension. Several lines of evidence support this link. Patients with hypertension invariably have some degree of atherosclerosis. Blood pressure has been shown to be an independent risk factor for cardiovascular disease (246). Furthermore, effective therapy for hypertension has been associated with reduced cardiovascular disease, as shown both in interventional trials and in countries where the use of antihypertensive therapy has become commonplace (246). Systolic blood pressure, in particular, has been associated with increased atherogenesis and with decreased large-vessel compliance (247). Another piece of evidence linking atherosclerosis and hypertension is the presence of endothelial dysfunction in both diseases (120,121). Rodriguez-Porcel et al (248) studied the effects of hypercholesterolemia (as a model for atherosclerosis), renovascular hypertension, or both in pigs. They found that endothelial dysfunction as measured by changes in renal perfusion pressure in response to acetylcholine or nitroprusside was worst in the pigs with both hypertension and hypercholesterolemia but was depressed in the other two experimental groups as well. These changes were paralleled by a decrease in oxygen radical scavengers. suggesting that hypertension and hypercholesterolemia can damage endothelial cells but that the two together can act synergistically to cause greater damage (248).

Clinical factors predicting the presence of renal injury in the setting of hypertension include microalbuminuria and increased serum creatinine at presentation. Microalbuminuria is associated with increased risk for cardiovascular disease (249). However, it is also recognized as an early sign for renal disease in the setting of hypertension (71–73,250). Progression to macroalbuminuria may signal the onset of glomerular disease (73,250) owing to either endothelial injury with dysfunction or to glomerular hyperfiltration. Pathologically one may find the solidified type of glomeruli. Vikse et al (251) performed a retrospective study with a 13-year follow-up on 102 patients who had a renal biopsy that confirmed the diagnosis of hypertensive nephrosclerosis. Proteinuria (>1 g/24 hours) and doubling of serum creatinine had a significant risk of progression to ESRD over the 13 years of follow-up. Each time the serum creatinine doubled, the relative risk of progressing to ESRD increased by 2.6 times. Likewise, each time the proteinuria increased by 1 g/24 hours, the relative risk of ESRD increased by 1.4 times. Patients with increased systolic blood pressure were at increased risk for ESRD during the first 3 years of the follow-up. In severe levels of hypertension, the serum creatinine level at the time of diagnosis has been a good indication of the outcome with regard to chronic renal function. In one study, patients with serum creatinine levels greater than 3.3 mg/100 mL had a poor outcome (252).

## SECONDARY HYPERTENSION AND ITS CAUSES

Most instances of hypertension (>90%) have no known underlying cause and are thus called *primary* or *essential hypertension.* However, many different conditions may be associated with secondary hypertension. Examples of these conditions are listed in Table 21.2. . Certain circumstances should prompt consideration of secondary forms of hypertension including rapid onset, severity of hypertension, resistance to antihypertensive drug therapy, absence of family history, signs of vascular disease elsewhere, onset after 60 years of age or before age 30 years (253). Recommended routine laboratory evaluation for secondary forms of hypertension includes hematocrit, serum potassium, serum creatinine, blood urea nitrogen, urinalysis, urinary albumin excretion, fasting blood glucose, serum cholesterol, plasma triglycerides, plasma renin activity, urinary sodium and potassium, electrocardiography, and possibly echocardiography (50). Additional studies are necessary for diagnosis of hypertension resulting from renal artery stenosis or catecholamine-secreting tumors.

## Prevalence of Secondary Hypertension

Secondary hypertension represents only a small percentage of cases of hypertension, reported in various studies from 5% to 21% (Table 21.3) (13,254–259). These apparent differences undoubtedly are owing to variation in referral patterns to hypertension study centers where the studies are performed. The frequency of secondary hypertension also depends on the demographics of the population studied. Anderson et al (13) showed that the prevalence of secondary hypertension increased with advancing age and prevalence of atherosclerosis. The leading causes were renal artery stenosis and renal parenchymal disease. Dluhy (260) found primary hypothyroidism was also a common cause of secondary hypertension in the elderly. Discrimination between renal vascular disease and renal parenchymal disease is often not possible clinically (261). The most frequent causes of secondary hypertension in children are neurofibromatosis (262) and unilateral renal artery stenosis (263).

The prevalence of secondary causes of hypertension is also greater in patients with malignant hypertension. A study performed by Sinclair et al (259) in Australia examined 83 patients with malignant hypertension. These authors (259) found that 80% of their group had secondary hypertension, with 65% related to renal parenchymal disease and 13% owing to renovascular disease. Lip et al (61) studied 242 patients with malignant hypertension over a 23-year period. These investigators found that secondary causes of hypertension were present in 40% of their patients. Secondary causes included chronic renal failure of unknown origin, pyelonephritis, glomerulonephritis, polycystic kidney disease, renal artery stenosis, primary aldosteronism, and pheochromocytoma. These studies indicate that some patients with malignant hypertension, at least those with renal artery stenosis, may have a potentially curable lesion.

## Renal Artery Stenosis—Atherosclerotic Renovascular Disease

Many conditions are recognized as causes of renal artery stenosis (Table 21.4). By far the most common are atherosclerosis, which occurs in 70% to 90% of cases, and fibromuscular dysplasia, which is seen in 10% to 30% of cases (264). Atherosclerotic renovascular disease and associated findings such as cholesterol emboli are sufficiently common to warrant detailed discussion. I will then comment on the other causes of renal artery stenosis including fibromuscular dysplasia, renal artery aneurysms, and Takayasu's disease.

### Clinical Features

Atherosclerotic renovascular disease (atherosclerotic renal artery stenosis, ARAS) is a disease of aging and is more common in those with evidence of atherosclerosis affecting extrarenal vessels as well (265–268). In autopsy studies, the prevalence of significant renal artery stenosis ranges

## TABLE 21.3

**FREQUENCY OF SECONDARY FORMS IN PATIENTS WITH HYPERTENSION**

| Authors | Number of Patients | Secondary Hypertension % | Renal Parenchymal Disease (%) | Renovascular Disease (%) | Other (%) | Oral Contraceptives (%) |
|---|---|---|---|---|---|---|
| Danielson and Dammstrom (256) | 1000 | 4.7 | 2.1 | 1 | 0.8 | 0.8 |
| Berglund et al (255) | 689 | 5.8 | 3.6 | 0.6 | 1.6 | — |
| Sinclair et al (259) | 3783 | 7.9 | 5.6 | 0.7 | 0.6 | 1 |
| Gifford (257) | 4939 | 11.1 | 5.2 | 5.1 | 0.8 | — |
| Bech and Hilden (254) | 482 | 20.7 | 12.6 | 5 | 1.6 | 1.5 |
| Anderson et al (13) | 4429 | 10.7 | 1.8 | 3.1 | 5.8 | — |
| Omura et al (258) | 1020 | 9.1 | 0[a] | 0.5 | 8.6 | — |

[a]Excluded patients with renal failure.

## TABLE 21.4
## CAUSES OF RENAL ARTERY STENOSIS

Atherosclerosis
Renal artery dysplasia
Dissecting aneurysms of either aorta or renal artery
Other aneurysms
Takayasu's arteritis
Other arteritides
Neurofibromatosis
Thromboemboli
Narrowing of anastomosis in renal transplantation
Moyamoya disease
Direct compression by tumor
Irradiation
Trauma
Arteriovenous fistulas

between 5% and 42% depending on age (265,268,269). A population-based study of 800 people older than 65 years without known kidney disease was 6.8% (more than 60% occlusion based on Doppler study) (270). The prevalence of ARAS in patients undergoing angiographic studies of other vessels such as coronary angiography ranges between 14% and 28% (268). Patients with extensive peripheral vascular disease have prevalence rates of renal artery involvement as high as 50% (261). The prevalence of bilateral renal artery disease in patients with coronary angiography is 4% (253). Bilateral renal artery stenosis may be present in 33% to 39% of cases with ARAS (259). Clearly, patients with bilateral involvement have a higher incidence of renal failure. Other investigators have emphasized that renal artery stenosis may be present in patients with normal blood pressure (269). Renal artery stenosis is more often seen in men than in women (267).

Certain features of the clinical presentation in patients with hypertension suggest the possible presence of renal artery stenosis. These include malignant or accelerated hypertension with loss of blood pressure control or grade 3 to 4 retinopathy, atherosclerotic vascular disease, and especially abdominal or flank bruits (271). In addition, the presence of resistant hypertension, proteinuria, absence of family history of hypertension, and hypokalemia also suggest the presence of ARAS (253,265,272). On occasion patients will present with "flash" pulmonary edema (265,268). Predictors of renal artery stenosis include older age, peripheral vascular disease, congestive heart disease, increased serum creatinine, dyslipidemias, diabetes, and a history of smoking (267,271).

A common complication of atherosclerosis is the occurrence of atheroemboli. This syndrome may occur spontaneously; however, it is most frequently seen during, immediately after, or within several months of angiographic or surgical procedures involving vessels (273). Other risk factors include male gender, aortic surgery, thrombolytic therapy, oral anticoagulants, and abdominal aortic aneurysms (274). The frequency of symptomatic multiple cholesterol syndrome has been reported to be between 0.08% and 0.8% after angiography (274). A clinical syndrome has been associated with the showering of multiple cholesterol emboli into the renal vessels and other major branches of the aorta (273–275). Clinical signs include livedo reticularis, acute renal failure, hypertension, leg pain, gastrointestinal symptoms, and vision loss (274). Peripheral eosinophilia and decreased serum complement have also been associated with this syndrome. The prevalence of these various manifestations is difficult to establish because many cases of atheroembolic disease may not be detected clinically (273). Spontaneous atheroembolism may present as unexplained renal failure or as de novo onset of hypertension (273,276).

Hypertension in adolescents is usually owing to essential hypertension. However, in younger children and neonates, secondary forms of hypertension predominate (277,278). The most frequent causes vary somewhat by age but in general, the most common form of secondary hypertension in children is chronic renal parenchymal diseases followed by coarctation of the aorta and endocrine causes (278). Neurofibromatosis is the most common cause of renal artery stenosis in children and adolescents (278). In the neonate, thrombotic events secondary to umbilical artery catheterization are most frequent (277).

### Diagnostic Tests

The number and variety of tests used to assess the presence and extent of renal vascular lesions are beyond the scope of this chapter and are reviewed elsewhere (264,279). The gold standard among imaging techniques is intra-arterial digital subtraction angiography. Several noninvasive tests are now available such as magnetic resonance angiography, computed tomographic angiography, and color-aided duplex ultrasonography (264). The advantage of the noninvasive tests is that they also allow an evaluation of function.

### Pathologic Findings

#### Renal Artery
The atherosclerotic plaque is usually present in the portion of the renal artery nearest the aorta, or it may be in the aorta and override the ostium of the renal artery. This lesion is recognized by abdominal aortography (Fig. 21.28). If the vessel is severely narrowed, poststenotic dilatation is also present.

The changes are the same as those seen in systemic atherosclerosis and are characterized by the presence of a fibrous plaque, usually in the proximal third of the renal artery. Cross section shows the fibrous plaque as an

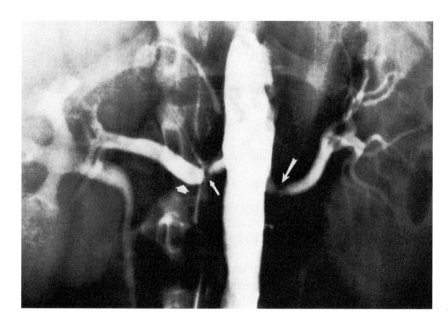

**Figure 21.28** Abdominal aortogram showing severe stenosis (*short white arrow*) with post-stenotic dilatation (*white arrowhead*) of the early part of the right main renal artery. Stenosis is less severe (*long white arrow*) in the proximal part of the left main renal artery. (Courtesy of Dr. Olga Gatewood, Department of Radiology, Johns Hopkins Hospital, Baltimore, MD.)

eccentric thickening of the intima (Fig. 21.29). The thickened intima contains amorphous material with lipid-laden macrophages, myofibroblasts, and various matrix proteins. The endothelium is usually intact, but if it becomes disrupted, then platelet aggregation and thrombosis may ensue. The media underlying the plaque is frequently thinned relative to the uninvolved portion of the vessel. Major complications include saccular or dissecting aneurysm formation and the occurrence of cholesterol emboli. Both events are discussed later, but suffice it to say, their incidence is increased when a catheter has been placed into the renal artery. The atherosclerotic lesion is most frequently single;

however, on occasion, multiple plaques are present, or a greater length of artery may be involved. Ostial plaques have a similar histologic appearance, but they are not as amenable to percutaneous angioplasty as intrarenal artery lesions.

### Ipsilateral Kidney

The changes seen in kidneys distal to renal artery stenosis vary with the age of the patient. In addition, the location of the narrowing is important. If the main renal artery is involved, then the whole kidney will show ischemic changes. On the other hand, if a segmental branch of the renal artery is affected, that portion of the kidney supplied by that vessel will be ischemic, and the rest of the kidney will show changes consistent with exposure to higher systemic pressures, as described earlier.

In young patients, purer ischemic changes are present. Thus, the kidney is uniformly reduced in size, with a smooth surface with tubular atrophy as the predominant alteration. Two types of atrophic tubules are seen in the patient with hypertension. The "classic" atrophic tubules with thickened basement membranes derive from the proximal tubules and are thought to result from repeated tubular injury, with regeneration causing the multiple layers of tubular basement membrane (280). A second type of atrophic tubule is the so-called endocrine form, first described by Selye and Stone (281) in hypertensive rats. In this form, the tubules have clear epithelial cells and narrow lumina, and they occur in clusters. They are usually derived from distal tubules (280). They are seen in association with ischemia. The glomeruli appear normal, but they are closer together than usual because of the tubular atrophy. These glomeruli may be atubular, as discussed below. Although the interstitium may appear normal, a connective tissue stain demonstrates diffuse but fine fibrosis.

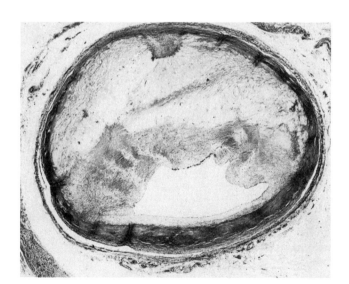

**Figure 21.29** Section through the origin of a renal artery to show occlusion of the lumen by atherosclerosis, from a 50-year-old man with severe hypertension. (H&E, ×13.) (From Heptinstall RH. In: Mostofi FK, Smith DE, eds. Vascular Diseases of the Kidney. International Academy of Pathology Monograph Series. Baltimore: Williams & Wilkins, 1966.)

In elderly patients, these changes are usually superimposed on those of both aging and atherosclerosis. Thus, such kidneys are often small, have a granular surface, and sometimes, larger scars, which may represent remote infarcts. Light microscopic examination reveals predominantly classic tubular atrophy and loss, with more interstitial fibrosis than seen in younger patients. Glomeruli may be normal, or they may show wrinkling and either partial or complete collapse of capillary loops. Simplification of the glomerular tuft is present with an apparent increase in Bowman's space. Vessels show a spectrum of changes, from hyaline arteriolosclerosis to fibrous intimal thickening in larger arteries. These changes were confirmed in a study by Marcussen (282) in which he examined kidneys removed for renal artery stenosis. The ipsilateral kidneys from patients with renal artery stenosis were reduced in size; most were less than half the normal weight. Juxtaglomerular hyperplasia was only mild to moderate. Tubular atrophy was prominent, accompanied by interstitial fibrosis and crowding of the glomeruli. Sometimes, Bowman's space was so dilated as to form microcysts. Marcussen (282) documented the presence of atubular glomeruli, which are defined as glomeruli with open capillary loops that, on serial sectioning, are not attached to a tubule. As a further comparison of the control kidneys with those from the patients with renal artery stenosis, he noted that the mean glomerular volume and number of glomeruli tended to be larger in the controls. In the controls, 95.9% of glomeruli were connected to proximal tubules, 1.5% were connected to atrophic tubules, and 2.5% were atubular. In contrast, in the patients with renal artery stenosis, 8.1% of glomeruli were connected to proximal tubules, 39.9% were connected to atrophic tubules, and 52.0% were atubular. Thus, in these patients, most glomeruli were either atubular or were connected to atrophic tubules. This investigator also found that proximal tubules were more frequently atrophic.

The study by Grone et al (283) examined the potential reversibility of tubular atrophy using an experimental model of ischemic injury. These investigators defined the term *hibernation* as a state of reduced organ function at rest that can be reversed by improving blood flow or increasing work load. As has been observed, renal artery stenosis leads to a reduction in the size of the kidney and atrophy, partly because of reduction of the blood flow. In some cases, revascularization of the kidney may result in return of at least some function to the kidney, but currently, investigators have no certain way of distinguishing between those individual patients who will improve with surgical treatment and those who will not. Results of studies with generalizations about prognostic features may be seen below in the Therapy section. In this study, the authors induced renal ischemia in rats using a clip on the renal artery. This procedure resulted in atrophy, which reversed with reestablishment of blood flow. Some of the animals received ACE inhibitors to induce renal tubular atrophy. All of the groups receiving ACE inhibitors had tubular atrophy predominantly in the proximal tubules with reduction in renal function. The tubules showed a loss of morphologic differentiation and decrease in the activity of various lysosomal and brush border enzymes. Atrophy was reversible after 14 days of ischemia even in those groups with more severe atrophy induced by the addition of ACE inhibitors. These researchers suggested that the presence of atubular glomeruli may be a useful prognosticator of potential irreversibility of renal injury in this setting (283).

## Cholesterol Emboli

Cholesterol emboli have been reported in renal vessels at autopsy (274) with an incidence ranging from 0.1% to 3.3%. However, if one looks only at the population at risk, the frequency is much higher; such emboli are present at autopsy in 31.0% of patients with aortic aneurysms and in 77.3% of patients dying during or shortly after surgical procedures involving the abdominal aorta (274). Involved vessels may range from arcuate arteries to glomerular capillary loops. Cholesterol emboli may also be found in kidneys removed for renovascular hypertension. These emboli are characterized by needlelike spaces representing the cholesterol crystals embedded in amorphous debris. The clefts are quickly surrounded by giant cells and incite a fibrous reaction (Fig. 21.30). Polarized light of unstained sections may be used to accentuate the cholesterol emboli. The emboli are frequently present at bifurcations. The renal parenchyma beyond the affected vessels shows alterations

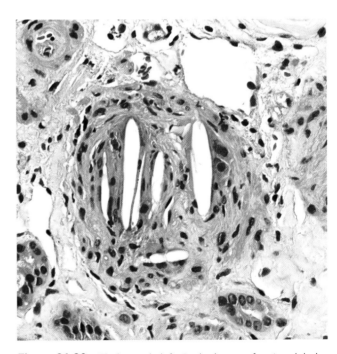

**Figure 21.30**  Cholesterol clefts in the lumen of an interlobular artery. Cholesterol is dissolved during the processing of the section, leaving characteristic clefts. (H&E, ×365.)

resulting from ischemia with atrophy predominant over infarcts.

## Etiology and Pathogenesis

Goldblatt et al (284) showed that constriction of one artery in the dog led to persistent elevation in blood pressure, a model analogous to unilateral renal artery stenosis. It was later found that the initial elevation was owing to increased plasma renin activity and peripheral resistance. In humans it has been found that a critical stenosis of 80% occlusion is required to reduce blood flow and produce the hypoperfusion that activates the pressor mechanisms (285). Increased AII leads to increase in aldosterone, which results in volume retention, hypervolemia, and increased cardiac output. In the experimental model with normal kidneys at the outset, within a few days the plasma renin activity, aldosterone, and cardiac output returned to normal with increased peripheral resistance maintaining the hypertension (286). However, in humans with ARAS, the kidney is not without blemish. Rather, the atherosclerosis has developed gradually on an aging kidney, which is often further compromised by smoking, obesity, or diabetes. Thus, there are multiple layers of repeated small injury to the kidney (261). The vessels are not able to autoregulate, and when the "critical stenosis" occurs, the structural changes in the vessels such as remodeling have already begun and are able to maintain the hypertension. The reduced perfusion leads to apoptosis, shrinkage, and atrophy. Furthermore, activation of the renin-angiotensin system activates oxidative stress mechanisms that lead to interstitial fibrosis. Textor (261) suggests that these repeated small injuries set the substrate for progressive renal injury. Furthermore, the extent of this underlying renal parenchymal injury may predict the response to revascularization. This aspect will be discussed below in the section on therapy.

## Differential Diagnosis

### Renal Artery Dysplasia

Renal artery dysplasia, sometimes referred to as fibromuscular dysplasia, is the second most common cause of renal artery stenosis. This disease affects a younger population, usually women, with the usual age of presentation in the second and third decades (287–289) compared with atherosclerosis, which presents in patients beyond the fourth decade. However, renal artery dysplasia has been described in the elderly as well (290). It may account for up to 2% of all cases of hypertension in a referral population.

*Pathologic Findings.* The classification of the lesions of renal artery dysplasia as described by Harrison and McCormack (291,292) has not been further refined. The

classification based on the layer of the vessel wall affected is as follows:

I. Intimal fibroplasia
II. Medial types

    A. Medial hyperplasia
    B. Medial fibroplasia with aneurysms
    C. Perimedial fibroplasia
    D. Medial dissection

III. Adventitial fibroplasia

Determination of the type of renal artery dysplasia requires both longitudinal and cross sections of the involved vessels so all the layers of the vessel wall can be evaluated. Trichrome and elastic stains such as Verhoeff–van Gieson are particularly useful in the assessment of these lesions.

*Intimal fibroplasia* is rare, accounting for only 1% to 2% of all cases of renal artery dysplasia (293). The involved vessels show a circumferential accumulation of loose, moderately cellular fibrous tissue inside the internal elastic lamina (Fig. 21.31). Neither lipid nor inflammatory cells are noted. Radiographic studies show a smooth, segmental, stenotic lesion. This lesion may affect other major branches of the aorta and is often bilateral. Intimal fibroplasia may also be seen in the other forms of renal artery dysplasia as a secondary change.

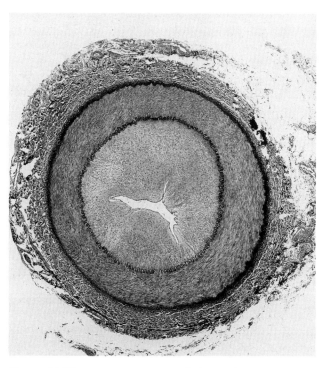

**Figure 21.31** Transverse section of the renal artery with primary intimal fibroplasia. The lumen is severely reduced by accumulation of loose cellular material. (H&E, ×25.) (Courtesy of Dr. L. McCormack.)

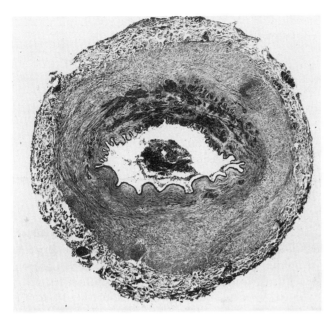

**Figure 21.32** Transverse section of the renal artery to show medial hyperplasia characterized by a random disorganized increase in muscle cells in the media with a reduction of the lumen. (H&E, ×25.) (Courtesy of Dr. T. A. Stamey.)

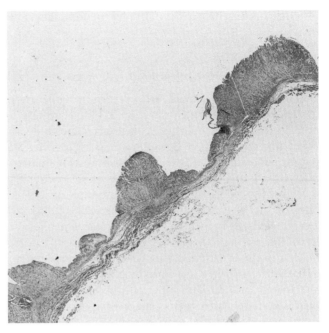

**Figure 21.33** Medial fibroplasia with multiple aneurysms with alternating segments of increased musculofibrous tissue and marked attenuation of the muscularis. Longitudinal section. (H&E, ×6.) (Courtesy of Dr. J. C. Hunt.)

*Medial hyperplasia* is characterized by true hyperplasia of the smooth muscle cells of the media (Fig. 21.32). This condition results in narrowing of the lumen, which radiographically is manifested as a smooth, linear stenosis without aneurysm. This type accounts for 5% to 15% of cases and is detected most commonly in the second decade in women and in men between the ages of 35 and 45 years (293).

*Medial fibroplasia with aneurysms* is the most common form, accounting for 60% to 70% of cases (293). It occurs in the distal two thirds of the renal artery and its major branches, in women aged 25 to 50 years, and is bilateral in 60% of cases. Thus, it is also the most common form to show bilateral disease. The lesion is characterized by thickened ridges caused by replacement of smooth muscle by collagen. Aneurysms form as a result of loss of smooth muscle and a deficient elastic lamina. In involved segments, the stenoses correlate with the ridges and alternate with areas of thinning, which represent the aneurysms (Fig. 21.33). Thrombosis or rupture occur only rarely. The typical radiographic picture resembles a string of beads or sausages (Fig. 21.34).

*Perimedial fibroplasia* is the second most common type of dysplasia, accounting for 15% to 25% of renal artery dysplasia. It occurs most commonly in women between the ages of 15 and 30 years. The lesion is characterized by replacement of the outer two thirds of the media by dense collagen (Fig. 21.35). The multifocal stenoses produce irregular beading such that, on radiographic examination, the beads are smaller than the vessel diameter (293). Rapid

increase in hypertension is frequently seen. Thrombosis is more common in this form than in the other types of renal artery dysplasia. The Masson trichrome stain is particularly helpful in distinguishing this form of dysplasia from the other forms.

*Medial dissection* accounts for 5% to 10% of cases. The channel forms in the outer one third of the vessel wall. The initial defect is thought to lie in the internal elastic lamina and provides an access for blood to enter the media (292). Intimal fibroplasia may occur in this lesion in the area of the dissection. Renal infarcts are more common in this lesion than in the other types of renal artery dysplasia.

*Periarterial fibroplasia* is rare and accounts for less than 1% of all types. It is manifested by dense collagen surrounding the vessel that penetrates the fibrofatty tissue. Similar lesions may be seen outside the renal arteries elsewhere in vessels of the same size. It has also been compared to idiopathic retroperitoneal fibrosis (291).

**Pathogenesis.** The pathogenesis of these lesions continues to be unknown. No relationship has been found with the use of oral contraceptives of alterations in sex hormones. However, genetic factors may be important as there is an increased risk of the disease in first-degree relatives (288,294).

As described earlier, these lesions, including all histologic types, are most often found in the main renal artery. However, other major branches of the aorta as well as other vascular beds may be involved (288,295,296). Luscher

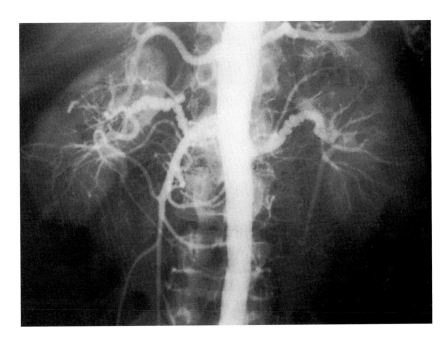

**Figure 21.34** Aortogram to show a sausage string, or string of beads, appearance of both main renal arteries in a case of medial fibroplasia with multiple aneurysms. Such a case would exhibit the pathologic features shown in Fig. 21.33. (Courtesy of the Department of Radiology, Johns Hopkins Hospital, Baltimore, MD.)

et al (296), in a cooperative study, found that renal arteries were involved in 89% of patients, with other sites including carotid (26%), cerebral (26%), intestinal (9%), subclavian (9%), and iliac (5%) arteries. Multiple sites in one patient were present in 28%, with renal and carotid arteries most commonly affected together. One study suggests that intrarenal vessels may also be involved (297). These investigators presented a case of a 58-year-old male patient with medial fibroplasia with aneurysms who required nephrec-

tomy. Examination of the intrarenal vessels demonstrated continuation of the variation in medial thickness to the arcuate arteries and into some interlobular arteries. These authors suggested that such involvement could account for hypertension after correction of renal artery lesions.

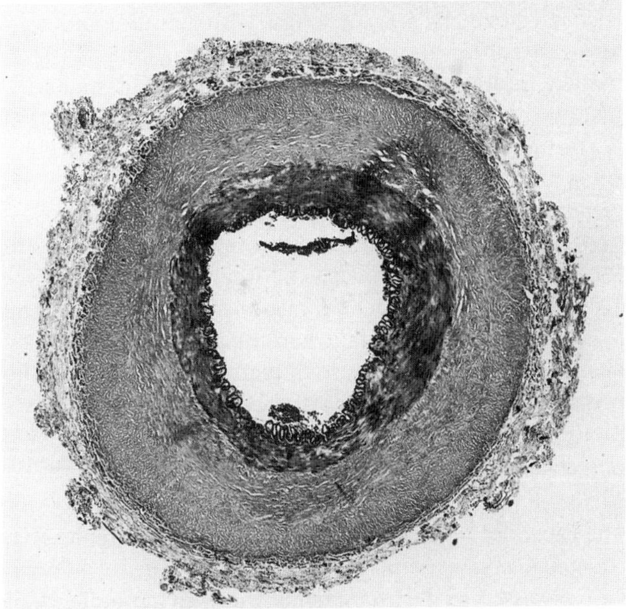

*Clinical Course and Therapy.* Several studies using repeated angiograms have been performed on patients with various forms of renal artery dysplasia. Two such studies showed that many patients progress with narrowing of their renal arteries when followed up to 10 years by angiographic techniques (287,298). Percutaneous transluminal renal angioplasty (PTRA) is the current treatment of choice for this condition (299). Alhadad et al (299) completed a retrospective study of 69 patients with renal artery dysplasia, 59 of whom had PTRA. The procedure was technically successful in 95% of the patients. Follow-up with a mean of 7 years showed cure in 24% with long-term benefit in up to 63% of patients. Patients with longer periods of hypertension prior to the procedure had the poorer outcomes. Carmo et al (300) used surgical revascularization for those patients who failed PTRA, and with a one-year follow-up, show similar results with 24% cure of hypertension and 64% with benefit.

### Renal Artery Aneurysms

Bulbul and Farrow (301), in a review of renal artery aneurysms, found that the incidence varied between 0.01% and 0.1%. Browne et al (302) found a prevalence of 1% for renal artery aneurysms during a retrospective review of contrast enhanced magnetic resonance angiography in screening for suspected renovascular disease. Bulbul and Farrow studied 67 patients with renal artery aneurysms

**Figure 21.35** Perimedial fibroplasia type of renal artery dysplasia in which the outer half to two thirds of the media is replaced by fibrous tissue. (H&E, ×32.)

and found a slight male predominance (3:2), with a range in age of 20 to 76 years. The presentation included hypertension (55%), hematuria (30%), flank pain (21%), and in one patient each, gastrointestinal bleeding, polyarteritis nodosa, and renal failure. Ninety-two percent of these aneurysms occurred in the extrarenal portion of the renal artery, with 70% saccular, 22.5% fusiform, and 7.5% dissecting aneurysms. All but seven were less than 2 cm in diameter. Most were noncalcified. Twenty percent were associated with medial hyperplasia. Rupture of these aneurysms is rare, particularly if they measure less than 1 cm, except that there is an increased risk of rupture during pregnancy (301,302). Indications for surgical repair include refractory hypertension, severe hematuria, pain, and size >1 cm.

Dissections of the aorta may extend into the renal artery and may result in either hypertension or renal failure. Dissections of the renal artery may also occur after trauma, renal artery catheterization, or spontaneously. In the study conducted by Bulbul and Farrow (301), three of the five dissecting aneurysms were associated with catheterization. The presenting symptoms included the sudden onset of flank pain and hypertension.

## Takayasu's Disease

Takayasu's disease affects the aorta and its major branches by an ill-defined inflammatory process. Criteria for its diagnosis include onset at or before 40 years of age, claudication of an extremity, decrease in brachial pulse, more than 10 mm Hg difference in systolic blood pressure between arms, bruit over the subclavian artery, and narrowing or occlusion of the aorta, its primary branches, or major arteries of the extremities (303). The presence of three of these six criteria is highly specific and sensitive for the disease. The disease may be restricted to the arch of the aorta, it may involve the entire aorta, or it may be present in the abdominal aorta or its branches (304,305). Hypertension, when present, is owing to either coarctation of the aorta or renal artery stenosis (Fig. 21.36). This disease is most commonly found in Japan, Southeast Asia, India, and Mexico rather than in the West, but a review of 32 patients at the Mayo Clinic included 23 North American Caucasians (306). In this study, Takayasu's disease was shown to affect young women, with a mean age of 31 years (range, 15 to 48 years) and an incidence rate of 2.6 per million. The clinical features included myalgia (6%), claudication (47%), fever (44%), dizziness (41%), bruits (94%), absent pulses (50%) and hypertension (41%). All patients had angiographic abnormalities, including occlusion, stenosis, irregularity of the lumen, or ectasia or aneurysm, often involving multiple sites. Nineteen patients had renal artery involvement, with 15 having bilateral disease and a slight predominance on the right side. A study in South Africa (305) reviewed 272 patients with a mean age at presentation of 25 years and a female predominance. Most were of

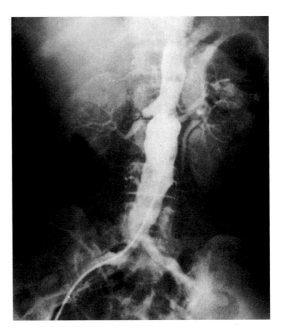

**Figure 21.36** Abdominal aortogram from a 45-year-old woman with Takayasu's syndrome showing aneurysmal dilatation of the abdominal aorta. Marked narrowing in the proximal part of the right renal artery is demonstrated. The right kidney is smaller than the left, indicating the hemodynamic severity of the arterial stenosis. (Courtesy of Dr. T. Ideura.)

mixed race or Asian background (62%) with 30% black and 8% white. Hypertension was the most common presenting sign and 40% had renal artery stenosis. PTRA was used in 10 patients with good results in only 3.

The pathologic characteristics of the lesion have been described by several authors (304,306). Takayasu disease is characterized by an acute phase with granulomatous arteritis that affects the media and adventitia with an inflammatory infiltrate composed of lymphocytes, plasma cells, histiocytes, and occasional giant cells. Neovascularization is a prominent feature from the intima to the vasa vasorum. Sclerosis then ensues with intimal hyperplasia, medial degeneration, and adventitial fibrosis. Disruption of the elastic lamellae may be seen, and thrombosis and aneurysm formation have been noted as in other forms of vasculitis. The result of these structural alterations may be so severe as to cause virtual coarctation of the aorta. The histologic changes are similar to those of giant cell aortitis, but the prevalence of abdominal aortic and renal artery involvement is typical of Takayasu's disease (304,306).

## Miscellaneous Causes

The causes of renal artery stenosis are listed in Table 21.4. *Neurofibromatosis* (von Recklinghausen's disease) is occasionally associated with hypertension with a prevalence of 18.5%, usually because of renal artery stenosis, although coarctation of the aorta may also occur (307). The mean age at which hypertension appears in such cases is 11 years

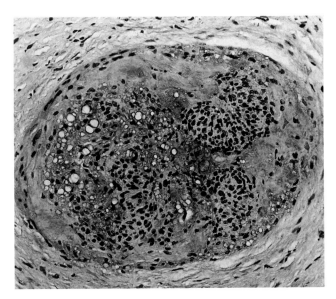

**Figure 21.37** Intima of the small arcuate or large interlobular artery completely replaced by small cells with dense nuclei and by mucinous connective tissue. (H&E, ×203.) (Courtesy of Dr. Gary S. Hill.)

(308). Renal artery stenosis is usually secondary to adventitial compression secondary to proliferation of Schwann cells accompanied by fibrosis, although this change has also been demonstrated in the intima (309). Smaller vessels show mesodermal dysplasia, a nodular proliferation of cells demonstrated by immunohistochemistry and electron microscopy to be smooth muscle cells (310). These nodules may be present in the media or in the intima and may result either in stenosis or occlusion (Fig. 21.37). These proliferative nodules are common in neurofibromatosis, appearing in 7 of 18 autopsies of patients with this disease (311). Hypertension in neurofibromatosis may also be owing to these proliferative lesions in the aorta, lesions that cause coarctation of that vessel. In addition, patients with neurofibromatosis have an increased incidence of pheochromocytomas, which may also cause hypertension (308).

*Thrombosis superimposed on an atherosclerotic plaque* causes additional narrowing in a vessel with pre-existing stenosis because of the plaque, thus worsening the ischemia and increasing the level of hypertension. Furthermore, the shedding of atheroemboli to smaller vessels may result, aggravating the hypertension. Hypertension in the setting of renal transplantation occurs in three situations: as a complication of cyclosporine or FK506 (see Chapters 24 and 28), from narrowing of the anastomosis of the renal allograft, or secondary to renal parenchymal disease (in either the native kidney or the allograft). Occasional technical problems with the renal artery anastomosis are reported to occur between 2.7% and 6.8% of the time (312).

*Moyamoya disease* is a condition first described in Japan that affects the carotid arteries and its branches (313). It is characterized by occlusions or stenoses of these vessels with the formation of netlike vessels. The carotid arteries show fibrointimal thickening and medial thinning. A study in children has reported a prevalence of renovascular hypertension in 8.3% of children with moyamoya disease (314). Intimal fibroplasias was seen in a specimen taken from one of the children.

Hypertension caused by *direct compression of the renal artery by neoplasms* is discussed later. Effects of *radiation* on the kidney are discussed in Chapter 16. *Trauma* and *arteriovenous fistulas* have also been associated with hypertension.

## Clinical Course, Prognosis, and Therapy

### Clinical Course and Prognosis

The diagnosis of renovascular disease depends on the radiologic demonstration of stenotic lesions and on proof that these lesions are responsible for the loss of renal function. As stated earlier, the prevalence of significant renal artery stenosis has been shown to range between 15% and 22%. A review of autopsies not selected for vascular disease was undertaken by Holley et al (269). These investigators, using as a cutoff diastolic blood pressure of 100 mm Hg, found that 22.5% of those patients with lower diastolic pressures had 50% stenosis of at least one renal artery whereas the group with higher diastolic blood pressures had a similar degree of stenosis in 53% of the patients (269). Angiography of patients with renal artery stenosis showed concomitant coronary or peripheral vascular disease in 85% of those studied (315).

Numerous studies have examined the progression of stenosis in renal arteries using various radiologic techniques. None of these studies have provided follow-up data on unselected patients, however, so the frequency and rate of progression are difficult to establish. One typical study from the Cleveland Clinic (287) examined 85 patients who had had at least two angiograms over a period of 4 years. Forty-four percent showed progression, with 16% going on to complete occlusion of the vessel. The latter occurred in the first 13 months in the patients with the most severe narrowing at the beginning of the study. It required up to 5 years for complete occlusion in patients with less severe narrowing. Kidney size was reduced more frequently in those patients who had progressive renal artery narrowing. The narrowing occurred in 62% of patients despite good control of blood pressure (287). The chief conclusion from most of the studies was that renal artery stenosis is a progressive disease, with occlusion occurring more commonly in those vessels with more severe degrees of intimal disease at the beginning of the study.

Rimmer and Gennari (315) reviewed five such studies. In the combined data, 237 patients were considered, of whom 49% showed worsening only, whereas 14%

progressed to occlusion during a follow-up period of 6 to 180 months. Furthermore, these investigators found that control of hypertension had little effect on progression, and serum creatinine did not accurately predict progression. They calculated that the rate of progression fell in a range of 0.4% to 1.5% additional stenosis per month (315). Conlon et al (253) have also reviewed the various studies as well as completing one of their own. In their study of patients undergoing coronary angiography, they found that 6.5% of patients showed progression of the lesion at 1 year and 25% at 6 years. However, they have been unable to show a relationship between the severity of the renal vascular lesion and the degree of renal dysfunction. Another study showed a higher rate of progression with overall cumulative incidence of progression 35% at 3 years and 51% at 5 years (316). This can also be interpreted to show that 50% did not progress over 5 years. Those patients with more severe disease at baseline were more likely to progress. The presence of nephrotic-range proteinuria predicts a poor prognosis (272). Since these patients inevitably have atherosclerosis affecting other vascular beds, they have considerable risk for cardiovascular mortality as well as for end-stage renal disease (317).

## Therapy

Treatment of hypertension associated with renal artery stenosis has evolved over the years. Surgical revascularization is still performed, although percutaneous transluminal angioplasty (PTRA) is used more frequently with stent placement. Noninvasive radiologic techniques are being developed that may be more accurate in assessment of renal function. However, the question of medical management versus surgery or angioplasty is still undecided. The major issue is the high mortality in these patients because of comorbidities.

Numerous studies have been undertaken over the last 30 years comparing various treatment modalities and differing measures of outcome. Review of these studies is beyond the scope of this chapter. Rather, I will discuss several papers that have compared the results of several studies and then provide current recommendations for therapy. Hollenberg (318) compiled the results of 11 studies, including 1310 patients with atherosclerotic renal artery stenosis treated with surgical revascularization. The results showed that 45% of patients were cured, 29% showed improvement, and 24% experienced no change or a worsening of their condition. Nine percent died after the surgical procedure.

Numerous investigators have examined the effects of renal angioplasty on renal artery stenosis. In one such study, Jensen et al (319) examined the results of percutaneous transluminal renal angioplasty in 180 arteries in 137 patients. Fibromuscular dysplasia was present in 22% of the patients and 78% had arteriosclerosis. Technical success beyond 1 year was present in 97% of patients with fibro-

muscular dysplasia and in 82% of those with arteriosclerosis. Relief of hypertension was noted in 86% of patients with fibromuscular dysplasia and in 64% of those with arteriosclerosis. As expected, patients with pre-existing renal failure were not as likely to show improvement in the GFR. Stenosis recurred in 6.7% of patients with fibromuscular dysplasia and in 15.0% of those with arteriosclerosis. Rimmer and Gennari (315) compared the results of angioplasty with those of surgical revascularization in a review of seven reports of these procedures. With angioplasty, 43% of patients improved, 57% were the same or worse, and 5% died. Renal revascularization produced similar results in this study, with 55% of patients improving, 31% remaining stable, and 14% becoming worse; 6% died. Weaver et al (320) reviewed their experience with 51 patients with renovascular hypertension over a period of 8 years. Most of their patients had atherosclerosis, but other conditions, including Takayasu's disease, fibromuscular dysplasia, renal artery dissection, trauma, and aneurysm, were also noted. The efficacy of treatment depended on the original cause of the renal artery stenosis. Seventeen percent of the patients with atherosclerosis and 9% of those with Takayasu's disease showed no improvement, whereas all other patients were cured or at least showed an improvement in their level of hypertension.

The placement of stents during angioplasty was introduced in the 1990s to prevent repeated stenosis of the renal artery. The stents are particularly useful when the narrowing is at the ostium, a location with a higher failure rate using PTRA. MacLeod et al (321) used the Palmaz stent in 29 patients with renal artery stenosis in whom previous angioplasty had been unsuccessful. Twenty-two patients had disease at the ostium. All patients showed immediate technical success. Follow-up data were available in 24 patients, and only 4 had recurrent stenosis within a mean period of 7 months. Hypertension was not cured in any of these patients, but blood pressure decreased in 44% and remained the same in 56%. Dorros et al (322) followed 146 patients who had undergone stent placement for 6 months to 4 years and found a reduction in blood pressure on average and easier control of blood pressure in most patients. Creatinine was decreased or stable in more than two thirds of patients. However, survival was poor (52% at 3 years) in those patients with creatinine greater than 2.0 mg/dL at baseline.

Few studies have compared these various techniques to medical management. Noordman et al (323) performed a meta-analysis comparing the effects of angioplasty with medical therapy in patients with renal artery stenosis. They concluded that angioplasty was more effective in lowering blood pressure than was medical therapy but that no difference was seen in renal function. Losito et al (317) examined the course of disease in 195 patients who had angiographically demonstrated renal artery stenosis. Angioplasty and/or stent placement was used in 136 patients. Medical treatment was also used as appropriate during the follow-up period. Fifty-four patients received only medical therapy. Various antihypertensive agents were used including ACE inhibitors, beta-blockers and calcium channel blockers. The mean follow-up time was 54 months. Multivariate analysis showed no difference in mortality or renal survival between the two treatment groups. Angioplasty was associated with better control of blood pressure, a finding repeated in many studies. Patients who received ACE inhibitors, across treatment groups, showed longer survival compared with other antihypertensive agents. Baseline serum creatinine was the only predictor of progression to end-stage renal disease.

In summary, ARAS is associated with increased mortality chiefly because of cardiovascular causes when compared with populations without such lesions. The reason is that such patients have atherosclerotic disease beyond the renal artery lesions that cause their premature deaths. Although angioplasty or surgical revascularization have been shown to be effective in enabling better control of blood pressure, there is no consistent evidence that these techniques improve the final end points of ESRD or death. Within the large groups of patients are three subsets. In one analysis, it was shown that 27.3% of patients showed improvement in renal function in long-term follow-up, 52.6% showed no change, but 20.1% had worsened renal function, likely owing to showers of atheroemboli (261). The problem is that no one knows how to determine how individual patients will fare with angioplasty. A therapeutic algorithm has been provided in one recent review (324) to help while we wait for more definitive trials.

## Chronic Renal Parenchymal Disease

Chronic renal parenchymal disease is the most common cause of secondary hypertension in all series reviewed in Table 21.3. Hypertension may complicate any form of glomerular disease, as shown in several reviews (157,325,326). Some of the more common causes of renal parenchymal hypertension have included postinfectious glomerulonephritis, focal segmental glomerulosclerosis (FSGS), IgA nephropathy, vasculitis, diabetes, crescentic glomerulonephritis, systemic lupus erythematosus, polycystic kidney disease, and chronic interstitial nephritis. Higher serum creatinine levels and proliferative forms of glomerulonephritis were associated with higher blood pressure in one study (325). FSGS and membranoproliferative glomerulonephritis are particularly prone to an association with hypertension (157).

Potential mechanisms for hypertension owing to chronic renal parenchymal disease include sodium retention leading to volume expansion, increase in pressor activity (either the renin–angiotensin system or endothelin), decrease in release of vasodepressor substances, and activation of the sympathetic nervous system (326). The first

of these mechanisms has been well studied in patients in long-term dialysis programs. These patients have higher exchangeable sodium, plasma volume, and extracellular fluid volume (327). Furthermore, blood pressure in these patients can be modified by removing salt and water by dialysis (328). Thus, the increased volume results in increased cardiac output leading to higher blood pressure usually accompanied by increased peripheral resistance. However, some patients have elevated levels of plasma renin. In such patients, dialysis does not control their hypertension, a finding pointing to a volume-independent mechanism (328).

## Tumors and Other Conditions Associated With Hypertension

### Pheochromocytoma

Pheochromocytoma is a tumor of chromaffin tissues that is most often seen in the adrenal glands (80% to 85%), but it can also occur in the organ of Zuckerkandl, the urinary bladder, or the parasympathetic chain (329,330). This tumor affects the two sexes equally and has a peak incidence in the fifth decade. The prevalence of this tumor in patients with hypertension is 0.1% to 0.6% (329). These tumors may be part of one of several familial syndromes as described below.

#### Familial Syndromes

Familial forms of pheochromocytoma were unusual findings until the familial clusters of endocrine tumors, known as multiple endocrine neoplasia (MEN) syndromes, were identified. The first of these syndromes to be described was reported by Sipple (331) and included the association of carcinoma of the thyroid and pheochromocytoma. Pheochromocytoma is part of MEN, type 2, an autosomal dominant syndrome. There are two variants: type 2A includes medullary thyroid carcinoma with pheochromocytomas and parathyroid hyperplasia as well as cutaneous lichen amyloidosis. Type 2B refers to the combination of medullary thyroid carcinoma, pheochromocytomas, mucosal neuromas, and a marfanoid habitus (329). The tumors in these patients produce both epinephrine and norepinephrine, but the epinephrine predominates. Most patients have bilateral tumors, but malignancy is rare (329). Mutations in the RET proto-oncogene, a receptor tyrosine kinase, have been found in both MEN 2A and MEN 2B (332). A single point mutation has been found in 95% of all cases of MEN 2B studied, whereas several different missense mutations have been found for MEN 2A (332).

Pheochromocytoma may also be associated with von Hippel-Lindau disease, another familial syndrome (329,333). The syndrome consists of various combinations of renal cell carcinomas and cysts, CNS and retinal hemangioblastomas, pheochromocytomas, pancreatic tumors and cysts, endolymphatic tumors, and epididymal cysts (329). Pheochromocytomas are present in about 20% of patients with the syndrome. Malignancy is present in only about 5% of patients. Germ-line mutations in the *VHL* gene on chromosome 3 are responsible for this syndrome (329). In addition, pheochromocytomas have been reported in patients with neurofibromatosis (von Recklinghausen's disease) (329) with the responsible gene being *NF1* and its protein neurofibromin. The most recent addition to the hereditary causes of pheochromocytoma are mutations in the succinate dehydrogenase family. These involve paragangliomas of the head, chest, and abdomen with a higher rate of malignancy (up to 50%) (329).

### Clinical Features and Diagnostic Tests

Patients with pheochromocytomas represent 0.1% to 0.6% of all those with hypertension (329). Variable clinical manifestations have been reported, but the characteristic presentation owing to the actions of the secreted catecholamines includes headache, hypertension, tachycardia, pallor, diaphoresis, and feelings of anxiety. These symptoms may last for only a few minutes or for hours. Other less well-defined presenting symptoms and signs include cardiomyopathy, psychosis, pyrexia, malignant hypertension, hypotension, wasting, acute abdominal pain, and labile hypertension (334). Hypertension is present in more than 90% of patients with pheochromocytomas and is frequently paroxysmal (329,330). The degree of hypertension does not necessarily correlate with the size of the tumor or the concentration of the metabolites (334).

Because hypertension in pheochromocytomas results from release of catecholamines into the circulation, useful diagnostic findings include a marked elevation of serum or urinary catecholamines and their metabolites. These tumors can synthesize and secrete catecholamines more rapidly than the adrenal medulla can. The most sensitive techniques currently used are measurements of plasma-free metanephrines or urinary-fractionated metanephrines. The sensitivity is 99% and specificity is 89% for the plasma measurement and 97% and 69% respectively for the urinary determination (329,335). A clonidine suppression test can be used to eliminate false-positives (329,335). Pheochromocytomas can also make and secrete other functional hormones such as adrenocorticotropic hormone (ACTH), growth hormone–releasing factor, vasoactive intestinal peptide, and parathormone (336). Once the diagnosis of pheochromocytoma has been made based on secretion of catecholamines, localization of the tumor must be made using computed tomography (CT) or magnetic resonance imaging. These techniques are especially useful in finding extra-adrenal tumors. Scintigraphy using metaiodobenzylguanidine (MIBG), an analog that resembles norepinephrine, can complement the use of CT (335).

Most pheochromocytomas are benign, but malignant tumors represent 5% to 26% of these neoplasms (337). Benign tumors may be cured by surgical excision, although recurrence has been reported (336). Patients with malignant tumors have a 5-year survival rate of 44%, but some patients have survived for 20 years. In general, however, the tumors respond poorly to chemotherapy or irradiation (336).

### Pathologic Findings

*Gross Appearance.* Pheochromocytomas are typically located within the medulla of the adrenal gland. Smaller tumors are surrounded by a rim of yellow cortex. The tumor itself is grayish pink. Larger tumors may be hemorrhagic and necrotic. Malignant tumors tend to be larger, contain more necrosis, and invade local tissues. When pheochromocytomas are fixed in formalin and then are exposed to light, they turn a light brown. However, tumors fixed in a bichromate solution turn dark brown.

*Microscopic Findings.* Most pheochromocytomas are composed of large, pink, polygonal cells, often arranged in a trabecular, organoid or alveolar pattern within a thin vascular stroma (Fig. 21.38). The typical arrangement forms so-called *Zellballen*. On occasion, the cells are smaller. At other times, the cells are spindled. The tumor is usually surrounded by a thin capsule. Brown granules may be identified in those tumors that have been fixed in bichromate containing fixatives. In malignant tumors, greater cellular polymorphism is noted and more necrosis is present. Other investigators suggest that malignant tumors also show ganglioneuroma-type differentiation and immunostaining for dopamine, but suggest that cellular

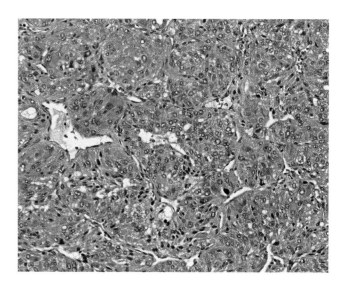

**Figure 21.38** Pheochromocytoma showing nests of cells in vascular stroma. The tumor cells contain ample granular cytoplasm. (H&E, ×260.)

polymorphism is not a differentiating characteristic. The distinction between benign and malignant is often difficult and may require the presence of metastases (337).

The ultrastructure of pheochromocytomas is characterized by the presence of dense core neurosecretory granules with the typical appearance of either epinephrine or norepinephrine granules or sometimes both within the same cell. Immunohistologic studies have shown the presence of chromogranin, neuron-specific enolase, dopamine, ACTH, vasoactive intestinal polypeptide (VIP), calcitonin, and somatostatin.

## Conditions Associated With Adrenal Cortical Lesions

### Hyperaldosteronism

Hypertension may result from the excess production of aldosterone, as first shown by Conn (338) in relation to removal of an adrenal cortical tumor. Hypertension is accompanied by hypokalemia, muscular weakness, decreased plasma renin concentration or activity, and increased plasma aldosterone. The diagnosis of hyperaldosteronism relies on the presence of hypokalemia, decreased plasma renin during sodium restriction, and high urinary and plasma aldosterone after sodium repletion (339). Primary aldosteronism is the cause of hypertension in only a few cases (between 0.05% and 2%) (340). Gordon et al (341) report a higher incidence of hyperaldosteronemia if all hypertensive patients are screened for an aldosterone-to-renin ratio. However, others dispute this finding (342).

The causes of increased aldosterone secretion include adrenal cortical adenoma, hyperplasia, or carcinoma, various genetic causes, and functional ovarian tumors, or other ectopic sites of production (339,343,344). Adenoma of the adrenal cortex is most commonly seen and accounts for 57% to 67% of cases, with hyperplasia of the zona glomerulosa the next most common cause, seen in up to 40% of cases (345). Hypertension in most of these is volume dependent with increased blood volume and cardiac output, although increased peripheral resistance eventually becomes predominant.

Numerous mendelian forms of human hypertension associated with hyperaldosteronism and low renin have now been described. These have been reviewed by several authors (111,344,346). They are listed in Table 21.5 and will be briefly described below. In glucocorticoid-remediable aldosteronism, a chimeric gene of aldosterone synthase and 11β-hydroxylase is expressed in the zona fasciculata under control of ACTH. The resulting synthesis of aldosterone is not suppressed by AII, and its secretion is unrestrained (344). Liddle's syndrome is caused by mutations in the epithelial sodium channel leading to increased numbers of channels at the cell surface. This process results

| TABLE 21.5 |
| --- |
| **LOW-RENIN HYPERTENSION WITH HYPERALDOSTERONISM** |

Glucocorticoid-remediable aldosteronism

Chimeric gene with promoter of 11β-hydroxylase and structural portion of aldosterone synthase

Liddle's syndrome
   β-Subunit of epithelial sodium channel
   γ-Subunit of epithelial sodium channel

Apparent mineralocorticoid excess
   11β-hydroxysteroid dehydrogenase type II

Pseudohypoaldosteronism type II (Gordon's syndrome)
   Increased expression of WNK1
   Loss of function of WNK4

Hypertension exacerbated in pregnancy
   Ligand binding domain of mineralocorticoid receptor

11β-Hydroxylase and 17α-hydroxylase deficiencies

Familial hyperaldosteronism type II
   Candidate-regulatory subunit of protein kinase A

in increased salt and water reabsorption independent of mineralocorticoid levels (111). The syndrome of apparent mineralocorticoid excess is characterized by the deficiency of an isoform of the enzyme 11β-hydroxysteroid dehydrogenase, which catalyzes the interconversion of hormonally active cortisol to inactive cortisone and dictates specificity for the mineralocorticoid receptor (111). This receptor binds aldosterone and cortisol with equal affinity. Normally, this enzyme is expressed in the kidney, with resulting inactivation of cortisol and greater access of aldosterone to the receptor. However, when this enzyme is deficient, more cortisol is bound to the receptor in preference to aldosterone. Cortisol is both more potent and present in greater concentration than is aldosterone, and its binding to the receptor results in an apparent mineralocorticoid excess (111). Pseudohypoaldosteronism type II (Gordon's syndrome) is associated with mutations in either WNK1 or WNK4 kinases. Both mutations lead to increased activity of the thiazide-sensitive sodium chloride cotransporter (347). Hypertension exacerbated in pregnancy results from a missense mutation in the mineralocorticoid receptor, which presents with hypertension before age 20 years (111). The hypertension is exacerbated during pregnancy because steroids lacking 21-hydroxyl groups, such as progesterone, which is elevated during pregnancy, are agonists of the mutant receptor. A second form of familial hyperaldosteronism, which cannot be suppressed by glucocorticoids, has been described and a possible candidate gene, which encodes a regulatory subunit of protein kinase A, identified (346). These patients have either adrenal cortical hyperplasia or aldosterone-producing tumors.

## Cushing's Syndrome and Related Conditions

*Congenital Adrenal Hyperplasia.* Congenital adrenal hyperplasia syndromes are autosomal recessive conditions resulting from a defect in one of the five steps in biosynthesis of cortisol. Deficiency of 21-hydroxylase accounts for most cases. Patients may present with hypertension, salt wasting, adrenal insufficiency, or sexual development anomalies. More than 40 mutations of 11-β hydroxylase (*CYP11B1*) have been found that result in a deficiency of 11β-hydroxylase that prevents production of cortisol even in the face of elevation of ACTH (346). Similarly mutations of 17-α hydroxylase (*CYP17*) result in deficiency of 17α-hydroxylase, which is also critical for the production of cortisol (346). In both cases the increased ACTH leads to increased deoxycortisol and deoxycorticosterone that produce sodium retention, hypervolemia, and hypertension. Both mutations lead to congenital adrenal hyperplasia. However, the children with 11β-hydroxylase deficiency present with virilization whereas 17α-hydroxylase deficiency results in undervirilization in males and lack of pubertal development in females (346).

*Cushing's Syndrome.* Cushing's syndrome is caused by an excess of cortisol. It is manifested clinically by hypertension, truncal obesity, characteristic facies, hirsutism, disturbed glucose tolerance, easy bruisability, and osteoporosis (339,348,349). It may result from the administration of exogenous steroids, from the release of ACTH from pituitary tumors (Cushing's disease) or from other tumors (ectopic ACTH), or from synthesis within various tumors of the adrenal cortex (339,348). Differentiation of the various causes of Cushing's syndrome may be accomplished by various tests, using a flow chart as provided by Orth (350).

*Cushing's Disease and Ectopic ACTH Syndrome.* Cushing's disease is found most often in young women, usually in association with a small tumor of the pituitary gland composed of either basophils or chromophobes (351). Ectopic production of ACTH may be seen in several different tumors, including small cell carcinomas of the lung, carcinoid tumors, islet cell tumors of the pancreas, medullary carcinoma of the thyroid, and pheochromocytoma (339,352). The result of increased serum ACTH is hyperplasia of the adrenal cortex accompanied by increased plasma cortisol and increased excretion of 17-hydroxysteroids and 17-ketosteroids.

## Pathologic Findings

*Adrenal Hyperplasia.* As many as one third of cases of hyperaldosteronism result from hyperplasia of the zona glomerulosa (353,354). Such hyperplasia is characterized by increased width of the cortex and may be accompanied by either large or small nodules.

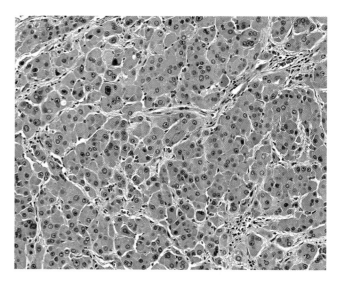

**Figure 21.39**    Adrenal cortical adenoma with large pink cells with ample cytoplasm and vesicular nuclei. An area with nuclear pleomorphism is present in the upper left portion of the micrograph. (H&E, ×260.)

*Adrenal Adenoma.* Grossly, adenomas are yellow, circumscribed, and usually small. Frequently they are single, but they may be multiple and associated with hyperplasia of the zona glomerulosa (354). The cells of the tumor have several different appearances. The most common is a large polygonal cell with clearing of the cytoplasm similar to that seen in normal zona fasciculata (Fig. 21.39). The cells are frequently present in cords. Other cell types include a hybrid form of small, lipid-rich cells resembling a mixture of cells from zona glomerulosa and zona fasciculata, cells resembling those of the zona glomerulosa alone, and some that are similar to those of the zona reticularis. Necrosis and hemorrhage may occur. Ultrastructural studies in tumors that produce aldosterone show the typical cytoplasmic features of cells of the zona glomerulosa (355). These changes include mitochondria with plate-like cristae, smooth endoplasmic reticulum, lipid droplets, polyribosomes, and Golgi complex. In addition, spironolactone bodies may be identified by the concentric, dense lamellae, which resemble myelin figures. High concentrations of aldosterone are present within these tumors (356), but, on occasion, renin (357) or atrial natriuretic peptide (358) can also be detected. Furthermore, nonaldosterone mineralocorticoids such as deoxycorticosterone may also be produced by these tumors (359).

The percentage of adrenal cortical tumors that produce corticosteroids has varied from 37.5% in one study to 74% in another (360,361). Within the group of functioning adrenal cortical neoplasms, most patients had either Cushing's syndrome or Cushing's syndrome with virilization (360–362); however, children more frequently showed virilization alone (362). Increasing use of CT and MRI has resulted in the finding of "incidental" adrenal tumors. The incidence of these tumors is 3% to 4%, and up to 20% of them produce glucocorticoids (363).

Surgical removal of these tumors frequently results in cure, unlike the results of adrenalectomy in cases of pure hyperplasia (353). Unilateral adenoma can be reliably differentiated from diffuse hyperplasia by adrenal vein sampling (364). Predictors of cure include young age, ability to localize aldosterone secretion to one side, and lower plasma renin activity. Expression of CYP11B2, which indicates aldosterone production, in a dominant nodule is also predictive of cure (365).

*Adrenal Carcinoma.* Aldosterone-producing adrenal cortical carcinomas are extremely rare. In a study from Italy, only 1 of 26 functioning adrenal cortical carcinomas was associated with hyperaldosteronism (360). The remainder were associated with Cushing's syndrome. In general, adenomas tend to be smaller and have fewer mitoses and a small nest growth pattern with larger, foamier cytoplasm (366). Necrosis is also more prominent in malignant tumors. A high mitotic rate seems to be the best single predictor of aggressive tumor behavior (354,366). In general, tumors greater than 6 cm in diameter are carcinomas (339). Carcinomas may produce different steroids at various times during their development (339).

## Bartter's Syndrome

### Clinical Features

Bartter's syndrome (367) is characterized by hypotension or normal blood pressure despite biochemical and hormonal changes that would suggest that hypertension could be present. Bartter's syndrome presents in children with hypokalemia, hyperreninemia, high AII, hyperaldosteronemia, hypercalciuria, and hypokalemic alkalosis. This syndrome occurs in an autosomal recessive pattern and is owing to a mutation in any one of three genes involved in salt resorption in the thick ascending limb of Henle (111). Loss-of-function mutations may be found in the Na-K-2Cl cotransporter resulting in severe salt wasting (111). Loss-of-function mutations may also be found in the apical potassium channels or in the basolateral voltage-dependent chloride channels (368). These also lead to marked salt wasting. The increased sodium delivery to the distal tubule results in hypokalemic alkalosis. The faulty sodium chloride reabsorption causes volume depletion activating the renin–angiotensin system (368).

### Pathologic Findings

The characteristic finding is extensive enlargement of the juxtaglomerular apparatus (JGA) (Fig. 21.40). In some cases, the macula densa is more prominent, but usually the entire apparatus is enlarged. Morphometry of the JGA

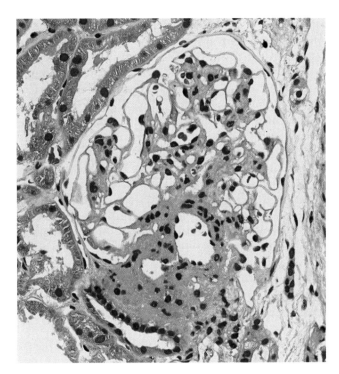

**Figure 21.40** Hyperplastic juxtaglomerular apparatus (JGA) from a patient with Bartter's syndrome. Every JGA in this biopsy showed similar changes. The average JGA shows approximately eight cells and is smaller in area as well. (H&E, ×330.)

in Bartter's syndrome has shown that the JGA may be increased in area by more than 50% above normal. Immunocytochemical techniques demonstrate increased numbers of cells containing renin, especially in the afferent arterioles (369). Electron microscopy of the JGA in Bartter's syndrome shows evidence of increased protein synthesis as manifested by increased rough endoplasmic reticulum with dilated cisterns, abundant free ribosomes, enlarged Golgi apparatus, and granules in different stages of development (369).

Other changes have been recorded. Afferent arteriolar thickening is not constant. Vacuolar change has been noted in the proximal convoluted tubular epithelial cells that may be owing to the hypokalemia. PAS positive granules have been observed in medullary collecting ducts and in interstitial cells identical to those seen in potassium-depleted rats (370).

## Hypertension Associated With Assorted Tumors

### Juxtaglomerular Cell Tumors

In 1967, Robertson et al (371) reported the first case of a juxtaglomerular cell tumor, although they described it as a hemangiopericytoma. This tumor contained a pressor substance considered to be renin. The 16-year-old patient presented with malignant hypertension (250/150 mm Hg), papilledema, and low serum potassium. Histologically, the tumor had sheets of large epithelioid cells with prominent vascular spaces. The tumor cells converged into the muscular walls of the arterioles within the substance of the tumor. Granules present in the cells stained with the Bowie stain, a finding indicative of renin.

A recent review of the world's literature showed a total of 66 cases of juxtaglomerular cell tumor with an age range of 6 to 69 years, with most of the adults in the third decade (372). A female predominance is noted. The presenting symptom of half of the patients was headache in an earlier review (373). All patients became hypertensive, usually at malignant levels, at some time during their course. Hypokalemia owing to the hyperaldosteronism was also present in all patients at some time in the course of this disease. Polyuria and proteinuria were noted in 10 of the 38 patients (373). Other findings included left ventricular hypertrophy, cerebrovascular accidents, nocturia, dizziness, and retinopathy (372,373). The renin secretion from these tumors is autonomous such that the hypertension may be difficult to control (374). Surgery is usually curative (372,374).

Grossly, these tumors are usually less than 5 cm in diameter, circumscribed, and gray or yellow white (372,375). They are well-circumscribed tumors characterized by sheets of polygonal cells within a vascular stroma. At times, the arteries can show intimal thickening and may become hyalinized (372,376) (Fig. 21.41). Electron microscopy demonstrates the typical paracrystalline rhombi seen in the JGA (372,376). Renin has been detected in the tumor cells using both immunohistologic and immunoelectron microscopic techniques (376,377). In situ hybridization demonstration of renin mRNA has proved that the tumor is synthesizing this product (378). Immunoperoxidase techniques show positivity for actin and CD34 (372). These tumors are considered benign.

### Neuroblastoma

Mason et al (379) reported the first case of hypertension-related neuroblastoma in which blood pressure decreased on removal of the tumor. Weinblatt et al (380) noted similar cases of neuroblastoma, ganglioneuroma, and ganglioneuroblastoma also associated with hypertension. Most of these patients excreted epinephrine, norepinephrine, or their metabolites in the urine. However, most patients with neuroblastoma are not hypertensive, yet they excrete these metabolites in the urine. Thus, either inappropriate storage or degradation to an inactive form by the tumor is believed to occur (381).

### Nephroblastoma (Wilms Tumor)

The first report of an association between hypertension and nephroblastoma was published in 1937 (382). Hypertension in patients with nephroblastoma is fairly common and is usually secondary to intrarenal ischemia owing to compression on the renal vessels by the tumor (383). Mitchell et al (384) demonstrated elevated plasma renin in a child with nephroblastoma, and the renin level returned to normal on surgical excision of the tumor. Assay of the tumor showed renin, whereas the adjacent kidney did not contain any renin. Lindop et al (385) found renin production with elevated plasma renin activity in 10 of 19 nephroblastomas. Usually, this form of renin was inactive. Immunohistochemical examination revealed renin in ovoid cells near tumor vessels in areas of well-differentiated mesenchyme, a finding suggesting that the tumor cells themselves produced the renin.

### Renal Cell Carcinoma

Renal cell carcinoma has also been associated with hypertension. In some reports reduction in blood pressure followed nephrectomy (386,387). Steffens et al (388) studied 129 patients with renal cell carcinoma. Forty-one had hypertension; however, resection of the tumors led to normalization of blood pressure in only six of these patients. These six patients also had high plasma renin activity in the ipsilateral renal vein and higher renin levels in the tumor tissue than in the remaining kidney. Furthermore, no evidence of compression of the renal arteries was seen in any of these six patients. These investigators suggested three possible mechanisms of hypertension in the 41 patients with elevation of blood pressure. These were tumor compression of the renal artery, arteriovenous fistula within the tumor producing ischemia of renal tissue, or, as found in the foregoing six patients, autonomous renin production by the tumor itself. Histochemical studies suggested that renin production occurred in endothelial cells within

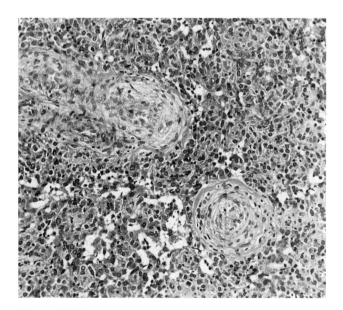

**Figure 21.41**   Renin-secreting tumor made up of polygonal cells. Several small arteries show considerable intimal thickening. (H&E, ×144.) (Courtesy of Dr. A. M. Jackson.)

the tumor. No staining for renin was seen in the other 123 cases.

## Miscellaneous Tumors

Various other tumors have also been reported to be associated with hypertension chiefly through the production of renin. These include carcinoma of the lung (389), stromal cell tumor of the ovary (390), epithelioid sarcoma of the soft tissues (378), liver hamartoma, hemangiopericytoma, and pancreatic carcinoma (374). Other mechanisms for the association between tumors and hypertension have also been described. As noted in the previous paragraph, large renal cell carcinomas may compress the renal artery and may produce stenosis. Tsuchida et al (391) reported a case of congenital mesoblastic nephroma in a 39-day-old boy with elevated plasma renin activity and total renin concentration. His mild hypertension returned to normal after extirpation of the tumor. Immunoperoxidase studies showed renin in the JGA of glomeruli trapped within the tumor, rather than in the tumor cells. Neilly et al (392) described two patients with non-Hodgkin's lymphoma with hypertension thought to be secondary to a lymphomatous infiltrate in the kidney that produced ischemia. The blood pressure returned to normal with successful treatment, as manifested by reduction in kidney size.

## Angiolymphoid Hyperplasia With Eosinophilia

The condition of angiolymphoid hyperplasia with eosinophilia is characterized by subcutaneous nodules with vessels that have enlarged and proliferating endothelial cells with an inflammatory infiltrate composed of lymphocytes, lymphoid follicles, and eosinophils. Fernandez et al (393) described a case in which excision of two such nodules was associated with reduction of hypertension. Renin was identified in cells surrounding the vessels. Six of eight other cases also showed renin-containing cells.

## Oral Contraceptive Agents and Hypertension

The recognition that oral contraceptives could induce hypertension in women was made in 1967 by Laragh et al (394). Stopping administration of the birth control pill reduced blood pressure, and reintroduction raised blood pressure once again. Several other authors reported similar observations (395–397). More recently, however, the degree of blood pressure elevation or the frequency of its appearance in association with oral contraceptives has decreased with the introduction of newer formulations (398–400). To date, no adverse effects on blood pressure have been related to the use of estrogen replacement therapy (401,402). However, oral contraceptives do pose a risk for uncontrolled elevations in blood pressure in patients with previous history of hypertension (403). Stopping oral contraceptives in hypertensive patients lowered the systolic blood pressure by 15.1 mm Hg and the diastolic pressure

by 10.4 mm Hg (404). A progestogen-only pill is a possible option for women who develop hypertension on other formulations or who are hypertensive prior to treatment. A review of several clinical trials showed no association between high blood pressure and the use of progestogen-only pills (405).

More recent formulations with lower conjugated estrogens and newer progesterones with antimineralocorticoid effects have lessened both the frequency and the severity of elevations in blood pressure associated with the use of these agents. Endrikat et al (398), in a study using a combination of ethinylestradiol and gestodene, found no hypertension in 479 women taking the preparation for a total of 4991 cycles. Fuchs et al (399), using monophasic gestodene in 1930 women, found that 5% showed an increase in blood pressure, but only 1.35% had pressures higher than 140/90 mm Hg; 3.5% actually lowered previously elevated blood pressures. In a study from China, Shen et al (406) compared blood pressure in a group of women taking oral contraceptives with that in a group of women using Norplant implants or intrauterine devices. These women had only a 1-mm Hg rise in diastolic pressure, which was considered clinically unimportant. Other authors have reported occasional significant rises in blood pressure. In the foregoing study of Fuchs et al (399), 0.67% of patients showed an increase of 20 mm Hg or more in systolic blood pressure or 15 mm Hg of more in diastolic blood pressure; however, only 4 of the 1930 women studied dropped out of the trials because of problems with blood pressure control.

Several possible mechanisms have been suggested for the hypertension induced by oral contraceptives. The two most widely held include effects on the renin–angiotensin system and on the insulin resistance syndrome (407). In the first of these, it is well known that estrogens increase the synthesis of the renin substrate in the liver, a change that may result in mild hyperaldosteronemia. This condition leads to sodium retention. In addition, the older progesterones also had mineralocorticoid actions, which enhanced this effect (407). The insulin resistance syndrome is characterized by hyperinsulinemia, impaired glucose tolerance, hypertriglyceridemia, reduced high-density lipoprotein, and hypertension (400). These disorders can all be induced by various formulations of oral contraceptives. Intravascular coagulation may also be important, as confirmed by the occasional occurrence of the hemolytic uremic syndrome. This issue is discussed by Stadel (408).

## REFERENCES

1. Chobanian AV, Bakris GL, Black HR, et al. Seventh report of the Joint National Committee on Prevention, Detection, Evaluation, and Treatment of High Blood Pressure. Hypertension 2003;42:1206.

2. Fields LE, Burt VL, Cutler JA, et al. The burden of adult hypertension in the United States 1999–2000: A rising tide. Hypertension 2004;44:398.

3. Qureshi AI, Suri FK, Kirmani JF, et al. Prevalence and trends of prehypertension and hypertension in United States: National Health and Nutrition Examination Surveys 1976 to 2000. Med Sci Monit 2005;11:CR403.

4. Carretero OA, Oparil S. Essential hypertension. Part I. definition and etiology. Circulation 2000;101:329.

5. Perneger TV, Klag MJ, Feldman HI, et al. Projections of hypertension-related renal disease in middle-aged residents of the United States. JAMA 1993;269:1272.

6. Bao W, Threefoot SA, Srinivasan SR, et al. Essential hypertension predicted by tracking of elevated blood pressure from childhood to adulthood: The Bogalusa Heart Study. Am J Hypertens 1995;8:657.

7. Manalich R, Reyes L, Herrera M, et al. Relationship between weight at birth and the number and size of renal glomeruli in humans: A histomorphometric study. Kidney Int 2000;58:770.

8. Pharoah POD, Stevenson CJ, West CR. Association of blood pressure in adolescence with birthweight. Arch Dis Child Fetal Neonatal 1998;79:F114.

9. Thame M, Osmond C, Wilks RJ, et al. Blood pressure is related to placental volume and birth weight. Hypertension 2000;35:662.

10. Woods LL, Weeks DA, Rasch R. Programming adult blood pressure by maternal protein restriction: Role of nephrogenesis. Kidney Int 2004;65:1339.

11. Whelton PK. Hypertension curriculum review: Epidemiology and the prevention of hypertension. J Clin Hypertens (Greenwich) 2004;6:636.

12. Franklin SS. New interpretation of blood pressure: The importance of pulse pressure. In: Oparil S, Weber MA, eds. Hypertension. Philadelphia: Elsevier-Saunders, 2005:230.

13. Anderson GH Jr, Blakeman N, Streeten DH. The effect of age on prevalence of secondary forms of hypertension in 4429 consecutively referred patients. J Hypertens 1994;12:609.

14. Mo R, Omvik, P. , Lund-Johansen P. The Bergen Blood Pressure Study: Offspring of two hypertensive parents have significantly higher blood pressures than offspring of one hypertensive and one normotensive parent. J. Hyperten. 1995;13:1614.

15. Carmelli D, Cardon LR, Fabsitz R. Clustering of hypertension, diabetes, and obesity in adult male twins: Same genes or same environments? Am J Hum Genet 1994;55:566.

16. Rostand SG. Hypertension and renal disease in blacks: Role of genetic and/or environmental factors? Adv Nephrol Necker Hosp 1992;21:99.

17. Hamet P. Genes and hypertension: Where we are and where we should go. Clin Exp Hypertens 1999;21:947.

18. Staessen JA, Wang J, Bianchi G, et al. Essential hypertension. Lancet 2003;361:1629.

19. Luft FC. Geneticism of essential hypertension. Hypertension 2004;43:1155.

20. Corvol P, Persu A, Gimenez-Roqueplo AP, et al. Seven lessons from two candidate genes in human essential hypertension: Angiotensinogen and epithelial sodium channel. Hypertension 1999;33:1324.

21. Smithies O, Kim HS, Takahashi N, et al. Importance of quantitative genetic variations in the etiology of hypertension. Kidney Int 2000;58:2265.

22. Jeunemaitre X, Soubrier F, Kotelevtsev YV, et al. Molecular basis of human hypertension: Role of angiotensinogen. Cell 1992;71:169.

23. Hopkins PN, Lifton RP, Hollenberg NK, et al. Blunted renal vascular response to angiotensin II is associated with a common variant of the angiotensin gene and obesity. J Hypertens 1996;14:199.

24. Castellano M, Glorioso N, Cusi D, et al. Genetic polymorphism of the renin-angiotensin-aldosterone system and arterial hypertension in the Italian population: The GENIPER Project. J Hypertens 2003;21:1853.

25. Saeed Mahmood M, Saboohi K, Osman Ali S, et al. Association of the angiotensin-converting enzyme (ACE) gene G2350A dimorphism with essential hypertension. J Hum Hypertens 2003;17:719.

26. Thomas GN, Young RP, Tomlinson B, et al. Renin-angiotensin-aldosterone system gene polymorphisms and hypertension in Hong Kong Chinese. Clin Exp Hypertens 2000;22:87.

27. Benjafield AV, Wang WY, Speirs HJ, et al. Genome-wide scan for hypertension in Sydney Sibships: The GENIHUSS study. Am J Hypertens 2005;18:828.

28. Caulfield M, Munroe P, Pembroke J, et al. Genome-wide mapping of human loci for essential hypertension. Lancet 2003;361:2118.

29. de Lange M, Spector TD, Andrew T. Genome-wide scan for blood pressure suggests linkage to chromosome 11, and replication of loci on 16, 17, and 22. Hypertension 2004;44:872.

30. Mein CA, Caulfield MJ, Dobson RJ, et al. Genetics of essential hypertension. Hum Mol Genet 2004;13 Spec No 1:R169.

31. Schwartz F, Duka A, Sun F, et al. Mitochondrial genome mutations in hypertensive individuals. Am J Hypertens 2004;17:629.

32. Cvetkovic B, Sigmund CD. Understanding hypertension through genetic manipulation in mice. Kidney Int 2000;57:863.

33. Friese RS, Mahboubi P, Mahapatra NR, et al. Common genetic mechanisms of blood pressure elevation in two independent rodent models of human essential hypertension. Am J Hypertens 2005;18(Pt 1):633.

34. Graham D, McBride MW, Brain NJ, et al. Congenic/consomic models of hypertension. Methods Mol Med 2005;108:3.

35. Matayoshi T, Kamide K, Takiuchi S, et al. The thiazide-sensitive Na(+)-Cl(−) cotransporter gene, C1784T, and adrenergic receptor-beta3 gene, T727C, may be gene polymorphisms susceptible to the antihypertensive effect of thiazide diuretics. Hypertens Res 2004;27:821.

36. Spiering W, Kroon AA, Fuss-Lejeune MJ, et al. Genetic contribution to the acute effects of angiotensin II type 1 receptor blockade. J Hypertens 2005;23:753.

37. Williams TA, Mulatero P, Filigheddu F, et al. Role of HSD11B2 polymorphisms in essential hypertension and the diuretic response to thiazides. Kidney Int 2005;67:631.

38. Hamilton M, Pickering GW, Fraser-Roberts JA, Sowry GSC. The aetiology of essential hypertension. I. The arterial pressure in the general population. Clin Sci 1954;13:11.

39. Tyroler HA, Heyden S, Hames CG. Weight and hypertension: Evans County studies of blacks and whites. In: Paul O, ed. Epidemiology and Control of Hypertension. New York: Stratton, 1975:177.

40. He J, Whelton PK. What is the role of dietary sodium and potassium in hypertension and target organ injury? Am J Med Sci 1999;317:152.

41. Miall WE, Oldham PD. Factors influencing arterial blood pressure in the general population. Clin Sci 1958;17:409.

42. Calhoun DA, Oparil S. Racial differences in the pathogenesis of hypertension. Am J Med Sci 1995;310(suppl 1):S86.

43. Hamet P, Pausova Z, Adarichev V, et al. Hypertension: Genes and environment. J Hypertens 1998;16:397.

44. Toto RD. Hypertensive nephrosclerosis in African Americans. Kidney Int 2003;64:2331.

45. Parmer RJ, Stone RA, Cervenka JH. Renal hemodynamics in essential hypertension: Racial differences in response to changes in dietary sodium. Hypertension 1994;24:752.

46. Suthanthiran M, Li B, Song JO, et al. Transforming growth factor-beta 1 hyperexpression in African American hypertensives: A novel mediator of hypertension and/or target organ damage. Proc Natl Acad Sci U S A 2000;97:3479.

47. Marcantoni C, Ma L-J, Federspiel C, et al. Hypertensive nephrosclerosis in African Americans versus Caucasians. Kidney Int 2002;62:172.

48. Hughson M, Farris AB III, Douglas-Denton R, et al. Glomerular number and size in autopsy kidneys: The relationship to birth weight. Kidney Int 2003;63:2113.

49. Keller G, Zimmer G, Mall G, et al. Nephron number in patients with primary hypertension. N Engl J Med 2003;348:101.

50. Krakoff LR. Diagnosis: Initial evaluation and follow-up assessment. In: Oparil S, Weber MA, eds. Hypertension. Philadelphia: Elsevier-Saunders, 2005:295.

51. He J, Whelton PK. Elevated systolic blood pressure as a risk factor for cardiovascular and renal disease. J Hypertens 1999;17 (suppl 2):S7.

52. Kannel WB. Coronary atherosclerotic sequelae of hypertension. In: Oparil S, Weber MA, eds. Hypertension. Philadelphia: Elsevier-Saunders, 2005:237.

53. Lip GYH. Target organ damage and the prothrombotic state in hypertension. Hypertension 2000;36:975.

54. Diamond JA, Phillips RA. Left ventricular hypertrophy, congestive heart failure, and coronary flow reserve abnormalities in hypertension. In: Oparil S, Weber MA, eds. Hypertension. Philadelphia: Elsevier-Saunders, 2005:250.

55. Leoncini G, Ratto E, Viazzi F, et al. Metabolic syndrome is associated with early signs of organ damage in nondiabetic, hypertensive patients. J Intern Med 2005;257:454.

56. Mimran A, Ribstein, J. Microalbuminuria in essential hypertension. Clin Exp Hyperten 1993;15:1061.

57. Mujais SK, Emmanouel DS, Kasinath BS, et al. Marked proteinuria in hypertensive nephrosclerosis. Am J Nephrol 1985;5:190.

58. Bianchi S, Bigazzi R, Campese VM. Microalbuminuria in essential hypertension: Significance, pathophysiology, and therapeutic implications: Am J Kidney Dis 1999;34:973.

59. Segura J, Campo C, Ruilope LM. Effect of proteinuria and glomerular filtration rate on cardiovascular risk in essential hypertension. Kidney Int 2004;92(suppl):S45.

60. Vidt DG. Management of hypertensive emergencies and urgencies. In: Oparil S, Weber MA, ed. Hypertension. Philadelphia: Elsevier-Saunders, 2005:826.

61. Lip GY, Beevers M, Beevers G. The failure of malignant hypertension to decline: A survey of 24 years' experience in a multiracial population in England. J Hypertens 1994;12:1297.

62. Lip GYH, Beevers M, Beevers DG. Do patients with de novo hypertension differ from patients with previously known hypertension when malignant phase hypertension occurs? Am J Hypertens 2000;13:934.

63. Thakur V, Godley C, Weed S, et al. Case reports: Cocaine-associated accelerated hypertension and renal failure. Am J Med Sci 1996;312:295.

64. Scarpelli PT, Gallo M, De Cesaris F, et al. Continuing follow-up of malignant hypertension. J Nephrol 2002;15:431.

65. Webster J, Petrie JC, Jeffers TA, Lovell HG. Accelerated hypertension: Patterns of mortality and clinical factors affecting outcome in treated patients. Q J Med 1993;86:485.

66. Whitworth CE, Fleming S, Cumming AD, et al. Spontaneous development of malignant phase hypertension in transgenic Ren-2 rats. Kidney Int 1994;46:1528.

67. Whitworth CE, Fleming S, Kotelevtsev Y, et al. A genetic model of malignant phase hypertension in rats. Kidney Int 1995;47: 529.

68. Fleming S. Malignant hypertension—the role of the paracrine renin-angiotensin system. J Pathol 2000;192:135.

69. Parving HH, Mogensen CE, Jensen HA, et al. Increased urinary albumin-excretion rate in benign essential hypertension. Lancet 1974;1:1190.

70. Keane WF. Proteinuria: Its clinical importance and role in progressive renal disease. Am J Kidney Dis 2000;35(suppl 1):S97.

71. Mimran A, Ribstein J, DuCailar G. Is microalbuminuria a marker of early intrarenal vascular dysfunction in essential hypertension? Hypertension 1994;23(Pt 2):1018.

72. Pontremoli R, Leoncini G, Ravera M, et al. Microalbuminuria, cardiovascular, and renal risk in primary hypertension. J Am Soc Nephrol 2002;13(suppl 3):S169.

73. Rosa TT, Palatini P. Clinical value of microalbuminuria in hypertension. J Hypertens 2000;18:645.

74. Wang TJ, Evans JC, Meigs JB, et al. Low-grade albuminuria and the risks of hypertension and blood pressure progression. Circulation 2005;111:1370.

75. Freedman BI, Beck SR, Rich SS, et al. A genome-wide scan for urinary albumin excretion in hypertensive families. Hypertension 2003;42:291.

76. Fox CS, Yang Q, Guo C-Y, et al. Genome-wide linkage analysis to urinary microalbuminuria in a community based sample: The Framingham Heart Study. Kidney Int 2005;67:70.

77. Cottone S, Vadala A, Mangano MT, et al. Endothelium-derived factors in microalbuminuric and nonmicroalbuminuric essential hypertensives. Am J Hypertens 2000;13:172.

78. Barisoni L, Yun, S, DeVita, M, et al. Nephrotic proteinuria in hypertensive nephrosclerosis. J Am Soc Nephrol 1994;5:556.

79. Harvey JM, Howie AJ, Lee SJ, et al. Renal biopsy findings in hypertensive patients with proteinuria. Lancet 1992;340: 1435.

80. Pedrinelli R, Giampietro O, Carmassi F, et al. Microalbuminuria and endothelial dysfunction in essential hypertension. Lancet 1994;344:14.

81. Kario K, Matsuo T, Kobayashi H, et al. Factor VII hyperactivity and endothelial cell damage are found in elderly hypertensives only when concomitant with microalbuminuria. Arterioscler Thromb Vasc Biol 1996;16:455.

82. Kincaid-Smith P, McMichael J, Murphy E A. The clinical course and pathology of hypertension with papilloedema (malignant hypertension). QJ Med. 1958;27:117.

83. Kaplan C, Pasternack B, Shah H, et al. Age-related incidence of sclerotic glomeruli in human kidneys. Am J Pathol 1975;80:227.

84. McManus JFA, Lupton, CH Jr. Ischemic obsolescence of renal glomeruli: The natural history of the lesions and their relation to hypertension. Lab Invest 1960;9:413.

85. Bohle A, Ratschek M. The compensated and the decompensated form of benign nephrosclerosis. Pathol Res Pract 1982;174:357.

86. Bohle A, Wehrmann M, Greschniok A, et al. Renal morphology in essential hypertension: Analysis of 1177 unselected cases. Kidney Int 1998;54(suppl):S205.

87. Kincaid-Smith P. Hypothesis: Obesity and the insulin resistance syndrome play a major role in end-stage renal failure attributed to hypertension and labelled 'hypertensive nephrosclerosis'. J Hypertens 2004;22:1051.

88. Hughson MD, Johnson K, Young RJ, et al. Glomerular size and glomerulosclerosis: Relationships to disease categories, glomerular solidification, and ischemic obsolescence. Am J Kidney Dis 2002;39:679.

89. Sommers SC, Melamed, J. Renal pathology of essential hypertension. Am J Hyperten 1990;3:583.

90. Heptinstall RH. Malignant hypertension: A study of fifty-one cases. J Pathol 1953;65:423.

91. Jones DB. Arterial and glomerular lesions associated with severe hypertension. Light and electron microscopic studies. Lab Invest 1974;31:303.

92. Ono H, Ono Y. Nephrosclerosis and hypertension. Med Clin North Am 1997;81:1273.

93. Grund KE, Mackensen S, Gruner J, et al. Renal insufficiency in nephrosclerosis (benign nephrosclerosis resp. transition from benign to secondary malignant nephrosclerosis) correlations between morphological and functional parameters. Klin Wochenschr 1978;56:1147.

94. Fogo A, Breyer JA, Smith MC, et al. Accuracy of the diagnosis of hypertensive nephrosclerosis in African Americans: A report from the African American Study of Kidney Disease (AASK) Trial. Kidney Int 1997;51:244.

95. Intengan HD, Schiffrin EL. Structure and mechanical properties of resistance arteries in hypertension: Role of adhesion molecules and extracellular matrix determinants. Hypertension 2000;36:312.

96. Volhard F, Fahr, T. Die Brightsche Nierenkrankheit. Berlin: Springer, 1914.

97. Burchfiel CM, Tracy RE, Chyou PH, Strong JP. Cardiovascular risk factors and hyalinization of renal arterioles at autopsy. The Honolulu Heart Program. Arterioscler Thromb Vasc Biol 1997;17:760.

98. Tracy RE, Parra D, Eisaguirre W, et al. Influence of arteriolar hyalinization on arterial intimal fibroplasia in the renal cortex of subjects in the United States, Peru, and Bolivia, applicable also to other populations. Am J Hypertens 2002;15:1064.

99. Hughson MD, Harley RA, Henninger GR. Cellular arteriolar nodules. Their presence in heart, pancreas, and kidneys of

patients with malignant nephrosclerosis. Arch Pathol Lab Med 1982;106:71.

100. Fahr J. Uber Nephrosklerose. Virchows Arch 1919;226:119.
101. Bohle A, Helmchen U, Grund KE, et al. Malignant nephrosclerosis in patients with hemolytic uremic syndrome (primary malignant nephrosclerosis). Curr Top Pathol 1977;65:81.
102. Gamble C. The pathogenesis of hyaline arteriolosclerosis. Am J Pathol 1986;122:410.
103. Shigematsu H, Dikman SH, Churg J, et al. Glomerular injury in malignant nephrosclerosis. Nephron 1978;22:399.
104. Nagle RB, Kohnen PW, Bulger RE, et al. Ultrastructure of human renal obsolescent glomeruli. Lab Invest 1969;21:519.
105. Thoenes W, Rumpelt HJ. The obsolescent renal glomerulus–collapse, sclerosis, hyalinosis, fibrosis. A light- and electron microscopical study on human biopsies. Virchows Arch A Pathol Pathol Anat 1977;377:1.
106. Hsu H, Churg J. The ultrastructure of mucoid "onionskin" intimal lesions in malignant nephrosclerosis. Am J Pathol 1980; 99:67.
107. Gabbiani G, Badonnel MC, Rona G. Cytoplasmic contractile apparatus in aortic endothelial cells of hypertensive rats. Lab Invest 1975;32:227.
108. Still WJ, Dennison S. The arterial endothelium of the hypertensive rat: A scanning and transmission electron microscopical study. Arch Pathol 1974;97:337.
109. Ookawa K, Sato M, Ohshima N. Morphological changes of endothelial cells after exposure to fluid imposed shear stress: Differential responses induced by extracellular matrices. Biorheology 1993;30:131.
110. Ott MJ, Olson JL, Ballermann BJ. Chronic in vitro flow promotes ultrastructural differentiation of endothelial cells. Endothelium 1995;3:21.
111. Lifton RP, Gharavi AG, Geller DS. Molecular mechanisms of human hypertension. Cell 2001;104:545.
112. Struijker Boudier HAJ, le Noble JL, Messing MW, et al. The microcirculation and hypertension. J Hyperten 1992;10 (suppl): S147.
113. Johnson RJ, Rodriguez-Iturbe B, Kang DH, et al. A unifying pathway for essential hypertension. Am J Hypertens 2005;18: 431.
114. Izzo JL Jr. The sympathetic nervous system in acute and chronic blood pressure elevation. In: Oparil S, Weber MA, eds. Hypertension. Philadelphia: Elsevier-Saunders, 2005:60.
115. Grisk O, Rettig R. Interactions between the sympathetic nervous system and the kidneys in arterial hypertension. Cardiovasc Res 2004;61:238.
116. Navar LG. The role of the kidneys in hypertension. J Clin Hypertens (Greenwich) 2005;7:542.
117. Aneja A, El-Atat F, McFarlane SI, et al. Hypertension and obesity. Recent Prog Horm Res 2004;59:169.
118. Hall JE. The kidney, hypertension, and obesity. Hypertension 2003;41(Pt 2):625.
119. Hall JE, Brands MW, Henegar JR. Angiotensin II and long-term arterial pressure regulation: The overriding dominance of the kidney. J Am Soc Nephrol 1999;10(suppl 12):S258.
120. Luscher TF. The endothelium in hypertension: Bystander, target or mediator? J Hypertens Suppl 1994;12:S105.
121. Endemann DH, Schiffrin EL. Endothelial dysfunction. J Am Soc Nephrol 2004;15:1983.
122. Li LJ, Geng SR, Yu CM. Endothelial dysfunction in normotensive Chinese with a family history of essential hypertension. Clin Exp Hypertens 2005;27:1.
123. Baylis C, Mitruka B, Deng A. Chronic blockade of nitric oxide synthesis in the rat produces systemic hypertension and glomerular damage. J Clin Invest 1992;90:278.
124. Raij L, Baylis C. Glomerular actions of nitric oxide. Kidney International 1995;48:20.
125. Knowles RG, Moncada S. Nitric oxide synthases in mammals. Biochem J 1994;298(Pt 2):249.
126. Dzau VJ, Gibbons GH, Morishita R, et al. New perspectives in hypertension research. Potentials of vascular biology. Hypertension 1994;23(Pt 2):1132.
127. Huang A, Sun D, Kaley G, et al. Superoxide released to high intra-

128. Rodrigo R, Passalacqua W, Araya J, et al. Homocysteine and essential hypertension. J Clin Pharmacol 2003;43:1299.
129. Touyz RM, Schiffrin EL. Role of endothelin in human hypertension. Can J Physiol Pharmacol 2003;81:533.
130. Reiter L, Brown MA, Edmonds J. Familial hyperuricemic nephropathy. Am J Kidney Dis 1995;25:235.
131. Sundstrom J, Sullivan L, D'Agostino RB, et al. Relations of serum uric acid to longitudinal blood pressure tracking and hypertension incidence. Hypertension 2005;45:28.
132. Mazzali M, Hughes J, Kim YG, et al. Elevated uric acid increases blood pressure in the rat by a novel crystal-independent mechanism. Hypertension 2001;38:1101.
133. Watanabe S, Kang DH, Feng L, et al. Uric acid, hominoid evolution and the pathogenesis of salt sensitivity. Hypertension 2002;40:355.
134. Brenner BM, Chertow GM. Congenital oligonephronia and the etiology of adult hypertension and progressive renal disease. Am J Kidney Dis 1994;23:171.
135. Epstein M. Aldosterone and the hypertensive kidney: Its emerging role as a mediator of progressive renal dysfunction: A paradigm shift. J Hypertens 2001;19:829.
136. Freel EM, Connell JMC. Mechanisms of hypertension: The expanding role of aldosterone. J Am Soc Nephrol 2004;15:1993.
137. Wilson C, Byrom FB. Renal changes in malignant hypertension: Experimental evidence. Lancet 1939;1:136.
138. Heptinstall RH, Hill GS. Steroid-induced hypertension in the rat. A study of the effects of renal artery constriction on hypertension caused by deoxycorticosterone. Lab Invest 1967;16:751.
139. Hill GS. Studies on the pathogenesis of hypertensive vascular disease. Effect of high-pressure intra-arterial injections in rats. Circ Res 1970;27:657.
140. Olson JL, Wilson SK, Heptinstall RH. Relation of glomerular injury to preglomerular resistance in experimental hypertension. Kidney Int 1986;29:849.
141. Fujihara CK, Michellazzo SM, de Nucci G, et al. Sodium excess aggravates hypertension and renal parenchymal injury in rats with chronic NO inhibition. Am J Physiol 1994;266(Pt 2):F697.
142. Byrom FB. The Hypertensive Vascular Crisis. New York: Grune & Stratton, 1969.
143. Dworkin LD, Hostetter TH, Rennke HG, et al. Hemodynamic basis for glomerular injury in rats with desoxycorticosterone-salt hypertension. J Clin Invest 1984;73:1448.
144. Hostetter TH, Olson JL, Rennke HG, et al. Hyperfiltration in remnant nephrons: A potentially adverse response to renal ablation. Am J Physiol 1981;241:F85.
145. Takenaka T, Forster H, De Micheli A, et al. Impaired myogenic responsiveness of renal microvessels in Dahl salt-sensitive rats. Circ Res 1992;71:471.
146. Palmer BF. Impaired renal autoregulation: Implications for the genesis of hypertension and hypertension-induced renal injury. Am J Med Sci 2001;321:388.
147. Sharma K, Cook A, Smith M, et al. TGF-beta impairs renal autoregulation via generation of ROS. Am J Physiol Renal Physiol 2005;288:F1069.
148. Griffin KA, Picken MM, Bidani AK. Deleterious effects of calcium channel blockade on pressure transmission and glomerular injury in rat remnant kidneys. J Clin Invest 1995;96:793.
149. Abu-Amarah I, Bidani AK, Hacioglu R, et al. Differential effects of salt on renal hemodynamics and potential pressure transmission in stroke-prone and stroke-resistant spontaneously hypertensive rats. Am J Physiol Renal Physiol 2005;289:F305.
150. Griffin KA, Picken MM, Bidani AK. Blood pressure lability and glomerulosclerosis after normotensive 5/6 renal mass reduction in the rat. Kidney Int 2004;65:209.
151. Tanaka M, Schmidlin O, Olson JL, et al. Chloride-sensitive renal microangiopathy in the stroke-prone spontaneously hypertensive rat. Kidney Int 2001;59:1066.
152. Chander PN, Rocha R, Ranaudo J, et al. Aldosterone plays a pivotal role in the pathogenesis of thrombotic microangiopathy in SHRSP. J Am Soc Nephrol 2003;14:1990.
153. Mori T, Cowley AWJ. Role of pressure in angiotensin II-induced

renal injury: Chronic servo-control of renal perfusion pressure in rats. Hypertension 2004;43:752.

154. Long DA, Price KL, Herrera-Acosta J, et al. How does angiotensin II cause renal injury? Hypertension 2004;43:722.

155. Hostetter TH. Hyperfiltration and glomerulosclerosis. Semin Nephrol 2003;23:194.

156. Klahr S. The role of nitric oxide in hypertension and renal disease progression. Nephrol Dial Transplant 2001;16(suppl 1):60.

157. Ljutic D, Kes P. The role of arterial hypertension in the progression of non-diabetic glomerular diseases. Nephrol Dial Transplant 2003;18(suppl 5):v28.

158. Camp TM, Smiley LS, Hayden MR, et al. Mechanism of matrix accumulation and glomerulosclerosis in spontaneously hypertensive rats. J Hypertens 2003;21:1719.

159. Donnelly R, Collinson DJ, Manning G. Hypertension, matrix metalloproteinases and target organ damage. J Hypertens 2003; 21:1627.

160. Kretzler M, Koeppen-Hagemann I, Kriz W. Podocyte damage is a critical step in the development of glomerulosclerosis in the uninephrectomized-desoxycorticosterone hypertensive rat. Virchows Arch 1994;425:181.

161. Durvasula RV, Petermann AT, Hiromura K, et al. Activation of a local tissue angiotensin system in podocytes by mechanical strain. Kidney Int 2004;65:30.

162. Kasiske BL. Relationship between vascular disease and age-associated changes in the human kidney. Kidney Int 1987;31: 1153.

163. Kappel B, Olsen S. Cortical interstitial tissue and sclerosed glomeruli in the normal human kidney, related to age and sex. A quantitative study. Virchows Arch Pathol Anat Histol 1980; 387:271.

164. Smith SM, Hoy WE, Cobb L. Low incidence of glomerulosclerosis in normal kidneys. Arch Pathol Lab Med 1989;113:1253.

165. Aviv A, Hollenberg NK, Weder AB. Sodium glomerulopathy: Tubuloglomerular feedback and renal injury in African Americans. Kidney Int 2004;65:361.

166. Kotchen TA, Piering AW, Cowley AW, et al. Glomerular hyperfiltration in hypertensive African Americans. Hypertension 2000;35:822.

167. Hill G, Heudes D, Bariety J. Morphometric study of arterioles and glomeruli in the aging kidney suggests focal loss of autoregulation. Kidney Int 2003;63:1027.

168. Rostand SG. Oligonephronia, primary hypertension and renal disease: Is the child father to the man?' Nephrol Dial Transplant 2003;18:1434.

169. Moritz AR, Oldt MR. Arteriolar sclerosis in hypertensive and nonhypertensive individuals. Am. J. Pathol. 1937;13:679.

170. Tracy RE, Strong JP, Newman WP, et al. Renovasculopathies of nephrosclerosis in relation to atherosclerosis at ages 25 to 54 years. Kidney Int 1996;49:564.

171. Biava CG, Dyrda I, Genest J, Bencosme S. A. Renal hyalin arteriolosclerosis. An electron microscope study. Am J Pathol 1964; 44:349.

172. Williams B, Baker AQ, Gallacher B, et al. Angiotensin II increases vascular permeability factor gene expression by human vascular smooth muscle cells. Hypertension 1995;25:913.

173. Tracy RE, Malcom GT, Oalmann MC, et al. Renal microvascular features of hypertension in Japan, Guatemala, and the United States. Arch Pathol Lab Med 1992;116:50.

174. Kloczko J, Wojtukiewicz MZ, Bielawiec M, et al. von Willebrand factor antigen and fibronectin in essential hypertension. Thromb Res 1995;79:331.

175. Hayden PS, Iyengar SK, Schelling JR, et al. Kidney disease, genotype and the pathogenesis of vasculopathy. Curr Opin Nephrol Hypertens 2003;12:71.

176. Reidy MA, Schwartz SM. A technique to investigate surface morphology and endothelial cell replication of small arteries: A study in acute angiotensin-induced hypertensive rats. Microvasc Res 1982;24:158.

177. Schulze P, Lee R. Oxidative stress and atherosclerosis. Curr Atherosclerosis Rep 2005;7:242.

178. Thuillez C, Richard V. Targeting endothelial dysfunction in hypertensive subjects. J Hum Hypertens 2005;19(suppl 1):S21.

179. Fisher AB, Chien S, Barakat AI, et al. Endothelial cellular response to altered shear stress. Am J Physiol Lung Cell Mol Physiol 2001;281:L529.

180. Lehoux S, Tedgui A. Signal transduction of mechanical stresses in the vascular wall. Hypertension 1998;32:338.

181. Kanai AJ, Strauss HC, Truskey GA, et al. Shear stress induces ATP-independent transient nitric oxide release from vascular endothelial cells, measured directly with a porphyrinic microsensor. Circ Res 1995;77:284.

182. Uematsu M, Ohara Y, Navas JP, et al. Regulation of endothelial cell nitric oxide synthase mRNA expression by shear stress. Am J Physiol 1995;269(Pt 1):C1371.

183. Awolesi MA, Sessa WC, Sumpio BE. Cyclic strain upregulates nitric oxide synthase in cultured bovine aortic endothelial cells. J Clin Invest 1995;96:1449.

184. Osanai T, Saitoh M, Sasaki S, et al. Effect of shear stress on asymmetric dimethylarginine release from vascular endothelial cells. Hypertension 2003;42:985.

185. Li JM, Shah AM. Endothelial cell superoxide generation: Regulation and relevance for cardiovascular pathophysiology. Am J Physiol Regul Integr Comp Physiol 2004;287:R1014.

186. Short D. Morphology of the intestinal arterioles in chronic human hypertension. Br Heart J 1966;28:184.

187. Izzard AS, Heagerty AM. Hypertension and the vasculature: Arterioles and the myogenic response. J Hypertens 1995;13:1.

188. Mulvany MJ. Resistance vessel structure and the pathogenesis of hypertension. J Hypertens Suppl 1993;11:S7.

189. Christensen KL. Reducing pulse pressure in hypertension may normalize small artery structure. Hypertension 1991;18:722.

190. Baumbach GL, Heistad DD. Remodeling of cerebral arterioles in chronic hypertension. Hypertension 1989;13(Pt 2):968.

191. Heagerty AM, Aalkjaer C, Bund SJ, et al. Small artery structure in hypertension. Dual processes of remodeling and growth. Hypertension 1993;21:391.

192. Schiffrin EL. Remodeling of resistance arteries in essential hypertension and effects of antihypertensive treatment. Am J Hypertens 2004;17:1192.

193. Simon G. Pathogenesis of structural vascular changes in hypertension. J Hypertens 2004;22:3.

194. Schiffrin EL, Park JB, Intengan HD, et al. Correction of arterial structure and endothelial dysfunction in human essential hypertension by the angiotensin receptor antagonist losartan. Circulation 2000;101:1653.

195. Rizzoni D, Porteri E, Guefi D, et al. Cellular hypertrophy in subcutaneous small arteries of patients with renovascular hypertension. Hypertension 2000;35:931.

196. Morishita R, Gibbons GH, Ellison KE, et al. Evidence for direct local effect of angiotensin in vascular hypertrophy. In vivo gene transfer of angiotensin converting enzyme. J Clin Invest 1994;94:978.

197. Sventek P, Turgeon A, Garcia R, et al. Vascular and cardiac overexpression of endothelin-1 gene in one-kidney, one clip Goldblatt hypertensive rats but only in the late phase of two-kidney, one clip Goldblatt hypertension. J Hypertension 1996;14:57.

198. Rizzoni D, Porteri E, Boari EM, et al. Prognostic significance of small artery structure in hypertension. Circulation 2003;108: 2230.

199. Skov K, Mulvany MJ. Structure of renal afferent arterioles in the pathogenesis of hypertension. Acta Physiol Scand 2004; 181:397.

200. O'Callaghan CJ, Williams B. Mechanical strain-induced extracellular matrix production by human vascular smooth muscle cells: Role of TGF-beta(1). Hypertension 2000;36:319.

201. Spiers JP, Kelso EJ, Siah WF, et al. Alterations in vascular matrix metalloproteinase due to ageing and chronic hypertension: Effects of endothelin receptor blockade. J Hypertens 2005; 23:1717.

202. Schiffrin EL. Vascular stiffening and arterial compliance: Implications for systolic blood pressure. Am J Hypertens 2004;17 (Pt 2):39S.

203. Mahmud A, Feely J. Arterial stiffness and the renin-angiotensin-aldosterone system. J Renin Angiotensin Aldosterone Syst 2004; 5:102.

204. Yasmin, Falzone R, Brown MJ. Determinants of arterial stiffness in offspring of families with essential hypertension. Am J Hypertens 2004;17:292.

205. D'Armiento J. Decreased elastin in vessel walls puts the pressure on. J Clin Invest 2003;112:1308.

206. Ledingham JM, Laverty R. Effects of nitric oxide synthase inhibition and low-salt diet on blood pressure and mesenteric resistance artery remodelling in genetically hypertensive rats. Clin Exp Pharmacol Physiol 2001;28:761.

207. Ledingham JM, Laverty R. Fluvastatin remodels resistance arteries in genetically hypertensive rats, even in the absence of any effect on blood pressure. Clin Exp Pharmacol Physiol 2002; 29:931.

208. Ledingham JM, Laverty R. Renal afferent arteriolar structure in the genetically hypertensive (GH) rat and the ability of losartan and enalapril to cause structural remodelling. J Hypertens 1998;16(Pt 2):1945.

209. Notoya M, Nakamura M, Mizojiri K. Effects of lisinopril on the structure of renal arterioles. Hypertension 1996;27:364.

210. Pu Q, Touyz RM, Schiffrin EL. Comparison of angiotensin-converting enzyme (ACE), neutral endopeptidase (NEP) and dual ACE/NEP inhibition on blood pressure and resistance arteries of deoxycorticosterone acetate-salt hypertensive rats. J Hypertens 2002;20:899.

211. Rizzoni D, Rossi GP, Porteri E, et al. Bradykinin and matrix metalloproteinases are involved the structural alterations of rat small resistance arteries with inhibition of ACE and NEP. J Hypertens 2004;22:759.

212. Sanchez-Losada LG, Tapia E, Santamaria J, et al. Mild hyperuricemia induces vasoconstriction and maintains glomerular hypertension in normal and remnant kidney rats. Kidney Int 2005;67:237.

213. Kang DH, Nakagawa T, Feng L, et al. A role for uric acid in the progression of renal disease. J Am Soc Nephrol 2002;13:2888.

214. Rocha R, Chander PN, Zuckerman A, Stier CT Jr. Role of aldosterone in renal vascular injury in stroke-prone hypertensive rats. Hypertension 1999;33(Pt 2):232.

215. Touyz RM. Recent advances in intracellular signalling in hypertension. Curr Opin Nephrol Hypertens 2003;12:165.

216. Touyz RM, Schiffrin EL. Reactive oxygen species in vascular biology: Implications in hypertension. Histochem Cell Biol 2004;122:339.

217. Mai M, Geiger H, Hilgers KF, et al. Early interstitial changes in hypertension-induced renal injury. Hypertension 1993;22:754.

218. Johnson RJ, Gordon KL, Giachelli C, et al. Tubulointerstitial injury and loss of nitric oxide synthases parallel the development of hypertension in the Dahl-SS Rat. J Hypertens 2000;18:1497.

219. Folkow B. Early structural changes in hypertension: Pathophysiology and clinical consequences. J Cardiovasc Pharmacol 1993;22(Suppl 1):S1.

220. Gobe G, Browning J, Howard T, et al. Apoptosis occurs in endothelial cells during hypertension-induced microvascular rarefaction. J Struct Biol 1997;118:63.

221. Ying WZ, Wang PX, Sanders PW. Induction of apoptosis during development of hypertensive nephrosclerosis. Kidney Int 2000;58:2007.

222. Nakagawa T, Kang DH, Ohashi R, et al. Tubulointerstitial disease: Role of ischemia and microvascular disease. Curr Opin Nephrol Hypertens 2003;12:233.

223. Thomas SE, Anderson S, Gordon KL, et al. Tubulointerstitial disease in aging: Evidence for underlying peritubular capillary damage, a potential role for renal ischemia. J Am Soc Nephrol 1998;9:231.

224. Zheng F, Plati AR, Banerjee A, et al. The molecular basis of age-related kidney disease. Sci Aging Knowledge Environ 2003; 2003:PE20.

225. Nochy D, Daugas E, Droz D, et al. The intrarenal vascular lesions associated with primary antiphospholipid syndrome. J Am Soc Nephrol 1999;10:507.

226. Nzerue CM, Hewan-Lowe K, Pierangeli S, et al. "Black swan in the kidney": Renal involvement in the antiphospholipid antibody syndrome. Kidney Int 2002;62:733.

227. Tektonidou MG, Sotsiou F, Nakopoulou L, et al. Antiphospho-

lipid syndrome nephropathy in patients with systemic lupus erythematosus and antiphospholipid antibodies. Arth Rheum 2004;50:2569.

228. Perneger TV, Whelton PK, Klag MJ. History of hypertension in patients treated for end-stage renal disease. J Hypertens 1997; 15:451.

229. Perera G. Hypertensive vascular disease: Description and natural history. J Chronic Dis 1955;1:33.

230. Scarpelli PT, Livi R, Caselli G-M, et al. Accelerated (malignant) hypertension: A study of 121 cases between 1974 and 1996. J Nephrol 1997;10:207.

231. Edmunds E, Beevers DG, Lip GY. What has happened to malignant hypertension? A disease no longer vanishing. J Hum Hypertens 2000;14:159.

232. McClellan WM. Epidemiology and risk factors for chronic kidney disease. Med Clin NA 2005;89:419.

233. Toto RD, Mitchell HC, Smith RD, et al. "Strict" blood pressure control and progression of renal disease in hypertensive nephrosclerosis. Kidney Int 1995;48:851.

234. Hsu CY, McCulloch CE, Darbinian J, et al. Elevated blood pressure and risk of end-stage renal disease in subjects without baseline kidney disease. Arch Intern Med 2005;165:923.

235. Walker WG. Hypertension-related renal injury: A major contributor to end-stage renal disease. Am J Kid Dis 1993;22:164.

236. Puttinger H, Soleiman A, Oberbauer R. Regression of hypertensive nephropathy during three years of optimal blood pressure control. Wien Klin Wochenschr 2003;115:429.

237. Fliser D, Ritz E. Does essential hypertension cause progressive renal disease? J Hypertens 1998;16(suppl 4):S13.

238. Ruilope LM, Alcazar JM, Rodicio JL. Renal consequences of arterial hypertension. J Hypertens 1992;10(suppl):S85.

239. Pillay VK, Wang F, Gandhi VC, et al. Uraemia from benign hypertension. S Afr Med J 1974;48:953.

240. Mallamaci F, Zuccala A, Zoccali C, et al. The deletion polymorphism of the angiotensin-converting enzyme is associated with nephroangiosclerosis. Am J Hypertens 2000;13:433.

241. Pontremoli R, Ravera M, Viazzi F, et al. Genetic polymorphism of the renin-angiotensin system and organ damage in essential hypertension. Kidney Int 2000;57:561.

242. Fabris B, Bortoletto M, Candido R, et al. Genetic polymorphisms of the renin-angiotensin-aldosterone system and renal insufficiency in essential hypertension. J Hypertens 2005;23:309.

243. Peterson JC, Adler S, Burkart JM, et al. Effects of blood pressure control on progressive renal disease in blacks and whites. Hypertension 1997;30(Pt 1):428.

244. Susic D, Frohlich ED. Nephroprotective effect of antihypertensive drugs in essential hypertension. J Hypertens 1998;16:555.

245. Taal MW, Brenner BM. Renoprotective benefits of RAS inhibition: From ACEI to angiotensin II antagonists. Kidney Int 2000; 57:1803.

246. Lithell H. Pathogenesis and prevalence of atherosclerosis in hypertensive patients. Am J Hypertens 1994;7(Pt 2):2S.

247. Mancia G, Giannattasio C, Failla M, et al. Systolic blood pressure and pulse pressure: Role of 24-h mean values and variability in the determination of organ damage. J Hypertens 1999;17 (suppl 5):S55.

248. Rodriguez-Porcel M, Krier JD, Lerman A, et al. Combination of hypercholesterolemia and hypertension augments renal function abnormalities. Hypertension 2001;37(Pt 2):774.

249. Borch-Johnsen K, Feldt-Rasmussen B, Strandgaard S, et al. Urinary albumin excretion: An independent predictor of ischemic heart disease. Arterioscler Thromb Vasc Biol 1999;19:1992.

250. Bakris GL. Implications of albuminuria on kidney disease progression. J Clin Hypertens (Greenwich) 2004;6(suppl 3):18.

251. Vikse BE, Aasarod K, Bostad L, et al. Clinical prognostic factors in biopsy-proven benign nephrosclerosis. Nephrol Dial Transplant 2003;18:517.

252. Yu SH, Whitworth JA, Kincaid-Smith PS. Malignant hypertension: Aetiology and outcome in 83 patients. Clin Exp Hypertens A 1986;8:1211.

253. Conlon PJ, O'Riordan E, Kalra PA. New insights into the epidemiologic and clinical manifestations of atherosclerotic renovascular disease. Am J Kidney Dis 2000;35:573.

254. Bech K, Hilden T. The frequency of secondary hypertension. Acta Med Scand 1975;197:65.

255. Berglund G, Andersson O, Wilhelmsen L. Prevalence of primary and secondary hypertension: studies in a random population sample. Br Med J 1976;2:554.

256. Danielson M, Dammstrom B. The prevalence of secondary and curable hypertension. Acta Med Scand 1981;209:451.

257. Gifford RW Jr. Evaluation of the hypertensive patient with emphasis on detecting curable causes. Milbank Mem Fund Q 1969;47:170.

258. Omura M, Yamaguchi K, Kakuta Y, et al. Prospective study on the prevalence of secondary hypertension among hypertensive patients visiting a general outpatient clinic in Japan. Hypertens Res 2004;27:193.

259. Sinclair AM, Isles CG, Brown I, et al. Secondary hypertension in a blood pressure clinic. Arch Intern Med 1987;147:1289.

260. Dluhy RG. Uncommon forms of secondary hypertension in older patients. Am J Hypertens 1998;11(Pt 2):52S.

261. Textor SC. Ischemic nephropathy: Where are we now? J Am Soc Nephrol 2004;15:1974.

262. McTaggart SJ, Gelati S, Walker RG, et al. Evaluation and long-term outcome of pediatric renovascular hypertension. Pediatr Nephrol 2000;14:1022.

263. Shahdadpuri J, Frank R, Gauthier BG, et al. Yield of renal arteriography in the evaluation of pediatric hypertension. Pediatr Nephrol 2000;14:816.

264. Leiner T, de Haan MW, Nelemans PJ, et al. Contemporary imaging techniques for the diagnosis of renal artery stenosis. Eur Radiol 2005;15:2219.

265. Connolly JO, Woolfson RG. Renovascular hypertension: Diagnosis and management. BJU Int 2005;96:715.

266. Kalra PA, Guo H, Kausz AT, et al. Atherosclerotic renovascular disease in United States patients aged 67 years or older: Risk factors, revascularization, and prognosis. Kidney Int 2005;68:293.

267. Textor SC. Atherosclerotic renal artery stenosis: How big is the problem, and what happens if nothing is done? J Hypertens 2005;23(suppl 3):S5.

268. Zalunardo N, Tuttle KR. Atherosclerotic renal artery stenosis: Current status and future directions. Curr Opin Nephrol Hypertens 2004;13:613.

269. Holley KE, Hunt JC, Brown AL Jr, et al. Renal artery stenosis, a clinical-pathological study in normotensive and hypertensive patients. Am J Med 1964;37:14.

270. Hansen KJ, Edwards MS, Craven TE, et al. Prevalence of renovascular disease in the elderly: A population based study. J Vasc Surg 2002;36:443.

271. Albers FJ. Clinical characteristics of atherosclerotic renovascular disease. Am J Kidney Dis 1994;24:636.

272. Halimi JM, Ribstein J, Du Cailar G, et al. Nephrotic-range proteinuria in patients with renovascular disease. Am J Med 2000;108:120.

273. Vidt DG. Cholesterol emboli: A common cause of renal failure. Annu Rev Med 1997;48:375.

274. Hauben M, Norwich J, Shapiro E, et al. Multiple cholesterol emboli syndrome–six cases identified through the spontaneous reporting system. Angiology 1995;46:779.

275. Tamura K, Umemura M, Yano H, et al. Acute renal failure due to cholesterol crystal embolism treated with LDL apheresis followed by corticosteroid and candesartan. Clin Exp Nephrol 2003;7:67.

276. Hara S, Asada Y, Fujimoto S, et al. Atheroembolic renal disease: Clinical findings of 11 cases. J Atheroscler Thromb 2002;9:288.

277. Flynn JT. Neonatal hypertension: Diagnosis and management. Pediatr Nephrol 2000;14:332.

278. Varda NM, Gregoric A. A diagnostic approach for the child with hypertension. Ped Nephrol 2005;20:499.

279. Pedersen EB, Madias NE, Aurell M, et al. New tools in diagnosing renal artery stenosis. Kidney Int 2000;57:2657.

280. Nadasdy T, Laszik Z, Blick KE, et al. Tubular atrophy in the end-stage kidney—a lectin and immunohistochemical study. Human Pathol. 1994;25:22.

281. Selye H, Stone H. Pathogenesis of the cardiovascular and re-nal changes which usually accompany malignant hypertension. J Urol 1946;56:399.

282. Marcussen N. Atubular glomeruli in renal artery stenosis. Lab Invest 1991;65:558.

283. Grone HJ, Warnecke E, Olbricht CJ. Characteristics of renal tubular atrophy in experimental renovascular hypertension: A model of kidney hibernation. Nephron 1996;72:243.

284. Goldblatt H, Lynch J, Hanzal RF, et al. Studies on experimental hypertension. I. The production of persistent elevation of systolic blood pressure by means of renal ischemia. J Exp Med 1934;59:347.

285. Simon G. What is critical renal artery stenosis? Implications for treatment. Am J Hypertens 2000;13:1189.

286. Romero JC, Feldstein AE, Rodriguez-Porcel MG, et al. New insights into the pathophysiology of renovascular hypertension. Mayo Clin Proc 1997;72:251.

287. Schreiber MJ, Pohl MA, Novick AC. The natural history of atherosclerotic and fibrous renal artery disease. Urol Clin North Am 1984;11:383.

288. Slovut DP, Olin JW. Fibromuscular dysplasia. N Engl J Med 2004;350:1862.

289. Sos TA, Pickering TG, Sniderman K, et al. Percutaneous transluminal renal angioplasty in renovascular hypertension due to atheroma or fibromuscular dysplasia. N Engl J Med 1983;309:274.

290. Pascual A, Bush HS, Copley JB. Renal fibromuscular dysplasia in elderly persons. Am J Kidney Dis 2005;45:e63.

291. Harrison EG Jr, McCormack LJ. Pathologic classification of renal arterial disease in renovascular hypertension. Mayo Clin Proc 1971;46:161.

292. McCormack JJ. Morphologic abnormalities of the renal artery associated with hypertension. In: Onesh G, Kim KE, eds. High Blood Pressure. New York: Grune and Stratton, 1973.

293. Youngberg SP, Sheps SG, Strong CG. Fibromuscular disease of the renal arteries. Med Clin North Am 1977;61:623.

294. Pannier-Moreau I, Grimbert P, Fiquet-Kempf B, et al. Possible familial origin of multifocal renal artery fibromuscular dysplasia. J Hypertens 1997;15(Pt 2):1797.

295. Boutouyrie P, Gimenez-Roqueplo AP, Fine E, et al. Evidence for carotid and radial artery wall subclinical lesions in renal fibromuscular dysplasia. J Hypertens 2003;21:2287.

296. Luscher TF, Keller HM, Imhof HG, et al. Fibromuscular hyperplasia: Extension of the disease and therapeutic outcome. Results of the University Hospital Zurich Cooperative Study on Fibromuscular Hyperplasia. Nephron 1986;44(suppl 1):109.

297. Holm-Bentzen M, Gerstenberg T, Horn T, et al. Medial fibroplasia: Involvement of renal artery and small renal arteries in renal vascular hypertension. Scand J Urol Nephrol 1993;27:263.

298. Goncharenko V, Gerlock AJ Jr, Shaff MI, et al. Progression of renal artery fibromuscular dysplasia in 42 patients as seen on angiography. Radiology 1981;139:45.

299. Alhadad A, Mattiasson I, Ivancev K, et al. Revascularisation of renal artery stenosis caused by fibromuscular dysplasia: Effects on blood pressure during 7-year follow-up are influenced by duration of hypertension and branch artery stenosis. J Hum Hypertens 2005;19:761.

300. Carmo M, Bower TC, Mozes G, et al. Surgical management of renal fibromuscular dysplasia: Challenges in the endovascular era. Ann Vasc Surg 2005;19:208.

301. Bulbul MA, Farrow GA. Renal artery aneurysms. Urology 1992;40:124.

302. Browne RF, Riordan EO, Roberts JA, et al. Renal artery aneurysms: Diagnosis and surveillance with 3D contrast-enhanced magnetic resonance angiography. Eur Radiol 2004;14:1807.

303. Arend WP, Michel BA, Bloch DA, et al. The American College of Rheumatology 1990 criteria for the classification of Takayasu arteritis. Arthritis Rheum 1990;33:1129.

304. Johnston SL, Lock RJ, Gompels MM. Takayasu arteritis: A review. J Clin Pathol 2002;55:481.

305. Mwipatayi BP, Jeffery PC, Beningfield SJ, et al. Takayasu arteritis: Clinical features and management: Report of 272 cases. ANZ J Surg 2005;75:110.

306. Hall S, Barr W, Lie JT, et al. Takayasu arteritis. A study of 32 North American patients. Hypertension 1984;6(Pt 2):III87.

307. Fossali E, Signorini E, Intermite RC, et al. Renovascular disease and hypertension in children with neurofibromatosis. Pediatr Nephrol 2000;14:806.

308. Han M, Criado E. Renal artery stenosis and aneurysms associated with neurofibromatosis. J Vasc Surg 2005;41:539.

309. Huppman JL, Gahton V, Bowers VD, et al. Neurofibromatosis and arterial aneurysms. Am Surg 1996;62:311.

310. Finley JL, Dabbs DJ. Renal vascular smooth muscle proliferation in neurofibromatosis. Hum Pathol 1988;19:107.

311. Salyer WR, Salyer DC. The vascular lesions of neurofibromatosis. Angiology 1974;25:510.

312. Tilney NL, Rocha A, Strom TB, et al. Renal artery stenosis in transplant patients. Ann Surg 1984;199:454.

313. Ohtoh T, Iwasaki Y, Namiki T, et al. Hemodynamic characteristics of the vertebrobasilar system in moyamoya disease: A histometric study. Hum Pathol 1988;19:465.

314. Choi Y, Kang BC, Kim KJ, et al. Renovascular hypertension in children with moyamoya disease. J Pediatr 1997;131:258.

315. Rimmer JM, Gennari FJ. Atherosclerotic renovascular disease and progressive renal failure. Ann Int Med 1993;118:712.

316. Caps MT, Zierler RE, Polissar NL, et al. Risk of atrophy in kidneys with atherosclerotic renal artery stenosis. Kidney Int 1998;53:735.

317. Losito A, Errico R, Santirosi P, et al. Long-term follow-up of atherosclerotic renovascular disease. Beneficial effect of ACE inhibition. Nephrol Dial Transplant 2005;20:1604.

318. Hollenberg NK. The treatment of renovascular hypertension: Surgery, angioplasty, and medical therapy with converting-enzyme inhibitors. Am J Kidney Dis 1987;10(suppl 1):52.

319. Jensen G, Zachrisson BF, Delin K, et al. Treatment of renovascular hypertension: One year results of renal angioplasty. Kidney Int 1995;48:1936.

320. Weaver FA, Kuehne JP, Papanicolaou G. A recent institutional experience with renovascular hypertension. Am Surg 1996;62:241.

321. MacLeod M, Taylor AD, Baxter G, et al. Renal artery stenosis managed by Palmaz stent insertion: Technical and clinical outcome. J Hypertens 1995;13:1791.

322. Dorros G, Jaff M, Mathiak L, et al. Four-year follow-up of Palmaz-Schatz stent revascularization as treatment for atherosclerotic renal artery stenosis. Circulation 1998;98:642.

323. Noordmann AJ, Woo KS, Parkes R, et al. Balloon angioplasty or medical therapy for hypertensive patients with arteriosclerotic renal artery stenosis? Am J Med 2003;114:44.

324. Mwipatayi BP, Beningfield SJ, White LE, et al. A review of the current treatment of renal artery stenosis. Eur J Vasc Endovasc Surg 2005;29:479.

325. Kheder MA, Ben Maiz H, Abderrahim E, et al. Hypertension in primary chronic glomerulonephritis analysis of 359 cases. Nephron 1993;63:140.

326. Preston RA, Singer I, Epstein M. Renal parenchymal hypertension: Current concepts of pathogenesis and management. Arch Intern Med 1996;156:602.

327. Dathan JR, Johnson DB, Goodwin FJ. The relationship between body fluid compartment volumes, renin activity and blood pressure in chronic renal failure. Clin Sci 1973;45:77.

328. Vertes V, Cangiano JL, Berman LB, et al. Hypertension in end-stage renal disease. N Engl J Med 1969;280:978.

329. Lenders JWM, Eisenhofer G, Mannelli M, et al. Phaeochromocytoma. Lancet 2005;366:665.

330. Lucon AM, Pereira MA, Mendonca BB, et al. Pheochromocytoma: Study of 50 cases. J Urol 1997;157:1208.

331. Sipple JH. The association of pheochromocytoma with carcinoma of the thyroid gland. Am J Med 1961;31:163.

332. Peczkowska M, Januszewicz A. Multiple endocrine neoplasia type 2. Familial Cancer 2005;4:25.

333. Atuk NO, McDonald T, Wood T, et al. Familial pheochromocytoma, hypercalcemia, and von Hippel-Lindau disease: A ten year study of a large family. Medicine (Baltimore) 1979;58:209.

334. Stein PP, Black HR. A simplified diagnostic approach to pheochromocytoma. A review of the literature and report of one institution's experience. Medicine (Baltimore) 1991;70:46.

335. Westphal SA. Diagnosis of pheochromocytoma. Am J Med Sci 2005;329:18.

336. Bravo EL, Gifford RW Jr. Pheochromocytoma. Endocrinol Metab Clin North Am 1993;22:329.

337. Eisenhofer G, Bornstein SR, Brouwers FM, et al. Malignant pheochromocytoma: Current status and initiatives for future progress. Endocr Relat Cancer 2004;11:423.

338. Conn JW. Primary aldosteronism. J Lab Clin Med 1955;45:661.

339. Vaughn ED. Diseases of the adrenal gland. Med Clin North Am 2004;88:443.

340. Melby JC. Primary aldosteronism. Kidney Int 1984;26:769.

341. Gordon RD, Stowasser M, Klemm SA, et al. Primary aldosteronism: Some genetic, morphological, and biochemical aspects of subtypes. Steroids 1995;60:35.

342. Padfield PL. Primary aldosteronism, a common entity? The myth persists. J Hum Hypertens 2002;16:159.

343. Ferriss JB, Beevers DG, Brown JJ, et al. Clinical, biochemical and pathological features of low-renin ("primary") hyperaldosteronism. Am Heart J 1978;95:375.

344. Luft FC. Mendelian forms of human hypertension and mechanisms of disease. Clin Med Res 2003;1:291.

345. Abdelhamid S, Muller-Lobeck H, Pahl S, et al. Prevalence of adrenal and extra-adrenal Conn syndrome in hypertensive patients. Arch Intern Med 1996;156:1190.

346. New MI, Geller DS, Fallo F, et al. Monogenic low renin hypertension. Trends Endocrinol Metab 2005;16:92.

347. Xu BE, Lee BH, Min X, et al. WNK1: Analysis of protein kinase structure, downstream targets, and potential roles in hypertension. Cell Res 2005;15:6.

348. Aron DC. Cushing's syndrome: Current concepts in diagnosis and treatment. Compr Ther 1987;13:37.

349. Scott HW Jr, Abumrad NN, Orth DN. Tumors of the adrenal cortex and Cushing's syndrome. Ann Surg 1985;201:586.

350. Orth DN. Identifying Cushing's syndrome and its causes. N Engl J Med 1995;332:791.

351. Aron DC, Findling JW, Tyrrell JB. Cushing's disease. Endocrinol Metab Clin North Am 1987;16:705.

352. Gomez-Sanchez CE. Cushing's syndrome and hypertension. Hypertension 1986;8:258.

353. Blumenfeld JD, Sealey JE, Schlussel Y, et al. Diagnosis and treatment of primary hyperaldosteronism. Ann Intern Med 1994;121:877.

354. Neville AM, O'Hare MJ. Histopathology of the human adrenal cortex. Clin Endocrinol Metab 1985;14:791.

355. Erlandson RA. Diagnostic Electron Microscopy of Tumors. New York: Raven Press, 1994.

356. Kaplan NM. The steroid content of adrenal adenomas and measurements of aldosterone production in patients with essential hypertension and primary aldosteronism. J Clin Invest 1967;46:728.

357. Mizuno K, Ojima M, Hashimoto S, et al. Multiple forms of immunoreactive renin in human adrenocortical tumour tissue from patients with primary aldosteronism. Clin Sci 1987;72:699.

358. Schaff Z, Racz K, Gutkowska J, et al. Immunohistochemical localization of atrial natriuretic peptide in primary aldosteronism. J Exp Pathol 1987;3:229.

359. Azar ST, Melby JC. 19-Nor-deoxycorticosterone production from aldosterone-producing adenomas. Hypertension 1992;19:362.

360. Boscaro M, Fallo F, Barzon L, et al. Adrenocortical carcinoma: Epidemiology and natural history. Minerva Endocrinol 1995;20:89.

361. Evans HL, Vassilopoulou-Sellin R. Adrenal cortical neoplasms: A study of 56 cases. Am J Clin Pathol 1996;105:76.

362. Mendonca BB, Lucon AM, Menezes CA, et al. Clinical, hormonal and pathological findings in a comparative study of adrenocortical neoplasms in childhood and adulthood. J Urol 1995;154:2004.

363. Sippel RS, Chen H. Subclinical Cushing's syndrome in adrenal incidentalomas. Surg Clin North Am 2004;84:875.

364. Doppman JL, Gill JR Jr. Hyperaldosteronism: Sampling the adrenal veins. Radiology 1996;198:309.

365. Enberg U, Volpe C, Hamberger B. New aspects on primary aldosteronism. Neurochem Res 2003;28:327.

366. Medeiros LJ, Weiss LM. New developments in the pathologic diagnosis of adrenal cortical neoplasms: A review. Am J Clin Pathol 1992;97:73.

367. Bartter FC, Pronove P, Gill JR Jr, MacCardle RC. Hyperplasia of the juxtaglomerular complex with hyperaldosteronism and hypokalemic alkalosis. Am J Med 1962;33:811.

368. Hatta S, Sakamoto J, Horio Y. Ion channels and diseases. Med Electron Microsc 2002;35:117.

369. Taugner R, Waldherr R, Seyberth HW, et al. The juxtaglomerular apparatus in Bartter's syndrome and related tubulopathies: An immunocytochemical and electron microscopic study. Virchows Arch A Pathol Anat Histopathol 1988;412:459.

370. France R, Shelley WM, Gray ME. Abnormal intracellular granules of the renal papilla in a child with potassium depletion (Bartter's syndrome) and renal tuberous sclerosis. Johns Hopkins Med J 1974;135:274.

371. Robertson PW, Klidjian A, Harding LK, et al. Hypertension due to a renin-secreting renal tumour. Am J Med 1967;43:963.

372. Martin SA, Mynderse LA, Lager DJ, et al. Juxtaglomerular cell tumor: A clinicopathologic study of four cases and review of the literature. Am J Clin Pathol 2001;116:854.

373. McVicar M, Carman C, Chandra M, et al. Hypertension secondary to renin-secreting juxtaglomerular cell tumor: Case report and review of 38 cases. Pediatr Nephrol 1993;7:404.

374. Corvol P, Pinet F, Plouin PF, et al. Renin-secreting tumors. Endocrinol Metab Clin North Am 1994;23:255.

375. Furusato M, Hayashi H, Kawaguchi N, et al. Juxtaglomerular cell tumor. With special reference to the tubular component in regards to its histogenesis. Acta Pathol Jpn 1983;33:609.

376. Camilleri JP, Hinglais N, Bruneval P, et al. Renin storage and cell differentiation in juxtaglomerular cell tumors: An immunohistochemical and ultrastructural study of three cases. Hum Pathol 1984;15:1069.

377. Hermus AR, Pieters GF, Lamers AP, et al. Hypertension and hypokalaemia due to a renin-secreting kidney tumour: Primary reninism. Neth J Med 1986;29:84.

378. Bruneval P, Fournier JG, Soubrier F, et al. Detection and localization of renin messenger RNA in human pathologic tissues using in situ hybridization. Am J Pathol 1988;131:320.

379. Mason GA, Hart-Mercer J, Millar EJ, et al. Adrenaline-secreting neuroblastoma in an infant. Lancet 1957;2:322.

380. Weinblatt ME, Heisel MA, Siegel SE. Hypertension in children with neurogenic tumors. Pediatrics 1983;71:947.

381. Voorhess ML. Neuroblastoma-pheochromocytoma: products and pathogenesis. Ann N Y Acad Sci 1974;230:187.

382. Pincoffs MC, Bradley JE. The association of adenosarcoma of the kidney (Wilms' tumor) with arterial hypertension. Trans Assoc Am Physicians 1937;53:320.

383. Wong W, Mauger D. Treatment of Wilms tumor-related hypertension with losartan and captopril. Pediatr Nephrol 2004;19:805.

384. Mitchell JD, Baxter, TJ, Blair-West, JR, and McCredie, DA Renin levels in nephroblastoma (Wilms' tumor): Report of a renin secreting tumour. Arch Dis Child 1970;45:376.

385. Lindop GB, Fleming S, Gibson AA. Immunocytochemical localisation of renin in nephroblastoma. J Clin Pathol 1984;37:738.

386. Lampe WT II, Crovatto AC. Renal adenocarcinoma producing hypertension: Diagnosis by radioactive renogram and aortography. J Urol 1965;93:673.

387. Lindop GB, Leckie B, Winearls CG. Malignant hypertension due to a renin-secreting renal cell carcinoma: An ultrastructural and immunocytochemical study. Histopathology 1986;10:1077.

388. Steffens J, Bock R, Braedel HU, et al. Renin-producing renal cell carcinomas–clinical and experimental investigations on a special form of renal hypertension. Urol Res 1992;20:111.

389. Genest J, Rojo-Ortega JM, Kuchel O, et al. Malignant hypertension with hypokalemia in a patient with renin-producing pulmonary carcinoma. Trans Assoc Am Physicians 1975;88:192.

390. Tetu B, Lebel M, Camilleri JP. Renin-producing ovarian tumor. A case report with immunohistochemical and electron-microscopic study. Am J Surg Pathol 1988;12:634.

391. Tsuchida Y, Shimizu K, Hata J, et al. Renin production in congenital mesoblastic nephroma in comparison with that in Wilms' tumor. Pediatr Pathol 1993;13:155.

392. Neilly IJ, Bennett NB, Dawson AA, et al. Systemic hypertension: An unusual presentation of T-cell lymphoma. Clin Lab Haematol 1994;16:75.

393. Fernandez LA, Olsen TG, Barwick KW, et al. Renin in angiolymphoid hyperplasia with eosinophilia. Its possible effect on vascular proliferation. Arch Pathol Lab Med 1986;110:1131.

394. Laragh JH, Sealey JE, Ledingham JG, et al. Oral contraceptives. Renin, aldosterone, and high blood pressure. JAMA 1967;201:918.

395. Boyd WN, Burden RP, Aber GM. Intrarenal vascular changes in patients receiving oestrogen-containing compounds: A clinical, histological and angiographic study. Q J Med 1975;44:415.

396. Crane MG, Harris JJ, Winsor WD. Hypertension, oral contraceptive agents, and conjugated estrogens. Ann Intern Med 1971;74:13.

397. Harris PW. Malignant hypertension associated with oral contraceptives. Lancet 1969;2:466.

398. Endrikat J, Jaques MA, Mayerhofer M, et al. A twelve-month comparative clinical investigation of two low-dose oral contraceptives containing 20 micrograms ethinylestradiol/75 micrograms gestodene and 20 micrograms ethinylestradiol/150 micrograms desogestrel, with respect to efficacy, cycle control and tolerance. Contraception 1995;52:229.

399. Fuchs N, Dusterberg B, Weber-Diehl F, et al. The effect on blood pressure of a monophasic oral contraceptive containing ethinylestradiol and gestodene. Contraception 1995;51:335.

400. Godsland IF, Crook D. Update on the metabolic effects of steroidal contraceptives and their relationship to cardiovascular disease risk. Am J Obstet Gynecol 1994;170(Pt 2):1528.

401. Nabulsi AA, Folsom AR, White A, et al. Association of hormone-replacement therapy with various cardiovascular risk factors in postmenopausal women. N Engl J Med 1993;328:1069.

402. Pfeffer RI, Kurosaki TT, Charlton SK. Estrogen use and blood pressure in later life. Am J Epidemiol 1979;110:469.

403. Lubianca JN, Faccin CS, Fuchs FD. Oral contraceptives: A risk factor for uncontrolled blood pressure among hypertensive women. Contraception 2003;67:19.

404. Lubianca JN, Moreira LB, Gus M, et al. Stopping oral contraceptives: An effective blood pressure lowering intervention in women with hypertension. J Hum Hypertens 2005;19:451.

405. Hussain SF. Progestogen-only pills and high blood pressure: Is there an association? A literature review. Contraception 2004;69:89.

406. Shen Q, Lin D, Jiang X, et al. Blood pressure changes and hormonal contraceptives. Contraception 1994;50:131.

407. Kaplan NM. The treatment of hypertension in women. Arch Intern Med 1995;155:563.

408. Stadel BV. Oral contraceptives and cardiovascular disease. N Engl J Med 1981;305:672.

409. Lanzani C, Citterio L, Jankaricova M, et al. Role of the adducin family genes in human essential hypertension. J Hypertens 2005;23:543.

410. Wang J-G, Staessen JA, Barlassina C, et al. Association between hypertension and variation in the alpha- and beta-adducin genes in a white population. Kidney Int 2002;62:2152.

411. Kumar NN, Benjafield AV, Lin RC, et al. Haplotype analysis of aldosterone synthase gene (CYP11B2) polymorphisms shows association with essential hypertension. J Hypertens 2003;21:1331.

412. Giner V, Poch E, Bragulat E, et al. Renin-angiotensin system genetic polymorphisms and salt sensitivity in essential hypertension. Hypertension 2000;35(Pt 2):512.

413. Higaki J, Baba S, Katsuya T, et al. Deletion allele of angiotensin-converting enzyme gene increases risk of essential hypertension in Japanese men. The Suita Study. Circulation 2000;101:2060.

414. Jain S, Li Y, Patil S, et al. A single-nucleotide polymorphism in

human angiotensinogen gene is associated with essential hypertension and affects glucocorticoid induced promoter activity. J Mol Med 2005;83:121.

415. Baudin B. Polymorphism in angiotensin II receptor genes and hypertension. Exp Physiol 2005;90:277.

416. Bhavani AB, Sastry KB, Reddy NK, et al. Lipid profile and apolipoprotein E polymorphism in essential hypertension. Indian Heart J 2005;57:151.

417. Cui J, Melista E, Chazaro I, et al. Sequence variation of bradykinin receptors B1 and B2 and association with hypertension. J Hypertens 2005;23:55.

418. Zhou XF, Cui J, DeStefano AL, et al. Polymorphisms in the promoter region of catalase gene and essential hypertension. Dis Markers 2005;21:3.

419. Abe M, Wu Z, Yamamoto M, et al. Association of dopamine beta-hydroxylase polymorphism with hypertension through interaction with fasting plasma glucose in Japanese. Hypertens Res 2005;28:215.

420. Chen W, Srinivasan SR, Li S, et al. Gender-specific influence of NO synthase gene on blood pressure since childhood: The Bogalusa Heart Study. Hypertension 2004;44:668.

421. Hannila-Handelberg T, Kontula K, Tikkanen I, et al. Common variants of the beta and gamma subunits of the epithelial sodium channel and their relation to plasma renin and aldosterone levels in essential hypertension. BMC Med Genet 2005;6:4.

422. Motone M, Katsuya T, Ishikawa K, et al. Association between hepatocyte growth factor gene polymorphism and essential hypertension. Hypertens Res 2004;27:247.

423. Kokubo Y, Inamoto N, Tomoike H, et al. Association of genetic polymorphisms of sodium-calcium exchanger 1 gene, NCX1, with hypertension in a Japanese general population. Hypertens Res 2004;27:697.

424. Newhouse SJ, Wallace C, Dobson R, et al. Haplotypes of the WNK1 gene associate with blood pressure variation in a severely hypertensive population from the British Genetics of Hypertension study. Hum Mol Genet 2005;14:1805.

# Pyelonephritis and Other Infections, Reflux Nephropathy, Hydronephrosis, and Nephrolithiasis

*Mark Weiss*    *Helen Liapis*
*John E. Tomaszewski*    *Lois J. Arend*

## PYELONEPHRITIS AND OTHER INFECTIONS

### Urinary Tract Infection

Strictly speaking, urinary tract infections (UTIs) include not only those occurring at any point from the kidney to the urethral meatus but also those in adjacent structures, such as the prostate and epididymis (1,2). However, this account will be confined to the former types. Most cases are merely incapacitating, but their very frequency is responsible for much time spent away from school or work as well as for considerable expenditures of money in their investigation and treatment. This is particularly true for such conditions as acute urethral syndrome in females (3) and many cases of cystitis. The kidneys may be involved in the infective process, with the chance of ensuing hypertension or renal failure. Although it is self-evident, it is important to emphasize that the term *bacteriuria* does not necessarily imply infection of the kidney. *Bacteriuria* simply means that there are organisms in the specimen of urine tested, and it may be found not only in patients whose kidneys are infected but also in those whose infection is confined to the lower urinary tract. It also must be appreciated that organisms may appear in a specimen of urine as a result of contamination during collection, and this possibility must be clearly differentiated from a genuine UTI.

Most UTIs are caused by Gram-negative enteric organisms, and the most common form of renal involvement is *pyelonephritis*. This is best defined as a bacterial infection of the kidney that affects the parenchyma, calices, and pelvis. It occurs in two forms, *acute* and *chronic*, and may be found with or without obstruction to the urinary tract. The infecting organisms reach the kidney from the lower urinary tract by an ascending route, and because vesicoureteral reflux (VUR) is the mechanism by which this happens in a substantial number of cases, the name *reflux nephropathy* has been given to those cases in which parenchymal scarring is found (4).

Another pattern of renal infection is that found with blood-borne invasion by such organisms as *Staphylococcus aureus*. This infection consists of vast numbers of minute abscesses scattered throughout the parenchyma, particularly the cortex. The names *multiple cortical abscesses*, *diffuse suppurative nephritis*, and *diffuse bacterial nephritis* are used for this picture. It should not be confused with acute pyelonephritis. The nomenclature used in renal infections is discussed in greater detail in subsequent sections.

## Urinary Contamination and the Concept of Significant Bacteriuria

It is clear that if a specimen of urine is taken by catheter to determine whether the bladder urine is infected, there is the likelihood that organisms residing in the urethra will be pushed up into the bladder and be present in the urine sampled. The same is true for samples of urine passed naturally, since they must traverse the urethra. As might be expected, the portion of the specimen most likely to be contaminated is that passed at the beginning of micturition. Midstream specimens of urine are unlikely to be tainted in this way and are therefore heavily relied on by clinicians to determine whether the bladder urine is infected. Suprapubic aspiration of urine from the bladder using a needle avoids contamination by the urethral flora; it is an invasive procedure, although it is frequently employed in infants.

To distinguish between genuinely infected urine and urine that contains contaminants, it is necessary to perform quantitative bacterial counts. Kass (5) demonstrated that bacterial counts of more than 100,000 colony-forming units (cfu) per milliliter of urine usually represent genuine infection. This is referred to as *significant bacteriuria*. Kass was careful to point out that a lower figure could indicate true infection under such conditions as rapid urinary flow, when urine pH is low, or when bacteriostatic drugs are being used. To these can be added other circumstances (2,6), but over the years, the figure of 100,000 cfu/mL of urine has provided a workable basis for the determination of significant bacteriuria, although a figure of 100 cfu/mL has been proposed for the specific instance of women with acute dysuria and frequency (7).

There is an increased prevalence of bacteriuria in older patients that is particularly apparent in men. Sobel (8) lists prostatic enlargement and loss of bactericidal activity of prostatic secretions as potent factors in men, while poor emptying of the bladder resulting from uterine prolapse and cystocele formation is considered important in women. Neuromuscular disease, increased instrumentation, and catheter use contribute in both sexes. He also considers that increased receptivity of vaginal, periurethral, and uroepithelial cells might be an important factor.

## Asymptomatic, or Covert, Bacteriuria

In certain people, particularly females, significant numbers of bacteria are found in the urine on routine testing despite the fact that there are no clear clinical manifestations (9,10). The name *asymptomatic bacteriuria* has been given to this situation, although the name has been challenged on the ground that symptoms referable to the lower urinary tract can often be found. The name *covert bacteriuria* has been suggested instead (11). It has been studied extensively in several groups of patients because of its relationship to UTIs in general, its origin, the future clinical course of patients in whom it is found, its relationship to hypertension, and its

effect on the mother and fetus in the context of pregnancy. The entire matter was covered in considerable detail in the fourth edition of this book, and that edition should be consulted for commentary and references by those interested in this subject. Important clinical aspects of bacterial UTIs in adults are addressed in recent review articles (12–15), and those that focus on UTI during pregnancy (16,17) and in persons with diabetes (18,19) should be consulted.

### Kidney Involvement in Urinary Tract Infection

Acute infections of the urinary tract and the causative role of what is now called *Escherichia coli* were established some 100 years ago, and the terms *cystitis* and *pyelitis* were introduced (20,21). The important observation of Thiemich (22) that the renal parenchyma was frequently infected in what had previously been regarded as pyelitis gave birth to the concept of acute pyelonephritis.

A full appreciation of the side effects of acute infection of the kidney came later, for although in 1882 Wagner (23) had recorded cases of contracted kidneys with features that we now associate with chronic pyelonephritis, it was not until 1917 that Löhlein (24) defined the clinical and pathologic features of the pyelonephritic contracted kidney in three young women who died in uremia, two of them with hypertension. Other influential articles on the clinical and pathologic features of chronic pyelonephritis appeared over the next three decades, chief among them those of Gibson (25), Staemmler and Dopheide (26), Longcope and Winkenwerder (27), Weiss and Parker (28), and Raaschou (29). Recognition of a unilateral form and its ability to produce hypertension (see Pickering and Heptinstall [30] for references) firmly established chronic pyelonephritis as an important disease entity.

Regrettably, during the 1950s and 1960s, many pathologists diagnosed chronic pyelonephritis with such profligacy that it became the most abused term in the whole of renal medicine. The diagnosis was frequently made purely on histologic changes in the parenchyma, few of which were specific for the sequelae of infection, and the essential "pyelo-" part of the term was completely ignored. It was not until pathologists, including Heptinstall (31,32), took notice of the radiologic observations of Hodson (33) that sanity was restored and stricter criteria for the diagnosis of chronic pyelonephritis imposed. While refinement of our criteria for its diagnosis has been aided by a better understanding of the ways in which organisms reach the kidney and the pattern of infection produced, these findings, in turn, have led to problems in nomenclature.

There are various terms over which there is no disagreement. *Pyelonephritis* is used to define a bacterial infection of the kidney that involves the parenchyma, calices, and pelvis. It is broken down into those types that have obstruction (*obstructive pyelonephritis*) and those that do not (*nonobstructive pyelonephritis*). Both can be subdivided into *acute* and *chronic* forms. The chronic nonobstructive form is the one that gave rise to so much confusion in the past, but the realization that vesicoureteral reflux (VUR) and infection are the initial events leading to parenchymal damage, coupled with the character of this damage, has given us a much clearer understanding of this condition. At the same time, the concept of reflux has resulted in problems in terminology.

In the first place, the possibility that reflux of sterile urine can initiate renal scarring has called into question the use of the term *chronic nonobstructive pyelonephritis*, which by definition implies an infective origin. Second, it has led to the introduction of the term *reflux nephropathy* (4) to describe the kidney with discrete focal scars in a lobar distribution, a term that is rapidly displacing "chronic pyelonephritis," specifically the nonobstructive form. The fact that the term does not specify the origin of the scars speaks in its favor, so that it could embrace potential cases of sterile reflux. It is also more appropriate as a description of the kidney with severe reflux in which there is generalized pelvic and caliceal dilatation, the so-called *back-pressure* type. The argument against its use is the exclusive emphasis placed on the mechanism whereby urine reaches the kidney, as though denying infection any role in scar formation. Infection, as we have seen, is the essential ingredient in the genesis of the vast majority of discrete lobar scars.

Furthermore, it is by no means certain that reflux is an invariable prerequisite for the development of renal scars, and there is increasing evidence to support this skepticism. First, several studies have indicated that scar formation can follow febrile UTIs in the apparent absence of reflux (34–36), particularly when P-fimbriated strains of *E. coli* are involved. Second, studies using dimercaptosuccinic acid (DMSA) scans have verified the presence of acute pyelonephritic lesions in the absence of reflux, followed at a later time by the development of discrete scars (37,38).

The type of renal involvement caused by blood-borne infections also presents problems with regard to nomenclature. Certain organisms, such as *S. aureus*, have the ability to localize, proliferate, and incite an acute inflammatory reaction in an unobstructed kidney. The resultant picture consists of vast numbers of minute abscesses situated mainly in the cortex. In contrast, no or only trivial inflammatory changes are found in the pelvis and calices; those that are present are secondary to the parenchymal infection. The picture is quite different from acute nonobstructive pyelonephritis caused by reflux of infected urine and from acute obstructive pyelonephritis; in both of these there is severe inflammation of pelvis and calices—the primary event—as well as of the parenchyma. Although many authors include the picture produced by blood-borne infection in the absence of obstruction under the heading of *pyelonephritis*, it is more accurate to use the terms *multiple cortical abscesses, diffuse suppurative nephritis,* or *diffuse bacterial nephritis* for this situation.

## Clinical Presentation of Renal Infection

### Acute Pyelonephritis

In a classic case in the adult, the onset is acute, with chills, fever, lumbar tenderness and pain, together with dysuria and frequency of micturition when infection of the lower urinary tract is present. Hypertension is usually absent. Renal function may be temporarily disturbed, and acute renal failure has been noted occasionally (39). While bacteremia is the cause of the chills, it very seldom leads to more serious side effects, such as disseminated intravascular coagulation. Blood cultures are positive in about a quarter or more of the cases of severe uncomplicated and complicated acute pyelonephritis (40). The urine contains organisms in excess of 100,000 cfu/mL, and white blood cells and white blood cell casts are present in the sediment. White blood cell casts are particularly important, implying that inflammation is taking place in the kidney itself. Proteinuria may or may not be present and is seldom heavy; hematuria, macroscopic or microscopic, may be found and is the result of the small hemorrhages in the renal pelvis or bladder. The initial symptoms in infants and young children consist of fever, vague abdominal complaints, and vomiting. Sometimes there is merely a failure to thrive. The pattern of early features in older children is closer to that in adults.

It must be appreciated that these features are relatively crude and imprecise and, in particular, that it is often impossible to distinguish on purely clinical grounds between acute pyelonephritis and infections confined to the lower urinary tract (41). This has led to the introduction of various ancillary laboratory tests to localize the site of infection more accurately, including tests for impairment of concentration of the urine, raised serum antibody levels to the offending organism, raised serum levels of antibody to Tamm-Horsfall protein, the presence of antibody-coated organisms in the urine, raised serum levels of C-reactive protein, and estimation of the lactic dehydrogenase levels in the urine. Even these tests have their shortcomings, which, along with their merits, were discussed in detail in Chapter 21 in the fourth edition of this book and will not be repeated.

Various imaging techniques add precision to the diagnosis. Ultrasonography (increased renal size), intravenous urography (renal enlargement with reduced nephrogram), and radionuclide methods using gallium-67-citrate and iodine-131-hippuran (defective uptake) have been used with varying degrees of success, but the most reliable results have come from dimercaptosuccinic acid (DMSA) scintigraphy. It is important to note that experimental studies in the pig (42,43) have established convincing correlations between focal areas of absent or decreased uptake of DMSA and the histologic picture of acute pyelonephritis. Several studies in humans (37,38,44–47) have used this technique and have demonstrated the same focal areas of impaired uptake of DMSA, which, as noted in some of the publications, have progressed over time to scar formation. Thus, DMSA scintigraphy provides the most reliable test at the present time for the diagnosis of acute pyelonephritis (48). In the normal situation, DMSA becomes fixed in the cells of the proximal convoluted tubule and upper part of the loop of Henle, reaching these cells by the peritubular capillaries or by tubular reabsorption following glomerular filtration (48). The pathophysiologic mechanism explaining the scanning abnormalities in acute pyelonephritis is probably diminished uptake of DMSA by the tubules as a result of decreased intrarenal blood flow and changes in tubular cell membrane transport function (49).

VUR is also commonly found in patients with acute pyelonephritis, and the importance of this phenomenon in causing bacterial invasion of the kidney is discussed later in the chapter. In an appreciable number of patients, acute pyelonephritis develops in the apparent absence of reflux (36–38,46,47), although tests for the detection of VUR are far from infallible.

### Multiple Cortical Abscesses, Diffuse Suppurative Nephritis, Diffuse Bacterial Nephritis

This is the type of renal lesion that is caused by blood-borne infection of the kidney, as opposed to ascending infection. Its prototype is the lesion caused by S. aureus, an organism that can localize in the absence of obstruction, and the usual context is septicemia. It may also be seen with E. coli bacteremia, but only when there is obstruction to urinary outflow.

In patients with staphylococcal septicemia, colonization of the kidney usually occur through the hematogenous route, the source of infection is often nosocomial, and S. aureus is the most common agent. Immunosuppressed patients are particularly vulnerable to staphylococcal infections (50,51). In the series of Moreno et al (50), of 75 episodes of bacteremia or fungemia in renal transplant recipients, the kidney and urinary tract were the site of infection in 21 cases (28%), and staphylococci were the most common infectious organisms. Patients present with fever, lumbar pain, symptoms of lower urinary tract infection, and renal insufficiency or renal failure (52). Staphylococci can be cultured from urine.

### Emphysematous Pyelonephritis

This rare condition, found predominantly in those with diabetes with or without urinary tract obstruction, consists of a severe suppurative infection of the kidney accompanied by gas formation in the pelvicaliceal region (emphysematous pyelitis), parenchyma, and sometimes in the perirenal tissue. Women are affected more often than men, with a mean age in the sixth decade. In most instances, only one kidney is involved, usually the left (53), although rarely both are affected (54,55). Nonspecific clinical features include chills, fever, pain in the flank, nausea and vomiting, abdominal pain and tenderness, pyuria, and glucose in the urine in those with diabetes. Thrombocytopenia, acute renal failure, disturbance of consciousness, and shock can be the initial presentation and are risk factors for poor outcome and mortality (56). Escherichia coli is the most common organism encountered, but others, such as Klebsiella pneumoniae, Enterobacter spp., Proteus mirabilis, Candida spp., and Cryptococcus neoformans, have been described (55,57). Diagnosis can be made by various imaging techniques, such as plain radiography and ultrasonography (53,57). However, computerized tomographic scans can not only confirm diagnosis, but also provide information that can be used to classify the extent of the intrarenal and extrarenal disease, which has both prognostic and therapeutic importance (56). It is a very serious condition that requires prompt and energetic treatment. The mortality rate with antibiotic treatment alone is high, particularly when gas is present in the perirenal tissue (57), and can be reduced considerably by a combination of antibiotics and surgical treatment in the form of drainage or nephrectomy (53–56).

### Pathologic Changes in Acute Infection of the Kidney

#### Acute Pyelonephritis

Virtually the only type of acute pyelonephritis seen by the pathologist is that accompanied by obstruction. Obstructive acute pyelonephritis shows evidence of an enlarged kidney with a bulging cut surface. The cortex has several swollen, whitish areas of acute infection, and between these more or less homogeneous areas are scattered, small, discrete, whitish-yellow abscesses with a hemorrhagic rim. These small abscesses, which may measure up to several millimeters in diameter across, are seen particularly well on the subcapsular surface (Fig. 22.1). These discrete cortical abscesses are indicative of a secondary blood-borne infection, because obstructive pyelonephritis in the acute stage very commonly gives rise to bacteremia.

In some cases, almost the entire cortex is white and swollen, suggesting that intrarenal reflux—the primary means of bacterial invasion—is taking place in all papillae. This is so because, in the presence of obstruction, even of short duration, it is possible for previously nonrefluxing papillae to be converted to a refluxing type (58). In addition to the cortical changes, the underlying medulla shows characteristic straight, whitish-yellow streaks that correspond to collecting ducts filled with pus (Fig. 22.2). Papillary necrosis may complicate the picture, and it is seen particularly in diabetic patients with severe, often terminal, acute renal infection. The pelvis and calices are dilated—a result of the obstruction—and the mucosal surfaces are often congested, with thickening of the pelvic wall. In cases where

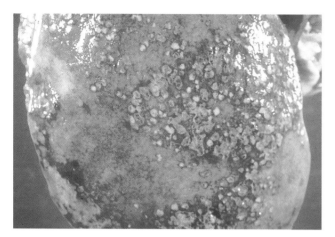

**Figure 22.1** Acute pyelonephritis. Cortical abscesses produce discrete or confluent, raised, yellowish-white, rounded nodules with surrounding hyperemia on the subcapsular surface.

there is severe obstruction, the renal parenchyma may be thinned with blunted papillae, and the pelvis filled with pus, a situation referred to as *pyonephrosis* (Fig. 22.3).

Regardless of whether it is the *obstructive* or *nonobstructive* type, the histologic picture in areas of acute infection is similar. Tubules are extensively destroyed by the acute inflammatory process, in which neutrophils predominate (Fig. 22.4). Glomeruli and blood vessels, such as arteries and arterioles, are surprisingly resistant to damage, and acute arteritis or arteriolitis is virtually unheard of. Although some glomeruli are secondarily involved by the inflammatory process—invasive glomerulitis (59)—the vast majority remain unscathed. Tubules that are not destroyed often contain large numbers of neutrophils, and breaches in the tubular epithelium are not uncommon (60). The collecting tubules in the medulla and cortex are filled with

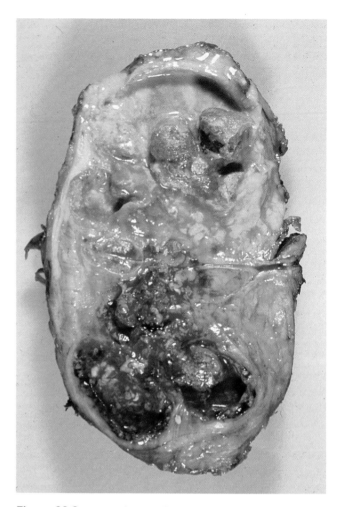

**Figure 22.3** Pyonephrosis. The kidney is converted into a pus-filled sac, with little identifiable parenchyma. The mucosa of the collecting system is focally hemorrhagic and covered by creamy exudate; it contains several calculi.

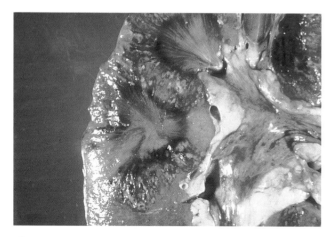

**Figure 22.2** Acute pyelonephritis. Abscesses are apparent on the cut surface of the cortex, and there are straight yellow streaks and hyperemia in the medulla. The pelvic mucosa is congested, granular, and dull.

neutrophils and correspond to the yellowish-white streaks seen grossly (Fig. 22.5).

Initially, the interstitial inflammatory exudate consists of neutrophils, with their presence first becoming apparent in the intertubular capillaries. This is followed by rupture of the capillary walls, with cellular and fluid leakage into the interstitial space (61). Chronic inflammatory cells, such as macrophages, lymphocytes, and plasma cells, soon appear, within a few days of the start of infection in the various species studied experimentally (43,58,62–64). Acute inflammatory changes are seen in relation to the pelvic and caliceal epithelium; they are generalized in the obstructive forms but restricted to the involved caliceal systems in those forms without obstruction. Although papillary necrosis is seen in some of the severe terminal renal infections with accompanying obstruction and diabetes (Fig. 22.6), it is an unlikely complication of acute nonobstructive pyelonephritis associated with VUR. An important

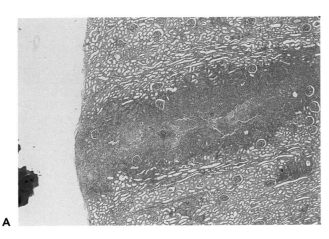
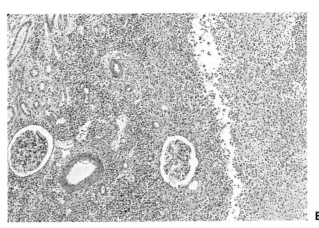

A

B

**Figure 22.4**    Acute pyelonephritis. **A:** Patchy suppurative inflammation extends to the capsular surface (*left*) and produces multiple confluent microabscesses. (hematoxylin & eosin [H&E; ×20.] **B:** The abscess (*right*) contains polymorphonuclear leukocytes and has tubular destruction with parenchymal liquefactive necrosis. Lymphocytes and plasma cells, which may appear after several days, are present in the adjacent cortex. Note the sparing of glomeruli, arteries, and arterioles. (H&E; ×100.)

feature of the acute nonobstructive form is the way in which large areas of the parenchyma are spared from infection.

## Multiple Cortical Abscesses, Diffuse Suppurative Nephritis, Diffuse Bacterial Nephritis

The kidneys are enlarged and are the site of abscess formation with intense inflammatory infiltration by large numbers of neutrophils. *Staphylococcus aureus* is the most common agent; both kidneys are affected and are enlarged to an equal degree. With *E. coli*, only the obstructed kidney is involved. The subcapsular surface is studded with vast numbers of whitish-yellow abscesses, often with red rims. The abscesses vary in size; some are as small as a pinhead, but others may measure up to half a centimeter across (Fig. 22.7). They are usually discrete, but some are confluent.

The cut surface bulges because of the accompanying interstitial edema and displays myriad small abscesses; some are rounded and similar to those seen on the subcapsular surface, but others are wedge-shaped with the apex pointing inward. The greatest numbers are present in the cortex, although some are situated in the medulla, particularly the outer part. Whitish streaking is often seen in the medulla; it represents collecting ducts filled with pus. The pelvis and calices are not usually dilated in the type associated with *S. aureus*, but they are dilated in the context of *E. coli*.

Microscopically, the gross abscesses consist of large numbers of neutrophils in the interstitium, with extensive destruction of tubules, particularly the proximal convoluted segments. Glomeruli, arteries, and arterioles are usually undamaged, although microabscesses may very

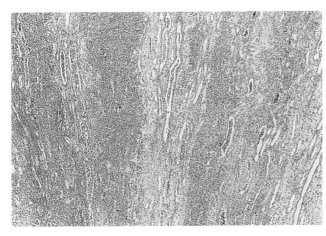

**Figure 22.5**    Acute pyelonephritis. The medullary infiltrate has a typical linear distribution, and collecting ducts are filled with polymorphonuclear leukocytes. (H&E; ×40.)

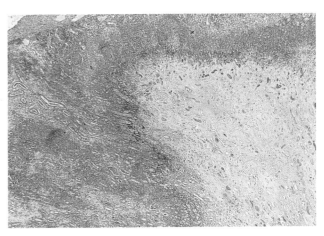

**Figure 22.6**    Acute pyelonephritis complicated by papillary necrosis. The necrotic papilla has the usual intense inflammatory border. (H&E; ×20.)

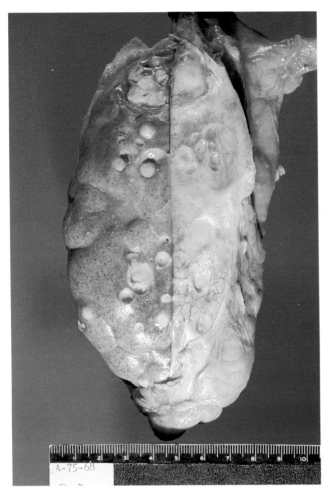

**Figure 22.7**   Diffuse suppurative nephritis. The subcapsular surface has numerous discrete and focally confluent, whitish-yellow abscesses of variable size.

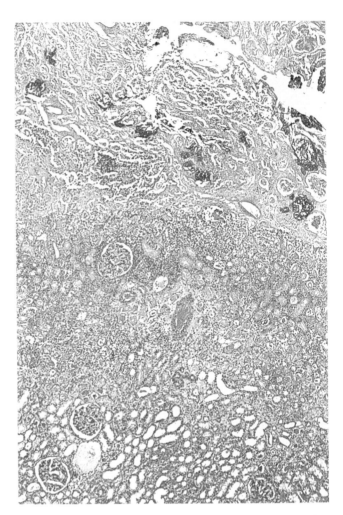

**Figure 22.8**   Cortical abscess caused by hematogenous staphylococcal infection. There is marked parenchymal necrosis involving glomeruli, and numerous bacterial colonies are present. (H&E; ×40.)

occasionally be seen in the glomerular capillary tufts (Fig. 22.8). Organisms are readily evident. In tubules that are not destroyed, the lumens may be filled with neutrophils, which account for the linear streaking seen grossly in the medulla. In contrast to acute pyelonephritis, there are no, or only a few, inflammatory cells beneath the caliceal and pelvic epithelium, and such changes as there are result from inflammation in the parenchyma (65).

### Emphysematous Pyelonephritis

Reviews of the pathologic lesions of the kidney (55–57) have described parenchymal abscesses and areas of infarction, with gas formation in the necrotic areas (Figs. 22.9 and 22.10); papillary necrosis is a typical finding, as are vascular thromboses. In some patients with diabetes, signs of that disease, such as glomerulosclerosis, were found. Obstruction was recorded in 40% of cases.

The pathogenesis of the condition is not clear, but many of the features are those described in the previous section and suggest a bloodborne infection. Four factors that may

be involved include gas-forming bacteria, high tissue glucose level, impaired tissue perfusion, and a defective immune response (56).

### Etiology and Pathogenesis

#### Organisms Involved

Most UTIs are caused by Gram-negative enteric organisms, of which *E. coli* is the most common, particularly in first and uncomplicated infections (66–68). Other organisms include *Klebsiella* sp., *Proteus* sp. (69), *Pseudomonas* sp., *Enterobacter* sp., *Serratia* sp., *Morganella morganii,* and rarely *Haemophilus influenzae* (70); these are found mainly in complicated cases in which instrumentation was used (1,69). Indwelling catheters are particularly troublesome. The spectrum of etiologic agents in UTIs is summarized in Table 22.1 (12).

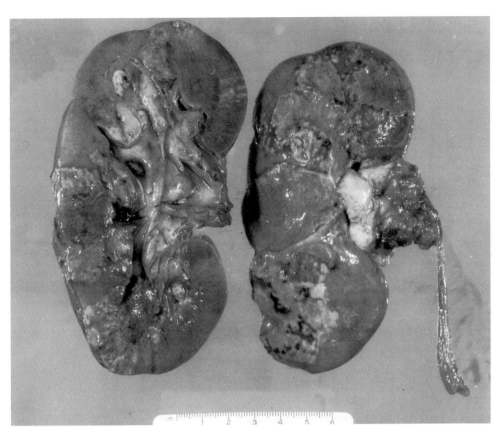

**Figure 22.9** Emphysematous pyelonephritis. The enlarged kidney has extensive necrosis with abscess formation and numerous cystic foci that are barely discernible to the naked eye.

## Source and Route of Entry of Organisms

Most infections of the urinary tract are considered to be caused by organisms originating in the feces. Thus, in a number of studies, the O serogroups of *E. coli* responsible for urinary infections were also present in the patients' fecal flora (71–74). The possibility that certain strains of *E. coli* are more likely than others to cause UTIs was raised by Rantz (75), who, in a study of 156 patients with such infections, found that certain O serotypes were isolated with disproportionate frequency. This observation has been repeatedly confirmed (73,76–78). There are two possible explanations for the small number of serotypes causing infections. On the one hand, it is possible that certain serotypes have a special propensity for the urinary tract; this is referred to as the *special pathogenicity theory* (see "Bacterial Virulence Factors"). The alternative explanation is that certain serotypes are found more commonly in UTIs because they occur more frequently than others in the feces, the natural reservoir of *E. coli*. This is called the *prevalence theory*.

To further develop the idea of an ascending route of infection for organisms originating in the feces, studies have been performed on the flora of the periurethral area. It has been noticed that the infrequency of the presence of Gram-negative bacteria in the vaginal vestibule of patients who do not have recurrent UTIs (79,80) contrasts sharply with the situation in females who do have such infections (80–83). These studies not only support the entry of organisms through the urethra but also emphasize the part played by the asymptomatic harboring of organisms in the vestibule in recurrent UTIs. A longitudinal prospective investigation of 40 women, 20 with and 20 without recurrent UTIs, confirmed the notion that women with recurrent UTIs have more frequent vaginal colonization than do comparable controls (84). Of relevance to this issue is the finding in females with recurrent UTIs of a greater binding capacity of *E. coli* to vaginal cells of women (85–87) and to periurethral cells of girls (88,89). Two other studies using the same approach as that of Stamey et al (83) confirmed that in certain women with recurrent UTIs, the infective episode is preceded by colonization of the periurethral area with the identical strain of *E. coli* (90,91).

While most studies have been carried out in females because of the greater frequency of UTIs, it has been shown in males (92,93) that a common cause of UTI is relapse of a chronic source of infection in the prostate. The importance of circumcision has also been noted (94), with the presence of a foreskin during the first 6 months of life associated with larger numbers of periurethral bacteria and a greater

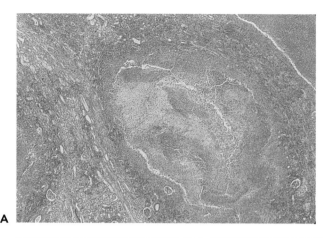

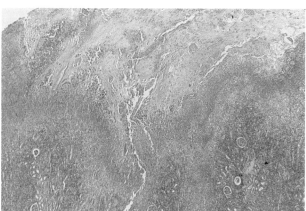

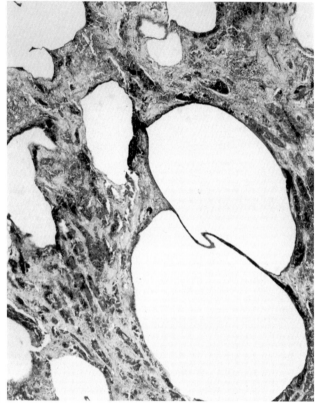

**Figure 22.10** Emphysematous pyelonephritis. **A:** A large cortical abscess is present. (H&E; ×20.) **B:** A triangular zone of cortical infarction is demarcated by a zone of hemorrhage and intense inflammation. (H&E; ×20.) **C:** Gas formation in necrotic tissue produces circular spaces resembling emphysema. (H&E; ×100.)

likelihood for the presence of potentially uropathogenic organisms.

## Host–Pathogen Interactions

The two main factors that determine the occurrence of a UTI are, first, the availability and virulence of infecting organisms, and, second, the various host defense mechanisms. Because the adherence of organisms to the mucosa of the urinary tract is central to the entire concept of UTIs, much of this section discusses adherence factors. Bacterial virulence factors are discussed to serve as an introduction to adherence, followed by accounts of host factors that predispose to infection and the several

defense mechanisms that protect the urinary tract from infection.

## Bacterial Virulence Factors

Reference was made earlier to the two theories put forward to account for the disproportionate frequency with which certain serotypes of *E. coli* are found in association with UTIs. Much evidence has accrued to give credence to the special pathogenicity theory, according to which some organisms have a greater ability than others to infect the urinary tract. This special propensity is brought about by certain properties of the organisms, collectively referred to as *virulence factors*. They are of several types.

## TABLE 22.1

### BACTERIAL ETIOLOGY OF URINARY TRACT INFECTION

| | Uncomplicated (%) | Complicated (%)[a] |
|---|---|---|
| **Gram-negative** | | |
| E. coli | 70–95 | 21–54 |
| P. mirabilis | 1–2 | 1–10 |
| Klebsiella sp. | 1–2 | 2–17 |
| Citrobacter sp. | <1 | 5 |
| Enterobacter sp. | <1 | 2–10 |
| P. aeruginosa | <1 | 2–19 |
| Other | <1 | 6–20 |
| **Gram-positive** | | |
| Coagulase-negative staphylococci | 5–10[b] | 1–4 |
| Enterococci | 1–2 | 1–23 |
| Group B streptococci | <1 | 1–4 |
| S. aureus | <1 | 1–2 |
| Other | <1 | 2 |

[a]Data from Hooton (12).
[b]S. saprophyticus.

*O, K, and H Serotypes.* The way in which certain O serotypes of *E. coli* have been found with disproportionate frequency in UTIs (73,76–78) was mentioned earlier. A limited number of O serotypes cause most of these infections, and the most prevalent types are O1, O2, O4, O6, O7, O8, O16, O16/72, O18, O25, O50, and O75 (76). In addition, these particular strains are found most commonly in patients with clinically diagnosed acute pyelonephritis, less commonly in cystitis, and least commonly in asymptomatic bacteriuria (77,95). Also, these UTI-associated O serotypes are less prevalent when acute pyelonephritis is found in the context of VUR than in those cases without reflux (77). The explanation for the uropathogenicity of the various O serotypes is not altogether clear, and whereas the O polysaccharides might interfere with complement-dependent bacterial killing, it may be that their virulence is related to other associated factors that will be discussed later in this section, such as P fimbriae, hemolysin, and serum resistance (76,78).

K antigens (capsular polysaccharides) have also been studied, and certain K types are found with undue frequency among isolates from patients with infections of the kidney and bladder (76). These include K1, K2, K3, K5, K12, K13, K20, and K51. Capsular polysaccharides are antiphagocytic and anticomplementary (76,96) and thereby elude elimination by the host. As with O serotypes, certain K strains are associated with other virulence factors, such as P fimbriae (76). Combinations of O, K, and H (flagellar) antigens might be expected to provide

more specific information on the relationships of strains to the clinical categories of UTI (pyelonephritis, cystitis, asymptomatic bacteriuria), but with the exception of one serotype, O75:K100:H5, which is uniquely associated with cystitis (76), the results are disappointing.

*Adherence Properties of Bacteria: The Role of Fimbriae.* Much attention has been given to the adhesion of bacteria to mucous membranes to explain colonization of the urinary tract. Adhesins include fimbriae, adherence pedestals (similar to fimbriae), and afimbrial adhesins, such as polymers, polysaccharides, lipoteichoic acid, and high–molecular-weight proteins. Whereas Gram-positive bacteria adhere more frequently via extracellular polysaccharides, adhesion occurs via fimbriae in the case of Gram-negative bacteria. This adhesion is effected by the interaction between receptors on the epithelial cell surface and hairlike appendages termed fimbriae or pili found on the surface of the infecting organism.

There are several genetically and chemically distinct forms of fimbriae. They are broadly divided into two main groups, depending on the ability of mannose to interfere with their ability to attach to receptors, and are accordingly designated *mannose sensitive* or *mannose resistant.* Type 1 fimbriae are mannose sensitive, while P fimbriae and X fimbriae are mannose resistant. P fimbriae (so called because they attach to a digalactoside residue [Gal–Gal] related to P blood group antigens on human erythrocytes and uroepithelial cells) appear to be the most important with regard to UTIs, especially with regard to renal involvement. The receptor binding adhesin at the tip of P fimbriae is pap G, and there are three classes of G-tip proteins (97). Class II–tip adhesin is associated with pyelonephritis and Class III–tip adhesin with cystitis.

In addition to their role in adherence, P fimbriae also contribute to the persistence of *E. coli* by enhancing the inflammatory response to infection (98). It was found that *E. coli* bacteria or isolated P fimbriae could induce mucosal cells to produce interleukin-6 (IL-6) and IL-8, which initiate a local inflammatory response. Interleukin-6 was considered to cause the fever and acute-phase response, which are part of UTIs, while IL-8 might act as a neutrophil chemoattractant (98).

### Other Virulence Factors

Many novel and putative virulence factors in uropathogenic *E. coli* have been identified using polymerase chain reaction (PCR) assays, including catecholate siderophore receptor (iroN), iron-regulated gene A homologue adhesin (iha), group II capsule (kpsMT), and outer membrane protease T (ompT) (99). Pathogenicity islands (defined blocks of DNA) present on the genomes of pathogenic strains are a mechanism of horizontal virulence factor gene transfers between the same or related species. A putative uropathogenic island including a gene-encoding, uropathogenic-specific protein (USP) has been identified in *E. coli* strains isolated from patients with pyelonephritis (99).

### Defense Mechanisms

*Extrinsic Bladder Mechanisms.* Various mechanisms operate to prevent the attachment of uropathogens to the epithelium of the vagina, periurethral region, and urethra. Natural endogenous bacteria, such as lactobacilli, protect by lowering local pH and also by interfering with attachment by such means as steric hindrance, competition for receptor sites, and inhibition of bacterial growth (100). As is mentioned later, the host's secretor status is clearly important in terms of shielding receptor sites (101). Surface mucosal antibodies also afford protection against colonization by pathogenic *E. coli*, and Stamey et al (102) have shown that cervicovaginal antibody is deficient in women with recurrent UTIs. Stamey et al have also shown the bactericidal properties of both human and canine prostatic fluid (103).

*Intrinsic Bladder Mechanisms.* The bladder is remarkably efficient in dealing with bacterial invasion. Urine supports the growth of such organisms as the *Enterobacteriaceae*, *Pseudomonas* sp., *Candida* sp., *Enterococcus* sp., and *S. aureus* (1), but because of its relatively low pH, relatively high osmolality, and high urea content, it is not the ideal culture medium (104). Clearly, when glucose is present in the urine, as in the context of diabetes mellitus, conditions are more propitious for bacterial growth. The mechanical act of voiding is also an important factor in preventing infection, and this becomes apparent when there is a breakdown in this mechanism, such as in obstruction of urinary outflow and in VUR.

Anti-adherence mechanisms abound in the bladder. First, there is a layer of glycosaminoglycans lining the urothelium (105), which prevents the attachment of pathogens. Second, there is the presence of oligosaccharides with the potential to detach epithelial-bound *E. coli* and to prevent bacterial attachment, presumably by competing with chemically similar cell surface receptors (106). Third, the so-called slime or uromucoid layer (now recognized to be Tamm-Horsfall protein), which lines the bladder, shows great avidity for *E. coli* bearing type 1 fimbriae and thereby protects the underlying mucosa (107). The urine itself may show anti-adherence properties, and immunoglobulins in the urine of patients with acute pyelonephritis have been found to be capable of reducing in vitro adherence of the infecting strain of *E. coli* to uroepithelial cells (108).

*Immune Mechanisms: Antibody Formation.* There is evidence from experimental studies that antibodies can have a protective role against bacteria invading the urinary tract, but their role in humans is more difficult to assess. Antibodies may be produced either locally or systemically (109,110). Experimental studies support the claims (111) that the finding of antibody-coated bacteria in the urine in human patients indicates an infection of the kidney, as opposed to an infection of the lower urinary tract.

In human acute pyelonephritis caused by *E. coli*, antibodies are produced against the O and K antigens (109) as well as against fimbriae (112,113), principally as a systemic response. Immunoglobulin M is dominant in the early stages, followed by IgG and IgA. The urine of patients with pyelonephritis also contains IgG and secretory IgA; the latter is probably produced by local mechanisms (8). The efficacy of these several antibodies in human patients is difficult to ascertain, but certainly their presence in the urine could explain the well-known fact that recurrent UTIs usually are caused by different strains, the original strains having been eradicated by antibodies.

### Factors Interfering with Host Defenses

*Increased Susceptibility to Bacterial Adherence.* The demonstration that vaginal, buccal, periurethral, and uroepithelial cells from patients with recurrent UTIs show greater adherence to standard strains of *E. coli* than do comparable cells from control patients was an early clue to the importance of host factors in UTI (85,88). Since that time, interest has centered on blood group antigens and secretor status. Secretors differ from nonsecretors in their ability to secrete water-soluble blood group antigens. An increased risk of recurrent UTIs was found among women of blood groups B and AB who were nonsecretors of blood group substance (114) and also in girls with the P1 blood group (115). It has also been shown that both girls (116) and women (117) who are nonsecretors in the ABH system are unduly prone to renal scarring following recurrent UTIs. Various explanations have been offered for these observations. Because uroepithelial cells from nonsecretors were found to adhere with greater avidity to uropathogenic strains of *E. coli* than were cells from secretors (101), it was suggested that the shielding of cell receptors by products under the control of the secretor gene was defective in the case of the nonsecretors. Claims have been made that the increased prevalence of renal scarring following recurrent UTIs in nonsecretors is a consequence of an elevated inflammatory response (118). The idea of an ineffective immune response in nonsecretors has received little support (119).

*Obstruction to Urinary Outflow.* Obstruction is a potent factor not only in initiating infection but also in causing it to persist and spread to the kidney. Obstruction below the bladder neck results in loss of the potent "flushing mechanism," which, together with incomplete emptying of the bladder, permits the multiplication of bacteria in the relatively static residual urine. The use of catheters in the context of obstruction is an additional hazard for introducing bacteria and, particularly in the case of indwelling catheters, for permitting bacterial growth. Spread of infection to the kidney is a particular danger, and this spread may come about in several ways. First, organisms may be carried to the kidney up the ureter through the intermediary of VUR, or, second, they may reach the kidney by a bloodborne route. It is an old observation that intravenously injected *E. coli* will not localize in the kidney in the absence of obstruction but will readily do so when the ureter is obstructed (63,120).

Moreover, release of the obstruction gives rise to healing of the inflammatory lesion produced, accompanied by scarring (63,120), whereas re-obstruction of the ureter in a rat with an almost completely healed infective lesion will lead to recrudescence of the infection (121). Even small intrarenal scars, by causing obstruction to a group of nephrons, may render that localized area more prone to bloodborne infection (122,123).

*Diabetes Mellitus.* Diabetes mellitus is invariably cited as a risk factor for UTIs and their side effects (18,19). Acute infections of the kidney are often claimed to be more common in diabetes (124), but this finding is based on autopsies performed on patients who died in large public hospitals (125,126) 50 years ago. However, claims for certain acute infections of the upper urinary tract stand on more solid foundations, and patients with diabetes are described as being more prone to cortical abscesses (124,127), perirenal abscesses (124), and emphysematous pyelonephritis (53,57). Finally, it should be added that there is little evidence of an increased prevalence of true chronic pyelonephritis in the diabetic population.

*Calculi.* Calculi affect the host's defense mechanism in several ways. First, they cause obstruction, either complete or partial, which may occur at various different levels. Second, they may serve as a nidus for the persistence of infection, either because they act as an irritant or because they may harbor organisms within their substance, rendering it difficult to completely eradicate the infection. Calculi are particularly troublesome, not only because they aggravate infections but also because they may, in the case of certain types of stone, be caused by them. This is particularly true of struvite stones, which form in the presence of urea-splitting bacteria such as *Proteus* sp.

## Route of Invasion of the Kidney

*Bloodborne Infection.* In certain situations, the bloodstream is undoubtedly the main route by which the kidney is infected. In experimental situations, *S. aureus* will cause a lesion in the unobstructed kidney following intravenous injection (128), and in humans, the kidney may become infected in staphylococcal endocarditis or as the result of

bacteremia from boils or carbuncles. Staphylococci cause renal infection because of several microbial factors: bacterial surface receptors that recognize fibrinogen; fibronectin, vitronectin, and laminin, which permit bacterial adherence to endothelial cells (129) and extracellular matrix (130); release of exotoxins (131), including pore-forming protein (132); various enzymes that interfere with structure and function of plasma membrane and degrade elastic tissue; and toxins that may function as superantigens (133). Staphylococci do not require obstruction of urine outflow for organisms to invade the kidneys.

Other infective agents that are able to colonize a healthy kidney following bloodstream invasion include *Actinomyces* sp., yeasts, filamentous fungi, *Mycobacterium tuberculosis*, and *Brucella* sp. In contrast, as described earlier, *E. coli* will not localize and proliferate in a healthy kidney after intravenous injection but will do so if the kidney is obstructed (63,120).

*Ascending or Upward Spread.* VUR is a well-authenticated way for organisms to pass up the ureter from the bladder to the pelvis of the kidney, gain access to the kidney parenchyma, and produce a lesion fulfilling the criteria of pyelonephritis with involvement of pelvis, calices, and parenchyma. It is probably the most important single factor by which infective organisms reach the kidney from the lower urinary tract.

Other ways have been proposed to explain ascending infections. Some old studies claiming that organisms can be carried up the ureter during its normal peristaltic contractions (134) received little recognition amid the great enthusiasm for reflux, but more recently the interest in fimbriated organisms has resurrected these notions. In monkeys, in whom organisms have been introduced into the bladder (135,136), and in humans (35,36,38,115), it has been claimed that pyelonephritis can occur in the absence of reflux when P-fimbriated strains of *E. coli* are involved. One sequence of events envisaged is that the organism attaches to receptor sites on the ureteral mucosa and by division creeps along the mucosa in the manner of ivy climbing up a wall (137). A further explanation, provided by Roberts (138), is that a certain strain of *E. coli*, later shown to be a P-fimbriated strain (36), had the ability to diminish peristalsis of the ureter of the stump-tailed monkey (*Macaca arctoides*) when instilled into the ureter. Infection of the kidney ensued in six of eight monkeys. The effect on the ureter amounted to an obstruction, and perfusion studies revealed that intraluminal pressure—which is transmitted back to the kidney—was elevated at normal urine flow.

The studies of infants and children by Winberg et al (36) are important with regard to ascending infections that occur in the apparent absence of VUR and further advanced the idea that ureteral infection with P-fimbriated organisms results in paralysis of the ureter, as a result of which pyelorenal backflow takes place at low pressures. This finding, coupled with the increasing numbers of cases of acute pyelonephritis diagnosed in the apparent absence of VUR by the much more reliable technique of DMSA renal scintigraphy (37,38,46,47), supports the idea that reflux is not the sole way in which organisms can reach the kidney by the ascending route.

## Clinical Course, Prognosis, and Therapy

A detailed discussion of clinical course, prognosis, and therapy of acute pyelonephritis is beyond the scope of this chapter, and recent reviews addressing long-term follow-up (139), prediction of mortality and treatment failure (140), and management of acute pyelonephritis in adults (40,141) should be consulted.

Outcome data and therapeutic approaches are influenced by the clinical syndromes, which can be differentiated as either "uncomplicated" or "complicated" pyelonephritis (Table 22.2). Patients with "complicated" pyelonephritis present with a wide range of structural or functional abnormalities of the urinary tract, with various underlying diseases that render them more susceptible to infection, or with a renal infection that follows urologic manipulation. A number of sequelae can further complicate the course of the disease, including infection stones, emphysematous pyelonephritis, papillary necrosis, pyonephrosis, perinephric abscess, and septicemia.

## Chronic Obstructive Pyelonephritis

### Pathologic Findings

#### Gross Appearance

Depending on the site of obstruction, one or both kidneys may be affected. For example, only one kidney will be affected if the obstruction is above the vesicoureteral junction, but both will be involved if the obstruction is below that level. With the renal capsule stripped, coarse, depressed scars are evident on the cortical surface (Fig. 22.11). There is dilatation of the pelvis and all the caliceal systems, and the pelvic wall is thickened and granular and often shows signs of congestion owing to active infection. Some of these cases are associated with stones, which may be found occupying the pelvis and calices.

As a consequence of generalized dilatation of the collecting system, it is common to find the parenchyma reduced in width, particularly in those parts that are in line with dilated calices (Fig. 22.12). Blunting of the papillae is almost invariably a feature. In some cases, it is possible to discern large, discrete scars, as in kidneys with the back-pressure type of reflux nephropathy. Often, however, scars are not apparent, and parenchymal thinning is uniform.

**TABLE 22.2**

## CLINICAL SYNDROMES OF ACUTE PYELONEPHRITIS IN ADULTS

**Uncomplicated pyelonephritis**
  **In women**
    Subclinical (silent) pyelonephritis[a]
    Acute symptomatic pyelonephritis (moderate or severe)
    Pyelonephritis in pregnant women[b]
    Recurrent pyelonephritis
  **In men (<50 years old)**
    Subclinical (silent) pyelonephritis[a]
    Acute symptomatic pyelonephritis (moderate or severe)

**Complicated pyelonephritis**
  **Structural or functional abnormalities**
    Prostate disease (benign prostatic hyperplasia, prostatitis)
    Obstruction
    Calculi
    Neurologic disease
    Vesicoureteral reflux

  **Urologic manipulation**
    Intubated drainage (bladder catheter)
    Urinary instrumentation (cystoscopy)
    Renal transplantation

  **Underlying disease**
    **Diabetes**
    Renal failure
    Immunosuppressed or immunodeficient
    Cystic renal disease

[a]Patients with clinically apparent cystitis may also have silent, invasive bacterial infection of the renal parenchyma.
[b]Many investigators would consider pyelonephritis in pregnancy as complicated pyelonephritis.
From Nickel JC. The management of acute pyelonephritis in adults. Can J Urol 2001;8:29.

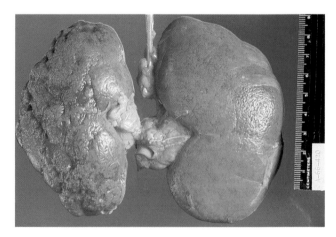

**Figure 22.11** Chronic pyelonephritis. Irregular, coarse, depressed scars on the cortical surface of the left kidney are easily appreciated with the capsule stripped.

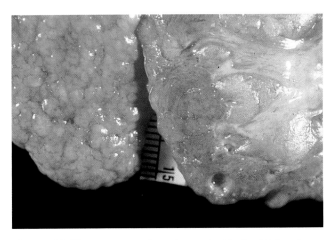

**Figure 22.12** Chronic pyelonephritis. The bivalved kidney has a characteristic, discrete, corticomedullary scar overlying a deformed calix.

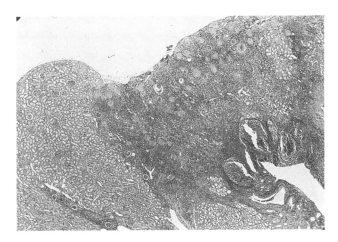

**Figure 22.14** Chronic pyelonephritis. A flat, depressed scar is sharply demarcated from the uninvolved, normal-appearing cortex. Marked interstitial chronic inflammation persists, and lymphoid follicles surround the deformed upper pole calix. (H&E; ×20.)

## Microscopic Findings

Unlike the nonobstructive (reflux nephropathy) type, chronic obstructive pyelonephritis shows changes in virtually the whole of the parenchyma. They are similar to those in the scars of chronic nonobstructive pyelonephritis, with the following exceptions: tubular atrophy with zones of thyroidization are not so well developed; chronic inflammatory cells are more plentiful; neutrophils are commonly seen in the interstitium, within tubules, and under the pelvic and caliceal mucosa (Figs. 22.13 to 22.16); and in those cases seen outside childhood, histologic features of renal dysplasia are lacking. Lymphoid follicles are present in the parenchyma and under the epithelium of the pelvis and calices. In those cases in which not all of the parenchyma shows evidence of chronic infection, there may be obstructive atrophy with a paucity of inflammatory cells.

## Etiology and Pathogenesis

The parameters that are required for renal parenchymal scarring to develop following UTI remain elusive. The persistence of uropathic bacteria in the kidney, able to engage with the host immune system to initiate the inflammatory response, explains most of the known clinical risk factors for chronic pyelonephritis. Genetic variability in the function of the host immune system, e.g., as mirrored by cytokines, cytokine receptors, chemokines, cell adhesion molecules, and growth factors, may determine whether lesions progress to renal scarring (142).

Urinary tract obstruction is clearly an adverse factor. In addition, the way in which it can convert nonrefluxing papillae to a type that refluxes is also of great importance.

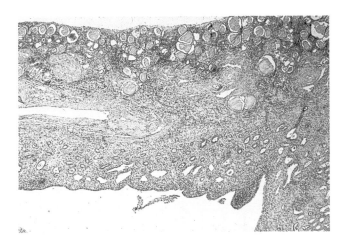

**Figure 22.13** Chronic pyelonephritis. The thinned, chronically inflamed cortex has variable interstitial fibrosis with prominent "thyroidized" tubules; the medulla is also fibrotic. This corticomedullary scar overlies a dilated calix, having a chronically inflamed mucosa. (H&E; ×20.)

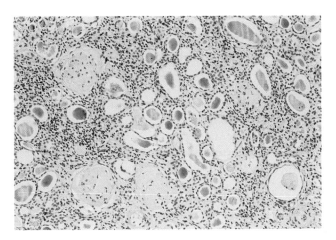

**Figure 22.15** Zone of "thyroidization" in chronic pyelonephritis. Atrophic, shrunken, or dilated tubules with flattened epithelium contain eosinophilic, waxy casts. A variable lymphoplasmacytic infiltrate, sclerotic arterioles, and obsolescent glomeruli, which focally merge with the fibrotic interstitium, are present. (H&E; ×100.)

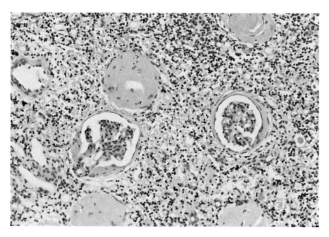

**Figure 22.16** Variable glomerular alterations within pyelonephritic scar. There is focal thickening of Bowman's capsule and periglomerular fibrosis, ischemic collapse with collagen deposited internal to Bowman's capsules, and global hyalinization. (H&E; ×200.)

## Specific Forms of Chronic Pyelonephritis

### Xanthogranulomatous Pyelonephritis

Xanthogranulomatous pyelonephritis is a chronic infective condition of the kidney that is becoming increasingly well recognized. Until 1973, the number of recorded cases was on the order of 100 (143), but since that time several large series have been reported (142–146).

#### Clinical Presentation

Xanthogranulomatous pyelonephritis occurs most often in adult females by a ratio of almost 4:1. The peak incidence is in the fifth and sixth decades. However, it may appear at any age, and patients as young as 2 months (149) and as old as 94 years (145) have been reported. Appreciable numbers of cases have been recorded in childhood (150) and even in infancy (145). Of the more than 400 cases published by 1996, approximately one-fourth occurred in children (151). Among children with xanthogranulomatous pyelonephritis, boys and girls are affected with equal frequency. In general, it is a unilateral disease, and both right and left kidneys are involved with equal frequency (146,148); occasionally, it is bilateral (147,148,152). Usually the whole of the kidney is involved (the generalized form), but restricted focal forms are not uncommon and have been found in children (153) and in adults (148,154). The once-held belief that the focal variant was the most common type of xanthogranulomatous pyelonephritis in childhood (155,156) is no longer credible (150,151, 157–159).

Xanthogranulomatous pyelonephritis manifests with various combinations of pain in the flank, malaise, weight loss, fever, and sometimes nausea and vomiting. There is frequently a palpable mass, tenderness in the loin,

anemia, leukocytosis, raised erythrocyte sedimentation rate, proteinuria, and pus cells in the urine, and miscellaneous organisms may be cultured from the urine. These organisms include *E. coli*, *Proteus* sp., *Klebsiella* sp., *P. aeruginosa*, and *Enterococcus faecalis*. At one time, it was believed that the most commonly found organism was *Proteus* sp., but *E. coli* has predominated in several large series (147,148). In an appreciable number of cases, the urine is sterile (146,148). Because renal involvement is predominantly unilateral, significant renal failure is rare. Hepatic dysfunction has been reported (160). The reason for this hepatic dysfunction is not clear, but abnormal test results often return to normal following removal of the damaged kidney.

Imaging techniques used to assist in diagnosis have included plain radiographs, intravenous urography, angiography (to rule out parenchymal neoplasms), sonography, computed tomography, and magnetic resonance imaging. Enlargement of the kidney, presence of stones or tumors in the renal pelvis, infected areas, and spread of infection to perinephric tissue may all be detected with one or another of these techniques. A particularly high degree of diagnostic precision has been achieved with computed tomography (161).

It is important to note that urinary obstruction is an almost invariable feature, and stones figure prominently as a cause. In two of the largest series to date, stones were found in 76% (147) and in 78% (148) of cases. Stones are frequently of the large staghorn type. Other causes of obstruction include transitional cell tumors of the renal pelvis, congenital pelviureteric stenosis, tumors of the ureter, and postirradiation stricture. In some cases, no cause for the obstruction is apparent (148).

#### Pathologic Findings

On macroscopic examination, the kidney is enlarged, and in severe cases, the infection may have spread outside the kidney. Adhesions to surrounding renal tissue and much perirenal fibrosis are common. The pelvis is dilated and frequently contains stones of the staghorn variety, in addition to necrotic material and pus. The calices are also dilated and the papillae lost, and the expanded calices are lined by a yellowish zone that is friable on the inner aspect (Figs. 22.17 and 22.18). The parenchyma contains similar foci of yellowish material, while the rest of it is brownish and firm owing to fibrosis and cellular infiltration. In those cases with much pelvicaliceal dilatation, there may be considerable cortical thinning.

Microscopic examination shows that the yellow areas consist of an admixture of large, finely granular foam cells and smaller macrophages containing coarser granules (Fig. 22.19). The large foam cells contain lipid, which consists of neutral fat and cholesterol ester (162). Periodic acid-Schiff (PAS)–positive granules may be thinly scattered throughout the foam cells, but they are larger and more prominent

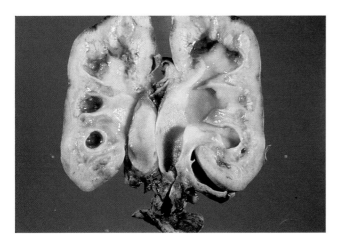

**Figure 22.17** Xanthogranulomatous pyelonephritis. Friable, yellow tissue surrounds the dilated calices.

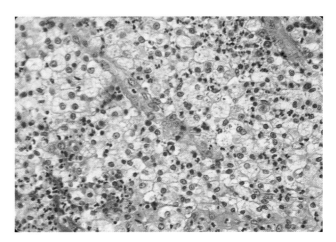

**Figure 22.19** Xanthogranulomatous pyelonephritis characterized by large, finely granular foam cells. (H&E; ×400.)

in the smaller macrophages mentioned earlier. In the outer parts of the yellow zone and in the adjacent parenchyma are mononuclear cells, plasma cells, eosinophils, and fibroblasts. Some fibrosis is present in these outer areas, which may also contain foreign-body giant cells. Some, but not all, of these giant cells are found in proximity to cholesterol crystals, which are seen in some cases.

On the inside of the yellow zone, nearest the calix, there is much necrotic debris with many neutrophils. Foci of calcification are not uncommon. The overlying cortex shows changes of chronic inflammation and, in some kidneys, microabscesses. Tubular loss is profound, and those tubules that remain are sometimes dilated, with amorphous hematoxyphilic material, cholesterol clefts, and fragmented inflammatory cells in the lumen. The interstitium shows signs

of fibrosis and contains many chronic inflammatory cells, among which plasma cells often predominate, and lymphoid follicles are frequent. Glomeruli are often remarkably normal, but in some cases, they may show evidence of sclerosis. Thrombosis with recanalization of large veins has been reported in the parenchyma between the yellow areas and the cortex, and a pathogenic role for venous obstruction has been suggested (145).

With the focal variant, which may be mistaken grossly for a clear cell renal cell carcinoma, the xanthogranulomatous process is restricted to a portion of the kidney, such as one or the other pole, with the rest of the kidney appearing normal. These localized areas of involvement show pathologic features identical to those described for the generalized form and are often related to a stone that has formed either in a single dilated calix or in the ureter in the case of a duplicated collecting system (154). Segmental resection has been shown to be curative in the focal form (154).

### Etiology and Pathogenesis

Xanthogranulomatous pyelonephritis is clearly of infective origin and probably assumes its particular appearance because of massive parenchymal necrosis and interference with urinary drainage, with resulting accumulation of foam cells. Ultrastructural studies of the lipid-laden macrophages, which are typically PAS-negative or only weakly PAS-positive, have demonstrated intracellular bacteria (163,164).

### Malakoplakia

Malakoplakia is an unusual inflammatory condition that can occur not only in the urinary tract but also at such sites as the gastrointestinal tract (mainly the large intestine), testis, prostate, vagina, lung, bone, brain, and skin (165). Another feature is the way in which it can manifest

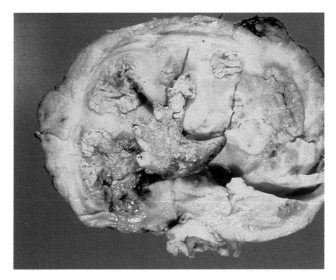

**Figure 22.18** Xanthogranulomatous pyelonephritis. A staghorn calculus is present in the dilated pelvis. Fibrotic renal parenchyma and perirenal tissue are adherent.

when the immune system is suppressed. Credit for the first description is given to von Hansemann (166), although two cases had apparently been described earlier by Michaelis and Gutmann (167). Malakoplakia is well known to urologists, who are very familiar with the characteristic small, discrete, yellowish-brown plaques or nodules seen on the bladder mucosa during cystoscopy. Similar nodules are found less frequently in the ureter and renal pelvis and occasionally in the renal parenchyma, where they are much larger and may extensively involve the entire organ.

## Clinical Presentation

A review of renal malakoplakia in 1993 by Dobyan et al (168) reported that 62 cases had been recorded at that time. Females are affected more often than males; there is a 4:1 ratio for malakoplakia in general (169) and 3:1 for the renal form (168). For the renal form, the age range is from childhood to the ninth decade, with a mean age for women of 45 years and a peak incidence in the sixth decade for men (168). Since the time of the review of Dobyan et al, several case reports have been published, including one in an 8-week-old infant (170). Unlike xanthogranulomatous pyelonephritis, which it resembles in many ways, malakoplakia quite often affects both kidneys, and it has assumed a bilateral form in 33% (168) to 50% of cases (171).

Clinically, in those cases affecting the kidney, there is a history of UTI, usually with pain in the flank. Fever and rigors are common, and signs of perinephric abscess may be noted. The urine contains protein in variable amounts, leukocytes, and sometimes red blood cells. Because bilateral involvement is not uncommon, renal failure may be present in a significant number of cases (168,172,173). It is a rare cause of acute renal failure (174). Culture of the urine reveals *E. coli* in most cases, and urinary cytologic study contributes to the diagnosis (175). Rao (176), for example, was able to make the diagnosis on the case he described by demonstration of the characteristic polygonal granular cells and Michaelis-Gutmann bodies in particles obtained from bladder washings. Various imaging techniques are employed, and they were considered by Dobyan et al (168) in their review. These authors also discussed the role of the renal biopsy and pointed out that of the 62 published cases of renal malakoplakia, 18 were accurately diagnosed by either open or needle biopsy. Renal malakoplakia has traditionally been associated with a substantial mortality rate (70%) and poor recovery of renal function (174). However, early diagnosis by renal biopsy, along with prompt and prolonged used of appropriate antibiotics such as fluoroquinolone, significantly reduces the mortality rate (174).

## Pathologic Findings

Pathologic changes have been studied at autopsy, in surgically excised kidneys, and in biopsy specimens. As stated earlier, one or both kidneys may be affected, with bilat-

eral involvement occurring in a significant proportion of cases. On macroscopic examination, the kidney may show the effects of obstruction caused by foci of ureteric malakoplakia. In this instance, the pelvis and calices are dilated, with pus in the pelvic cavity and thinning of the renal parenchyma. It is striking that, in contrast to xanthogranulomatous pyelonephritis, calculi are seldom noted in the pelvis and calices. Perinephric abscesses are not uncommon; they were documented in 18% of the 62 cases reviewed by Dobyan et al (168).

Parenchymal involvement consists of yellowish or tan nodules of variable size, which may remain discrete, coalesce to involve much of the renal substance, or undergo suppuration with abscess formation. The nodules are clearly visible on the subcapsular surface, while on the cut surface they can be seen extending down to the papilla. The lesions are sometimes confined to the papilla, which may show necrosis (177), and although yellow areas lining a dilated calix are sometimes evident, they are not recorded with the same frequency as in cases of xanthogranulomatous pyelonephritis. As is true of the latter condition, malakoplakia may take a diffuse or a focal form. The diffuse variant is much more common, which, coupled with the fact that significant numbers of cases are bilateral, explains why so many patients have renal failure. In the focal form, there is a single focus, which may be mistaken for tumor.

On microscopic inspection, the lesion consists of clusters of moderately large polygonal cells, which have a foamy eosinophilic cytoplasm and rather compact, densely staining nuclei (Fig. 22.20). Within the cytoplasm of these cells may be seen granules that stain positively with the PAS method and larger inclusions, 4 to 10 μm in diameter, that stain strongly with hematoxylin. These larger inclusions—which may be homogeneous or laminated—are called *Michaelis-Gutmann bodies*. In most instances,

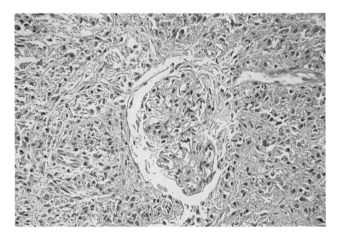

**Figure 22.20**   malakoplakia. Tubules are destroyed by an interstitial inflammatory infiltrate composed of histiocytes with granular eosinophilic cytoplasm. (H&E; ×160.)

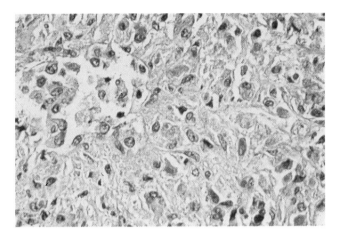

**Figure 22.21**   malakoplakia. Intracytoplasmic Michaelis-Gutman bodies. (Periodic acid-Schiff [PAS]; ×400.)

they show positive staining with PAS (maintained after treatment with diastase; Fig. 22.21), von Kossa for calcium, and the Prussian blue reaction for iron; less consistently, positive staining is obtained with oil red O, alizarin red, and Sudan black B (165). Other inflammatory cells—mononuclear cells and plasma cells—contribute to the reaction, and the component structures of the parenchyma, particularly the tubules, are severely damaged. These changes are accompanied by an interstitial fibroblastic and collagenous reaction, which may be fine or coarse with a superficial resemblance to a connective tissue neoplasm. Unless Michaelis-Gutmann bodies are diligently sought, the diagnosis of malakoplakia may be overlooked. In those cases attended by much pelvicaliceal dilatation, the parts of the parenchyma not affected by malakoplakia formation may show the changes of obstructive atrophy.

### Etiology and Pathogenesis

The macrophages with PAS-positive granules and the Michaelis-Gutmann bodies have been studied extensively with the electron microscope in both renal and nonrenal cases (163,168–180), with more or less consistent findings. The PAS-positive granules in the macrophages correspond to phagolysosomes, which contain complex membranous whorls. Bacteria in various stages of breakdown have also been recorded in phagolysosomes (163,179,180), and it is likely that the membranous structures represent degraded bacteria. The most constant picture of the Michaelis-Gutmann body is a central core (often containing crystals), an adjacent lighter zone in which crystals are scant or absent, and one or more exterior lamellar rings in which crystals are often found. Complex membranous whorls may be seen at the periphery.

It is therefore believed that the Michaelis-Gutmann body is formed by aggregation of crystals upon a nidus of breakdown products of bacteria contained in phagolysosomes. A bacterial origin is supported by studies in rats,

and injection of a lipopolysaccharide extract of cell walls of *E. coli* (Boivin antigen) into the kidney or testis reproduces many of the features of human malakoplakia (181). It was found that low concentrations of extract resulted in the formation of macrophages with a granular cytoplasm, while greater concentrations produced, in addition, structures similar to human Michaelis-Gutmann bodies.

While it is accepted that malakoplakia is of infective origin, it is not clear why it should take on its unique appearance. Because a large number of cases of malakoplakia have been associated with various abnormalities of the immune system or with the administration of immunosuppressive agents (169), the idea has arisen that there are deficiencies in the ability to dispose of bacteria. Much attention has been paid to defects in leukocytes. For example, a study of four patients in whom immunosuppressive agents had been used (182) revealed that leukocytes were unable to kill *S. aureus* and *E. coli*. When the immunosuppressive agents were withdrawn, malakoplakia improved. In the study of Abdou et al (183), it was found that monocytes derived from a hypogammaglobulinemic patient with widespread malakoplakia had diminished bactericidal activity against *E. coli*. These cells had low levels of cyclic guanosine monophosphate, and it was proposed that the low levels resulted in decreased lysosomal degradation and an inability of the cells to release lysosomal enzymes. Whereas cholinergic agonists were able to reverse the defects in the monocytes in this study (183), they had no beneficial effect on the bacterial killing ability of leukocytes in the other study quoted (182). McClure (165) has reviewed the various studies designed to test the idea of leukocyte abnormalities, with the conclusion that whereas a small number of patients with extensive malakoplakia may have defective monocyte bacterial function, most patients with the localized forms of the disease do not.

The similarity of malakoplakia to xanthogranulomatous pyelonephritis is apparent, and several authors have commented on the overlap (153,163,178). It has been speculated that the formation of the Michaelis-Gutmann body is related to the rate at which a nidus is cleared from a focus of infection and that malakoplakia might simply represent a xanthogranulomatous reaction in which bacterial degradation is abnormal. The same overlap is seen in megalocytic interstitial nephritis, which is described in the next section.

## Megalocytic Interstitial Nephritis

Megalocytic interstitial nephritis is a rare condition with many of the features of malakoplakia. It may involve the kidney diffusely, with multiple grayish foci of various sizes (184), or it may appear as a solitary cortical nodule (185) resembling a tumor. Histologic characteristics are large numbers of polygonal cells with a coarsely granular eosinophilic cytoplasm, the granules staining strongly with the PAS method. Esparza et al (178) have discussed how some authors have emphasized the absence of Michaelis-Gutmann bodies in megalocytic interstitial nephritis as a point of differentiation from malakoplakia and how some regard it as a prediagnostic phase of malakoplakia.

## Other Infections

Renal infections are a major cause of morbidity and mortality, particularly in immunocompromised and transplant recipients (51). During the early posttransplantation period, common bacteria and fungi are the most common causative agents (50,186); in the late period, viruses and tuberculosis predominate (187).

## Mycobacterial Infections

After continued decline for three decades, pulmonary tuberculosis is again increasing and remains the leading cause of death worldwide from infectious disease (186–189). Extrapulmonary tuberculosis declined less rapidly than pulmonary tuberculosis, and its prevalence has remained relatively constant in Western countries (188–190). In a survey of inner-city hospitals in Boston, extrapulmonary tuberculosis accounted for 4.5% of all new cases of active tuberculosis, and genitourinary involvement accounted for 20% of cases of extrapulmonary disease (193). However, involvement of the kidneys varies. In Western countries, the prevalence of renal involvement among patients with tuberculosis is around 5% (190,191). The review of Corbishley et al indicated that the most common form of nonpulmonary tuberculosis, however, is genitourinary disease, accounting for 27% of nonpulmonary cases (range 14% to 41%) (191). In African countries, the prevalence of renal tuberculosis is probably higher. In Nigeria, the prevalence of renal tuberculosis among patients with pulmonary tuberculosis was found to be 9.5% if diagnosed using urine Ziehl-Nielsen stains, but the prevalence rate rose to 14% if a combination of urine stains, sterile pyuria, and tissue histology was used (190). Therefore, it is evident that the diagnostic methods clearly influence the prevalence rate. Newer, more sensitive methods, including PCR, may improve the diagnostic accuracy. Males are affected twice as often as females (186), and most commonly, the disease occurs between the ages of 15 and 60 years.

Although *M. tuberculosis* is the most common agent of renal infection, other mycobacteria, such as *M. bovis*, *M. kansasii*, *M. avium-intracellulare* (194), and *M. leprae*, can also cause renal infection. For example, of 1392 isolates of mycobacteria obtained from urine and the genitourinary tracts of patients in southeast England from 1980 to 1989, 753 were positive for *M. tuberculosis*, 45 for *M. bovis*, and 4 for *M. africanum*; the remainder were positive for environmental mycobacteria, and they were of no apparent clinical significance (195). Immunosuppressed patients are more vulnerable to infections by mycobacteria (190,191,194,196). Transplantation is a risk factor for the development of tuberculosis, particularly in developing countries and East Asia (191,197). The epidemic of HIV infection has a particular relevance on the spread of tuberculosis worldwide, particularly in Africa (191). Approximately 10% of all cases of tuberculosis worldwide were HIV related, but in certain regions in sub-Saharan Africa, the percentage was as high as 60%.

There are two main types of renal tuberculosis: miliary and cavitary (197,198).

### Miliary Tuberculosis of the Kidney (Disseminated Infection)

Renal involvement may result from hematogenous dissemination of a primary tuberculous infection, from an active pulmonary lesion, or from reactivation of a healed tuberculous lesion. Miliary tuberculosis of the kidneys is often clinically silent (199) and overshadowed by clinical manifestations of the systemic infection (186). Grossly, the kidneys show white nodules (i.e., tubercles) about 1 mm in diameter, which occur more often in the cortex than in the medulla (200). Microscopically, the early tubercle is a caseating granuloma that consists of epithelioid cells and neutrophils and has central caseous necrosis. Organisms are usually found in such lesions. Often a mononuclear cell infiltrate of lymphocytes, monocytes, and plasma cells is also present. The tubercle may be contained and heal, or the infection may expand and, if in the renal medulla, may reach the renal pelvis, allowing release of microorganisms into the urinary tract. In patients who died of pulmonary tuberculosis, renal tubercles were found in more than 60% of autopsy cases (200).

### Cavitary Tuberculosis of the Kidney (Localized Urinary Tract Infection)

A high proportion of men have associated genital tuberculosis, particularly affecting the epididymis and, less frequently, the prostate. Genital tuberculosis is less common in women (if present, it is usually in the fallopian tubes). The lower urinary tract is commonly affected in cavitary renal tuberculosis. Therefore, the possibility of ascending infection from the urogenital tract arises. However, there is agreement that it is much more likely that the primary lesion is in the kidney and the infection spreads downstream to the urinary tract. The site of preference is the renal medulla, where confluent epithelioid caseating granulomas will form larger and larger cavities, frequently associated with papillary necrosis. In the cavitary form of renal tuberculosis, also called caseous and ulcerative, most of the symptoms result from involvement of the lower urinary tract (193), particularly the urinary bladder, and manifest as frequency, dysuria, and hematuria. Common urinary findings include sterile pyuria and microscopic hematuria (186,193). Infection confined to the kidney is usually clinically silent (199). Because involvement is usually unilateral, renal function is well preserved, and chronic renal failure develops in only a small proportion of patients (12% in one series) (186). In 4% to 12% of patients, renal tuberculosis is complicated by hypertension (153). The diagnosis of renal tuberculosis requires a positive culture for mycobacteria, and culture of the first-voided urine specimen, obtained for 3 to 5 consecutive days, has been recommended (201). More sensitive methodologies, including urine PCR for mycobacteria, may improve the diagnostic accuracy. Clinically, renal cavitary tuberculosis usually presents as a unilateral disease, but autopsy studies indicate that even in these instances, the contralateral kidney is also involved to some degree (197,198).

Grossly, the kidneys may be enlarged or decreased in size, and the surface shows irregular scarring. On cut section, the calices and the pelvis are dilated or deformed, pelvic-ureteric constriction may occur, and parenchymal atrophy and foci of calcification are apparent. The lesion often begins in the renal medulla with involvement of the papilla by caseation necrosis. Extension of infection into the perinephric tissues may simulate invasive renal cell carcinoma (202). When ureteral involvement occurs, segmental strictures can be demonstrated. A combination of caseous necrosis of the pelvis and caliceal systems with ureteral stenosis leads to tuberculous pyonephrosis (Fig. 22.22). When this occurs, the renal parenchyma is replaced by caseous material, leaving rims of fibrous tissue that give a loculated appearance to the organ. This condition is also known as "cement," "putty," or "chalk" kidney.

Microscopically, the center of such lesions shows typical caseous material, and the peripheral portions demonstrate a granulomatous reaction (Fig. 22.23). Mycobacteria are found in peripheral portions of areas of caseation or cavitary lesions. Less involved areas surrounding foci of caseation necrosis may show variable interstitial inflammation with lymphocytes and plasma cells amidst calcific foci, probably representing calcified tubercles.

In renal biopsies, particularly in developed countries, tuberculosis is rarely seen. However, it is imperative to request a mycobacterial stain (acid fast blue or Ziehl-Nielsen) if granulomas are present in the biopsy specimen, particularly if the patient's immune system is compromised. Also, it is important to remember that in immunocompromised patients, atypical mycobacteriosis can occur, including infections with *M. avium-intracellulare*, which does not form typical granulomas, but abundant mycobacteria are present in foamy-appearing macrophages.

### Renal Infection Caused by *Mycobacterium leprae*

Visceral involvement is more common, and the presence and degree of involvement greater, in the lepromatous forms than in the tuberculoid forms of leprosy (203). The tuberculoid pole is characterized by granuloma

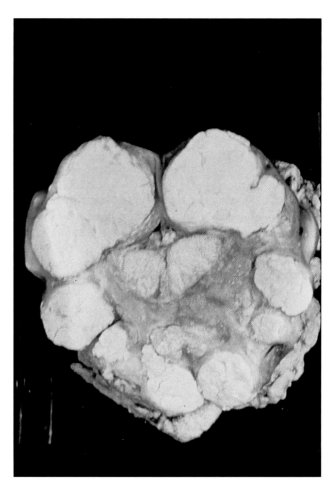

**Figure 22.22** Tuberculous pyonephrosis. With secondary involvement of the ureter and resulting urinary tract obstruction, this hydronephrotic kidney has become filled with cheesy material.

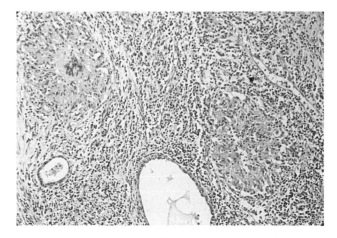

**Figure 22.23** Renal tuberculosis. Caseating granulomas are composed of epithelioid histiocytes and multinucleated giant cells. The surrounding parenchyma has a dense lymphocytic infiltrate with loss of tubules and interstitial fibrosis. (H&E; ×100.)

formation, whereas in the lepromatous pole there is a tendency toward a more diffuse infiltration of macrophages and foamy bacilli-laden cells. Renal injury seems to be more common in patients with erythema nodosum leprosum (203).

Renal lesions are found in approximately 70% of autopsied patients with leprosy (204,205). Although renal involvement by *M. leprae* more often results in glomerular pathology (e.g., glomerulonephritis, amyloidosis), chronic tubulointerstitial nephritis has been observed in patients with lepromatous or tuberculoid leprosy in 3.8% to 54% of cases (205). Organisms are not detected in the kidney. The inflammatory infiltrate is mononuclear, and there is associated interstitial fibrosis and tubular atrophy. Renal infection appears to occur in patients who have undergone prolonged chemotherapy for leprosy. Leproma caused by direct invasion of the renal parenchyma by *M. leprae* is rare; when present, bacteria can be identified in aggregations of macrophages or giant cells (206). In the series of Jayalakshmi et al (204), renal failure developed in 6 of 35 patients with renal leprosy (17%).

## Fungal Infections

Primary infections of the kidney by fungi are rare. The most common offending agents are *Candida* and *Torulopsis*. Such agents infect the lower urinary tract and may involve the kidneys through the ascending route. More often, fungal infections of the kidney result from systemic fungemia, and the source may be nosocomial (207).

Fungal infections of the kidney almost invariably occur in immunocompromised patients, particularly in patients undergoing cytostatic treatment for malignancies. Renal infection in such cases is part of the systemic fungal sepsis. Numerous fungi, including *Candida, Torulopsis, Aspergillus, Cryptococcus, Histoplasma, Coccidioides, Blastomyces, Paracoccidioides*, and Mucorales, have been reported to invade the kidney. Interstitial nephritis secondary to fungal infections is usually found during autopsies, and the morphology of the inflammation is not different from that secondary to fungal infections in other organs. Detection of fungi in renal biopsy specimens is very unusual and happens only in immunocompromised patients. However, it is important to emphasize that fungal infections may cause granulomatous inflammation; therefore, in any granulomatous inflammation of the kidney, a fungal infection should be considered in the differential diagnosis. Importantly, the PAS reaction should be part of the routine stains used during renal biopsy workup. PAS is an excellent fungal stain; therefore, the presence of fungi in the renal biopsy should not be missed if a kidney biopsy is appropriately worked up. We strongly recommend that the PAS reaction should be always performed in every renal allograft biopsy as well.

## Candidiasis

Most infections by *C. albicans* are opportunistic and originate from mucosal surfaces of the oral cavity, upper respiratory tract, digestive tract, and vagina, followed by hematogenous dissemination. Neonates (208), granulocytopenic patients (209,210), and immunosuppressed patients (210,211) are at risk, and the source of infection often is nosocomial (50,212).

The incidence of candidiasis varies. Of 75 episodes of bacteremia or fungemia in renal transplant recipients, *C. albicans* was detected in only 2 (2.6%) (50), and of 102 episodes of nosocomial fungemia, *C. albicans* was detected in 76 (74.5%) (207). In Paya's series (213), fungal infections occurred in 5% and 40% of kidney and liver transplant recipients, respectively, and *Candida* and *Aspergillus* were the commonest fungi. In two series of systemic candidiasis, renal involvement was reported to be 52% (211) and 82% (209).

Presenting symptoms are those of severe renal infection, with low-grade fever, flank pain, tenderness at the costovertebral angle, hematuria, hypotension, progressive loss of renal function, and acute renal failure (52). Fungus balls may develop in the pelvis and calices (214), and their passage may result in ureteral colic. Anuria occurs when fungus balls obstruct both ureters (214,215) or the ureter of a single functioning kidney (216). Recovery of *Candida* from urine specimens, together with positive blood culture, suggests disseminated infection, and detection of *Candida* casts in urine is diagnostic of renal involvement (217).

The kidneys may show little or no inflammatory response; alternatively, there may be extensive necrosis, miliary abscesses (Figs. 22.24 and 22.25), and papillary necrosis (206,208) (Fig. 22.26). In one series (208), papillary necrosis was present at autopsy in 9 (21%) of 42 patients who had had systemic candidiasis. In those with

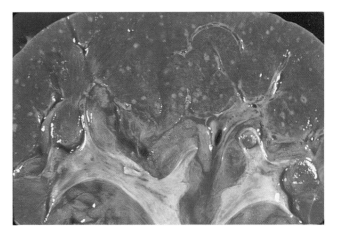

**Figure 22.24** *Candida* septicopyemia with diffusely scattered small, discrete, yellow-white miliary abscesses. (This is the same case as that seen in Fig. 22.25.)

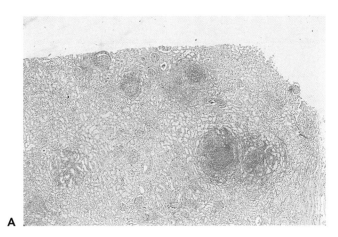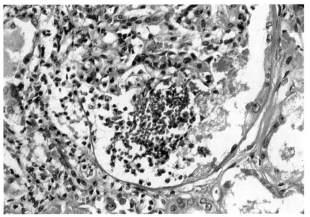

A                                                                                                                         B

**Figure 22.25**   Renal candidiasis. **A:** Many cortical abscesses are centered around and destroy glomeruli. (H&E; ×20.) **B:** *Candida* yeast can be identified within glomerular capillaries. (H&E; ×400.)

diabetes, *C. albicans* infection may result in emphysematous pyelonephritis (218). Mycotic aneurysms may be present in glomerular capillaries and arterioles. However, in comparison with other fungi, invasion of blood vessels by *Candida* is less common, and cortical infarction is rare (206). In tissue sections, pseudohyphae and rounded yeast forms, 2 to 4 μm in diameter, predominate. Although *Candida* can be seen in sections stained with hematoxylin and eosin, they are more readily identified with PAS or Grocott's methenamine silver stains. Systemic candidiasis has a fatality rate of 70% to 79% (206,219).

To colonize surface epithelia, *Candida* organisms adhere to epithelial cells through mannoproteins and hydrophobic forces (220) and through proteins that bind iC3b receptors (221). Unless phagocytosed, *Candida* organisms reach the subepithelial layer, and through surface receptors (CR3-like protein), they bind to extracellular matrix components with arginine-glycine-aspartate

(RGD) sequences common to collagens, fibronectin, laminin, and vitronectin (222). During colonization and penetration, an epithelial reaction (proliferation) and an inflammatory reaction (T-cell–based) are elicited. Patients with defective T-cell function or immunosuppression may not mount an adequate cellular reaction to contain the fungus.

Vascular invasion follows and probably involves enzymes with collagenolytic properties. *Candida* organisms adhere to endothelial cells through a complement receptor (221) present in mannoproteins (222), and endothelial injury requires phagocytosis of live fungus, a process that, for *C. albicans*, is microfilament and microtubule dependent (223). Colonization of endothelial and vascular walls, unchecked by leukocytes, provides foci for hematogenous dissemination. Cytokines such as tumor necrosis factor-alpha (TNFα) may attenuate the effects of systemic candidiasis (224).

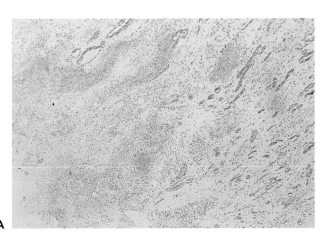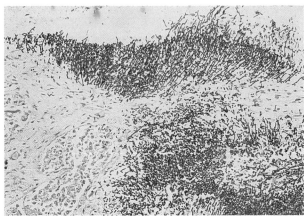

A                                                                                                                         B

**Figure 22.26**   Renal candidiasis. **A:** The necrotic papilla of this renal allograft contains large numbers of fungal organisms, which fill collecting ducts and invade the interstitium. An inflammatory response is lacking. (H&E; ×40.) **B:** Yeast and pseudohyphae are clearly demonstrated. (PAS; ×100.)

## Torulopsosis

*Torulopsis glabrata*, the agent of torulopsosis, is an opportunistic yeastlike fungus present in the normal microflora of the oral pharynx, gastrointestinal tract, skin, urethra, and vagina. Of low virulence, *T. glabrata* is the second most common fungal pathogen of the urinary tract (206). The kidneys are usually involved as part of disseminated infections, but they also can be the site of a primary infection through the ascending route (225), particularly in diabetic patients (225,226). Torulopsosis also is an important cause of nosocomial infection. Of 102 episodes of nosocomial fungemia reported by Taylor et al (207), *T. glabrata* accounted for 8 and was second only to *C. albicans*. Presenting symptoms are comparable to those caused by infection with *C. albicans*.

Nearly 50% of patients with disseminated infection have renal involvement that often is microscopic. In severe cases, miliary or extensive abscess formation (227), papillary necrosis (225,228), and perinephric abscess formation have been described (225,229). Inflammatory changes resemble those caused by *Candida* infection. *Torulopsis glabrata* organisms may be seen in tissue sections as 2- to 4-μm, budding, round to oval, nonencapsulated, yeastlike organisms demonstrable by Grocott's methenamine silver stain.

The outcome of patients with torulopsosis is poor. Of 27 patients with clinically significant fungemia reported by Berkowitz et al (227), 10 died. Low-grade, persistent fever, underlying disease, neoplasia, and coexistent bacterial infection were the most important factors responsible for death.

Cytokines appear to be important in the pathogenesis of torulopsosis. In the study of Kowanko et al (230), granulocyte-macrophage colony-stimulating factor increased fungal killing by neutrophils by enhancing respiratory burst and degranulation.

## Aspergillosis

Aspergillosis can be caused by various species of aspergilli, but the most common pathogen is *A. fumigatus*. The organism is present in nature, and the portal of entry to the host is usually the respiratory tract and mucosal surfaces, cutaneous wounds, or intravenous access lines (210). Renal aspergillosis is frequently the result of hematogenous dissemination, usually from invasive bronchial infection, necrotizing pneumonitis, or infarct by aspergilli, particularly in patients receiving corticosteroids, patients who become neutropenic (210), patients with diabetes (231,232), and immunocompromised patients (51,219, 233). Less frequently, the kidneys may be involved through the ascending route (231). Renal parenchymal infections may produce symptoms comparable to those of acute pyelonephritis (231,232). The urinary tract may be obstructed by growth of mycelium, and fungus balls may be passed into the urine (231).

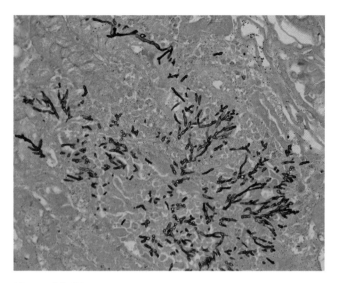

**Figure 22.27** Renal aspergillosis. Large numbers of branching, septate hyphae are illustrated. (Methenamine silver; ×380.)

Renal involvement occurs in 30% to 40% of the patients who die of disseminated aspergillosis (206). The involvement may be bilateral in systemic infections and in the isolated type of renal involvement (232). In the series of Young et al (234), the kidneys were involved in 12 of 34 cases of disseminated infection. Multiple small abscesses, a few millimeters in diameter and each surrounded by a red rim, are the most common lesions. However, extensive abscess formation with vascular invasion, thrombosis, and infarction also occurs and is more common in the medulla than in the cortex (234). Microscopic examination reveals inflammation with mononuclear cells and neutrophils and abscesses and infarcts containing typical septate branching hyphae. The fungus takes the form of branching septate hyphae 3 to 5 μm wide that can be demonstrated with PAS or Grocott's methenamine silver stain (Fig. 22.27). The histologic diagnosis of aspergillosis should consider members of the genera *Fusarium* and *Pseudoallescheria*, which can be excluded using antibody specific to *Aspergillus* (206).

The mechanism of infection by aspergilli appears to involve adherence to epithelial surfaces and production and release of proteases, including elastase and phospholipases (235), some of which may facilitate vascular invasion and thrombosis. The mechanism by which killing of *Aspergillus* takes place has not been elucidated (236). Some evidence suggests that priming of neutrophils by formylated tripeptide followed by IL-8 enhances phagocytosis of serum opsonized conidia from 15% to 55% (237).

## Cryptococcosis

*Cryptococcus neoformans*, the agent of cryptococcosis, is a yeastlike fungus with worldwide distribution encountered in avian habitats, particularly those contaminated with

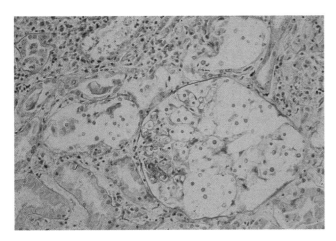

**Figure 22.28** Renal involvement in systemic cryptococcosis. Yeast within glomeruli and tubules are separated by clear halos corresponding to their thick capsule. (H&E; ×200.)

pigeon droppings (206). The portal of entry to the host is the respiratory tract, and pulmonary infection is common, particularly in immunosuppressed (210) and neutropenic patients (210,238). Hematogenous dissemination results in fungal localization to the central nervous system and various organs, including the kidneys. In renal transplant recipients, the incidence of cryptococcal infection in one series was 7.7% (238). Renal involvement may be clinically silent, or it may manifest with costovertebral angle tenderness, pyuria, and gross hematuria. Yeast forms can be cultured from the urine (239) and can be recognized in the urinary sediment by negative staining with India ink (240,241).

Renal involvement is found in about 50% of patients who die of disseminated cryptococcosis (206). In the series of Salyer and Salyer (239), the kidneys were affected in 20 (51.3%) of 39 cases of systemic cryptococcal infection. Small parenchymal abscesses, or granulomas, with central necrosis involving the cortex and medulla have been described (206,239,241). Papillary necrosis may occasionally be found (241). The organism may elicit little inflammatory reaction despite causing extensive tubular destruction. Cryptococci can be identified in tissue sections as spherical structures, 4 to 20 μm in diameter, with a polysaccharide capsule (Fig. 22.28). The capsule is distinctive and stains intensely with mucicarmine, Alcian blue, and PAS. Renal impairment was described in some patients by Salyer and Salyer (239) but was attributed to coexistent disease.

The process of elimination of cryptococci from sites of infection involves growth inhibition, a process that depends on nitric oxide production by phagocytes (242) and phagocytosis by macrophages, a complement-dependent mechanism that is modulated by cytokines (243).

## Histoplasmosis

Histoplasmosis, caused by *H. capsulatum*, is endemic in South and Central America and in the Ohio River and Mississippi River valleys in the United States (206). Infection is caused by inhalation of dust particles containing conidia forms from soil contaminated with bird or bat droppings containing the fungus. The initial presentation resembles pulmonary tuberculosis. Disseminated histoplasmosis may result from a primary infection or from a reactivated, healed lesion during immunosuppression (210). The disease is not contagious. Renal involvement is usually clinically silent (244), and compromise of renal function is uncommon.

The kidneys are involved in about 40% of patients as a result of progressive disseminated histoplasmosis (244). Less commonly, infection may be acquired during graft implantation (245). Grossly, the lesions range from one or more firm or soft, usually well-circumscribed nodules to diffuse inflammation and necrosis involving most of the kidney. Papillary necrosis also has been described (244,246). Microscopically, small aggregates of yeast-laden macrophages may be present in all renal compartments, usually associated with granulomas at various stages (244) (Fig. 22.29). In the series of Goodwin et al (244), 10% of patients with disseminated histoplasmosis showed focal lesions consisting of aggregations of macrophages accompanied by focal necrosis in the medulla. Parasitized macrophages show large numbers of round or oval, tiny yeast forms up to 5 μm in diameter, usually identifiable with Grocott's methenamine silver stain (Fig. 22.30). The histologic diagnosis of histoplasmosis can be confirmed by immunofluorescence using antibody to the wall polysaccharide antigens of serotypes of *H. capsulatum* (206).

Conidia, the infectious form, enter macrophages, multiply within lysosomes, and kill macrophages. Dissemination of infection is probably facilitated by proteinases with collagenolytic activity secreted by the fungus (247). Killing of infectious forms requires T-cell and macrophage activation by TNFα (248).

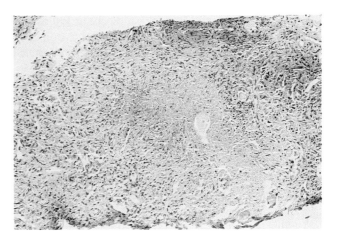

**Figure 22.29** Histoplasmosis in a renal allograft. Parenchymal necrosis and mild chronic inflammation are present. (H&E; ×100.)

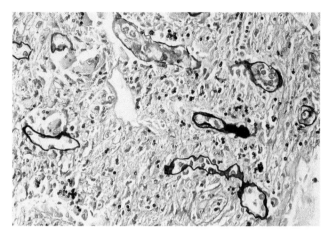

**Figure 22.30**  Histoplasmosis in a renal allograft. Macrophages contain yeast forms of *H. capsulatum*. (Methenamine silver; ×400.)

## Coccidioidomycosis

Coccidioidomycosis, caused by *C. immitis*, is endemic in the southwest and western United States. However, sporadic cases of disseminated coccidioidomycosis have been reported in nonendemic areas in 35 states (249). The fungus exists in nature in a mycelial form, but it produces arthroconidia, which is the infective form. Inhalation of arthrospores results in asymptomatic pulmonary infection in most patients or symptomatic infection in about 10% of patients. Progressive pulmonary infections are rare, and systemic dissemination in fewer than 1% of cases usually affects immunosuppressed (210,250) and diabetic patients or pregnant women (251,252). Although it is not contagious, coccidioidomycosis is transmissible during autopsy procedures, presumably through aerosolization of endospores (253).

The kidneys are involved in one third of patients who die of disseminated infection (206). Grossly, minute granulomas and multiple abscesses are present. The granulomas show caseous or suppurative necrosis, and *C. immitis* organisms are easily found in active lesions within macrophages or giant cells as thick-walled spherules, about 100 mm in diameter, containing endospores that are 5 to 30 mm in diameter (206). Progression of the disease has been equated with attenuation of cellular immunity from antigen overload, suppressor cells, immune complexes, and immunosuppressive factors released from the fungus (254).

Arthrospores and endospores are engulfed by macrophages but are not killed, because they block fusion of phagosome and lysosome (255,256). The release of endospores from spherules is associated with peak proteinase activity with elastolytic activity, which facilitates tissue invasion and destruction and endospore dissemination (257). Containment of infection depends on development of cellular immunity that, through release of lymphokines, enhances phagosome–lysosome fusion and killing of the fungus (255).

## Blastomycosis

North American blastomycosis, caused by *B. dermatitidis*, is endemic in the Ohio River and Mississippi River valleys and the southeastern United States (206). The fungus is a saprophytic budding yeast found in soils. Infection results from inhalation of infectious forms. Blastomycosis is prevalent among immunosuppressed patients (210). It is found four times more frequently in males than in females, and in most patients, involvement occurs between the ages of 30 and 50 years (206). In north central Wisconsin, the annual rate of infection ranged from 40.4 to 101.3 cases per 100,000 persons (258). Primarily a pulmonary infection (258), it disseminates through blood to various organs, including the kidneys. Renal involvement is usually clinically silent. In severe infections, fever, weight loss, chest pain, cough, costovertebral angle tenderness, flank pain, renal insufficiency, and chronic discharging sinuses or subcutaneous abscesses have been reported (259). The diagnosis can be established through culture of urine or discharging fluids or by characteristics of the organism in fluids and tissue sections (260). Blastomycosis is not a transmissible disease.

Renal blastomycosis is estimated to occur in 25% of systemic infections; involvement is often bilateral and varies from small circumscribed nodules to diffuse inflammation and necrosis involving the whole kidney (206). The cortex is more often affected than the medulla, and extension of the infection through the capsule results in perinephric abscesses and discharging sinuses. In tissue sections, granulomatous and suppurative lesions are seen. In some patients, microabscess formation and epithelioid and giant cell granulomas, some with caseation resembling tuberculosis, develop. *Blastomyces dermatitidis* can be detected in either type of lesion; yeast cells with a double-contoured appearance, 8 to 15 mm in diameter, and broad-based branching daughter cells provide the diagnostic features. Although organisms can be easily seen in sections stained with hematoxylin and eosin, the Grocott's methenamine silver stain facilitates their detection. Antibodies against the cell wall polysaccharide antigen of *B. dermatitidis* are available and can be used for organism identification (206). Blastomycosis tends to recur in 10% to 15% of patients and has a mortality rate of 90% (260).

A 120-kD glycoprotein antigen expressed in *B. dermatitidis* has a 25–amino acid repeat that is an immunodominant B-cell epitope and a carboxy terminus that promotes adhesion of the yeast to host cells and to extracellular matrix proteins. This antigen is the target of cellular and humoral immune response in human infections (261).

## Paracoccidioidomycosis

Paracoccidioidomycosis (i.e., South American blastomycosis), caused by *P. brasiliensis*, is a chronic pulmonary disease endemic to Mexico and South and Central America.

Pulmonary infection caused by inhalation of spores from *P. brasiliensis* tends to be progressive and to be followed by dissemination to mucous membranes, lymph nodes, and various organs. Although the presenting symptoms are usually pulmonary, the disease is often manifested by dissemination.

The kidneys are involved in 10% to 15% of cases of disseminated infection, and typical lesions consist of miliary granulomas, a few millimeters in size and often with necrotic centers, involving the cortex and medulla (206). The microorganism, found in areas of inflammation at the periphery of necrotic granulomas and within giant cells, is easily identified in sections stained with hematoxylin and eosin, but details are brought out by Grocott's methenamine silver stain. Nonbudding forms, about 10 mm in diameter, predominate, but multiple buds from a single cell, 10 to 60 mm in diameter and resembling the steering wheel of a ship, are diagnostic, although they are less common (206). Progression of the disease and dissemination are associated with depressed cell-mediated responses (262).

The initial response to yeast forms of the fungus is inflammatory infiltration with neutrophils and macrophages, recruited to sites of fungal infections by β-glucan in the cell wall of the fungus (263). Neutrophils are gradually replaced with macrophages, with formation of epithelioid granulomas; antibodies and a cell-mediated immune reaction are present by 15 days, peak at 30 days, and decline thereafter (264). Yeast forms of the fungus bind laminin through a 43-kD glycoprotein, a virulence factor thought to facilitate spreading and dissemination (265). Phagocytosed *P. brasiliensis* can multiply within macrophages;

however, activation of macrophages by gamma interferon inhibits fungal growth by 65% to 95% (266).

## Mucormycosis

Mucormycosis (i.e., zygomycosis) is an opportunistic infection of lungs and upper respiratory tract caused by fungi of the order Mucorales, whose most common pathogen is *Rhizopus oryzae*. Infection is acquired by inhalation of airborne spores. Disseminated infection occurs in immunocompromised (210,238,267,268) and diabetic patients (267). Rarely, isolated mucormycosis may involve the kidney only (267). *Rhizopus oryzae* frequently invades blood vessels and disseminates through the hematogenous route. In the report of Morrison and McGlave (268), of 1500 bone marrow transplant recipients, mucormycosis occurred in 13 (0.9%), with kidney involvement in a single patient. Involvement of the urinary tract may be clinically silent or manifest by signs and symptoms of renal infarction, including flank pain, dysuria, gross hematuria, and acute renal failure (52,206).

Renal involvement occurs in 50% of patients dying of disseminated mucormycosis (206). Thrombosis of several vessels may occur and results in segmental or subtotal renal infarction. Involvement can be unilateral (269) or bilateral (270). Microscopically, there is suppurative, necrotizing inflammation with thrombosis of interlobar and arcuate arteries. Granulomatous inflammation, fibrosis, and Langerhans-type multinucleated giant cells are seen. Hyphae can be detected in areas of acute inflammation or infarction. In tissue sections, the fungus consists of a broad, nonseptate hyphae that shows right-angle branching (Fig. 22.31). Organisms can be identified with the use

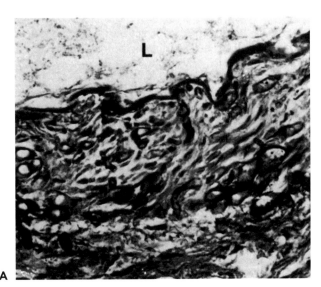
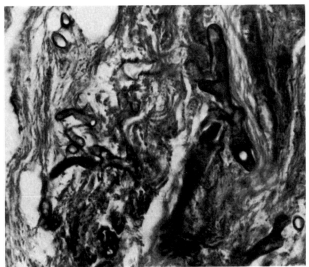

**Figure 22.31**  Renal mucormycosis involving a small artery. **A:** Hyphal forms with extensive invasion of the media. L, arterial lumen. (H&E; ×425.) **B:** Right-angle branching and the nonseptate character of hyphae are better seen in this illustration of adventitia and adjacent tissue. (H&E; ×600.)

of Grocott's methenamine silver stain or fluoresceinated antibodies (206).

## Viral Nephropathies

### Polyoma Virus Infection and BK Nephropathy

BK virus (BKV) is a member of the polyoma subgroup of papovaviruses. BK virus was named in 1971 after the initials of a transplant patient with ureteral obstruction secondary to a virally induced distal ureteral mass. The virus recovered from this mass, while structurally similar to simian virus 40 (SV40), was recognized as being antigenically distinct and hence was recognized as a new pathogen. Today BKV is recognized as one of the three small DNA viruses which can be tropic for the kidney including BKV, JC virus, and SV40.

BK virus is a small, nonenveloped DNA virus measuring approximately 45 nm with circular, double-stranded DNA. BK virus infection is acquired most often in childhood through primary pulmonary infection. Pulmonary symptoms include fever and nonspecific upper respiratory findings. In the United States, serologic evidence of infection ranges from 60% to 100%. Hematogenous spread of the primary infection carries BKV to the kidney and urothelium, where the virus enters latency. BK virus can also infect leukocytes, tonsils, and brain. Latent virus can be recovered from kidney, peripheral blood leukocytes, urothelium, endothelial cells, ependymal cells, and astrocytes. Reactivation occurs with immunodeficiency, which is predominantly cellular immunodeficiency. As such, organ transplant patients, HIV-infected patients, and patients with hematologic malignancies are at substantial risk for reactivation of BKV infection and productive infection. Patients with lesser degrees of immunosuppression, such as pregnant women, diabetic patients, and the elderly, may also be at risk for increased virus replication and shedding in the urine.

The cellular receptor for BKV in not known; however, gangliosides type II are known to play an important role in the binding of cells to virions (271). BK virus enters cells through caveola-mediated endocytosis (272). Following internalization, the viral genome is delivered to the nucleus. The genome of polyoma virus in infected cells can be divided into early and late regions. The early region is the part of the genome transcribed early after the virus enters the cell. The late region of the genome is effectively expressed only after viral DNA replication begins. The early regions encode the T antigens (large T and small t). The late regions encode the viral capsid proteins VP1, VP2, and VP3. A sixth gene, agnogene, is thought to participate in the assembly of viral proteins. The viral DNA in latency is most likely episomal. In latency, early genes are expressed at a low level and late genes are repressed by cellular factors. Kraus et al (273) hypothesized that in a latently infected cell, under appropriate stimuli, the BKV early promoter is activated, whereas the late genes remain quiescent. When the early gene product of large T antigen has accumulated to sufficient levels, it binds to the DNA replication region (0ri). This represses transcription of the early promoter and initiates replication of the genome. Once the amplification of the genome has achieved sufficiently high levels, repression of the late promoter is relieved by the release of repressors. Nuclear factor 1 family members mediate repression of the BK virus late promoter (273). Loss of latency repressors allows transcription from the promoter, synthesis of the capsid proteins, and assemblage of the viral genomes into virions.

The stimuli that allow for the switch from latency to a lytic productive infection are not well defined. Some postulated factors include the status of the host's antiviral immune system, the amount of virus present, the effects of the immunosuppressives being used, allogeneic stimulation from histoincompatibility, and the nature of the virus itself. Sequence variations in transcription factor–binding sites could facilitate viral replication and productive infection. Randhawa has shown substantial sequence heterogeneity in the regulatory regions of BKV in patients with BK nephropathy (274).

*BKV in Transplantation: BK Nephropathy.* The clinical renal and urinary tract findings in BKV reactivation infection include asymptomatic hematuria, hemorrhagic and nonhemorrhagic cystitis, ureteral stenosis, and renal allograft dysfunction with BK nephropathy (BKN). The pathologic lesions of BKN in transplantation have received most attention.

The clinical features of BKN closely resemble those of rejection. BK virus reactivation infection occurs in 10% to 60% of renal transplants. One percent to 5% of renal allografts develop BK nephropathy (275,276). The median time for urinary virus shedding after engraftment is 16 weeks; viremia develops a median of 23 weeks after engraftment, and BKN takes 28 weeks to develop (275). Multiple clinical features have been evaluated for their ability to predict BKN. Positive associations with BKN have been suggested for male sex, age over 60, use of tacrolimus and mycophenolate mofetil (277), previous rejection episodes, and seroconversion for BKV at transplant. The strengths of these clinical features as risk factors for BKN are disputed.

In reactivation infection, intermittent viruria generally precedes persistent viruria, which in turn generally precedes viremia. These principles guide the relative utilities of screening tests for the recognition of BKN.

The "decoy cell" in urinary cytology refers to productively infected inclusion-bearing cells that mimic urothelial carcinoma in situ because of the cellar hyperchromasia. Urine cytology is a sensitive method for identifying urinary tract BKV infection, with nearly 100% sensitivity

(275); however, the specificity is low, with a positive predictive value below 20% for BKN (278). In a prospective study, Hirsch et al (275) found that, of the 30% of patients with urine cytology that was positive for decoy cells, only 6% had BKN.

Urine measurements of viral large T copy number are 100- to 1000-fold higher than in plasma, and thresholds can be chosen to distinguish shedding from active viral replication and BKN (279). Since VP1 is the major capsid protein whose transcription and translation is dependent on viral DNA replication, it is found only in productive infection. Tests have also been developed for VP1 mRNA in urine (280) in which a copy number of $6.5 \times 10^5$ predicted BKN with a sensitivity of 93.8% and a specificity of 93.9%.

Plasma viral loads are thought to be the best correlate of BKN. Sensitivity of 100% and specificity of 88% with a positive predictive value of 50% have been reported (275). This study showed plasma viral copy numbers of more than 7700/mL in BKN, which was 14 times that of patients without BKN. Plasma viral loads decrease with graft nephrectomy, suggesting origin of the infection from the kidney. Genomic variations in BKV can create false-negative results.

Algorithms based on the urine and plasma screening for BKV DNA have been used to diagnosis and manage renal transplant patients (275,281). Agha and Brennan (282) divided patients into the following groups: (a) patients with intermittent viruria of fewer than 3 weeks' duration, (b) those with sustained viruria without viremia, and (c) those with viremia. Their data indicated that surveillance and preemptive reduction of immunosuppression may be effective in prevention of BKN.

Renal biopsy is the most definitive method of establishing a diagnosis of BKN. The clinical settings in which both renal allograft rejection and BKN can occur substantially overlap, and both conditions must be considered in biopsy evaluation. To complicate matters, some histopathologic features are shared between these two conditions, and careful attention to feature differences is important in distinguishing rejection from BKN. The fundamental features of BKN include intranuclear inclusions, tubular necrosis, and interstitial inflammation.

Nickeleit et al (283) enumerated four different varieties of intranuclear inclusion bodies, which can be seen in any part of the nephron. Type 1 inclusions are the classic basophilic inclusions. These have an amorphous, ground-glass appearance with peripheral chromatin rimming (Fig. 22.32). This type of inclusion is most frequent in BKN. Type 1 inclusions are found in the urothelium lining the

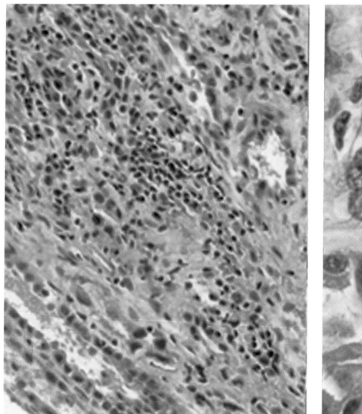
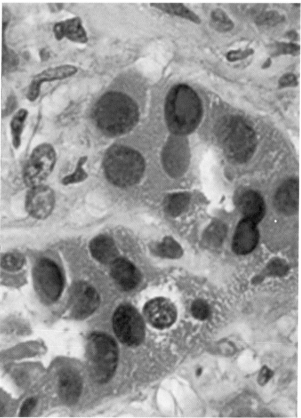

**Figure 22.32**  BK nephropathy. **A:** Interstitial inflammation in BK nephropathy composed mostly of lymphocytes. (×13.) **B:** A tubule with multiple basophilic type 1 intranuclear inclusions. (×67.)

renal pelvis. Type 2 inclusions are eosinophilic and granular and surrounded by an incomplete halo. Type 3 inclusions are finely granular and lack a halo. Type 4 inclusions have a markedly enlarged nucleus with clumped irregular chromatin and prominent nucleoli. Sometimes type 4 inclusions are difficult to distinguish from reparative tubular epithelial atypia, and confirmatory immunohistochemical stains may be necessary to recognize infection. Infected cells are seen only occasionally in the glomerular epithelium. Endothelial cells, mesenchymal cells, and inflammatory cells are not infected. BK virus–infected cells with targetoid inclusions are not cytomegalic and do not have cytoplasmic inclusions; as such, they can be distinguished from cytomegalovirus (CMV). The inclusions of adenovirus are more irregularly smudged than the basophilic inclusions of BK. The multinucleation and molding of herpesvirus are not found in BK inclusions. If there is doubt about the nature of an inclusion, immunohistochemistry may be of help (see following). Ultrastructural examination of tissue with BKN is adjunctive. The virions measure approximately 40 nm in diameter.

Necrotic and infected tubular epithelial cells are often most prominent in the medulla. Cells round up and are extruded into the tubular lumens, forming cellular casts and leaving the tubular basement membranes denuded. This pattern of tubular necrosis can be a clue to search for diagnostic inclusion-bearing cells.

Interstitial inflammation is a hallmark of BKN (283,284). The inflammation is generally mild in intensity (Fig. 22.32). The cell types are heterogeneous and composed of lymphocytes, macrophages, and occasional plasma cells and neutrophils. The major challenge is to distinguish this interstitial inflammation from rejection. Tubulitis in BKN is inconspicuous. Cellular rejection and BKN can coexist. Nickeleit (283) found up-regulation of tubular MHC II in rejection but not in BKN. Likewise, C4d is expressed on peritubular capillaries in rejection but not in BKN (285).

Immunohistochemistry for BKV can confirm suspected inclusion disease. Antibodies to the large T antigen of SV40 have crossreactivity with the large T antigen of BK and JC viruses (Fig. 22.33). Co-infection with BK and SV40 can occur, and more BK-specific reagents may be useful (286).

Early detection of BKN by surveillance biopsy may be associated with less severe inflammation, less tubular atrophy, and less interstitial fibrosis as compared to biopsies

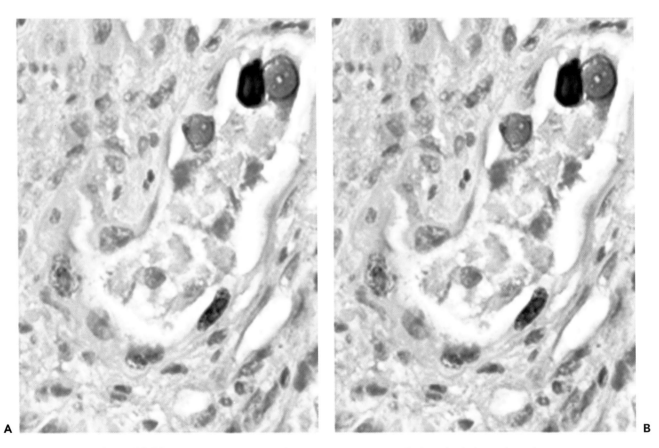

**Figure 22.33** BK nephropathy. **A:** Uniform nuclear decoration of infected tubular nuclei with antibody Pab 597 (provided by Dr. Jennifer Gordon, Temple University, Philadelphia) against polyoma virus (including BK, JC, and SV40). **B:** SV40 stain (Calbiochem, LaJolla, CA) showing variable labeling of inclusion-bearing tubular nuclei. (×27.)

obtained in response to an increase in creatinine. Patients with BKN diagnosed in a surveillance biopsy program more frequently have stable serum creatinine after 6 months of follow-up (287).

## The Biology of Epstein-Barr Virus Infection

Epstein-Barr virus (EBV) infection in nonimmunosuppressed hosts is common. Most adults have serologic evidence of past infection. Primary infections may be manifested as infectious mononucleosis. Primary infections may also be silent, with little in the way of clinical signs and symptoms. The major target is the B cell. The EBV attaches to cells for which it is tropic through the CD21 receptor. In infected cells, the EBV virus may exist in a latent or lytic state. During early latency, EBV nuclear antigen 2 activates B lymphocytes through induction of CD23. Also in latency, the EBV late membrane protein induces expression of CD23, intercellular adhesion molecule 1, and leukocyte factor antigen-3. The most frequent RNA in late latency is Epstein-Barr early antigen. Latently infected cells can be switched into a productive or lytic phase by a number of environmental stresses. The immediate early gene of the latent to lytic switch is BZLF-1. GP-350 is expressed in the late lytic phase.

## Posttransplant Lymphoproliferative Disorders and Epstein-Barr Virus Infection

In latently infected immunocompetent hosts, B-cell proliferation is kept in check by cytotoxic T cells that recognize and kill infected B cells. In patients with a compromised T-cell immune system, EBV-activated B cells may proliferate without regulation, resulting in B-cell expansions and neoplasia. Posttransplant lymphoproliferative disorders (PTLD) are lymphoid proliferations that occur in immunosuppressed patients, including bone marrow and solid organ transplant recipients, patients treated with immunosuppression for autoimmune disease, and patients with inherited immune deficiencies. Among solid organ transplant recipients, patients receiving renal allografts have the lowest frequency of PTLD (<1%). Cardiac allografts (1% to 2%) and heart-lung or liver-bowel (5%) have increased frequencies of PTLD. More than 80% of PTLD cases are associated with EBV infection. In solid organs, most PTLD cases are of host cell origin, with fewer than 10% of donor origin. There are multiple risk factors for PTLD. The most important is seronegativity for EBV, which conveys a 24-fold risk. Other risk factors include CMV serologic mismatch and prior therapy with orthoclone (OKT3). A patient with all of these factors is estimated to have a 654-fold risk over the reference transplant population for the development of PTLD.

The lesions of PTLD are categorized by the World Health Organization (288) according to Table 22.3. Because some of the histopathologic features of rejection can overlap with PTLD in kidney tissue, particular attention

### TABLE 22.3

**WORLD HEALTH ORGANIZATION CATEGORIES OF POSTTRANSPLANT LYMPHOPROLIFERATIVE DISORDER LESIONS**

**Early lesions**
  Reactive plasmacytic hyperplasia
  Infectious mononucleosis-like

**Polymorphic posttransplant lymphoproliferative disorders**
**Monomorphic posttransplant lymphoproliferative disorders**

B-cell neoplasms
  Diffuse large B-cell lymphoma
  Burkitt/Burkitt-like lymphoma
  Plasma cell myeloma
  Plasmacytoma-like lesions

T-cell neoplasms
  Peripheral T-cell lymphoma
  Other types

**Hodgkin lymphoma**

to the morphology of "early lesions" and polymorphous PTLD is warranted. "Early lesions" are characterized by either marked plasmacytosis (in the absence of substantial chronicity) or by an infectious mononucleosis-like reaction, with a brisk lymphoid proliferation showing a mixture of small lymphoid cells, plasma cells, and immunoblasts (Fig. 22.34). In "polymorphous PTLD," the mixed morphotype of the infectious mononucleosis–type reaction is repeated but with a greater number of immunoblasts, occasional atypical immunoblasts, cells with irregular nuclei resembling centrocytes, increased mitoses, and frequently necrosis (Fig. 22.35). Posttransplant lymphoproliferative disorder involving renal allografts does not show the lymphocytic tubulitis or vasculitis of cellular rejection.

### Renal Involvement in PTLD

In a representative series of 36 renal transplant (31) and/or renal/pancreas (4) transplant patients with a diagnosis of PTLD from the University of Pennsylvania (289), PTLD was diagnosed from 6 days to 10 years after engraftment (mean 509 days). Fourteen patients (40%) had been given 10- to 20-day courses of OKT3 or ALG prior to PTLD diagnosis. All 14 of these patients developed PTLD within 6 weeks of transplantation. Seven of 10 patients tested showed recent EBV infection, and 7 of 15 patients tested had active CMV infection at the time of PTLD diagnosis.

Essentially all of the morphologies listed in Table 22.3 have been described in renal allografts. Recognition of the early lesions and polymorphic histologies of PTLD is particularly critical to the practicing nephropathologist in that the distinction from rejection is challenging. Furthermore, the therapeutic approaches to rejection and PTLD

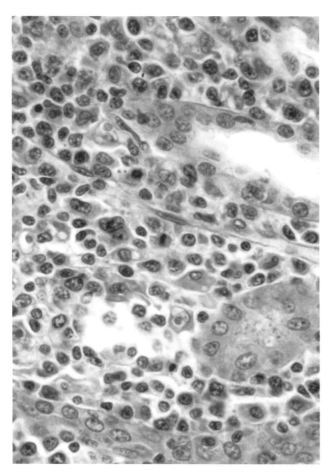

**Figure 22.34** Early mononucleosis–like infiltrate of PTLD. The interstitial infiltrate is mostly mature lymphocytes. Only rare immunoblasts are seen. (×27.)

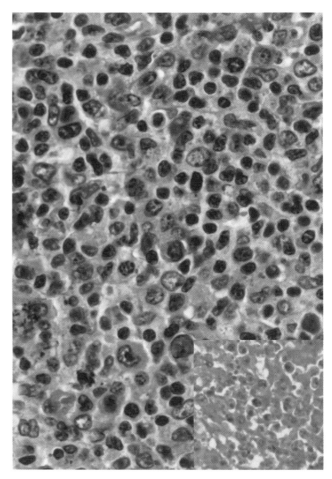

**Figure 22.35** Polymorphous PTLD. The number of transformed cells is increased, with many immunoblasts. Focal necrosis is seen (insert). (×27.)

are markedly different, making the distinction between the two conditions all the more important. In the University of Pennsylvania series (289) the initial PTLD diagnosis was classified as "early" lesions (13), polymorphic PTLD (P-PTLD) (11), and monomorphic PTLD (M-PTLD) (12). Thirty-three lesions were B-cell proliferations, whereas the remaining two lesions were γ-δ T-cell lymphomas. Two patients who initially presented with early lesions rapidly progressed to P-PTLD then to M-PTLD. Thirty-two of the PTLDs, all of which were B-cell in phenotype, were EBV positive by in situ hybridization. Seventeen patients (49%) presented with PTLD in the allograft. Of the 17 patients who presented with allograft PTLD, 9 showed moderate to marked interstitial hemorrhage. Six of these patients had renal biopsies prior to PTLD diagnosis. The renal biopsies prior to PTLD were all classified as moderate to severe acute rejection. While these biopsies showed acute rejection (tubulitis, vasculitis, and/or interstitial hemorrhage), closer examination also showed transformed lymphocytes, lymphocyte mitoses, and focal immunoblasts in three patients. In situ hybridization showed EBV in these three biop-

sies. Thus, very early PTLD in allografts may coexist with rejection.

Posttransplant lymphoproliferative disorders can present in renal allografts and may be confused with allograft rejection. Careful examination of the histology and EBV studies may be needed to distinguish PTLD from rejection. Allograft biopsies with dense lymphoid infiltrates should be evaluated for transformed lymphocytes, lymphoid mitoses, and immunoblasts. These findings may precede PTLD development. Allograft involvement by PTLD is also often associated with interstitial hemorrhage, a finding that is also seen in humoral rejection. Further analysis for PTLD, including studies for EBV and C4d, should be undertaken in renal allograft recipients with dense lymphoid infiltrates showing atypia and/or in suspected vascular rejection.

Most cases of PTLD in renal transplants regress with reduction of immunosuppression; however, a minority of cases can progress to lethal lymphoma. The time from infection to fatal disease progression can be as little as a few weeks. The early recognition and diagnosis of PTLD can offer an opportunity for reduction of immunosuppression and reconstitution of the host immune system, which is necessary for control of the EBV infection.

## Cytomegalovirus Nephritis

Some 20% to 60% of renal transplant recipients may suffer CMV disease with clinical signs of fever, leukopenia, and organ dysfunction (290). Cytomegalovirus infection in a renal allograft recipient may be a primary infection, a re-activation infection, or a reinfection. Primary infections occur in previously uninfected patients who are seronegative for CMV. Blood products or the donated allograft are the usual sources of infection. Re-activation infection occurs in previously infected recipients who re-activate latent infections. Re-infection occurs when a seropositive recipient acquires a new strain of latent virus from a seropositive donor, which subsequently becomes reactivated. The most significant risk factor for primary CMV infection is receipt of a seropositive donor allograft by a seronegative recipient (D+R−) (291). Children are at the highest risk for primary infection. The extent of immunosuppression is the other risk factor for CMV infection. The total amount of immunosuppressive therapy and, in particular, the use of antilymphocyte antibodies enhance the risk for CMV infection.

The histopathologic changes associated with CMV infection vary. A seminal article by Richardson et al (292) described a glomerulopathy in renal allografts with endothelial swelling, hypertrophy, and necrosis; obliteration of the capillary lumens; fibrillar deposits in the glomerular capillaries; mild segmental hypercellularity; a mononuclear cell infiltration; and no CMV inclusions. Because most of these patients had CMV viremia or CMV infection without viremia, the authors associated this pathology with CMV infection and not rejection. Tauzon et al (293) described similar cases and noted a predominance of CD8+ cells in the glomeruli. Rao et al (294) described a case of de novo immunotactoid glomerulopathy with resolution after recovery from a CMV infection. Others have questioned the causative role of CMV infection in such cases. Herrera et al (295), in studying immunosuppressed patients with CMV infection, found histologic lesions similar to those described by Richardson; however, no parenchymal evidence for CMV infection of the kidney was found by immunofluorescence or electron microscopy. The authors raised the possibility of damage secondary to anti-endothelial antibodies and vascular rejection. Anderson et al (296), using immunohistochemistry and in situ hybridization from CMV viremic allograft recipients with glomerulopathy, found no evidence of CMV antigens or DNA. Rubin (297) has suggested that CMV-mediated injury may be indirect. Pro-inflammatory cytokines such as γ interferon can up-regulate MHC in kidney. CMV infection may also increase both Class I and II MHC. Immunologically mediated injury resulting from enhanced MHC ex-

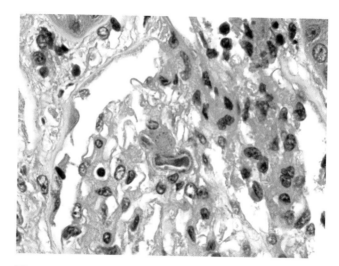

**Figure 22.36** Cytomegalovirus glomerulitis with productive infection, as demonstrated by classic intranuclear and cytoplasmic CMV inclusions. (×67.)

pression and increased targeting may produce the lesions associated with CMV glomerulopathy.

A second mechanism for CMV damage of the kidney is more clearly related to direct viral infection. Payton et al (298) described CMV inclusions in glomerular and peritubular capillary endothelial cells as well as in tubular epithelial cells (Fig. 22.36). Cameron et al (299) described CMV inclusions in tubular epithelial cells in the absence of rejection. Birk and Chavers (300) reported CMV inclusion glomerulopathy in a young transplant patient. Such cases, while rare, document productive CMV infection in both glomerular and tubulointerstitial compartments in a small subset of patients. Pathognomonic viral cytopathic changes include marked cellular enlargement, large pleomorphic nuclei containing eosinophilic intranuclear inclusions with a surrounding clear halo, and smaller basophilic cytoplasmic inclusions.

Cytomegalovirus infection may be diagnosed by serology, tissue examination through histology with immunofluorescence or immunohistochemistry, or CMV-PCR of buffy coat or tissue. Quantitative buffy coat CMV-PCR does not correlate well with the tissue presence of CMV inclusions (301); however, the frequency of discovering CMV infection in renal allografts may be increased by CMV-PCR techniques.

## Hantavirus Infection

Hantaviruses belong to the family Bunyaviridae. Hantaviruses chronically infect rodents and spread by aerosolized excreta to humans. Two main syndromes are associated with clinical Hantavirus infection: hemorrhagic fever with renal syndrome (HFRS) and Hantavirus pulmonary syndrome. We will focus only on HFRS in this section.

Hemorrhagic fever with renal syndrome is dominant in Asia, including China, Korea, and eastern Russia, with more than 100,000 cases annually caused by Hantaan virus carried by the striped field mouse *(Apodemus agrarius)*. Dobravirus carried by the yellow-necked field mouse *(Apodemus flavicollis)* is the usual cause of severe HFRS in the Balkans. Puumala virus carried by the bank vole *(Clethrionomys glareolus)* is found in Scandinavia, Western Russia, and the Balkans and causes less severe disease. Seoul virus from the gray rat *(Rattus norvegicus)* is worldwide in distribution. In the United States, the most likely causative virus of HFRS is the Seoul virus. The incidence of HFRS in the United States is not well known. The prevalence of positive serum antibodies for Seoul virus in urban U.S. residents is less than 1%.

Clinically, HFRS is typically divided into four phases: a febrile period lasting 3 to 5 days, a hypotensive phase lasting a few hours to 2 days, an oliguric phase lasting a few days to 2 weeks, and a polyuric recovery phase (302). Symptoms include fever and chills, myalgias, nausea and vomiting, thirst, abdominal pain, photophobia, and periorbital edema. Petechiae, thrombocytopenia, and disseminated intravascular coagulation are common. There is an extensive vascular leak syndrome with hemoconcentration and postural hypotension. Back pain may be associated with retroperitoneal fluid accumulation. Severe hypotension and shock follow. Proteinuria is marked and urine specific gravity falls, followed by oliguria. The more severe cases of Hantaan virus infection in Asia or Dobrava virus infection in the Balkans have case fatality rates of 5% to 15%. The less severe forms of HFRS from Seoul or Puumala virus infection usually do not display the full spectrum of clinical manifestations and have a case fatality rate of less than 1%. Human leukocyte antigen associations with severe disease have been described (303).

Physiologically, the acute phase of HFRS is characterized by a markedly decreased glomerular filtration rate and increased glomerular permeability, with impairment of both the size- and charge-selectivity properties of the glomerular filter (304).

The most common renal biopsy findings in acute hantavirus infection are acute interstitial nephritis with dominant lymphocytic inflammation accompanied by acute interstitial hemorrhage and tubular necrosis (305,306). No viral inclusions are present. Biopsies taken later in the course may show interstitial fibrosis. Glomerular changes in these cases are limited to some mild mesangial hypercellularity. A small number of cases show diffuse proliferative glomerulonephritis (307), sometimes with a pattern of membranoproliferative glomerulonephritis (308). The fine ultrastructure of the family Bunyaviridae (309) is that of a round or oval shape, about 100 nm in diameter, with a two-layer lipid envelope from which spikes protrude. The nucleocapsid of the virus appears to be hollow microfilaments or dense granules. The infected cells display an enlarged and proliferating Golgi apparatus.

Interferon is thought to play a role in the cellular defenses against hantavirus infection at an early stage (310). The major pathogenetic mechanisms may be related to the immune system's response to the virus. In part, the damage in hantavirus disease results from the elimination of the virus with subsequent necrosis. T-cell–mediated responses, including the T-cell cytokines TNFα and γ-interferon, are prominent in hantavirus disease (311).

## Syphilis

Renal syphilis occurs in the tertiary stage of the disease, and its manifestations usually reflect glomerular involvement. In congenital syphilis, the nephrotic syndrome secondary to membranous nephropathy is common (312). In contrast, tubulointerstitial involvement by gumma is rare (313).

Thompson (313) reviewed 7 instances of gumma and 16 instances of tubulointerstitial nephritis among 220 autopsies of syphilitic patients. Similarly, dense infiltration of the interstitium by mononuclear cells, including a large number of plasma cells, and associated interstitial fibrosis was reported by Rich (314) in 13 of 200 patients with documented tertiary syphilis. Rich (314) also described tubulointerstitial nephritis with mononuclear cells forming nodules that herniated into the tubular lumen. Levy et al (315) reported one patient with syphilis, membranous glomerulonephritis, and tubulointerstitial nephritis with granular deposits of immunoglobulin and complement in tubular basement membrane (TBM). The researchers did not report whether such deposits contained *Treponema pallidum* antigen.

Endothelial cells are probably the site of the initial lesion induced by *Treponema*, and attachment of spirochete to endothelial cells is facilitated by fibronectin molecules bound to the surface of the microorganism (316). The spirochetes elicit humoral and cell-mediated immune responses. The mononuclear cell infiltrate has the characteristics of a delayed-type hypersensitivity reaction and, based on experimental studies using animals, is thought to be more important than antibodies in containing the initial infection (317). Antibodies and complement (C3) opsonize the bacterium and facilitate phagocytosis by macrophages, which kill and degrade the microorganisms. Lymphocytes also secrete soluble factors that kill *T. pallidum*.

## Actinomycosis

Actinomycosis is an opportunistic infection caused by *Actinomyces* organisms, filamentous bacteria that reside in the mouth and throat of healthy individuals. The most common agent is the bacterium *A. israelii*. Systemic infection results from penetration of mucosal defects usually associated with other bacterial infections. Kidney involvement is rare. In Brown's series (318) of 181 patients with actinomycosis, disseminated infection occurred in 18 patients and renal involvement in 1 patient. Renal involvement also may result from contiguous spread from an abdominal site of infection (319) and may be confused with neoplasia (320). Sulfur granules can be detected in the urine (321). Renal infection results in suppurative, necrotizing pyelonephritis, with multiple abscess formation (206). Actinomycosis is recognized by the presence of sulfur granules in fluid draining from a sinus tract or by intraoperative biopsy (320). Sulfur granules can easily be seen in sections stained with hematoxylin and eosin, and the filaments, about 1 mm in diameter, are Gram and methenamine silver positive. They also can be identified by fluoresceinated antibodies to *Actinomyces* (206).

## Nocardiosis

The most common agent of nocardiosis is *Nocardia asteroides*, a filamentous bacteria that is present in nature. However, the incidence of infections with *N. farcinica* is rising, and this agent, indistinguishable from *N. asteroides* by routine laboratory methods, is not sensitive to most antimicrobial agents (322). The bacteria are found in soils, and infection results from inhalation of infective forms or their introduction into soft tissue through trauma. Kidney involvement is rare and occurs as part of hematogenous dissemination, usually a pulmonary infection in immunocompromised patients (240,324–326) or in patients receiving corticosteroids (324). Hematogenous dissemination may be complicated by vascular thromboses (324). Renal infection results in single (324) or multiple small abscesses (324) or diffuse pyelonephritis, often with draining sinus tracts (206). Identification of *Nocardia* must rely on Gram, PAS, or Grocott's methenamine silver. Branched filaments, about 1 mm in diameter, can be demonstrated in the inflammatory infiltrate. *Nocardia* can also grow in large colonies, forming massive granules (i.e., mycetomas).

## Rickettsial Infections

Rickettsial infections are transmitted through several vectors and caused by obligatory intracellular microorganisms. All rickettsioses are zoonoses, and all rickettsia are found in arthropods; humans are accidental hosts that do not maintain these organisms in nature (325). All rickettsioses cause significant clinical disease, and most cause renal involvement, some with mild renal insufficiency and some with acute renal failure and fatal outcomes.

### Rocky Mountain Spotted Fever

Rocky Mountain spotted fever, caused by *Rickettsia rickettsii*, is transmitted by bites of ticks, and small mammals function as reservoirs. In a survey (326), this condition was

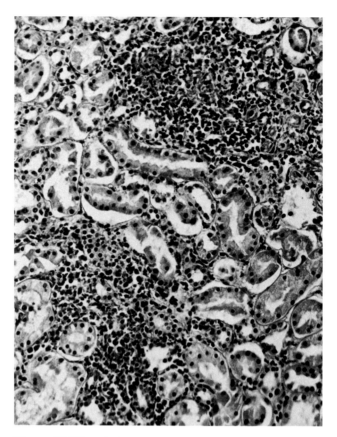

**Figure 22.37** Tubulointerstitial nephritis caused by *R. rickettsii* infections is characterized by multifocal inflammatory infiltration of the tubules and interstitium with mononuclear cells. The collection at the top of the section gives the impression that it is centered on a capillary inflammatory focus. (H&E; ×238.)

reported in 46 states, of which four (i.e., North Carolina, Oklahoma, Tennessee, and South Carolina) accounted for 48% of the cases. Patients present with fever, headache, myalgia, nausea, and vomiting, followed by a rash; history of exposure to habitats containing ticks is a key epidemiologic factor (326,327).

Disseminated rickettsia infection results in increased vascular permeability, hypotension, and shock, with attendant prerenal azotemia or acute tubular necrosis. Some patients develop acute renal failure (327–329) and on biopsy show inflammatory infiltration with mononuclear cells and neutrophils, edema, and necrosis of tubular cells. The inflammation is seen more frequently around vessels and has a predilection for the outer medulla and the corticomedullary junction. Figure 22.37 depicts a specimen from a patient who died of Rocky Mountain spotted fever. Endothelial necrosis can be seen, and immunofluorescence studies have identified *Rickettsia* antigens in the capillary endothelium (329). Figure 22.38 shows rickettsia antigen within endothelial cells. Thrombosis of small capillaries may occur (330). Although the diagnosis can be made by serologic tests, immunopathologic identification of the agent in skin lesions is the only approach that results in

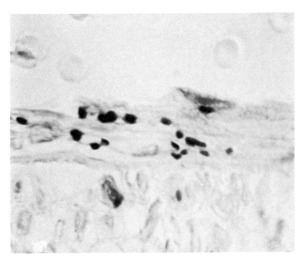

**Figure 22.38** Tubulointerstitial nephritis caused by *R. rickettsii* is detected with an immunoperoxidase preparation using a polyvalent antiserum against *R. rickettsii* in the same kidney as shown in Figure 22.37. Dark-staining areas in the endothelium of a small blood vessel of the kidney indicate sites of rickettsiae antigen. (×1475.) (Courtesy of Dr. Steven Dumler.)

a timely diagnosis during the acute phase of the disease (327,328).

Renal failure and tubulointerstitial nephritis may resolve or may contribute to death (297). Other risk factors associated with death include older age, delay in treatment, or no treatment. The case-fatality ratio for 1981 and 1992 was 4.0% (326).

### Mediterranean Spotted Fever

*Rickettsia conorii*, the etiologic agent of Mediterranean spotted fever, also causes tubulointerstitial nephritis, and the infection can manifest with acute renal failure (331,332). In the report of Shaked et al (333), 5 of 31 patients with this condition developed renal impairment, and in 3, the renal tissues showed multifocal perivascular tubulointerstitial nephritis. The inflammatory infiltrate consists of lymphocytes and histiocytes. Features of acute tubular necrosis also can be found and are thought to result from fluid loss owing to vascular leakage and fever. Yagupsky and Wolach (332) described three children with this condition; all had renal failure, and all died within 24 hours. Rash was seen in only one patient.

### Scrub Typhus

Scrub typhus, caused by *R. tsutsugamushi* and transmitted by mites, presents with a primary lesion (i.e., eschar), generalized lymphadenopathy, fever, rash, and myalgia. Renal involvement is infrequent and is comparable to that of other rickettsial infections but milder; vascular necrosis and thrombosis are rare. The inflammatory infiltrate is vasocentric, predominantly interstitial, and consists of lymphocytes and histiocytes, and there is associated edema and enlarge-

ment of tubular cells (334). Acute renal failure is rare but does occur (335).

### Epidemic Typhus

Epidemic typhus, caused by *R. prowazekii*, is transmitted by body lice and usually occurs under conditions of crowding and of poor hygiene or sanitation. Patients present with fever, myalgia, hypotension, petechiae, jaundice, proteinuria, hematuria, and pyuria (336). The diagnosis can be made by various serologic and other tests or by PCR (336). The inflammatory infiltration is vasocentric and consists of mononuclear cells in the interstitium forming typhus nodules. Vasculitis and endothelial cells containing rickettsiae are common. Schumann et al (337) reported a case of epidemic typhus with fever, renal insufficiency, high titer of antibodies to *R. prowazekii* and *R. mooseri*, and relevant epidemiologic data in a 58-year-old woman. This patient was treated with doxycycline with improvement, but she developed acute renal failure 5 days after treatment was instituted. Her renal biopsy findings, 8 days after antibiotic treatment, demonstrated granulomatous tubulointerstitial nephritis. Continued treatment with doxycycline resulted in improvement of renal function and a decline in the titer of antibodies to *R. prowazekii*.

Rickettsiae enter cells by receptor-mediated endocytosis through the cholesterol receptor; once endocytosed, they leave the endocytic vacuole and multiply in the cytosol. Injury to endothelial cells is mediated, at least in part, by superoxide radicals (338). Endothelial cells, smooth muscle cells, or both are infected, resulting in an increase in vascular permeability, vasculitis, thrombosis, and hemorrhages. Vasculitis requires adhesion of neutrophils to endothelial cells and depends on E-selectin expression (339). Thrombosis appears to result from enhanced tissue factor expression by endothelial cells (330) and from release of von Willebrand factor from Weibel-Palade bodies (340). Infected and injured endothelial cells detach from the vascular wall and circulate in the blood. They can be captured and used as targets for the diagnosis of rickettsial infection (341).

## Leptospirosis

Several species of *Leptospira* can cause human infections: *L. icterohaemorrhagiae* (i.e., Weil's disease), *L. pomona*, *L. bataviae*, *L. shermani*, and *L. grippotyphosa*. Among 50 patients reported by Lecour et al (342), *L. icterohaemorrhagiae*, *L. canicola*, and *L. grippotyphosa* were responsible for infections in 39, 6, and 2 patients, respectively. Patients present with renal dysfunction or acute renal failure (52) and, in the case of Weil's disease, jaundice (342).

Leptospirosis is a ubiquitous enzootic disease. Animal reservoirs include rodents, skunks, foxes, livestock, ducks, and frogs. The animals usually exhibit a prolonged urinary shedding of the organism. Humans may acquire the microorganism when they are in direct contact with the infected tissues or fluids or with contaminated water. Renal involvement, particularly early involvement, is very common and occurs in 44% to 67% of patients (343). Tubulointerstitial nephritis is the main pattern of renal injury in leptospirosis.

In Weil's disease, the kidneys are enlarged, edematous, and brownish yellow, and they demonstrate acute tubular necrosis; inflammatory infiltrate including lymphocytes, monocytes, plasma cells, and neutrophils; petechial hemorrhages; and foci of vasculitis (344,345). The interstitial inflammatory cell infiltrate is frequently associated with prominent acute tubular injury (346,347). Leptospira may be detected in tissue section with the Levaditi stain, but the method is tedious and may require multiple sections (342).

The pathogenesis of the inferred interstitial nephritis may be secondary to the direct infection of the renal parenchyma by the microorganism. There is recent evidence that the outer membrane protein of leptospira has an important pathogenic role (343,348). The outer membrane protein activates nuclear factor κB and downstream stimulates inducible nitric oxide, monocyte chemoattractant protein-1, and TNFα expression (348).

The outcome of the disease, even if untreated, is relatively good; however, in elderly patients the mortality is higher. Antibiotic therapy, particularly penicillin, is effective.

## Parasitic Infections

Granulomatous tubulointerstitial nephritis caused by parasites may result from their localization in the kidney (e.g., filaria) or from renal localization of their eggs (e.g., schistosomiasis). In malaria, the parasite is found in parasitized red blood cells in the kidney, but tubulointerstitial lesions may reflect complex interactions of various factors, including inflammatory mediators and ischemia (349).

### Malarial Infection

Malaria is commonly transmitted by the bite of mosquitoes infected with *Plasmodium*, but organ transplantation can also be a vehicle for malaria infection (350). Glomerular involvement may result in proteinuria, hematuria, and nephrotic syndrome (349,351,352). This chronic glomerular disease is classically associated with *P. malariae* infection (quartan malarial nephropathy) (see "Miscellaneous Infectious Causes of Nephrotic Syndrome"). *Plasmodium malariae* and *P. falciparum* cause tubulointerstitial injury related to hypotensive or ischemic insult (352–355). Patients develop a form of hemoglobinuric acute renal failure known as *blackwater fever* because the urine passed is dark owing to the presence of large amounts of hemoglobin. Acute renal failure complicates *P. falciparum* infection in 1% to 4% of patients in endemic areas (352). Interestingly, acute renal failure is much more common in Eu-

ropeans who are infected and do not live in the endemic areas. Reported figures indicate a 25% to 30% incidence of acute renal failure among Europeans infected with malaria (352).

The histologic picture in malaria-associated acute renal failure is usually that of an acute tubular necrosis; however, interstitial nephritis is a well-recognized complication (352). There is interstitial edema, tubular dilation, focal tubular cell necrosis (354), hemoglobin casts, and hemosiderin in tubules; interstitial edema and mononuclear cell infiltration, mainly lymphocytes, may be present (351). In two patients infected with *P. vivax* and *P. ovale*, respectively, during renal implantation, fever and renal dysfunction coincided with parasitemia on days 20 and 8 after transplantation (350). In the patient infected with *P. vivax*, a renal biopsy demonstrated intense tubulointerstitial nephritis with mononuclear cell infiltration; in both patients, renal function returned to normal with antimalarial therapy. Dialysis has led to considerable improvement in the outcome of patients with malaria-related tubulointerstitial disease, and overall mortality caused by renal failure has decreased from 30% to 10% (351). No deaths from renal failure were observed among 42 patients treated by Stone et al (355). However, other reports indicate much more serious complications, with a reported mortality rate between 15% and 45% (352).

Acute renal failure is thought to result from blockade of the microcirculation by parasitized cells and from nonspecific inflammatory factors (351,352,354). Circulatory impedance, or vascular occlusion, is caused by endothelial attachment of parasitized red blood cells through a histidine-rich protein.

### Schistosomiasis

Four major species of *Schistosoma* affect humans, and two cause significant renal disease. Infection with *S. mansoni* results in glomerulonephritis (356–358) attended by proteinuria or nephrotic syndrome, whereas infection with *S. haematobium* produces obstructive uropathy owing to inflammatory and fibrotic reaction to egg localization in tissues, usually in the excretory system (359).

Three types of interstitial inflammation occur in schistosomal nephropathy. The first is a granulomatous reaction to egg localization to the kidney (360). The granulomatous response is modulated by cytokines released in response to egg-soluble antigens (361). Eggshells can be readily identified in tissues: those of *S. mansoni* and *S. japonicum* are acid-fast; those of *S. haematobium* are not. The second, more common response is an inflammatory infiltration with mononuclear cells and interstitial fibrosis associated with obstructive uropathy (359). The third is an interstitial inflammation and fibrosis accompanying schistosomal glomerulopathy, as occurs with other forms of chronic glomerular diseases (358,360).

### Filariasis

Microfilariae may cause granulomatous inflammation in glomeruli (362) and in the interstitium. Severe tubulointerstitial mononuclear cell infiltration with lymphocytes, plasma cells, and eosinophils, independent of granuloma, also has been described (363).

### Microsporidiosis

Microsporidia, which belong to the genus Encephalitozoon, are obligate intracellular protozoa. Five microsporidia are reported to infect patients with AIDS—*E. bieneusi*, *S. intestinalis*, *E. hellem*, *Pleistophora*, and *E. cuniculi*. *E. cuniculi*, the prototypic species of this genus, targets the central nervous system and kidneys with involvement of macrophages, epithelium and endothelium. In hematoxylin and eosin sections, the oval to slightly elongated, 1- to 2-$\mu$m spores have a blue staining outline and either a central blue band or a dense blue pole opposite a clear polar vacuole. Spore detection is enhanced by Gram staining, polarization, and fluorescence chitin stains. Morphologic speciation is imprecise and requires antigenic and molecular studies, including polymerase chain reaction.

Tubulointerstitial nephritis can occur with disseminated *S. intestinalis*. Mertens et al (364) reported necrotizing microsporidiosis of the kidney caused by *E. cuniculi*. Although the glomeruli contained occasional microsporidial spores, infection was concentrated in the distal nephron, especially in the medulla. Parasitophorous vacuoles expanded the cytoplasm of attached and sloughed tubular epithelial cells. Tubular lumina also contained spore-laden macrophages, cellular debris, and free spores. Progressive destruction of tubules led to microabscess-like foci rich in macrophages, debris, spores, and scattered neutrophils. Some infected pyramids were necrotic.

### Amoebiasis

Amoebiasis is a protozoal infection caused by *Entamoeba histolytica*. Renal involvement is very rare; however, in invasive infections, the kidney is the fifth most common site of abscess localization (365). Trophozoites can be found within foci of liquefaction necrosis and abscess formation.

### Hydatidosis

Cystic hydatid disease is caused by the larval form of *Echinococcus granulosus*. It is endemic in parts of Africa, Latin America, Mediterranean, the southeast, and Turkey. Renal involvement comprises 2% to 4% of all cases (366). The kidney is usually involved as part of disseminated disease. Echinococcal larvae may reach the kidneys through the bloodstream, via the lymph glands, or by direct invasion. Isolated renal echinococcosis is extremely rare (366). The most common symptoms are palpable mass, flank pain, hematuria, malaise, and fever. Hydatiduria is a pathognomonic sign involving passage of a typical grapelike material in the urine but occurs in only 5% to 25% of cases (366). Treatment is mainly surgical; partial nephrectomy and percutaneous drainage carry the risk of dissemination and fatal anaphylactic reaction.

## Miscellaneous Infectious Causes of Nephrotic Syndrome

There is a spectrum of renal diseases associated with parasitic diseases (367), and these manifestations are summarized in Table 22.4. Most of the glomerular lesions are proliferative, i.e., membranoproliferative or mesangioproliferative. However, membranous nephropathy, focal segmental glomerulosclerosis, and minimal change nephrotic syndrome are sometimes seen. The clinical spectrum ranges from isolated proteinemia or hematuria to nephrotic syndrome, nephritic syndrome, renal insufficiency, and rapidly progressive glomerulonephritis.

### Malarial Infections

Malaria is responsible for certain forms of renal disease, but only *P. malariae* is associated with nephrotic syndrome. In contrast to infection with *P. malariae*, there is little to suggest that glomerulonephritis is commonly a dominant and sole lesion in the context of *P. falciparum*. In patients with *P. falciparum*, urinary abnormalities have been associated with glomerular mesangial and endothelial proliferation and mesangial deposits of IgM and C3 with or without IgG, but these histologic findings are apparently reversible, for they were not present on second biopsy taken 6 weeks after the first (368).

In countries where quartan malaria *(P. malariae)* is endemic, a different spectrum of causes of nephrotic syndrome is experienced. Good accounts of the historic and geographic aspects have been given on several occasions (369,370), and from these reports, various important facts emerge. First, nephrotic syndrome is much more common in such countries as Nigeria and Uganda than in other parts of Africa and in nontropical countries (371). Thus, when new hospital admissions of patients with nephrotic syndrome were expressed as a percentage of total medical admissions, rates of 2.4% (Nigeria) and 2.0% (Uganda) were found, compared with 0.15% in Zimbabwe and 0.12% and 0.03% in two hospitals in North America. Second, whereas minimal change nephrotic syndrome is the most common cause of nephrotic syndrome among children in the United States and also occurs in adults in appreciable numbers, it is extremely rare in Nigeria, Kenya, Uganda, and the Ivory Coast (372–375). As is described later, glomerular changes attributed to infection with *P. malariae* make a significant contribution to the pool of cases of nephrotic syndrome.

## TABLE 22.4

## RENAL MANIFESTATIONS ASSOCIATED WITH PARASITIC DISEASES

| Parasite (Disease) | Clinical Manifestations | Renal Lesions | Pathogenesis |
|---|---|---|---|
| *Plasmodium malariae* (quartan malaria) | Proteinuria to nephrotic syndrome | Mesangioproliferative GN, membranoproliferative GN | IC, autoimmune component |
| | Nephrotic syndrome | Minimal change nephrotic syndrome (rare) | |
| | Nephrotic syndrome | Focal segmental glomerulosclerosis (rare) | |
| | Nephrotic syndrome | Membranous GP (rare) | IC, autoimmune component |
| **Plasmodium falciparum** (tertian malaria) | Acute renal failure | Tubulointerstitial damage | Hemolysis and hypoperfusion |
| | Proteinuria to nephrotic syndrome (rare) | Mesangioproliferative GN, membranoproliferative GN (rare) | IC, coagulopathy |
| *Schistosoma haematobium* | Chronic renal failure | Hydronephrosis and pyelonephritis | Vesicoureteral fibrosis and reflux |
| *Schistosoma mansoni* | Proteinuria | Mesangioproliferative GN Membranoproliferative GN | IC, autoimmune component, portal shunting |
| | Nephrotic syndrome | Focal segmental glomerulosclerosis | |
| | Nephrotic syndrome | Membranous GP | |
| | Nephrotic syndrome | Amyloidosis (rare) | |
| | Acute renal failure | Crescentic GN (rare) | |
| **Leishmania donovani** (kala-azar) | Proteinuria | Mesangioproliferative GN Amyloidosis | IC, autoimmune component, coagulopathy |
| | Nephrotic syndrome | | |
| *Trypanosoma brucei rhodesiense, Trypanosoma brucei gambiense* | Proteinuria | Mesangioproliferative GN (rare) | IC |
| *Toxoplasma gondii* | Proteinuria to nephritic syndrome | Membranoproliferative GN | IC, coagulopathy |
| | Nephrotic syndrome | Focal segmental glomerulosclerosis (rare) | Congenital toxoplasmosis |
| | Acute renal failure | Tubulointerstitial nephritis | Sulfadiazine crystal deposition |
| *Trichinella spiralis* | Proteinuria | Mesangioproliferative GN, membranoproliferative GN | IC, coagulopathy |
| | Mild renal failure | Tubular necrosis | Hypovolemia and myoglobinuria |
| *Babesia bovis, Babesia divergens, Babesia microti* | Acute renal failure | Tubular necrosis | Shock and hemolysis |
| *Echinococcus granulosus* (hydatid disease) | Nephrotic syndrome | Membranous GP (rare) Membranoproliferative GN (rare) | IC |
| | Nephrotic syndrome | Minimal change nephrotic syndrome (rare) | |
| | Mass effect | Cyst (generally solitary) | |
| *Wuchereria bancrofti, Brugia malayi* (lymphatic filariasis) | Proteinuria to nephritic syndrome | Mesangioproliferative GN, membranoproliferative GN | IC |
| *Onchocerca volvulus* (river blindness), *Loa loa* | Nephrotic syndrome | Amyloidosis (rare) | |
| | Renal failure | Interstitial nephritis (rare) | |
| *Wuchereria bancrofti* | Nephritic syndrome | Acute GN (rare) | |
| *Loa loa* | Nephrotic syndrome | Membranous GP | IC |
| | Nephrotic syndrome | Minimal change nephrotic syndrome | |
| | Nephrotic syndrome | Focal segmental glomerulosclerosis (rare) | |

GN, glomerulonephritis; GP, glomerulopathy; IC, immune complexes.
Modified from Velthuysen M-L, Florquin S. Glomerulopathy associated with parasitic infections. Clin Microbiol Rev 2000;13:55.

The evidence for the role of *P. malariae* as a cause of the nephrotic syndrome and the associated pathologic picture has been summarized (374,376) and includes (a) a highly significant selective increase in *P. malariae* parasitemia in children with nephrotic syndrome compared with children from the same population who are ill but without nephrotic syndrome or who are healthy, (b) the demonstration that the specific antibody and antigen are present in the glomeruli of patients with the pathologic changes attributed to infection with *P. malariae*, and (c) the production of nephrotic syndrome in *Aotus* monkeys by infection with quartan malaria. It should be added that many of the pathologic features seen in quartan malarial nephropathy in humans (described later in this section) can be reproduced in *Aotus* monkeys by the injection of *P. malariae* (377).

### Clinical Presentation

Clinical findings are similar in cases reported from Uganda and Nigeria (371,378,379). The condition occurs in both children and adults, but among children, the average age was higher than in children with nephrotic syndrome in the United States and in Europe. This higher age coincides with the peak incidence of malarial infection among children. Malarial antibody titers of high levels were found in a greater proportion, even allowing for the fact that antibodies were lost in the urine in the population with nephrotic syndrome. In general, the clinical presentation was no different from that seen in temperate climates. Proteinuria was poorly selective, and the response to steroids was generally not good.

### Pathologic Findings

The pathologic changes in patients with malaria and the nephrotic syndrome vary from country to country. In the cases reported from Uganda (371,380) the diagnoses were as follows. Of the 77 patients studied by renal biopsy (31 children and 46 adults), 55 showed signs of proliferative glomerulonephritis, and 16 of these 55 had a diffuse increase in nuclei and a secondary increase in basement membrane fibrils. Three had a similar type of change, but with an accentuated lobular pattern; 11 had a focal form, in which less than 50% of the glomeruli were involved, with a localized or segmental pattern of involvement. Eight had a more chronic form, and 17 had a mild form of focal glomerular change. The remaining 22 patients had a variety of symptoms, the largest group consisting of 9 who had diffuse thickening of the capillary walls with no proliferative element. It was stated that in 31 patients there was evidence of quartan malaria and that all but 1 showed signs of the proliferative type of lesion on histology.

Of the cases reported from Nigeria (369,379), all 63 were in children; most of the renal biopsies showed a combination of findings unlike those seen in a group of children with nephrotic syndrome from tem-

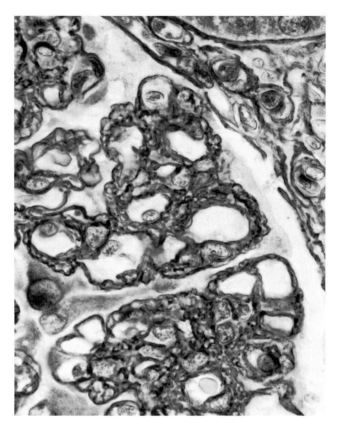

**Figure 22.39** Double-contour and plexiform arrangement of glomerular capillary walls in a patient with malarial nephrosis. (Silver impregnation; ×1080.) (Courtesy of Dr. L. Morel-Maroger.)

perate climates. They were designated *quartan malarial nephropathy* (QMN). One characteristic of QMN was a thickening of the glomerular capillary walls, which, in the earliest cases, was segmental and involved only a few glomeruli. This change affected more and more capillaries as the disease progressed, and narrowing of the capillary lumina took place. The thickening involved the subendothelial aspects of the capillary wall and consisted of a double-contour or plexiform arrangement of PAS-positive or argyrophilic fibrils (Fig. 22.39). This process, together with a concomitant sclerosis of the mesangium, led initially to a segmental type of glomerular sclerosis; it later became more extensive and involved the entire tufts.

Cellular proliferative changes were not a feature of QMN, except for localized islands of mesangial hypercellularity in a few cases. Tubular atrophy and interstitial round-cell infiltration were proportionate to the degree of glomerular involvement. With the electron microscope, effacement of foot processes and a thickening of the capillary basement membrane were evident, caused by an increase in subendothelial basement membrane–like material of varying density. Small lacunae in the basement membrane were invariable features, and these often contained material of an electron density comparable to that of the basement membrane. Immunofluorescence studies revealed one of three patterns. The first consisted of coarse, medium-sized granular deposits along capillary walls with antisera directed against IgG, IgM, or C3; the second showed very small, fine deposits homogeneously distributed along capillary walls with IgG and, in one case of seven, with C3; the third pattern was a mixture of the first two. *Plasmodium malariae* antigen was detected in one of three biopsies tested, but *P. falciparum* antigen was never found. Quartan malarial parasites were discovered in the blood in 38 of 51 patients with QMN.

Other histologic pictures encountered in the total group of patients with nephrotic syndrome were minimal change nephrotic syndrome, membranoproliferative glomerulonephritis, focal glomerular sclerosis, and amyloidosis. It is noteworthy that 7 of 12 patients with these abnormalities had quartan malaria parasitemia.

The differences in the histologic appearances of the glomeruli between the Ugandan cases (371,380) and the Nigerian cases (369,379) are difficult to reconcile. The complexity of renal disease in tropical settings is further emphasized by the observations of Morel-Maroger et al (381) on the nephrotic syndrome in Senegal, where the prevalence of *P. malariae* is low. On renal biopsy, a picture similar to that of QMN was found on light microscopy, namely, fibrillary changes in the glomerular capillary wall and progressive segmental sclerosis. The immunofluorescence picture, however, was different, in that there was no diffuse deposition of immunoglobulins. Serologic evidence of malaria was lacking in a third of the cases in children, and in most of the remainder, titers against *P. falciparum* were higher than those against *P. malariae*. Attempts to demonstrate the presence of *P. falciparum* antigen in the glomeruli were unsuccessful in the six cases in which it was sought. Because of the uncertainty of the source, the authors used the noncommittal term *tropical nephropathy* for this entity.

### Etiology and Pathogenesis

From the evidence available, it appears that quartan malaria can produce nephrotic syndrome and that immunologic injury plays a part. Fluorescent antibody studies on the Ugandan cases (382) support the idea of an immune complex disease, and additional studies from Nigeria (372,383,384) reinforce this view. Houba et al (385,386) have discussed the evidence for an immune complex pathogenesis for the renal lesions associated with malaria. He points out that immune complexes, preformed in the circulation, localize in glomeruli and initiate the changes. In acute lesions, such as are experienced with *P. falciparum*, the deposition of complexes is found shortly after infection. In these cases, glomerular injury is reversible, and the response to antimalarial therapy is good. In chronic lesions, such as are associated with *P. malariae*, the changes are progressive and do not respond to antimalarial treatment.

At the beginning of the process, malarial antigen is present in the lesion, but progression of the disease process does not appear to be caused by a constant supply of malarial antigen. Houba (385,386) raises the possibility that in these chronic cases, immune complexes trigger a sequence that could be autoimmune in nature. This issue also was addressed by Goldman et al (376), who considered that polyclonal activation of B cells might be a pathogenetic factor in malarial nephropathy. The role of anti-DNA autoantibodies (387,388) and cellular factors (389) in the pathogenesis of the glomerular lesion in malaria infection is suggested by clinical studies that demonstrate a variety of autoantibodies in patients with malaria, including anti-DNA antibodies, and experimental studies in murine models of malaria.

## Schistosomal Infection

There are three major species of human schistosomes—*S. mansoni*, *S. haematobium*, and *S. japonicum*. Only *S. mansoni* causes glomerular disease by what is thought to be immune complex deposition, and these patients have initial signs of proteinuria and the nephrotic syndrome. *Schistosoma mansoni* infection occurs in most African countries south of the Sahara, Egypt, Libya, some Arabian countries, Brazil, and a few other countries in South America (370). The adult worms live in the hepatic portal system, and most of the associated pathologic lesions occur in the liver and spleen. The eggs have a lateral spine and are passed in the feces.

The main renal manifestation is *glomerulonephritis*, and there is good evidence that it is mediated by immune complexes. The prevalence of glomerulonephritis in *S. mansoni* infection shows considerable geographic variation, but the contributions of geography and other factors, including hepatic fibrosis and intercurrent infections with hepatitis B (390) and salmonellosis, leading to overt glomerular disease, are incompletely understood (391). *Schistosoma mansoni* infection was implicated in nephrotic syndrome in 42.5% of the cases in an endemic area (392), and prospective clinical studies have reported evidence of overt renal disease in 15% of patients with hepatosplenic schistosomiasis (393,394). Among 240 patients with active *S. mansoni* infection but no symptoms of glomerular disease, 48 had proteinuria (dipstick). Eight of 15 renal biopsies showed early signs of glomerular lesions, comprising focal mesangial proliferation and immunofluorescent deposits, mainly IgM and C3 (395). In contrast, only 1 of 58 Sudanese patients hospitalized for advanced hepatosplenic schistosomiasis had significant proteinuria, and 5 had microscopic hematuria. Intraoperative renal biopsies performed during portal decompression showed no evidence of glomerulonephritis by light fluorescence and electron microscopy (396).

Studies have provided strongly suggestive evidence for a cause-and-effect relationship between *S. mansoni* infection and glomerular lesions. It was shown that (a) schistosomal antigen is present in the glomeruli (397–399), (b) antibody reactive with adult worm antigen can be eluted from kidneys with glomerular lesions (398,399), (c) circulating immune complexes have been detected in patients with *S. mansoni* infection (400), and (d) glomerular lesions can be produced in a variety of animals by injection of *S. mansoni* (401). These various findings suggest an immune complex pathogenesis for the glomerular lesions. The dominance of IgA in the glomerular deposits of the more chronic and progressive forms of glomerular pathologic lesions has suggested that altered hepatic clearance of IgA aggregates or immune complexes from the circulation can contribute to glomerular immune injury in the absence of active infection. This may explain the poor response of the renal lesion to antischistosomal drugs (391).

## Clinical Presentation

The clinical picture varies. The patients are usually young adults, and many have the nephrotic syndrome (394,397). Others have asymptomatic proteinuria (394,397). The proteinuria is usually of a poorly selective type, with IgM, $\alpha_2$-macroglobulins, and lipoproteins appearing in the urine (402). Hepatosplenomegaly is commonly detected (394), and worm eggs are usually found in the stool.

## Pathologic Findings

The pathologic appearances are also varied (393). On light microscopic examination, membranoproliferative glomerulonephritis (370,394,399,402) (Figs. 22.40 and 22.41) and focal segmental glomerulosclerosis (399,402) are the glomerular lesions most frequently associated with clinical symptoms and the nephrotic syndrome. In what were regarded as early cases, mesangial proliferative glomerulonephritis was the most common lesion (397). Membranous glomerulonephritis (397,399) and amyloidosis (393) are described less often. Exudative glomerulonephritis with endocapillary neutrophils, monocytes, platelets, fibrin, and proliferating mesangial and endothelial cells has been reported in patients with hepatosplenic schistosomiasis complicated by salmonella infection (393). These patients have hypocomplementemia. In most accounts, there is no mention of the status of the tubules and interstitium.

Immunofluorescence microscopy reveals granular deposits of IgM and C3 in the mesangium (Fig. 22.42) and

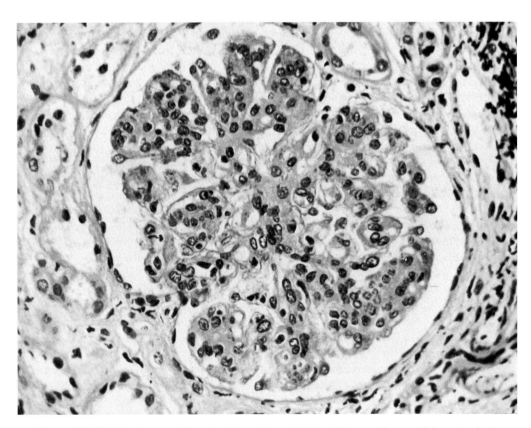

**Figure 22.40** Membranoproliferative glomerulonephritis in a 25-year-old man with hepatosplenic schistosomiasis caused by *S. mansoni*. There is centrolobular (mesangial) hypercellularity and localized thickening of the glomerular capillary walls (better seen in Fig. 22.41). (H&E; ×500.) (From Andrade ZA, et al. Schistosomal nephropathy. In: Kibukamusoke JW, ed. Tropical Nephrology. Canberra: Citforge, 1984.)

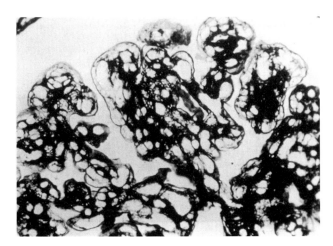

**Figure 22.41** Membranoproliferative glomerulonephritis in *S. mansoni* infection. Double contours are clearly visible, explaining the localized thickening of the capillary wall. The mesangium is expanded. (Methenamine silver/PAS; ×240.)

along the capillary walls in cases diagnosed as membranoproliferative glomerulonephritis, IgM and C3 in a focal and segmental distribution in cases with focal and segmental glomerular sclerosis (397), and endocapillary granular deposits of C3 in cases with exudative glomerulonephritis (393). Barsoum and colleagues (391) have emphasized the prominence of mesangial deposits of IgA in both the membranoproliferative and focal segmental sclerosis forms of glomerular involvement. This finding suggests that the underlying hepatic pathologic condition contributes to the pathogenesis of the glomerular lesion. Serum IgA antigliadin and anti-DNA antibodies, and glomerular IgA deposits, are markers of significant renal involvement in patients with hepatosplenic schistosomiasis. Schistosomal antigen has been found to be present in the mesangium and

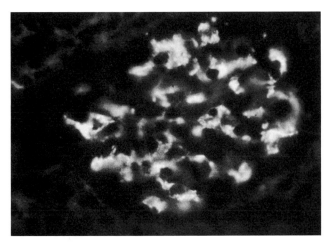

**Figure 22.42** *Schistosoma mansoni* glomerulonephritis shows IgG deposition in the mesangium and, to a lesser extent, in the capillary wall.

capillary walls (393,397,399). Electron microscopic techniques reveal electron-dense deposits in the mesangium and on the epithelial side of glomerular basement membranes (402).

### Clinical Course, Prognosis, and Therapy

The natural history of the condition is difficult to determine from most published accounts, but Rocha and Martinelli (403) consider that the overall courses of the membranoproliferative and focal segmental glomerular sclerosis variants are comparable to those of the idiopathic forms with these two histologic pictures. At the end of 5 years of follow-up of 25 patients with *S. mansoni*–related membranoproliferative glomerulonephritis, renal function was normal in 7, renal insufficiency was present in 11, and end-stage renal disease was seen in 7. Of 25 patients with *S. mansoni*–related focal and segmental glomerular sclerosis followed for 5 years, 17 had normal renal function, 4 had renal insufficiency, and 4 had end-stage renal disease. In a prospective study, 12 patients with hepatosplenic schistosomiasis, the nephrotic syndrome, and focal segmental glomerulosclerosis (FSGS) were followed up for more than 12 years (125 ± 9.1 months) (404). Four patients were in complete remission with normal renal function, and one was in relapse; seven patients had persistent proteinuria, with progression to renal insufficiency in six and to end-stage renal disease in three. That end-stage kidney disease is common is apparent from other accounts (399). Response to treatment with antischistosomal drugs is poor (405–407).

### Echinococcal Infection (Hydatid Disease)

Most reports of hydatid disease and renal involvement concern renal cysts. A few cases of glomerular lesions have been reported, and the histologic changes have included minimal change nephrotic syndrome, membranous nephropathy, and membranoproliferative glomerulonephritis (367,408). In most cases, the glomerular lesions are reported to be reversible by treating the infection. In one patient with membranous nephropathy, echinococcal antigens and antibodies were eluted from renal tissue, supporting an immune complex–mediated pathogenesis.

### Filarial Infection

Glomerulonephritis is a well-known complication of filarial infections, including *Wucheria bancrofti*, *Onchocerca volvulus*, and *Loa loa* (367,409). A clear association is often difficult to establish because of frequent coinfections (hepatitis B and malaria). Parasitic antigens were demonstrated in 9 of 18 patients with proliferative glomerular disease owing to onchocerciasis, supporting an immune complex pathogenesis (410). Membranoproliferative glomerulonephritis as well as membranous nephropathy and minimal change nephrotic syndrome have been reported in patients with filariasis (367,409). The usual clinical presentation of filarial-associated glomerulonephritis is with proteinuria, often in the nephrotic range, with hypertension in some 75% and severe impairment of renal function in 48% of patients (410).

## REFLUX NEPHROPATHY

Urine reflux constitutes chronic nonobstructive backflow of urine from the lower to the upper urinary tract. Urine reflux can be congenital (primary) or acquired and unilateral or bilateral. Primary reflux is caused by incompetence of the vesicoureteric junction (VUJ) at the point of the ureteral orifice. The normal ureter enters the urinary bladder obliquely and extends into the submucosa at a length that in adults averages 1.3 cm and in children 0.5 cm (411). Physiologic VUJ function requires correct insertion angle, an adequately long intramural ureteral segment, and contraction of the longitudinal muscle of the submucosal ureter. The support by the bladder detrusor muscle at the trigone is very important for the valve mechanism to operate promptly. Forward flow of urine is also influenced by ureteral peristalsis. Reversal of urine flow into the ureter, renal pelvis, and calices may cause dilation and damage the renal parenchyma, both via increased fluid pressure and/or through contamination by pathogenic organisms present in the bladder urine. The combination of VUR and renal scarring was previously known as *atrophic* or *chronic nonobstructive pyelonephritis*. These terms erroneously considered all scarred kidneys in VUR to have had infections and are now replaced by the term *reflux nephropathy* (RN), which was first introduced in 1973 by Bailey (412). Reflux nephropathy is distinguished from pyelonephritis, which implies inflammation of the renal pelvis secondary to infection irrespective of reflux, and from kidney hydronephrosis, a term that describes urine accumulation in the renal pelvis and calices secondary to physical or functional obstruction (obstructive nephropathy). Secondary VUR in children can be the result of congenital anomalies associated with incompetent VUJ, for example, duplicate ureters, megaureter, urethral cysts, crossed renal ectopia, or pelvic (horseshoe) kidney. In adults, neurogenic bladder and repeated urinary tract infections that cause VUJ inflammation and edema are frequent causes of reflux. Occasionally, reflux occurs in the transplanted kidney. Radiologists and urologists tend to use the anatomic term VUR, which focuses on the underlying structural abnormality that may be treated with surgery. *Reflux nephropathy* to clinicians simply describes renal scars, irrespective of pathology. However, kidney specimens have a broad spectrum of gross and histologic findings that differ based on whether VUR is congenital or acquired, as described below.

### Incidence and Clinical Presentation

Prenatal ultrasound detects some degree of ureter or renal pelvis dilation in approximately 1% of live births (413,414). Of these, at least 25% have VUR postnatally. Siblings of affected children are at high risk, with an incidence that varies from 4.7% to over 50% (415–417). Most cases of VUR are mild (about 66%) and, according to the most recent studies, resolve within 2 years. It was a held belief that the majority of babies with reflux diagnosed in utero are boys with usually severe bilateral disease. This view is now revised, with most children having unilateral disease; VUR in girls has a frequency estimated to be 1 in 100 (418).

Clinical presentation is dependent on age and presence of UTIs (419,420). Congenital reflux in infants and young children may be asymptomatic, or they may present with nonspecific lower urinary tract symptoms, including dysuria, flank pain and tenderness, and fever. In fact, temperature above 38.5°C was the predominant feature in young children with reflux in a 350-patient series (419). Many of these children carried a diagnosis from fetal ultrasound and had affected siblings. Vesicoureteral reflux is found in about 50% of children investigated for UTIs and in 15% to 34% of children with asymptomatic bacteriuria worldwide.

In recent decades, a relatively common nonanatomic but functional disorder of the lower urinary tract characterized by abnormal holding of urine and disturbed voiding patterns has been recognized (421,422). Both boys and girls are affected, and the condition enters the differential diagnosis in children undergoing screening for VUR and/or infection. This category of reflux is collectively called *dysfunctional elimination syndrome* to include terms such as *vesical sphincter dyssynergia, nonneurogenic neurogenic bladder dysfunction, uninhibited pediatric bladder,* and *irritable bladder syndrome.* According to the International Reflux Study in Children (421), dysfunctional elimination syndrome accounts for as many as 18% of children with reflux. The diagnosis is made by establishing a history of wetting and voiding cystourethrography.

### Radiologic Evaluation

Diagnosis of RN is made with imaging studies. Ultrasound and voiding cystourethrography are the primary tests to establish the diagnosis of VUR. Ultrasound is safe and noninvasive and therefore the most frequent in-office test for patient follow-up or initial assessment. However, although it is convenient and free of ionizing radiation, this test too frequently gives false-positive results, particularly if reflux is of low grade. Voiding cystourethrography utilizes fluoroscopy to delineate the bladder outline, bladder neck, and urethral anatomy and provides a good estimate of the bladder capacity. Urine reflux may occur during bladder filling or during voiding. Radionuclide cystography with technetium 99 is an enhancing test for children that requires repeated testing annually and screening for siblings. Involvement of the upper urinary tract was historically evaluated by excretory urography (IVP), a test that is particularly suited for children with febrile UTIs. Up to 85% of children undergoing IVP who do not have evidence of obstruction, but have parenchymal scars, may be found to have VUR (420). One or more scars, defined as focal thinning of the renal cortex, often overlying a dilated calix, may be identified, depending on the severity of reflux.

Focal scarring is explained by the microscopic anatomy of the papillae, which was first studied in piglets and later confirmed in humans by Ransley and Risdon (423). There are two types of papillae: simple and compound. Simple papillae are dome shaped and contain ducts of Bellini that open up onto the surface through slitlike orifices. Compound papillae have a flat surface and consist of two or three fused pyramids. Openings of ducts of Bellini in these are larger and round. Injection of contrast media in the ureter is taken up by the compound papillae, which are situated at the poles of the kidneys, but not simple papillae, which are found mainly in the mid-zone. It is thought that backward pressure of urine forces the slitlike collecting duct orifices in simple papillae closed, but not the large openings in compound papillae, suggesting that the latter are susceptible to intrarenal urine dispersion. Autopsy studies have confirmed that humans tend to have more scars at the poles of the kidney, indicating that compound papillae are more vulnerable to reflux. However, humans appear to have more simple than compound papillae compared to the pig, which confers a natural protection against intrarenal reflux. A radiographically small atrophic kidney represents end-stage disease.

## Grading of Reflux

Early in 1980, the International Reflux Study Group classified reflux into five grades:

- Grade I: Reflux into the ureter only
- Grade II: Reflux into the ureter and the renal pelvis
- Grade III: Reflux into the ureter and pelvis with mild to moderate tortuosity of both
- Grade IV: Reflux grade III plus complete obliteration of the caliceal fornices
- Grade V: Reflux into the ureter, pelvis, and calices with tortuosity of the ureter and gross dilation of the pelvis and calices with visible papillary impressions (Fig. 22.43)

High-grade reflux, often referred to as the "back-pressure type," is most frequently the type associated with cortical scars.

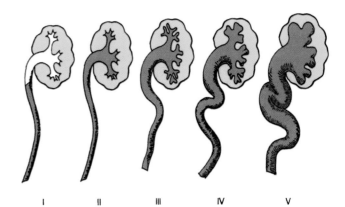

**Figure 22.43** Grades of VUR. (modified from medical versus surgical treatment of primary vesicoureteral reflux: A prospective international reflux study in children. J Urol 1981;125:277–283.)

## Pathology

### Gross Pathology and Light Microscopy

Gross pathology of severe congenital VUR is a frequent fetal autopsy finding. In bilateral VUR, the ureters are dilated often to their full length, connecting to either normal or malformed kidneys. An example of bilateral VUR in a female fetus is shown in Figure 22.44. Kidneys are normally lobulated, with mild hydronephrosis. The urinary bladder is dilated. Upon dissection, no anatomic obstruction was found. In other cases, ureters may be tortuous or have a thick, muscular wall. The kidneys are usually smaller than normal, segmentally or diffusely scarred, or cystic (Fig. 22.45). Bladder outlet obstruction, valves in the posterior urethra, bladder diverticula, ureteroceles (paraureteric saccules), and duplicate ureters are the most common concurrent entities (listed in Table 22.5). An example

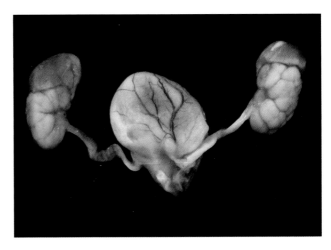

**Figure 22.44** Bilateral vesicoureteral reflux; 18-week female fetus with dilation of ureters and mild hydronephrosis. The kidneys are normally lobulated, with no evidence of dysplasia.

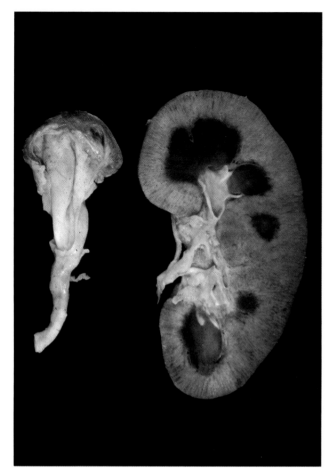

**Figure 22.45**   Unilateral reflux; 8-month-old girl with hypoplastic (pea size) left kidney and ipsilateral reflux caused by stenotic posterior urethral valve. The contralateral kidney appears grossly normal with no evidence of hydronephrosis.

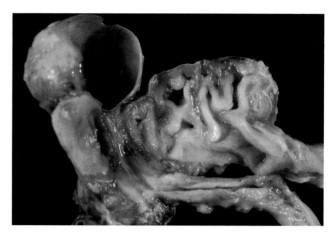

**Figure 22.46**   Dysplastic kidney is grossly cystic and atrophic. Notice the double ureters.

of VUR-associated with duplicate ureters in shown in Figure 22.46. Histologically, these grossly malformed kidneys or atrophic small kidneys are almost always dysplastic. Renal dysplasia typically consists of immature glomeruli and collecting ducts, with the latter encircled in smooth muscle whorls known as fibromuscular collars (Fig. 22.47). Islands of cartilage are found in about one third of renal dysplasias (for details on renal dysplasia, see Chapter 26).

An alternative pattern of RN consists of renal cortical scars sharply demarcated from adjacent normal parenchyma. Scars contain sclerotic glomeruli, atrophic tubules, and chronic inflammatory cells but lack the changes of renal dysplasia. Radiologically, these scars may look very similar to renal dysplasia; therefore the term *renal scarring* is used indiscriminately by clinicians to describe both. Histology in primary and secondary RN is similar, and it should be noted that there is often an overlap with obstructive nephropathy. Clinical and animal studies

---

### TABLE 22.5
## ETIOLOGY OF REFLUX NEPHROPATHY

Primary
   Lateral ectopia of the ureter
   Dysfunctional elimination syndrome

Secondary
   Posterior urethral valves
   Bladder diverticula
   Ureteroceles
   Duplicate ureters
   Neuropathic bladder
   Chronic infection that involves the vesicoureteral junction
   Transplant kidney

Physiologic
   Pregnancy

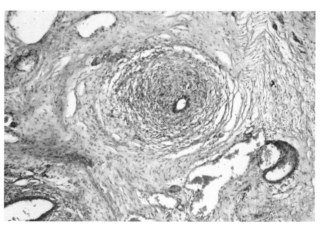

**Figure 22.47**   Renal dysplasia in reflux. Primitive ducts encircled by fibromuscular collars are characteristic of renal dysplasia. (H&E; ×400.) Islands of cartilage in other areas were also present (not shown).

reveal that renal scarring develops in the areas where intrarenal urine reflux occurs, which can be visualized radiologically by flattened or irregular papillae. The role of superimposed UTI on the pathogenesis of VUR scarring has been debated extensively. Most investigators to date agree that repeated UTIs impose a significant risk and determine prognosis postnatally, but there is still ambiguity as to how best to explain scarring and occasionally progressive disease in children who have no history of documented infection but are thought to have sterile reflux. Histology of the vesicoureteral valve is very rarely examined in routine pathologic evaluation. In a detailed study of 27 patients who had documented VUR prior to surgery, resected VUJ valves were serially sectioned and examined histologically. Fifteen of 27 valves were found to have either a single or a double flap. The muscle of the unobstructed segment of ureter distal to the valve appeared normal, in contrast to a hypertrophic muscle of the obstructed proximal segment (424). Evaluation of the anatomy of the vesicoureteral valve is best done radiologically. Congenital malimplantation, lateral ectopias of the ureteral orifice, short or duplicate ureters, and abnormal shape and diameter of the ureteral orifice may be identified in association with various grades of reflux. In about 4% of VUR, the ureteral orifice appears normal.

Beyond the two most common pathologic patterns of renal dysplasia and cortical atrophy without dysplasia, there are additional clinically and or pathologically distinct types of reflux. These include the so-called Ask-Upmark kidney (segmental renal atrophy with urine reflux), hereditary reflux, reflux in the allograft kidney, glomerulonephritis-associated with reflux, sterile reflux, and reflux in pregnant women.

## Distinct Types of Reflux

### Ask-Upmark Kidney

In 1929 Eric Ask-Upmark first described a renal abnormality characterized by segmental atrophy in six patients who presented with malignant hypertension. Seventy-five years later, more than 175 cases have been reported in the literature. Ask-Upmark kidney may be unilateral or bilateral, found both in children and adults, and occur in males and females, with a preponderance for women (425–430). We have seen four unreported cases in the last 10 years. Three were girls. Grossly, the affected kidney was reduced in size, with one or more sharply separated hypoplastic segments overlying elongated and dilated calices. Histologically, the thin segment contains atrophic tubules with thyroidization, thick vessels, and no glomeruli (Fig. 22.48A). Absence of glomeruli is characteristic and contrasts with the sclerotic glomeruli seen in other types of cortical atrophy. Severe hypertension is seen in most children and 60% of adults

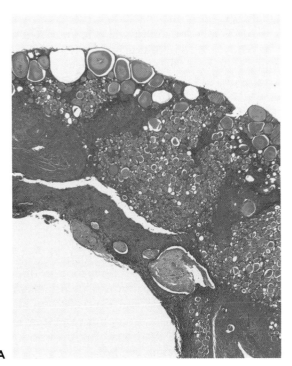

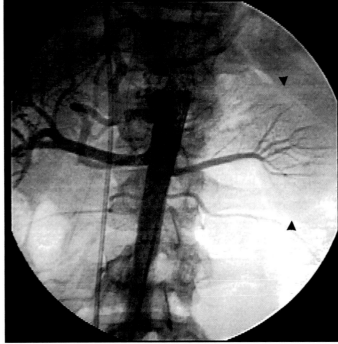

**Figure 22.48** Ask-Upmark kidney from a 6-year-old girl. **A:** The renal cortex is thin above dilated calix. The scar consists of atrophic tubules with thyroidization and chronic inflammatory cells. There are no glomeruli within the scarred area. (H&E; ×100.) **B:** Renal artery angiography shows small left kidney without renal artery stenosis. The contralateral right kidney was intact.

and may be the presenting symptom. Other symptoms include recurrent UTI, proteinuria, or decreased renal function (425). Ask-Upmark kidney was originally described as a congenital anomaly, but most investigators now consider segmental atrophy to be secondary to parenchymal pressure owing to reflux of urine and infection (428). Others have shown that the atrophic segment is irrigated by a small renal artery branch, and therefore the lesion is attributed to a developmental defect of the renal vasculature (427). The debate on whether the kidney "scar" is caused by urine backflow and superimposed inflammation or by a vascular anomaly started with early investigators, who argued that maldevelopment of the kidney was unlikely to be caused by inflammatory destruction and postulated an ischemic process. Subsequent studies demonstrated that some patients with Ask-Upmark kidney had renin-dependent hypertension, substantiating the ischemic hypothesis. In fact, many of the recent reports demonstrate segmental renal artery stenosis, which occurs either as an isolated renal finding or with extrarenal vascular aneurysms (427,430). The precise origin and role of renin in this form of hypertension are still under investigation. Some have suggested that the hypoplastic areas may not release renin because of the absence of glomeruli and juxtaglomerular cells and that increased plasma renin may be derived by adjacent tissue. However, it should be noted that many patients have normal plasma renin, and no evidence of arterial stenosis. For example, in the case depicted in Figure 22.48B, angiography shows a small left kidney but no evidence of renal artery stenosis. Plasma renin was normal in this patient. Nonetheless, nephrectomy typically cures hypertension.

The natural history of segmental hypoplasia in Ask-Upmark kidney is little known. In a study of nine children that initially had normally functioning kidneys, scars were evaluated radiographically and histologically (428). Mean time from discovery of reflux to renal scar was 6.1 years, and the onset of hypertension in six patients was 7.8 years. Resected kidneys had lobar atrophy, atrophic tubules, and segmental loss of nephrons. These findings reveal that renal scarring in Ask-Upmark kidney is a progressive as opposed to a static lesion, despite correction of the reflux or prevention of UTI, suggesting optimization of clinical management and timing for surgical intervention. Contralateral or extrarenal vascular anomalies should be ruled out. An association with contralateral fibromuscular dysplasia of the renal artery has also been reported (430).

Because the Ask-Upmark entity may have overlapping angiography with isolated stenosis of the renal artery or its branches and renin-dependent hypertension, some cases may have been interpreted solely on the finding of stenosis. For example, in a case report of an infant with reflux, emphasis was placed on the stenotic arterial segment associated with severe hypertension. Parenchymal scarring was present, but the connection to the entity of Ask-Upmark was not made (431).

### Hereditary Reflux

The high frequency of reflux in siblings and ureteral or renal anomalies in first degree relatives of patients with reflux implies that genetic factors may play important roles in this disease. For example, there is familial occurrence of double ureters, and nearly 500 families with reflux and affected members in three to four generations have been described worldwide (432,433). Very few of these families had genetic analysis. Modes of inheritance include autosomal dominant, X-linked, and polygenetic inheritance. One study showed a balanced translocation in chromosome 6p, another showed association with human leukocyte antigen types, and a third reported an association of reflux with PAX2 mutations (434–436). The PAX2 gene is located in chromosome 10q. Mutations of PAX2 cause the renal-coloboma syndrome (optic nerve coloboma, renal anomalies, and VUR) (436). In a study of seven European families, a dominant mode of inheritance was found, with more women than men affected. Vesicoureteral reflux in these families mapped on chromosome 1, but specific mutations were not identified (437). No mutations in 6p or 10q, where PAX2 is located, were found in these families either. The greater severity in males is proposed to be caused by a linkage-disequilibrium phenomenon or an X-linked transmission pattern.

Reflux in the spectrum of renal tract malformations has been linked to gene mutations of the angiotensin II receptor type 2 (AT2) located on Xq, which in knock-out mice induces VUR. A 1332G transition in the AT2 receptor gene was found in primary obstructive megaureter and ureteropelvic junction (UPJ) obstruction but not in humans with primary VUR (438). The authors proposed that whereas AT2 is crucial for the normal development of the ureter, it does not appear to contribute to the processes that lead to VUR, which they consider primarily an abnormality in the bladder trigone. Similarly, screening of families for uroplakin III, a gene associated with abnormal ureteral orifice in mice revealed no mutations in humans (439,440). It was concluded that such mutations may be lethal in humans. The BMP4 and FOXC1 genes are two other genes that in mice are shown to participate in ureter morphogenesis. Screening for mutations in BMP4 and FOXC1 genes in humans so far has identified a mutation in three of seven patients with complex malformations including VUR (441). Vesicoureteral reflux is also associated with heritable syndromes such as Hirschsprung's disease, Apert's syndrome, branchiootorenal syndrome, Townes-Brocks syndrome, and renal-coloboma syndrome, suggesting that mutations in diverse genes may give rise to the same clinical condition (VUR and RN) and that interaction with more than one gene may be required (442,443). In humans, VUR is highly likely to be a genetically heterogeneous entity.

## Reflux in the Allograft Kidney

Allograft kidneys are not known to be associated with RN. The ureter is usually simply implanted by a new ureterocystostomy. The question was recently examined in 146 consecutive allograft nephrectomies (444). Four adult cases were identified in this population that had characteristic sharply demarcated cortical scars with tubular thyroidization, global glomerulosclerosis, and significant chronic inflammation. All four patients had recurrent infection, and two were radiologically confirmed using dimercaptosuccinic acid (DMSA) scans. Donor kidneys at the time of implantation were normal; therefore, these scars were attributed to intrarenal reflux in the allograft kidney. In this series, at least one of four patients had hilar FSGS. Two children transplanted for renal dysplasia were retrospectively found to have sustained at least one UTI, but one (a boy) had not been on antibiotic prophylaxis for more than 3 years, while the second (a girl) was on chemoprophylaxis for more than 3 years after her infections. Both had evidence of VUR in the transplanted kidney, and DMSA scan and cystogram showed de novo reflux.

## Sterile Reflux

Sterile reflux was described by Hodson and Edwards in 1960 (445). They performed their studies in the multipapillary piglet model and based their conclusions on radiologic evidence of renal scarring induced by sterile reflux. Subsequently, Ransley and Risdon argued against a role for sterile reflux in the same model, because they found that scarring occurred only when infection was present (423). It was also shown that children with reflux in utero and renal scarring at birth do not develop new scars unless infections intervene. Others argue that the absence of documented infection in humans is not proof of absence of infection, and it is highly likely that brief periods of infection would never be documented. Nonetheless, the question of whether VUR without infection may cause renal damage does not appear to have been completely resolved to this day, perhaps because VUR is not always easily demonstrable in children and/or because of how clinicians worldwide may define VUR. Renal biopsies from children presumed to have sterile reflux are unlikely to be performed, unless reflux is complicated by significant proteinuria. In the latter case, biopsy may reveal minimal inflammation, multifocal interstitial fibrosis, and tubular atrophy with globally or segmentally sclerotic glomeruli (Fig. 22.49). If VUR, including sterile reflux, presents with nephrotic syndrome, it is prudent to consider secondary FSGS, known as hyperfiltration FSGS caused by reflux.

## Reflux in Pregnancy

The existence of physiologic reflux in normal individuals, for example, pregnant women, has been investigated and thought to be caused by hydrodynamic changes. Most in-

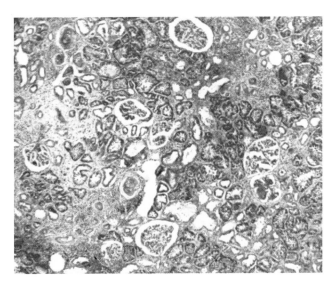

**Figure 22.49** Wedge biopsy from a 6-year-old girl with known VUR and negative UTI history who presented with nephrotic syndrome. The renal cortex has minute but multifocal interstitial fibrosis. Atrophic tubules and globally sclerosed glomeruli are noted. Focal segmental glomerulosclerosis is present in a minority of glomeruli, suggestive of hyperfiltration FSGS. (Trichrome stain; ×20.)

vestigators currently conclude that reflux does not occur in normal individuals.

During pregnancy, physiologic hormonal changes may alter ureteral peristalsis and tortuosity and cause lateral displacement of the intravesical portion of the ureter by the gravid uterus and urine reflux. Asymptomatic bacteriuria affects 7% of pregnant women, and pyelonephritis is reported in as many as 20% to 40%. Women with pre-existing reflux and a history of childhood UTIs are at higher risk for developing symptomatic bacteriuria and pyelonephritis versus those without reflux, and they have an increased risk of fetal loss. In a series of 345 pregnancies, 137 women had reflux (about 40%) (446). Twelve percent of these had fetal loss, and 39% had maternal complications with increased serum creatinine beyond 1.2 mg/dL. The risk was related to renal scarring, while women with VUR and no scars had insignificant complications. These studies suggest that in girls with reflux and identifiable renal scars in childhood, surgical repair during adolescence may be a good option.

## Reflux and Proteinuria

Occasionally, patients with VUR will develop glomerular proteinuria. Renal biopsy may reveal FSGS, and the question may be whether this is coincidental or a consequence of reflux. A histologic review of 86 pediatric nephrectomy specimens from patients with VUR found perihilar FSGS in 20% (447). The controls in this study were 40 hypoplastic kidneys and 70 nephrectomy specimens, none of which had FSGS. Whether 20% represents a true frequency of FSGS in VUR is difficult to answer; however, multiple clinical and experimental studies in the 1970s and 1980s documented the role of reflux in glomerulosclerosis (448). Recently, a Japanese study revealed a moderate increase in glomerular capillary length in children with VUR and FSGS that had good prognosis and a threefold increase in capillary length in cases with poor prognosis, suggesting that marked lengthening of glomerular capillaries in young patients with VUR is a compensatory reaction to hyperfiltration. Tuft adhesions to Bowman's capsule and podocyte detachment were primarily found in patients with poor prognosis (449). (Focal segmental glomerulosclerosis is discussed in Chapter 5.)

## Pathogenesis

Study of VUR pathogenesis in the last 20 years has shifted from clinical and experimentally induced VUR in animals to molecular genetic studies in genetically engineered mice and co-cultures of metanephric mesenchyme and ureteral bud tissue. Embryogenesis of the ureter cannot be separated from kidney development, but this discussion will focus on the development of the ureter, its orifice, and the detrusor muscle at the trigone (450–455).

## Development of the Ureter

The ureter is a derivative of the ureteric bud that in the human embryo develops at about 5 weeks of gestation from the base of the mesonephric (Wolffian) duct. The ureters are initially connected to the bladder via the Wolffian duct, but prior to sexual differentiation the ureteral orifices undergo maturation, detach from the Wolffian duct, and establish direct connection with the bladder (Fig. 22.50). The "ureteric bud" arises from its distal end of the Wolffian duct as an unbranched diverticulum. Normally, only one ureteric bud forms from each Wolffian duct, thought to be restrained by lateral inhibition. These crucial first steps are mediated by complex signaling involving at least five important genes: PAX2, cRET, GDNF (glial-derived nerve factor), WT1, and EYA-1 (451,452). PAX2 is highly expressed in the mouse mesonephric mesenchyme and thought to be responsible for development of the mesonephric duct. Mice with homozygous PAX2 null mutation lack ureters, kidneys, and a genital tract, and heterozygous mice have small kidneys. cRET is a tyrosine kinase receptor that first appears in the pre-bud phase in wild type mice. Later, cRET is expressed at the tip of the ureteric bud. In PAX2 mutant mice, the caudal end of the Wolffian duct does not develop and cRET is absent. As soon as the ureteric bud forms, it invades the surrounding mass of mesenchymal cells, and epithelial components start forming simultaneously with induced dichotomous branching of the ureteric buds. Ureteric bud outgrowth requires WT1 expressed by the metanephric mesenchyme. Absence of WT1 results in renal agenesis. Ureteric buds from cRET –/– null mice fail to branch when co-cultured with metanephric mesenchyme (blastema). However, branching is restored

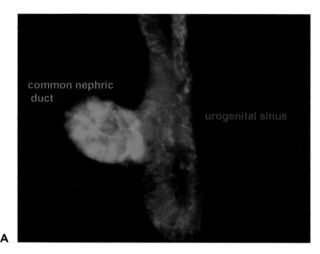

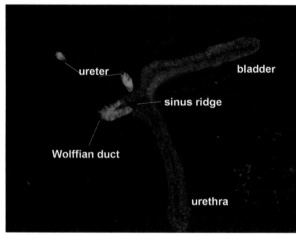

**Figure 22.50** Development of the ureter in the Hoxb7-Gfp mouse that expresses green fluorescence protein (Gfp) in excretory duct epithelia. **A:** E11 mouse: the common nephric duct (stained green with Gfp) appears as a short extension of mesenchymal cells connected to the early urogenital sinus (stained red with E-cadherin). **B:** E13 mouse. A normal ureter is initially connected to the Wolffian duct (urothelium, ureter, and Wolffian duct are stained green with Gfp). As formation of the bladder proceeds, the ureter separates. The figure illustrates the close interaction between the Wolffian duct, the ureter, and the sinus ridge, the raised portion of the dorsal urogenital sinus where insertion of the ureter takes place (Courtesy of Cathy Mendelsohn, Columbia University, New York.)

by GDNF and/or a transcription factor expressed in the mesenchyme called EYA-1, which is thought to drive GDNF expression. As the ureteric bud continues to branch many more molecules coordinate proper contact with the mesenchyme and new nephrons form at the tip of the branching segments. These molecules bring both inductive and inhibitory signals and include WNT-11, which regulates GDNF; EMX-2; members of the transforming growth factor β (TGFβ) superfamily, such as TGFβ1; bone morphogenetic protein 2 (BMP2), and bone morphgenetic protein 4 (BMP4). BMP4 is highly expressed in the mesenchyme surrounding the trunk and major branches of the ureteric bud, but it is not expressed at the periphery. Mice with null BMP4 mutations develop duplicate ureters and

VUJ obstruction as well as hypodysplastic kidneys. BMP4 is thus thought to facilitate proper ureteric bud branching and inhibit ectopic or duplicate ureters.

Other genes that assist in the process are those involved in program cell death, for example, Bcl-2 and AT2 (452). In vivo and in vitro studies have shown that AT2 promotes apoptosis of the undifferentiated cells that surround the branching ureteric bud. Mice with AT2 null mutations develop VUR and duplicate ureters associated with renal malformation. It is proposed that AT2 mutation leads to inappropriate apoptosis in the mesenchyme and misguided caudal or lateral ectopias of the ureteric bud, that cause VUR. These studies are influenced by the hypothesis known as the "bud theory" proposed by Mackie and Stephens, which postulated that VUR may be caused by ectopic launching of the ureteric bud and loss of the right tract, which would allow the developing ureter to enter correctly into the corner of the bladder base, the trigone (452). By day 33 of gestation in humans, the Wolffian duct below the ureteric bud dilates and becomes the common excretory duct (urethra). The origin of the ureteric bud enters directly into the bladder by day 37, to become the ureteric orifice. Thereafter, the orifices migrate cranially and laterally to later be absorbed in the bladder at the primitive trigone.

The bud theory assumes that a single embryonic mistake may explain both VUR and associated renal malformations, collectively called CACUT (congenital anomalies of the kidney and the urinary tract). Summarizing the fact that anomalies such as duplex ureters, incompetent vesicoureteral orifice, and anomalies of the bladder and urethral valves are often accompanied by hypoplastic and dysplastic kidneys and the fact that these anomalies have a familial pattern of incomplete or complete penetrance, Ichikawa et al speculated that the spectrum of CACUT may have a common pathogenesis (452).

## Development of the Bladder Trigone

The portion of the ureteric bud that lies outside the kidney will become the ureter. Distal ureters join the bladder at the trigone, defined as the triangular region of the mucosa and muscular wall of the bladder that includes the ureteral orifice. The primitive trigone forms at about 4 weeks of gestation, but ureter development will continue for weeks; between 10 and 14 weeks of gestation the ureter becomes a muscular tube. During the end of this process, the submucosal course into the bladder begins.

There is little known of the molecular signaling that underlines the initial process of the trigone, which precedes vesicoureteral valve formation. A role for retinoic acid receptors a or b (RARa, RARb) and vitamin A is suggested from work in RARa -/- and RARb -/- null mice that develop incorrectly positioned distal ureters, hydronephrosis, and megaureters. Vitamin A regulates branching morphogenesis through the tyrosine kinase receptor RET, which, as

mentioned earlier, is important for urinary bladder branching. In RARa -/- and RARb -/- mice, vitamin A and RET mediate displacement of the urinary bladder by controlling epithelial expansion of the base of the Wolffian ducts. It is proposed that Vitamin A and cRET signaling modulate the formation of the "trigonal wedge" (453). Independent studies in the HoxB7/RET transgenic mouse have confirmed the significance of cRET in distal ureter morphogenesis (454). Thirty percent of these mice that overexpress RET have VUR at postnatal day 1 and a shorter intravesical portion of the ureter compared to wild type mice. Ureters are grossly dilated and kidneys are small.

In contrast to the remainder of the bladder that derives from ectoderm (epithelial and mesenchymal cells of the urogenital sinus), the trigone is thought to derive from precursors of the mesoderm via the mesonephric duct and epithelial cells of the ureteric bud. Tissue recombination experiments show that stromal-epithelial interactions underlie formation of the trigone, but it is not yet clear which precise cell types are required for proper induction (455). The processes underscoring distal ureter and trigone development continue to be investigated by developmental biologists, providing fascinating and continuously advancing insights that hold great promise to ultimately answer clinically important questions.

## Clinical Management, Prognosis, and Therapy

The main issues in the clinical management of patients with VUR is the avoidance of new renal scarring. The cornerstone of therapy has traditionally consisted of long-term antibacterial prophylaxis, and determination of the need for surgery. Recent studies question the progressive nature of reflux nephropathy and therefore the need for either prophylactic antibiotics or surgery.

### Reflux and Urinary Tract Infections

The frequent association of RN with UTIs has generated much discussion and numerous publications regarding the overall contribution of infection to progressive renal disease and how best to select patients that need prophylaxis and long-term management. About 30% to 60% of children who present with UTIs have VUR, but the true incidence of reflux in asymptomatic children is lower than 1%. Reflux nephropathy is reportedly responsible for 5% to 40% of end-stage renal disease (ESRD) in children less than 16 years of age and 5% to 20% of ESRD in adults under 50 years of age (416). These numbers are difficult to interpret, as often there is not enough information provided to distinguish the contribution of true pyelonephritis. However, in a long-term study of 226 adults, in which the outcome of reflux was studied 10 to 41 years after initial diagnosis, 63% remained free of UTI. Reflux persisted in 63% and had resolved in 69% of 169 medically treated children (456). About 7.5% of adults had hypertension meriting treatment and/or increased serum creatinine. Sixteen (8%) had scarred kidneys. Progressive kidney disease was predictable based on the type of scars and clinical presentation in childhood. Renal growth was not affected by severity of initial reflux and/or persistence of VUR. No new scars developed after puberty. Those with VUR who were managed carefully during childhood had good prognoses. Adults with extensive scarring in childhood and/or hypertension had worse prognoses. The greatest proportion of children in this study were patients with moderate to severe congenital reflux (grades III to V). Only 13 patients had acquired disease. The study revealed that even moderately severe reflux in the absence of obstructive hydronephrosis and chronic intrarenal reflux had a good prognosis. The study also revealed that girls had more frequent UTI and less severe reflux, compared to boys, who tended to have severe bilateral reflux. Similar differences between reflux in boys and girls were reported by the Italian Registry on Reflux, which recognizes two distinct long-term prognostic categories (457): (a) progressive disease for boys with severe reflux, and (b) milder disease in girls, who tend to have repeated UTIs.

Overall, it appears that a relatively small number of children with VUR have concomitant infection, ranging between 7.5% and 12%. In most cases (58%), reflux resolves with medical management (458). Persistence of reflux is directly related to the grade of reflux at the time of initial diagnosis. Severity of disease depends on laterality (unilateral versus bilateral). Antibiotics are recommended in children with reflux that fails to resolve (459). In high-grade reflux (grade V and above) medical management has been less successful than surgery (460). However, the literature is unclear on whether surgery prevents ESRD in severe cases (461). It is concluded that most children with ESRD have severe disease in infancy, and no surgery or medical management can prevent ultimate progression. Reflux-associated ESRD accounts for about 25% of all children with ESRD, but one must not lose sight of the fact that most children diagnosed with reflux have a good prognosis and rarely need surgical intervention or even antibiotic prophylaxis (458–462).

The perplexing role of infection as a diminishing risk of acute renal scarring after infancy has also been addressed in experimental models using piglets and adult pigs subjected to experimental reflux with *E. coli*–infected urine. Both piglets and adult pigs that sustained persistent urine infections for 3 weeks developed parenchymal renal scars, supporting the theory that kidney maturation does not prevent scarring, as was previously thought.

In summary, it seems that children who sustain scars in infancy have an inherent susceptibility and are born with risk factors that allow them to develop scars when very young. O'Donnell's review on the aforementioned issues, which are of great interest to the urology and pediatric nephrology community, gives an account of the reflux literature that spans two centuries and has seen many concepts originally thought true fade away in the light of new discoveries (418), including the fallacy that RN is rare. It is not. Second, it was believed that reflux was a progressive disease and always bilateral. In reality, only very severe congenital reflux is progressive, often in association with other urogenital anomalies and renal dysplasia. Unilateral and mild or moderate VUR in children is, rather, regressive instead of progressive.

## HYDRONEPHROSIS AND OBSTRUCTIVE NEPHROPATHY

*Hydronephrosis* describes pelvic dilation caused by physical blockage of urine flow and back pressure of accumulated urine that distends the pelvis and or the calices secondary to obstruction. In contrast to reflux nephropathy (RN), which is defined as reversal of urine flow mainly because of incompetent vesicoureteral junction (VUJ), congenital or acquired urine flow obstruction may be functional or physical at any level along the length of the ureter or at the ureteropelvic junction (UPJ). A narrow UPJ may occur as an isolated defect or coexist with stenotic posterior urethral valves, incompetent VUJ, and duplicate or crossed ureters. Ureteropelvic junction obstruction is the most common cause of hydronephrosis in children. Other moieties in children or adults (Table 22.6) may include ureteral diaphragms (false valves); polyps in the renal pelvis and/or renal stones; tumors derived from transitional epithelium anywhere in the genitourinary system; inflammation, such as ureteritis, urethritis, and prostatitis; pregnancy; or spinal cord damage (neurogenic bladder paralysis). Hydronephrosis may be unilateral or bilateral, complete or incomplete, and occasionally functional and not physical in nature. If acute obstruction is relieved (for example, stone removal), recovery is complete. If obstruction is sustained for long time periods, it leads to compression

| TABLE 22.6 |
| --- |
| **ETIOLOGY OF OBSTRUCTIVE NEPHROPATHY** |
| Ureteropelvic junction obstruction |
| Fibroepithelial polyps in pelvis or ureter |
| Ureteral valves |
| Bladder outlet obstruction |
| Posterior urethral valves |
| Neurogenic bladder obstruction |
| Bladder tumors, benign or malignant retroperitoneal fibrosis |
| Prostatitis |
| Ureteritis |
| Granulomas abscesses |
| Stones |
| Pregnancy |

of the pelvis, calices, and renal cortex. The damage to the kidney when this happens is referred to as obstructive nephropathy.

## Ureteropelvic Junction Obstruction

### Incidence, Diagnosis, and Clinical Presentation

The incidence of UPJ obstruction is estimated to be 1 in 500 fetuses (463). Most children with UPJ obstruction are now diagnosed by maternal ultrasound. Excretory urography was one of the tests to evaluate obstructive nephropathy postnatally but is rarely used today. Nuclear scanning in addition to ultrasound is useful in assessing renal function and washout of urine from the kidney. Most reports find UPJ obstruction more commonly in boys and on the left side. The most common presenting sign is pain followed by infection and hematuria. Hematuria after minor trauma is a classic presentation, but rupture of the kidney following forceful blunt trauma is known to happen. Repair of the ruptured kidney to salvage function may be attempted. About 10% of kidneys diagnosed with UPJ obstruction have poor function at presentation, and a nephrectomy is performed. Fifteen percent to 30% of children demonstrate UPJ obstruction in both kidneys. Hypertension accompanies severe UPJ obstruction in anecdotal reports, but there are no large series to confirm a clinical association between a severely obstructed kidney and hypertension.

### Gross Pathology and Histology

The normal renal pelvis is grossly funnel shaped and microscopically composed of an orderly arranged muscle layer and submucosal collagen. Kidneys with UPJ obstruction are invariably hydronephrotic. Above the narrow UPJ, only the renal pelvis may be dilated initially, which is thought to provide more compliance to the accumulating pressure and preserve function of the kidney (Fig. 22.51). In severe cases, the entire kidney becomes atrophic (Fig. 22.52). Histologically, early lesions show tubular dilation, followed by atrophy and fibrosis of the interstitium with apparent glomerulosclerosis. Inflammation is invariably present, but there are no grossly visible cysts. Presence of cystic lesions is suggestive of renal dysplasia developing on the grounds of congenital UPJ obstruction. At the time of pyeloplasty, tissue from obstructed UPJ examined histologically shows disarrayed smooth muscle fibers and chronic inflammation (Fig. 22.53). Smooth muscle abnormalities appear to be important in the pathogenesis of UPJ and were experimentally studied by inducing partial UPJ obstruction in the rabbit. Obstruction increases muscular thickness and the collagen-to-muscle ratio at this site (464). Reversal of partial obstruction normalizes the ratio. In summary, pelvic and calyceal dilatation are the predom-

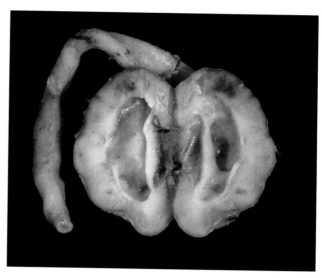

**Figure 22.51** Unilateral hydronephrosis in a 3-month boy with UPJ obstruction and posterior urethral valves. The pelvis is dilated, compressing the renal cortex. The ureter is dilated and has a thick muscular wall.

inant features in UPJ. Renal dysplasia may be present histologically, particularly in kidneys with multiple cysts.

Below the narrow UPJ opening, the ureter may and often does assume a normal caliber, except when other concurrent anomalies are present, for example, obstruction by posterior urethral valves. An example of UPJ associated with posterior urethral valves is shown in Fig. 22.54. Ureters appear thickened. The posterior urethra was not patent to probing.

The examples presented in the previous figures represent the most severe end of the spectrum in UPJ obstruction. However, mild or moderate obstruction is more frequent and of great interest to pediatric urologists, who have long sought objective criteria for surgical intervention. It appears that a worldwide consensus may have been reached

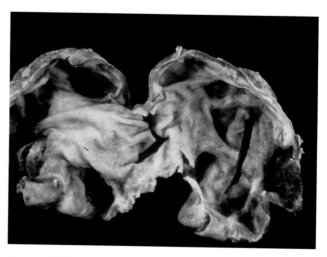

**Figure 22.52** Ureteropelvic junction obstruction with massive pelvic dilation and flattening of the caliceal system. The renal cortex is extremely thin.

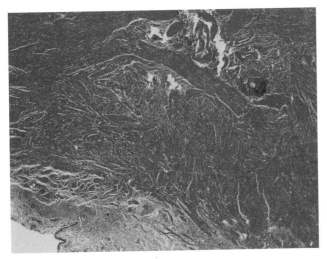

**Figure 22.53** Light microscopy of obstructed UPJ. The muscle layer is thick, and smooth muscle fibers are randomly arranged. (H&E; ×200.)

recently that defined a sonographically determined 10-mm dilation as the most reliable measurement of neonatal anteroposterior renal pelvis for predicting significant UPJ obstruction in the third trimester and at birth (465). Histologic assessment to provide the surgeon with histologic prognostic criteria at the time of pyeloplasty has been sought by some surgeons who procure renal tissue during pyeloplasty. Four histologic grades have been devised (466):

- Grade 1: No histologic abnormality
- Grade 2: Occasional glomerulosclerosis and minimal tubular atrophy

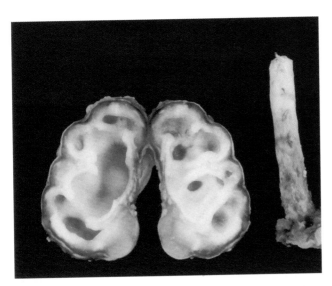

**Figure 22.54** Five-month-old boy with left kidney hydronephrosis because of posterior urethral valves. The renal pelvis and calices are both dilated, and the cortex is thin. The ureter appears short with a thick wall.

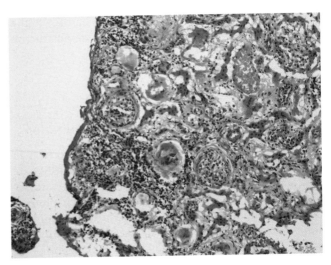

**Figure 22.55** This renal biopsy was submitted during a pyeloplasty and was performed to assess prognosis. There is mild fibrosis, mild chronic inflammation and tubular atrophy, and several globally sclerosed glomeruli. The findings are consistent with UPJ grade 3. (H&E; ×200.)

- Grade 3: Variable, but generally limited, glomerulosclerosis and moderate interstitial fibrosis and tubular atrophy
- Grade 4: Severe changes, including findings of renal dysplasia, more than 20% glomerulosclerosis, and extensive tubular atrophy and fibrosis

Grades 1 and 2 have excellent prognoses and correlate with good renal function assessed by radionuclide studies. Grade 3 has the poorest correlation, perhaps because biopsies in this category have great histologic variability. Grade 4 biopsies predict poor function. An example of Grade 3 histology in a patient with UPJ pyeloplasty is shown in Fig. 22.55.

## Differential Diagnosis

Occasionally, obstruction in the renal pelvis will not be caused by UPJ obstruction but by the presence of fibroepithelial polyps. These polyps are detected radiologically and appear as solitary, cylindric, sessile, or frondlike tumors (Fig. 22.56). Rare cases of multiple and bilateral lesions have been reported (467). Polyps are usually smaller than 5 cm and benign, but larger polyps with malignant transformation have been reported. It is thought that fibroepithelial polyps are either congenital or acquired lesions that develop as a result of chronic uroepithelial infection, inflammation, or obstruction. Similar to UPJ obstruction, the most common presenting signs and symptoms are hematuria and/or flank or abdominal pain. Urinary frequency, dysuria, and pyuria are less common findings. Fibroepithelial polyps can occur in newborns and adults older than 70 years but commonly present in the third to fourth decade, with a male/female ratio of 3:2. Approximately 62% of ureteral fibroepithelial polyps occur at the

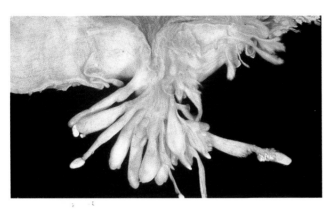

**Figure 22.56** Fibroepithelial polyp. The proximal ureter contains a polypoid intraluminal mass with multiple fingerlike projections.

ureteropelvic junction or upper ureter, but they may also be found in the lower ureter, the posterior urethra, or bladder. Polyps in the renal pelvis have a female preponderance and more commonly occur on the right side, in contrast to polyps in the proximal ureter, which have a predilection for men and the left side (467). Fibroepithelial polyps of the lower urinary tract occur most commonly in the posterior urethra and more often in children. Histologically, fibroepithelial polyps are dense fibrous or fibrovascular lesions covered by transitional epithelium.

Other benign lesions of the upper urinary tract that may enter the differential diagnosis of UPJ obstruction in adults include endometriomas, fibromas, leiomyomas, granulomas, neurofibromas, hemangiomas, and lymphangiomas.

Hydronephrosis may also be caused by ureteral valves (Fig. 22.57). These appear as translucent membranes and are thought to be embryonic remnants of incomplete recanalization of the ureter. In human 28- to 41-week embryos, during normal UPJ and proximal ureter development, ureters undergo temporary luminal obstruction,

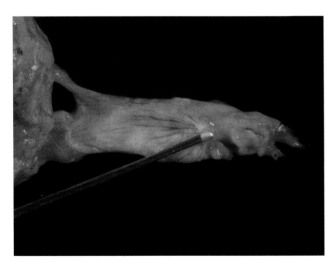

**Figure 22.57** Ureteral valve in the midportion of the ureter, from a 1-year-old girl with multicystic dysplastic right kidney.

which subsequently resolves with recanalization of the ureter (468). At 35 weeks, the entire length of the ureter is patent, while the cloaca is imperforate at this time, presumably to facilitate withdrawal of mesonephric urine. Between 37 and 47 days' gestation, a membrane temporarily occludes the junction between the ureter and bladder, and the ureter becomes occluded through its entire length. The recanalization process appears to begin in the middle third of the ureter and, temporarily, it seems related to the longitudinal growth of the ureter. These processes and muscularization of the ureter are not entirely understood. Muscularization is discontinuous and multicentric, appearing to be induced by metanephric urine production. This complicated path to ureter maturation seems to cause incomplete resolution of temporary physiologic obstruction in individuals with ureteral valves.

## Pathogenesis

The UPJ forms in utero at about 18 weeks' gestation. During the perinatal period, the kidney becomes the only organ for nitrogenous waste removal and increases its urine production by about 50-fold. The renal pelvis develops rapidly then to accommodate the increased demand for urine removal by acquiring smooth muscle layers that provide adequate structural support and contractibility. Studies in mice show that the funnel-shaped renal pelvis starts developing right after birth. In wild type mice, the UPJ is situated outside of the kidney proper (Fig. 22.58A). In a recombinant mouse carrying a conditional null mutation for calcineurin b isoform 1 (Cnb1), the PAX3-Cre-Cnb1 recombinant mouse, calcineurin function was deleted selectively in mesenchyme and smooth muscle cells of the developing kidney (469). Mutant mice have hydronephrosis and a flat, not a funnel-shaped, UPJ and lack the muscular renal pelvic extension. The UPJ is still tucked in the hilum (Fig. 22.58B). The funnel-shaped pelvis fails to develop in the mutants at any age. Examination of cell proliferation in the renal pelvic wall reveals a decrease in proliferation rate in the mesenchyme, where the smooth muscle cells and their progenitors reside. This study demonstrates that calcineurin is required for the proliferation of the urinary tract mesenchymal cells for the proper formation of the renal pelvis. Disruption of calcineurin function in these structures can result in malformation of the renal pelvis and ureter, leading to defective pyeloureteral peristalsis and obstructive nephropathy. At day 12, these mice are obviously hydronephrotic, and renal parenchyma has features of obstructive nephropathy. The study is also an example of functional obstruction and emphasizes the role of the UPJ as a pelvic "pacemaker" for peristaltic movement of the ureter (470).

Pathogenesis of obstructive nephropathy has for many decades been studied by experimental ureteral ligation in rodents, marsupials, and mammals (471). Histopathologic

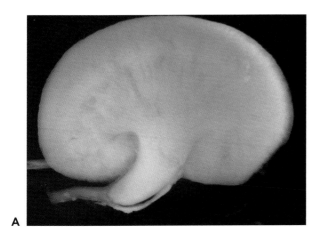
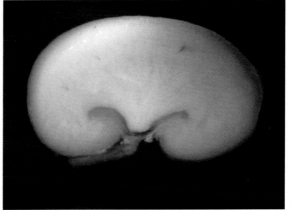

**Figure 22.58** Control and mutant calcineurin b isoform 1 (Cnb1) mouse. **A:** UPJ in the wild type mouse is funnel-shaped. **B:** Mutant mouse has UPJ still tucked in the renal hilum 12 days after birth. The model demonstrates that calcineurin b1 is important in muscle development of the UPJ. (Courtesy of Feng Chen, PhD, Washington University, St. Louis, Missouri.)

features of congenital obstructive nephropathy in experimental animals include tubular cell apoptosis, mesenchymal expansion and transformation to myocytes, infiltration of the renal interstitium by macrophages, and glomerular injury. The pathogenesis of obstructive nephropathy in adult animals may share some of the mechanisms seen in newborn animals, such as apoptosis, interstitial fibrosis, and glomerulosclerosis (472). Congenital obstruction is unique in that it disrupts active renal growth and causes renal maldevelopment. It will be discussed in detail in Chapter 26 in the section on pathogenesis of renal malformations. Beyond ureteral ligation, molecular pathogenesis in animals with spontaneous mutations that develop obstructive nephropathy—and more recently in genetically engineered mice—has shown complex interactions. Signaling molecules, including growth factors and cytokines that mediate tubular epithelial cell apoptosis, fibroblast proliferation and interstitial scarring and ultimately nephron loss are altered with obstruction (473–475). Because of certain overlap between studies in neonatal and adult animals, the diverse conditions encountered in obstructive nephropathy in adult humans, and limited space in this chapter, pathogenesis of obstructive nephropathy in adult rodents will not be discussed.

### Clinical Course and Prognosis

A significant 39% of infants with mild to moderate fetal pyelectasis may evolve to severe hydronephrosis. The converse is also true that severe fetal hydronephrosis can resolve with no long-term renal effect. Ultrasound is an excellent screening tool with high sensitivity and negative predictive value, thereby helping avoid unjustified surgical treatment and unnecessary follow-up in neonates with two negative ultrasound scans. Those who ultimately require surgery are now successfully treated in more than 90% to

95% of the cases (463). Minimally invasive procedures introduced in 1990 have further decreased postsurgical complications by approaching correction of the obstructed UPJ endoscopically or laparoscopically. However, not all cases recover renal function, and for these there is a great need to understand the pathogenesis of progression of obstructive nephropathy and to identify novel, perhaps medical, therapies. Underscoring these open questions is the uncertainty regarding which infants should undergo early pyeloplasty for UPJ obstruction. It appears that urologists may have come closer to agree on a threshold of 10 mm of pelvic diameter at birth or the third trimester (465). Even after successful surgery for congenital obstructive nephropathy, all patients should be followed for hypertension, proteinuria, or renal deterioration (463).

## HYPERCALCEMIA

Hypercalcemia is found in a large number of conditions (Table 22.7), many of which are associated with renal functional and morphologic lesions. With the exception of rare entities, such as familial hypocalciuric hypercalcemia, hypercalcemia almost always implies *hypercalciuria*—the excretion of excess quantities of calcium in the urine. This excretion, in turn, often leads to deposition of calcium within the renal parenchyma, termed *nephrocalcinosis*, or the development of renal stones, called *nephrolithiasis*, and sometimes both. Nephrocalcinosis can be seen on occasion without hypercalcemia, as, for example, in the case of secondary hyperparathyroidism, and as detailed in the section on nephrolithiasis. Hypercalcemia is only part of the story in renal stone disease. Nephrocalcinosis is often a more pernicious condition than nephrolithiasis since its presentation is nonspecific and may not be apparent until significant renal parenchymal damage and loss of function have

## TABLE 22.7
### CAUSES OF HYPERCALCEMIA

Primary hyperparathyroidism
Malignancy-related hypercalcemia
   Humoral
   Skeletal metastases
Genetic Causes
   Mutations of the calcium-sensing receptor
      Familial hypocalciuric hypercalcemia
      Neonatal severe hyperparathyroidism
   Williams' syndrome
   Bartter's syndrome
Infantile or neonatal conditions
   Iatrogenic
   Secondary hyperparathyroidism
   Subcutaneous fat necrosis of the newborn
Vitamin A or D excess
Sarcoidosis
Milk-alkali syndrome
Thyrotoxicosis
Immobilization
Medications

occurred. Renal stones come to the fore early and usually before any significant injury because of their propensity to cause pain.

## Clinical Features of Hypercalcemia

Symptoms vary depending on the degree and duration of hypercalcemia (476,477). With mild hypercalcemia, patients may be asymptomatic. Higher levels of serum calcium can cause nausea and vomiting. With acute elevations in serum calcium, the patient may show confusion and obtundation with extracellular volume contraction and renal failure, constituting a medical emergency. There may be problems with cardiac arrhythmias, depression and psychosis, and rarely, skeletal manifestations, such as osteitis fibrosa cystica. Defects in the ability to concentrate urine are perhaps the earliest manifestations, and indeed may be the only recognizable abnormality in asymptomatic patients whose hypercalcemia is incidentally recognized during examination for another problem. In acute hypercalcemia, as, for example, in multiple myeloma, the severity of renal insufficiency tends to parallel the degree of hypercalcemia and severity of the resulting dehydration (478). Chronic calcium nephropathy can present as interstitial nephritis, with polyuria, little proteinuria, and a bland urinary sediment. Hypercalcemia may be marked by various acid-base disorders, notably both proximal and distal renal tubular acidosis (479,480). There is also salt wasting (481), potassium (479) and magnesium (482,483) wasting, as well as aminoaciduria (484).

## Causes of Hypercalcemia

The causes of hypercalcemia are listed in Table 22.7. Hyperparathyroidism is the cause in approximately 55% of cases of hypercalcemia. Hypercalcemia associated with malignancy (humoral or osteolytic), accounting for approximately 35%, is the most important category in terms of clinical symptoms and numbers of affected patients. After malignancy, the incidence of conditions associated with hypercalcemia declines rapidly. Other causes such as vitamin toxicity, milk-alkali syndrome, granulomatous diseases, and drugs account for less than 10% of cases. In some cases, hypercalcemia is clearly owing to deossification of the skeleton, particularly in hyperparathyroidism and malignancy. Some conditions can be categorized as representing increased intestinal absorption of calcium. In other instances, however, the source of hypercalcemia is not clear.

## Primary Hyperparathyroidism

Primary hyperparathyroidism is characterized by spontaneous, unregulated oversecretion of parathyroid hormone. Benign adenomas (single gland or multiple gland involvement) are the underlying cause in 85%, hyperplasia in 15%, and carcinoma in less than 1% of cases. The prevalence of primary hyperparathyroidism is estimated to be 25 to 30 cases per 100,000 people in the general population (485,486). Women outnumber men 3:1, with a peak incidence during the fifth decade. In one study of postmenopausal women undergoing mammography, 2.1% were found to have hyperparathyroidism (487). The cause is usually sporadic, though primary hyperparathyroidism can also be found in some inherited syndromes, such as multiple endocrine neoplasia (MEN) 1 and 2, hyperparathyroidism-jaw tumor syndrome, and familial isolated hyperparathyroidism.

Patients with primary hyperparathyroidism are typically asymptomatic, with elevated serum calcium detected on routine screening. Serum calcium concentrations at the time of diagnosis are usually less than 1 mg/dL above normal. Nearly 75% of patients have no signs or symptoms attributable to the parathyroid abnormality. Bone, kidney, and other related changes are becoming rare. When primary hyperparathyroidism was initially described in the 1920s, patients typically were diagnosed with severe bone disease, *osteitis fibrosa cystica*, and pronounced hypercalcemia. These patients were rare then and are very rare today, particularly in developed countries (488,489).

### Clinical Features

In symptomatic cases, the clinical features of primary hyperparathyroidism include nonspecific symptoms owing to hypercalcemia such as thirst, polyuria, muscular weakness, and gastrointestinal symptoms such as constipation;

various manifestations of myocardial failure and renal impairment may also occur. More specific symptoms are related to passage of a stone and those referable to bony involvement. Classic bony involvement in severe hypercalcemia is characterized by pain and tenderness, with radiographic findings of osteitis fibrosa cystica, including subperiosteal resorption of the phalanges and fraying of the distal phalanges, occasionally with true cyst formation and the formation of brown tumors (490–492), although these florid manifestations of hyperparathyroidism are seldom seen since patients tend to be recognized on routine screening when they are still asymptomatic. Even mild asymptomatic hyperparathyroidism can be associated with an increased risk of fractures, however, with a prevalence as high as 5% (493,494). Bone resorption is most prominent in the distal third of the radius, whereas the cancellous bone of the lumbar spine is minimally reduced.

### Renal Function

Important functional renal manifestations of hyperparathyroidism include decreased glomerular filtration rate and abnormalities in tubular function leading to decreased concentrating ability. Stones remain the most common renal manifestation of primary hyperparathyroidism. Hypercalciuria is seen in approximately 40% of patients. Nephrocalcinosis also occurs, but the incidence is difficult to determine without biopsy.

### Physiology of Parathyroid Hormone

Parathyroid hormone (PTH) secretion by the parathyroid glands is regulated in a negative feedback fashion by serum concentrations of ionized calcium (496,497). Regulation of parathyroid hormone is through the calcium-sensing receptor located on the surface of parathyroid cells (498,499). PTH is produced as a preprohormone and is then proteolytically converted to the active 84 amino acid molecule (497,500,501). The intact hormone has a molecular weight (MW) of 9500, but it is rapidly metabolized in the liver, kidneys, and bone into two fragments. The smaller fragment (MW 3500) comes from the amino-terminal portion of the hormone and contains the biologic activity, whereas the larger, MW 5500 carboxy-terminal end has no activity. Both the intact hormone and the amino-terminal fragment are rapidly removed from the circulation, whereas the carboxy-terminal fragment has a longer half-life (90 minutes).

### Stone Disease in Primary Hyperparathyroidism

The action of PTH to increase intestinal absorption of calcium through vitamin D is of primary importance in the development of stones in hyperparathyroidism. Bone resorption is also a contributing factor. Hypercalciuria, which is the most clearly defined risk factor for nephrolithiasis in primary hyperparathyroidism (488,502), ensues secondarily to the hypercalcemia and increased filtered load of cal-

cium (503,504). Since PTH has a direct effect to increase reabsorption of filtered calcium in the renal tubule, enhanced tubular reabsorption contributes to the hypercalcemia.

### Diagnosis

The diagnosis of primary hyperparathyroidism is made by immunoassay of serum PTH levels with antibody against the full-length active molecule (peptides 1 to 84) (505,506). In the presence of hypercalcemia, elevated intact PTH confirms the diagnosis of primary hyperparathyroidism, whereas in hypercalcemia of malignancy, PTH levels are suppressed or within the normal range. In idiopathic hypercalciuria, serum calcium levels are normal and PTH levels are normal, but urinary excretion of calcium is very high. In familial hypocalciuric hypercalcemia (FHH), which can be confused with primary hyperparathyroidism, PTH can be elevated or normal, but calcium excretion is very low; FHH patients also typically present at a younger age and usually with a family history. Neonatal severe hyperparathyroidism is associated with extremely high serum calcium and PTH levels, at odds with the findings in other conditions associated with elevated PTH.

### Treatment and Outcome

In symptomatic patients, surgical removal of the parathyroid glands is recommended and highly successful. In many asymptomatic patients, however, medical management is recommended. A National Institutes of Health (NIH) consensus conference in 2002 (507) developed guidelines for surgery in asymptomatic hyperparathyroidism. Surgery should be considered only in patients with one of the following: serum calcium greater than 1 mg/dL above normal, calciuria greater than 400 mg/day, markedly reduced bone density (T score less than −2.5), creatinine clearance reduced below 30% of normal (age and sex matched), or the patient is younger than 50 years of age. In approximately 25% of patients followed conservatively over 10 years, the criteria will be met for surgical intervention, but in the remainder, all parameters remain unchanged (508).

### Pathology

A single parathyroid adenoma is responsible for hyperparathyroidism in 85 to 90% of patients (509,510). Adenomas occur in a single gland, vary in size from less than a gram to more than 100 g, and are made up most frequently of chief cells. Oncocytic/oxyphil cells, transitional cells, water–clear cells, or a mixture of cells make up the remainder of adenomas. A rim of normal parathyroid tissue admixed with adipose tissue cells can be seen compressed around the edge of the adenoma nodule. No adipose tissue is found within the adenoma. In very rare cases, multiple adenomas may be found. In parathyroid hyperplasia, there also is little or no adipose tissue, and any or all cell types normally found in parathyroid are present. Four-gland hyperplasia constitutes most of the cases.

Most show chief or oncocytic cell hyperplasia, diffuse or nodular (510), with nodular hyperplasia predominating in older patients. Water–clear cell hyperplasia has always been an infrequent finding, usually in cases with marked hypercalcemia (510). Parathyroid carcinomas make up a minority, less than 1%, of parathyroid lesions. Similar to adenomas, they may produce a mass, but unlike adenomas, it is generally ill-defined rather than a distinct nodule and shows infiltrative growth and capsular invasion. They are best recognized not simply from nuclear pleomorphism, which may be seen in benign lesions, but from the infiltrative growth pattern and evidence of metastasis.

In bone, the pathologic features of osteitis cystica fibrosa are very seldom seen today (511). In most patients with hyperparathyroidism, osteopenia is found, particularly in cortical bone in the forearm, hip, and spine.

Little information is available in the recent literature on histology of the kidney in hyperparathyroidism. The principal lesions described in older reports were those owing to nephrocalcinosis, such as might be seen with hypercalcemia of any cause, not simply that related to hyperparathyroidism (504). The most important renal lesion in hyperparathyroidism is development of renal stones and their consequences, such as infection and obstruction. Secondary pathology related to the obstructive nature of stones is described in the section on hydronephrosis.

## Hypercalcemia of Malignancy

### Humoral Hypercalcemia of Malignancy

Hypercalcemia in association with malignancy has long been recognized and was traditionally thought to be primarily related to bone erosion by metastatic deposits. However, many patients with malignancy are hypercalcemic in the absence of any significant bony metastases (512–514). In these cases, parathyroid hormone–related peptide (PTHrP) is responsible for the hypercalcemia. PTHrP has been isolated from tumors in patients with humoral hypercalcemia. It behaves very much like PTH; it interacts with parathyroid hormone receptors, leads to bone resorption, and causes a rise in urinary cyclic adenosine monophosphate (cAMP) that triggers increased tubular reabsorption of calcium (512,515,516). PTHrP shares structural homology with the amino terminus of PTH (residues 1 to 13), but thereafter it diverges (512,513) while retaining the ability to regulate calcium handling by binding to the same receptor as PTH (517). In addition to being found in tumors, PTHrP is also found in normal keratinocytes, lactating breast tissue, the brain, lung, parathyroid glands, and other sites (512,518,519).

Studies in patients with humoral hypercalcemia of malignancy reveal that the levels of PTHrP are elevated to an average of ten times normal values and are associated with a parallel rise in urinary cAMP excretion (512,520). The levels of PTHrP tend to broadly parallel the degree of hypercalcemia, but they may be elevated in some normocalcemic patients (514,521,522). By contrast, patients with hypercalcemia owing to osteolytic metastases, primary hyperparathyroidism, and various other causes have normal or only slightly raised levels of PTHrP (512).

Several types of tumors have been proven to produce PTHrP. Breast carcinoma has attracted the most attention (521–523). Levels tend to be greater in patients with bony metastases, and there is some evidence that PTHrP may predispose to bone metastasis (524). Other tumors reported to have an association with elevated PTHrP are squamous cell carcinoma, renal cell carcinoma, bladder carcinoma, prostate cancer, pheochromocytoma, pancreas cancer, lung cancer, and some lymphoid malignancies (512,525–532). Mesoblastic nephroma, the most common renal tumor in neonates, manifests humoral hypercalcemia and seems likely to make PTHrP, although it has not yet been documented (533). Malignant rhabdoid tumor of the kidney, which in an early study (534) showed immunoreactivity for PTH (in less specific assays), probably also elaborates PTHrP.

Although PTHrP is responsible for most cases of humoral hypercalcemia of malignancy, true PTH has been recognized on at least two occasions, one an ovarian carcinoma (535) and the other a small cell carcinoma of the lung (536). Osteolytic hypercalcemia does, indeed, occur on occasion as well, particularly in breast carcinoma (512,513). It can be distinguished from the humoral variant by normal levels of PTHrP and also by a failure of cAMP excretion to rise (512). Cases of concurrent primary hyperparathyroidism and cancer with elevation of both PTH and PTHrP have also been reported (537).

Nephrocalcinosis can result from tumor-related hypercalcemia, and renal failure may take place (538). There appears to be no consistent site of deposition of calcium, and any segment of the nephron may be affected. In some instances, the disparity between the morphologic damage and the degree of renal failure may be impressive, with only very scanty calcification (538). Bisphosphonates are used to treat hypercalcemia of malignancy, but some have been shown to cause glomerular disease (539) or acute tubular necrosis (540).

### Osteolytic Hypercalcemia of Malignancy

Approximately 20% of cases of cancer-related hypercalcemia are related to local osteolysis by the tumor. Generally, these are hematologic malignancies, lymphomas, and, most frequently and notably, multiple myeloma (514). In multiple myeloma, hypercalcemia can be extreme, constituting a medical emergency. No evidence has been adduced to date that the hypercalcemia is other than osteolytic in origin. There is experimental evidence, however, that hypercalcemia may markedly worsen Bence Jones cast nephropathy (541), and it is equally recognized that dehydration and hypercalcemia may trigger acute renal failure in patients with myeloma (542,543). Nephrocalcinosis does develop, but it tends to be fairly mild and is usually overshadowed by cast nephropathy, light-chain deposition, or both.

## Neonatal or Infantile Hypercalcemia

Infantile hypercalcemia is a rare condition, but can have serious renal complications. Chronic renal insufficiency may result either from nephrocalcinosis leading to tubular dysfunction or from nephrolithiasis. Several disorders of calcium regulation in infancy are recognized. The most common cause of infantile hypercalcemia is iatrogenic, often owing to intravenous administration of calcium usually from parenteral nutrition, and is alleviated by cessation of the infusion. Idiopathic infantile hypercalcemia (IIH) was first described by Lightwood in the 1950s (544) and was primarily caused by administration of high doses of vitamin D. Infants present with thirst, dehydration, and polyuria and can develop nephrocalcinosis (544,545). In some cases, either a dysregulation of renal vitamin D metabolism or increased sensitivity to vitamin D in the intestine seems to be causative (546). The hypercalcemia usually resolves, and prognosis for recovery in these cases is good.

### Williams' Syndrome

Previously known as severe idiopathic infantile hypercalcemia (IIH), Williams' syndrome is a multisystem genetic disorder caused by a contiguous deletion in the long arm of chromosome 7, affecting a large number of genes known to include elastin and LIM 1 kinase (547,548). The approximate incidence is 1 per 20,000 births worldwide, and it is mainly a sporadic defect with a few reported cases of apparent autosomal dominant transmission (549). Various features distinguish Williams' syndrome from IIH. Patients are born small for gestational age with a characteristic facies, develop hypercalcemia and nephrocalcinosis (550), have neurodevelopmental defects that affect hearing and speech (551,552), and have very distinctive personalities (553). Approximately 10% to 15% of these patients have hypercalcemia that often resolves in the first year (554,555), although the hypercalcemia has been reported to recur in adulthood (556). Approximately 30% of the affected individuals have hypercalciuria (553). The exact genetic cause underlying each of the various abnormalities is largely unknown.

### Primary or Secondary Hyperparathyroidism

Neonatal severe hyperparathyroidism (primary) is very rare and is caused in most cases by an inactivating mutation of the calcium-sensing receptor (557). This entity is discussed in the section on familial hypocalciuric hypercalcemia. Secondary hyperparathyroidism may occur in an infant whose mother's calcium metabolism goes awry during gestation. Complications occur in up to 80% of affected fetuses and include growth retardation and preterm delivery (558). At least one report suggests serious consequences such as seizure may result (559). During pregnancy, surgical removal of a maternal parathyroid adenoma may be indicated to avoid fetal demise. Infants usually require only supportive treatment in the neonatal period until the hypercalcemia resolves (546).

### Subcutaneous Fat Necrosis of the Newborn

In this rare disease, there are plaques of fat necrosis, often in the buttocks, in the wake of which hypercalcemia develops (560). This condition occurs most often in neonates who experienced a complicated delivery (561) and usually presents in the first week of life. Characteristic nodules are seen on the buttocks, trunk, arms, and cheeks. Histologically, the lesions consist of fat necrosis with a granulomatous inflammation including histiocytes, giant cells, and needle-shaped clefts in fat cells (562). The condition usually has a benign course with resolution of the skin lesions, though hypercalcemia may develop up to several months later and can be a cause of significant morbidity and mortality (561,563,564). The underlying mechanism of the hypercalcemia is not clear, but may involve release of $1,25(OH_2)D_3$ from the granulomatous areas of inflammation, leading to increased intestinal uptake of calcium (564).

## Disorders of the Calcium-Sensing Receptor

The calcium-sensing receptor (CaR) is located on a number of cell types throughout the body including the parathyroid gland, certain cells in the kidney, osteoclasts, and some cells in the brain (565–569). The CaR located on parathyroid cells regulates the release of PTH. High calcium activates the CaR, which inhibits PTH release, leading to a reduction in serum calcium. In the kidney, CaR molecules in the thick ascending limb sense elevated calcium levels in the peritubular capillaries and reduce calcium reabsorption (498,570). Changes in water permeability of the collecting duct may also be mediated through the CaR, allowing for polyuria and less concentrated urine to help prevent calcium precipitation and the formation of urinary stones (571). Several disease conditions have been associated with mutations of the CaR gene (572–574).

### Familial Hypocalciuric Hypercalcemia (FHH)

Heterozygous loss-of-function mutations result in FHH. This disorder has an autosomal dominant inheritance. FHH is usually asymptomatic, characterized by hypercalcemia, hypocalciuria, mild to moderate hypermagnesemia, mild hypophosphatemia, and normal to slightly increased PTH values (not suppressed as would be expected with hypercalcemia) (575,576). The mutation in the CaR results in a decreased sensitivity of the receptor to calcium levels in the serum so that a higher calcium concentration is required for its activation, leading in most cases to mild hypercalcemia. A lack of the normal inhibition of PTH secretion by the CaR also contributes to hypercalcemia. The mutation is also responsible for the paradoxical hypocalciuria, owing to a lack of thick ascending limb CaR response to the hypercalcemia. Calcimimetics may have some utility in stimulating the receptor pharmacologically (577).

### Severe Neonatal Hyperparathyroidism

Homozygous loss-of-function mutations in the CaR result in this life-threatening form of hypercalcemia (557,572) characterized by failure to thrive and fractures owing to undermineralization of the skeleton. The total lack of CaR in the parathyroid gland leads to markedly elevated PTH. Parathyroidectomy may be necessary for survival.

### Gain-of-Function CaR Mutations

Individuals with inactivating mutations (heterozygous or homozygous) of the CaR do not typically develop nephrocalcinosis or nephrolithiasis, despite the hypercalcemia. Alternatively, gain-of-function CaR mutations lead to hypocalcemia and hypercalciuria owing to hypoparathyroidism (578–582). These mutations have been found to cause autosomal dominant as well as sporadic cases of hypoparathyroidism (583). In individuals with gain-of-function mutations, the hypercalciuria leads to an increased tendency toward developing nephrocalcinosis and nephrolithiasis (581,582). Other symptoms vary by patient; some have asymptomatic hypocalcemia whereas others present in infancy with hypocalcemic seizures (578–580,583).

## Vitamin A or D Excess

Prolonged ingestion of large amounts of vitamin A (in excess of 50,000 IU per day) or administration of retinoic acid as treatment for various malignancies has been shown to result in bone resorption and hypercalcemia (584–587).

Hypercalcemia caused by vitamin D excess has been documented to occur in several ways. Cases of ingestion of excessively fortified milk have been reported (588,589), with some individuals developing hypercalcemia. Some hematologic malignancies are associated with elevated levels of circulating $1,25(OH_2)D_3$ (590–592). Whether the lymphomatous cells themselves produce the excess vitamin D, or whether, as suggested by Hewison et al (593), the vitamin D is produced by tumor-adjacent macrophages remains to be determined.

Pathologic descriptions of vitamin D excess in the older literature depict kidneys that are normal in size or enlarged, pale, swollen, and yellow. Calcification takes place in all segments of the tubules, and foreign-body giant cells are sometimes seen. Tubular loss, lymphocytic infiltration of the interstitium, periglomerular fibrosis, and sclerosis may all be present (594). Metastatic calcification may be evident in the heart, arteries, lung, and stomach. Calcification may also occur around joints, sometimes in the form of calcium-containing cysts.

## Granulomatous Diseases

Sarcoidosis and other granulomatous diseases, such as tuberculosis, Crohn's disease, and leprosy, can be a cause of hypercalcemia and hypercalciuria owing to excess vitamin D from extrarenal conversion of $1,25(OH_2)D_3$ (595–597). In one study, nephrocalcinosis was found in 22% of patients with chronic sarcoidosis (598).

## Milk-Alkali Syndrome

This syndrome was formerly a complication of peptic ulcer disease in patients who took large quantities of milk and absorbable alkali as therapy, which led to hypercalcemia and alkalosis (599). Nephrocalcinosis ensued, leading to renal insufficiency in some patients (599,600). With the advent of histamine blockers, the classic milk-alkali syndrome became rare; however, cases of milk-alkali syndrome associated with the use of calcium carbonate to treat osteoporosis or chronic renal failure became more common (476,601–603). Renal pathologic descriptions are scanty, but they document foci of calcification in the tubules and interstitium with interstitial fibrosis and inflammation (599,600).

## Defects of Tubular Handling

Although not always associated with hypercalcemia, several disorders of tubular handling are associated with nephrocalcinosis and/or nephrolithiasis owing to hypercalciuria. Abnormalities have been identified in paracellin, a tight junction protein, and in potassium channels and chloride channels. These disorders have been meticulously reviewed elsewhere (498,572,604–616). Familial hypomagnesemic hypercalciuria, autosomal dominant hypoparathyroidism, antenatal Bartter's syndrome (or hyperprostaglandin E syndrome), and classic Bartter's syndrome all have in common hypercalciuria, which likely predisposes to nephrocalcinosis and nephrolithiasis.

## Other Causes of Nephrocalcinosis

Nephrocalcinosis has been linked to a wide variety of disorders (Table 22.8), including primary hyperoxaluria, distal tubular acidosis, and various disorders of tubular transport involving chloride, phosphate, magnesium, calcium, and sodium (604,617–621). Rare causes include reactions to certain drugs and a very rare condition known as amelogenesis imperfecta (622,623).

| TABLE 22.8 |
| --- |
| **CAUSES OF NEPHROCALCINOSIS** |

Hypercalcemic/hypercalciuric states
Acquired immune deficiency syndrome
Primary hyperaldosteronism
Cystic fibrosis
Medications
  Acetazolamide
  Oral phosphate solutions
  Mercuric chloride
Cortical necrosis
Transplant rejection
Renal vein thrombosis
Renal tubular acidosis, type 1
Other

## Acquired Immunodeficiency Syndrome

Several reports have described nephrocalcinosis in cases of AIDS (624–626). In many instances, nephrocalcinosis is but one manifestation of multiorgan calcification in the liver, spleen, adrenals, and lymph nodes during the course of disseminated infection with *Pneumocystis carinii* organisms (625,626).

## Adrenal Disorders

Nephrocalcinosis has been described in primary hyperaldosteronism (627), and a form of adenoma producing excess aldosterone and testosterone was described in a young boy (628), leading to significant hypertension and nephrocalcinosis. Both persisted despite removal of the tumor.

## Cystic Fibrosis

Approximately 35% of patients with cystic fibrosis have hypercalciuria (629,630), and one study demonstrated that more than 90% of cystic fibrosis patients have nephrocalcinosis at autopsy (629). There is also an increased incidence of nephrolithiasis. Bentur et al (631), however, found that only 4 of their 34 patients had hypercalciuria and that there was only sparse nephrocalcinosis at autopsy in these patients, no more than in controls in their estimation. In 2005, Hoppe et al (632) demonstrated that absorptive hyperoxaluria owing to the malabsorptive state of cystic fibrosis, and hypocitraturia are the main causes of the increased incidence of nephrocalcinosis and nephrolithiasis.

## Renal Parenchymal Injury

Under appropriate circumstances, any cause of extensive renal parenchymal damage may occasionally lead to nephrocalcinosis. Severe acute tubular necrosis induced by toxic agents such as mercuric chloride may be followed by calcification (633). Calcium is deposited in the tubules that have undergone necrosis—usually the proximal tubules, because this is the segment most frequently damaged. Tubular cal-

cifications have been described after ingestion of uranium nitrate, acetazolamide, and certain medications that cause tubular injury (622,634,635). Finally, renal vein thrombosis with renal parenchymal calcification has been found antenatally by ultrasound (636).

Cases of extensive dystrophic tubular calcification can occur in the wake of transplantation of a kidney in which there was significant perioperative acute tubular necrosis. In at least some cases of delayed graft function, high intracellular calcium, rather than nephrocalcinosis per se, may be the cause of reduced function (637). Nephrocalcinosis may also be found in association with rejection (638,639). Severe dystrophic calcification may follow renal cortical necrosis (640). Similarly, cortical calcification has been described in severe hemolytic uremic syndrome with prolonged anuria (and presumably severe tubular damage) (641).

## Nephrocalcinosis Associated with Bowel-Cleansing Agents

Cases of renal failure with biopsy-proven acute tubular necrosis and nephrocalcinosis following the use of oral sodium phosphate solutions prior to colonoscopy have been reported (642,643). Deposition of nonpolarizable calcium phosphate crystals are found in patients without hypercalcemia or other risk factor for the development of nephrocalcinosis (Fig. 22.59). Most of these patients have normal renal function prior to the procedure and develop acute renal failure following the colonoscopy. In addition to calcium deposits, tubular atrophy and associated

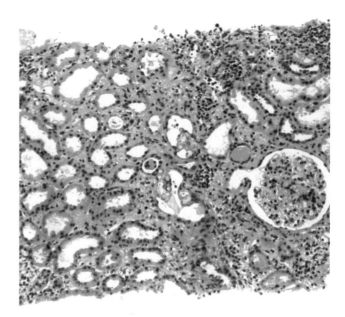

**Figure 22.59** Nephrocalcinosis associated with oral phosphate bowel-cleansing agents. Acute tubular necrosis develops along with deposition of nonpolarizable calcium phosphate crystals. Tubular atrophy and interstitial fibrosis are also present. (H&E, ×100.)

interstitial fibrosis are present. Many of the affected patients were hypertensive before the incident and being treated with agents that are known to reduce perfusion pressure or had other conditions that could be associated with reduction in perfusion pressure, such as dehydration or use of diuretics. Unfortunately, in most cases, the decline in renal function appears to be chronic.

### Renal Tubular Acidosis

Any condition resulting in distal, or type 1, renal tubular acidosis is associated with an increased incidence of nephrocalcinosis and/or nephrolithiasis (644). These conditions include primary hereditary disorders causing a defect of the anion exchanger AE1 on intercalated cells of the collecting duct, or of the distal tubule apical proton pump or $H^+$-$K^+$ATPases (645–647), autoimmune diseases such as systemic lupus or Sjögren's (648), and certain drugs. See also the section on renal tubular acidosis and nephrolithiasis.

## Experimental Studies on Hypercalcemia, Nephrocalcinosis, and Nephrolithiasis

### Physiologic Effects of Hypercalcemia

Mild hypercalcemia rarely results in renal functional abnormalities. Defects in urinary concentrating ability are among the manifestations of more pronounced hypercalcemia. In part, this appears to be related to a reduction in sodium chloride reabsorption in the thick ascending limb (649). The glomerular filtration rate is frequently reduced (650), perhaps as a result of calcium-induced preglomerular vasoconstriction. In the rat, there is a decrease in the glomerular ultrafiltration coefficient—a determinant of the single-nephron filtration rate—owing to an alteration of electrophysical forces at the filtration barrier (651). There is evidence in some models of increased medullary blood flow, with washout of the concentration gradient (652). Inhibition of vasodilator prostaglandins may restore urinary concentrating ability (653), although in the context of chronic hypercalcemia, the net effect may be a diminution in renal function owing to ischemic damage (654).

### Animal Models

Animal models, principally rats, have been used for decades to study the physiologic, morphologic, and pathogenetic features of hypercalcemia, including nephrocalcinosis and nephrolithiasis. Rosen et al (654) studied prolonged hypercalcemia over 8 weeks by repeated injections of vitamin $D_2$ in the rat. They confirmed the observation that there is a marked rise in plasma calcium and a sustained diminution of urine-concentrating ability without any reduction in creatinine clearance. Lesions developed in the inner stripe of the outer medulla where thick ascending limbs (mTALs)

showed various degrees of collapse and atrophy associated with basal lamina calcification and focal cell necrosis. The most seriously damaged tubules were those farthest from the vasa recta, a pattern consistent with hypoxic injury. Ultrastructural examination showed calcified mitochondria and basal lamina in the damaged tubules. Corresponding to the tubular damage, there was an increase in the medullary interstitial tissue with spotty inflammation. In the cortex, lesions were fewer, with only a few areas of focal tubular necrosis and calcification. There was significant interstitial fibrosis and loss of tubules. The renal papillae showed virtually no lesions, even adjacent to the inner stripe lesions just above. Parathyroidectomy partially protected against the lesions owing to vitamin $D_2$, apparently by preventing hypercalcemia.

In an acute model of nephrocalcinosis, using isolated perfused rat kidneys, the authors had previously noted augmentation of medullary hypoxic injury by calcium, particularly to the mTALs (652). On the basis of the combined studies, they suggested that because of its selective occurrence in zones of poorest oxygen supply, this inner stripe, calcium-related injury may derive from vulnerability to hypoxia. Other authors have described selective inner medullary lesions in experimental studies of hypercalcemia (650,655,656) and magnesium deficiency that leads to hypercalcemia (657). Predominantly medullary calcification is also seen in nephrocalcinosis in humans (521,658).

At the ultrastructural level, studies have given somewhat equivocal results, perhaps owing to the different agents used to induce hypercalcemia. Calcification of mitochondria seems to be a lesion common to many models, although it may be relatively inconspicuous in some (654,659,660). In one study using PTH in the rat (660), there was a reduction in mitochondria together with calcification of the tubular basement membrane (TBM). Hyaline bodies then appeared within the cells, bursting into the lumen to act as foci of precipitation for stone formation (an appearance reminiscent of some cases of early calcium deposition in humans).

In an interesting study in the mouse, two different methods of inducing hypercalcemia produced totally different lesions (638). PTH led to apatite formation in mitochondria, vacuoles, and the tubular cytoplasm in the distal portion (pars recta) of the proximal tubule. Calcium gluconate, by contrast, generated calcium carbonate deposits in the TBMs of the pars convoluta of the proximal tubule. Clearly, the type and site of calcium deposition may vary widely according to the cause of the hypercalcemia. Rats, particularly female rats, are subject to spontaneous nephrocalcinosis, with deposition of calcium salts in the corticomedullary region (523,661,662). Nephrocalcinosis in a similar distribution can be found in streptozotocin-induced diabetic rats on a low-zinc diet (663). Cockell and Belonje (664) showed that rats fed a standard chow developed nephrocalcinosis at a high incidence compared with rats fed a diet with a higher phosphorous content and lower calcium phosphate product. This result seems to contradict studies that show diets low in magnesium (which lead to hypercalcemia), high in calcium, and high in phosphorus all augment nephrocalcinosis (523,661,665). In the latter instance, the higher the phosphate excretion, the greater the nephrocalcinosis (666), and the same observations appear to hold true for children with hypophosphatemic rickets (665). By contrast, diets high in protein are associated with only minimal nephrocalcinosis. All maneuvers that increase nephrocalcinosis also increase the urinary excretion of albumin and elevate plasma urea levels (523,661).

Bushinsky et al (667–669) and Hoopes et al (670) have developed a rat model for idiopathic hypercalciuria. The rats excrete excessive amounts of urinary calcium owing in part to increased intestinal calcium absorption. Even in the presence of a low-calcium diet, however, calcium excretion is elevated, suggesting a renal and/or bone abnormality as well. These rats have high numbers of vitamin D receptors in the gut, bone, and kidney. When fed standard chow, the animals form calcium phosphate stones, but when provided an increase in dietary hydroxyproline, they form calcium oxalate stones (671). Sections of kidneys from these animals demonstrate formation of crystalline deposits located within the urinary space, closely apposed to the urothelium of the pelvis, without calcium deposition in the kidney parenchyma.

In previous studies in rats with intraperitoneal administration of sodium oxalate, Khan (672) found calcium oxalate crystals in the lumens of proximal tubules as well as in collecting ducts in the cortex and papilla. Renal papillary tips and calyceal surfaces were a preferential site for crystal retention, and papillary epithelium exhibited injury. Epithelium of the proximal tubule also showed changes, with formation of apical blebs and focal loss of the brush border. Other evidence of epithelial injury included cytoplasmic vacuolation and increased mitotic activity (673). It is unclear whether cellular injury occurs prior to or as a result of crystal formation.

### Cell Culture Studies
Cultured epithelial cells have been used extensively to study the role tubular epithelium plays in calcium crystallization and nephrolithiasis. Proximal tubule cells are often used to study oxalate transport (674,675), whereas cells derived from more distal nephron segments are studied for the interaction of crystals with renal epithelium (676–679).

Madin-Darby canine kidney (MDCK) cells used as a model of distal nephron cells take up and subsequently release calcium oxalate crystals (677). When incubated with potassium oxalate or calcium oxalate, MDCK cells become injured and can detach from the monolayer (676). Lieske et al (678) demonstrated that anionic surface molecules function as a site for adhesion of calcium oxalate microcrystals, which could result in formation of calculi. Other cell-surface characteristics have also been shown to be important for attachment of crystals to the epithelium, such as heparan sulphate (680) or certain lipids (681). One study comparing primary cell cultures with various cell lines (682) found that nondividing, differentiated cells are more protected from crystal attachment, suggesting that tubular cells in individuals prone to nephrolithiasis may have dedifferentiated or lost an inhibitory factor characteristic of mature cells (683). Various molecules have been identified as modulators of stone formation (684), such as glycosaminoglycans, citrate, uropontin, nephrocalcin, and Tamm-Horsfall protein (see Inhibitors of Stone Formation).

## Pathology of Renal Calcification

### Isolated Calcium Concretions

These basophilic structures may be seen in many conditions not primarily associated with nephrocalcinosis and nephrolithiasis. They may be present in patients with significant proteinuria of various causes, following ischemic tubular injury, as well as in aging kidneys. They are associated with little morphologic damage and do not seem to have any functional significance. In one study, nearly all kidneys at autopsy had isolated interstitial calcific deposits (685).

Typically, the earliest structures are intracytoplasmic, but they erode into the lumen at an early stage or less frequently expand, pushing the tubular cytoplasm before them to reduce the lumen to a small crescent, effectively occluding the tubule. In the early stages, the structures are pale to clear with rounded or somewhat irregular contours (Fig. 22.60).

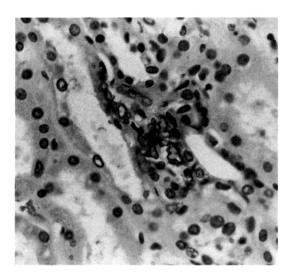

**Figure 22.60** Isolated tubular concretions. The calcifications have a laminated quality and appear to originate in the tubular cytoplasm. (H&E, ×525.)

As they grow, they progressively calcify and become basophilic, often with a faintly lamellar appearance, resembling miniature psammoma bodies. The tubular cytoplasm, if it persists, becomes flattened and pale, but often it is eroded completely away. These isolated concretions are usually confined to the tubule without surrounding inflammation. Occasionally, they may rupture through the TBM into the interstitium with resulting inflammatory response.

## Tubular Accumulations of Oxalate Crystals

These accumulations are also fairly typical and are often found in end-stage kidneys and in transplanted kidneys. Isolated oxalate crystals do not necessarily imply significant damage; renal insufficiency of any nature can lead to accumulations of oxalate. However, with extensive deposits of oxalate, the hyperoxaluric conditions should be considered (see Hyperoxaluria). Histologically, calcium oxalate crystals are either yellowish-white or display a wide range of colors, appear fan shaped, radially arranged or spiculated, and are birefringent on polarization as opposed to calcium phosphate crystals that do not polarize (Fig. 22.61). Acute and chronic tubular injury can occur with inflammation early on, sometimes including a giant cell reaction and later progressing to tubular atrophy with interstitial fibrosis.

## Renal Papillary Calcifications and Randall's Plaques

Foci of calcification are quite commonplace in renal papillae, usually in the absence of stone formation; however, these calcifications are believed to be the initial site of stone formation in susceptible individuals. One

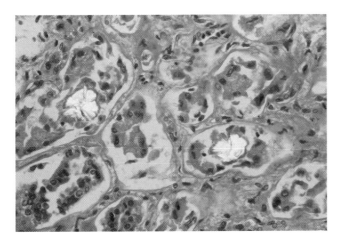

**Figure 22.61** Cortex of kidney with calcium oxalate crystals, photographed under half-polarized light. The crystals occupy the lumens of tubules. (H&E, ×100.)

careful study using stereomicroscopy of renal papillae at autopsy (686) disclosed externally visible foci in 201 of 372 kidneys (54.0%). An incidence of 22.2% was found in one early study (687). Calcifications took the form of tiny round deposits along the sides of the papillae, linear deposits coursing longitudinally along the papillae and appearing to outline the tubules, or larger plaques. The plaques were variably distributed along the sides of the papilla, as a ring around the tip, surrounding the openings of the ducts of Bellini, or as Randall's plaques covering the tip with irregular pitting of the surface. Randall's plaques were found in 27.9% of cases. Small calculi were found in 30 of 272 cases (8.1%), either attached to or embedded in the side of the papilla (Fig. 22.62) or lying free in the renal calyces.

Randall's plaques as originally described by Randall et al. (688) were believed to be papillary calcifications that presumably eroded outward and projected from the surface to act as a nidus for crystal formation. Randall et al (688) believed that calcium phosphate, calcium oxalate, and uric acid stones began in this manner. Indeed, many common calcium oxalate stones appear to develop from Randall's plaques, as demonstrated in a study by Evan et al (689). Biopsies from kidneys of patients undergoing nephrolithotomy or other surgical procedures unrelated to stone disease were examined. The authors found microscopic deposits (as small as 50 nm) almost exclusively along basement membranes of thin limbs of the loop of Henle (Fig. 22.63). These initial sites of crystal deposition were found only in patients who were known idiopathic hypercalciuric calcium oxalate stone formers. No plaques were identified in patients with a history of stones following intestinal bypass, or in individuals with no history of stones. The mechanism of action put forward by Randall et al (688) does therefore explain the formation of some stones; however, other mechanisms seem likely to be operative as well.

## Nephrocalcinosis

Nephrocalcinosis is a disorder of increased calcium content and deposition within the renal parenchyma. Diffuse tubular injury, both acute and chronic, along with numerous tubular calcium deposits occurs. It may be found as an isolated condition or associated with nephrolithiasis. Unlike nephrolithiasis, nephrocalcinosis may not produce any identifiable signs or symptoms until a considerable amount of parenchymal damage has occurred and renal function is compromised.

The term *nephrocalcinosis* was coined by Albright et al in 1934 (690) to describe the radiologic appearance of primary hyperparathyroidism. The general histologic picture in established nephrocalcinosis—for example, that seen in primary hyperparathyroidism—consists of alternating areas of normal parenchyma and wedge-shaped scars

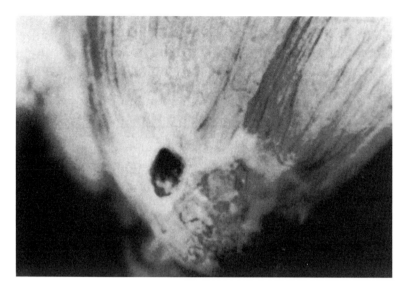

**Figure 22.62** Stereomicroscopic photograph of a renal papilla with a small calculus adherent to the side near the tip. (From Abrahams C. Stereopathy of the renal papilla: A stereomicroscopic autopsy study. Hum Pathol 1985;16:488.) Extensive tubular basement membrane (TBM) calcifications in experimental phosphate deficiency in the rat. The TBM calcifications show multiple areas of fracture, probably artifactual. Despite calcification, the tubular cytoplasm is still viable in most tubules. (PAS, ×295.)

(Fig. 22.64). The latter areas show tubular atrophy and loss as well as glomeruli with varying degrees of collapse and sclerosis of the sort seen in ischemia. There is usually little vascular narrowing, however. The most prominent change is calcification of TBMs, particularly in the proximal con-

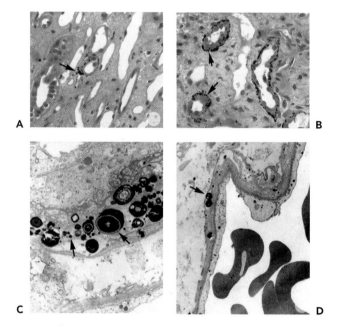

**Figure 22.63** Initial sites of crystal deposition. This set of illustrations shows the initial sites and size of calcium deposition in the papillary tissue of a calcium oxalate patient as seen by light (**A** and **B**) and transmission electron (**C** and **D**) microscopy. Sites of crystalline material (arrows) are noted in the basement membranes near the collagen of the thin loops of Henle (**A–C**) and to a lesser degree in the basement membranes of vas recta (**D**). (**A:** ×900, **B:** ×1000, **C:** ×15,600, **D:** ×5500. (From Evan AP, Lingeman JE, Coe FL, et al. Randall's plaque of patients with nephrolithiasis begins in basement membranes of thin loops of Henle. J Clin Invest 2003;111:607.)

voluted tubules, although other segments may be affected. This calcification shows up as a purplish tinge or stippling on routine hematoxylin-eosin sections; it is particularly well brought out by the von Kossa stain (Fig. 22.65), which reveals dark-staining rings in the cortex. TBM calcification involves not only atrophic but also ostensibly intact tubules in both scarred and nonscarred areas. As calcification becomes more widespread, it may also involve Bowman's capsules and eventually sclerotic glomeruli.

Tubular concretions similar to those described above are present in variable numbers. They appear to involve every level of the nephron, although in individual instances identifiable epithelium disappears. There may be large purplish concretions in the tubular lumina, particularly in the collecting tubules, at all levels from the cortex to the papilla. These concretions are more often seen in the areas of scarring, and the impression is that there has been obstruction to the larger collecting tubules in these areas with consequent atrophy of the overlying cortex. Calcium may also be deposited in the interstitium, usually just outside tubules (Fig. 22.66); some of the deposits are dense and basophilic, whereas others are finer and less darkly staining. Arteries may show medial calcification, usually without any significant compromise of the lumen until the deposits become massive. Similar deposits are found in arteries elsewhere in the body, and there is calcification as well in the pulmonary alveolar septa, in the myocardium, and in the gastric mucosa, all traditional sites of metastatic calcification.

In different variants of nephrocalcinosis, the distribution of lesions may be different. For example, in some forms of infantile hypercalcemia, calcification is confined to the medulla, particularly the outer medulla (691), and parallels that seen in experimental hypercalcemia (654). In medullary sponge kidney, nephrocalcinosis develops

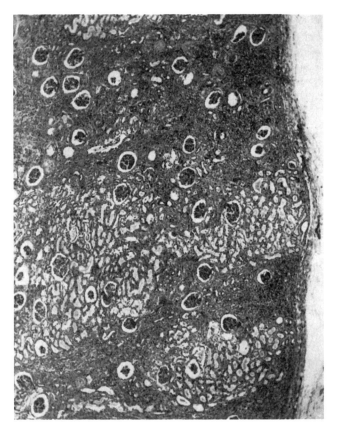

**Figure 22.64** The kidney from a 58-year-old woman with primary hyperparathyroidism shows alternating areas of normal and scarred parenchyma. (H&E, ×29.)

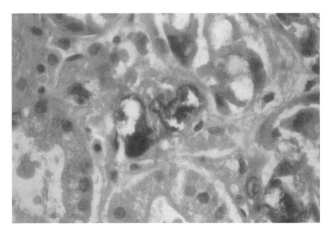

**Figure 22.66** Interstitial and tubule-associated basophilic concretions of calcium. (H&E, ×400.)

in the pyramids (692,693). In other forms, such as that following severe renal tubular damage or renal cortical necrosis (640), the calcification is primarily dystrophic in nature and follows the distribution of the necrotic tubules.

In the study by Evan et al (689), intestinal bypass patients who develop hyperoxaluria tended to have apatite

(calcium phosphate) crystal deposition in the lumens of inner medullary collecting ducts, not in the interstitium or loop of Henle basement membrane, compared with those patients who develop idiopathic calcium oxalate stones. Randall identified similar deposits in a follow-up to his seminal study describing Randall's plaques and termed these type 2 deposits (694). Sayer et al (605) speculate that this may be the mechanism underlying nephrocalcinosis development. However, in a 1981 study by Ibels et al (695), 57 of 59 end-stage kidneys from various diseases showed calcium deposition in cortical tubule cells, basement membranes, and the interstitium.

## NEPHROLITHIASIS

Renal stone disease (nephrolithiasis) is an important source of morbidity in the United States, with a lifetime prevalence of 3% to 5% (696,697). The annual incidence may be as high as 1 or 2 per 1000 individuals (669,697,698). These figures probably underestimate the actual incidence, because many cases never come to medical attention. Some estimates are as high as 10% of the population in industrialized regions (698).

Four of every five patients with nephrolithiasis are men; most stones in women are due to either metabolic defects such as cystinuria, or infection. Men have a much higher incidence of uric acid calculi (699). The peak age at first episode is approximately 30 to 40 years with a later initial presentation in females (700,701). Up to 75% of patients will have recurrent stones, sometimes ten or more over their lifetime (495).

Urinary calculi are more common in whites compared with nonwhites (702). North American Indians, Hispanics, blacks in both America and Africa, Asians, and native-born Israelis have fewer stones (699,702). Stone composition varies somewhat by ethnicity, with calcium oxalate stones being much more common in whites; uric acid, struvite,

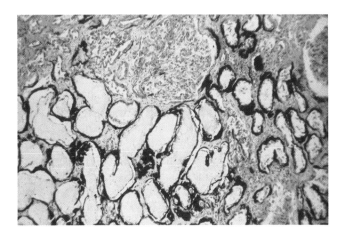

**Figure 22.65** Calcification in the basement membranes of nonatrophic tubules and focally in Bowman's capsule. (von Kossa, ×100.)

and matrix stones are slightly more common in nonwhites (702). The underlying etiology of stone formation is similar, except that whites appear to have a higher incidence of hypercalciuria; the incidence of hypocitraturia, hyperuricosuria, hyperoxaluria, and other metabolic abnormalities are similar among the various ethnic groups studied (702). Geography and temperature seem to have a relationship to nephrolithiasis in that there is a noticeable increase in urinary calculi in mountainous areas, and there is also a tendency in a given region for the highest incidence of stones to occur in the warmer months (699,701). These observations suggest that a balance of fluid intake, perspiration, and urinary output is important, and therefore, increasing fluid intake in an attempt to defend against recurrences of renal stones is universally recommended.

Urinary calculi often make their presence known by an episode of ureteral colic when they become entrapped. There are five typical locations. Stones may become impacted in a renal calyx, at the ureteropelvic junction, at the pelvic brim where the ureter arches over the iliac vessels, in the posterior pelvis where the ureter is crossed anteriorly by pelvic vessels, or at the ureterovesical junction. Congenital or acquired anomalies of the urinary tract may influence the location of stone formation and passage. Ordinarily, small stones are passed spontaneously. Beyond a certain size (703), however, the stone is too large to pass and remains in the renal pelvis, where it usually continues to grow. Eventually, particularly with struvite or infection stones, they may completely fill the renal pelvis and calyces, creating the staghorn calculus (Fig. 22.67). These stones may create a situation of chronic partial obstruction with hydronephrosis and slowly declining renal function. Often, the situation can be complicated by infection. Even those stones not owing to infection by urea-splitting organisms not infrequently become secondarily infected, as does the overlying kidney. In such instances, there may be sepsis, shock, and precipitous renal failure. The kidney itself shows varying mixtures of acute and chronic pyelonephritis. One

### TABLE 22.9
### RELATIVE FREQUENCY OF KIDNEY STONES

| Composition | % of All Stones |
|---|---|
| Calcium, oxalate and/or phosphate | 70–80 |
| Struvite | 10 |
| Uric acid | 5–10 |
| Cystine | 1 |
| Other (xanthine, matrix, medications, etc.) | |

distinctive form particularly associated with renal calculi is xanthogranulomatous pyelonephritis, and one case of purely granulomatous pyelonephritis resembling tuberculosis has been described in association with nephrolithiasis (704).

The great majority of stones in humans, 70% to 80%, are composed of calcium oxalate or calcium phosphate (Table 22.9). Other calculi are made up of struvite (magnesium ammonium phosphate) in infection stones (10%), uric acid (5% to 10%), cystine (<1%), xanthine (<1%), and more rarely, other substances (698,705–707). Since treatment varies depending mainly on the type of stone, evaluation of stone composition radiologically and biochemically is important.

## Mechanisms of Stone Formation

The physicochemical mechanisms of action underlying crystal formation and the ultimate development of calculi can be broken into three interrelated components: (a) the degree of saturation of the urine with respect to the crystal system in question; (b) the presence of conditions permitting nucleation, or growth of crystals, which in most instances means heterogeneous nucleation—the growth of crystals of one type on a crystalline nidus of different composition; and (c) the presence and level of inhibitors of stone formation (684,698,708,709). A brief discussion of each of these major components of stone formation follows.

### Saturation of Urine

For a stone to form, an absolute prerequisite is that the urine must be supersaturated for the precipitating crystalline phase (669,709–712). The state of saturation for any potential crystal system, as, for example, calcium oxalate, depends on several variables, including the concentration of the solutes, pH, ionic strength, and "complexation." The solubility product of a salt is dependent on the pH of the solution, and the ionic strength, principally from the monovalent ions in the urine, effectively determines the concentration of calcium and oxalate needed to saturate the

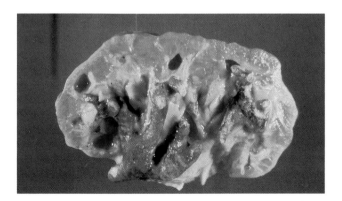

**Figure 22.67** Multiple staghorn calculi filling the pelvis and extending into calyces. Early hydronephrosis and cortical scarring are appearing on the right pole.

urine for the crystalline phase. Normally, approximately 50% of the calcium and approximately 50% of the oxalate in the urine are available in free ionic form (709). The term *complexation* refers to the ability of such compounds as citrate and magnesium to form soluble complexes with calcium or oxalate, respectively, and effectively reduce the free ion concentration of each. Supersaturation of the urine for salts is a common occurrence, but formation of the solid phase occurs only in certain individuals, suggesting that substances are present that modify the ability of crystals to form in a saturated urine, some of which are absent or abnormal in stone formers. Inhibitors of stone formation have been identified and are discussed later.

## Nucleation

Heterogeneous nucleation is the common in vivo mechanism for stone formation. This form of nucleation is based on the presence of debris or other crystals that serve as a nidus for development of crystals (667). Heterogeneous nucleation occurs at a lower level of saturation than homogeneous nucleation and therefore requires less energy thermodynamically. Spontaneous, or homogeneous, nucleation is uncommon, principally because of the large expenditure of energy required to initiate it. One example of heterogeneous nucleation is provided by monosodium urate and uric acid, which are excellent heterogeneous nuclei for calcium oxalate (713). Heterogeneous nucleation is thought to form the link between hyperuricosuria and calcium oxalate stones.

## Inhibitors of Stone Formation

There is a large body of evidence that inhibitors of stone formation exist in the urine (679,684,714–719). Among known inhibitors are citrate, uropontin, nephrocalcin, Tamm-Horsfall protein, glycosaminoglycans, prothrombin F1 peptide, and bikunin (uronic acid–rich protein). The mechanism of action in inhibiting stone formation is not entirely clear for most of these factors, but may involve the ability either to provide a barrier on the epithelial surface whereby cell–crystal interaction is minimized, or to cover the crystals with an organic material to reduce their ability to interact with cells or debris. Some of these putative inhibitors are reviewed briefly.

## Citrate

Hypocitraturia is recognized in 20% to 50% of patients with calcium oxalate stones (503,710). The main function of citrate is to reduce supersaturation by forming a complex with calcium. It may also reduce aggregation of calcium oxalate crystals (720), though one study has failed to show an effect of citrate on aggregation (714).

## Uropontin/Osteopontin

In vitro studies show that uropontin inhibits aggregation, as well as nucleation and growth (721–723) of calcium oxalate and calcium phosphate crystals (724). Hoyer et al (725) isolated uropontin, which is a form of osteopontin, from human urine. Subsequently, Lieske et al (726) demonstrated that calcium oxalate crystals stimulate production of uropontin by epithelial cell lines at the mRNA level. Studies in stone-forming rats show an increase in uropontin mRNA in distal tubule and collecting ducts (727). In mice deficient in osteopontin, a hyperoxaluric diet resulted in numerous intrarenal calcium oxalate crystals whereas wild-type mice had no calcium crystals (719). Osteopontin has been identified within calcium stones, leading to speculation that it may also be capable of paradoxically promoting stone formation (728).

## Nephrocalcin

Nephrocalcin, a glycoprotein, has also been isolated from calcium stones (729) and is known to inhibit nucleation, growth, and aggregation of crystals. Molecular abnormalities in nephrocalcin have been identified in stone-forming individuals that appear to involve alterations in its phosphorylation and amino acid sequence (730,731).

## Tamm-Horsfall Protein

Aggregation of calcium oxalate and hydroxyapatite crystals can be inhibited *in vitro* by Tamm-Horsfall protein (THP) but THP does not appear to inhibit nucleation or growth (732,733). The function of THP may lie in its ability to self-aggregate, as abnormal self-aggregation in one kindred resulted in a decreased ability of their urine to inhibit crystal aggregation (734).

## Prothrombin F1 Peptide

In 1995, Ryall et al (735) demonstrated that the F1 fragment of prothrombin (PF1) is a potent inhibitor of calcium oxalate crystallization. PF1 is produced by the action of thrombin on prothrombin and is then filtered into urinary filtrate, but can also be synthesized in the kidney (736). In addition to inhibiting stone formation, PF1 may aid in removal or detachment of crystals from tubular epithelium (737).

## Summary

These three factors—supersaturation, heterogeneous nucleation, and reduction of inhibitors of stone formation—play varying roles in each of the major variants of calcium nephrolithiasis, being paramount in some and negligible in others. By definition, *supersaturation* is a necessary but not sufficient condition for the development of any stone, and it is the major driving force in some disease processes. *Heterogeneous nucleation* is thought to be important in calcium oxalate stone formation and probably also occurs in hyperparathyroidism. *Reduced inhibitors* of stone formation are clearly important, although much more research is needed to clarify their mechanisms.

## Causes of Calcium Nephrolithiasis

### Idiopathic Hypercalciuria

Table 22.10 lists etiologic factors in stone disease. Approximately 95% of idiopathic nephrolithiasis is owing to idiopathic hypercalciuria. Patients with idiopathic hypercalciuria have a normal serum calcium level but have hypercalciuria, defined as the urinary excretion of more than 300 mg calcium per day in men or more than 250 mg per day in women or more than 4 mg/kg/day (503). Idiopathic hypercalciuria is found in 40% to 50% of patients with calcium oxalate nephrolithiasis (739,740). It is clear that there is a genetic component in at least some individuals; early studies found that 12 to 20% of all patients with stones had a positive family history of stone formation (740,741). Pak et al (742), examining one group of patients with idiopathic hypercalciuria, found that 44.7% of those with absorptive idiopathic hypercalciuria and 38.5% of those with renal idiopathic hypercalciuria

### TABLE 22.10
### ETIOLOGY OF STONE DISEASE

Hypercalcemic states
Hypercalciuric states
Renal tubular disorders
    Renal tubular acidosis
    Distal tubule defects
        Chloride channel mutations
        Disorders of magnesium handling
        Mutations of the calcium-sensing receptor
    Cystinuria
Hyperuricosuria
    Idiopathic
    Gout
    Low urine pH and/or low urine volume
    High-protein diet
    Malignancy
    Purine metabolism defects
Hyperoxaluria
    Primary
    Secondary
Hypocitraturia
Xanthinuria
Medications
Deficiency in inhibitors of stone formation
Other
    Infection urolithiasis
    Obstruction urolithiasis
    Urinary diversion
    Medullary sponge kidney, cystic disease
    Foreign chemicals and compounds

had a family history of stone formation. This tendency was thought to be inherited as an autosomal dominant trait, but now a polygenic mode of inheritance is favored in many instances. It is likely that a combination of factors are at play. Although current evidence has failed to show that mutations in the calcium-sensing receptor are the cause of idiopathic hypercalciuria, polymorphisms in the receptor may play a role (743–745). Hypercalcemia, vitamin D excess, hyperthyroidism, malignant neoplasm, and sarcoidosis must be excluded to allow a diagnosis of idiopathic hypercalciuria (746).

#### Pathophysiology
Theories to explain idiopathic hypercalciuria include abnormalities in handling of calcium in the kidney, intestines, or bone leading to an increase in calcium excretion. Mechanisms include decreased tubular reabsorption, increased calcium absorption by the intestines, or an increase in bone mineral resorption (669,747). Some authors believe individual patients may have abnormalities in one specific organ of calcium regulation and have divided patients into absorptive, renal, or resorptive types (698,748). Categorization of patients into these groups is difficult clinically because of rapid metabolic corrections that offset the initial dysregulation, although the distinction between absorptive and renal hypercalciuria is one worth making in therapeutic terms, since renal hypercalciuria appears to respond to thiazide therapy, whereas absorptive hypercalciuria does not (749). In addition, in some pedigrees with a severe form of absorptive hypercalciuria, there appears to be a role for the soluble adenylate cyclase gene, providing a possible future avenue for treatment (750,751).

#### Therapy
The primary therapy in idiopathic hypercalciuria aims at reducing urinary calcium by two approaches, both of which work to decrease supersaturation (503,710,752). There is general agreement that thiazide diuretics are effective in mitigating idiopathic hypercalciuria, reducing recurrent stone formation by approximately 50% over an extended period (751). Increased fluid intake, such that urine output reaches 2 L per day, is prescribed in combination with diuretic therapy. In addition, limiting protein and sodium intake is generally accepted as a means to decrease calcium excretion (753). Calcium restriction, which has been suggested in the past, induces increased intestinal absorption of oxalate and carries a risk of increased bone resorption in patients with already decreased bone density (747,754).

### Primary Hyperparathyroidism

The incidence of renal stones in primary hyperparathyroidism is between 15% and 20% (488). Conversely, in patients with stone disease, primary hyperparathyroidism is found in up to 10% (488,504,755). Patients with primary hyperparathyroidism typically form calcium oxalate or mixed calcium oxalate–calcium phosphate stones (488,755), although the fraction of calcium phosphate in the stones is generally greater in primary hyperparathyroidism than in patients with idiopathic hypercalciuric stone formation (504).

## Chloride Channel Mutations

At least three types of hypercalciuric nephrolithiasis are linked to mutations in the *CLCN5* gene, which codes for the ClC-5 chloride channel on the short arm of the X chromosome (617,756). X-linked recessive nephrolithiasis, Dent's disease, and recessive hypophosphatemic rickets are lumped together under the name *Dent's disease complex* and share features of low–molecular-weight proteinuria, hypercalciuria, and other tubular abnormalities leading to Fanconi-type syndromes, and nephrocalcinosis, nephrolithiasis, or both (756). The ClC-5 chloride channel is a voltage-gated channel expressed in proximal tubules, thick ascending limb of Henle's loop, and alpha-intercalated cells of collecting ducts (757). There are several theories for the mechanism by which mutation of the chloride channel results in hypercalciuria and the other abnormalities of Dent's disease, most of which are unproven. The ClC5 channel may be important in endocytosis in the proximal tubule, providing a possible explanation for its role in proteinuria. The loss of other electrolytes in the urine by faulty tubular reabsorption may influence handling of calcium by the kidney and allow for hypercalciuria. Other genes may also be responsible in some individuals with features of Dent's disease, as demonstrated in a study by Hoopes et al (758), who reported no mutation in the *CLCN5* gene in 13 patients, suggesting genetic heterogeneity.

The symptoms of Dent's disease appear in childhood, with males affected more than females. Renal failure can occur and may be related to the development of nephrocalcinosis. Nonspecific histologic features of tubular atrophy, interstitial fibrosis, and glomerulosclerosis have been reported (759,760).

## Hyperuricosuria

Coe (761) was the first to point out the high incidence of uricosuria, 26.3% overall, among calcium stone formers. In 14.6% of these patients, it arose on its own, in the absence of any sign of hypercalciuria. More recent studies find an even higher incidence of hyperuricosuria in calcium oxalate stone formers, up to 41% (762). It has been suggested that uric acid crystals or other urates act as the nidus for heterogeneous nucleation of calcium oxalate (763–765). Others have suggested that perhaps colloidal urates adsorb one or more of the inhibitors of stone formation, thus permitting stone formation. Alternatively, urate salts may re-

duce the solubility of calcium oxalate (766). Regardless of the underlying pathophysiologic factors, the causal association between hyperuricosuria and calcium nephrolithiasis is attested to by the efficacy of allopurinol to limit recurrence of stones in these patients (767). A low-purine diet, alkalinization of the urine, and increased fluid intake are also means of reducing uricosuria.

## Hyperoxaluria

Despite the fact that oxalate is the most common component of calcium stones, many stone formers excrete normal amounts of oxalate (495). Increased oxalate excretion does, however, occur in some people, and this increase raises the saturation of the urine with respect to calcium oxalate. Hyperoxaluria in and of itself has been found experimentally to lead to stone formation, the severity of which is related to the level of oxalate administration (768). Hyperoxaluria can be divided into primary (metabolic overproduction) and secondary forms; of the latter, the most important are the various forms of enteric oxalate hyperabsorption (Table 22.11).

### Primary Hyperoxaluria

There are two forms of hereditary hyperoxaluria. Primary hyperoxaluria type 1 (PH1) is caused by a deficiency in alanine glyoxylate aminotransferase (AGT), leading to decreased conversion of glyoxylate to glycine, allowing excess oxalate synthesis from glyoxylate oxidation. PH2 results from an abnormality in glyoxylate reductase, also leading to increased conversion of glyoxylate to oxalate. Both PH1 and PH2 are autosomal recessive conditions. Numerous mutations in both genes have been identified (769).

---

**TABLE 22.11**

**CAUSES OF HYPEROXALURIA**

Primary hyperoxaluria
    Type 1    deficiency of alanine glyoxylate aminotransferase
    Type 2    deficiency of glyoxylate reductase
Secondary hyperoxaluria
    Enteric hyperoxaluria
        Crohn's disease
        Celiac sprue
        Pancreatic insufficiency
        Small intestine bypass or ileal resection
    Other
        Overingestion of oxalate-containing foods
        Absence of enteric oxalate-degrading bacteria
        Pyridoxine (vitamin B$_6$) deficiency
        Excess ascorbic acid ingestion
        Ethylene glycol ingestion
        Methoxyflurane anesthesia in susceptible individuals
        Glycol irrigation in prostatectomy
        Aspergillosis

Aberrant splicing appears to underlie at least some of the defects in PH2 (770). Patients with PH1 tend to have a more severe phenotype and develop nephrocalcinosis, leading to renal failure, as well as nephrolithiasis. Stone disease is more common than nephrocalcinosis in PH2 (698); thus there is typically a milder course.

Primary hyperoxaluria typically makes its appearance in early childhood, in either sex, with recurrent calcium oxalate nephrolithiasis and renal failure related to obstruction, infection, and oxalate deposition within the kidney. In some patients, the disease does not manifest until adult life (771), and in these patients, the renal disease progresses at a slower pace. The kidney is the only route of excretion of oxalate, so that when renal function declines below the level at which oxalate can be completely filtered (with a small portion excreted by the tubules), oxalate begins to accumulate in the kidney. The kidneys may show widespread deposition of crystals in the tubular lumens, some of which are dilated and others atrophic, as well as in tubular cytoplasm. The crystals can readily be seen by examination under polarized light because of their birefringence (see Fig. 22.61).

With the advent of renal failure, deposits of oxalate begin to appear elsewhere in the body, notably in the myocardium (particularly in the conduction system), retina, skin, central nervous system, bone marrow, and blood vessels (772). With survival extended by dialysis, these deposits pose clinical problems in the form of cardiac arrhythmias, cardiomyopathies, erosive synovitis, digital gangrene, and mononeuritis multiplex, with elevated mortality rates. Combined hepatic and renal transplantation has been used in an attempt to correct both the enzymatic defect and the renal failure, with variable success (771,773,774). It is recommended that in patients with primary hyperoxaluria, transplantation be carried out much earlier than in other renal diseases, because oxalate deposits in other organs do not seem to accumulate until renal failure supervenes. Some patients respond favorably to pyridoxine, an enzyme cofactor for the defective enzyme in type 1 hyperoxaluria, that, when given in pharmacologic doses, attenuates the enzymatic defect in some patients (775).

### Secondary Hyperoxaluria

Enteric hyperoxaluria is the most important variant of secondary hyperoxaluria. It is caused by hyperabsorption of oxalate by the gut in various disorders and situations, including Crohn's disease, celiac sprue, pancreatic insufficiency, and small intestinal bypass surgery for obesity (776–778). All of these conditions have in common fat malabsorption with steatorrhea, which increases oxalate absorption from the small intestine and, to a lesser extent, the colon. In the case of jejunoileal bypass, symptomatic stone disease usually appears within 2 years of the operative procedure, requiring lithotomy in about one fifth of patients (779). There also appears to be a direct correlation between the absence of intestinal, oxalate-degrading bacteria such as *Oxalobacter formigenes* and hyperoxaluria (780–782).

Other causes of hyperoxaluria are much more rare and include ethylene glycol intoxication, adverse reaction to methoxyflurane, and excess intake of ascorbic acid (vitamin C) or foods rich in oxalate such as cocoa, spinach, beet greens, and rhubarb (778,783).

### Hypocitraturia

The role of citrate in preventing stone formation is not entirely clear, but it is known that increasing urinary citrate excretion is beneficial, at least in part because citrate complexes calcium and lessens free calcium ion activity. Citrate likely acts as an inhibitor of stone formation through decreased crystal growth and aggregation (720,784) (see Inhibitors of Stone Formation). Hypocitraturia is found in many calcium stone formers, ranging from 13% to 63% of patients (785,786). Estrogen increases citrate excretion and may play a part in reducing stone formation in women. Siener et al (762) found hypocitraturia in 57% of calcium oxalate stone formers, although intake of a standardized diet including increased intake of fluid reduced both the urinary abnormality and stone formation. Hypocitraturia can be caused by stimulation of its reabsorption in renal tubules owing to intracellular acidosis, as is found in distal renal tubular acidosis, a high protein diet, chronic diarrhea, or with potassium depletion (669,787). Administration of alkalinizing agents can correct the acidosis and restore citrate levels in the urine.

### Renal Tubular Acidosis

With rare exceptions, stone formation and nephrocalcinosis in renal tubular acidosis (RTA) are limited to patients with type 1, classic distal RTA. Approximately 75% of patients with type 1 RTA develop nephrocalcinosis, nephrolithiasis, or both (644). Type 1 RTA may be inherited as an autosomal dominant disorder or may occur sporadically without associated disease (650,711). It may also be acquired in conjunction with other systemic diseases, such as dysproteinemias, Sjögren's syndrome, Wilson's disease, primary biliary cirrhosis, lymphocytic thyroiditis, and intestinal bypass surgery, as well as with the use of certain drugs, including amphotericin B, lithium, and toluene (502,503). Carbonic anhydrase inhibitors, which produce a clinical picture of RTA type 2, paradoxically result in stone formation (788,789).

Patients with RTA have renal tubular cell acidosis, which results in increased calcium and phosphorus excretion, decreased citrate excretion, and a high urine pH, all of which are conditions that raise the likelihood of crystal formation. Therapy consists of alkali administration to acidify the urine, reduce calcium excretion, and increase urinary citrate, slowing the pace of nephrolithiasis and nephrocalcinosis. Treatment with potassium citrate tablets has been shown to be effective and is better tolerated than sodium bicarbonate (790,791).

## Noncalcium Stones

### Infection (Struvite) Stones

Infection stones are calculi composed of magnesium ammonium phosphate ($MgNH_4PO_4 \cdot 6H_2O$), or struvite, usually admixed with carbonate apatite ($Ca_{10}(PO_4)6 \cdot CO_3$) (746,792,793). They are also known as struvite, urease, or triple-phosphate stones and account for 10% to 15% of urinary calculi. These stones may form initially as matrix stones, composed in part of glycocalyx of bacterial origin, plus Tamm-Horsfall urinary mucoprotein and other mucoid components (698,793). Over time, struvite and carbonate apatite fill in and replace the matrix with the evolution of a dense, radiopaque stone. Struvite stones form most often in the presence of infection by urea-splitting bacteria, usually *Proteus* organisms. The presence of urease can elevate the concentration of ammonium ion, $NH_4$, and the urine pH and carbonate concentrations sufficiently high for crystallization of struvite to occur (793). Once infection is well established, the stones can grow and branch rapidly, forming staghorn calculi. Microscopic urinalysis demonstrates very characteristic crystals with a "coffin lid" or quartz crystal appearance. Histologically, there may be advanced chronic changes of tubular atrophy and interstitial fibrosis owing in part to the infectious process and to obstruction or compression of parenchyma.

*Proteus vulgaris*, *Proteus mirabilis*, *Morganella morgagnii*, and *Providencia rettgeri* are the most frequent offenders. However, other urease-producing species of *Providencia*, *Klebsiella pneumoniae*, *Serratia marcescens*, *Enterobacter aerogenes*, *Ureaplasma urealyticum*, and even staphylococci have been identified (793–795).

Many of these stones form in individuals who have a primary condition predisposing them to stone formation. Smith (709) found that there were underlying metabolic disorders in 70 of 114 consecutive patients (61%) with infected stones, most frequently idiopathic hypercalciuria, primary hyperparathyroidism, and gout, with calcium oxalate or uric acid serving as the nidus from which the struvite stone formed. Aside from the context of other primary stone diseases, infection stones are seen in situations in which urinary tract infections are more often present: vesicoureteral reflux, obstructive uropathy, neurogenic bladder, and ileal diversion of the ureter (796). Infection stones affect 8% of patients with spinal cord injury, and struvite stones develop in up to 30% of patients with ileal loops (793).

One of the most pernicious aspects of these stones arises from the fact that the bacteria are incorporated into the substance of the stone and, once there, are largely invulnerable to antibiotics; organisms may remain viable despite literally years of continuous antibiotic coverage (796). It is this aspect that renders treatment difficult by any of the current modes of therapy, including extracorporeal shock wave lithotripsy (ESWL). Percutaneous nephrolithotomy may be necessary to completely remove struvite stones. In many instances "infection stones" are really "infected stones," i.e., stones of other origin that have become secondarily infected.

## Uric Acid Stones

About 5% to 10% of renal stones are uric acid stones (746,797,798) (Fig. 22.68). There is a higher incidence of uric acid stone formation among patients with gout; from 10% to 50% form uric acid stones, the variation being a result of differences in rate of uric acid excretion (799,800).

Uric acid crystals develop in urine of low pH, especially when the uric acid content is high (698). However, low urine pH and low urine volume are more important than the absolute content of uric acid in the development of stones in patients with gout as well as those with idiopathic uric acid stones (698). Idiopathic uric acid stone formers tend to excrete less ammonia, leading to the low urine pH values found (698). Those patients with gout who form stones also tend to have low urinary pH values, suggesting a defect in ammonia production in this group as well (746). The higher prevalence of uric acid stones in some countries, such as the middle eastern countries (40% or more), testifies to the role of dehydration in formation of these type of stones.

Low-carbohydrate, high-protein diets also tend to reduce urine pH, increasing the risk for urolithiasis (801). A connection between insulin resistance and uric acid nephrolithiasis has been suggested, since individuals with

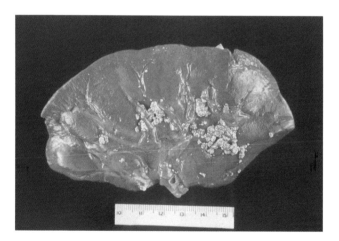

**Figure 22.68** Uric acid nephrolithiasis. Multiple small, pale yellow uric acid stones.

gout share features of the metabolic syndrome and there is a higher incidence of uric acid stone formation in type 2 diabetic stone formers (802–804). Insulin resistance is also associated with an acidic urine (803), the condition most favorable for uric acid stone formation.

A smaller group of uric acid stone formers consists of those patients in whom there is overproduction of uric acid. The simplest examples of overproduction of uric acid are malignancies, primarily lymphoproliferative and myeloproliferative disorders, in which increased nucleotide catabolism generates excess purines and hence excess uric acid. Chemotherapy, with abrupt tumor necrosis, may lead to the same result, with stone formation and even obstruction. Polycythemia, hemolytic anemia, and sickle cell disease can all increase uric acid formation. Enzyme defects, all of which are rare, may also lead to hyperuricemia. Among others, these conditions include hypoxanthine-guanine phosphoribosyltransferase deficiency (Lesch-Nyhan syndrome), adenine phosphoribosyltransferase deficiency, elevated phosphoribosylpyrophosphate synthetase activity, decreased phosphoribosylpyrophosphate substrate utilization, and type 1 glycogen storage disease (698).

Gouty microtophi can be identified in individuals with gout. In renal biopsies, uric acid crystals are seen as clear "needles" within the interstitium, usually surrounded by an inflammatory reaction that can contain giant cells (Fig. 22.69).

## Cystinuria

Cystinuria is a hereditary disorder of tubular transport which results in the excretion of abnormally large amounts of cystine, as well as other dibasic amino acids, in the urine and ultimately the development of recurrent cystine stones (669,698,746). The disease is inherited in most cases as an autosomal recessive trait (type 1) or incomplete recessive (types 2 and 3). The incidence varies from 1 in 2500 to 1 in 15,000 (805). Renal stones typically begin to form in the second or third decade, but they may appear earlier or later. Cystine stones constitute approximately 2% of all urinary stones (746,798). The typical hexagonal crystals are usually readily recognized in the urine, particularly a concentrated early-morning urine.

The genetic defect in type 1 is a mutation in the gene SLC3A1 (solute-linked carrier 3A1), whereas types 2 and 3 are associated with mutations in SLC7A9. These genes code for cystine, dibasic, and amino acid transporters (329–331).

The renal calculi that form may appear as multiple small stones or large staghorn calculi; radiographically, they can be of two types, with either a smooth or a rough surface (698). Radiographically, they are radiopaque because of the sulfur-containing molecules, but are less so than calcium-containing stones. Although cystine stones in general are more resistant than other stones to shock wave lithotripsy, those with a rough surface have been found to be more susceptible to this treatment (809). Grossly, they are granular and often sand-colored to yellow-brown. Cystine may be admixed with oxalate, phosphate, and struvite in some patients. The risk in these patients, as with other forms of nephrolithiasis, is secondary infection and obstruction

Cystinuria should be distinguished from *cystinosis*. In that condition, also a rare hereditary enzymatic disorder, there is widespread *intracellular* accumulation of cystine, with extensive damage, particularly in the kidney, and ensuing renal failure. In *cystinuria*, by contrast, renal parenchymal deposits are all extracellular, in the tubular lumens and renal pelvis.

Treatment involves increasing fluid intake, alkalinization of the urine and reducing sodium intake (502). Drugs that act to reduce free cysteine (cystine is formed by disulfide linkage of two cysteine molecules), such as penicillamine, mercaptopropionylglycine, tiopronin, and captopril, show some promise in treatment of cystine stones (810,811).

## Miscellaneous Stones

### Xanthinuria

Xanthinuria is a rare hereditary disorder, transmitted as an autosomal recessive trait (812). There is a deficiency of xanthine dehydrogenase, an enzyme responsible for the oxidation of hypoxanthine and xanthine to uric acid, such that xanthine and hypoxanthine appear in the urine in greatly increased quantities. Conversely, serum urate and urinary uric acid levels are very low. Radiolucent xanthine stones are found in about one third of patients with this disorder. On occasion, xanthine stones are also seen as a

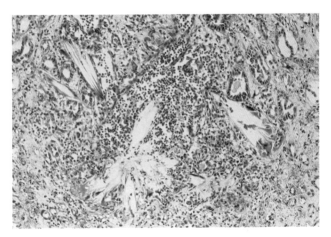

**Figure 22.69** Microtophi in a patient with gout. Needle-shaped clear spaces in the interstitium surrounded by an intense inflammatory reaction. (H&E, x 200.)

complication of allopurinol therapy for hyperuricemia, since allopurinol blocks xanthine oxidase (709).

### Matrix Stone

A rare type of stone consisting almost entirely of a noncrystalline matrix has been described in patients on maintenance dialysis (813), and in the presence of urinary tract infections (814,815). Matrix is a substance composed of a carbohydrate material (often mucopolysaccharide) plus protein (such as mucoprotein). These stones are somewhat gelatinous or claylike and can have a laminated appearance. Matrix stones, unlike crystalline stones, do not calcify, though some authors believe they may be a nidus for calcium stone formation. Because of their physical and radiologic properties, they may be mistaken for renal tumors (816).

### Medication-Related Stones

Individuals who ingest large amounts of ephedrine or guaifenesin have been found to produce stones with a large component of these chemicals (598,705,706). In some individuals, these compounds had been abused as stimulants. Alkalinization of the urine was successful in treating most cases.

## Treatment of Stones by Lithotripsy

Most stones will pass spontaneously and do not require intervention (703,817,818). Stones that are 4 to 5 mm have a 40% to 50% chance of spontaneously passing in the urine. For those stones that are greater than 5 mm, spontaneous passage is less likely and further intervention is necessary. Stones in the middle to distal ureter have a greater chance of passage than those in the proximal ureter or calyces. Shock wave lithotripsy (ESWL) has revolutionized the management of urinary calculi (809,819), although for distal calculi, some authors recommend ureteroscopy over SWL for the overall higher success rate and reduced need for secondary interventions or retreatment (820).

In ESWL, shock waves are created by the lithotriptor and focused on the stone, such that the stone disintegrates as a result of erosion at the points of entry and exit of the shock waves. In addition, the stone shatters owing to buildup of a pressure gradient when the focused shock waves encounter solids of different acoustic properties than the surrounding tissues and water whose acoustic properties are similar (819). The overall stone-free rate at 3 months following ESWL is nearly 75%. With stones smaller than 1.5 cm, the stone-free rate is approximately 90%. Indications for ESWL include large stones with a risk of obstruction, smaller stones in the proximal ureter, and any stones in the distal ureter (809).

Despite the success of ESWL to eliminate stones, this treatment is not without complications (821,822). Most patients will experience minimal morbidity from ESWL; however, a few notable complications have occurred. Perirenal hematoma and pain complicates approximately 0.1% to 0.3% of cases (823). Cases of post–shock wave hypertension owing to compression of the kidney by perirenal hemorrhage have been reported (824), although one study found no difference between SWL and other treatment types (825) and another found no difference in blood pressure changes between a control group of patients and an ESWL-treated group (826).

In animal experiments, ESWL to canine kidneys produced renal trauma that appeared to be dose related according to the number of shocks delivered (827,828). There were intraparenchymal and perirenal hemorrhages and interstitial edema along the shock wave path. The small veins seemed to be particularly vulnerable to rupture and thrombosis (827,828), and there was tubular dilatation and cast formation (probably related to tubular epithelial damage). Newman et al (828) reported fibrosis, with scars extending from the cortex to the medulla and with loss of both tubules and glomeruli.

Although there are issues related to the use of SWL, many stones are treated with lithotripsy as a first attempt. Most stones smaller than 2 cm will be successfully removed by this technique. Larger stones may need to be approached by ureterostomy or percutaneous nephrolithotomy. In the setting of urinary tract anomalies, complex stones or those in the distal ureter, or in select groups of patients such as children or the obese, SWL is not the treatment of choice (710,809). Absolute contraindications to ESWL are distal obstruction, infection, pregnancy, and coagulopathy. Cystine, calcium oxalate monohydrate, and matrix stones are more refractory to treatment by SWL than are other stones, such as those formed from uric acid, and may require ureterostomy or percutaneous nephrolithotomy (809,819).

## REFERENCES

1. Kunin CM. Detection, Prevention, and Management of Urinary Tract Infections, 4th ed. Philadelphia: Lea & Febiger, 1987.
2. Maskell R. Recurrent urinary tract infections including covert bacteriuria. In: Catto GRD, ed. Urinary Tract Infection. Dordrecht, Netherlands: Kluwer, 1989:1.
3. Stamm WE, Wagner KF, Amsel R, et al. Causes of the acute urethral syndrome in women. N Engl J Med 1980;303:409.
4. Bailey RR. The relationship of vesicoureteric reflux to urinary tract infection and chronic pyelonephritis-reflux nephropathy. Clin Nephrol 1973;1:132.
5. Kass EH. Chemotherapeutic and antibiotic drugs in the management of infections of the urinary tract. Am J Med 1955;18:764.
6. Kass EH. Personal perspectives on bacteriuria and pyelonephritis in relation to the Fourth Symposium. In: Kass EH, Svanborg Edén C, eds. Host–Parasite Interactions in Urinary Tract Infections. Chicago: University of Chicago Press, 1989:2.
7. Platt R. Quantitative definition of bacteriuria. Am J Med 1983;75(suppl 1B):44.
8. Sobel JD. Pathogenesis of urinary tract infections: Host defenses. Infect Dis Clin North Am 1987;1:751.

9. Kass EH. Asymptomatic infections of urinary tract. Trans Assoc Am Physicians 1956;69:56.

10. Kass EH. Pyelonephritis and bacteriuria: A major problem in preventive medicine. Ann Intern Med 1962;56:46.

11. Medical Research Council Bacteriuria Committee. Recommended terminology of urinary-tract infection. Br Med J 1979; 2:717.

12. Hooton TM. The current management strategies for community-acquired urinary tract infection. Infect Dis Clin North Am 2003; 017:303.

13. Bass PF III, Jarvis JAW, Mitchell CK. Urinary tract infections. Prim Care 2003;30:41.

14. Miller O II, Hemphill RR. Urinary tract infection and pyelonephritis. Emerg Med Clin North Am 2001;19:655.

15. Wagenlehner FME, Naber KG. Uncomplicated urinary tract infections in women. Curr Opin Urol 2001;11:49.

16. Gilstrap LC, Ramin SM. Urinary tract infections during pregnancy. Obstet Gynecol Clin North Am 2001;28:581.

17. Connolly A, Thorp JM Jr. Urinary tract infections in pregnancy. Urol Clin North Am 1999;26:779.

18. Hoepelman AIM, Meiland R, Geerlings SE. Pathogenesis and management of bacterial urinary tract infections in adult patients with diabetes mellitus. Int J Antimicrob Agents 2003;22 Suppl 2:35.

19. Ronald A, Ludwig E. Urinary tract infections in adults with diabetes. Int J Antimicrob Agents 2001;17:287.

20. Escherich T. Ueber Cystitis bei Kindern hervorgerufen durch das *Bact. coli* commune: Vortrag geh. am 26 Februar 1894 im Verein der Aerzte in Steiermark. Quoted by Trumpp J. Über Colicystitis im Kindersalter. Jahrb Kinderheilkd 1897;44:268.

21. Göppert F II. Über die eitrigen Erkrankungen der Harnwege im Kindersalter: Pyelitis, Pyelocystitis und Cystitis. Ergeb Inn Med Kinderheilkd 1908;2:30.

22. Thiemich M. Über die eitrigen Erkrankungen der Nieren und Harnwege im Säuglingsalter. Jahrb Kinderheilkd 1910;72:243.

23. Wagner EL. Handbuch der Krankheiten des Harnapparates. I. Hälfte: Der Morbus Brightii. In: von Ziemssen HW, ed. Handbuch der speciellen Pathologie und Therapie, vol 9, part 1, 3rd ed. Leipzig: Vogel, 1882:309.

24. Löhlein M. Über Schrumpfnieren. Beitr Pathol Anat 1917;63: 570.

25. Gibson AG. Pyelitis and pyelonephritis. Lancet 1928;2:903.

26. Staemmler M, Dopheide W. Die Pyelonephritische Schrumpfniere. Virchows Arch A Pathol Anat Histopathol 1930; 277:713.

27. Longcope WT, Winkenwerder WL. Clinical features of the contracted kidney due to pyelonephritis. Bull Johns Hopkins Hosp 1933;52:255.

28. Weiss S, Parker F Jr. Pyelonephritis: Its relation to vascular lesions and to arterial hypertension. Medicine (Baltimore) 1939;18: 221.

29. Raaschou F. Studies of Chronic Pyelonephritis with Special Reference to the Kidney Function. Copenhagen: Munksgaard, 1948.

30. Pickering GW, Heptinstall RH. Nephrectomy and other treatment for hypertension in pyelonephritis. Q J Med 1953;22:1.

31. Heptinstall RH. The limitations of the pathological diagnosis of pyelonephritis. In: Black DAK, ed. Renal Disease, 2nd ed. Oxford: Blackwell, 1967:350.

32. Smith JF. The diagnosis of the scars of chronic pyelonephritis. J Clin Pathol 1962;15:522.

33. Hodson CJ. The radiological diagnosis of pyelonephritis. Proc R Soc Med 1959;5:669.

34. Lomberg H, Hanson LA, Jacobsson B, et al. Correlation of P blood group, vesicoureteral reflux, and bacterial attachment in patients with recurrent pyelonephritis. N Engl J Med 1983; 308:1189.

35. Meyrier A, Condamin M-C, Fernet M, et al. Frequency of development of early cortical scarring in acute primary pyelonephritis. Kidney Int 1989;35:696.

36. Winberg J, Bollgren I, Källenius G, et al. Clinical pyelonephritis and focal renal scarring: A selected review of pathogenesis, prevention, and prognosis. Pediatr Clin North Am 1982;29:801.

37. Benador D, Benador N, Slosman DO, et al. Cortical scintigraphy in the evaluation of renal parenchymal changes in children with pyelonephritis. J Pediatr 1994;124:17.

38. Majd M, Rushton HG, Jantausch B, Wiedermann BL. Relationship among vesicoureteral reflux, P-fimbriated *Escherichia coli*, and acute pyelonephritis in children with febrile urinary tract infection. J Pediatr 1991;119:578.

39. Kooman JP, Barendregt NM, vander Sande FM, van Suylen R-J. Acute pyelonephritis: A cause of acute renal failure? Neth J Med 2000;57:185.

40. Nickel JC. The management of acute pyelonephritis in adults. Can J Urol 2001;8(suppl 1):29.

41. Busch R, Huland H. Correlation of symptoms and results of direct bacterial localization in patients with urinary tract infections. J Urol 1984;132:282.

42. Risdon RA, Godley ML, Parkhouse HF, et al. Renal pathology and the $^{99m}$Tc-DMSA image during the evolution of the early pyelonephritic scar: An experimental study. J Urol 1994;151:767.

43. Rushton HG, Majd M, Chandra R, Yim D. Evaluation of $^{99m}$technetium-dimercapto-succinic acid renal scans in experimental acute pyelonephritis in piglets. J Urol 1988;140(5 Pt 2): 1169.

44. Jakobsson B, Nolstedt L, Svensson S, et al. $^{99m}$Technetium-dimercaptosuccinic acid scan in the diagnosis of acute pyelonephritis in children: Relation to clinical and radiological findings. Pediatr Nephrol 1992;6:328.

45. Jantausch BA, Wiedermann BL, Hull SI, et al. *Escherichia coli* virulence factors and $^{99m}$Tc-dimercaptosuccinic acid renal scan in children with febrile urinary tract infection. Pediatr Infect Dis J 1992;11:343.

46. Rosenberg AR, Rossleigh MA, Brydon MP, et al. Evaluation of acute urinary tract infection in children by dimercaptosuccinic acid scintigraphy: A prospective study. J Urol 1992;148(5 Pt 2): 1746.

47. Tappin DM, Murphy AV, Mocan H, et al. A prospective study of children with first acute symptomatic E. coli urinary tract infection: early $^{99m}$technetium dimercaptosuccinic acid scan appearances. Acta Paediatr Scand 1989;78:923.

48. Goldraich NP, Goldraich IH. Update on dimercaptosuccinic acid renal scanning in children with urinary tract infection. Pediatr Nephrol 1995;9:221.

49. Rushton HG, Majd M. Dimercaptosuccinic acid renal scintigraphy for the evaluation of pyelonephritis and scarring: A review of experimental and clinical studies. J Urol 1992;148:1726.

50. Moreno A, Mensa J, Almela M, et al. Estudio de 138 episodios de bacteriemia o funguemia en pacientes con transplante de órgano sólido (renal o hepático). Med Clin (Barc) 1994;103:161.

51. Scroggs MW, Wolfe JA, Bollinger RR, Sanfilippo F. Causes of death in renal transplant recipients: A review of autopsy findings from 1966 through 1985. Arch Pathol Lab Med 1987;111:983.

52. Wiecek A, Zeier M, Ritz E. Role of infection in the genesis of acute renal failure. Nephrol Dial Transplant 1994;9suppl 4:40.

53. Pontin AR, Barnes RD, Joffe J, Kahn D. Emphysematous pyelonephritis in diabetic patients. Br J Urol 1995;75:71.

54. Lowe BA, Poage MD. Bilateral emphysematous pyelonephritis. Urology 1991;37:229.

55. Michaeli J, Mogle P, Perlberg S, et al. Emphysematous pyelonephritis. J Urol 1984;131:203.

56. Huang J-J, Tseng C-C. Emphysematous pyelonephritis: Clinico-radiological classification, management, prognosis, and pathogenesis. Arch Intern Med 2000;160:797.

57. Evanoff GV, Thompson CS, Foley R, Weinman EJ. Spectrum of gas within the kidney: Emphysematous pyelonephritis and emphysematous pyelitis. Am J Med 1987;83:149.

58. Ransley PG, Risdon RA. Reflux nephropathy: Effects of antimicrobial therapy on the evolution of the early pyelonephritic scar. Kidney Int 1981;20:733.

59. Kimmelstiel P, Wilson C. Inflammatory lesions in the glomeruli in pyelonephritis in relation to hypertension and renal insufficiency. Am J Pathol 1936;12:99.

60. Iványi B, Rumpelt HJ, Thoenes W. Acute human pyelonephritis: Leukocytic infiltration of tubules and localization of bacteria. Virchows Arch A Pathol Anat Histopathol 1988;414:29.

61. Iványi B, Thoenes W. Microvascular injury and repair in acute

human bacterial pyelonephritis. Virchows Arch A Pathol Anat Histopathol 1987;411:257.

62. Heptinstall RH. Experimental pyelonephritis: Bacteriological and morphological studies on the ascending route of infection in the rat. Nephron 1964;1:73.

63. Heptinstall RH, Gorrill RH. Experimental pyelonephritis and its effect on the blood pressure. J Pathol 1955;69:191.

64. Hodson CJ, Maling TMJ, McManamon PJ, Lewis MG. The pathogenesis of reflux nephropathy (chronic atrophic pyelonephritis). Br J Radiol 1975;13(suppl):1.

65. Heptinstall RH. Experimental pyelonephritis: A comparison of blood-borne and ascending patterns of infection. J Pathol 1965;89:71.

66. Bergström T, Lincoln K, Redin B, Winberg J. Studies of urinary tract infections in infancy and childhood. X. Short- or long-term treatment in girls with first- or second-time urinary tract infections uncomplicated by obstructive urological abnormalities. Acta Paediatr Scand 1968;57:186.

67. Freedman LR. Prolonged observations on a group of patients with acute urinary tract infections. In: Quinn EL, Kass EH, eds. Henry Ford Hospital Symposium on Biology of Pyelonephritis. Boston: Little, Brown, 1960:345.

68. Winberg J, Andersen HJ, Bergström T, et al. Epidemiology of symptomatic urinary tract infection in childhood. Acta Paediatr Scand 1974;252(suppl):1.

69. Coker CC, Poore CA, Li X, Mobley HLT. Pathogenesis of Proteus mirabilis urinary tract infection. Microbes Infect 2000;2:1497.

70. Demetrios P, Constantine B, Demetrios S, Nikolaos A. Haemophilus influenza acute pyelonephritis in the elderly. Intern Urol Nephrol 2002;34:23.

71. Källenius G, Möllby R, Svenson SB, et al. Occurrence of P-fimbriated Escherichia coli in urinary tract infections. Lancet 1981;2:1369.

72. Roberts AP, Linton JD, Waterman AM, et al. Urinary and faecal Escherichia coli O-serogroups in symptomatic urinary-tract infection and asymptomatic bacteriuria. J Med Microbiol 1975;8:311.

73. Vosti KL, Goldberg LM, Monto AS, Rantz LA. Host–parasite interaction in patients with infections due to Escherichia coli. I. The serogrouping of E. coli from intestinal and extraintestinal sources. J Clin Invest 1964;43:2377.

74. Wold AE, Caugant DA, Lidin-Janson G, et al. Resident colonic Escherichia coli strains frequently display uropathogenic characteristics. J Infect Dis 1992;165:46.

75. Rantz LA. Serological grouping of Escherichia coli: Study in urinary tract infection. Arch Intern Med 1962;109:37.

76. Johnson JR. Virulence factors in Escherichia coli urinary tract infection. Clin Microbiol Rev 1991;4:80.

77. Lomberg H, Hellström M, Jodal U, et al. Virulence-associated traits in Escherichia coli causing first and recurrent episodes of urinary tract infection in children with and without vesicoureteral reflux. J Infect Dis 1984;150:561.

78. Väisänen V, Elo J, Tallgren LG, et al. Mannose-resistant haemagglutination and P antigen recognition are characteristics of Escherichia coli causing primary pyelonephritis. Lancet 1981;2:1366.

79. Fair WR. Observations on the origin of urinary tract infections. In: Kincaid-Smith P, Fairley KF, eds. Renal Infection and Renal Scarring. Melbourne: Mercedes, 1970:89.

80. Stamey TA, Sexton CC. The role of vaginal colonization with Enterobacteriaceae in recurrent urinary infections. J Urol 1975;113:214.

81. Cox CE, Lacy SS, Hinman F Jr. The urethra and its relationship to urinary tract infection. II. The urethral flora of the female with recurrent urinary infection. J Urol 1968;99:632.

82. Gower PE. A study of the vestibular flora in women with symptoms of recurrent acute lower urinary infections. In: Kincaid-Smith P, Fairley KF, eds. Renal Infection and Renal Scarring. Melbourne: Mercedes, 1970:103.

83. Stamey TA, Timothy M, Millar M, Mihara G. Recurrent urinary infections in adult women: The role of introital enterobacteria. Calif Med 1971;115:1.

84. Stamm WE, Hooton TM, Johnson JR, et al. Urinary tract infec-

tions: From pathogenesis to treatment. J Infect Dis 1989;159:400.

85. Fowler JE Jr, Stamey TA. Studies on introital colonization in women with recurrent urinary infections. VII. The role of bacterial adherence. J Urol 1977;117:472.

86. Kozody NL, Harding GKM, Nicolle LE, et al. Adherence of Escherichia coli to epithelial cells in the pathogenesis of urinary tract infection. Clin Invest Med 1985;8:121.

87. Schaeffer AJ, Jones JM, Dunn JK. Association of in vitro Escherichia coli adherence to vaginal and buccal epithelial cells with susceptibility of women to recurrent urinary-tract infections. N Engl J Med 1981;304:1062.

88. Källenius G, Winberg J. Bacterial adherence to periurethral epithelial cells in girls prone to urinary-tract infections. Lancet 1978;2:540.

89. Svanborg-Edén C, Jodal U. Attachment of Escherichia coli to urinary sediment epithelial cells from urinary tract infection–prone and healthy children. Infect Immun 1979;26:837.

90. Brumfitt W, Gargan RA, Hamilton-Miller JMT. Periurethral enterobacterial carriage preceding urinary infection [erratum appears in Lancet 1987 Apr 25;1:994]. Lancet 1987;1:824.

91. Kunin CM, Polyak F, Postel E. Periurethral bacterial flora in women: Prolonged intermittent colonization with Escherichia coli. JAMA 1980;243:134.

92. Fair WR, Stamey TA. Bactericidal properties of prostatic fluid. In: Stamey TA, Hinman F, Sanford JP, eds. Proceedings of a Workshop on Urinary Infections in the Male. Washington, D.C.: National Academy of Sciences, National Research Council, 1969:199.

93. Stamey TA, Govan DE, Palmer JM. The localization and treatment of urinary tract infections: The role of bactericidal urine levels as opposed to serum levels. Medicine (Baltimore) 1965;44:1.

94. Wiswell TE, Miller GM, Gelston HM Jr, et al. Effect of circumcision status on periurethral bacterial flora during the first year of life. J Pediatr 1988;113:442.

95. Hanson LA, Ahlstedt S, Jodal U, et al. The host–parasite relationship in urinary tract infections. Kidney Int 1975;8(suppl 4):S28.

96. Svanborg Edén C, de Man P. Bacterial virulence in urinary tract infection. Infect Dis Clin North Am 1987;1:731.

97. Roberts JA. Tropism in bacterial infections: Urinary tract infections. J Urol 1996;156:1552.

98. Svanborg C, Agace W, Hedges S, et al. Bacterial adherence and mucosal cytokine production. Ann N Y Acad Sci 1994;730:162.

99. Kanamaru S, Kurazono H, Ishitoya S, et al. Distribution and genetic association of putative uropathogenic virulence factors iroN, iha, kpsMT, ompT and USP in Escherichia coli isolated from urinary tract infections in Japan. J Urol 2003;17:2490.

100. Svanborg C. Resistance to urinary tract infection. N Engl J Med 1993;329:802.

101. Lomberg H, Cedergren B, Leffler H, et al. Influence of blood group on the availability of receptors for attachment of uropathogenic Escherichia coli. Infect Immun 1986;51:919.

102. Stamey TA, Wehner N, Mihara G, Condy M. The immunologic basis of recurrent bacteriuria: Role of cervicovaginal antibody in enterobacterial colonization of the introital mucosa. Medicine (Baltimore) 1978;57:47.

103. Stamey TA, Fair WR, Timothy MM, Chung HK. Antibacterial nature of prostatic fluid. Nature 1968;218:444.

104. Miller TE, North JDK. Host response in urinary tract infections. Kidney Int 1974;5:179.

105. Parsons CL. Pathogenesis of urinary tract infections: Bacterial adherence, bladder defense mechanisms. Urol Clin North Am 1986;13:563.

106. Järvinen A-K, Sandholm M. Urinary oligosaccharides inhibit adhesion of E. coli onto canine urinary tract epithelium. Invest Urol 1980;17:443.

107. Orskov I, Orskov F, Birch-Andersen A. Comparison of Escherichia coli fimbrial antigen F7 with type 1 fimbriae. Infect Immun 1980;27:657.

108. Svanborg Edén C, Svennerholm AM. Secretory immunoglobulin A and G antibodies prevent adhesion of Escherichia coli to human urinary tract epithelial cells. Infect Immun 1978;22:790

109. Hanson LA, Fasth A, Jodal U, et al. Biology and pathology of urinary tract infections. J Clin Pathol 1981;34:695.

110. Hjelm EM. Local cellular immune response in ascending urinary tract infection: Occurrence of T-cells, immunoglobulin-producing cells, and Ia-expressing cells in rat urinary tract tissue. Infect Immun 1984;44:627.

111. Thomas VL, Forland M. Antibody-coated bacteria in urinary tract infections. Kidney Int 1982;21:1.

112. de Ree JM, van den Bosch JF. Serological response to the P fimbriae of uropathogenic Escherichia coli in pyelonephritis. Infect Immun 1987;55:2204.

113. Rene P, Silverblatt FJ. Serological response to Escherichia coli pili in pyelonephritis. Infect Immun 1982;37:749.

114. Kinane DF, Blackwell CC, Brettle RP, et al. ABO blood group, secretor state, and susceptibility to recurrent urinary tract infection in women. Br Med J 1982;285:7.

115. Lomberg H, Hanson LA, Jacobsson B, et al. Correlation of P blood group, vesicoureteral reflux, and bacterial attachment in patients with recurrent pyelonephritis. N Engl J Med 1983; 308:1189.

116. Lomberg H, Hellström M, Jodal U, Svanborg Edén C. Secretor state and renal scarring in girls with recurrent pyelonephritis. FEMS Microbiol Immunol 1989;47:371.

117. Jacobson SH, Lomberg H. Overrepresentation of blood group non-secretors in adults with renal scarring. Scand J Urol Nephrol 1990;24:145.

118. Lomberg H, Jodal U, Leffler H, et al. Blood group non-secretors have an increased inflammatory response to urinary tract infection. Scand J Infect Dis 1992;24:77.

119. Blackwell CC, May SJ, Maccallum CJ, et al. Secretor state and susceptibility to recurrent urinary tract infections. In: Kass EH, Svanborg Edén C, eds. Host–Parasite Interactions in Urinary Tract Infections. Chicago: University of Chicago Press, 1989:234.

120. Mallory GK, Crane AR, Edwards JE. Pathology of acute and of healed experimental pyelonephritis. Arch Pathol 1940;30:330.

121. Heptinstall RH, Brumfitt W. Experimental pyelonephritis: Reactivation of the healing lesion by ureteric occlusion. Br J Exp Pathol 1960;41:381.

122. Beeson PB, Rocha H, Guze LB. Experimental pyelonephritis: Influence of localized injury in different parts of the kidney on susceptibility to hematogenous infection. Trans Assoc Am Physicians 1957;70:120.

123. De Navasquez S. Further studies in experimental pyelonephritis produced by various bacteria, with special reference to renal scarring as a factor in pathogenesis. J Pathol 1956;71:27.

124. Patterson JE, Andriole VT. Bacterial urinary tract infections in diabetes. Infect Dis Clin North Am 1995;9:25.

125. Edmondson HA, Martin HE, Evans N. Necrosis of renal papillae and acute pyelonephritis in diabetes mellitus. Arch Intern Med 1947;79:148.

126. Robbins SL, Tucker AW Jr. The cause of death in diabetes: A report on 307 autopsied cases. N Engl J Med 1944;231:865.

127. Bevan JS, Griffiths GJ, Williams JD, Gibby OM. Bilateral renal cortical abscesses in a young woman with type 1 diabetes. Diabet Med 1989;6:454.

128. De Navasquez S. Experimental pyelonephritis in the rabbit produced by staphylococcal infection. J Pathol 1950;62:429.

129. Cheung AL, Krishnan M, Jaffe EA, Fischetti VA. Fibrinogen acts as a bridging molecule in the adherence of Staphylococcus aureus to cultured human endothelial cells. J Clin Invest 1991;87:2236.

130. Lopes JD, dos Reis M, Brentani RR. Presence of laminin receptors in Staphylococcus aureus. Science 1985;229:275.

131. Iandolo JJ. Genetic analysis of extracellular toxins of Staphylococcus aureus. Annu Rev Microbiol 1989;43:375.

132. Bhakdi S, Tranum-Jensen J. Alpha-toxin of Staphylococcus aureus. Microbiol Rev 1991;55:733.

133. Swaminathan S, Furey W, Pletcher J, Sax M. Crystal structure of staphylococcal enterotoxin B, a superantigen. Nature 1992;359: 801.

134. Shapiro AH. Pumping and retrograde diffusion in peristaltic waves. In: Glenn JF, ed. Proceedings of a Workshop on Ureteral Reflux in Children. Washington, DC: National Academy of Sciences, National Research Council, 1967:109.

135. Roberts JA, Marklund B-I, Ilver D, et al. The Gal(a1–4) Gal-specific tip adhesin of Escherichia coli P-fimbriae is needed for pyelonephritis to occur in the normal urinary tract. Proc Natl Acad Sci U S A 1994;91:11889.

136. Roberts JA, Suarez GM, Kaack B, et al. Experimental pyelonephritis in the monkey. VII. Ascending pyelonephritis in the absence of vesicoureteral reflux. J Urol 1985;133:1068.

137. Discussion on fimbriated organisms. Contrib Nephrol 1984;39: 281.

138. Roberts JA. Experimental pyelonephritis in the monkey. III. Pathophysiology of ureteral malfunction induced by bacteria. Invest Urol 1975;13:117.

139. Raz R, Sakran W, Chazan B, et al. Long-term follow-up of women hospitalized for acute pyelonephritis. Clin Infect Dis 2003;37:1014.

140. Efstathiou SP, Pefanis AV, Tsioulos DI, et al. Acute pyelonephritis in adults: Prediction of mortality and failure of treatment. Arch Intern Med 2003;163:1206.

141. Roberts JA. Management of pyelonephritis and upper urinary tract infections. Urol Clin North Am 1999;26:753.

142. Webb NJA, Brenchley PEC. Cytokines and cell adhesion molecules in the inflammatory response during acute pyelonephritis. Nephron Exp Nephrol 2004;96:e1.

143. Gingell JC, Roylance J, Davies ER, Penry JB. Xanthogranulomatous pyelonephritis. Br J Radiol 1973;46:99.

144. Chuang C-K, Lai M-K, Chang P-L, et al. Xanthogranulomatous pyelonephritis: Experience in 36 cases. J Urol 1992;147:333.

145. McDonald GSA. Xanthogranulomatous pyelonephritis. J Pathol 1981;133:203.

146. Rosi P, Selli C, Carini M, et al. Xanthogranulomatous pyelonephritis: Clinical experience with 62 cases. Eur Urol 1986;12:96.

147. Grainger RG, Longstaff AJ, Parsons MA. Xanthogranulomatous pyelonephritis: a reappraisal. Lancet 1982;1:1398.

148. Parsons MA, Harris SC, Longstaff AJ, Grainger RG. Xanthogranulomatous pyelonephritis: A pathological, clinical and aetiological analysis of 87 cases. Diagn Histopathol 1983;6:203.

149. Clapton WK, Boucaut HAP, Dewan PA, et al. Clinicopathological features of xanthogranulomatous pyelonephritis in infancy. Pathology 1993;25:110.

150. Hammadeh MY, Nicholls G, Calder CJ, Buick RG, Gornall P, Corkery JJ. Xanthogranulomatous pyelonephritis in childhood: Pre-operative diagnosis is possible. Br J Urol 1994;73:83.

151. Gregg CR, Rogers TE, Munford RS. Xanthogranulomatous pyelonephritis. Current Clin Topics Infect Dis 1999;19:287.

152. Husain I, Pingle A, Kazi T. Bilateral diffuse xanthogranulomatous pyelonephritis. Br J Urol 1979;51:162.

153. Cohen MS. Granulomatous nephritis. Urol Clin North Am 1986; 13:647.

154. Elder JS, Marshall FF. Focal xanthogranulomatous pyelonephritis in adulthood. Johns Hopkins Med J 1980;146:141.

155. Abbate AC, Meyers J. Xanthogranulomatous pyelonephritis in children. J Urol 1976;116:231.

156. Klugo RC, Anderson JA, Reid R, et al. Xanthogranulomatous pyelonephritis in children. J Urol 1977;117:350.

157. Braun G, Moussali L, Balanzar JL. Xanthogranulomatous pyelonephritis in children. J Urol 1985;133:236.

158. Watson AR, Marsden HB, Lendon M, Morris Jones PH. Renal pseudotumours caused by xanthogranulomatous pyelonephritis. Arch Dis Child 1982;57:635.

159. Bingol-Kologlu M, Ciftci AO, Senocak ME, et al. Xanthogranulomatous pyelonephritis in children: Diagnostic and therapeutic aspects. Eur J Pediatr Surg 2002;12:42.

160. Malek RS, Greene LF, DeWeerd JH, Farrow GM. Xanthogranulomatous pyelonephritis. Br J Urol 1972;44:296.

161. Zorzos I, Moutzouris V, Korakianitis G, Katsou G. Analysis of 39 cases of xanthogranulomatous pyelonephritis with emphasis on CT findings. Scand J Urol Nephrol 2003;37:342.

162. Saeed SM, Fine G. Xanthogranulomatous pyelonephritis. Am J Clin Pathol 1963;39:616.

163. Kelly DR, Murad TM. Megalocytic interstitial nephritis, xanthogranulomatous pyelonephritis, and malakoplakia: An ultrastructural comparison. Am J Clin Pathol 1981;75:333.

164. Khalyl-Mawad J, Greco MA, Schinella RA. Ultrastructural

demonstration of intracellular bacteria in xanthogranulomatous pyelonephritis. Hum Pathol 1982;13:41.
165. McClure J. Malakoplakia. J Pathol 1983;140:275.
166. Von Hansemann D. Über Malakoplakie der Harnblase. Virchows Arch A Pathol Anat Histopathol 1903;173:302.
167. Michaelis L, Gutmann C. Über Einschlüsse in Blasentumoren. Z Klin Med 1902;47:208.
168. Dobyan DC, Truong LD, Eknoyan G. Renal malacoplakia reappraised. Am J Kidney Dis 1993;22:243.
169. Stanton MJ, Maxted W. Malacoplakia: A study of the literature and current concepts of pathogenesis, diagnosis and treatment. J Urol 1981;125:139.
170. Saleem MA, Milford DV, Raafat F, White RHR. Renal parenchymal malakoplakia: A case report and review of the literature. Pediatr Nephrol 1993;7:256.
171. Hartman DS, Davis CJ Jr, Lichtenstein JE, Goldman SM. Renal parenchymal malacoplakia. Radiology 1980;136:33.
172. Cadnapaphornchai P, Rosenberg BF, Taher S, et al. Renal parenchymal malacoplakia: An unusual cause of renal failure. N Engl J Med 1978;299:1110.
173. Mokrzycki MH, Yamase H, Kohn OF. Renal malacoplakia with papillary necrosis and renal failure. Am J Kidney Dis 1992;19:587.
174. Tam VKK, Kung WH, Li R, Chan KW. Renal parenchymal malakoplakia: A rare cause of acute renal failure with review of recent literature. Am J Kidn Dis 2003;41:E13.
175. Melamed MR. The urinary sediment cytology in a case of malakoplakia. Acta Cytol (Baltimore) 1962;6:471.
176. Rao NR. Malacoplakia: Report of a case with observations on experimental production of the lesion. J Urol 1971;105:611.
177. Bowers JH, Cathey WJ. Malakoplakia of the kidney with renal failure. Am J Clin Pathol 1971;55:765.
178. Esparza AR, McKay DB, Cronan JJ, Chazan JA. Renal parenchymal malacoplakia: Histologic spectrum and its relationship to megalocytic interstitial nephritis and xanthogranulomatous pyelonephritis. Am J Surg Pathol 1989;13:225.
179. Lou TY, Teplitz C. Malacoplakia: Pathogenesis and ultrastructural morphogenesis. A problem of altered macrophage (phagolysosomal) response. Hum Pathol 1974;5:191.
180. McClurg FV, D'Agostino AN, Martin JH, Race GJ. Ultrastructural demonstration of intracellular bacteria in three cases of malacoplakia of the bladder. Am J Clin Pathol 1973;60:780.
181. Garrett IR, McClure J. Renal malakoplakia: Experimental production and evidence of a link with interstitial megalocytic nephritis. J Pathol 1982;136:111.
182. Biggar WD, Crawford L, Cardella C, et al. Malakoplakia and immunosuppressive therapy: Reversal of leukocyte abnormalities after withdrawal of prednisone and azathioprine. Am J Pathol 1985;119:5.
183. Abdou NI, NaPombejara C, Sagawa A, et al. Malakoplakia: Evidence for monocyte lysosomal abnormality correctable by cholinergic agonist in vitro and in vivo. N Engl J Med 1977;297:1413.
184. Ravel R. Megalocytic interstitial nephritis: An entity probably related to malakoplakia. Am J Clin Pathol 1967;47:781.
185. Jander HP, Pujara S, Murad TM. Tumefactive megalocytic interstitial nephritis. Radiology 1978;129:635.
186. Simon HB, Weinstein AJ, Pasternak MS, et al. Genitourinary tuberculosis: Clinical features in a general hospital population. Am J Med 1977;63:410.
187. Deen JL, Blumberg DA. Infectious disease considerations in pediatric organ transplantation. Semin Pediatr Surg 1993;2:218.
188. Bloom BR, Murray CJL. Tuberculosis: Commentary on a reemergent killer. Science 1992;257:1055.
189. Reichman LB. The U-shaped curve of concern. Am Rev Respir Dis 1991;144:741.
190. Chijioke A. Current views on epidemiology of renal tuberculosis. West Afr J Med 2001;20:217.
191. Corbishley CM, Eastwood JB, Grange JM. Tuberculosis and the kidney. J Am Soc Nephrol 2001;12:1307.
192. Petersen L, Mommsen S, Pallisgaard G. Male genitourinary tuberculosis: Report of 12 cases and a review of the literature. Scand J Urol Nephrol 1993;27:425.
193. Alvarez S, McCabe WR. Extrapulmonary tuberculosis revisited: A review of experience at Boston City and other hospitals. Medicine (Baltimore) 1984;63:25.
194. Spence RK, Dafoe DC, Rabin G, et al. Mycobacterial infections in renal allograft recipients. Arch Surg 1983;118:356.
195. Grange JM, Yates MD. Survey of mycobacteria isolated from urine and the genitourinary tract in south-east England from 1980 to 1989. Br J Urol 1992;69:640.
196. Lenk S, Oesterwitz H, Scholz D. Tuberculosis in cadaveric renal allograft recipients: Report of four cases and review of the literature. Eur Urol 1988;14:484.
197. Kretschmer HL. Tuberculosis of the kidney, a critical review based on a series of 221 cases. N Engl J Med 202:660.
198. Auerback O, Greenberger ME, Wershub LP. The incidence of renal tuberculosis in five hundred autopsies for pulmonary and extrapulmonary tuberculosis. JAMA 104:726.
199. Benn JJ, Scoble JE, Thomas AC, Eastwood JB. Cryptogenic tuberculosis as a preventable cause of end-stage renal failure. Am J Nephrol 1988;8:306.
200. Medlar EM. Cases of renal infection in pulmonary tuberculosis: Evidence of healed tuberculous lesions. Am J Pathol 1926;2:401.
201. Weinberg AC, Boyd SD. Short-course chemotherapy and role of surgery in adult and pediatric genitourinary tuberculosis. Urology 1988;31:95.
202. Njeh M, Jemni M, Abid R, et al. La tuberculose rénale à forme pseudo-tumorale: à propos d'un cas. J Urol (Paris) 1993;99:150.
203. Klioze AM, Ramos-Caro FA. Visceral leprosy. Intern J Dermatol 2000;39:641.
204. Jayalakshmi P, Looi LM, Lim KJ, Rojogopalan K. Autopsy findings in 35 cases of leprosy in Malaysia. Int J Lepr Other Mycobact Dis 1987;55:510.
205. Nakayama EE, Ura S, Fleury RN, Soares V. Renal lesions in leprosy: A retrospective study of 199 autopsies. Am J Kid Dis 2001;38:26.
206. Sinniah R, Churg J, Sobin LH. Renal Disease: Classification and Atlas of Infectious and Tropical Diseases. Chicago: ASCP Press, 1988.
207. Taylor GD, Buchanan-Chell M, Kirkland T, et al. Trends and sources of nosocomial fungaemia. Mycoses 1994;37:187.
208. Tomashefski JF Jr, Abramowsky CR. Candida-associated renal papillary necrosis. Am J Clin Pathol 1981;75:190.
209. Myerowitz RL, Pazin GJ, Allen CM. Disseminated candidiasis: Changes in incidence, underlying diseases, and pathology. Am J Clin Pathol 1977;68:29.
210. Samonis G, Bafaloukos D. Fungal infections in cancer patients: An escalating problem. In Vivo 1992;6:183.
211. Hughes WT. Systemic candidiasis: A study of 109 fatal cases. Pediatr Infect Dis 1982;1:11.
212. Carlotti A, Zambardi G, Couble A, et al. Nosocomial infection with *Candida albicans* in a pancreatic transplant recipient investigated by means of restriction enzyme analysis. J Infect 1994;29:157.
213. Paya CV. Fungal infections in solid-organ transplantation. Clin Infect Dis 1993;16:677.
214. Biggers R, Edwards J. Anuria secondary to bilateral ureteropelvic fungus balls. Urology 1980;15:161.
215. Eckstein CW, Kass EJ. Anuria in a newborn secondary to bilateral ureteropelvic fungus balls. J Urol 1982;127:109.
216. Levin DL, Zimmerman AL, Ferder LF, et al. Acute renal failure secondary to ureteral fungus ball obstruction in a patient with reversible deficient cell-mediated immunity. Clin Nephrol 1975;4:202.
217. Navarro EE, Almario JS, King C, et al. Detection of *Candida* casts in experimental renal candidiasis: Implications for the diagnosis and pathogenesis of upper urinary tract infection. J Med Vet Mycol 1994;32:415.
218. Jemal S, Bahloul A, Jelidi R, Mhiri MN. Pyélonéphrite emphysémateuse à *Candida albicans*: A propos d'un nouveau cas. J Urol (Paris) 1994;100:159.

219. Rantala A. Postoperative candidiasis. Ann Chir Gynaecol 1993; 205(suppl):1.
220. Odds FC. Pathogenesis of *Candida* infections. J Am Acad Dermatol 1994;31(3 Pt 2):S2.
221. Pendrak ML, Klotz SA. Adherence of *Candida albicans* to host cells. FEMS Microbiol Lett 1995;129:103.
222. Calderone RA, Braun PC. Adherence and receptor relationships of *Candida albicans*. Microbiol Rev 1991;55:1.
223. Filler SG, Swerdloff JN, Hobbs C, Luckett PM. Penetration and damage of endothelial cells by *Candida albicans*. Infect Immun 1995;63:976.
224. Louie A, Baltch AL, Smith RP, et al. Tumor necrosis factor alpha has a protective role in a murine model of systemic candidiasis. Infect Immun 1994;62:2761.
225. Khauli RB, Kalash S, Young JD Jr. *Torulopsis glabrata* perinephric abscess. J Urol 1983;130:968.
226. Kauffman CA, Tan JS. Torulopsis glabrata renal infection. *Am J Med* 1974;57:217.
227. Berkowitz ID, Robboy SJ, Karchmer AW, Kunz LJ. *Torulopsis glabrata* fungemia: A clinical pathological study. Medicine (Baltimore) 1979;58:430.
228. Vordermark JS II, Modarelli RO, Buck AS. *Torulopsis* pyelonephritis associated with papillary necrosis: A case report. J Urol 1980;123:96.
229. High KP, Quagliarello VJ. Yeast perinephric abscess: Report of a case and review. Clin Infect Dis 1992;15:128.
230. Kowanko IC, Ferrante A, Harvey DP, Carman KL. Granulocyte-macrophage colony-stimulating factor augments neutrophil killing of *Torulopsis glabrata* and stimulates neutrophil respiratory burst and degranulation. Clin Exp Immunol 1991;83:225.
231. Flechner SM, McAninch JW. Aspergillosis of the urinary tract: Ascending route of infection and evolving patterns of disease. J Urol 1981;125:598.
232. Warshawsky AB, Keiller D, Gittes RF. Bilateral renal aspergillosis. J Urol 1975;113:8.
233. Meyohas MC, Roux P, Poirot JL, Meynard JL, Frottier J. Aspergillose au cours du syndrome d'immunodéficience acquise. Pathol Biol (Paris) 1994;42:647.
234. Young RC, Bennett JE, Vogel CL, Carbone PP, DeVita VT. Aspergillosis: The spectrum of the disease in 98 patients. Medicine (Baltimore) 1970;49:147.
235. Vartivarian SE. Virulence properties and nonimmune pathogenic mechanisms of fungi. Clin Infect Dis 1992;14(suppl 1):S30.
236. Latgé JP, Paris S, Sarfati J, Debeaupuis JP, Diaquin M, Girardin H. Outils, progrès et questions dans l'étude moléculaire de *Aspergillus fumigatus* et de l'aspergillose invasive. Pathol Biol (Paris) 1994;42:632.
237. Richardson MD, Patel M. Stimulation of neutrophil phagocytosis of *Aspergillus fumigatus* conidia by interleukin-8 and N-formylmethionyl-leucylphenylalanine. J Med Vet Mycol 1995;33:99.
238. Reis MA, Costa RS, Ferraz AS. Causes of death in renal transplant recipients: A study of 102 autopsies from 1968 to 1991. J R Soc Med 1995;88:24.
239. Salyer WR, Salyer DC. Involvement of the kidney and prostate in cryptococcosis. J Urol 1973;109:695.
240. Hellman RN, Hinrichs J, Sicard G, et al. Cryptococcal pyelonephritis and disseminated cryptococcosis in a renal transplant recipient. Arch Intern Med 1981;141:128.
241. Randall RE Jr, Stacy WK, Toone EC, et al. Cryptococcal pyelonephritis. N Engl J Med 1968;279:60.
242. Lee SC, Dickson DW, Brosnan CF, Casadevall A. Human astrocytes inhibit Cryptococcus neoformans growth by a nitric oxide-mediated mechanism. J Exp Med 1994;180:365.
243. Kozel TR. Opsonization and phagocytosis of Cryptococcus neoformans. Arch Med Res 1993;24:211.
244. Goodwin RA Jr, Shapiro JL, Thurman GH, et al. Disseminated histoplasmosis: Clinical and pathologic correlations. Medicine (Baltimore) 1980;59:1.
245. Watanabe M, Hotchi M, Nagasaki M. An autopsy case of disseminated histoplasmosis probably due to infection from a renal allograft. Acta Pathol Jpn 1988;38:769.

246. Superdock KR, Dummer JS, Koch MO, et al. Disseminated histoplasmosis presenting as urinary tract obstruction in a renal transplant recipient. Am J Kidney Dis 1994;23:600.
247. Okeke CN, Müller J. Production of extracellular collagenolytic proteinases by Histoplasma capsulatum var.duboisii and Histoplasma capsulatum var. capsulatum in the yeast phase. Mycoses 1991;34:453.
248. Wu-Hsieh BA, Lee GS, Franco M, Hofman FM. Early activation of splenic macrophages by tumor necrosis factor alpha is important in determining the outcome of experimental histoplasmosis in mice [erratum appears in Infect Immun 1992;60:5324]. Infect Immun 1992;60:4230.
249. Jones JL, Fleming PL, Ciesielski CA, et al. Coccidioidomycosis among persons with AIDS in the United States. J Infect Dis 1995;171:961.
250. Ampel NM, Dols CL, Galgiani JN. Coccidioidomycosis during human immunodeficiency virus infection: Results of a prospective study in a coccidioidal endemic area. Am J Med 1993; 94:235.
251. Barbee RA, Hicks MJ, Grosso D, Sandel C. The maternal immune response in coccidioidomycosis: Is pregnancy a risk factor for serious infection? Chest 1991;100:709.
252. Peterson CM, Schuppert K, Kelly PC, Pappagianis D. Coccidioidomycosis and pregnancy. Obstet Gynecol Surv 1993;48:149.
253. Kohn GJ, Linné SR, Smith CM, Hoeprich PD. Acquisition of coccidioidomycosis at necropsy by inhalation of coccidioidal endospores. Diagn Microbiol Infect Dis 1992;15:527.
254. Stevens DA. Coccidioidomycosis. N Engl J Med 1995;332:1077.
255. Beaman L, Benjamini E, Pappagianis D. Activation of macrophages by lymphokines: enhancement of phagosome-lysosome fusion and killing of Coccidioides immitis. Infect Immun 1983; 39:1201.
256. Murphy JW. Mechanisms of natural resistance to human pathogenic fungi. Annu Rev Microbiol 1991;45:509.
257. Resnick S, Pappagianis D, McKerrow JH. Proteinase production by the parasitic cycle of the pathogenic fungus *Coccidioides immitis*. Infect Immun 1987;55:2807.
258. Baumgardner DJ, Buggy BP, Mattson BJ, et al. Epidemiology of blastomycosis in a region of high endemicity in north central Wisconsin. Clin Infect Dis 1992;15:629.
259. Busey JF. Blastomycosis: I. A review of 198 collected cases in Veterans Administration Hospitals. Blastomycosis Cooperative Study of the Veterans Administration. Am Rev Respir Dis 1964;89:659.
260. Eickenberg H-U, Amin M, Lich R Jr. Blastomycosis of the genitourinary tract. J Urol 1975;113:650.
261. Klein BS, Hogan LH, Jones JM. Immunologic recognition of a 25–amino acid repeat arrayed in tandem on a major antigen of *Blastomyces dermatitidis*. J Clin Invest 1993;92:330.
262. Brummer E, Castaneda E, Restrepo A. Paracoccidioidomycosis: An update. Clin Microbiol Rev 1993;6:89.
263. Silva CL, Alves LM, Figueiredo F. Involvement of cell wall glucans in the genesis and persistence of the inflammatory reaction caused by the *fungus Paracoccidioides brasiliensis*. Microbiology 1994;140:1189.
264. Defaveri J, Rezkallah-Iwasso MT, de Franco MF. Experimental paracoccidioidomycosis in mice: Morphology and correlation of lesions with humoral and cellular immune response. Mycopathologia 1982;77:3.
265. Vicentini AP, Gesztesi J-L, Franco MF, de Souza W, et al. Binding of *Paracoccidioides brasiliensis* to laminin through surface glycoprotein gp43 leads to enhancement of fungal pathogenesis. Infect Immun 1994;62:1465.
266. Moscardi-Bacchi M, Brummer E, Stevens DA. Support of *Paracoccidioides brasiliensis* multiplication by human monocytes or macrophages: inhibition by activated phagocytes. J Med Microbiol 1994;40:159.
267. Levy E, Bia MJ. Isolated renal mucormycosis: Case report and review. J Am Soc Nephrol 1995;12:2014.
268. Morrison VA, McGlave PB. Mucormycosis in BMT population. Bone Marrow Transplant 1993;11:383.
269. Vesa J, Bielsa O, Arango O, Lladó C, Gelabert A. Massive renal infection due to mucormycosis in an AIDS patient. Infection 1992;20:234.

270. Dansky AS, Lynne CM, Politano VA. Disseminated mucormycosis with renal involvement. J Urol 1978;119:275

271. Sinibaldi L, Goldoni P, Pietropaulo V, et al. Involvement of gangliosides in the interaction between BK virus and Vero cells. Arch Virol 1990;113:291.

272. Eash S, Querbes W, Atwood WJ. Infection in Vero cells by BK virus is dependent on caveolae. J Virol 2004;78:11583.

273. Kraus RJ, Shadley L, Mertz JE. Nuclear factor 1 family members mediate repression of the BK virus late promoter. Virology 2001;287:89.

274. Randhawa P, Zygmunt D, Shapiro R, et al. Viral regulatory region sequence variations in kidney tissue obtained from patients with BK virus nephropathy. Kidney Int 2003;64:743.

275. Hirsch HH, Knowles W, Dickenmann M, et al. Prospective study of polyomavirus type BK replication and nephropathy in renal-transplant recipients. N Engl J Med 2002;347:488.

276. Nickeleit V, Klimkait T, Binet IF, et al. Testing for polyomavirus type BK DNA in plasma to identify renal-allograft recipients with viral nephropathy. N Engl J Med 2002;342:1309.

277. Mengel M, Marwedel M, Radermacher J, Eden G. Incidence of polyomavirus-nephropathy in renal allografts: Influence of modern immunosuppressive drugs. Nephrol Dial Transplant 2003;18:1190.

278. Nickeleit V, Hirsch HH, Binet IF, et al. Polyomavirus infection of renal allograft recipients. From latent infection to manifest disease. J Am Soc Nephrol 1089;10:1080.

279. Hirsch HH. Polyomavirus BK nephropathy: A (re)emerging complication in renal transplantation. Am J Transplant 2002;2:25.

280. Ding R, Medeiros M, Dadhania D, et al. Noninvasive diagnosis of BK virus nephritis by measurement of messenger RNA for BK virus VP-I in urine. Transplantation 2002;74:987.

281. Nickeleit V, Steiger J, Mihatsch MJ. BK virus infection after kidney transplantation. Graft 2002;5:S46.

282. Agha IA, Brennan DC. BK virus and current immunosuppressive thereapy. Graft 2002;5:S65.

283. Nickeleit V, Hirsch HH, Zeiler M, Gudat F, Prince O, Thiel G, Mihatsch MJ. BK-virus nephropathy in renal transplants—Tubular necrosis, MHC-class II expression and rejection in a puzzling game. Nephrol Dial Transplant 2000;15:324.

284. Randhawa PS, Finkelstein S, Scantlebury V, et al. Human polyomavirus–associated interstitial nephritis in the allograft kidney. Transplantation 1999;67:103.

285. Nickeleit V, Mihatsch MJ. The pathologist's approach to therapeutic decision making in renal transplantation. Transplantation 2002;74:181.

286. Li RM, Mannon RB, Kleiner D, et al. BK virus and SV40 co-infection in polyoma virus nephropathy. Transplantation 2002;74:1497.

287. Buehrig CK, Lager DJ, Stegall MD, et al. Influence of surveillance renal allograft biopsy on diagnosis and prognosis of polyomavirus-associated nephropathy. Kidney Int 673;64:665.

288. Harris NL, Swerdlow SH, Frizerra G, Knowles DM. Posttransplant lymphoproliferative disorders. In: Jaffe E, ed. World Health Organization Classification of Tumours, vol 3: Pathology and Genetics of Tumours of Haematopoietic and Lymphoid Tissues. IARC Press, 2001:264.

289. Montone KT, Hodinka RL, Tomaszewski JE. Post-transplant lymphoproliferative disorders following renal and renal/pancreas transplantation: Frequent presentation in the allograft. (unpublished data)

290. Hibberd PL, Tolkoff-Rubin NE, Cosimi AB, et al. Symptomatic cytomegalovirus disease in the cytomegalovirus antibody seropositive renal transplant recipient treated with OKT3. Transplantation 1992;53:68.

291. Farrugia E, Schwab T. Management and prevention of cytomegalovirus infection after renal transplantation. Mayo Clin Proc 1992;67:879.

292. Richardson WP, Colvin RB, Cheeseman SH, et al. Glomerulopathy associated with cytomegalovirus viremia in renal allografts. N Engl J Med 1981;305:57.

293. Tauzon TV, Scheneeberger EE, Bahn AK, et al. Mononuclear cells in acute allograft glomerulopathy. Am J Pathol 132;129:119.

294. Rao KV, Hafner GP, Crary GS, et al. De-novo immunotactoid glomerulopathy of the renal allograft: Possible association with cytomegalovirus infection. Am J Kidney Dis 1994;24:97.

295. Herrera GA, Alexander RW, Cooley CF, et al. Cytomegalovirus glomerulopathy: A controversial lesion. Kidney Int 1986;29:725.

296. Anderson CB, Ladefoged SD, Lauritsen HK, et al. Detection of CMV and CMV antigens in renal allograft biopsies by in situ hybridization and immunohistochemistry. Nephrol Dial Transplant 1990;5:1045.

297. Rubin RH. Impact of cytomegalovirus infection on organ transplant recipients. Rev Infect Dis 1990;12(suppl):S754.

298. Payton D, Thorner P, Eddy A, et al. Demonstration by light microscopy of cytomegalovirus in a renal biopsy of a renal allograft recipient: Confirmation by immunohistochemistry and in situ hybridization. Nephron 1987;47:205.

299. Cameron J, Rigby RJ, van Deth AG, Petrie JJB. Severe tubulointerstitial disease in a renal allograft due to cytomegalovirus infection. Clin Nephrol 1982;8:321.

300. Birk PE, Chavers BM. Does cytomegalovirus cause glomerular injury in renal allograft recipients? J Am Soc Nephrol 1997;8:1801.

301. Liapis H, Storch GA, Hill DA, et al. CMV infection of the renal allograft is much more common than the pathology indicates: A retrospective analysis of qualitative and quantitative buffy coat CMV-PCR, renal biopsy pathology and tissue CMV-PCR. Nephrol Dial Transplant 2003;18:397.

302. Peters CJ, Simpson GL, Levy H. Spectrum of hantavirus infection: Hemorrhagic fever with renal syndrome and hantavirus pulmonary syndrome. Annu Rev Med 1999;50:531.

303. Mustonen J, Partanen J, Kanerva M, et al. Genetic susceptibility to severe course of nephropathica epidemica caused by Puumala hantavirus. Kidney Int 1996;49:217

304. Ala-Houhala I, Koskinen M, Ahola T, et al. Increased glomerular permeability in patients with nephropathia epidemica caused by Puumala hantavirus. Nephrol Dial Transplant 2002;17:246.

305. Bren AF, Pavlovcic SK, Koselj M, et al. Acute renal failure due to hemorrhagic fever with renal syndrome. Renal Failure 1996;18:635.

306. Mustonen J, Helin H, Pietila K, et al. Renal biopsy findings and clinicopathologic correlations in nephropathia epidemica. Clin Nephrol 1994;41:121.

307. Grcevska L, Polenakovic M, Oncevski A, et al. Different pathohistological presentations of acute renal involvement in Hantaan virus infection: Report of two cases. Clin Nephrol 1990;34:197.

308. Mustonen J, Makela S, Helin H, et al. Mesangiocapillary glomerulonephritis caused by Puumala hantavirus infection. Nephron 2001;89:402.

309. Wang S, Zang L, Feng M, Liang Z, et al. Transmission electron microscopic study of the hemorrhagic spots in patients with epidemic hemorrhagic fever in the early stage. Ultrastruct Pathol 1997;21:281.

310. Nam JH, Hwang KA, Yu CH, et al. Expression of interferon inducible genes following Hantaan virus infection as a mechanism of resistance in A549 cells. Virus Genes 2003;26:31.

311. Temonen M, Mustonen J, Helin H, et al. Cytokines, adhesion molecules, and cellular infiltration in nephropathia epidemica kidneys: An immunohistochemical study. Clin Immunol Immunopathol 1996;78:47.

312. Losito A, Bucciarelli E, Massi-Benedetti F, Lato M. Membranous glomerulonephritis in congenital syphilis. Clin Nephrol 1979;12:32.

313. Thompson L. Syphilis of the kidney. JAMA 1920;75:17.

314. Rich AR. The pathology of nineteen cases of a peculiar and specific form of nephritis associated with acquired syphilis. Bull Johns Hopkins Hosp 1932;50:357.

315. Levy M, Guesry P, Loirat C, et al. Immunologically mediated tubulo-interstitial nephritis in children. Contrib Nephrol 1979;16:132.

316. Thomas DD, Baseman JB, Alderete JF. Enhanced levels of attachment of fibronectin-primed *Treponema pallidum* to extracellular matrix. Infect Immun 1986;52:736.

317. Fitzgerald TJ. The Th1/Th2-like switch in syphilitic infection: Is it detrimental? Infect Immun 1992;60:3475.

318. Brown JR. Human actinomycosis: A study of 181 subjects. Hum Pathol 1973;4:319.

319. Weese WC, Smith IM. A study of 57 cases of actinomycosis over a 36-year period: A diagnostic "failure" with good prognosis after treatment. Arch Intern Med 1975;135:1562.

320. Khalaff H, Srigley JR, Klotz LH. Recognition of renal actinomycosis: Nephrectomy can be avoided. Can J Surg 1995;38:77.

321. Wajszczuk CP, Logan TF, Pasculle AW, Ho M. Intraabdominal actinomycosis presenting with sulfur granules in the urine. Am J Med 1984;77:1126.

322. Miralles GD. Disseminated *Nocardia farcinica* infection in an AIDS patient. Eur J Clin Microbiol Infect Dis 1994;13:497.

323. Frazier AR, Rosenow EC III, Roberts GD. Nocardiosis: A review of 25 cases occurring during 24 months. Mayo Clin Proc 1975;50:657.

324. Yenrudi S, Shuangshoti S, Pupaibul K. Nocardiosis: Report of 2 cases with review of literature in Thailand. J Med Assoc Thai 1991;74:47.

325. Walker DH, Fishbein DB. Epidemiology of rickettsial diseases. Eur J Epidemiol 1991;7:237.

326. Dalton MJ, Clarke MJ, Holman RC, et al. National surveillance for Rocky Mountain spotted fever, 1981–1992: Epidemiologic summary and evaluation of risk factors for fatal outcome. Am J Trop Med Hyg 1995;52:405.

327. Walker DH. Rocky Mountain spotted fever: A seasonal alert. Clin Infect Dis 1995;20:1111.

328. Green WR, Walker DH, Cain BG. Fatal viscerotropic Rocky Mountain spotted fever: Report of a case diagnosed by immunofluorescence. Am J Med 1978;64:523.

329. Walker DH, Mattern WD. Acute renal failure in Rocky Mountain spotted fever. Arch Intern Med 1979;139:443.

330. Sporn LA, Haidaris PJ, Shi R-J, et al. Rickettsia richettsii infection of cultured human endothelial cells induces tissue factor expression. Blood 1994;83:1527.

331. Galicia MA, Fort J, de Torres I, et al. Tubulointerstitial nephritis and Mediterranean spotted fever. Nephron 1991;58:128.

332. Yagupsky P, Wolach B. Fatal Israeli spotted fever in children. Clin Infect Dis 1993;17:850.

333. Shaked Y, Shpilberg O, Samra Y. Involvement of the kidneys in Mediterranean spotted fever and murine typhus. Q J Med 1994;87:103.

334. Hwang T-S, Chu Y-C, Kim Y-B, et al. Pathologic study of mice infected with *Rickettsia tsutsugamushi* R19 strain. J Korean Med Sci 1993;8:437.

335. Hsu GJ, Young T, Peng M-Y, et al. Acute renal failure associated with scrub typhus: Report of a case. J Formos Med Assoc 1993;92:475.

336. Perine PL, Chandler BP, Krause DK, et al. A clinico-epidemiological study of epidemic typhus in Africa. Clin Infect Dis 1992; 14:1149.

337. Schumann V, Fritschka E, Helmchen U, et al. Interstitielle Nephritis bei Fleckfieber. Dtsch Med Wochenschr 1993;118:893.

338. Santucci LA, Gutierrez PL, Silverman DJ. *Rickettsia rickettsii* induces superoxide radical and superoxide dismutase in human endothelial cells. Infect Immun 1992;60:5113.

339. Sporn LA, Lawrence SO, Silverman DJ, Marder VJ. E-selectin dependent neutrophil adhesion to *Rickettsia rickettsii*-infected endothelial cells. Blood 1993;81:2406.

340. Sporn LA, Shi R-J, Lawrence SO, et al. *Rickettsia rickettsii* infection of cultured endothelial cells induces release of large von Willebrand factor multimers from Weibel-Palade bodies. Blood 1991;78:2595.

341. Drancourt M, George F, Brouqui P, et al. Diagnosis of Mediterranean spotted fever by indirect immunofluorescence of *Rickettsia conorii* in circulating endothelial cells isolated with monoclonal antibody-coated immunomagnetic beads. J Infect Dis 1992;166:660.

342. Lecour H, Miranda M, Magro C, et al. Human leptospirosis: A review of 50 cases. Infection 1989;17:8.

343. Losuwanrak K, Kanjanabuch T, Sitprija V. Leptospiral nephropathy. Semin Nephrol 2003;23:42.

344. Arean VM. The pathologic anatomy and pathogenesis of fatal human leptospirosis (Weil's disease). Am J Pathol 1962;40:393.

345. Feigin RD, Anderson DC. Human leptospirosis. Crit Rev Clin Lab Sci 1975;5:413.

346. Lai KN, Aarons I, Woodroffe AJ, Clarkson AR. Renal lesions in leptospirosis. Aust N Z J Med 1982;12:276.

347. Sitprija V, Evans H. The kidney in human leptospirosis. Am J Med 1970;49:780.

348. Yang CW, Wu MS, Pan MJ. Leptospirosis renal disease. Nephrol Dial Transplant 2001;5:73.

349. Barsoum RS. Malarial nephropathies. Nephrol Dial Transplant 1998;13:1588.

350. Lee PC, Lee PY, Lei HY, et al. Malaria infection in kidney transplant recipients. Transplant Proc 1994;26:2099.

351. Sitprija V. Nephropathy in falciparum malaria. Kidney Int 1988;34:867.

352. Barsoum R. Malarial acute renal failure. J Am Soc Nephrol 2000; 11:2147.

353. Mukherjee AP, White JC, Lau KS. Falciparum malaria associated with jaundice, renal failure and anemia. Trans R Soc Trop Med Hyg 1971;65:808.

354. Rosen S, Hano JE, Inman MM, et al. The kidney in blackwater fever: Light and electron microscopic observations. Am J Clin Pathol 1968;49:358.

355. Stone WJ, Hanchett JE, Knepshield JH. Acute renal insufficiency due to falciparum malaria: Review of 42 cases. Arch Intern Med 1972;129:620.

356. Andrade ZA, Rocha H. Schistosomal glomerulopathy. Kidney Int 1979;16:23.

357. Barsoum RS. Schistosomal glomerulopathies. Kidney Int 1993; 44:1.

358. Falcão HA, Gould DB. Immune complex nephropathy in schistosomiasis. Ann Intern Med 1975;83:148.

359. Barsoum RS. Schistosomiasis and the kidney. Semin Nephrol 2003;23:34.

360. Andrade ZA, Andrade SG, Sadigursky M. Renal changes in patients with hepatosplenic schistosomiasis. Am J Trop Med Hyg 1971;20:77.

361. Chensue SW, Warmington K, Ruth J, et al. Cytokine responses during mycobacterial and schistosomal antigen-induced pulmonary granuloma formation: Production of Th1 and Th2 cytokines and relative contribution of tumor necrosis factor. Am J Pathol 1994;145:1105.

362. Date A, Gunasekaran V, Kirubakaran MG, Shastry JCM. Acute eosinophilic glomerulonephritis with *Bancroftian filariasis*. Postgrad Med J 1979;55:905.

363. Sitprija V, Boonpucknavig V. Renal involvement in parasitic diseases. In: Tisher CC, Brenner BM, eds. Renal Pathology with Clinical and Functional Correlations, Vol 1. Philadelphia: JB Lippincott, 1994:626.

364. Mertens RB, Didier ES, Fishbein MC, et al. Encephalitozoon cuniculi microsporidiosis: Infection of the brain, heart, kidneys, trachea, adrenal glands, and urinary bladder in a patient with AIDS. Mod Pathol 1997;10:68.

365. Guvel S, Kilinc F, Kayaselcuk FK, et al. Emphysematous pyelonephritis and renal amoebiasis in a patient with diabetes mellitus. Int J Urol 2003;10:404.

366. Gogus C, Safak M, Baltaci S, Turkolmez K. Isolated renal hydatidosis: Experience with 20 cases. J Urol 2003;169:186.

367. Velthuysen M-L F, Florquin S. Glomerulopathy associated with parasitic infections. Clin Microbiol Rev 2000;13:55.

368. Rath RN, Patel DK, Das PK, et al. Immunopathological changes in kidney in *Plasmodium falciparum* malaria. Indian J Med Res 1990;91:129.

369. Hendrickse RG, Adeniyi A. Quartan malarial nephrotic syndrome in children. Kidney Int 1979;16:64.

370. Kibukamusoke JW. Tropical Nephrology. Canberra: Citforge, 1984.

371. Kibukamusoke JW, Hutt MS, Wilks NE. The nephrotic syndrome in Uganda and its association with quartan malaria. Q J Med 1967;36:393.

372. Abdurrahman MB, Aikhionbare HA, Babaoye FA, et al.

Clinicopathological features of childhood nephrotic syndrome in northern Nigeria. Q J Med 1990;75:563.

373. Hendrickse RG. Epidemiology and prevention of kidney disease in Africa. Trans R Soc Trop Med Hyg 1980;74:8.

374. Hutt MS. Renal disease in a tropical environment. Trans R Soc Trop Med Hyg 1980;74:17.

375. Hutt MSR, Burkitt DP. The Geography of Noninfectious Disease. Oxford, England: Oxford University Press, 1986:72.

376. Goldman M, Baran D, Druet P. Polyclonal activation and experimental nephropathies. Kidney Int 1988;34:141.

377. Aikawa M, Broderson JR, Igarashi I, et al. An Atlas of Renal Disease in Aotus Monkeys with Experimental Plasmodial Infection. Arlington, VA: American Institute of Biological Sciences, 1988.

378. Adeniyi A, Hendrickse RG, Houba V. Selectivity of proteinuria and response to prednisolone or immunosuppressive drugs in children with malarial nephrosis. Lancet 1970;1:644.

379. Hendrickse RG, Adeniyi A, Edington GM, et al. Quartan malarial nephrotic syndrome: Collaborative clinicopathological study in Nigerian children. Lancet 1972;1:1143.

380. Kibukamusoke JW, Hutt MS. Histological features of the nephrotic syndrome associated with quartan malaria. J Clin Pathol 1967;20:117.

381. Morel-Maroger L, Saimot AG, Sloper JC, et al. "Tropical nephropathy" and "tropical extramembranous glomerulonephritis" of unknown aetiology in Senegal. Br Med J 1975;1:541.

382. Ward PA, Kibukamusoke JW. Evidence for soluble immune complexes in the pathogenesis of the glomerulonephritis of quartan malaria. Lancet 1969;1:283.

383. Allison AC, Hendrickse RG, Edington GM, et al. Immune complexes in the nephrotic syndrome of African children. Lancet 1969;1:1232.

384. Soothill JF, Hendrickse RG. Some immunological studies of the nephrotic syndrome of Nigerian children. Lancet 1967;2:629.

385. Houba V. Immunologic aspects of renal lesions associated with malaria. Kidney Int 1979;16:3.

386. Houba V, Lambert PH, Voller A, Soyanwo MA. Clinical and experimental investigation of immune complexes in malaria. Clin Immunol Immunopathol 1976;6:1.

387. Lloyd CM, Collins I, Belcher AJ, et al. Characterization and pathological significance of monoclonal DNA-binding antibodies from mice with experimental malaria infection. Infect Immun 1994;62:1982.

388. Wozencraft AO, Lloyd CM, Staines NA, Griffiths VJ. Role of DNA-binding antibodies in kidney pathology associated with murine malaria infections. Infect Immunol 1990;58:2156.

389. Lloyd CM, Wozencraft AO, Williams DG. Cell-mediated pathology during murine malaria-associated nephritis. Clin Exp Immunol 1993;94:398.

390. Zeid AM, Hassan MM, Attia WM, et al. Hepatitis-B virus and schistosomiasis infections in childhood proteinuria. J Egypt Soc Parasitol 1994;24:371.

391. Barsoum R, Nabil M, Saady G, et al. Immunoglobulin-A and the pathogenesis of schistosomal glomerulopathy. Kidney Int 1996;50:920.

392. Ezzat E, Osman RA, Ahmet KY, Soothill JF. The association between Schistosoma haematobium infection and heavy proteinuria. Trans R Soc Trop Med Hyg 1974;68:315.

393. Barsoum RS. Schistosomal glomerulopathies. Kidney Int 1993;44:1.

394. Rocha H, Cruz T, Brito E, Susin M. Renal involvement in patients with hepatosplenic schistosomiasis mansoni. Am J Trop Med Hyg 1976;25:108.

395. Sobh M, Moustafa F, el-Arbagy A, et al. Nephropathy in asymptomatic patients with active Schistosoma mansoni infection. Int Urol Nephrol 1990;22:37.

396. Kaiser C, Doehring-Schwerdtfeger E, Abdel-Rahim IM, et al. Renal function and morphology in Sudanese patients with advanced hepatosplenic schistosomiasis and portal hypertension. Am J Trop Med Hyg 1989;40:176.

397. Sobh MA, Moustafa FE, Sally SM, et al. Characterization of kidney lesions in early schistosomal-specific nephropathy. Nephrol Dial Transplant 1988;3:392.

398. Hoshino-Shimizu S, De Brito T, Kanamura HY, et al. Human schistosomiasis: Schistosoma mansoni antigen detection in renal glomeruli. Trans R Soc Trop Med Hyg 1977;70:492.

399. Sobh MA, Moustafa FE, el-Housseini F, et al. Schistosomal specific nephropathy leading to end-stage renal failure. Kidney Int 1987;31:1006.

400. Bout D, Santoro F, Carlier Y, et al. Circulating immune complexes in schistosomiasis. Immunology 1977;33:17.

401. Houba V. Experimental renal disease due to schistosomiasis. Kidney Int 1979;16:30.

402. Andrade ZA, Rocha H. Schistosomal glomerulopathy. Kidney Int 1979;16:23.

403. Rocha H, Martinelli R. Parasitic glomerulonephritis. In: Brodehl J, Ehrich JHH, eds. Paediatric Nephrology. Berlin: Springer-Verlag, 1984:250.

404. Martinelli R, Pereira LJ, Brito E, Rocha H. Clinical course of focal segmental glomerulosclerosis associated with hepatosplenic schistosomiasis mansoni. Nephron 1995;69:131.

405. Martinelli R, Pereira LJ, Rocha H. The influence of anti-parasitic therapy on the course of the glomerulopathy associated with schistosomiasis mansoni. Clin Nephrol 1987;27:229.

406. Sobh MA, Moustafa FE, Sally SM, et al. Effect of anti-schistosomal treatment on schistosomal-specific nephropathy. Nephrol Dial Transplant 1988;3:744.

407. Sobh MA, Moustafa FE, Sally SM, et al. A prospective, randomized therapeutic trial for schistosomal specific nephropathy. Kidney Int 1989;36:904.

408. Gelman R, Brook G, Green J, et al. Minimal change glomerulonephritis associated with hydatid disease. Clin Nephrol 2000;53:152.

409. Hall CL, Stephens L, Peat D, Chiodini PL. Nephrotic syndrome due to loiasis following a tropical adventure holiday: A case report and review of the literature. Clin Nephrol 2001;56:247.

410. Ngu JL, Chatelanat R, Leke R, et al. Nephropathy in Cameroon: Evidence for filarial derived immune complex pathogenesis in some cases. Clin Nephrol 1985;24:128.

411. Hutch JA. Theory of maturation of the intravesical ureter. J Urol 1961;86:534.

412. Dillon MJ, Goonasekera CD. Reflux nephropathy. J Am Soc Nephrol 1998;9:2377.

413. Scott JE, Renwick M. Antenatal diagnosis of congenital abnormalities in the urinary tract: Results from the Northern Region Fetal Abnormality Survey. Br J Urol 1988;62:295.

414. Elder J. Antenatal hydronephrosis: Fetal and neonatal management. Pediatr Clin North Am 1997;44:1299.

415. Orellana P, Baquedano P, Rangarajan V, et al. Relationship between acute pyelonephritis, renal scarring, and vesicoureteral reflux: Results of a coordinated research project. Pediatr Nephrol 2004;19:1122.

416. Ataei N, Madani A, Esfahani ST, et al. Screening for vesicoureteral reflux and renal scars in siblings of children with known reflux. Pediatr Nephrol 2004;19:1127.

417. Lama G, Tedesco MA, Graziano L, et al. Reflux nephropathy and hypertension: Correlation with the progression of renal damage. Pediatr Nephrol 2003;18:241.

418. O'Donnell B. Reflections on reflux. J Urol 2004;172:1635.

419. Woodard JR, Holden S. The prognostic significance of fever in childhood urinary infections: Observations in 350 consecutive patients. Clin Pediatr (Phila) 1976;15:1051.

420. Smellie JM, Normand IC. Bacteriuria, reflux, and renal scarring. Arch Dis Child 1975;50:581.

421. van Gool J, Hjalmas, K, Tamminen-Mobius, et al. Historical clues to the complexity of dysfunctional voiding, urinary tract infection and vesicoureteral reflux. The International Reflux Study in Children. J Urol 1992;148:1699.

422. Chen JJ, Mao W, Homayoon K, et al. A multivariate analysis of dysfunctional elimination syndrome and its relationships with gender, urinary tract infection and vesicoureteral reflux in children. J Urol 2004;171:1907.

423. Ransley PG, Risdon RA. Renal papillae and intrarenal reflux in the pig. Lancet 1974;2:1114.

424. Maizels M, Stephens FD. Valves of the ureter as a cause of primary obstruction of the ureter: Anatomic, embryologic and clinical aspects. J Urol 1980;123(5):742.

425. Babin J, Sackett M, Delage C, et al. The Ask-Upmark kidney: A curable cause of hypertension in young patients. J Hum Hypertens 2005;19:315.

426. Becu L, Quesada EM, Medel R, et al. Small kidney associated with primary vesicoureteral reflux in children. A pathological overhaul. Eur Urol 1988;14:127.

427. Marwali MR, Rossi NF. Ask-Upmark kidney associated with renal and extrarenal arterial aneurysms. Am J Kidney Dis 1999; 33:e4.

428. Arant BS Jr, Sotelo-Avila C, Bernstein J. Segmental "hypoplasia" of the kidney (Ask-Upmark). J Pediatr 1979;95:931.

429. Shindo S, Bernstein J, Arant BS Jr. Evolution of renal segmental atrophy (Ask-Upmark kidney) in children with vesicoureteric reflux: Radiographic and morphologic studies. J Pediatr 1983;102:847.

430. Bonsib SM, Meng RL, Johnson FP Jr. Ask-Upmark kidney with contralateral renal artery fibromuscular dysplasia. Am J Nephrol 1985;5:450.

431. Muchant DG, Gloor JM, Norling LL. Persistent severe hypertension in an infant with posterior urethral valves. Pediatr Nephrol 1996;10:764.

432. Atwell JD, Cook PL, Strong L, Hyde I. The interrelationship between vesico-ureteric reflux, trigonal abnormalities and a bifid pelvicalyceal collecting system: A family study. Br J Urol 1977;49:97.

433. Heale WF. Hereditary vesicoureteric reflux: Phenotypic variation and family screening. Pediatr Nephrol 1997;11:504.

434. Groenen PM, Vanderlinden G, Devriendt K, et al. Rearrangement of the human CDC5L gene by a t(6;19)(p21;q13.1) in a patient with multicystic renal dysplasia. Genomics 1998;49:218.

435. Mackintosh P, Almarhoos G, Heath DA. HLA linkage with familial vesicoureteral reflux and familial pelvi-ureteric junction obstruction. Tissue Antigens 1989;34:185.

436. Sanyanusin P, Schimmenti LA, McNoe LA, et al. Mutation of the PAX2 gene in a family with optic nerve colobomas, renal anomalies and vesicoureteral reflux. Nat Genet 1995;9:358.

437. Feather SA, Malcolm S, Woolf AS, et al. Primary, nonsyndromic vesicoureteric reflux and its nephropathy is genetically heterogeneous, with a locus on chromosome 1. Am J Hum Genet 2000;66:1420.

438. Hohenfellner K, Hunley TE, Yerkes E, et al. Angiotensin II, type 2 receptor in the development of vesico-ureteric reflux. BJU Int 1999;83:318.

439. Jiang S, Gitlin J, Deng FM, et al. Lack of major involvement of human uroplakin genes in vesicoureteral reflux: Implications for disease heterogeneity. Kidney Int 2004;66:10.

440. Kelly H, Ennis S, Yoneda A, et al. Uroplakin III is not a major candidate gene for primary vesicoureteral reflux. Eur J Hum Genet 2005;13(4):500.

441. Nakano T, Niimura F, Hohenfellner K, et al. Screening for mutations in BMP4 and FOXC1 genes in congenital anomalies of the kidney and urinary tract in humans. Tokai J Exp Clin Med 2003;28:121.

442. Pierides AM, Athanasiou Y, Demetriou K, et al. A family with the branchio-oto-renal syndrome: Clinical and genetic correlations. Nephrol Dial Transplant 2002;17:1014.

443. Woolf AS. A molecular and genetic view of human renal and urinary tract malformations. Kidney Int 2000;58:500.

444. Howie AJ, Buist LJ, Coulthard MG. Reflux nephropathy in transplants. Pediatr Nephrol 2002;17:485.

445. Hodson CJ, Edwards D. Chronic pyelonephritis and vesicoureteric reflux. Clin Radiol 1960;11:219.

446. el-Khatib M, Packham DK, Becker GJ, Kincaid-Smith P. Pregnancy-related complications in women with reflux nephropathy. Clin Nephrol 1994;41:50.

447. Cotran RS. Nephrology forum. Glomerulosclerosis in reflux nephropathy. Kidney Int 1982;21:528.

448. Hinchliffe SA, Kreczy A, Ciftci AO, et al. Focal and segmental glomerulosclerosis in children with reflux nephropathy. Pediatr Pathol 1994;14(2):327.

449. Tada M, Jimi S, Hisano S, et al. Histopathological evidence of poor prognosis in patients with vesicoureteral reflux. Pediatr Nephrol 2001;16:482.

450. Thomas JC, Demarco RT, Pope JC. Molecular biology of ureteral bud and trigonal development. Curr Urol Rep 2005;6:146.

451. Glassberg KI. Normal and abnormal development of the kidney: A clinician's interpretation of current knowledge. J Urol 2002;167:2339.

452. Ichikawa I, Kuwayama F, Pope JC IV, et al. Paradigm shift from classic anatomic theories to contemporary cell biological views of CAKUT. Kidney Int 2002;61:889.

453. Batourina E, Choi C, Paragas N, et al. Distal ureter morphogenesis depends on epithelial cell remodeling mediated by vitamin A and Ret. Nat Genet 2002;32:109.

454. Yu OH, Murawski IJ, Myburgh DB, Gupta IR. Overexpression of RET leads to vesicoureteric reflux in mice. Am J Physiol Renal Physiol 2004;287:F1123.

455. Hayward SW. Approaches to modeling stromal-epithelial interactions. J Urol 2002;168:1165.

456. Smellie JM, Prescod NP, Shaw PJ, et al. Childhood reflux and urinary infection: A follow-up of 10-41 years in 226 adults. Pediatr Nephrol 1998;12:727.

457. Ardissino G, Avolio L, Dacco V, et al. Long-term outcome of vesicoureteral reflux associated chronic renal failure in children. Data from the ItalKid Project. J Urol 2004;172:305.

458. Brophy MM, Austin PF, Yan Y, Coplen DE. Vesicoureteral reflux and clinical outcomes in infants with prenatally detected hydronephrosis. J Urol 2002;168:1716.

459. Thompson RH, Chen JJ, Pugach J, et al. Cessation of prophylactic antibiotics for managing persistent vesicoureteral reflux. J Urol 2001;166:1465.

460. Austin JC, Cooper CS. Vesicoureteral reflux: Surgical approaches. Urol Clin North Am 2004;31:543.

461. Fanos V, Cataldi L. Antibiotics or surgery for vesicoureteric reflux in children. Lancet 2004;364:1720.

462. Coulthard MG, Flecknell P, Orr H, et al. Renal scarring caused by vesicoureteric reflux and urinary infection: A study in pigs. Pediatr Nephrol 2002;17:481.

463. Steinhardt GF. Ureteropelvic junction obstruction. In: Gonzales ET, Bauer SB, eds. Pediatric Urology Practice. Philadelphia: Lippincott Williams & Wilkins, 1999:181.

464. Cheng EY, Maizels M, Chou P. Response of the newborn ureteropelvic junction complex to induced and later reversed partial ureteral obstruction in the rabbit model. J Urol 1993;150:782.

465. Ismaili K, Avni FE, Wissing KM, Hall M. Long-term clinical outcome of infants with mild and moderate fetal pyelectasis: Validation of neonatal ultrasound as a screening tool to detect significant nephrouropathies. J Pediatr 2004;144:759.

466. Zhang PL, Peters CA, Rosen S. Ureteropelvic junction obstruction: Morphological and clinical studies. Pediatr Nephrol 2000;14:820.

467. Lam JS, Bingham JB, Gupta M. Endoscopic treatment of fibroepithelial polyps of the renal pelvis and ureter. Urology 2003; 62:810.

468. Alcaraz A, Vinaixa F, Tejeno-Mateu A, et al. Obstruction and recanalization of the ureter during embryonic development. J Urol 1991;145:410.

469. Chang CP, McDill BW, Neilson JR, et al. Calcineurin is required in urinary tract mesenchyme for the development of the pyeloureteral peristaltic machinery. J Clin Invest 2004;113: 1051.

470. Mendelsohn C. Functional obstruction: The renal pelvis rules. J Clin Invest 2004;113:957.

471. Peters CA. Animal models of fetal renal disease. Prenat Diagn 2001;21:917.

472. Klahr S, Morrissey J. Obstructive nephropathy and renal fibrosis. Am J Physiol Renal Physiol 2002;283:F861.

473. Liapis H. Biology of congenital obstructive nephropathy. Nephron Exp Nephrol 2003;93:e87.

474. Woolf AS. Congenital obstructive nephropathy gets complicated. Kidney Int 2003;63:761.

475. Chevalier RL. Biomarkers of congenital obstructive nephropathy: Past, present and future. J Urol 2004;172:852.

476. Weiss-Guillet EM, Takala J, Jakob SM. Diagnosis and management of electrolyte emergencies. Best Pract Res Clin Endocrinol Metab 2003;17:623.

477. Bilezikian JP. Clinical review 51: Management of hypercalcemia. J Clin Endocrinol Metab 1993;77:1445.

478. Lins LE. Reversible renal failure caused by hypercalcemia. A retrospective study. Acta Med Scand 1978;203:309.

479. Ferris T, Kashgarian M, Levitin H, et al. Renal tubular acidosis and renal potassium wasting acquired as a result of hypercalcemic nephropathy. N Engl J Med 1961;265:924.

480. Muldowney FP, Carroll DV, Donohoe JF, Freaney R. Correction of renal bicarbonate wastage by parathyroidectomy. Implications in acid-base homeostasis. Q J Med 1971;40:487.

481. Transbol I, Hornum I, Dawids S. Hypercalcaemia and sodium-losing renal disease. Studies on the renal handling of calcium and sodium. Scand J Urol Nephrol 1970;4:125.

482. Sutton RA. Plasma magnesium concentration in primary hyperparathyroidism. Br Med J 1970;1:529.

483. Sutton RA, Wong NL, Quamme GA, Dirks JH. Renal tubular calcium transport: Effects of changes in filtered calcium load. Am J Physiol 1983;245:F515.

484. Cusworth DC, Dent CE, Scriver CR. Primary hyperparathyroidism and hyperaminoaciduria. Clin Chim Acta 1972;41:355.

485. Adami S, Marcocci C, Gatti D. Epidemiology of primary hyperparathyroidism in Europe. J Bone Miner Res 2002;17(Suppl 2):N18.

486. Melton LJ 3rd. The epidemiology of primary hyperparathyroidism in North America. J Bone Miner Res 2002;17(Suppl 2):N12.

487. Lundgren E, Rastad J, Thrufjell E, et al. Population-based screening for primary hyperparathyroidism with serum calcium and parathyroid hormone values in menopausal women. Surgery 1997;121:287.

488. Broadus AE. Primary hyperparathyroidism. J Urol 1989;141 (Pt 2):723.

489. Bilezikian JP, Brandi ML, Rubin M, Silverberg SJ. Primary hyperparathyroidism: New concepts in clinical, densitometric and biochemical features. J Intern Med 2005;257:6.

490. Sugden CJ, Laird BJ. Hammers and nails: A report. Palliat Med 2004;18:734.

491. Gal-Moscovici A, Popovtzer MM. New worldwide trends in presentation of renal osteodystrophy and its relationship to parathyroid hormone levels. Clin Nephrol 2005;63:284.

492. Walsh MD Jr, Chan K, Travers S, McIntyre RC Jr. Destructive maxillomandibular brown tumor in severe hyperparathyroidism. J Am Coll Surg 2005;201:315.

493. Khosla S, Melton LJ 3rd, Wermers RA, et al. Primary hyperparathyroidism and the risk of fracture: A population-based study. J Bone Miner Res 1999;14:1700.

494. Di Monaco M, Vallero F, Di Monaco R, et al. Primary hyperparathyroidism in elderly patients with hip fracture. J Bone Miner Metab 2004;22:491.

495. Asplin J, Favus M, Coe F. Nephrolithiasis. In: Brenner B, ed. Brenner and Rector's The Kidney, 5th ed. Philadelphia: WB Saunders, 1996:1983.

496. Chen R, Goodman W. Role of the calcium-sensing receptor in parathyroid gland physiology. Am J Physiol Renal 2004;286:F1005.

497. Moe S. Core curriculum in nephrology: Disorders of calcium, phosphorus, and magnesium. Am J Kidney Dis 2005;45:213.

498. Brown EM, Gamba G, Riccardi D, et al. Cloning and characterization of an extracellular Ca(2+)-sensing receptor from bovine parathyroid. Nature 1993;366:575.

499. Muff R, Nemeth EF, Haller-Brem S, Fischer JA. Regulation of hormone secretion and cytosolic Ca2+ by extracellular Ca2+ in parathyroid cells and C-cells: Role of voltage-sensitive Ca2+ channels. Arch Biochem Biophys 1988;265:128.

500. Younes NA, Shafagoj Y, Khatib F, Ababneh M. Laboratory screening for hyperparathyroidism. Clin Chim Acta 2005;353:1.

501. Gensure RC, Gardella TJ, Juppner H. Parathyroid hormone and parathyroid hormone-related peptide, and their receptors. Biochem Biophys Res Commun 2005;328:666.

502. Coe FL, Parks JH, Asplin JR. Pathogenesis and treatment of kidney stones. N Engl J Med 1992;327:1141.

503. Parks JH, Coe FL. Pathogenesis and treatment of calcium stones. Semin Nephrol 1996;16:398.

504. Peacock M. Primary hyperparathyroidism and the kidney: Biochemical and clinical spectrum. J Bone Miner Res 2002;17(Suppl 2):N87.

505. Martin KJ, Akhtar I, Gonzalez EA. Parathyroid hormone: New assays, new receptors. Semin Nephrol 2004;24:3.

506. Gao P, D'Amour P. Evolution of the parathyroid hormone (PTH) assay–importance of circulating PTH immunoheterogeneity and of its regulation. Clin Lab 2005;51:21.

507. Bilezikian JP, Potts JT Jr, Fuleihan Gel H, et al. Summary statement from a workshop on asymptomatic primary hyperparathyroidism: A perspective for the 21st century. J Bone Miner Res 2002;17(Suppl 2):N2.

508. Silverberg SJ, Shane E, Jacobs TP, et al. A 10-year prospective study of primary hyperparathyroidism with or without parathyroid surgery. N Engl J Med 1999;341:1249.

509. Pyrah LN, Hodgkinson A, Anderson CK. Primary hyperparathyroidism. Br J Surg 1966;53:245.

510. Tominaga Y, Grimelius L, Johansson H, et al. Histological and clinical features of non-familial primary parathyroid hyperplasia. Pathol Res Pract 1992;188:115.

511. Silverberg SJ, Bilezikian JP. Evaluation and management of primary hyperparathyroidism. J Clin Endocrinol Metab 1996;81:2036.

512. Burtis WJ, Brady TG, Orloff JJ, et al. Immunochemical characterization of circulating parathyroid hormone-related protein in patients with humoral hypercalcemia of cancer. N Engl J Med 1990;322:1106.

513. Martin TJ. Properties of parathyroid hormone-related protein and its role in malignant hypercalcaemia. Q J Med 1990;76:771.

514. Stewart A. Hypercalcemic and hypocalcemic states. In: Giebisch GH, ed. The Kidney: Physiology and Pathophysiology, 2nd ed. New York: Raven Press, 1992:2431.

515. Syed MA, Horwitz MJ, Tedesco MB, et al. Parathyroid hormone-related protein-(1–36) stimulates renal tubular calcium reabsorption in normal human volunteers: Implications for the pathogenesis of humoral hypercalcemia of malignancy. J Clin Endocrinol Metab 2001;86:1525.

516. Strewler GJ. The physiology of parathyroid hormone-related protein. N Engl J Med 2000;342:177.

517. Kemp BE, Moseley JM, Rodda CP, et al. Parathyroid hormone-related protein of malignancy: Active synthetic fragments. Science 1987;238:1568.

518. Hastings RH. Parathyroid hormone-related protein and lung biology. Respir Physiol Neurobiol 2004;142:95.

519. Danks JA, Ebeling PR, Hayman J, et al. Parathyroid hormone-related protein: Immunohistochemical localization in cancers and in normal skin. J Bone Miner Res 1989;4:273.

520. Burtis WJ, Wu T, Bunch C, et al. Identification of a novel 17,000-dalton parathyroid hormone-like adenylate cyclase-stimulating protein from a tumor associated with humoral hypercalcemia of malignancy. J Biol Chem 1987;262:7151.

521. Bundred NJ, Ratcliffe WA, Walker RA, et al. Parathyroid hormone related protein and hypercalcaemia in breast cancer. BMJ 1991;303:1506.

522. Grill V, Ho P, Body JJ, et al. Parathyroid hormone-related protein: Elevated levels in both humoral hypercalcemia of malignancy and hypercalcemia complicating metastatic breast cancer. J Clin Endocrinol Metab 1991;73:1309.

523. Ritskes-Hoitinga J, Lemmens AG, Beynen AC. Nutrition and kidney calcification in rats. Lab Anim 1989;23:313.

524. Powell GJ, Southby J, Danks JA, et al. Localization of parathyroid hormone-related protein in breast cancer metastases: Increased incidence in bone compared with other sites. Cancer Res 1991;51:3059.

525. Stewart AF, Hoecker JL, Mallette LE, et al. Hypercalcemia in pheochromocytoma. Evidence for a novel mechanism. Ann Intern Med 1985;102:776.

526. Asadi F, Kukreja S. Parathyroid hormone-related protein in prostate cancer. Crit Rev Eukaryot Gene Expr 2005;15:15.

527. Matsen SL, Yeo CJ, Hruban RH, Choti MA. Hypercalcemia and pancreatic endocrine neoplasia with elevated PTH-rP: Report of two new cases and subject review. J Gastrointest Surg 2005;9: 270.

528. Moseley JM, Kubota M, Diefenbach-Jagger H, et al. Parathyroid hormone-related protein purified from a human lung cancer cell line. Proc Natl Acad Sci U S A 1987;84:5048.

529. Kounami S, Yoshiyama M, Nakayama K, et al. Severe hypercalcemia in a child with acute nonlymphocytic leukemia: The role of parathyroid hormone-related protein and proinflammatory cytokines. Acta Haematol 2004;112:160.

530. Fan K, Smith DJ. Hypercalcemia associated with renal cell carcinoma: Probable role of neoplastic stromal cells. Hum Pathol 1983;14:168.

531. Budayr AA, Nissenson RA, Klein RF, et al. Increased serum levels of a parathyroid hormone-like protein in malignancy-associated hypercalcemia. Ann Intern Med 1989;111:807.

532. Henderson JE, Shustik C, Kremer R, et al. Circulating concentrations of parathyroid hormone-like peptide in malignancy and in hyperparathyroidism. J Bone Miner Res 1990;5: 105.

533. Rousseau-Merck MF, Nogues C, Roth A, et al. Hypercalcemic infantile renal tumors: Morphological, clinical, and biological heterogeneity. Pediatr Pathol 1985;3:155.

534. Mayes LC, Kasselberg AG, Roloff JS, Lukens JN. Hypercalcemia associated with immunoreactive parathyroid hormone in a malignant rhabdoid tumor of the kidney (rhabdoid Wilms' tumor). Cancer 1984;54:882.

535. Nussbaum SR, Gaz RD, Arnold A. Hypercalcemia and ectopic secretion of parathyroid hormone by an ovarian carcinoma with rearrangement of the gene for parathyroid hormone. N Engl J Med 1990;323:1324.

536. Yoshimoto K, Yamasaki R, Sakai H, et al. Ectopic production of parathyroid hormone by small cell lung cancer in a patient with hypercalcemia. J Clin Endocrinol Metab 1989;68:976.

537. Casez J, Pfammatter R, Nguyen Q, et al. Diagnostic approach to hypercalcemia: Relevance of parathyroid hormone and parathyroid hormone-related protein measurements. Eur J Intern Med 2001;12:344.

538. Sanderson PH. Hypercalcaemia and renal failure in multiple secondary carcinoma of bone: Report of a case. Br Med J 1959;5147:275.

539. Schwimmer JA, Markowitz GS, Valeri A, Appel GB. Collapsing glomerulopathy. Semin Nephrol 2003;23:209.

540. Markowitz GS, Fine PL, Stack JI, et al. Toxic acute tubular necrosis following treatment with zoledronate (Zometa). Kidney Int 2003;64:281.

541. Smolens P, Barnes JL, Kreisberg R. Hypercalcemia can potentiate the nephrotoxicity of Bence Jones proteins. J Lab Clin Med 1987;110:460.

542. Basic-Jukic N, Kes P, Labar B. Myeloma kidney: Pathogenesis and treatment. Acta Med Croatica 2001;55:169.

543. McCarthy CS, Becker JA. Multiple myeloma and contrast media. Radiology 1992;183:519.

544. Lightwood R, Stapleton T. Idiopathic hypercalcaemia in infants. Lancet 1953;265:255.

545. Rhaney K, Mitchell RG. Idiopathic hypercalcaemia of infants. Lancet 1956;270:1028.

546. Rodd C, Goodyer P. Hypercalcemia of the newborn: Etiology, evaluation, and management. Pediatr Nephrol 1999;13:542.

547. Osborne LR, Martindale D, Scherer SW, et al. Identification of genes from a 500-kb region at 7q11.23 that is commonly deleted in Williams syndrome patients. Genomics 1996;36:328.

548. Donnai D, Karmiloff-Smith A. Williams syndrome: From genotype through to the cognitive phenotype. Am J Med Genet 2000;97:164.

549. Pankau R, Siebert R, Kautza M, et al. Familial Williams-Beuren syndrome showing varying clinical expression. Am J Med Genet 2001;98:324.

550. Pankau R, Partsch CJ, Winter M, et al. Incidence and spectrum of renal abnormalities in Williams-Beuren syndrome. Am J Med Genet 1996;63:301.

551. Pagon RA, Bennett FC, LaVeck B, et al. Williams syndrome: Features in late childhood and adolescence. Pediatrics 1987;80:85.

552. Schlesinger BE, Butler NR, Black JA. Severe type of infantile hypercalcaemia. Br Med J 1956;127.

553. Morris CA, Mervis CB. Williams syndrome and related disorders. Annu Rev Genomics Hum Genet 2000;1:461.

554. Cagle AP, Waguespack SG, Buckingham BA, et al. Severe infantile hypercalcemia associated with Williams syndrome successfully treated with intravenously administered pamidronate. Pediatrics 2004;114:1091.

555. Amenta S, Sofocleous C, Kolialexi A, et al. Clinical manifestations and molecular investigation of 50 patients with Williams syndrome in the Greek population. Pediatr Res 2005;57:789.

556. Morris CA, Leonard CO, Dilts C, Demsey SA. Adults with Williams syndrome. Am J Med Genet Suppl 1990;6:102.

557. Gunn IR, Gaffney D. Clinical and laboratory features of calcium-sensing receptor disorders: A systematic review. Ann Clin Biochem 2004;41(Pt 6):441.

558. Schnatz PF, Curry SL. Primary hyperparathyroidism in pregnancy: Evidence-based management. Obstet Gynecol Surv 2002; 57:365.

559. Jaafar R, Yun Boo N, Rasat R, Latiff HA. Neonatal seizures due to maternal primary hyperparathyroidism. J Paediatr Child Health 2004;40:329.

560. Fernandez-Lopez E, Garcia-Dorado J, de Unamuno P, et al. Subcutaneous fat necrosis of the newborn and idiopathic hypercalcemia. Dermatologica 1990;180:250.

561. Fenniche S, Daoud L, Benmously R, et al. Subcutaneous fat necrosis: Report of two cases. Dermatol Online J 2004;10:12.

562. Mahe E, Descamps V, Belaich S, Crickx B. Cytosteatonecrosis of the newborn infant [in French]. Presse Med 2002;31:612.

563. Dudink J, Walther FJ, Beekman RP. Subcutaneous fat necrosis of the newborn: Hypercalcaemia with hepatic and atrial myocardial calcification. Arch Dis Child Fetal Neonatal Ed 2003;88: F343.

564. Tran JT, Sheth AP. Complications of subcutaneous fat necrosis of the newborn: A case report and review of the literature. Pediatr Dermatol 2003;20:257.

565. Garrett JE, Tamir H, Kifor O, et al. Calcitonin-secreting cells of the thyroid express an extracellular calcium receptor gene. Endocrinology 1995;136:5202.

566. Rogers KV, Dunn CK, Hebert SC, Brown EM. Localization of calcium receptor mRNA in the adult rat central nervous system by in situ hybridization. Brain Res 1997;744:47.

567. Lloyd SE, Gunther W, Pearce SH, et al. Characterisation of renal chloride channel, CLCN5, mutations in hypercalciuric nephrolithiasis (kidney stones) disorders. Hum Mol Genet 1997;6:1233.

568. Cheng I, Klingensmith ME, Chattopadhyay N, et al. Identification and localization of the extracellular calcium-sensing receptor in human breast. J Clin Endocrinol Metab 1998;83:703.

569. Kameda T, Mano H, Yamada Y, et al. Calcium-sensing receptor in mature osteoclasts, which are bone resorbing cells. Biochem Biophys Res Commun 1998;245:419.

570. Brown EM, Hebert SC. A cloned Ca(2+)-sensing receptor: A mediator of direct effects of extracellular Ca2+ on renal function? J Am Soc Nephrol 1995;6:1530.

571. Sands JM, Naruse M, Baum M, et al. Apical extracellular calcium/polyvalent cation-sensing receptor regulates vasopressin-elicited water permeability in rat kidney inner medullary collecting duct. J Clin Invest 1997;99:1399.

572. Pollak MR, Brown EM, Chou YH, et al. Mutations in the human Ca(2+)-sensing receptor gene cause familial hypocalciuric hypercalcemia and neonatal severe hyperparathyroidism. Cell 1993;75:1297.

573. Chou YH, Pollak MR, Brandi ML, et al. Mutations in the human Ca(2+)-sensing-receptor gene that cause familial hypocalciuric hypercalcemia. Am J Hum Genet 1995;56:1075.

574. Pearce SH, Thakker RV. The calcium-sensing receptor: Insights into extracellular calcium homeostasis in health and disease. J Endocrinol 1997;154:371.

575. De Luca F, Baron J. Molecular biology and clinical importance of the Ca(2+)-sensing receptor. Curr Opin Pediatr 1998;10: 435.

576. Heath H 3rd. Familial benign (hypocalciuric) hypercalcemia. A troublesome mimic of mild primary hyperparathyroidism. Endocrinol Metab Clin North Am 1989;18:723.

577. Brown EM. Mutations in the calcium-sensing receptor and their clinical implications. Horm Res 1997;48:199.

578. Pollak MR, Brown EM, Estep HL, et al. Autosomal dominant hypocalcaemia caused by a Ca(2+)-sensing receptor gene mutation. Nat Genet 1994;8:303.

579. Baron J, Winer KK, Yanovski JA, et al. Mutations in the Ca(2+)-sensing receptor gene cause autosomal dominant and sporadic hypoparathyroidism. Hum Mol Genet 1996;5:601.

580. Pearce SH, Williamson C, Kifor O, et al. A familial syndrome of hypocalcemia with hypercalciuria due to mutations in the calcium-sensing receptor. N Engl J Med 1996;335:1115.

581. Mancilla EE, De Luca F, Ray K, et al. A Ca(2+)-sensing receptor mutation causes hypoparathyroidism by increasing receptor sensitivity to Ca2+ and maximal signal transduction. Pediatr Res 1997;42:443.

582. Lienhardt A, Bai M, Lagarde JP, et al. Activating mutations of the calcium-sensing receptor: Management of hypocalcemia. J Clin Endocrinol Metab 2001;86:5313.

583. De Luca F, Ray K, Mancilla EE, et al. Sporadic hypoparathyroidism caused by de novo gain-of-function mutations of the Ca(2+)-sensing receptor. J Clin Endocrinol Metab 1997; 82:2710.

584. Ragavan VV, Smith JE, Bilezikian JP. Vitamin A toxicity and hypercalcemia. Am J Med Sci 1982;283:161.

585. Bergman SM, O'Mailia J, Krane NK, Wallin JD. Vitamin-A-induced hypercalcemia: Response to corticosteroids. Nephron 1988;50:362.

586. Sakakibara M, Ichikawa M, Amano Y, et al. Hypercalcemia associated with all-trans-retinoic acid in the treatment of acute promyelocytic leukemia. Leuk Res 1993;17:441.

587. Villablanca JG, Khan AA, Avramis VI, Reynolds CP. Hypercalcemia: A dose-limiting toxicity associated with 13-cis-retinoic acid. Am J Pediatr Hematol Oncol 1993;15:410.

588. Jacobus CH, Holick MF, Shao Q, et al. Hypervitaminosis D associated with drinking milk. N Engl J Med 1992;326:1173.

589. Blank S, Scanlon KS, Sinks TH, et al. An outbreak of hypervitaminosis D associated with the overfortification of milk from a home-delivery dairy. Am J Public Health 1995;85:656.

590. Davies M, Mawer EB, Hayes ME, Lumb GA. Abnormal vitamin D metabolism in Hodgkin's lymphoma. Lancet 1985;1: 1186.

591. Adams JS. Extrarenal production and action of active vitamin D metabolites in human lymphoproliferative diseases. In: Feldman D, Glorieux FH, Pike JW, eds. Vitamin D. San Diego: Academic Press, 1997:903.

592. Moore JJ, Isbister JP, Clifton-Bligh P, Eckstein RP. Calcitriol mediated hypercalcaemia in a T-cell rich B-cell lymphoma. Aust N Z J Med 1998;28:479.

593. Hewison M, Kantorovich V, Liker HR, et al. Vitamin D-mediated hypercalcemia in lymphoma: Evidence for hormone production by tumor-adjacent macrophages. J Bone Miner Res 2003;18: 579.

594. Stickler G, Hagge W. Hypocalcemia, hypercalciuria, and renal disease. In: Edelman C, ed. Pediatric Kidney Disease. Boston: Little, Brown and Company, 1978:907.

595. Bushinsky DA, Monk RD. Electrolyte quintet: Calcium. Lancet 1998;352:306.

596. Porter N, Beynon HL, Randeva HS. Endocrine and reproductive manifestations of sarcoidosis. Q J Med 2003;96:553.

597. Tuohy KA, Steinman TI. Hypercalcemia due to excess 1,25-dihydroxyvitamin D in Crohn's disease. Am J Kidney Dis 2005; 45:e3.

598. Bergner R, Hoffmann M, Waldherr R, Uppenkamp M. Frequency of kidney disease in chronic sarcoidosis. Sarcoidosis Vasc Diffuse Lung Dis 2003;20:126.

599. Randall RE Jr, Strauss MB, McNeely WF. The milk-alkali syndrome. Arch Intern Med 1961;107:163.

600. Junor BJ, Catto GR. Renal biopsy in the milk-alkali syndrome. J Clin Pathol 1976;29:1074.

601. Abreo K, Adlakha A, Kilpatrick S, et al. The milk-alkali syndrome. A reversible form of acute renal failure. Arch Intern Med 1993;153:1005.

602. Kleinig TJ, Torpy DJ. Milk-alkali syndrome: Broadening the spectrum of causes to allow early recognition. Intern Med J 2004;34:366.

603. Fiorino AS. Hypercalcemia and alkalosis due to the milk-alkali syndrome: A case report and review. Yale J Biol Med 1996;69:517.

604. Konrad M, Weber S. Recent advances in molecular genetics of hereditary magnesium-losing disorders. J Am Soc Nephrol 2003;14:249.

605. Sayer JA, Carr G, Simmons NL. Nephrocalcinosis: Molecular insights into calcium precipitation within the kidney. Clin Sci (Lond) 2004;106:549.

606. Simon DB, Lu Y, Choate KA, et al. Paracellin-1, a renal tight junction protein required for paracellular Mg2+ resorption. Science 1999;285:103.

607. Weber S, Schneider L, Peters M, et al. Novel paracellin-1 mutations in 25 families with familial hypomagnesemia with hypercalciuria and nephrocalcinosis. J Am Soc Nephrol 2001;12: 1872.

608. Blanchard A, Jeunemaitre X, Coudol P, et al. Paracellin-1 is critical for magnesium and calcium reabsorption in the human thick ascending limb of Henle. Kidney Int 2001;59:2206.

609. Hebert SC. Extracellular calcium-sensing receptor: Implications for calcium and magnesium handling in the kidney. Kidney Int 1996;50:2129.

610. Vargas-Poussou R, Huang C, Hulin P, et al. Functional characterization of a calcium-sensing receptor mutation in severe autosomal dominant hypocalcemia with a Bartter-like syndrome. J Am Soc Nephrol 2002;13:2259.

611. Seyberth H, Soergel M, Koeckerling A. Hypokalaemic tubular disorders: The hyperprostaglandin E syndrome and Gitelman-Bartter syndrome. In: Davison AM, Cameron JS, Grünfeld JP, et al, eds. Oxford Textbook of Clinical Nephrology. Oxford, UK: Oxford University Press, 1998:1085.

612. Simon DB, Karet FE, Hamdan JM, et al. Bartter's syndrome, hypokalaemic alkalosis with hypercalciuria, is caused by mutations in the Na-K-2Cl cotransporter NKCC2. Nat Genet 1996;13: 183.

613. Simon DB, Karet FE, Rodriguez-Soriano J, et al. Genetic heterogeneity of Bartter's syndrome revealed by mutations in the K+ channel, ROMK. Nat Genet 1996;14:152.

614. Bartter FC, Pronove P, Gill JR Jr, Maccardle RC. Hyperplasia of the juxtaglomerular complex with hyperaldosteronism and hypokalemic alkalosis. A new syndrome. Am J Med 1962;33:811.

615. Konrad M, Vollmer M, Lemmink HH, et al. Mutations in the chloride channel gene CLCNKB as a cause of classic Bartter syndrome. J Am Soc Nephrol 2000;11:1449.

616. Simon DB, Bindra RS, Mansfield TA, et al. Mutations in the chloride channel gene, CLCNKB, cause Bartter's syndrome type III. Nat Genet 1997;17:171.

617. Lloyd SE, Pearce SH, Fisher SE, et al. A common molecular basis for three inherited kidney stone diseases. Nature 1996;379: 445.

618. Bruce LJ, Unwin RJ, Wrong O, Tanner MJ. The association between familial distal renal tubular acidosis and mutations in the red cell anion exchanger (band 3, AE1) gene. Biochem Cell Biol 1998;76:723.

619. Nicoletta JA, Schwartz GJ. Distal renal tubular acidosis. Curr Opin Pediatr 2004;16:194.

620. Laing CM, Toye AM, Capasso G, Unwin RJ. Renal tubular acidosis: Developments in our understanding of the molecular basis. Int J Biochem Cell Biol 2005;37:1151.

621. Milliner DS. The primary hyperoxalurias: An algorithm for diagnosis. Am J Nephrol 2005;25:154.

622. Markowitz GS, Perazella MA. Drug-induced renal failure: A focus on tubulointerstitial disease. Clin Chim Acta 2005;351:31.

623. Normand de la Tranchade I, Bonarek H, Marteau JM, et al. Amelogenesis imperfecta and nephrocalcinosis: A new case of this rare syndrome. J Clin Pediatr Dent 2003;27:171.

624. Feuerstein IM, Francis P, Raffeld M, Pluda J. Widespread visceral calcifications in disseminated *Pneumocystis carinii* infection: CT characteristics. J Comput Assist Tomogr 1990;14:149.

625. Radin DR, Baker EL, Klatt EC, et al. Visceral and nodal calcification in patients with AIDS-related *Pneumocystis carinii* infection. AJR Am J Roentgenol 1990;154:27.

626. Seney FD Jr, Burns DK, Silva FG. Acquired immunodeficiency syndrome and the kidney. Am J Kidney Dis 1990;16:1.

627. Yang CW, Kim SY, Kim YS, et al. Nephrocalcinosis associated with primary aldosteronism. Nephron 1994;68:507.

628. Schmitt K, Frisch H, Neuhold N, et al. Aldosterone and testosterone producing adrenal adenoma in childhood. J Endocrinol Invest 1995;18:69.

629. Katz SM, Krueger LJ, Falkner B. Microscopic nephrocalcinosis in cystic fibrosis. N Engl J Med 1988;319:263.

630. Ozcelik U, Besbas N, Gocmen A, et al. Hypercalciuria and nephrocalcinosis in cystic fibrosis patients. Turk J Pediatr 2004;46:22.

631. Bentur L, Kerem E, Couper R, et al. Renal calcium handling in cystic fibrosis: Lack of evidence for a primary renal defect. J Pediatr 1990;116:556.

632. Hoppe B, von Unruh GE, Blank G, et al. Absorptive hyperoxaluria leads to an increased risk for urolithiasis or nephrocalcinosis in cystic fibrosis. Am J Kidney Dis 2005;46:440.

633. Siegel FL, Bulger RE. Scanning and transmission EM of rat kidney following low dose mercuric chloride administration. Beitr Pathol 1975;156:313.

634. Evans BM, Macpherson CR. Some observations on acetazolamide-induced nephrocalcinosis in the rat. Br J Exp Pathol 1956;37:533.

635. Parikh JR, Nolan RL, Bannerjee A, Gault MH. Acetazolamide-associated nephrocalcinosis in a transplant kidney. Transplantation 1995;59:1742.

636. Sanders LD, Jequier S. Ultrasound demonstration of prenatal renal vein thrombosis. Pediatr Radiol 1989;19:133.

637. Boom H, Mallat MJ, de Fijter JW, et al. Calcium levels as a risk factor for delayed graft function. Transplantation 2004;77:868.

638. Ferguson RK, Reed DM, Barber KG, et al. Sodium-losing nephropathy and nephrocalcinosis after transplantation. Am J Kidney Dis 1985;5:206.

639. Harrison RB, Vaughan ED Jr. Diffuse cortical calcification in rejected renal transplants. Radiology 1978;126:635.

640. Smith LE, Adelman RD. Early detection of renal cortical calcification in acute renal cortical necrosis in a child. Nephron 1981;29:155.

641. Pereira S, Marwaha RK, Pereira BJ, et al. Haemolytic uraemic syndrome with prolonged anuria and cortical calcification: A case report. Pediatr Nephrol 1990;4:65.

642. Desmeules S, Bergeron MJ, Isenring P. Acute phosphate nephropathy and renal failure. N Engl J Med 2003;349:1006.

643. Markowitz GS, Nasr SH, Klein P, et al. Renal failure due to acute nephrocalcinosis following oral sodium phosphate bowel cleansing. Hum Pathol 2004;35:675.

644. Brenner RJ, Spring DB, Sebastian A, et al. Incidence of radiographically evident bone disease, nephrocalcinosis, and nephrolithiasis in various types of renal tubular acidosis. N Engl J Med 1982;307:217.

645. Karet FE, Gainza FJ, Gyory AZ, et al. Mutations in the chloride-bicarbonate exchanger gene AE1 cause autosomal dominant but not autosomal recessive distal renal tubular acidosis. Proc Natl Acad Sci U S A 1998;95:6337.

646. Karet FE, Finberg KE, Nelson RD, et al. Mutations in the gene encoding B1 subunit of H+-ATPase cause renal tubular acidosis with sensorineural deafness. Nat Genet 1999;21:84.

647. Smith AN, Skaug J, Choate KA, et al. Mutations in ATP6N1B, encoding a new kidney vacuolar proton pump 116-kD subunit, cause recessive distal renal tubular acidosis with preserved hearing. Nat Genet 2000;26:71.

648. Buckalew VM Jr. Nephrolithiasis in renal tubular acidosis. J Urol 1989;141(Pt 2):731.

649. Peterson LN. Vitamin D-induced chronic hypercalcemia inhibits thick ascending limb NaCl reabsorption in vivo. Am J Physiol 1990;259(Pt 2):F122.

650. Epstein FH, Beck D, Carone FA, et al. Changes in renal concentrating ability produced by parathyroid extract. J Clin Invest 1959;38:1214.

651. Humes HD, Ichikawa I, Troy JL, et al. Influence of calcium on the determinants of glomerular ultrafiltration. Trans Assoc Am Physicians 1977;90:228.

652. Brunette MG, Vary J, Carriere S. Hyposthenuria in hypercalcemia. A possible role of intrarenal blood-flow (IRBF) redistribution. Pflugers Arch 1974;350:9.

653. Levi M, Peterson L, Berl T. Mechanism of concentrating defect in hypercalcemia. Role of polydipsia and prostaglandins. Kidney Int 1983;23:489.

654. Rosen S, Greenfeld Z, Bernheim J, et al. Hypercalcemic nephropathy: Chronic disease with predominant medullary inner stripe injury. Kidney Int 1990;37:1067.

655. Carone FA, Epstein FH, Beck D, Levitin. The effects upon the kidney of transient hypercalcemia induced by parathyroid extract. Am J Pathol 1960;36:77.

656. Epstein FH, Rivera MJ, Carone FA. The effect of hypercalcemia induced by calciferol upon renal concentrating ability. J Clin Invest 1958;37:1702.

657. Schneeberger EE, Morrison AB. The nephropathy of experimental magnesium deficiency: Light and electron microscopic investigations. Lab Invest 1965;14:674.

658. Burry AF, Axelsen RA, Trolove P, Saal JR. Calcification in the renal medulla; a classification based on a prospective study of 2261 necropsies. Hum Pathol 1976;7:435.

659. Caulfield JB, Schrag PE. Electron microscopic study of renal calcification. Am J Pathol 1964;44:365.

660. Engfeldt B, Gardell S, Hellstrom J, et al. Effect of experimentally induced hyperparathyroidism on renal function and structure. Acta Endocrinol (Copenh) 1958;29:15.

661. Ritskes-Hoitinga J, Lemmens AG, Danse LH, Beynen AC. Phosphorus-induced nephrocalcinosis and kidney function in female rats. J Nutr 1989;119:1423.

662. Anastasia JV, Braun BL, Smith KT. General and histopathological results of a two-year study of rats fed semi-purified diets containing casein and soya protein. Food Chem Toxicol 1990;28:147.

663. Minami T, Ichii M, Okazaki Y, et al. Renal changes of streptozotocin-induced diabetic rats fed a low-zinc diet. Ren Fail 1995;17:349.

664. Cockell KA, Belonje B. Nephrocalcinosis caused by dietary calcium:phosphorus imbalance in female rats develops rapidly and is irreversible. J Nutr 2004;134:637.

665. Alon U, Donaldson DL, Hellerstein S, et al. Metabolic and histologic investigation of the nature of nephrocalcinosis in children with hypophosphatemic rickets and in the Hyp mouse. J Pediatr 1992;120:899.

666. Ritskes-Hoitinga J, Mathot JN, Van Zutphen LF, Beynen AC. Inbred strains of rats have differential sensitivity to dietary phosphorus-induced nephrocalcinosis. J Nutr 1992;122:1682.

667. Bushinsky DA. Kidney stones. In: Schrier R, ed. Advances in Internal Medicine. Mosby, 2001:225.

668. Bushinsky DA, Asplin JR, Grynpas MD, et al. Calcium oxalate stone formation in genetic hypercalciuric stone-forming rats. Kidney Int 2002;61:975.

669. Bushinsky DA. Nephrolithiasis. J Am Soc Nephrol 1998;9:917.

670. Hoopes RR Jr, Reid R, Sen S, et al. Quantitative trait loci for hypercalciuria in a rat model of kidney stone disease. J Am Soc Nephrol 2003;14:1844.

671. Evan AP, Bledsoe SB, Smith SB, Bushinsky DA. Calcium oxalate crystal localization and osteopontin immunostaining in genetic hypercalciuric stone-forming rats. Kidney Int 2004;65:154.

672. Khan SR. Pathogenesis of oxalate urolithiasis: Lessons from experimental studies with rats. Am J Kidney Dis 1991;17:398.

673. Khan SR, Hackett RL. Urolithogenesis of mixed foreign body stones. J Urol 1987;138:1321.

674. Koul H, Ebisuno S, Renzulli L, et al. Polarized distribution of oxalate transport systems in LLC-PK1 cells, a line of renal epithelial cells. Am J Physiol 1994;266(Pt 2):F266.

675. Verkoelen CF, Romijn JC. Oxalate transport and calcium oxalate renal stone disease. Urol Res 1996;24:183.

676. Hackett RL, Shevock PN, Khan SR. Madin-Darby canine kidney cells are injured by exposure to oxalate and to calcium oxalate crystals. Urol Res 1994;22:197.

677. Verkoelen CF, Romijn JC, de Bruijn WC, et al. Association of calcium oxalate monohydrate crystals with MDCK cells. Kidney Int 1995;48:129.

678. Lieske JC, Leonard R, Swift H, Toback FG. Adhesion of calcium oxalate monohydrate crystals to anionic sites on the surface of renal epithelial cells. Am J Physiol 1996;270(Pt 2):F192.

679. Lieske JC, Toback FG. Renal cell-urinary crystal interactions. Curr Opin Nephrol Hypertens 2000;9:349.

680. Verkoelen CF, Vanderboom BG, Romijn JC, Schroder FH. Cell density dependent calcium oxalate crystal binding to sulphated proteins at the surface of MDCK cells. In: Pak CYC, Resnick MI, Preminger GM, eds. Urolithiasis. Dallas, TX: Millet, 1996: 208.

681. Bigelow MW, Wiessner JH, Kleinman JG, Mandel NS. Calcium oxalate-crystal membrane interactions: Dependence on membrane lipid composition. J Urol 1996;155:1094.

682. Bigelow MW, Wiessner JH, Kleinman JG, Mandel NS. Calcium oxalate crystal attachment to cultured kidney epithelial cell lines. J Urol 1998;160:1528.

683. Lieske JC, Deganello S, Toback FG. Cell-crystal interactions and kidney stone formation. Nephron 1999;81(Suppl 1):8.

684. Coe FL, Parks JH. New insights into the pathophysiology and treatment of nephrolithiasis: New research venues. J Bone Miner Res 1997;12:522.

685. Bruwer A. Primary renal calculi: Anderson-Carr-Randall progression? AJR Am J Roentgenol 1979;132:751.

686. Abrahams C. Stereopathy of the renal papilla: A stereomicroscopic autopsy study. Hum Pathol 1985;16:488.

687. Rosenow E. Renal calculi: A study of papillary calcification. J Urol 1940;44:19.

688. Randall A, Eiman J, Leberman P. Studies of the pathology of the renal papilla: relationship to renal calculus. J Am Med Assoc 1937;109:1698.

689. Evan AP, Lingeman JE, Coe FL, et al. Randall's plaque of patients with nephrolithiasis begins in basement membranes of thin loops of Henle. J Clin Invest 2003;111:607.

690. Albright F BP, Cope O, Bloomberg E. Studies on the physiology of the parathyroid glands. IV. Renal complications of hyperparathyroidism. Am J Med Sci 1934;187:49.

691. Lowe KG, Henderson JL, Park WW, McGreal DA. The idiopathic hypercalcaemic syndromes of infancy. Lancet 1954;267:101.

692. Patriquin HB, O'Regan S. Medullary sponge kidney in childhood. AJR Am J Roentgenol 1985;145:315.

693. Shultz PK, Strife JL, Strife CF, McDaniel JD. Hyperechoic renal medullary pyramids in infants and children. Radiology 1991;181:163.

694. Randall A. The aetiology of primary renal calculus. Int Abstr Surg 1940;71:209.

695. Ibels LS, Alfrey AC, Huffer WE, et al. Calcification in end-stage kidneys. Am J Med 1981;71:33.

696. Stamatelou KK, Francis ME, Jones CA, et al. Time trends in reported prevalence of kidney stones in the United States: 1976–1994. Kidney Int 2003;63:1817.

697. Smith LH. The medical aspects of urolithiasis: An overview. J Urol 1989;141(Pt 2):707.

698. Tiselius H-G. Aetiological factors in stone formation. In: Davison AM, Cameron JS, Grünfeld JP, et al, eds. Oxford Textbook of Clinical Nephrology, 2nd ed. Oxford, UK: Oxford University Press, 1998:1199.

699. Drach G. Urinary lithiasis. In: Stamey T, ed. Campbell's Urology. Philadelphia: WB Saunders, 1986:1094.

700. Griffin DG. A review of the heritability of idiopathic nephrolithiasis. J Clin Pathol 2004;57:793.

701. Parmar MS. Kidney stones. BMJ 2004;328:1420.

702. Maloney ME, Springhart WP, Ekeruo WO, et al. Ethnic background has minimal impact on the etiology of nephrolithiasis. J Urol 2005;173:2001.

703. Segura JW, Preminger GM, Assimos DG, et al. Ureteral Stones Clinical Guidelines Panel summary report on the management of ureteral calculi. The American Urological Association. J Urol 1997;158:1915.

704. Hoorens A, Van Der Niepen P, Keuppens F, et al. Pseudotuberculous pyelonephritis associated with nephrolithiasis. Am J Surg Pathol 1992;16:522.

705. Assimos DG, Langenstroer P, Leinbach RF, et al. Guaifenesin-and ephedrine-induced stones. J Endourol 1999;13:665.

706. Bennett S, Hoffman N, Monga M. Ephedrine- and guaifenesin-induced nephrolithiasis. J Altern Complement Med 2004;10:967.

707. Hoffman N, McGee SM, Hulbert JC. Resolution of ephedrine stones with dissolution therapy. Urology 2003;61:1035.

708. Ryall RL. Macromolecules and urolithiasis: Parallels and paradoxes. Nephron Physiol 2004;98:37.

709. Smith LH. The pathophysiology and medical treatment of urolithiasis. Semin Nephrol 1990;10:31.

710. Bihl G, Meyers A. Recurrent renal stone disease-advances in pathogenesis and clinical management. Lancet 2001;358:651.

711. Asplin J, Parks J, Coe FL. Dependence of upper limit of metastability on supersaturation in nephrolithiasis. Kidney Int 1997;52:1602.

712. Bushinsky DA, Parker WR, Asplin JR. Calcium phosphate supersaturation regulates stone formation in genetic hypercalciuric stone-forming rats. Kidney Int 2000;57:550.

713. Pak CY, Arnold LH. Heterogeneous nucleation of calcium oxalate by seeds of monosodium urate. Proc Soc Exp Biol Med 1975;149:930.

714. Hess B, Nakagawa Y, Coe FL. Inhibition of calcium oxalate monohydrate crystal aggregation by urine proteins. Am J Physiol 1989;257(Pt 2):F99.

715. Boeve ER, Cao LC, Deng G, et al. Effect of two new polysaccharides on growth, agglomeration and zeta potential of calcium phosphate crystals. J Urol 1996;155:368.

716. Verkoelen CF, Romijn JC, Cao LC, et al. Crystal-cell interaction inhibition by polysaccharides. J Urol 1996;155:749.

717. Grover PK, Ryall RL. Inhibition of calcium oxalate crystal growth and aggregation by prothrombin and its fragments in vitro: Relationship between protein structure and inhibitory activity. Eur J Biochem 1999;263:50.

718. Verkoelen CF, Schepers MS. Changing concepts in the aetiology of renal stones. Curr Opin Urol 2000;10:539.

719. Wesson JA, Johnson RJ, Mazzali M, et al. Osteopontin is a critical inhibitor of calcium oxalate crystal formation and retention in renal tubules. J Am Soc Nephrol 2003;14:139.

720. Kok DJ, Papapoulos SE, Blomen LJ, Bijvoet OL. Modulation of calcium oxalate monohydrate crystallization kinetics in vitro. Kidney Int 1988;34:346.

721. Worcester EM, Beshensky AM. Osteopontin inhibits nucleation of calcium oxalate crystals. Ann N Y Acad Sci 1995;760:375.

722. Asplin JR, Arsenault D, Parks JH, et al. Contribution of human uropontin to inhibition of calcium oxalate crystallization. Kidney Int 1998;53:194.

723. Hoyer JR, Asplin JR, Otvos L. Phosphorylated osteopontin peptides suppress crystallization by inhibiting the growth of calcium oxalate crystals. Kidney Int 2001;60:77.

724. Goldberg HA, Hunter GK. The inhibitory activity of osteopontin on hydroxyapatite formation in vitro. Ann N Y Acad Sci 1995;760:305.

725. Hoyer JR, Otvos L Jr, Urge L. Osteopontin in urinary stone formation. Ann N Y Acad Sci 1995;760:257.

726. Lieske JC, Hammes MS, Hoyer JR, Toback FG. Renal cell osteopontin production is stimulated by calcium oxalate monohydrate crystals. Kidney Int 1997;51:679.

727. Jiang XJ, Feng T, Chang LS, et al. Expression of osteopontin mRNA in normal and stone-forming rat kidney. Urol Res 1998;26:389.

728. Kohri K, Suzuki Y, Yoshida K, et al. Molecular cloning and sequencing of cDNA encoding urinary stone protein, which is identical to osteopontin. Biochem Biophys Res Commun 1992; 184:859.

729. Nakagawa Y, Ahmed M, Hall SL, et al. Isolation from human calcium oxalate renal stones of nephrocalcin, a glycoprotein inhibitor of calcium oxalate crystal growth. Evidence that nephrocalcin from patients with calcium oxalate nephrolithiasis is deficient in gamma-carboxyglutamic acid. J Clin Invest 1987;79:1782.

730. Nakagawa Y, Abram V, Parks JH, et al. Urine glycoprotein crystal growth inhibitors. Evidence for a molecular abnormality in calcium oxalate nephrolithiasis. J Clin Invest 1985;76:1455.

731. Nakagawa Y, Otsuki T, Coe FL. Elucidation of multiple forms of nephrocalcin by 31P-NMR spectrometer. FEBS Lett 1989;250:187.

732. Hess B. The role of Tamm-Horsfall glycoprotein and Nephrocalcin in calcium oxalate monohydrate crystallization processes. Scanning Microsc 1991;5:689; discussion 696.

733. Beshensky AM, Wesson JA, Worcester EM, et al. Effects of urinary macromolecules on hydroxyapatite crystal formation. J Am Soc Nephrol 2001;12:2108.

734. Hess B, Nakagawa Y, Parks JH, Coe FL. Molecular abnormality of Tamm-Horsfall glycoprotein in calcium oxalate nephrolithiasis. Am J Physiol 1991;260(Pt 2):F569.

735. Ryall RL, Grover PK, Stapleton AM, et al. The urinary F1 activation peptide of human prothrombin is a potent inhibitor of calcium oxalate crystallization in undiluted human urine in vitro. Clin Sci (Lond) 1995;89:533.

736. Stapleton AM, Timme TL, Ryall RL. Gene expression of prothrombin in the human kidney and its potential relevance to kidney stone disease. Br J Urol 1998;81:666; discussion 671.

737. Ryall RL, Fleming DE, Grover PK, et al. The hole truth: Intracrystalline proteins and calcium oxalate kidney stones. Mol Urol 2000;4:391.

738. Lerolle N, Lantz B, Paillard F, et al. Risk factors for nephrolithiasis in patients with familial idiopathic hypercalciuria. Am J Med 2002;113:99.

739. Baggio B. Genetic and dietary factors in idiopathic calcium nephrolithiasis. What do we have, what do we need? J Nephrol 1999;12:371.

740. Resnick M, Pridgen DB, Goodman HO. Genetic predisposition to formation of calcium oxalate renal calculi. N Engl J Med 1968;278:1313.

741. Favus MJ. Familial forms of hypercalciuria. J Urol 1989;141 (Pt 2):719.

742. Pak CY, Britton F, Peterson R, et al. Ambulatory evaluation of nephrolithiasis. Classification, clinical presentation and diagnostic criteria. Am J Med 1980;69:19.

743. Lerolle N, Coulet F, Lantz B, et al. No evidence for point mutations of the calcium-sensing receptor in familial idiopathic hypercalciuria. Nephrol Dial Transplant 2001;16:2317.

744. Petrucci M, Scott P, Ouimet D, et al. Evaluation of the calcium-sensing receptor gene in idiopathic hypercalciuria and calcium nephrolithiasis. Kidney Int 2000;58:38.

745. Vezzoli G, Tanini A, Ferrucci L, et al. Influence of calcium-sensing receptor gene on urinary calcium excretion in stone-forming patients. J Am Soc Nephrol 2002;132517.

746. Coe FL, Evan A, Worcester E. Kidney stone disease. J Clin Invest 2005;115:2598.

747. Monk RD, Bushinsky DA. Pathogenesis of idiopathic hypercalciuria. In: Coe F, Favus M, Pak C, eds. Kidney Stones: Medical and Surgical Management. New York: Raven Press, 1996: 759.

748. Pak CY. The spectrum and pathogenesis of hypercalciuria. Urol Clin North Am 1981;8:245.

749. Ohkawa M, Tokunaga S, Nakashima T, et al. Thiazide treatment for calcium urolithiasis in patients with idiopathic hypercalciuria. Br J Urol 1992;69:571.

750. Reed BY, Gitomer WL, Heller HJ, et al. Identification and characterization of a gene with base substitutions associated with the absorptive hypercalciuria phenotype and low spinal bone density. J Clin Endocrinol Metab 2002;87:1476.

751. Reed BY, Heller HJ, Gitomer WL, Pak CY. Mapping a gene defect in absorptive hypercalciuria to chromosome 1q23.3-q24. J Clin Endocrinol Metab 1999;84:3907.

752. Borghi L, Schianchi T, Meschi T, et al. Comparison of two diets for the prevention of recurrent stones in idiopathic hypercalciuria. N Engl J Med 2002;346:77.

753. Lewandowski S, Rodgers AL. Idiopathic calcium oxalate urolithiasis: Risk factors and conservative treatment. Clin Chim Acta 2004;345:17.

754. Curhan GC. Dietary calcium, dietary protein, and kidney stone formation. Miner Electrolyte Metab 1997;23:261.

755. Parks J, Coe F, Favus M. Hyperparathyroidism in nephrolithiasis. Arch Intern Med 1980;140:1479.

756. Scheinman SJ. X-linked hypercalciuric nephrolithiasis: Clinical syndromes and chloride channel mutations. Kidney Int 1998;53:3.

757. Thakker RV. Pathogenesis of Dent's disease and related syndromes of X-linked nephrolithiasis. Kidney Int 2000;57:787.

758. Hoopes RRJ, Raja KM, Koich A, et al. Evidence for genetic heterogeneity in Dent's disease. Kidney International 2004;65:1615.

759. Wrong OM, Norden AG, Feest TG. Dent's disease; a familial proximal renal tubular syndrome with low-molecular-weight proteinuria, hypercalciuria, nephrocalcinosis, metabolic bone disease, progressive renal failure and a marked male predominance. QJM 1994;87:473.

760. Igarashi T, Hayakawa H, Shiraga H, et al. Hypercalciuria and nephrocalcinosis in patients with idiopathic low-molecular-weight proteinuria in Japan: Is the disease identical to Dent's disease in United Kingdom? Nephron 1995;69:242.

761. Coe FL. Treated and untreated recurrent calcium nephrolithiasis in patients with idiopathic hypercalciuria, hyperuricosuria, or no metabolic disorder. Ann Intern Med 1977;87:404.

762. Siener R, Schade N, Nicolay C, et al. The efficacy of dietary intervention on urinary risk factors for stone formation in recurrent calcium oxalate stone patients. J Urol 2005;173:1601.

763. Coe FL, Lawton RL, Goldstein RB, Tembe V. Sodium urate accelerates precipitation of calcium oxalate in vitro. Proc Soc Exp Biol Med 1975;149:926.

764. Pak CY, Hayashi Y, Arnold LH. Heterogeneous nucleation with urate, calcium phosphate and calcium oxalate. Proc Soc Exp Biol Med 1976;153:83.

765. Tiselius HG. Effects of sodium urate and uric acid crystals on the crystallization of calcium oxalate. Urol Res 1984;12:11.

766. Grover PK, Ryall RL, Marshall VR. Calcium oxalate crystallization in urine: Role of urate and glycosaminoglycans. Kidney Int 1992;41:149.

767. Sorensen CM, Chandhoke PS. Hyperuricosuric calcium nephrolithiasis. Endocrinol Metab Clin North Am 2002;31:915.

768. Khan SR, Shevock PN, Hackett RL. Acute hyperoxaluria, renal injury and calcium oxalate urolithiasis. J Urol 1992;147:226.

769. Danpure CJ. Primary hyperoxaluria: From gene defects to designer drugs? Nephrol Dial Transplant 2005;20:1525.

770. Danpure CJ, Rumsby G. Molecular aetiology of primary hyperoxaluria and its implications for clinical management. Expert Rev Mol Med 2004;2004:1.

771. David-Walek T, Niederstadt C, Rob PM, et al. Primary hyperoxaluria type 1 causing end-stage renal disease in a 45-year-old patient. Nephron 2001;87:80.

772. Spiers EM, Sanders DY, Omura EF. Clinical and histologic features of primary oxalosis. J Am Acad Dermatol 1990;22(Pt 2):952.

773. Jamieson NV. The results of combined liver/kidney transplantation for primary hyperoxaluria (PH1) 1984–1997. The European PH1 transplant registry report. European PH1 Transplantation Study Group. J Nephrol 1998;11(Suppl 1):36.

774. Onaca N, Sanchez EQ, Melton LB, et al. Cadaveric orthotopic auxiliary split liver transplantation and kidney transplantation: An alternative for type 1 primary hyperoxaluria. Transplantation 2005;80:421.

775. Hoppe B, Langman CB. A United States survey on diagnosis, treatment, and outcome of primary hyperoxaluria. Pediatr Nephrol 2003;18:986.

776. Parks JH, Worcester EM, O'Connor RC, Coe FL. Urine stone risk factors in nephrolithiasis patients with and without bowel disease. Kidney Int 2003;63:255.

777. Hoppe B, Leumann E, von Unruh G, et al. Diagnostic and therapeutic approaches in patients with secondary hyperoxaluria. Front Biosci 2003;8:e437.

778. Williams HE. Oxalic acid and the hyperoxaluric syndromes. Kidney Int 1978;13:410.

779. Clayman RV, Williams RD. Oxalate urolithiasis following jejunoileal bypass. Surg Clin North Am 1979;59:1071.

780. Sidhu H, Schmidt ME, Cornelius JG, et al. Direct correlation between hyperoxaluria/oxalate stone disease and the absence of the gastrointestinal tract-dwelling bacterium *Oxalobacter formigenes*: Possible prevention by gut recolonization or enzyme replacement therapy. J Am Soc Nephrol 1999;10(Suppl 14):S334.

781. Troxel SA, Sidhu H, Kaul P, Low RK. Intestinal *Oxalobacter formigenes* colonization in calcium oxalate stone formers and its relation to urinary oxalate. J Endourol 2003;17:173.

782. Goldfarb DS. Microorganisms and calcium oxalate stone disease. Nephron Physiol 2004;98:48.

783. Brinkley LJ, Gregory J, Pak CY. A further study of oxalate bioavailability in foods. J Urol 1990;144:94.

784. Bek-Jensen H, Fornander AM, Nilsson MA, Tiselius HG. Is citrate an inhibitor of calcium oxalate crystal growth in high concentrations of urine? Urol Res 1996;24:67.

785. Nicar MJ, Skurla C, Sakhaee K, Pak CY. Low urinary citrate excretion in nephrolithiasis. Urology 1983;21:8.

786. Pattaras JG, Moore RG. Citrate in the management of urolithiasis. J Endourol 1999;13:687.

787. Hamm LL, Hering-Smith KS. Pathophysiology of hypocitraturic nephrolithiasis. Endocrinol Metab Clin North Am 2002;31:885, viii.

788. Tawil R, Moxley RT 3rd, Griggs RC. Acetazolamide-induced nephrolithiasis: Implications for treatment of neuromuscular disorders. Neurology 1993;43:1105.

789. LaRoche SM, Helmers SL. The new antiepileptic drugs: Scientific review. JAMA 2004;291:605.

790. Preminger GM, Sakhaee K, Skurla C, Pak CY. Prevention of recurrent calcium stone formation with potassium citrate therapy in patients with distal renal tubular acidosis. J Urol 1985;134:20.

791. Wilkinson H. Clinical investigation and management of patients with renal stones. Ann Clin Biochem 2001;38(Pt 3):180.

792. Cohen TD, Preminger GM. Struvite calculi. Semin Nephrol 1996;16:425.

793. Lerner SP, Gleeson MJ, Griffith DP. Infection stones. J Urol 1989;141(Pt 2):753.

794. Grenabo L, Hedelin H, Pettersson S. Urinary infection stones caused by *Ureaplasma urealyticum*: A review. Scand J Infect Dis Suppl 1988;53:46.

795. Dewan B, Sharma M, Nayak N, Sharma SK. Upper urinary tract stones & *Ureaplasma urealyticum*. Indian J Med Res 1997;105:15.

796. Hill G. Urinary tract infections: General considerations. In: Hill G, ed. Uropathology. New York: Churchill Livingstone, 1989:278.

797. Moe OW, Abate N, Sakhaee K. Pathophysiology of uric acid nephrolithiasis. Endocrinol Metab Clin North Am 2002;31:895.

798. Pak CY, Poindexter JR, Adams-Huet B, Pearle MS. Predictive value of kidney stone composition in the detection of metabolic abnormalities. Am J Med 2003;115:26.

799. Yu TF. Urolithiasis in hyperuricemia and gout. J Urol 1981;126:424.

800. Riese RJ, Sakhaee K. Uric acid nephrolithiasis: Pathogenesis and treatment. J Urol 1992;148:765.

801. Reddy ST, Wang CY, Sakhaee K, et al. Effect of low-carbohydrate high-protein diets on acid-base balance, stone-forming propensity, and calcium metabolism. Am J Kidney Dis 2002;40:265.

802. Pak CY, Sakhaee K, Moe O, et al. Biochemical profile of stone-forming patients with diabetes mellitus. Urology 2003;61:523.

803. Abate N, Chandalia M, Cabo-Chan AV Jr, et al. The metabolic syndrome and uric acid nephrolithiasis: Novel features of renal manifestation of insulin resistance. Kidney Int 2004;65:386.

804. Maalouf NM, Cameron MA, Moe OW, Sakhaee K. Novel insights into the pathogenesis of uric acid nephrolithiasis. Curr Opin Nephrol Hypertens 2004;13:181.

805. Saadi I, Chen X, Hediger M, et al. Molecular genetics of cystinuria: Mutation analysis of SLC3A1 and evidence for another gene in type I (silent) phenotype. Kidney Int 1998;54:48.

806. Calonge MJ, Gasparini P, Chillaron J, et al. Cystinuria caused by mutations in rBAT, a gene involved in the transport of cystine. Nat Genet 1994;6:420.

807. Bisceglia L, Purroy J, Jimenez-Vidal M, et al. Cystinuria type I: Identification of eight new mutations in SLC3A1. Kidney Int 2001;59:1250.

808. Schmidt C, Vester U, Wagner CA, et al. Significant contribution of genomic rearrangements in SLC3A1 and SLC7A9 to the etiology of cystinuria. Kidney Int 2003;64:1564.

809. Paterson RF, Lifshitz DA, Kuo RL, et al. Shock wave lithotripsy monotherapy for renal calculi. Int Braz J Urol 2002;28:291.

810. Sloand JA, Izzo JL Jr. Captopril reduces urinary cystine excretion in cystinuria. Arch Intern Med 1987;147:1409.

811. Purohit RS, Stoller ML. Stone clustering of patients with cystine urinary stone formation. Urology 2004;63:630; discussion 634.

812. Raivio K, Saksela M, Lapatto R. Xanthine oxidoreductase—Role in human pathophysiology and hereditary xanthinuria. In: Scriver C, Beaudet A, Sly W, Valle D, eds. The metabolic and molecular basis of inherited disease. New York: McGraw-Hill; 2001:2653

813. Bommer J, Ritz E, Tschope W, et al. Urinary matrix calculi consisting of microfibrillar protein in patients on maintenance hemodialysis. Kidney Int 1979;16:722.

814. Allen TD, Spence HM. Matrix stones. J Urol 1966;95:284.

815. Okochi H, Iiyama T, Kasahara K, et al. Renal matrix stones in an emphysematous pyelonephritis. Int J Urol 2005;12:1001.

816. Bani-Hani AH, Segura JW, Leroy AJ. Urinary matrix calculi: Our experience at a single institution. J Urol 2005;173:120.

817. Miller OF, Kane CJ. Time to stone passage for observed ureteral calculi: A guide for patient education. J Urol 1999;162(Pt 1):688 discussion 690.

818. Coll DM, Varanelli MJ, Smith RC. Relationship of spontaneous passage of ureteral calculi to stone size and location as revealed by unenhanced helical CT. AJR Am J Roentgenol 2002;178:101.

819. Marguet CG, Springhart WP, Auge BK, Preminger GM. Advances in the surgical management of nephrolithiasis. Minerva Urol Nefrol 2004;56:33.

820. Gettman MT, Segura JW. Management of ureteric stones: Issues and controversies. BJU Int 2005;95(Suppl 2):85.

821. Lingeman JE, Kim SC, Kuo RL, et al. Shockwave lithotripsy: Anecdotes and insights. J Endourol 2003;17:687.

822. Putman SS, Hamilton BD, Johnson DB. The use of shock wave lithotripsy for renal calculi. Curr Opin Urol 2004;14:117.

823. Sandhu C, Anson KM, Patel U. Urinary tract stones. II. Current status of treatment. Clin Radiol 2003;58:422.

824. Sasaguri M, Noda K, Matsumoto T, et al. A case of hyperreninemic hypertension after extracorporeal shock-wave lithotripsy. Hypertens Res 2000;23:709.

825. Strohmaier WL, Schmidt J, Lahme S, Bichler KH. Arterial blood pressure following different types of urinary stone therapy. Presented at the 8th European Symposium on Urolithiasis, Parma, Italy, 1999. Eur Urol 2000;38:753.

826. Elves AW, Tilling K, Menezes P, et al. Early observations of the effect of extracorporeal shockwave lithotripsy on blood pressure: A prospective randomized control clinical trial. BJU Int 2000;85:611.

827. Delius M, Jordan M, Eizenhoefer H, et al. Biological effects of shock waves: Kidney haemorrhage by shock waves in dogs–administration rate dependence. Ultrasound Med Biol 1988;14:689.

828. Newman R, Hackett R, Senior D, et al. Pathologic effects of ESWL on canine renal tissue. Urology 1987;29:194.

# Acute and Chronic Tubulointerstitial Nephritis

**23**

*Tibor Nadasdy    Daniel Sedmak*

## TERMINOLOGY

Cellular and fluid exudation in the interstitial tissue was noted by Councilman in 1898 while he studied kidneys of patients who died of scarlet fever and diphtheria (1). Councilman also determined that these kidneys did not contain bacteria (they were sterile). He called the condition acute interstitial nephritis. The term *interstitial nephritis* connotes predominant involvement of the renal interstitium and tubules by inflammatory cells, often with edema or fibrosis and tubular atrophy. Because interstitial nephritis is commonly accompanied by variable tubular damage, the term *tubulointerstitial nephritis*, or *tubulointerstitial nephropathy*, is preferable and is often used interchangeably with interstitial nephritis. Tubulointerstitial nephritis has two common clinical presentations: sudden onset and rapid decline in renal function—*acute tubulointerstitial nephritis*—and protracted onset and slow decline in renal function—*chronic tubulointerstitial nephritis*. Because chronic tubulointerstitial nephritis may present with prominent fibrosis and few inflammatory cells, the term *chronic tubulointerstitial fibrosis*, or *chronic tubulointerstitial nephropathy*, is used by many. *Tubulitis* refers to infiltration of the tubular epithelium by leukocytes, usually mononuclear cells. Obviously acute tubulointerstitial nephritis, with time, can turn into chronic tubulointerstitial nephritis; therefore, overlaps between these two entities often exist.

The term *primary tubulointerstitial nephritis* refers to cases where the inflammation is essentially limited to the tubules and interstitium; glomeruli and vessels are uninvolved or show minor changes. *Secondary tubulointerstitial nephritis* implies tubulointerstitial inflammation associated with a primary glomerular, vascular, or systemic disease. *Idiopathic tubulointerstitial nephritis* is a primary tubulointerstitial nephritis whose etiologic agent or cause is unknown.

*Reactive tubulointerstitial nephritis* connotes tubulointerstitial inflammation from the effects of systemic infections; the kidneys usually are sterile. *Infectious tubulointerstitial nephritis* denotes tubulointerstitial inflammation from the effects of localization of live micro-organisms in the kidney, where they can be identified and from which they often can be cultured.

Interstitial nephritis is commonly secondary to infection. These include acute and chronic pyelonephritis by bacteria or fungus, viral infection, and protozoal infections. Infection-associated interstitial nephritis is discussed in Chapter 22.

## INCIDENCE

The exact incidence of tubulointerstitial nephritis is unknown. Available figures vary and reflect differences in the populations considered. For unselected, asymptomatic individuals, Petterson et al (2) reported an incidence of 0.7 cases per 100,000 persons. For selected, asymptomatic individuals with abnormal urinalysis, the incidence in the same population was 1.2% (2). Among symptomatic patients with acute renal failure, the incidence ranged from 8% to 10.7% (3,4), and among symptomatic patients with chronic renal failure, the incidence ranged from about 22% to 33.5% (5,6). Among unselected patients with acute tubulointerstitial nephritis, 40% (12 of 30 patients) of cases were caused by drug reactions (7). Among unselected patients with chronic tubulointerstitial nephritis, 31%

(9 of 29 patients) of cases were caused by drugs and about 28% (8 of 29 patients) of cases were idiopathic (8).

It is important to establish the diagnosis of tubulointerstitial nephritis through kidney biopsy for the following reasons: (a) clinical and laboratory data alone often do not differentiate between tubulointerstitial nephritis and other renal diseases attended by renal insufficiency or renal failure; (b) most acute tubulointerstitial nephritides can be successfully treated; (c) untreated acute tubulointerstitial nephritis may result in interstitial fibrosis and irreversible renal disease (9); (d) the use of molecular and other techniques permits the disclosure of possible genetic abnormalities (10) and the underlying mechanisms of tissue injury (11).

## ETIOLOGIC AGENTS AND CAUSES

The etiologic agents and causes of tubulointerstitial nephritis are varied but can be grouped into broad categories. The classification that we follow in our outline has been modified from those of Churg et al (12) and Colvin and Fang (13). Some causes of tubulointerstitial nephritis including infectious etiologies are covered in other chapters. Tubulointerstitial nephritis is often multifactorial, and several etiologic agents or causes, such as concurrent infection and obstruction, may contribute to tubulointerstitial renal disease in the same patient (5). In a recent paper, Baker and Pusey (14) pooled their own data with two contemporary series from the literature (15,16). They found that based on recent data, the most frequent cause of interstitial nephritis is drug related (71.1%) with antibiotics accounting for about a third of these cases. Interstitial nephritis cases that were secondary to infection accounted for 15.6% and 7.8% were idiopathic. Tubulointerstitial nephritis and uveitis syndrome (TINU) was responsible for 4.7% of cases, and only 0.8% of the biopsies were diagnosed as sarcoidosis.

## CLINICAL FEATURES OF PRIMARY TUBULOINTERSTITIAL NEPHRITIS

Various nonspecific clinical and laboratory findings may occur. Acute interstitial nephritis may develop at any age and is associated with a variable degree of acute renal insufficiency. The acute renal failure tends to be more prominent in the elderly. Systemic manifestations of hypersensitivity, such as erythematosus, maculopapular skin rash, arthralgias, fever, and peripheral eosinophilia may occur primarily in drug-induced acute interstitial nephritis, but these findings are frequently absent. Urinalysis reveals usually microscopic hematuria. Very rarely, gross hematuria or red blood cell casts may be seen. Typically, these patients have white blood cells in the urine and urine cultures are negative (sterile pyuria). Eosinophils in the urine, particularly if this number is greater than 1% of the cells, is

thought to be a very characteristic finding in acute interstitial nephritis. Ruffing et al (17) addressed the diagnostic accuracy of this test. In a selected group of patients, in which the diagnosis of acute interstitial nephritis was suspected by the nephrologist, the sensitivity of eosinophiluria was 40% and the specificity was 72% with a positive predictive value of only 38%. The same authors also examined consecutive patients with white blood cells in the urine who did not have interstitial nephritis. Four of these patients had urinary eosinophils greater than 1%. Eosinophiluria is not uncommon in secondary forms of interstitial nephritis, particularly in those that are associated with crescentic glomerulonephritis (vasculitis).

Mild proteinuria, usually less than 1 g/24 hours, is frequently seen, but nephrotic-range proteinuria is rare. Nephrotic syndrome may occur if interstitial nephritis is associated with minimal change disease secondary to nonsteroidal anti-inflammatory drugs (NSAIDs). If the inflammation affects primarily the proximal tubule, it may result in renal glucosuria, aminoaciduria, phosphaturia, and uricosuria. If the distal tubule is primarily damaged, potassium secretion and sodium balance regulation suffer. Renal tubular acidosis may occur following the damage of both distal and proximal tubules. It is worth noting that in many instances, both the proximal and distal tubules are equally undergoing injury. Medullary inflammation may be associated with inappropriate urinary concentration and polyuria.

## PATHOLOGY OF PRIMARY TUBULOINTERSTITIAL NEPHRITIS

The details of gross and histologic features underlying the pathology of tubulointerstitial nephritides associated with various agents or conditions are provided in the following sections. In this section, we present an overview of the pathology of primary tubulointerstitial nephritis. Pyelonephritis and other infection-related interstitial nephritides are discussed in Chapter 22.

### Acute Tubulointerstitial Nephritis

Grossly, the kidneys are pale, edematous, and enlarged, with the degree of enlargement proportional to the extent of involvement. The external surface is smooth.

Microscopically, the cellular infiltration and edema are multifocal and vary in intensity. Although neutrophils are common in acute tubulointerstitial nephritis, mononuclear cells, including lymphocytes and macrophages, also participate and are usually the predominant cell types (Fig. 23.1). Drug reactions, such as those to antibiotics, are often associated with mononuclear cell infiltrates, including lymphocytes, and frequently eosinophils. Most mononuclear cells in the inflammatory infiltrate are T cells (Fig. 23.2) (18–20). Overall, CD4$^+$ T cells predominate relative

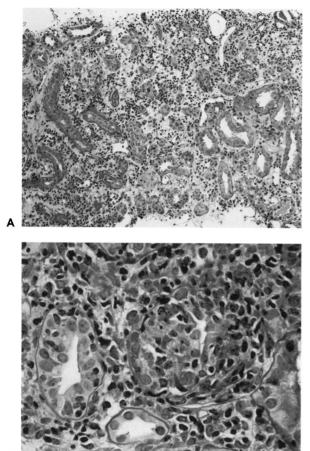

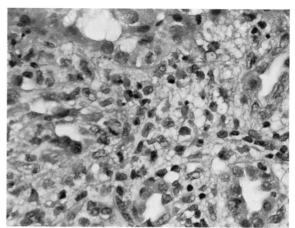

**Figure 23.1**   Interstitial nephritis in a 66-year-old patient who did not have any identifiable underlying etiology but had peripheral eosinophilia. **A:** Interstitial mononuclear cell infiltrate with edema. (PAS, ×100.) **B:** Focally large numbers of eosinophils were present in the interstitium. (H&E, ×400.) **C:** In several foci, the inflammatory cells infiltrated the tubular epithelium (tubulitis). (PAS, ×600.)

to CD8$^+$ T cells. However, in the report of Bender et al (18), nine patients with drug-induced tubulointerstitial nephritis had nephrotic-range proteinuria and predominance of CD8$^+$ T cells in the interstitial infiltrate. Similarly, in the report of D'Agati et al (21), CD8$^+$ T cells

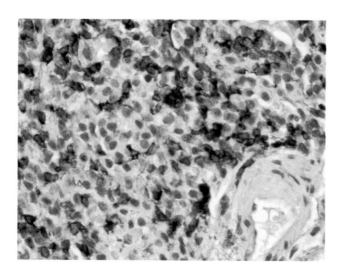

**Figure 23.2**   Immunohistochemistry reveals many T cells in the interstitial inflammatory cell infiltrate in this biopsy from a patient with Sjögren's syndrome. (Immunoperoxidase with an anti-CD3 antibody, ×400.)

outnumbered CD4$^+$ T cells in the interstitium of 22 of 26 biopsies of patients with lupus nephritis. In late stages of the disease, monocytes/macrophages tend to predominate (19,20). Eosinophils are common in drug-induced cases, but their absence does not exclude a drug-induced form of interstitial nephritis (22). After a few days or weeks have elapsed, a variable accumulation of plasma cells and histiocytes may be present (Fig. 23.3). Although not a common component of acute tubulointerstitial nephritis, granuloma formation may occur in drug reactions, sarcoidosis, and idiopathic forms (Fig. 23.4).

Tubular injury includes tubulitis (Fig. 23.1C), breaks of tubular basement membrane (TBM), necrosis of tubular cells and atrophy and loss of tubules, depending on the etiologic agent. According to Ivanyi et al (23), tubulitis more often involves the distal nephron. Biopsies taken several days after the initial insult show features of tubular cell regeneration manifest as flattening of the epithelial lining, cytoplasmic basophilia, and enlarged nuclei with frequent and prominent nucleoli. Although not a common component of acute tubulointerstitial nephritis, some interstitial fibrosis, as part of the reparative process, may be seen in late biopsies. The presence of monocytes/macrophages and granulomas and some degree of fibrosis encountered in some forms of acute tubulointerstitial nephritis emphasize the overlap that exists between acute and chronic

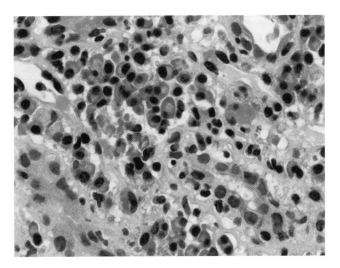

**Figure 23.3** Many plasma cells in an acute and chronic interstitial nephritis, in a patient with Sjögren's syndrome. (H&E, ×600.)

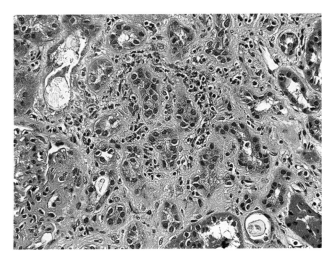

**Figure 23.5** Note the active appearing interstitial inflammatory cell infiltrate with eosinophils in the background of interstitial fibrosis and tubular atrophy. This patient had a long history of gout and multiple medication use. (H&E, ×200.)

tubulointerstitial nephritis (Figs. 23.3 to 23.5). Tamm-Horsfall protein (THP) may find its way into the interstitium following tubular rupture (Fig. 23.6). Interstitial THP is commonly found in nephron obstruction, but it is by no means a diagnostic finding of obstructive nephropathy.

Immunofluorescence and immunohistochemical techniques are rarely helpful in determining the underlying cause. Linear deposits of antibody and complement along the TBM suggest antibody directed to or cross-reactive with the TBM. Granular deposits of antibody and complement in the TBM, interstitium, or both suggest an immune complex pathogenesis. However, granular or linear TBM staining for complement (particularly C3) is a frequent nonspecific finding, especially in the basement membrane of atrophic tubules.

Electron microscopy is also of limited value. Ultrastructural examination may occasionally reveal electron-dense immune-type deposits along the TBM or in the interstitium, particularly if there is underlying systemic lupus erythematosus. Crystalline inclusions in tubular epithelial cells or finely granular electron-dense deposits along the TBM indicate monoclonal immunoglobulin deposition. Rarely, electron microscopy may be helpful in detecting viral particles in infected tubular epithelial cells.

In acute tubulointerstitial nephritis, the glomeruli are mostly spared. Arterial and arteriolar changes are usually absent. When present in older persons, they are unrelated to the primary tubulointerstitial process and reflect aging, associated hypertension, or both.

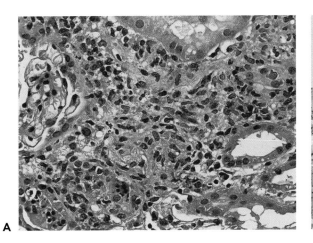

A

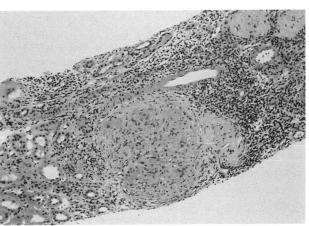

B

**Figure 23.4** Different appearances of granulomatous interstitial nephritis. **A:** Ill-defined interstitial granulomas in a biopsy from a patient who was treated with cephalosporin, vancomycin, and clindamycin because of a staphylococcal infection. (H&E, ×400.) **B:** Well-defined epithelioid granuloma in the renal biopsy of a patient with sarcoidosis. (H&E, ×100.)

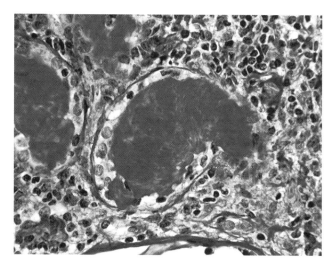

**Figure 23.6** Tubular rupture with expulsion of Tamm-Horsfall protein from the tubule into the interstitium. Note the interstitial inflammatory cell infiltrate around the Tamm-Horsfall protein. This is a nonspecific finding that can occur in any renal injury with tubular disruption and secondary interstitial Tamm-Horsfall protein deposits. (PAS, ×400.)

The morphology of acute interstitial nephritis is nonspecific, and only in rare instances is it possible to define the exact cause. If typical viral inclusions are present or other micro-organisms can be identified or if characteristic immune complex deposits are present, an etiologic diagnosis may be possible. A more detailed description of the morphologic findings will be given in this chapter in the section describing the different forms of acute interstitial nephritis.

## Chronic Tubulointerstitial Nephritis

Common causes of chronic tubulointerstitial nephritis are infections, drug reactions (e.g., analgesics, lithium), urinary tract obstruction and sterile reflux of urine, some forms of immune-mediated tubulointerstitial nephritis, plasma cell dyscrasias, metabolic disorders, exposure to heavy metals, hereditary diseases, and various chronic nephropathies, including idiopathic tubulointerstitial nephritis. Chronic tubulointerstitial nephritis always develops if a progressive chronic primary glomerular disease is present. It is also a common finding in systemic disorders involving the kidney, including systemic autoimmune diseases, monoclonal gammopathies, and metabolic diseases. Vascular diseases are also frequently associated with chronic tubulointerstitial nephritis, particularly vasculitis and chronic forms of thrombotic microangiopathies but also ischemia secondary to atherosclerosis, and hypertension can induce chronic tubulointerstitial injury with some degree of inflammation.

Grossly, kidneys with chronic tubulointerstitial nephritis become small, contracted, and pale. Variable papillary involvement, including papillary necrosis, sclerosis, and calcification may be evident. The external surface is usually scarred or finely granular from small vessel disease, compensatory hypertrophy of residual nephrons, or both. The corticomedullary junction is usually poorly demarcated. The intrarenal vessels are prominent and may have thickened walls.

Microscopically, the inflammatory cell infiltrate is made up of variable numbers of lymphocytes, monocytes/macrophages, and plasma cells. Granulomas may be seen in tubulointerstitial nephritis because of drugs; infections with mycobacteria, fungi, and parasites; sarcoidosis; and vasculitis. Some are idiopathic (24). Tubular atrophy and interstitial fibrosis are the histologic hallmarks of chronic interstitial nephritis, usually associated with some degree of interstitial mononuclear cell infiltrate. Tubular atrophy has three morphologic subtypes (25) (Fig. 23.7). The most common type is the "classic"-type atrophic tubule with prominently thickened, frequently wrinkled, and lamellated basement membrane. The "endocrine"-type atrophic tubule has a narrow lumen or no lumen at all, is usually prominently reduced in diameter, and has simplified epithelium and a thin basement membrane. These endocrine-type atrophic tubules usually occur in clusters. The "thyroid"-type atrophic tubule has only mildly thickened basement membrane, a simplified flattened epithelium, and a lumen filled with eosinophilic PAS positive homogenous proteinaceous material; therefore, the tubule resembles a thyroid follicle. These thyroid-type atrophic tubules also occur in clusters, and in occasional cases of renal scarring, the parenchyma resembles thyroid gland. The diagnostic significance of these different types of atrophic tubules is somewhat limited. The endocrine-type atrophic tubule is frequently seen in chronic ischemia, including renal artery stenosis. The thyroid-type atrophic tubule is a common finding in chronic pyelonephritic scars, but we have also frequently observed thyroidization of tubules in ischemic scars, including kidneys with interstitial fibrosis secondary to antiphospholipid antibodies.

In chronic tubulointerstitial injury, tubules frequently undergo compensatory hypertrophy, disregarding the cause. These hypertrophic tubules are lined usually with tall proximal-appearing tubular epithelial cells. The lumen is dilated and commonly irregular (Fig. 23.8). Microcystic dilatation of tubules in scarred interstitial areas may also occur. These microcystic tubules usually have a thin simplified epithelium and are filled by proteinaceous homogeneous material. Sometimes the microcysts may have a scalloped outline (Fig. 23.9).

Interstitial fibrosis, a characteristic feature of chronic tubulointerstitial nephritis, must be considered according to location. In the cortex, the interstitial volume is uniform and composes 7% of the cortical volume (26), whereas in the medulla, the interstitial space increases from the

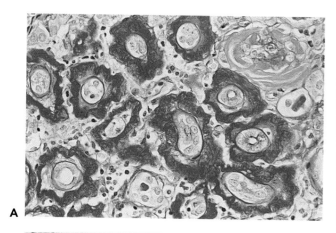

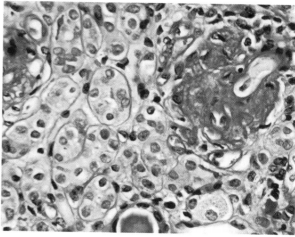

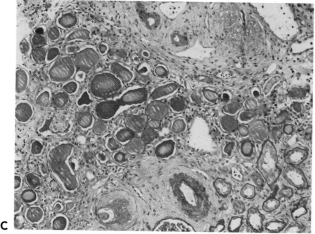

**Figure 23.7** Different histologic appearances of atrophic tubules. **A:** Prominently thickened and wrinkled PAS-positive basement membranes of so-called classic atrophic tubules. Note the simplified epithelium lining the atrophic tubules. The section was also stained with *Tetragonolobus purpuras* lectin (brown color along the apical cell membrane), a marker of proximal renal tubular epithelium, indicating proximal tubular origin of these tubules. (PAS with *Tetragonolobus purpuras*, lectin stain, ×400.) **B:** Endocrine-type atrophic tubules surrounding a sclerotic glomerulus. In this type of endocrine tubule, the basement membrane is thin and the epithelium is simplified with no or only very narrow lumen. These tubules resemble endocrine glands. (PAS, ×400.) **C.** Thyroidization of tubules in a scarred area of renal cortex. Thyroid-type atrophic tubules have flattened epithelium and PAS-positive proteinaceous filling the lumen, resembling thyroid follicles. (PAS, ×400.)

outer stripe of the inner medulla to the tip of the renal papilla. For example, in the rat the interstitial space at the base of the inner medulla is about 10% of the medullary space but attains 30% of the interstitial space at the tip of the papilla (27). Interstitial fibrosis may be multifo-

cal or diffuse, and the deposited extracellular matrix is a combination of various types of collagens, including types I, III, and V, derived from interstitial fibroblasts (28), and type IV, derived from endothelial and tubular epithelial cells (29). Interstitial fibrosis and tubular atrophy are

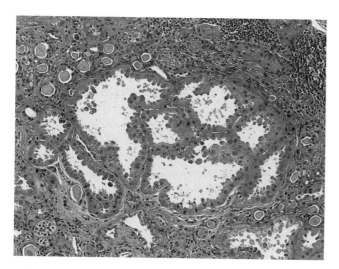

**Figure 23.8** It is common to see large hypertrophic tubules with thick, hypertrophic epithelial lining in any type of advanced chronic renal injury. (H&E, ×100.)

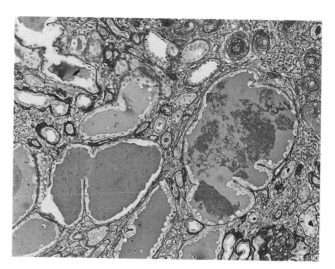

**Figure 23.9** Microcystic dilatation of tubules with scalloped outline. Such tubules can be seen in any kind of chronic tubulointerstitial injury. (PAS, ×100.)

cardinal features for the diagnosis of chronic tubulointerstitial nephritis because inflammatory cells may be scarce or absent.

Immunofluorescence and immunohistochemical techniques enable delineation of pathogenic mechanisms in a few cases, in a manner similar to that already described for acute tubulointerstitial nephritis. Granular deposits of immunoglobulin and complement along the TBM and interstitium may indicate tubulointerstitial injury mediated by immune complexes. But one has to remember that C3 deposition is a very common nonspecific finding in the basement membrane of atrophic tubules. Immunohistochemical techniques also can be used to identify the segment of the nephron that is involved (Fig. 23.7A) (30) to develop functional correlates of tissue injury (31). For example, when tubulointerstitial nephritis involves predominantly the proximal tubules, proximal renal tubular acidosis (type II) develops owing to loss of proximal tubule resorbate (e.g., glucose, phosphate, uric acid, organic acids, low–molecular-weight proteins), with or without Fanconi's syndrome. When distal tubules are predominantly involved, distal renal tubular acidosis (type I) ensues caused by failure to lower the urinary pH, with or without hyperkalemia and salt wasting. When collecting ducts and papillary involvement predominate, water conservation is compromised by the decreased ability to concentrate urine. Molecular techniques have enabled the detection of deletions of genetic material as a possible cause of tubulointerstitial nephritis (10,32).

Electron microscopy in chronic tubulointerstitial nephritis has limited diagnostic value, as indicated above in the discussion of acute interstitial nephritis. The basement membrane of atrophic tubules is not only thickened on ultrastructural examination, but is usually also lamellated. This lamellation is probably the result of repeated tubular epithelial injury and regeneration. The regenerating renal

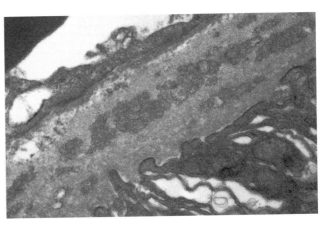

**Figure 23.11**  Deposits of granular to microspherical material in the tubular basement membrane is a common finding in atrophic tubules. Under low magnification, these structures may be misinterpreted as electron-dense immune-type deposits in the tubular basement membrane. (Uranyl acetate and lead citrate, ×20,000.)

epithelium probably creates newer and newer thin layers of basement membrane material, which will lend a lamellated pattern to the thickened tubular basement membrane (Fig. 23.10). Aggregates of granular to microspherical material in the thickened basement membranes of atrophic tubules are not uncommon (Fig. 23.11). This material should not be misinterpreted as immune complex deposition.

In contrast to acute tubulointerstitial nephritis, in which glomeruli are usually spared, glomeruli in chronic tubulointerstitial nephritis often show changes. These glomerular changes are frequently secondary to poor glomerular blood perfusion and include tuft wrinkling and collapse, thickening of Bowman's capsule, periglomerular fibrosis, and glomerular obsolescence. Occasionally, segmental glomerulosclerosis may develop. Arterial and arteriolar changes such as intimal thickening and medial hyperplasia are usually present and reflect aging and associated hypertension.

## PATHOGENESIS OF TUBULOINTERSTITIAL NEPHRITIS

The pathogenetic mechanisms operative in tubulointerstitial nephritides associated with various agents or conditions are provided in the sections to follow. In this section, we present a brief overview of pathogenetic mechanisms that are specific for certain tubulointerstitial nephropathies and that are common to most forms of chronic tubulointerstitial nephropathies.

*Reactive tubulointerstitial nephritis* appears to result from systemic release of lymphokines that are filtered and reabsorbed by the kidneys, thereby promoting chemoattraction and activation of mononuclear cells in the kidneys (1,13,33,34). *Infectious tubulointerstitial nephritis* results

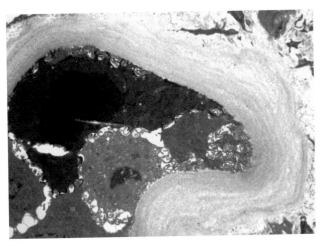

**Figure 23.10**  Thickened lamellated basement membrane of an atrophic tubule. (Uranyl acetate and lead citrate, ×3000.)

from three basic mechanisms of tissue injury (35): microbial release of degradative enzymes and toxic molecules; direct contact or penetration of host cells by the microbe; and the inflammatory response mediated by antibodies, T cells, or both. The pathogenesis of infectious tubulointerstitial nephritis and vesicoureteral reflux is covered in Chapter 22.

*Drug-induced tubulointerstitial nephritis* is most likely immunologically mediated. The most widely accepted theory is that drugs behave as haptens after binding to extrarenal proteins that later will be planted in the kidney, or to renal proteins (36). This will be discussed in detail in the following section of this chapter. Drug-induced acute interstitial nephritis occurs in only a small percentage of patients taking a medication, is not dose dependent, and exacerbation occurs after re-exposure to the drug. Also, systemic signs of hypersensitivity may be evident.

*Tubulointerstitial nephritis owing to anti-TBM antibodies* involves predominantly IgG antibodies directed against different autoantigens in basement membranes, including a 58-kDa protein called tubulointerstitial nephritis antigen (37–40). *Tubulointerstitial nephritis owing to immune complexes* involves predominantly IgG antibodies, but the nature of target antigens, with a few possible exceptions (41,42), is unknown. Tubulointerstitial injury may depend on complement activation by antibody (43,44), release of chemoattractants, and activation of leukocytes with release of chemokines, cytokines, proteases, and toxic oxygen radicals (34,45). In many forms of interstitial nephritis, eosinophils are prominent in the interstitium, which may be related to a chemotactic cytokine, eotaxin, produced locally by renal parenchymal cells (46). *Tubulointerstitial nephritis owing to cell-mediated mechanisms* encompasses two types of reactions. First, delayed-type hypersensitivity reaction, which requires prior sensitization and is caused by CD4$^+$ T cells and macrophages, results in production of various lymphokines and may induce a granulomatous reaction (11). Second, cytotoxic T-cell injury, which requires no prior sensitization, is mediated by CD4$^+$ and CD8$^+$ T cells (11).

*Tubulointerstitial inflammation, fibrosis, and tubular atrophy,* common to most chronic tubulointerstitial nephropathies, can be induced by various agents and causes. If the underlying cause is persistent and cannot be eliminated, eventually all etiologic agents will cause chronic tubulointerstitial injury. Various pathogenetic factors are involved in the generation of interstitial fibrosis and tubular atrophy including ischemia, reactive oxygen species, toxic agents, or immunologic injury. It is likely that an important role in the common final pathway leading to fibrosis can be attributed to the transforming growth factor beta (TGF-beta)/Smad3 signaling pathway (47–49). TGF-beta is up-regulated in response to injurious stimuli, by angiotensin II (49). This accounts, at least in part, for the beneficial effect of angiotensin convertase inhibition slow-

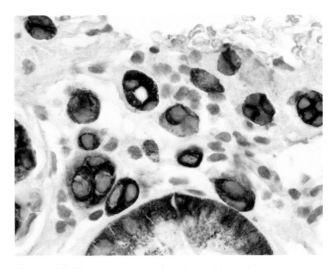

**Figure 23.12** Scattered cytokeratin-positive cells are commonly found in the fibrotic renal interstitium. It is theoretically possible that these cytokeratin-positive cells represent cells undergoing epithelial to mesenchymal transformation. (Immunoperoxidase, ×600.)

ing the progression of chronic renal injury. TGF-beta transmembrane receptors transduce downstream signals via cytoplasmic latent transcription factors called Smad proteins. Smad 2 and 3 are phosphorylated and they bind to Smad 4 and translocate to the nucleus where they act as transcriptional regulators of target genes. Disruption of the TGF-beta/Smad signaling pathway inhibits interstitial fibrosis in experimental animals (47). Connective tissue growth factor (CTGF) is a downstream mediator of the profibrotic effects of TGF-beta. Recent data indicate that CTGF may play a pivotal role in the pathogenesis of TGF-beta–dependent interstitial fibrosis (50). There is growing evidence that TGF-beta is also capable of inducing epithelial-myofibroblast transdifferentiation of renal tubular epithelial cells (51). This transdifferentiation process of the injured tubular epithelial cells may be a key pathogenetic step in the development of chronic interstitial nephritis (Fig. 23.12).

## TUBULOINTERSTITIAL NEPHRITIS ASSOCIATED WITH DRUG REACTIONS

The kidney is adversely affected by a wide range of therapeutic and diagnostic agents and toxic compounds. However, there are only a limited number of patterns of injury produced in the kidney. These may affect any of the compartments of the kidney including tubulointerstitial, glomerular, and vascular pathology (52–54). In the previous edition of this book, an entire chapter was devoted to all forms of renal injury caused by therapeutic and diagnostic agents (52). Now, in the following section, we will focus only on acute and chronic tubulointerstitial nephritis induced by drugs. Other patterns of renal injury associated with drug reactions, including acute tubular necrosis, glomerular changes, and vascular changes, will be discussed in other chapters.

It should be recognized that it is often difficult to establish a pathogenetic link between a pathologic lesion and a particular drug or toxin. Several factors contribute to this uncertainty, including concurrent factors that may produce renal injury such as administration of several potentially nephrotoxic drugs at the same time, lack of or inadequacy of morphologic data in reported cases of drug toxicity, and the fact that some drugs may have multiple effects. Moreover, experimental models of toxicity may not be relevant to a particular clinical context owing to interspecies variation and markedly different dosing of drugs in these models. In general, we limit our discussion to those drugs for which toxicity has been well documented in humans by disappearance of toxic effects when the drug is withdrawn, reoccurrence of symptoms on rechallenge, or both.

As pointed out earlier, today the most common form of interstitial nephritis is drug induced. Many drugs, including a range of widely used therapeutic agents, produce unpredictable idiosyncratic systemic reactions that may manifest in the kidney primarily as tubulointerstitial nephritis.

## Clinical Features

Tubulointerstitial nephritis caused by drug or toxin exposure develops in a few patients who receive the drug; reactions can sometimes be predicted if the patient has had a reaction to the same or a similar agent. The reaction is generally unrelated to the cumulative dose of the drug. Exposure to the offending agent typically occurs days to a few weeks before presentation (55). Patients may show signs of a systemic syndrome that include fever, skin rash, eosinophilia, and arthralgias. However, only a few patients will have this classic constellation of symptoms (16). Affected individuals may note fluid retention or a fall in urine output and occasionally patients may experience back or flank pain (56). Many patients show symptoms of acute renal failure (ARF).

Analysis of the urine typically reveals pyuria, with numerous mononuclear cells, including lymphocytes and monocytes. There may also be eosinophils, which researchers have touted as a specific marker for allergic interstitial nephritis (57). However, eosinophiluria is not specific for drug-induced interstitial nephritis (58). Eosinophils may best be detected by the use of special stains, such as the Hansel stain (59). Hematuria is not uncommon and is usually microscopic. Mild proteinuria may also be detected, and proteinuria may occasionally be in the nephrotic range, especially in those cases caused by drugs that also produce minimal change disease in the glomeruli; nonsteroidal anti-inflammatory drugs (NSAIDs) most commonly cause this constellation of symptoms. Urine cultures are routinely negative.

Because the interstitial inflammatory process can result in tubular injury, there may be evidence of tubular dysfunction. Patients may have glycosuria, aminoaciduria, and phosphaturia; occasionally, Fanconi's syndrome has been described. In addition, tubular acidosis, electrolyte losses, or concentrating defects may be documented. On ultrasound, the kidneys are seen to be of normal size or enlarged. The parenchyma is typically echogenic, a finding that has been correlated with the extent of inflammatory infiltrate (and with the development of long-term changes in the interstitium).

Patients may have renal dysfunction without other accompanying symptoms. Because drug-induced interstitial nephritis is eminently reversible in the early stages, it is important to recognize the etiologic agent so that long-term damage can be avoided. Some drugs produce more insidious changes, resulting in protracted injury without an obvious acute phase. Classic examples are lithium and analgesic compounds. These patients may show initial signs of salt wasting or acid-base imbalances and evidence of progressive tubular injury. In cases with sloughing of necrotic papillae, the initial symptoms are acute with renal colic.

## Pathology

### Gross Findings

In acute tubulointerstitial nephritis, the kidney is usually pale and swollen. Areas of congestion and hyperemia may be seen at the corticomedullary junction. In chronic tubulointerstitial nephritis, the kidney is smaller with thinning of the cortex. The surface of the kidney may become granular. Parenchymal cysts may develop as interstitial fibrosis progresses. The cortex may become pale owing to a combination of fibrosis and inflammatory cells.

### Light Microscopy

#### Glomeruli

Glomeruli are typically spared. Occasionally, the interstitial inflammatory infiltrate may breach Bowman's capsule. In later stages of chronic interstitial nephritis, glomeruli may show nonspecific ischemic collapse and sclerosing changes. Periglomerular fibrosis is common in chronic cases.

#### Interstitium

In acute interstitial nephritis (AIN), there are patchy or diffuse edema and inflammatory infiltrates. The infiltrate is predominantly mononuclear (Fig. 23.1). Both CD4$^+$ and CD8$^+$ T cells have been detected in varying proportions. B cells and monocyte/macrophages can also be found. Eosinophils typically make up 10% or less of the infiltrating cells. The eosinophils in the infiltrate may be focal and, rarely, they form clusters resembling a microabscess (Fig. 23.1B) (57). Eosinophils are typically seen in reactions to antibiotics, especially penicillins, sulfonamides, and rifampicin, more than in response to various other drugs. Neutrophils are usually rare. Basophils, which are difficult to detect without special stains, have been reported to constitute 1% to 2% of infiltrating cells (60). Steroid treatment may reduce the severity of the inflammation and, in particular, lessen accompanying edema.

Granulomatous features are seen in the inflammatory reaction to some drugs (Table 23.1; Fig. 23.4A). Granulomas, typically noncaseating and composed of epithelioid histiocytes, lymphocytes, and a few giant cells, are scattered in the interstitium. Penicillins, sulfonamides, polymyxin B, allopurinol (61), diuretics (62), rifampicin, acyclovir, NSAIDs, omeprazole (63), lamotrigine (64), levofloxacin (65), nitrofurantoin (66), and ciprofloxacin have all been reported to cause inflammatory infiltrates with granulomas.

In chronic drug-induced interstitial nephritis, the defining feature is interstitial fibrosis. An interstitial inflammatory infiltrate often persists, but it is usually mild and composed largely of nonactivated lymphocytes, plasma cells, and macrophages. These infiltrates are often nodular and localized to fibrotic areas. Although drug-induced acute tubulointerstitial nephritis occasionally may persist and lead to chronic interstitial nephritis, some drugs have a propensity to produce subclinical progression to chronic renal failure. These drugs include analgesics, lithium, and cyclosporine.

### Tubules

Accompanying acute tubulointerstitial nephritis, there may be evidence of tubular cell injury, with vacuolation, loss of brush border, and exfoliation and loss of tubular cells. The tubular epithelium is often infiltrated by inflammatory cells, usually lymphocytes (tubulitis) (Fig. 23.1C). Although these characteristics are often described in the proximal nephron, a few investigators have reported that tubular injury and tubulitis may be more severe in the distal nephron (22,23). With a severe inflammatory reaction, the TBM may be disrupted. In the circumstance of chronic interstitial nephritis, tubular atrophy is typically seen to be associated with fibrosis in the interstitium. Focal tubulitis may be present as well.

### Vessels

Vessels are usually uninvolved, though a few drugs may produce vasculitis.

## Immunopathology

Fibrin is often detected in the interstitium by immunofluorescence, reflecting interstitial edema. Immunoglobulin-G (IgG) and C3 have been reported to be deposited in a linear pattern along the TBM in some cases of apparent drug-induced interstitial nephritis, including cases induced by penicillins (57,67–69) and rifampicin (70). Minetti et al (71) have also reported granular peritubular IgG in one case owing to rifampicin. In cases of methicillin-induced AIN, a drug antigen has been immunolocalized along the TBM as well (67,68).

## Electron Microscopy

Ultrastructural examination is usually of limited informative value in drug-induced interstitial nephritis. Electron microscopy of the interstitium in cases of drug-induced interstitial nephritis reveals edema, infiltrating inflammatory cells, and tubulitis. Olsen et al (72) have described severe reduction of the proximal tubular brush border and proximal and distal tubular basolateral infoldings in this context, reflecting tubular injury. In some areas, there may be thinning or disruption of the TBM. Electron-dense immune-type deposits are usually not present in TBMs.

---

**TABLE 23.1**

### CAUSES OF GRANULOMATOUS INTERSTITIAL NEPHRITIS

Infection (see Chapter 22)
    Tuberculosis
    Fungal Infections
    Brucellosis
    Parasites

Drugs
    Sulfonamides (144)
    Penicillins (73,364)
    Fluoroquinolones (65,76,105)
    Vancomycin (148)
    Gentamicin (24)
    Nitrofurantoin (66)
    Allopurinol (61)
    Furosemide (62)
    Hydrochlorothiazide (501)
    Omeprazole (63)
    Lamotrigine (64)
    Nonsteroidal anti-inflammatory drugs (NSAIDs) (189)
    Bisphosphonates (Alendronate) (504)
    Diphenylhydantoin (245)
    Carbamazepine (503)
    Oxycodone (500)
Sarcoidosis (354–363)
Tubulointerstitial nephritis and uveitis syndrome (TINU) (499)
Granulomatous vasculitis (Wegener's) (24,364,365)
Oxalosis (Chapter 25)
Gout (Chapter 25)
Cholesterol granuloma (502)
Idiopathic (366–370)

## Etiology and Pathogenesis

Three major types of immune mechanisms may lead to tubulointerstitial nephritis in response to drugs. These include hypersensitivity/allergic, immune complex, and cell-mediated reactions. Each of these types is discussed in turn. In a few individual cases, mechanisms of action are clearly defined, but for others, pathogenetic mechanisms are assumed, often based on morphologic and clinical findings. It is possible that several mechanisms of action are at work in an individual patient.

Allergic-type hypersensitivity reactions are idiosyncratic and not related to dose. The reaction to the agent is presumably caused by previous sensitization, and, indeed, patients may give a history of exposure to the ingested drug or a similar drug. The reaction in the kidney is often part of a systemic hypersensitivity reaction, which may include fever, arthralgias, and skin rash. Eosinophils are often a significant component of cells in the inflammatory infiltrate, and, as noted earlier, there is often a peripheral eosinophilia as well.

Reactions involving immune complex deposition are of two types: those with formation of immune complexes that are deposited around tubules and those owing to formation of antibodies directed against antigens at or in the TBM. In a few cases, antigens from the drug have been immunolocalized to the TBM. The inciting drug may serve as a hapten, leading to antibody formation. In a few patients, anti-TBM antibodies have been found; Colvin and Fang (13), in one review, reported that these antibodies are frequently found in patients with different forms of AIN if they are sought. In many cases, however, it is unclear whether these antibodies are of clinical significance, and the specificity of the methodologies to detect these antibodies is not always high. The finding of linear staining for IgG along the TBM is not a specific test to detect anti-TBM antibodies; proof of presence of anti-TBM antibodies requires demonstration of the antibody in the serum or renal eluates. Complexing of antibody to antigen may lead to complement binding and activation, triggering a cascade of events that result in inflammatory infiltrates and tissue injury.

Cell-mediated immunity has also been implicated in the genesis of drug-induced interstitial nephritis. The presence of granulomas in the kidney, in a number of cases of interstitial inflammatory reaction to drugs, is consistent with delayed-type hypersensitivity. T-cell reactivity has been documented in some patients with drug-induced hypersensitivity reactions (73,74). Cytotoxic lymphocytes, which were reactive against autologous renal cell line, have been isolated from one patient being treated with recombinant interleukin 2 (IL2) (75).

Chronic interstitial nephritis with fibrosis resulting from a prolonged inflammatory process is likely mediated by inflammatory cells and the cytokines released by them. Some drugs appear to produce persistent tubulointersti-

tial damage without an acute injury phase. They include phenacetin-containing analgesics and lithium. Persistent changes produced by analgesics presumably result in part from ischemia produced by imbalances in the vasodilatory versus vasoconstrictor prostaglandins over a prolonged period (see later section on analgesics and nonsteroidal anti-inflammatory drugs). Chronic tubulointerstitial nephritis is associated with prominent loss of the peritubular capillaries, which may further aggravate the ischemic injury (76). As pointed out earlier, certain cytokines, such as TGF-beta, enhance production and release of matrix from epithelial and mesenchymal cells and likely also play a role in bringing about interstitial fibrosis through promoting epithelial-mesenchymal transdifferentiation of renal tubular epithelial cells (12,13).

## Clinical Course

Drug-induced interstitial nephritis is generally reversible by withdrawal of the offending agent. Steroid therapy may enhance the rate of recovery and is frequently given along with withdrawal of the drug. A typical and diagnostic feature of drug-induced interstitial nephritis is its recurrence on re-exposure to the drug or a related compound. Although recovery of renal function is the rule if the drug is withdrawn immediately, a study from Germany indicates that permanent renal insufficiency remained in 88% of drug-induced acute tubulointerstitial nephritis cases if the suspected drug was taken for more than a month before the diagnosis (77). Also, the same authors suggest that NSAID-induced interstitial nephritis has a worse outcome compared with other drug-induced forms.

## Specific Agents

### Antimicrobial Agents

#### Cephalosporins

The cephalosporin group of antibiotics comprises several generations of these useful agents, defined on the basis of antimicrobial activity. The first generation includes cefazolin, cephalothin, and cephalexin. Cefamandole, cefonicid, cefuroxime, cefaclor, cefoxitin, and cefotetan are second generation, whereas the third generation includes ceftazidime, cefotaxime, and ceftriaxone. Cefepime is a fourth-generation cephalosporin more resistant to beta-lactamases than the previous agents. These drugs may be nephrotoxic, particularly in patients with pre-existing renal insufficiency. Cephaloridine, the most toxic of the group, is no longer available in the United States, but is used experimentally for toxicity studies.

*Clinical Presentation.* The cephalosporins are most likely to produce renal failure in patients with pre-existing renal insufficiency (78,79), in those with drug overdose (80), and in those receiving other antibiotics (80). Patients simultaneously receiving furosemide (80) are also at increased risk, which is probably related to the ability of furosemide to prolong the half-life of the cephalosporins (81). Many of the patients reported to have nephrotoxicity because of cephalosporins are elderly and acutely ill with severe infections.

*Cephaloridine* has been reported to cause ARF, often as the result of oliguria (80,82). *Cephalothin* given alone (83,84) or with gentamicin, tobramycin (82,85), or other substances (86) can cause ARF in humans or can worsen pre-existing renal insufficiency (78,79). The ARF is usually reversible. *Cephalexin* is less likely to cause nephrotoxicity than cephaloridine or cephalothin, but hematuria, eosinophilia, and a transient rise in blood urea nitrogen (BUN) have been reported (87). Clinical features suggest an immunologic basis. Hypersensitivity reactions have been reported in patients treated with cephalothin as well (84,88). Rare cases of skin rash, eosinophilia, fever, and renal insufficiency with *ceftriaxone* have been reported (89).

**Pathology.** Renal biopsies have been obtained in relatively few cases of cephalosporin-induced renal injury, usually in those in which the older cephalosporins were given. Biopsies have shown a picture of interstitial edema with variable numbers of mononuclear cells, accompanied by a variable degree of acute tubular injury (82,90–92). No immunoglobulins or complement have been seen with immunofluorescence techniques.

**Pathogenesis.** Cephalosporins appear to be capable of producing direct toxic injury to tubular cells. Tune and Hsu (93) have shown that cephalosporins interfere with mitochondrial function in the renal tubule. Cephaloridine has structural homology to carnitine and it has toxic effects on carnitine transport and fatty acid metabolism in rabbit renal cortical mitochondria in vivo; in vitro effects on pyruvate metabolism have been seen, albeit at very high concentrations (93). Cephaloridine also produces lipid peroxidation and acylation and inactivation of some tubular cell proteins. Other cephalosporins, which lack cephaloridine's side group constituents, largely affect tubular cell proteins and especially mitochondrial anionic substrate transporters (93). In vitro, proximal tubular cells show evidence of cytotoxicity on exposure to cephaloridine, cephalexin, and cephalothin whereas distal tubules do not. These studies provide evidence of the role of oxidative stress, cytochrome P450 activation, and mitochondrial dysfunction in tubular cell toxicity (94). It is important to note that pre-existing chronic renal failure (the degree of which is not accurately represented by serum creatinine levels alone) is a very important risk factor for the development of progressive renal failure following the use of nephrotoxic medications.

In addition, cephalosporins are known to cause hypersensitivity reactions. In some cases, there has been resolution with drug withdrawal and, in a few cases, recurrence on rechallenge (90). The cephalosporins are structurally similar to the penicillins, which produce similar reactions (see later), and cross-reactivity may occur in 1% to 20% of patients (95,96). No specific cephalosporin is more likely than others to cause such a reaction.

### Fluoroquinolones

*Clinical Presentation.* Fluoroquinolones are relatively new antimicrobial agents. *Ciprofloxacin*, the most widely used of these drugs, has been reported to produce ARF. Levofloxacin, norfloxacin, and tosufloxacin have also been associated with interstitial nephritis (76,97,98). There is typically fever, eosinophilia, and skin rash (99–103), but systemic manifestations may not be present (104). Onset of symptoms is generally within 2 to 12 days of beginning either oral or intravenous therapy. Patients have responded to withdrawal of the drug and, generally, concomitant treatment with immunosuppressive agents.

*Pathology.* Renal biopsies in cases of fluoroquinolone-associated renal dysfunction have revealed interstitial nephritis. In a few cases there were granulomatous features in the interstitial inflammatory infiltrate (76,103,105). Shih et al (103) have reported a necrotizing vasculitis in the kidney in two patients being treated with ciprofloxacin. An interesting case from Japan was reported in which a patient developed crystal-forming chronic interstitial nephritis following long-term exposure to tosufloxacin (98). The crystals were present in interstitial macrophages, but the crystals did not contain immunoglobulin. The patient's renal function improved following discontinuation of the drug.

*Pathogenesis.* The mechanism of pathogenesis appears to be a hypersensitivity reaction, with evidence of a cell-mediated process in the few cases with granulomatous features. As with many drug reactions, the possibility that another drug or underlying disease process may have produced the renal effects cannot be ruled out in several of these cases.

### Penicillins

In the following section, adverse reactions to ampicillin, methicillin, and penicillin are discussed in detail. AIN has been reported with other penicillins as well, including *cloxacillin* (106) and *piperacillin* (107,108).

*Clinical Presentation.* Several cases are recorded in which ampicillin appears to have provoked renal dysfunction (109–112). Fever, skin rash, and eosinophilia may be found and may antedate renal symptoms. Renal manifestations may be mild, with hematuria and a small amount of proteinuria, or severe, with acute oliguric renal failure. Rapid recovery is the rule. Time to onset varies, but renal symptoms generally appear within a few days of administration of ampicillin; other manifestations, such as fever and skin rash, develop within 24 hours. In several cases, there had been prior treatment with penicillin, methicillin, or tetracycline.

There are many reports of renal damage caused by *methicillin*. Nephrotoxicity with methicillin is not dose dependent. Onset of toxic reactions usually begins between the 2nd and 37th day after initiation of the drug. Patients typically manifest fever and skin rash, and 73% of patients in a review of 68 patients were male (113). Patients of all ages are at risk, though renal failure appears to be more common in older patients. Eosinophilia is a typical feature and may reach very high levels (57). Hematuria may occur; it is often the first sign of renal involvement. Proteinuria is seen in some cases but is generally mild. White blood cells are frequently found in the urine, which is usually sterile, and eosinophils are present in the urine in a high proportion of patients (57,113). Azotemia occurs in over half of patients and oliguria in one third. Complete recovery of renal function is the rule, though azotemia may persist in less than 10% of patients (114).

*Penicillin* has been widely used for almost 50 years, and there have been few reports of nephrotoxicity ascribed to the drug. Appel and Neu (115) summarized the reported adverse reactions to penicillin under three main headings: various vascular and glomerular lesions, acute anuric renal failure after a single injection, and AIN. In a number of cases, there is fever, skin rash, and eosinophilia, suggesting a hypersensitivity reaction. The patients have hematuria with varying degrees of proteinuria, and renal failure may ensue.

*Pathology.* On *histology*, the predominant finding in cases associated with ampicillin is interstitial nephritis with edema and variable numbers of inflammatory cells. Tubules may show focal necrosis or degenerative changes, and calcification is occasionally reported (110). Glomeruli exhibit no changes, except for rare reports of mild hypercellularity (110,112) and minimal change disease (116). Immunofluorescence studies generally show negative results. Electron-dense fibrillar deposits and viruslike particles have been seen in basal areas of the distal convoluted tubules (112). The fibrillary densities are of unknown significance (probably nonspecific), but they are similar to those described after methicillin (109).

Pathologic findings have been reported in many cases of methicillin-induced nephrotoxicity. In most cases, the glomeruli are reported to be normal, but in one case described by Woodroffe et al (112), mild mesangial hypercellularity was recorded. Necrotizing and proliferative glomerulitis was reported in another case (117), but this patient had also received ampicillin. The main changes are

found in the tubules and interstitium. Tubules show various lesions, including necrosis, cell loss, regeneration, and in some cases, tubular atrophy. Desquamated cells and occasional polymorphonuclear leukocytes may be found in tubular lumens. Olsen and Asklund (69) have reported a predominance of involvement of distal tubules over proximal tubules. There is interstitial edema with variable numbers of inflammatory cells, including small lymphocytes, plasma cells, eosinophils, and polymorphonuclear leukocytes. They frequently surround tubules, suggesting a relationship to the tubular damage. Several authors have described epithelioid cells in the interstitium, sometimes forming granulomas (69,118,119). Although blood vessels are usually normal, vasculitis involving arterioles and small arteries has been recorded (57,117). Discontinuation of the drug is usually followed by resolution of the changes. In rare instances, a follow-up biopsy may show interstitial fibrosis (Figs. 23.8 to 23.12) (120).

Results of *immunofluorescence studies* in most patients with *methicillin*-induced lesions have been negative (57,69). In others, weak staining for C3 in glomeruli and focal peritubular IgG, IgA, and C3 have been reported (120). Some biopsies, however, have shown linear staining of the TBM for IgG (67,68,121,122) with or without C3 present in glomeruli. In two biopsies (67,68), dimethoxyphenyl penicilloyl (DPO), the major haptenic antigen determinant of methicillin, was found in a linear pattern in relation to TBMs; in one (67), IgG was also deposited in a linear pattern in the glomerular tufts. Prior absorption by DPO-amylamine or methicillin-treated rabbit red cells blocked the positive staining for DPO. In addition, anti-TBM antibody was demonstrable in the serum in a few cases (68,118); DPO in these cases may be acting as a hapten, binding to the TBM and inducing antibody formation (67). *Electron microscopy* in some cases has revealed loose fibrillar electron-dense deposits in glomerular epithelial cells and in tubular cells adjacent to the basement membrane (109). There were also small amounts of electron-dense material in TBMs and damage to the basal part of tubules, with insinuation of inflammatory cells between tubular cells (57).

The renal lesion on biopsy or at autopsy in *penicillin* nephrotoxicity is similar to that of methicillin; acute tubulointerstitial nephritis is found on histologic examination (60,67). Immunofluorescence studies in one report (60) revealed irregular fibrinogen or fibrin deposits, traces of IgG in the interstitium, and rare granular deposits of C3 near tubules. In that report, a rabbit antiserum to penicillin G bound diffusely in the interstitium and to tubular and glomerular basement membranes, but it also bound to normal autopsied kidneys from patients who had received penicillin and oxacillin with ampicillin or cephalothin for several days before death.

Based on the above, it is apparent that morphologic examination cannot differentiate between interstitial nephritides caused by different penicillins. In fact, the histology does not even tell whether the interstitial nephritis is secondary to penicillin or some other drug or injurious agent. Pirani et al (123) compared beta-lactam–induced interstitial nephritis with NSAID-induced interstitial nephritis and found that the beta-lactam–induced cases contained more eosinophils. Both types contained primarily mononuclear cells with some plasma cells in the infiltrate. Still, these are histologic findings of low specificity.

*Pathogenesis.* Nephrotoxicity of the penicillins is not dose dependent, and the clinical picture overall is that of a hypersensitivity reaction. In several studies, immunofluorescence microscopy provides evidence that anti-TBM antibodies may play a role (67,68,118,121). Cell-mediated mechanisms may also be involved in some cases, based on the nature of the inflammatory infiltrate and the absence of antibody and complement deposition. Gilbert et al (109) have reported exacerbation of the reaction to methicillin by inadvertent exposure to ampicillin, a closely related drug. In addition, some case histories suggest that ampicillin can trigger a hypersensitivity reaction in patients who might have been sensitized to other penicillins. In one of these cases, antibodies against ampicillin were detected in the patient's serum (111). In a few studies, hypocomplementemia provided additional evidence of an immune reaction (109,118).

## Rifampicin

*Clinical Presentation.* Rifampicin is a drug used in the treatment of tuberculosis. When it is given intermittently, it causes various adverse reactions, including fever, chills, dizziness, nausea, and diarrhea (124,125). There have been several reports of acute oliguric renal failure during intermittent rifampicin therapy (117,124–128). The most common clinical scenario is ARF following a single dose of rifampicin after a drug-free period. Most patients recover when the drug is withdrawn (125); a few cases have been reported to result in permanent renal damage (127,129).

*Pathology.* Renal biopsies in cases of rifampicin toxicity typically show interstitial edema with variable numbers of mononuclear cells, and eosinophils have also been found (70). Rarely, granulomas may be seen (130). There may be patchy necrosis of the tubular epithelium. Even patchy cortical necrosis has been described (129); in that case, there was residual renal dysfunction. However, the degree of tubular necrosis is often not severe, and in one case the tubules were described as unaffected (124). In addition, pigmented casts may be evident. Although glomeruli and vessels are usually normal, rarely glomerulonephritis, including crescentic and necrotizing glomerulonephritis, has been noted (70,125). On immunofluorescence microscopy, it has usually not been possible to establish the presence of immunoglobulins or complement (126–128), although C3 has been found in the mesangium and in the TBM (70,131) (common nonspecific findings).

*Pathogenesis.* Antibodies to rifampicin have been detected in patients (132,133); in one study, they were present in one third of 49 patients (132). The various adverse reactions reported in this series, including renal dysfunction, were found more commonly in patients with antibodies than in patients without them. These authors suggest that the drug acts as a hapten, which, after it has become bound to macromolecules in the plasma, becomes antigenic with the formation of antibodies. The antibodies are considered to be directed against the drug, with formation of hapten–antibody complexes when the drug is given again.

## Sulfonamides

The sulfonamides have been widely used, with relatively few renal complications. Alleged hypersensitivity reactions in the early days of their use were associated with polyarteritis or acute interstitial nephritis (134,135). However, acute interstitial nephritis secondary to sulfonamides has become a rare event and only a few cases have been reported (136,137). In one case, acute oliguric renal failure developed in a patient being treated with *sulfadiazine*. The patient recovered after 6 weeks of oliguria (137). *Cotrimoxazole* (sulfamethoxazole and trimethoprim) has occasionally been found to cause deterioration of renal function (138,139).

Patients in whom crystalline precipitates develop with the use of sulfonamides have microscopic or gross hematuria, crystalluria, and renal colic, and in some cases they become oliguric or anuric (115,140). Occasionally, urolithiasis may evolve. In one series of 40 patients, the urinary bladder was the most common location of stones (141). Sulfasalazine (a combination of 5-amino salicylic acid and sulfapyridine) has recently been reported to cause obstructive uropathy secondary to calculi (142). Less soluble forms, including sulfapyridine, sulfathiazole, and sulfadiazine, are most frequently associated with crystalline obstruction (143). Fortunately, this complication became rarer when sulfonamides of greater solubility became available. Rapid improvement may take place with discontinuation of the drug, fluid administration, and alkalinization of the urine.

The typical pathologic finding is interstitial nephritis. Eosinophils are a typical component of the infiltrate (136,139,144). Granulomas have occasionally been described (144). In patients with crystallization of sulfonamide in the kidney, some pathologic changes are owing to obstruction as a consequence of crystal formation.

## Vancomycin

Vancomycin is a glycopeptide antibiotic used increasingly to treat infections caused by organisms resistant to other antibiotics such as methicillin-resistant *Staphylococcus aureus*. Nephrotoxicity is a known complication of the drugs when given alone or in combination with other drugs, especially aminoglycosides (145,146). Pediatric patients may be less susceptible to the toxic effects of vancomycin combination therapy (147). Some patients have an associated rash and eosinophilia, suggesting a hypersensitivity reaction. In addition to these adverse renal effects, in some cases, patients have an anaphylactoid reaction to the drug, with generalized flushing—the so-called red-man syndrome.

Tubulointerstitial nephritis with many eosinophils has been documented in renal biopsies in a number of cases of vancomycin-associated renal toxicity (148–150). With increasing incidence of methicillin-resistant staphylococci, the use of vancomycin is becoming more and more widespread. Therefore we may encounter increasing numbers of renal biopsies with vancomycin-induced interstitial nephritis.

The pathogenesis of renal toxicity is not well defined clinically, but experimental studies suggest that it stems from tubular cell injury. In some patients, the constellation of clinical symptoms and pathologic features indicate a hypersensitivity reaction, but many patients do not develop such a syndrome. The potentiation of toxic reactions when vancomycin is used with aminoglycosides may be owing, at least in part, to enhancement of aminoglycoside binding to brush border and, presumably, its uptake into tubular cells, with subsequent cellular injury (151).

## Analgesics and Nonsteroidal Anti-Inflammatory Drugs

Anti-inflammatory agents can be classified as steroidal and nonsteroidal. However, by convention, the generic term *nonsteroidal anti-inflammatory drugs* (NSAIDs) has come to refer to specific prostaglandin (PG) synthase (cyclooxygenase) inhibitors, exclusive of aspirin. This causes some conceptual confusion because aspirin, in fact, is a PG synthase inhibitor. These drugs are used for their analgesic, antipyretic, and anti-inflammatory effects. Cyclooxygenase (COX) has two isoforms. COX-1 is the constitutive isoform normally expressed in the tissues, and COX-2 is the inducible isoform. The hypothesis was that COX-1–derived prostaglandins are responsible for regulating physiologic functions whereas COX-2–derived prostaglandins play a more important role in the pathogenesis of inflammation and tissue damage. The older generation of NSAIDs block both COX-1 and COX-2. A new generation of drugs selectively inhibits COX-2, and the assumption was made that these would not be associated with serious gastrointestinal and renal side effects. This led to the finding that constitutive tissue expression is present not only for COX-1 but also for COX-2. COX-2 has been detected in normal renal tissue in the medullary interstitial cells, in the macula densa, in the thick ascending limb of Henle, and also in smooth muscle cells and endothelial cells of arterioles and veins (152,153).

Importantly, more and more data indicate that renal toxicity, including ARF with interstitial nephritis and also heavy proteinuria, may be associated not only with conventional NSAIDs but also with COX-2 inhibitors (154–159). At the time of writing this chapter, there is considerable controversy about COX-2 inhibitors and their cardiovascular side effects, which resulted in the withdrawal of rofecoxib (Vioxx) from the market. The future of these otherwise promising anti-inflammatory medications is currently uncertain.

Under euvolemic conditions, renal prostaglandin (PG) synthesis is low; however, if the renal blood flow is compromised, PG exerts a compensating influence on renal function. Some PGs induce renal vasodilatation that counterbalances vasoconstrictor effects of angiotensin-II and norepinephrine. They also affect sodium excretion, and, as a consequence of renal vasodilatation, they may increase the filtered load of sodium. They also increase medullary blood flow and reduce hypertonicity of the loop of Henle. PGs also have natriuretic effect by direct inhibition of sodium transport in the loop of Henle and distal nephron, and they also oppose the hydro-osmotic effects of vasopressin (153). There are several different PGs with diverse effects. The above list of the actions of PGs is not complete, highlighting the complexity of their effect on renal function under normal and pathologic conditions.

Acetaminophen is frequently not classified as an NSAID because it has no anti-inflammatory effect, and it is not a PG synthase inhibitor. It is, however, one of the most widely used analgesic and antipyretic drugs and is discussed under the category of NSAIDs by many pharmacology textbooks. For convenience, we discuss acetaminophen with NSAIDs (Table 23.2). The gastrointestinal toxicity of these agents is well known, but their adverse effect on renal function became apparent only in the past three decades.

### Incidence

The incidence of NSAID nephrotoxicity is not well established. Taking into consideration their over-the-counter availability and the frequency with which people take them for pain relief or fever, the incidence appears to be rather low. On the other hand, because of their widespread use and availability, many patients with renal impairment have a history of NSAID use. In a number of such patients, the association of NSAIDs and renal failure is incidental. A causative relationship between NSAIDs and renal impairment should be considered if the initiation of NSAID therapy and the renal impairment show a close temporal association, if other etiologic factors can be excluded, and if renal function improves following discontinuation of NSAIDs.

Approximately 50 million Americans per year are likely to take NSAIDs, and some 500,000 (1%) of them are thought to experience renal side effects (160,161). Murray

## TABLE 23.2

### NONSTEROIDAL ANTI-INFLAMMATORY DRUGS[a]

Nonselective prostaglandin synthase inhibitors
  (COX-1 and -2) Carboxylic acids
  Salicylic acid derivatives
    Aspirin
    Salicylates
    Diflunisal
  Acetic acids
    Indomethacin
    Sulindac
    Tolmetin
    Diclofenac
    Etodolac
    Nabumetone
    Ketorolac
  Propionic acids
    Ibuprofen
    Naproxen
    Fenoprofen
    Ketoprofen
    Flurbiprofen
    Oxaprozin
  Fenamic acids
    Mefenamic
    Meclofenamic
    Flufenamic
  Enolic acids
    Oxicams
    Piroxicam

Selective COX-2 inhibitors
  Celecoxib
  Rofecoxib[b]
  Valdecoxib

Nonprostaglandin synthase inhibitors
  Para-aminophenols
  Acetaminophen
  Phenacetin[b]

---

[a]Specific anti–rheumatoid arthritis agents and antigout agents are not included.
[b]Withdrawn from the market.

and Brater (162), in a prospective study, found renal impairment in 18% of patients treated with ibuprofen. Kleinknecht et al (163), in a prospective study, collected 2160 cases of ARF, 146 of which (6.8%) were attributed to NSAIDs. ARF was defined as a greater than 50% rise in the serum creatinine level or an increase to greater than 2.4 mg/dL from the baseline value. Data from the Boston Drug Surveillance Program on 122,000 hospitalized patients taking NSAIDs indicate that the serum creatinine did not increase compared with levels in patients not receiving NSAIDs (164). A meta-analysis reviewing 1368 patients taking NSAIDs found only 3 patients in whom the serum creatinine concentration increased to greater than 2 mg/dL (165). Corwin and Bonventre (166) reviewed 26 patients with ARF owing to NSAID treatment. The serum

creatinine increased from a mean value of $1.6 \pm 0.1$ to $3.3 \pm 0.3$ mg/dL following $4.2 \pm 0.7$ days' mean duration of treatment, and the serum creatinine returned to normal following withdrawal of NSAIDs. They estimated the incidence of ARF, defined as the number of recognized cases per inpatient days of therapy, and found it to be 0.001, 0.0003, 0.0001, and 0.0001 for indomethacin, ibuprofen, zomepirac, and sulindac, respectively (166). The incidence may be overestimated in some of these studies because hospitalized patients already represent a selected population and may have risk factors for NSAID toxicity (see later).

### Clinical Presentation

*ARF* is the typical clinical presentation and may be accompanied by varying degrees of proteinuria (157,166–168). The condition usually develops within a few days to weeks after initiation of therapy. Sodium retention and edema may occur, and occasionally hyperkalemia may develop, presumably as the result of reduced renal PG production and a subsequent decrease in serum aldosterone (169,170). Calvo-Alen et al (171) found that prolonged use of NSAIDs leads to subclinical renal failure, which manifests first in decreased renal concentrating capacity and is correlated with the cumulative intake of the drug.

*Proteinuria* is common among patients with NSAID toxicity; with approximately 10% to 12% of patients with renal impairment owing to NSAIDs developing nephrotic-range proteinuria (172,173). A group of researchers from Chicago found that 9% of their adult cases of minimal change nephrotic syndrome were associated with NSAIDs (174). Patients usually take the drugs for several months before the nephrotic syndrome develops. It is worth noting that women appear to be more susceptible (173,174). Rarely COX-2 inhibitors may also induce nephrotic syndrome as has been reported with celecoxib (157). The proteinuria typically subsides within a few weeks after discontinuation of the NSAIDs, but may worsen with re-exposure to the drug. The usual glomerular lesion is minimal change disease and is discussed in Chapter 4.

The concurrence of renal insufficiency and severe proteinuria, particularly if the renal failure is nonoliguric, is strongly suggestive of AIN (172,173). Hypersensitivity symptoms (skin rash, eosinophilia) and fever are less frequently noted than in cases of antibiotic-induced AIN (123). Hematuria may also be present. The male-to-female ratio is 1:2. The symptoms usually appear weeks to months after initiation of NSAID therapy and may resolve within days or weeks afterwards (123,174,175). Recovery is not always the case for NSAID-associated AIN, and cases of patients who progress to end-stage renal disease have been reported (163,175,176). Approximately 20% of AIN cases are associated with acetic acid derivatives. However, other NSAIDs, including mefenamic acid, niflumic acid, and many others including COX-2 inhibitors, are reported to induce AIN (123,154–159,174–176).

Oligohydramnios with *congenital renal insufficiency* may follow *in utero* exposure of the fetus to NSAIDs, which also may cause bleeding diathesis, premature closure of the ductus arteriosus, and ileal perforation. Tubular dysgenesis with incomplete differentiation of the proximal tubules as well as tubular microcystic dilatation has been described (177–179), and the renal damage is severe and irreversible. Most reported cases are related to prolonged in utero indomethacin exposure (177,178).

### Risk Factors

NSAIDs do not alter the glomerular filtration rate (GFR) in healthy, euvolemic individuals (180), but they reduce the GFR in patients with chronic renal disease or with *pre-existing impaired renal function* (161,180,181). Elderly patients are particularly vulnerable to the toxic effects of NSAIDs (162,182), which can be explained by the fact that aging is associated with a progressive decline in the GFR and impaired pharmacokinetics of NSAIDs (168). *Dehydration and decreased cardiac output* are also associated with an increased risk of nephrotoxicity; diminished GFR may be the main risk factor in these conditions as well (58,166). Patients with *liver cirrhosis* are also at higher risk, which may be related, in part, to the impaired hepatic metabolism of NSAIDs and to renal impairment associated with chronic hepatic failure (168). In addition, cirrhotic patients have enhanced urinary PG-E production, which is vasodilatory and can be abolished by NSAID treatment (183).

Certain types of NSAIDs are more likely to cause renal injury than others. Approximately 20% of the cases of interstitial nephritis are related to indomethacin and other indoleacetic derivatives (176). Baisac and Henrich (184), in their review of 59 cases of NSAID-induced minimal change nephrotic syndrome, found that 28 of the 59 cases were related to fenoprofen. Whelton et al (170) found that in patients with asymptomatic renal failure, ibuprofen is more frequently associated with ARF than are sulindac and piroxicam. There are also data that suggest that sulindac has less nephrotoxic potential than other NSAIDs. Sulindac does not reduce the excretion of urinary PGs and appears to be a safe drug even in patients with pre-existing renal failure (168). The kidney has the ability to metabolize sulindac into an inactive sulfone metabolite, thus protecting its own PG metabolism against the drug (168). In spite of the occasional renal side effects, it appears that selective COX-2 inhibitors are perhaps less nephrotoxic than other NSAIDs; however, reliable epidemiologic data are not available yet. Acetaminophen and aspirin are usually not associated with acute renal injury, but large doses of these drugs may cause ARF (185–187).

### Pathology

In most patients with ARF, no renal biopsy is performed, and we can assume that in many of these cases the nephrotoxicity is functional (renal vasoconstriction) and that there

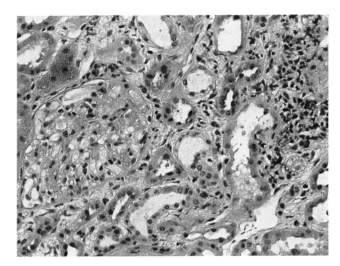

**Figure 23.13**   Mild interstitial edema and inflammation, associated with acute tubular injury, in a patient following NSAID administration. The glomerulus is unremarkable. This patient had nephrotic syndrome and acute renal failure. The renal failure and proteinuria reversed after discontinuation of NSAIDs. (H&E, ×200.)

are no, or only minor, light microscopic changes. *Acute tubular necrosis* may be present, but the tubular degenerative and regenerative changes are frequently coupled to interstitial nephritis, minimal change disease, or both (Fig. 23.13) (123).

The morphologic features of NSAID-associated *AIN* are similar to those of other interstitial nephritides and are characterized by a mononuclear interstitial infiltrate. However, minor differences do exist. Pirani et al (123) compared NSAID and beta-lactam antibiotic-associated renal changes and found that in NSAID-induced interstitial nephritis there is less intensive infiltrate and the proportion of eosinophils is substantially smaller. The paucity of eosinophilic cells in the infiltrate was also reported by Bender et al (18). It is worth noting that routine staining methods may not reveal degranulated eosinophils; thus, the actual number of eosinophils may be underestimated. There are also fewer plasma cells, and tubulitis as well as granulomatous features are less common (123). There is agreement that the infiltrate consists mainly of lymphocytes, primarily T lymphocytes, but plasma cells, B lymphocytes, and polymorphonuclear leukocytes may also be present in substantial numbers (17,123,188). There are few data regarding T-lymphocyte subsets, and these are controversial. Initial studies indicated a predominance of cytotoxic/suppressor T cells (17,176), but other researchers have found a helper/inducer cell predominance (188). The different types of antibodies used and the diverse methodologies, forms of fixation, and selection biases may account for the divergent results.

Occasionally, NSAID-associated interstitial nephritis may have granulomatous features (189). The condition has to be differentiated from sarcoidosis and infectious granulomatous interstitial nephritis, including tuberculosis. The differential diagnosis should not be based on the morphologic characteristics alone because the histologic changes are usually not distinctive. In NSAID-associated interstitial nephritis, the granulomas are usually, but not always, less distinct than in sarcoidosis. The clinical history is the most important factor in making the correct diagnosis. Discontinuation of NSAIDs usually leads to resolution (189).

Either the glomeruli show no changes on electron microscopy, or, if nephrotic-range proteinuria is present, *minimal change disease* can be seen with the effacement of podocyte foot processes (123,173,174,190,191). Baisac and Henrich (184) reviewed 59 cases of NSAID-induced minimal change nephrotic syndrome and found that interstitial nephritis was also present in 43 patients. Occasionally, glomerular lesions other than minimal change disease (e.g., membranous glomerulopathy) are reported. These NSAID-induced glomerular diseases are discussed in the appropriate chapters (Chapters 4 and 6).

### Pathogenesis

There is agreement that NSAIDs exert their toxic effect on the kidney through their interference with renal PG metabolism (152,153). $PGI_2$ is the most abundant PG in the cortex; it is produced primarily by arterioles and glomeruli. $PGE_2$ is the most abundant PG synthesized by the tubular epithelium, primarily in the distal nephron segments (distal tubules, collecting ducts) (192). Thromboxane $A_2$ is produced by the glomeruli, and $PGF2_{2\alpha}$ is produced by the tubules. The effect of PGs on the renal vasculature is primarily vasodilatory (193). Vasoconstrictive mediators, such as angiotensin II, sympathetic stimuli, norepinephrine, arginine vasopressin, and endothelin, also stimulate $PGI_2$ and $PGE_2$ synthesis, which, in turn, will counterbalance the vasoconstriction. PGs also inhibit tubular water and salt reabsorption (168). As mentioned earlier, NSAIDs do not alter the GFR in healthy, euvolemic individuals (180). In contrast, in conditions where the systemic hemodynamic conditions are compromised, NSAIDs may have a deleterious effect on the renal circulation. Owing to the inhibition of cyclooxygenase, the synthesis of vasodilatory $PGI_2$ and $PGE_2$ is diminished, and severe unbalanced renal vasoconstriction may develop, resulting in ARF (168,194).

The development of AIN is probably related to a delayed-type hypersensitivity response to NSAIDs, which is also reflected in the composition of the infiltrate (17,123). This suggestion is also supported by the prolonged exposure and the infrequency of hypersensitivity symptoms. This condition is somewhat different from antibiotic-associated interstitial nephritides, where hypersensitivity signs are more common and eosinophil cells are more prominent in the infiltrate.

The pathogenesis of NSAID-associated severe proteinuria is unclear. In fact, there is some evidence that NSAIDs may ameliorate glomerular proteinuria (195). Why in certain patients the opposite happens is unresolved. The fact that nephrotic-range proteinuria and interstitial nephritis are frequently present at the same time suggests the role of mediators such as lymphokines released from interstitial or circulating inflammatory cells, which could alter glomerular permeability. In addition, the inhibition of PG synthesis by NSAIDs may hamper the inhibitory effects of PGs on T-cell function, thus intensifying immune activation and cytokine release. The inhibition of cyclooxygenase may also result in a shift of arachidonic acid metabolism toward the lipoxygenase pathway, which may result in the enhanced production of proinflammatory leukotrienes (167,173).

## Analgesic Nephropathy

Analgesic nephropathy is a chronic progressive tubulointerstitial disease induced by the prolonged use (abuse) of analgesics and potentially addictive substances, such as caffeine or codeine. Analgesic nephropathy was first described in the 1950s (196) and was further characterized in the following decades. It became apparent that the chronic use of analgesics, primarily phenacetin, might be associated with the development of renal failure. However, larger case-control studies demonstrating this relationship were published only more recently (197–201). The definition of analgesic abuse is quite variable and arbitrary in the different studies, but the consumption of daily analgesics for 1 year or more or a cumulative intake greater than 1000 units (tablets) is the minimum criterion required by most investigators. However, true analgesic abuse and subsequent nephropathy is associated with higher cumulative intake (usually more than 5000 units).

### Incidence

The incidence varies greatly from study to study, depending primarily on the region or country where the investigation was performed. In Europe, the percentage of analgesic nephropathy among patients undergoing long-term dialysis secondary to end-stage renal disease (ESRD) varies widely, from only 0.1% in Ireland, Norway, Poland, and Hungary to 18.1% in Switzerland (202). According to the Analgesic Nephropathy Network of Europe study, the average European incidence of analgesic nephropathy among patients who were started on renal replacement therapy in 1991 to 1992 was 6.4% (198). In Australia and Canada, 11% and 2.5% incidence rates have been reported, respectively (203,204). In the United States, 1.7% to 10% of the ESRD cases are thought to be the result of analgesic nephropathy in various regions (199,205). These large geographic differences may be explained by differences in local habits, psychosocial factors, availability of these drugs, and probably also the frequency of correct diagnosis and reporting.

The removal of phenacetin from the market as well as other regulations (restricting over-the-counter sales and marketing smaller packages) resulted in a decline of the proportion of patients requiring dialysis therapy for analgesic nephropathy in Australia and Sweden, and in Berlin, Germany (204,206,207). Still, the incidence remains high in many countries, indicating that drugs other than phenacetin, such as acetaminophen and NSAIDs, are responsible for the development of the disease (197,206). Some authors believe that combination analgesics (acetaminophen and salicylates or aspirin) are more likely to induce analgesic nephropathy than single-drug usage (197). Recently Michielsen and Schepper (208) reviewed data on analgesic nephropathy in two highly endemic regions: Belgium and New South Wales, Australia. In Belgium, the sale of phenacetin was banned but other combined analgesics remained on the market. In contrast, in New South Wales, not only phenacetin but all combined analgesics were prohibited. Still, the downward trend and prevalence of analgesic nephropathy was very similar during the follow-up period, indicating that nonphenacetin mixed analgesics probably do not play a significant role in the development of analgesic nephropathy (208). The cumulative dose of analgesics appears to be an important factor. Perneger et al (199) have shown that the odds ratio of ESRD is 2.0 in patients with a cumulative dose of more than 1000 pills and 2.4 in patients taking more than 5000 pills of acetaminophen, compared with persons taking less than 1000 pills. They also found that the use of NSAIDs is associated with an increased risk of ESRD in patients taking more than 5000 pills of NSAIDs (odds ratio 8.8), whereas the use of aspirin is not. It appears that the absolute risk of developing ESRD in analgesic abusers is approximately 1.6 to 1.7 per 1000 per year (197). However, the true incidence of analgesic nephropathy is difficult to determine. The Ad Hoc Committee of the International Study Group on Analgesics and Nephropathy critically reviewed the available data of the association between NSAID and renal disease (209). They found that many studies on analgesic nephropathy are inconclusive because of sparse information and substantial methodologic problems. Also, they emphasized that the diagnosis of analgesic nephropathy in different studies can vary, and in many cases the diagnosis is based primarily on information about drug ingestion without any specific imaging or histologic studies. Therefore, the committee decided that there is no convincing evidence that nonphenacetin combined analgesics are truly associated with nephropathy (209).

Data from the physicians' health study recently indicated that analgesic use in healthy male patients is not associated with the risk of subsequent renal failure (210). The study involved 4772 healthy male physicians with normal serum creatinine levels in 1982. During a follow-up period of 14 years, there was no evidence of renal impairment in these patients, not even in those who consumed more than 7000 analgesic pills (210). This study somewhat contradicts previous data, but it emphasizes that a pre-existing underlying renal condition or other coexisting aggravating pathogenetic factors (such as hypertension, diabetes, obesity, and so on) may be important in the pathogenesis of analgesic nephropathy and analgesic intake by itself may not be deleterious to the kidney if no other coexistent or pre-existent pathologic factors are present (211). In spite of this contradictory data, considering the widespread use and abuse of analgesics, analgesic nephropathy has to be considered an important public health issue.

## Clinical Presentation

The typical patient is a middle-aged woman with various symptoms, frequently including headaches and some degree of acute and/or chronic renal failure. The decline in the GFR may be caused by vasoconstriction, vascular damage, or tubular obstruction (212). Tubular damage is reflected in defects of urinary concentration, acidification, and sodium retention. Microscopic hematuria occurs in 40% of patients (212). Gross hematuria with loin pain and ARF are suggestive of papillary necrosis (213). Occasionally, full-blown papillary necrosis occurs. If the necrotic papilla is sloughed into the renal pelvis, fragments of necrotic papilla segments may cause obstruction or be voided in the urine. Significant proteinuria (greater than 0.3 g/24 hours) is present in half of the patients, but nephrotic-range proteinuria is uncommon (212). Hypertension develops in a substantial number of patients.

The diagnosis of analgesic nephropathy should not be solely based on renal biopsy. Renal imaging techniques, such as sonography and particularly computed tomography, are the best methods for diagnosis in the appropriate clinical context (198). The Analgesic Nephropathy Network of Europe study showed that shrinkage of renal mass (sensitivity 96%, specificity 37%), bumpy renal contours (sensitivity 57%, specificity 92%), and the presence of papillary calcifications (sensitivity 85%, specificity 93%) are the most useful criteria in diagnosing analgesic nephropathy. The combination of these three criteria resulted in a sensitivity of 85% and a specificity of 93% (198). Radiocontrast examinations may be helpful in the diagnosis of papillary necrosis. The specificity and sensitivity of diagnostic imaging studies have been reviewed by De Broe and Elseviers (214).

## Pathologic Findings

*Gross Appearance.* In the full-blown form, both kidneys are somewhat contracted, and the subcapsular surface shows irregularly alternating depressed areas and raised nodules, the latter sometimes assuming a characteristic ridged form (215,216). The depressed areas correspond to atrophic, scarred portions of the cortex above a necrotic papilla. The nodular areas correspond to the hypertrophic

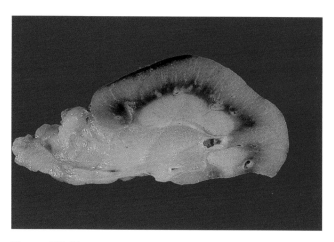

**Figure 23.14** Portion of a kidney with advanced analgesic nephropathy. Note the pale grey-white papilla, representing papillary sclerosis/necrosis.

areas of the cortex above the columns of Bertin. The papillae are shrunken and withered and may be pale or brown (Fig. 23.14). Calcification may be present, primarily in the medulla. In early-stage papillary necrosis, yellow stripes radiating outward from the tip of the medulla may be seen, separated by dark zones. This appearance may be confined to the tip or may extend through the entire papilla. Later, the yellow appearance becomes confluent and extends to the border of the inner and outer medullas. In some cases, only the tip of the papilla becomes necrotic;in others, the necrosis is found only in the central part of the papilla. Occasionally, the necrotic papillae become sequestered and may be found lying free in the pelvis. Soft phosphate stones may also be noted in the pelvis in association with papillary necrosis. A characteristic brown pigmentation of the pelvic mucosa may be observed, which is thought to be the result of lipid deposition (217,218).

*Light Microscopy.* The earliest change is the sclerosis (basement membrane thickening) of capillaries beneath the urothelial mucosa (Fig. 23.15) (216,218,219). This suburothelial capillary calcification was demonstrated in phenacetin abuse-associated analgesic nephropathy and it is not entirely clear whether non–phenacetin-related cases have the same capillary calcification. This capillary sclerosis increases in intensity toward the pelvic-ureteric junction, is most prominent in the proximal ureter, and then gradually decreases (216). At a more advanced stage (in early stages of papillary necrosis), the capillary sclerosis involves the peritubular capillaries in the papilla and inner medulla. The ascending loop of Henle also exhibits a substantially thickened basement membrane, but the basement membranes of the collecting ducts, descending loop of Henle, and vasa recta are not affected or are only mildly affected. The thickened basement membranes are PAS-positive and contain lipid as well as calcium deposits (Fig. 23.16). Ul-

trastructurally, this basement membrane thickening consists of numerous thin layers of basement membrane material (Fig. 23.15B), which probably forms as the result of repeated injury of the capillary endothelium and the epithelium of the thin limb of Henle (216,220). Early on, these changes are confined to the central part of the inner medulla, but as the disease progresses, the affected small foci become confluent and may involve the entire inner medulla.

As full-blown papillary necrosis develops, the collecting ducts and the vasa recta become necrotic as well, and a ghost outline of the original structure is present (Fig. 23.17). Renal papillary necrosis is not associated with the influx of neutrophils into the necrotic areas or the bordering preserved renal parenchyma. There may be focal collections of lymphocytes and macrophages. If the necrotic portion of the papilla sloughs into the lumen of the renal pelvis, the resulting cavity will re-epithelialize. The necrotic material may also remain in place, and in such cases calcification of the necrotic papilla is common, with possible bone formation (Fig. 23.18).

The cortical changes are thought to stem from the alterations in the papilla (221,222). The cortex may be normal in the early and intermediate forms. The cortical changes consist of tubular loss and tubular atrophy with interstitial fibrosis and a varying degree of interstitial infiltration of chronic inflammatory cells (Fig. 23.19). Lipofuscin accumulation is frequently noted in the epithelium of atrophic tubules. These are nonspecific changes and cannot be reliably differentiated from other forms of chronic tubulointerstitial injury. It appears that the necrotic papilla, in some ways analogous to obstructive nephropathy, is responsible for the cortical changes. This is also supported by the fact that the columns of Bertin are often spared.

The glomerular changes are presumably the result of the tubulointerstitial changes and are quite nonspecific as well. In the atrophic suprapapillary cortex, periglomerular fibrosis, glomerular ischemia, obsolescence, and sclerosis may occur. In the columns of Bertin, where compensatory hypertrophy is common, some glomeruli may undergo segmental hyalinosis and sclerosis (216,223). Zollinger (223) called this change "overload glomerulitis," which is in fact identical to glomerular hyperperfusion injury. Except for the medullary and pelvic capillary sclerosis, there are no vascular changes characteristic of analgesic nephropathy. Arteriolar hyalinosis and varying degrees of arterial intimal fibrosis may develop, particularly in older patients and in patients with arterial hypertension.

## Differential Diagnosis

The key to the differential diagnosis is the clinical history. From the point of view of morphology, the gross findings are at least as characteristic as the histologic appearance. The irregular bumpy cortical contours with underlying papillary necrosis and sclerosis are distinct from the medullary

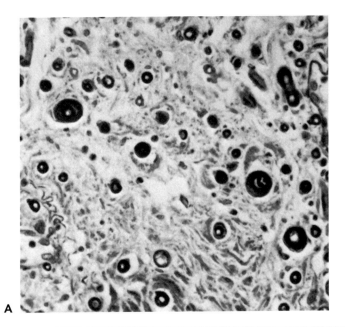

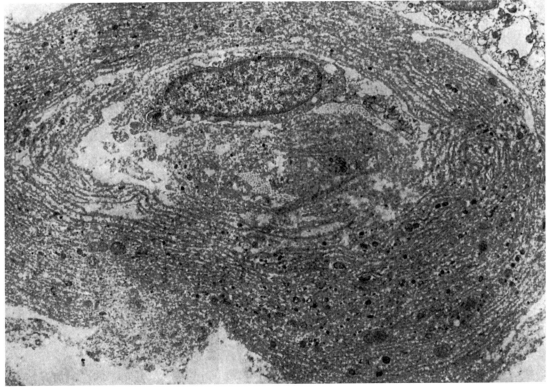

**Figure 23.15** Appearance of capillaries in the submucosa of the renal pelvis in analgesic nephropathy. **A:** A section of the submucosa at the upper end of the ureter from a patient who had abused analgesics shows extreme thickening of the capillary walls. It may be so pronounced as to render the capillaries solid. (PAS, ×350.) (Prepared from a slide supplied by Dr. H.U. Zollinger.) **B:** Electron micrograph of a capillary obtained by biopsy of the renal pelvis of a patient who had abused analgesics. Numerous new basement membrane lamellae have been formed, and the multilayering is responsible for the appearance in **(A)**. (×7050.) (From Mihatsch MJ, et al. The morphologic diagnosis of analgesic (phenacetin) abuse. *Pathol Res Pract* 1979;164:68.)

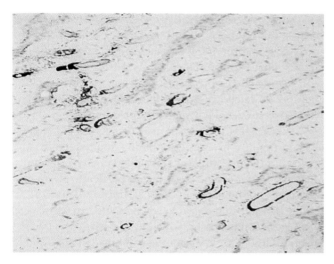

**Figure 23.16**   Calcium deposits in the basement membranes of the vasa recta in the renal papilla in analgesic nephropathy. (Von Kossa, ×200.)

and cortical scarring with caliceal deformities in chronic pyelonephritis/reflux nephropathy. Obstructive uropathy with renal pelvis dilatation and parenchymal atrophy is easy to recognize. However, analgesic nephropathy predisposes patients to infections, and both acute and chronic pyelonephritis are much more common than in the normal population (216). Diabetic nephropathy with papillary necrosis may have a similar gross and microscopic appearance with basement membrane thickening of the loop of Henle and peritubular capillaries. However, the capillary sclerosis beneath the urothelium is not seen. Papillary necrosis may occur in sickle cell disease and, rarely, in vasculitis and systemic lupus erythematosus (213). In these

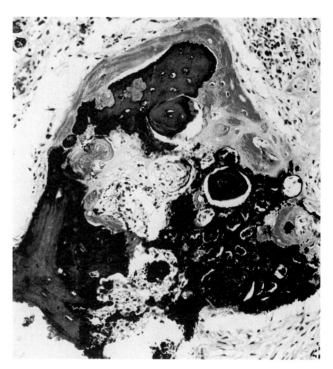

**Figure 23.18**   Bone formation in a necrotic papilla from a patient who had abused analgesics and who survived several years after the initial diagnosis. (H&E, ×145.)

conditions, as well as in diabetes, the characteristic features of the underlying disease assist in making the diagnosis.

## Pathogenesis

One theory is that the papillary changes are caused by insufficient blood supply (224,225). Lagergren and Ljungqvist (226) were unable to demonstrate the postglomerular vessels of juxtamedullary glomeruli, indicating

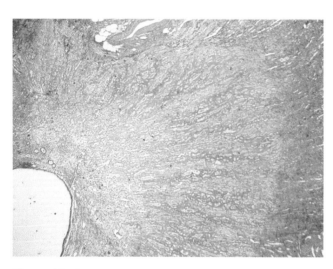

**Figure 23.17**   Low-magnification picture taken from the specimen shown in Figure 23.14. In analgesic nephropathy, typically there is no inflammatory reaction around a necrotic/sclerotic papilla. The ghost structure of the renal papilla is still recognizable. (H&E, ×10.)

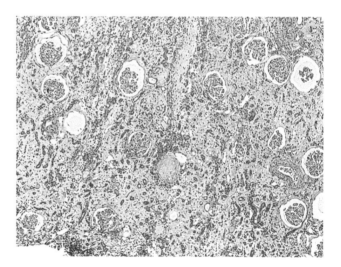

**Figure 23.19**   Interstitial fibrosis and tubular atrophy in the cortex of a kidney with analgesic nephropathy. Note that most glomeruli in this section are preserved; only scattered sclerotic glomeruli are seen. (H&E, ×40.)

decreased blood supply of the papilla. A reduction in number and dimension of the vasa recta in a rat model of analgesic nephropathy was noted by Kincaid-Smith et al as well (224). Molland (225) suggested that the reduced medullary blood flow in analgesic nephropathy is the consequence of disturbed autoregulation.

Certainly, capillary sclerosis can compromise the medullary blood flow, but it appears that capillary sclerosis itself is the consequence of toxic effects (227). The concentric lamellated ultrastructure of the thickened basement membranes of the peritubular and pelvic capillaries and the loop of Henle suggests repeated injury and subsequent repair of the capillary endothelium and loop of Henle's epithelium, respectively. Analgesic drugs are highly lipophilic, and they can easily diffuse out of the urine into the medullary and papillary interstitium and cause capillary damage. It has been shown that the concentration of analgesic substances in the renal medulla can be many times higher than in the blood (228). Thus, it appears that the topographic distribution of renal injury is related to the local concentration of analgesics and their metabolites. The primary injury appears to be toxic capillary damage, which in turn, through ischemia, aggravates the injury and leads eventually to papillary necrosis.

The natural history of the medullary/papillary changes is unclear. We had the opportunity to examine a cadaveric donor kidney from a semiprofessional athlete who died because of an automobile accident (Fig. 23.20). Organ dona-tion was considered, but the kidneys were not transplanted because of very poor perfusion on the perfusion pump. Gross examination of the kidney revealed prominent edematous renal papillae (Fig. 23.20A). Histologically, in the prominently edematous papilla, calcium deposits, including capillary calcification, were noted (Fig. 23.20B and C). Otherwise, the renal parenchyma, including the renal cortex, was normal and there was no evidence of renal impairment in the donor. After questioning family members, it turned out that the athlete had been taking large amounts of analgesics for several years before his death. There was no evidence of impairment of renal function. Therefore, it is quite possible that this kidney represented an early stage of analgesic nephropathy, which in this particular patient may have been secondary to the combined effect of periodic dehydration because of the strenuous exercise and the large doses of analgesics.

The pathogenesis of cortical changes is most likely secondary to medullary damage. The nephrons from the columns of Bertin drain into the forniceal region of the calyx, which explains their escape from obstruction and subsequent injury in papillary necrosis (215,222). Furthermore, cortical atrophy and chronic interstitial nephritis develop primarily in areas where the underlying papilla remains in situ and undergoes sclerosis with the obstruction of the urine flow. If the separation of the necrotic papilla ensues, the urine flow may persist and less cortical damage will develop (215,216,222). An alternate theory is that the

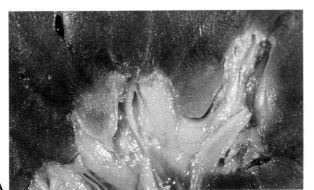

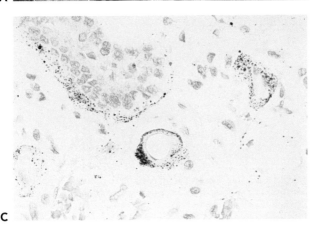

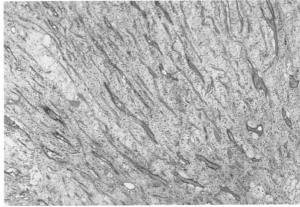

**Figure 23.20**    This is a nephrectomy specimen from a young athlete who used large doses of analgesic medications for many years and died of an automobile accident. **A:** Note the edematous papillae. **B:** Histologic examination revealed prominently edematous renal papillae with compression of the vasa recta. (H&E, ×100.) **C:** von Kossa stain revealed finely granular calcium deposits in the basement membranes of the vasa recta and collecting ducts. (×400.)

cortical atrophy in papillary sclerosis/necrosis may be the consequence of the interruption of the limbs of Henle, with subsequent atrophy of the distal and eventually the proximal nephron. The interruption of the peritubular capillaries and vasa recta, by interfering with the blood supply of the tubulointerstitium, may play an important role in the medullary changes and possibly in the cortical changes as well.

The exact pathogenesis of the toxicity of analgesic compounds and the primary target of the toxic reactions are unknown. Inhibition of PG synthesis and immunologic reactions are unlikely causes (216). It is possible that metabolites of phenacetin, aspirin, or paracetamol, under the influence of P450 mono-oxygenase, bind covalently to cellular proteins and cause toxic damage (212).

Another possible explanation is cellular glutathione depletion with subsequent lipid peroxide production (229). This theory is based on the observation that combination analgesics are more prone to cause damage. Acetaminophen becomes concentrated in the papillae and there undergoes oxidative metabolism, which turns it into a reactive quinone imine that becomes conjugated to glutathione. If acetaminophen is ingested alone, there is sufficient glutathione generated to detoxify the reactive metabolites. If acetaminophen is taken in combination with aspirin or salicylates (aspirin will be converted to salicylate as well), the papillary concentration of salicylates will also be very high. Salicylates potently deplete glutathione, probably through the inhibition of NADPH production. Thus, with the combination of acetaminophen and salicylates or aspirin, glutathione depletion in the papilla may ensue and result in the production of lipid peroxides by the reactive acetaminophen metabolites. This subsequently leads to local tissue damage, resulting in papillary necrosis (229).

There are a few animal models for analgesic nephropathy. Moeckel et al (230) administered COX-2 inhibitors to mice and found that COX-2 inhibition dramatically reduced osmolyte accumulation in medullary interstitial cells. Exogenous osmolytes reversed COX-2–induced cell death in cultured renal medullary cells. They proposed that the reduction of osmolytes may have a pathogenetic role in analgesic nephropathy (230). In another mouse model of acetaminophen-induced nephrotoxicity, a nitric oxide donor prevented renal injury as measured by blood urea nitrogen levels and renal pathology (interstitial congestion, proximal tubular cell degeneration, and necrosis) (231). The authors proposed that the protective mechanism is secondary to attenuation of lipid peroxidation in the kidney. Ahmed et al (232) described an animal model with nephropathy following the administration of phenacetin and chloroquine. The renal injury was prevented by the administration of the nitric oxide synthase inhibitor L-nitroarginine ethylester (L-NAME). A more recent experiment, however, indicated that COX-2 inhibitors may actually be protective against renal injury in an animal model. Administration of COX-2 inhibitor and then an angiotensin-1 receptor inhibitor prevented progressive renal injury in a 5/6 renal ablation model in the rat (233,233). However, there are clear differences in rodent and human responses to drugs. Chronic aspirin administration can cause renal papillary necrosis in rodents, which has not been reported in humans (234). Therefore, interpreting the somewhat controversial experimental data has to be done with caution. Perhaps nonrodent animals may provide a better model for human analgesic nephropathy.

### Urothelial Cancer and Analgesic Abuse

It is now widely accepted that there is an association between analgesic abuse and transitional cell carcinoma of the renal pelvis and urinary tract (235–237). The incidence is variable, and according to Mihatsch and Knüsli (236), it may occur in at least 10% of phenacetin abusers. The latent period can be two or more decades (237). With the decline of phenacetin abuse, the incidence of transitional cell carcinomas of the urinary tract appears to have declined in Australia and Sweden (235,237); however, longer followup is needed for definitive proof. Although renal papillary necrosis has been found in a high proportion of patients with transitional cell carcinoma associated with analgesic abuse, it is not a prerequisite for the development of these tumors. Occasional publications also implicate an increased number of renal cell carcinomas in analgesic abusers. However, a study from the National Cancer Institute did not confirm this finding (238).

### 5-Aminosalycilic Acid

5-Aminosalicylates are anti-inflammatory medications widely used for the treatment of inflammatory bowel disease. Two forms of these medications, mesalazine and sulfasalazine, are used. Based on data from the United Kingdom General Practice Research Database, it appears that the incidence of renal failure in patients on 5-aminosalicylic medications is low (0.17 cases per 100 patients per year) (239). This database indicates that the risk of renal failure is comparable with mesalazine and sulfasalazine use. Examining the renal side effects, Ransford and Langman (240) found that interstitial nephritis was described only following the use of mesalazine. This is intriguing because the difference between mesalazine and sulfasalazine is that in sulfasalazine, 5-amniosalycilic acid is combined with sulfapyridine (a sulfonamide). Therefore, theoretically one might expect a higher prevalence of interstitial nephritis with sulfasalazine. Arend and Springate (241) reviewed mesalazine-induced interstitial nephritis recently. They concluded that mesalazine-related renal insufficiency occurs in approximately 1 in 100 to 500 patients. In patients with biopsy-proven interstitial nephritis, the frequency of residual renal insufficiency is 61%, and 13% of patients develop end-stage renal disease despite discontinuation of the drug (241).

## Other Medications

### Diphenylhydantoin

The drug diphenylhydantoin (Dilantin) is used extensively for the treatment of seizures and arrhythmias. There are several side effects, but adverse reactions involving the kidney are rare. A few cases of oliguric ARF and interstitial nephritis have been reported (242–244). Hyman et al (243) described the case of an 8-year-old girl who showed cutaneous and systemic signs of hypersensitivity 22 days after starting a course of diphenylhydantoin. This was followed 10 days later by the appearance of nephrotic syndrome, hematuria, and azotemia. A renal biopsy revealed interstitial nephritis by light microscopy and linear deposits of IgG along TBMs on immunofluorescence. Diphenylhydantoin antigen was found along TBMs by immunohistochemistry. Anti-TBM antibody was present in the serum, and peripheral blood lymphocyte transformation was observed following incubation with diphenylhydantoin. The suggestion was made that cellular hypersensitivity to deposits of diphenylhydantoin on TBMs could have induced antigenic alterations, resulting in the production of anti-TBM antibody.

It is well known that vascular changes take place with the use of diphenylhydantoin, and granulomatous arteritis can be seen in patients hypersensitive to this drug (245). Gaffey et al (245) reviewed eight cases of vasculitis caused by hypersensitivity to Dilantin. The kidney was involved in six cases; three patients had granulomatous interstitial nephritis. Blood eosinophilia of more than 14% occurred in four patients.

### Lithium

The widespread use of lithium carbonate in psychiatric practice for the treatment of manic-depressive states has been associated with occasional cases of ARF, the more common occurrence of a diabetes insipidus-like state, and permanent impairment of renal function in others.

*Clinical Presentation.* Nephrogenic diabetes insipidus (polyuria, polydipsia, and impaired renal concentrating capacity) is the most usual renal complication of maintenance lithium therapy (246). Defective distal tubular acidification owing to low fractional excretion of bicarbonate, with normal serum levels of bicarbonate and phosphate and normal ammonia excretion, is also common. Hypercalcemia may also occur (247). These side effects are usually reversible; however, there are reports that chronic irreversible renal injury may develop following maintenance lithium therapy (248,249).

The frequency with which chronic renal insufficiency and permanent morphologic damage occur in patients receiving long-term lithium therapy has been considered by several authors (250–252). Walker and Edwards (252) summarized the results of seven longitudinal studies between 1981 and 1988 and found little potential for decreased GFR in lithium-treated patients. In a prospective study of 65 lithium-treated patients, Jorkasky et al (251) found a mild decline in the GFR in men but not in women. They questioned whether the reduction in the GFR was progressive and would lead to clinically significant renal insufficiency. A recent study from France indicates that the prevalence of lithium nephrotoxicity among end-stage renal disease patients is two per 1000 dialysis patients (247). They calculated that the lithium therapy duration until ESRD was 19.8 years and the estimated cumulative lithium salt given was 5231 grams per patient. Cases of the nephrotic syndrome have been rarely reported (247,253,254). Interestingly, a study from the Columbia University indicates that 25% of patients who underwent kidney biopsy and were diagnosed to have lithium nephrotoxicity also had nephrotic syndrome (254). These patients had the light microscopic pattern of focal segmental glomerular sclerosis. Lithium nephrotoxicity appears to be a slowly progressive disease, and discontinuation of lithium will result in improved renal function only if the chronic injury is relatively mild.

*Pathologic Findings.* The sparse reports on the renal pathologic features of acute lithium toxicity (255,256) have disclosed little apart from dilated convoluted tubules with some pyknotic nuclei, hyaline droplets, and vacuolated tubular epithelial cells. Chronic lithium nephrotoxicity is associated with progressive chronic tubulointerstitial nephritis.

The original concern about chronic renal disease was raised by the study on the pathologic characteristics of lithium-induced renal disease by Hestbech et al (249). In this study, renal biopsies were done on 14 patients receiving long-term treatment (1 to 15 years) with lithium carbonate for manic-depressive disease. Thirteen of the biopsies showed pronounced tubular atrophy, interstitial fibrosis, interstitial lymphocytes, and glomerular sclerosis. When the biopsies were assessed by morphometric methods and compared with an age-matched control group without renal disease (transplant donor kidneys for the most part), the lithium patients had twice the amount of interstitial connective tissue, three times the degree of tubular atrophy, and five times the number of sclerotic glomeruli. The intensity of interstitial mononuclear cell infiltrate was relatively mild, compared with the degree of interstitial fibrosis. In addition, two kidneys from patients taking lithium were seen at autopsy, and those had a granular surface and contained small cortical cysts. Renal cortical microcysts, along with fibrosis, have been described in patients on long-term lithium therapy (Fig. 23.21) (254,257). Markowitz et al (254), using nephron-specific markers, determined

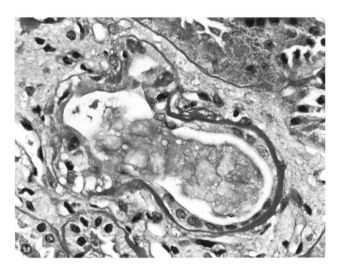

**Figure 23.21** Dilatation of a tubule with vacuolated epithelium, in the background of fibrosis, in a patient who developed chronic renal insufficiency following decades of lithium treatment. (PAS, ×400.)

that the microcysts are of distal nephron origin. Other investigators questioned the relevance of these findings (250,258,259). In spite of these controversial studies, there is now agreement that chronic lithium nephrotoxicity is a cause of chronic tubulointerstitial nephritis with the above described morphologic changes (247,254).

Kincaid-Smith et al (258) and Walker et al (260) described a peculiar tubular lesion in biopsies from patients treated with lithium. They found this lesion in the distal convoluted tubules and collecting ducts. It consists of cytoplasmic ballooning or vacuolation with strands of PAS-positive material in the vacuolated cytoplasm, sometimes radiating from the nucleus to the periphery of the cells. The change was regarded as unique; it appeared shortly after the start of lithium therapy and disappeared when treatment was stopped. Other investigators only rarely see this tubular lesion (254).

Glomerular changes are usually secondary and include scattered globally sclerotic glomeruli. Rare cases of minimal change disease and focal segmental glomerular sclerosis have been reported (253,261). Interestingly, Markowitz et al (254) found that 50% of their biopsies from patients with chronic lithium nephrotoxicity had the glomerular pattern of focal segmental glomerular sclerosis. Half of these patients also had nephrotic syndrome.

None of the above detailed morphologic changes appear to be specific. A characteristic finding is the microcystic dilatation of tubules, which is seen in most cases. One has to remember, however, that microcystic dilatation of the tubules is a nonspecific finding and is commonly seen in any chronic tubulointerstitial disorder. Therefore, obviously, chronic lithium nephrotoxicity is not a renal biopsy diagnosis and the correct diagnosis can be made only following careful correlation of the clinical and morphologic findings.

*Pathogenesis.* The pathogenesis of diabetes insipidus secondary to lithium treatment is most likely the result of the down-regulation of aquaporin-2 expression in the distal nephron (262). The pathogenesis of possible chronic tubulointerstitial injury is much more obscure; it is probably associated with a series of repeated acute injuries and repair. The nephrotic syndrome, seen only occasionally, could be the result of the interaction of lithium with anionic sites on the glomerular basement membranes (253).

### Proton-Pump Inhibitors

Proton-pump inhibitors are commonly used in the treatment of acid peptic disorders. More and more recent publications indicate that AIN may be a complication of these medications (263–267). Torpey et al (266) found that in 8 out of 14 drug-related acute interstitial nephritis cases at their institution, the etiologic agents were probably proton-pump inhibitors. AIN is diagnosed in and average of 2.7 months following administration of proton-pump inhibitors (263). Clinical presentation and the morphologic findings do not differ from other forms of drug-induced interstitial nephritides. Among the proton-pump inhibitors, Omeprazole appears to be the drug most commonly associated with AIN (263).

### Protease Inhibitors

Protease inhibitors have become the mainstay of current therapy in patients with AIDS. Renal complications, particularly crystalluria, were recognized early as a complication of these medications. However, recent reports indicate that acute interstitial nephritis may also be associated with protease inhibitors, primarily with indinavir (268,269). Two patients have been reported who developed acute interstitial nephritis with foreign body-type giant cells, presumably secondary to the crystalluria caused by indinavir (270). A case of interstitial nephritis with atazanavir has also been reported (271).

## TUBULOINTERSTITIAL NEPHRITIS MEDIATED BY IMMUNOLOGIC MECHANISMS

Tubulointerstitial nephritis owing to immune mechanisms may be mediated by antibodies, immune complexes, or T cells. Experimental aspects of tubulointerstitial nephritis have been reviewed by McCluskey (11), Kelly et al (45), and Wuthrick and Sibalic (272). A brief discussion of immune mechanisms and the various human interstitial nephritides in which such mechanisms are presumed to be operational is offered in this section. In most forms of acute and chronic tubulointerstitial nephritis, immunologic mechanisms are likely to play a pathogenic role, regardless of the initial inciting agent or cause of tissue injury.

## Tubulointerstitial Nephritis With Anti-Tubular Basement Membrane Antibodies

The presence of linear deposits of immunoglobulins and complement in TBM together with tubulointerstitial inflammation is presumptive evidence of anti-TBM antibody disease. However, the significance of TBM deposits of immunoglobulins or complement alone is difficult to ascertain, because such deposition can occur in diabetes (273) and other advanced chronic renal injuries with tubular atrophy. Complement (C3) may be focally present along the TBM even in normal human kidneys (274). Therefore, detection of circulating anti-TBM antibodies in the serum or elution of the antibodies from the renal tissue is important to prove the association with interstitial nephritis antibodies. Drug-induced tubulointerstitial nephritis with anti-TBM antibodies was discussed earlier in this chapter.

### Primary Anti-Tubular Basement Membrane Antibody Nephritis

Primary anti-TBM antibody nephritis is a form of tubulointerstitial nephritis with linear deposits of IgG and complement along the TBM, presence of anti-TBM antibodies in serum, mononuclear cell and neutrophilic infiltration of the interstitium and tubules, and edema and tubular cell injury. Glomeruli and vessels are normal or show nonspecific changes. Very few instances of primary anti-TBM nephritis have been reported. The two patients described by Clayman et al (275) and Brentjens et al (276) fulfill the criteria delineated earlier. One of the patients, a 27-year-old woman, presented with nausea, vomiting, fever, and generalized body aches. She became rapidly anuric, and a renal biopsy demonstrated intense inflammatory cell infiltrate in the interstitium with neutrophils and mononuclear cells and linear deposits of IgG, C3, and the terminal components of complement in the TBM. The glomeruli demonstrated no deposits of immunoreactants, and anti-TBM antibodies were detected in the serum. This patient recovered renal function after intensive steroid therapy, but features of renal tubular acidosis persisted. The other patient, a 36-year-old man, presented with end-stage renal disease. Both patients had circulating antibodies that were reactive with a 48- to 58-kDa TBM protein, and in both, this antibody activity could be inhibited with a rodent antibody to a cross-reactive antigen. This 58-kDa protein in the TBM was later called tubulointerstitial nephritis antigen (277). The case reported by Bergstein and Litman (278), also an instance of primary anti-TBM nephritis, describes a 6-year-old boy who presented with polydipsia, polyuria, microscopic hematuria, proteinuria, and glucosuria. The renal biopsy demonstrated mononuclear cell infiltrate with occasional lymphoid follicles, pronounced interstitial fibrosis, and tubular atrophy and loss (Fig. 23.22) associated with linear deposits of IgG and C3 in the TBM (Fig. 23.18). The

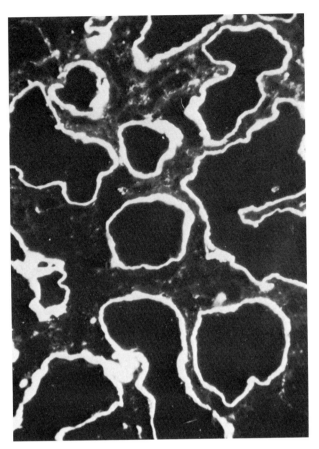

**Figure 23.22** Primary tubulointerstitial nephritis with anti-tubular basement membrane (TBM) antibodies is detected by linear fluorescence for IgG along the TBM. (From Bergstein J, Litman NN. Interstitial nephritis with anti-tubular basement membrane antibody. N Engl J Med 1975;292.)

glomeruli demonstrated no deposits of immunoreactants. Anti-TBM antibodies were demonstrated in the serum and were not reactive with glomerular basement membrane (GBM) antigens. The reports of Rakotoarivony et al (279), Laberke and Bohle (7), Freycon et al (280), and Helczynski and Landing (281) probably include instances of primary tubulointerstitial nephritis with anti-TBM antibodies.

### Secondary Anti-Tubular Basement Membrane Antibody Nephritis

Included in the category of secondary anti-TBM antibody nephritis are various types of primary glomerulonephritides and allograft nephropathy in which there is an associated component of tubulointerstitial nephritis with linear deposits of IgG and complement in the TBM.

### Anti-Glomerular Basement Membrane Antibody Disease

Anti-GBM antibody disease, with or without pulmonary hemorrhage, is an autoimmune disease owing to antibodies reactive exclusively, or principally, with the non-collagenous domain—NC1—of the α3 chain of type IV collagen (282). Anti-TBM antibodies are found in 50% (283) to 70% (284) of patients with anti-GBM nephritis. In general, tubular linear deposits are focal, they are less intense than deposits along the GBM, and they often involve proximal tubules. In the series of Lehman et al (274), 23 of 26 patients with Goodpasture's syndrome (88.4%) and 13 of 21 patients with anti-GBM antibody disease without pulmonary hemorrhage (61.9%) had linear TBM deposits of IgG, sometimes accompanied by C3. In the series of Graindorge and Mahieu (284a), 9 of 11 patients with linear deposits of immunoglobulins along the GBM had anti-TBM antibodies by radioimmunoassay (82%), and 8 of these 9 patients showed linear deposits of IgG along the TBM. Anti-TBM antibodies are detected more frequently in kidney eluates than in serum (274).

Although anti-TBM antibodies are usually of the IgG class, Border et al (285) reported anti-TBM antibodies of the IgA class in a patient with Goodpasture's syndrome. The specificity of anti-TBM antibodies in patients with Goodpasture's syndrome is unknown, but they probably are nephritogenic. Andres et al (283) investigated their relative role in the pathogenesis of tubulointerstitial nephritis in three groups of patients with crescentic glomerulonephritis: group 1 with anti-GBM and anti-TBM antibodies, group 2 with anti-GBM antibodies only, and group 3 with neither anti-GBM nor anti-TBM antibodies. Group 1 had the most severe, group 2 intermediate, and group 3 the mildest form of tubulointerstitial nephritis. In group 1, lymphocytes and macrophages predominated, but there was also a substantial number of neutrophils and plasma cells in the interstitium. Gaps or extensive destruction of TBM and interstitial giant cells also were observed. In groups 2 and 3, interstitial inflammatory changes were less impressive. These observations were interpreted to suggest that anti-TBM antibodies contribute to the development of tubulointerstitial nephritis in patients with anti-GBM antibody disease. Merkel et al (286) described autoreactive T cells that recognize the N-terminal NC1 domain of α3 chain of type IV collagen in patients with Goodpasture's syndrome. Whether T cells exert a pathogenic role in the tubulointerstitial nephritis of such patients is unknown.

### Membranous Glomerulopathy

Some patients with membranous glomerulopathy may show evidence of anti-TBM antibodies in kidney biopsies, serum, or both (287,288). Males are more often affected than females, and in most patients, the disease occurs before 5 years of age (289). HLA haplotypes B7 and DRw8 provide susceptibility to disease (288). In the publications of Levy et al (287), Katz et al (288), and Makker et al (289), patients presented with proteinuria or the nephrotic syndrome and tubular dysfunction with features of Fanconi's syndrome. Some cases have occurred in families

(280,281,290). In the report of Makker et al (289), the putative antigen in glomerular deposits was determined to be human gp330, the Heymann antigen, or megalin (291). However, in most cases, the target antigen in the TBM is the 58-kDa TIN antigen (288,289,292). The disease progresses to chronic renal failure (289,292). Ivanyi et al (292) reported a child who developed progressive membranous glomerulopathy with circulating antibodies to the TIN antigen. The patient did not develop recurrent disease in his allograft after a 2-year follow-up.

### Renal Allografts

Linear deposits of immunoglobulins and complement in TBM are found with variable frequency in patients with renal allografts. In the report by Rotellar et al (293), IgG and complement were present in 18 (2.7%) of 662 biopsies, and they occurred 3 to 13 months after transplantation. Of the 18 patients, circulating anti-TBM antibodies were detected in 10, and in 5 of these 10 patients, anti-TBM antibodies were detected in sera before linear TBM deposits could be found in renal biopsies. Linear deposits of IgG and C3 also were detected in patients who were clinically stable (not rejecting). In 10 of 15 patients who were subjected to sequential biopsies, linear TBM deposits disappeared. Overall, circulating anti-TBM antibodies were detected predominantly in the first 6 months after transplantation; they persisted for an average of 3 months and did not recur after they disappeared (293). Because graft survival was the same in patients with or without anti-TBM antibodies, the investigators (293) concluded that the presence of anti-TBM antibodies in renal allografts was not contributory to deterioration of graft function. Renal allograft recipients develop anti-TBM antibodies as a result of antigenic polymorphism, and the target antigen is the 48- to 58-kDa TBM protein (284,294,295). However, TBM staining for IgG and complement is a frequent nonspecific finding in renal allograft biopsies, particularly if chronic injury is already evident. Therefore, such TBM staining has to be interpreted with caution.

### Miscellaneous Diseases

Morel-Maroger et al (296) reported a patient with crescentic poststreptococcal glomerulonephritis, the nephrotic syndrome, and renal insufficiency. This patient underwent four renal biopsies within 28 weeks, but only the last biopsy revealed linear deposits of IgG and C3 along the TBM. There was also interstitial inflammation with mononuclear cells, tubular atrophy, and interstitial fibrosis. This patient's serum was reactive with TBM of one of his previous biopsies that had been found to be negative for TBM deposits. Anti-TBM antibodies also have been described in patients with systemic lupus erythematosus (297), Kimura disease (298), polyglandular autoimmune syndrome (299) and in isolated cases of IgA nephropathy, focal segmental glomerulosclerosis, lipoid nephrosis, and malignant hypertension (122).

## Pathologic Findings

The kidney size varies and shows multifocal or diffuse infiltration with mononuclear cells with occasional neutrophils, edema, and tubular cell injury. Most of the changes occur in proximal tubules (122,279,283). Depending on the time of the biopsy relative to the onset of disease, tubular atrophy and thickening and redundancy of TBM, with or without TBM disruption and associated interstitial fibrosis, also may be present. By immunofluorescence, linear deposits of IgG and rarely other immunoglobulins, often with complement, are detected along the TBM (Fig. 23.22) (122,274,276). In primary anti-TBM nephritis, glomeruli are normal or show nonspecific changes. In secondary anti-TBM nephritis, the glomerular changes vary and include crescentic (274,296), membranous (287,288,290,292), lupus (297), or mesangioproliferative glomerulonephritis or focal segmental glomerulosclerosis (122). Arteries and arterioles may show hypertensive or age-related changes. Electron microscopy does not reveal electron-dense immune-type deposits along the TBM.

## Etiology and Pathogenesis

To establish that tubulointerstitial nephritis is mediated by anti-TBM antibodies, it is necessary to demonstrate linear deposits of immunoglobulins, commonly IgG, and complement along the TBM (11); to detect antibodies specific for TBM antigens in the circulation (11); to demonstrate that antibodies are concentrated severalfold in renal eluates relative to their concentration in plasma; to demonstrate that the antibody activity can be abolished by incubation of plasma or eluate with TBM antigen; and to demonstrate that the antibodies have a pathogenic role, for example, by transferring tubulointerstitial nephritis to syngeneic recipients through injection of antibodies alone. Because only some of these requirements can be satisfied, the diagnosis of human tubulointerstitial nephritis associated with anti-TBM antibodies is inferential and by analogy to data derived from experimental models (11,272). The anti-TBM antibodies usually arise because of renal damage, and they recognize at least three major antigens present in collagenase digests of TBM.

1. The first antigen (or group of antigens), a 48- to 54-kDa (37,39) or 58-kDa protein (38), is the target of autoantibodies in idiopathic anti-TBM disease. The latter is called TIN antigen. Differences in reported size of glycoproteins may be owing to technical differences in Western blotting (284) or to multiple antigens sharing common nephritogenic epitopes (277). The antigen is

referred to as 48- to 54-kDa protein (37,39), 58-kDa protein (38), or 48- to 58-kDa protein (284) and as 3M-1 antigen (300). The antigen, isolated from collagenase solubilized TBM of rabbits, is localized predominantly on the abluminal surface of the TBM of the proximal tubules (300). According to Crary et al (38), antibodies raised against preparations containing the 58-kDa protein and other minor proteins (i.e., 300, 175, 160, 100, and 50 kDa) localize the referenced antigens to basement membranes of proximal tubules and other sites: distal tubules, Bowman's capsule, peritubular capillaries, small bowel, skin, and cornea, but not the GBM or mesangial matrix (38). Some of these minor proteins may represent higher–molecular-weight forms of the 58-kDa protein (288,301). Purified 3M-1 protein induces antibodies to TBM and tubulointerstitial nephritis in susceptible hosts; TBM preparations selectively depleted of 3M-1 protein do not (275). Studies by Yoshioka et al (300) demonstrated that sera from patients with anti-TBM nephritis bind to both 48- and 54-kDa antigens, and the studies of Miyazato et al (302) demonstrated that the 48- and 54-kDa glycoproteins share the same epitope but are encoded by different mRNA. The cDNA encoding the 58-kDa TBM antigen has been cloned (277). The predicted amino acid sequence contains a highly conserved epidermal growth factor-like repeat in the $NH_2$ terminus, common to several classes of extracellular matrix adhesive proteins, whereas extensive homology with the cathepsinlike family of cysteine proteinases is present in the carboxy terminus (277). The protein may contribute to basement membrane assembly and cellular adhesion (303) through interaction with $\alpha3\beta1$ and $\alpha v\beta3$ integrins (304) and also play an important role in renal development (305,306).

2. The second antigen, a 70-kDa protein, is the target of autoantibodies present in patients with anti-GBM nephritis and in some patients with lupus nephritis. This antigen is present in the GBM and TBM (274).

3. The third antigen, a 45- to 50-kDa protein, is target of autoantibodies in patients with anti-GBM disease (307) and of antibodies that developed in one patient with Alport's syndrome after renal transplantation (40). This antigen, distributed in various basement membranes (e.g., glomerular, tubular, alveolar, epidermal, placental), is absent in patients with Alport's syndrome because of mutations or deletions in the gene coding for the $\alpha5$ chain of collagen IV on the X chromosome.

The antibodies involved have been predominantly IgG and, rarely, other immunoglobulins (274,276). Interaction of antigen and antibody results in complement activation and deposition of C3 in TBM. That complement is required for inflammatory infiltration and tubular epithelial cell injury is indicated by the studies of Hatanaka et al (43). Decomplementation with cobra venom factor abrogates tubulointerstitial injury and leukocytic infiltration induced by anti-basement membrane antibodies. Leukocytic infiltration is preceded by enhanced expression of intercellular adhesion molecule-1 (ICAM-1) in renal tissue and β2-integrin in leukocytes, and by up-regulation of IL-1β, IL-6, TNFα, and monocyte chemotactic protein-1 (308). Tubulointerstitial injury results from release of proteases and reactive oxygen species; repair and fibrosis results from release of cytokines, growth factors, activation of fibroblasts, and collagen deposition (309).

## Tubulointerstitial Nephritis With Immune Complexes

Tubulointerstitial nephritis with immune complexes implies the presence of granular deposits of immunoglobulins and complement in the TBM, interstitium, or both. Deposits often are associated with an underlying renal disease, usually a form of glomerulonephritis mediated by immune complexes, and the incidence of tubulointerstitial immune complex deposits in renal biopsies varies: 1.5% (16 of 1100 biopsies) in the series of Orfila et al (122), 6.5% (13 of 200 biopsies) in the Lehman et al series (274), and 42.9% (6 of 14 biopsies) in the study of Levy et al (287). In these three series, the underlying conditions were various glomerulonephritides (e.g., lupus, membranous, cryoglobulinemic, membranoproliferative, focal proliferative, crescentic, postinfectious, shunt nephritis), minimal change glomerular disease, allograft rejection, graft versus host reaction, idiopathic tubulointerstitial nephritis, hepatitis B infection, and syphilis. We would like to reiterate that complement and even IgG staining may occur nonspecifically in the TBM, particularly if the tubules are atrophic and if the patient is diabetic. Granular or finely vacuolar deposits are commonly seen in the basement membranes of atrophic tubules by electron microscopy. On low magnification, these nonspecific deposits may appear as discrete immune-type electron-dense deposits. Therefore, before the diagnosis of immune complex deposits in the TBM is made, careful morphologic examination and correlation of the findings with laboratory results are necessary.

## Primary Tubulointerstitial Nephritis With Immune Complexes

Primary tubulointerstitial nephritis with immune complexes is rare. Klassen et al (294) reported the case of a 12-year-old boy who presented with fever, abdominal pain, rash, microscopic hematuria, and proteinuria. A renal biopsy showed focal interstitial infiltrates with lymphocytes and tubular atrophy associated with granular C3, C1q, and electron-dense deposits in the TBM of proximal tubules. Glomeruli were normal. Ellis et al (310) reported one patient with proximal tubule dysfunction and

tubulointerstitial nephritis with granular deposits of immunoglobulins and complement in tubules and interstitium; the glomeruli were normal.

Granular deposits of IgE have been detected in at least two patients with tubulointerstitial nephritis. The first patient was a 54-year-old woman who presented with anemia, diverticulitis, hypocomplementemia, eosinophilia, and renal insufficiency. The patient had no allergic or drug history and no evidence of systemic connective tissue disease. The kidney biopsy demonstrated tubulointerstitial nephritis with granular TBM deposits for IgE, IgG, IgM, and C3; deposits of IgE predominated (311). The second patient was a 72-year-old man who had a positive antinuclear antibody (ANA) assay but no evidence of systemic lupus erythematosus. The kidney biopsy demonstrated advanced tubulointerstitial nephritis with prominent granular IgE deposits (13).

Recently, Kambham et al (44) reported 8 patients who had interstitial nephritis in their renal biopsies associated with tubulointerstitial immune complex deposition and hypocomplementemia. They used the term "idiopathic hypocomplementemic interstitial nephritis" to designate this entity. None of these patients had evidence of SLE or Sjögren's syndrome. In six of their eight patients, complement levels were available. C3 and C4 levels were depressed in all patients except one, in whom C3 was normal and C4 levels were low. In one of their patients, the infiltrate was suggestive of a marginal zone lymphoma and heavy chain gene rearrangement studies indicated monoclonality (44). Immunofluorescence revealed granular tubular basement deposits for IgG in all cases. C1q was detected in six of eight cases and C3 in only four of the eight cases. Electron microscopy revealed discrete electron-dense immune-type deposits in all biopsies. In two cases, the tubular basement membrane deposits had a paracrystalline fingerprintlike substructure. Follow-up data were available in six of their patients, and five of them responded favorably to immunosuppressive medication. Immunosuppression included prednisone and a combination of tacrolimus, prednisone, and mycophenolate mofetil in the patient who had the monoclonal cell population (161). We have recently encountered a very similar case. The patient was a 52-year-old female with serum creatinine of 2.6 mg/dL, no proteinuria, and only very mild hematuria. She had a history of hypothyroidism, hypertension, obesity, and anemia. All serologies, including ANA, were negative. Both C3 and C4 were low. Light microscopy revealed moderate interstitial inflammatory cell infiltrate with focal plasma cell aggregate (Fig. 23.23A). By immunofluorescence, granular deposition of IgG, kappa and lambda light chains, and C3 were present along the tubular basement membrane and the interstitium (Fig. 23.23B). The deposits were not positive for IgA, IgM, and C1q. Ultrastructural examination revealed numerous electron-dense immune-type deposits in the tubular basement membranes and

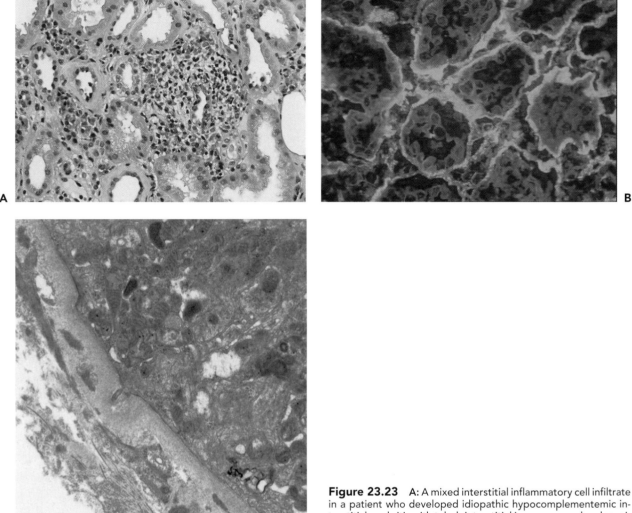

**Figure 23.23** **A:** A mixed interstitial inflammatory cell infiltrate in a patient who developed idiopathic hypocomplementemic interstitial nephritis with tubulointerstitial immune complex deposition. (H&E, ×200.) **B:** Immunofluorescence revealed widespread granular tubular basement membrane and interstitial immune complex deposits positive for IgG. (Immunofluorescence with anti–human IgG, ×400.) **C:** Electron microscopy revealed abundant electron-dense immune-type deposits along the tubular basement membranes. (Uranyl acetate and lead citrate, ×20,000.)

along peritubular capillaries (Fig. 23.23C). Only rare, small mesangial dense deposits were identified. No endothelial tubuloreticular inclusions were seen. Rare older and more recent case reports have been published describing very similar primary immune complex tubulointerstitial cases with hypocomplementemia (311–313).

Markowitz, et al (314) described a patient whose peculiar kidney biopsy showed polyclonal large electron-dense deposits along the tubular basement membranes between the tubular epithelial cells and the basement membrane. These deposits were IgG-positive and had a distinctive curvilinear substructure. The patient had underlying diabetic nephropathy, but it did not show evidence of active interstitial nephritis.

## Secondary Tubulointerstitial Nephritis With Immune Complexes

Included in the category of secondary tubulointerstitial nephritis with immune complexes are various glomerulonephritides and other renal diseases in which there is tubulointerstitial inflammation associated with granular deposits of immunoglobulins and complement in the interstitium or TBM.

### Systemic Lupus Erythematosus (SLE)

SLE is the most common form of tubulointerstitial disease associated with granular deposits of immunoglobulins and complement. Almost one half of the kidney biopsies from patients with SLE have such deposits. The inflammatory infiltrate is variable, but includes large numbers of mononuclear cells and occasional neutrophils (21,315,316). Deposits are predominantly found in proximal tubules, but can also be found in other segments of the nephron (317). The deposits include IgG, IgM, rarely IgA, and complement components C3 and C1q (318). The deposits can be found on various locations: interstitial side of the TBM, intramembranous, around peritubular capillaries, and in the interstitium. Rarely, tubulointerstitial immune complex disease may occur in patients with systemic lupus erythematosus in the absence of significant glomerular disease. Renal disease, including interstitial nephritis in SLE, is discussed in Chapter 12.

### Sjögren's Syndrome

Sjögren's syndrome is an immunologic disorder characterized by progressive destruction of the exocrine glands leading to mucosal and conjunctival dryness (i.e., sicca syndrome) associated with autoimmune disease affecting various organs. The disease is discussed in detail in Chapter 12.

Renal changes consist of interstitial inflammation with mononuclear cells including histiocytes, plasma cells, and lymphocytes. Plasma cells may occasionally be abundant (Fig. 23.3). Several cases have been reported in which immunofluorescence and electron microscopy revealed immune deposits along the tubular basement membranes. However, in our experience, and based on literature review, it appears that most cases do not have obvious tubulointerstitial immune complex deposits detectable by immunofluorescence and/or electron microscopy. Clinically, many patients present with renal failure and renal tubular acidosis. Patients with Sjögren's syndrome are prone to develop lymphoma, in particular, marginal zone lymphoma (mucosa-associated lymphoid tissue [MALT] lymphoma). The lymphoma primarily involves the salivary glands and head and neck lymph nodes. Involvement of the kidney by lymphoma in Sjögren's syndrome is exceptional (319). Steroid treatment is beneficial. For more details see Chapter 12.

### Membranoproliferative Glomerulonephritis

Membranoproliferative glomerulonephritis occasionally may manifest with granular deposits of immunoglobulins or complement in TBM. In type II membranoproliferative glomerulonephritis (dense-deposit disease), the characteristic very electron-dense ribbonlike deposits may occasionally be seen along the TBM as well.

### Mixed Cryoglobulinemia

Mixed cryoglobulinemia usually manifests with proliferative glomerulonephritis, and some patients can present with focal interstitial inflammation, including mononuclear cells, edema, and tubular cell injury associated with granular IgG and C3 deposits in the TBM (274). In our experience, TBM deposits in cryoglobulinemic glomerulonephritis are rare.

### Membranous Glomerulonephritis

A few patients with membranous glomerulonephritis have tubulointerstitial inflammation with monocytes, plasma cells and eosinophils, and granular deposits of immunoglobulins and complement in the TBM (122,310,320). In the series of Orfila et al (122), 2 of 57 patients with membranous glomerulonephritis had such deposits. In the patient reported by Douglas et al (321), granular GBM and TBM deposits were reactive with antiserum to FX1A. This antiserum recognizes antigens present in crude cortical extracts, including gp330 or megalin, one of the putative antigens in Heymann nephritis (322). The reactivity of circulating antibodies to tubular brush border antigen could be abolished by absorption with human FX1A antigenic preparation. More recently, Markowitz et al (323) reported three biopsies with membranous glomerulopathy and tubular basement membrane deposits. They were unable to detect autoantibodies to normal renal epithelial structures or matrix constituents using immunofluorescence and enzyme-linked immunosorbent assay (ELISA), respectively.

### Familial Immune Complex Tubulointerstitial Nephritis

Familial immune complex tubulointerstitial nephritis is a syndrome characterized by familial occurrence of tubulointerstitial immune complex disease, often with membranous glomerulopathy. Patients present with diarrhea, dermatitis, proteinuria or the nephrotic syndrome, and renal insufficiency (310). Tubulointerstitial nephritis is characterized by a mononuclear cell infiltrate, variable tubular atrophy, and interstitial fibrosis. By immunofluorescence, granular deposits of immunoglobulin and complement are found in the TBM. Chronic tubulointerstitial disease and villous atrophy of the small intestine were found in two first cousins (310). Both had proximal tubule dysfunction and malabsorption syndrome with granular deposits of IgG and C3 in intestinal epithelial cells, and their sera (IgG) were reactive with intestinal epithelial antigen. Membranous glomerulopathy was detected in only one of these patients; the other had normal glomeruli.

### Other Miscellaneous Diseases

Patients with various types of crescentic glomerulonephritis (283,287,294), graft versus host reaction (324), autoimmune pancreatitis (326) postinfectious glomerulonephritis, shunt nephritis, hepatitis B, syphilis (287), or fibrillary glomerulonephritis (325) may show tubulointerstitial nephritis with granular deposits of immunoglobulins or complement in the interstitium, the TBM, or both.

## Pathology of Tubulointerstitial Nephritis With Immune Complexes

The kidney size varies and may be normal, enlarged, or reduced, depending on whether tubulointerstitial nephritis is acute or chronic. The interstitial infiltrate is multifocal or diffuse and is composed predominantly of lymphocytes, monocytes, and plasma cells (Fig. 23.23A) (287). Neutrophils may be present. By immunofluorescence, granular deposits of immunoglobulins, often with complement, are seen in the TBM, the interstitium, or both (Fig. 23.23B) (122,287). By electron microscopy, dense deposits are usually present in the same location (Fig. 23.23C). Overall, dense deposits are more frequently seen in biopsies of patients with systemic lupus erythematosus. We would like to reiterate that one has to be careful evaluating the immunofluorescence and electron microscopy findings for TBM deposits because C3 deposits are commonly seen along the TBM, particularly in biopsies with chronic injury and tubular atrophy. Also, granular cell debris in the tubular basement membrane may mimic electron-dense immune-type deposits on electron microscopy if the TBM is examined only under low magnification (Fig. 23.11).

Tubular atrophy and interstitial fibrosis are usually absent from early lesions, but are present in patients with chronic renal insufficiency. In primary tubulointerstitial nephritis, glomeruli are normal or show nonspecific changes. In secondary tubulointerstitial nephritis, glomeruli may show crescentic, membranous, proliferative, exudative, or segmental changes according to the primary disease. Arteries and arterioles are normal or show hypertensive or age-related changes.

## Pathogenesis of Tubulointerstitial Nephritis With Immune Complexes

To establish that tubulointerstitial nephritis is mediated by immune complexes, the same basic requirements delineated for anti-TBM nephritis apply, except that deposits of antibody, usually IgG, and complement have a granular configuration and localize in the TBM and interstitium, and antigen targets differ and are essentially unknown. Because only some of the requirements can be satisfied, the diagnosis of human tubulointerstitial nephritis with immune complexes also is inferential and based on data derived from experimental models.

In one experimental model of Heymann nephritis, the putative antigen, gp330 or megalin, is present in the GBM (291) and in the brush border of proximal tubules (326). Immune complexes formed in the GBM result in membranous nephropathy and the nephrotic syndrome (327); passive transfer of antibodies to brush border antigens result in complement-independent tubular cell injury (328). Douglas et al (321) provided evidence that, in some patients with membranous nephropathy, an antigen related to or comparable to Heymann antigen may be involved.

In another experimental model developed by Hoyer (329), the putative antigen is Tamm-Horsfall glycopro-

tein, synthesized and secreted by epithelial cells of the thick ascending limb of Henle. Rats and mice immunized with Tamm-Horsfall glycoprotein develop granular TBM deposits of immunoglobulins and complement, electron-dense deposits along the base of tubular cells of thick ascending limb of loops of Henle, and tubulointerstitial mononuclear cell infiltration (329–331). The distribution of Tamm-Horsfall protein varies with species, and in mice immune deposits also are formed in the TBM of distal convoluted tubules (330). Deposits are formed in situ by interaction of circulating antibodies with antigen present in the abluminal side of the tubular cells. Ureteral obstruction in mice promotes the localization of such deposits in extratubular sites and apparently contributes to interstitial inflammation and scarring (332). Tamm-Horsfall glycoprotein does elicit weak antibody response in humans (333), and a component of interstitial inflammation may be related to extravasation of this glycoprotein into the interstitium. Antibodies to *E. coli* that are cross-reactive with Tamm-Horsfall glycoprotein (334) and some anti-DNA antibodies cross-reactive with heparan sulfate (335) provide examples in which autoimmunity may contribute to tubulointerstitial nephritis mediated by immune complexes. Heymann nephritis is an accepted animal model of human membranous nephropathy (322), but whether Hoyer's animal model has a human counterpart is unknown (336).

In human tubulointerstitial nephritis with immune complexes, antigens involved, with few possible exceptions (41,42), are unknown. Antibodies are usually of the IgG class and, less frequently, of other classes (274). Immune deposits may result from immune complexes formed in the circulation, or they may result from local interaction between free antibody and antigen in tissues. Both mechanisms may be operational in systemic lupus erythematosus, in which immune complexes activate complement, as judged by the presence of C3 and terminal components of complement in electron-dense deposits (318). Complement also can be activated by mechanisms other than those involving immune complexes. For example, ammonia can trigger the alternative pathway of complement activation and cause tubulointerstitial inflammation and injury (337). Based on experimental models, some forms of tubulointerstitial nephritis may require complement activation by antibody, release of chemoattractants, activation of leukocytes, and release of proteases and toxic oxygen radicals (45). Whether such mechanisms play a pathogenic role in human tubulointerstitial nephritis with immune deposits awaits demonstration.

## Tubulointerstitial Nephritis With T-Cell Mechanisms

Tubulointerstitial nephritis in which T-cell mechanisms have been implicated are probably more common than appreciated and include drug reactions; reactions to allograft antigens; systemic disease with renal involvement; reactions to renal localization of various micro-organisms, foreign bodies, and crystals; renal involvement in sarcoidosis; and most forms of progressive renal disease.

## Primary Tubulointerstitial Nephritis With T-Cell Mechanisms

### Allograft Rejection

Most allograft rejections represent a form of tubulointerstitial nephritis that results from disparity between major histocompatibility complex (MHC) antigens between the recipient and the donor. Allograft rejection is covered in Chapter 28.

### Tubulointerstitial Nephritis With Uveitis

The syndrome of tubulointerstitial nephritis with uveitis was described in 1975 by Dobrin et al (338). The two patients reported presented with acute renal failure owing to tubulointerstitial nephritis, with predominance of eosinophils in the infiltrate associated with anterior uveitis and granulomas in bone marrow and lymph nodes. These patients were Caucasian females, 14 and 17 years of age. Both recovered renal function, but one required treatment with corticosteroids for about 1 year. The syndrome has been reported mainly in children (339–343), rarely in adults (344,345). It may occur in siblings with identical haplotypes (346) and monozygotic twins (343). Females are affected more often than males.

Patients may present with one or more of the following features: proximal tubule dysfunction, including Fanconi's syndrome, renal insufficiency and proteinuria, renal failure, and ocular symptoms (341,347). Uveitis may precede or follow renal dysfunction or acute renal failure.

The kidney shows inflammatory infiltrates comprising mononuclear cells, including many lymphocytes and fewer plasma cells and macrophages. Eosinophils, prominent in the initial cases presented by Dobrin, are less commonly seen by others. By immunofluorescence, immunoreactants usually are not found in the TBM, and repeat or late biopsies may show variable amounts of interstitial fibrosis and fewer inflammatory cells. Inflammatory cells are mostly T cells, but the predominance of a CD4+ or CD8+ phenotype varies (341,347–350). The proximal tubules show the greatest degree of alterations, with circular arrays of infiltrating mononuclear cells. Acute tubular endothelial injury and flattening of the tubular epithelium often occur. Noncaseating granulomas may be found in bone marrow, lymph nodes, and the kidneys (338).

Morino et al (346) reported two sisters with tubulointerstitial nephritis and chronic sialoadenitis, one of them with recurrent uveitis; this patient also had an immune complex–mediated glomerulonephritis, which is not a component of the syndrome. It is conceivable that the syndrome encompasses other manifestations, as reported, or that the referenced patient had an overlap syndrome with features of Sjögren syndrome. Recovery by spontaneous remission (338,341,345,351) or in response to corticosteroids (348) does occur in children. Some degree of permanent renal dysfunction may remain in adults (344).

The cause of the disease is unknown, but an autoimmune pathogenesis is suspected. Although uveitis appears to be mediated by immune complexes (346,351), possibly formed locally (351), the interstitial inflammation in the kidney has the characteristics of a T-cell–mediated reaction. Lymphocyte reactivity has been detected against antigens from renal tubular epithelia using an assay of inhibition of leukocyte migration (352). One case report describes a patient who had circulating antibodies to a 125-kDa protein localized to the cytoplasm of renal cortical tubular epithelial cells (342). A genetic predisposition to an autoimmune pathogenesis also finds support in the observation that the syndrome has been reported in identical twins (353) and in siblings with identical haplotypes (346).

### Sarcoidosis

Sarcoidosis is a chronic disorder, involving multiple systems and characterized by accumulation of lymphocytes and other mononuclear cells forming noncaseating epithelioid granulomas. Most patients present with enlarged lymph nodes, cough, weight loss, fever, dyspnea, polyuria, increased serum calcium concentrations, and occasionally with proteinuria and microscopic hematuria (354–356). Sarcoidosis is more common in males and in blacks, and the peak incidence occurs in the second and third decades of life (356). Serum levels of angiotensin-converting enzyme (ACE) are frequently high. Renal involvement, manifested by renal dysfunction, is rare and occurs in only 1% to 2% of all patients with sarcoidosis. For example, of 75 cases of sarcoidosis reviewed by Richmond et al (357), only 1 patient had tubulointerstitial nephritis (1.3%). However, this low incidence of clinically manifest renal disease is misleading, because in autopsy series an incidence of 9% to 25% has been reported (356,358,359). A more recent publication from Heidelberg, Germany, describes 46 patients with sarcoidosis and 48% of them had renal abnormalities (359). The patients underwent renal biopsies—6 of these 10 patients had nephrocalcinosis and only 3 patients had interstitial nephritis; 1 patient had IgA nephropathy. Five of the six patients with nephrocalcinosis had hypercalcemia. These authors found a positive correlation between serum ACE levels and granuloma formation in the renal tissue (359). The most common renal complication in patients with sarcoidosis is related to disturbance in calcium metabolism. Hypercalciuria is present in 50% to 60% of patients with sarcoidosis, and 10% to 20% of them also have hypercalcemia (172,360).

In renal sarcoidosis, granulomas are abundant and are sharply delineated with many epithelioid cells and many giant cells (Fig. 23.4B). The granulomas are associated with an inflammatory infiltrate of mononuclear cells, including many plasma cells and lymphocytes (24,172,360,361). Differentiation of sarcoid granulomas from other granulomas causing granulomatous interstitial nephritis, such as drug-induced granulomas, can be difficult; however, drug-induced granulomas are usually less distinct (Fig. 23.4A). Also, granulomas may be missed in a kidney biopsy specimen and sometimes just an interstitial mononuclear cell infiltrate is seen. ACE levels are often high in many patients' sera, and they can also be detected in the giant cells and epithelioid cells in the granulomas. Unfortunately, this methodology is not commonly used by renal pathologists to differentiate granulomas in sarcoidosis; we could find only one case report describing ACE-positive epithelioid granulomas in a renal biopsy from a patient with sarcoidosis (362). For the same reason, the specificity of this methodology in renal biopsies cannot be assessed. Renal function may improve after early corticosteroid therapy; however, serum creatinine rarely returns to normal, and long-term follow-up has shown that some patients develop permanent renal dysfunction (363) or chronic renal failure (172,354,355,360,361). Current views on the pathogenesis of sarcoidosis implicate an immune mechanism whereby T cells and macrophages are involved (24,360).

### Granulomatous Tubulointerstitial Nephritis

A list of agents and conditions that can be associated with granulomatous interstitial pathogenic nephritis is given in Table 23.1. This list is always incomplete because additional causes of granulomatous interstitial nephritis are constantly reported. All these causes should be carefully considered in the differential diagnosis, but one has to remember that, occasionally, granuloma formation can probably be associated with any etiologic agent causing interstitial nephritis.

The most common cause of granulomatous tubulointerstitial nephritis is exposure to drugs. This was discussed previously in this chapter. For example, in the report by Mignon et al (364) of 32 patients studied, 28% were owing to drugs, 16% to Wegener's granulomatosis, and 9% each to tuberculosis and sarcoidosis. Most infectious granulomatous tubulointerstitial nephritides are caused by infection with bacteria, fungi, or parasites and are discussed in chapter 22.

Oxalosis or hyperoxaluria after small intestine bypass is associated with granulomatous reaction to deposited oxalate crystals. In general, the inflammatory reaction is discrete and granulomas are few and are of the giant cell foreign body type. Other particles or crystals, as may occur in intravenous drug abuse and gout, also can result in granulomatous tubulointerstitial nephritis. In granulomatous tubulointerstitial nephritis associated with Wegener's granulomatosis, the number of granulomas varies, but in general, few are found in kidney biopsies (365). The granulomas in vasculitis (such as Wegener's granulomatosis) are usually localized around crescent damage and/or involve arteries.

Several cases of so-called idiopathic granulomatous interstitial nephritis have been reported (366–370). Some authors consider granulomatous idiopathic interstitial nephritis with sarcoid features as cases of isolated renal sarcoidosis (368,369). They base their assumption on elevated ACE levels in some patients and a positive response to steroids. However, steroid treatment is not always successful in idiopathic granulomatous interstitial nephritis (369). Interestingly, a recent report describes a good response and recovery of renal function following treatment with an antibody to tumor necrosis factor alpha (infliximab) (370).

## Secondary Tubulointerstitial Nephritis With T-Cell Mechanisms

### Tubulointerstitial Nephritis Associated With Progressive Nephropathies

Chronic interstitial disease is present in almost all forms of progressive glomerular and vascular disease of the kidney. This subject has been reviewed by Pichler et al (371), Strutz and Neilson (372), and Dodd (373) and is considered here because cell-mediated immunity appears to play a major role in its pathogenesis. Tubulointerstitial nephritis accompanying various renal diseases progresses from an inflammatory to a fibrotic phase.

During the inflammatory phase, inflammatory cells accumulate in the interstitium in response to deposition or local formation of immune complexes or in response to cytokines and other mediators released from injured glomeruli into the filtrate and subsequently to the tubules. Cytokines may also exit the glomeruli through Bowman's capsule, the vascular pole, and the efferent arteriole (371). In response to cytokines and other mediators, adhesion molecules (374) and growth factors (375) are expressed or overexpressed, and inflammatory cells, mostly lymphocytes and macrophages, accumulate in the interstitium.

## Pathology of Tubulointerstitial Nephritis With T-Cell Mechanisms

The kidneys are usually enlarged and show variable edema, and the inflammatory infiltrate consists of lymphocytes, plasma cells, and few eosinophils. Lymphocytes account for more than 50% of the infiltrating cells, and monocytes/macrophages and plasma cells account for most of the remainder (376,377). Neutrophils may be seen, but they are infrequently present in large numbers. Granulomas may be found (see above). Tubulitis, tubular cell injury, regenerative epithelial changes, and variable numbers of casts are seen. Tubular atrophy and interstitial fibrosis are variable and more likely to be present in patients who have biopsies late in the course of their disease or in chronic forms. By immunofluorescence, deposits of immune complexes are absent from glomeruli or tubules. Vessels are normal or show hypertension and age-related changes. In secondary tubulointerstitial nephritis with T-cell mechanisms, the glomeruli or vessels may show active, healing, or healed lesions characteristic of the underlying glomerulonephritis and vasculitis.

## Pathogenesis of Tubulointerstitial Nephritis With T-Cell Mechanisms

The mechanism by which inflammatory cells induce fibrosis has been reviewed (47,48,372) and will be discussed here briefly. To establish that tubulointerstitial nephritis is mediated by cellular mechanisms, it is necessary to demonstrate that the transfer of T cells, but not of serum, from a donor with tubulointerstitial nephritis to a normal syngeneic recipient results in tubulointerstitial nephritis in the recipient of T cells (11) or that neonatal thymectomy obviates the expression of tubulointerstitial nephritis (378). Because studies of this type cannot be performed with humans, the diagnosis of cell-mediated tubulointerstitial nephritis is inferential and based on animal models in which T cells have been demonstrated to have a pathogenic role.

Mononuclear cells can mediate tubulointerstitial nephritis by two types of reactions (379). The first, delayed-type hypersensitivity, involves prior exposure and sensitization of the host and is caused by CD4+ T cells and macrophages resulting in production of various lymphokines and a granulomatous reaction. Interstitial lymphocytes interact with monocytes/macrophages, endothelial cells, and possibly with tubular epithelial cells (380) in antigen presentation, resulting in a delayed-type cell-mediated reaction. IFN-γ augments but is not a necessary requirement for up-regulation of class I and class II molecule expression in renal tubules (381). Some drug reactions and sarcoidosis appear to result from this mechanism. The second, cytotoxic T-cell injury, requires no prior sensitization and involves CD4+ T cells and CD8+ T cells. Whether a diffuse cellular infiltrate or a granulomatous inflammation develops is also determined by the interplay of cytokines brought into the interstitial microenvironment by T cells (378).

The mechanism of interstitial inflammation involves several biologic events, as discussed previously. Briefly, CD4+ T cells become activated by cells expressing class II MHC antigens (382), including tubular epithelial cells (383). Activated T cells, monocytes/macrophages, and renal tubular epithelial cells release chemokines and cytokines (e.g., macrophage colony-stimulating factor [M-CSF], platelet-derived growth factor [PDGF], TGFβ)

that induce chemotaxis of cells to inflammatory sites (299,305,313,375,384,385) and various enzymes that degrade collagens and facilitate fibroblast motility (386). It is now evident that renal tubular epithelial cells are a major site of M-CSF production. Therefore, activated/injured tubular epithelial cells in interstitial nephritis, in turn, may further attract macrophages into the kidney and interstitium, aggravating the disease process (33,34). TGFβ and PDGF activate fibroblasts (387,388), enhance collagen deposition, and promote fibrogenesis (47–49). TGFβ also appears to have an important role in the induction of tubular epithelial cell/myofibroblast transdifferentiation, which is increasingly recognized and accepted as an important pathogenetic factor in progressive interstitial fibrosis (51). Other cytokines (IL-1, TNFα, IFN-γ), modulate inflammation and fibrogenesis (389–391).

## TUBULOINTERSTITIAL NEPHROPATHY ASSOCIATED WITH METABOLIC DISORDERS OR MONOCLONAL GAMMOPATHIES

Tubulointerstitial nephropathy associated with metabolic disorders is reviewed in Chapter 25. Tubulointerstitial nephropathy associated with monoclonal gammopathies is reviewed in Chapter 19.

## TUBULOINTERSTITIAL NEPHROPATHY ASSOCIATED WITH HEAVY METAL EXPOSURE

Exposure to heavy metals results in tubular dysfunction and acute or chronic renal disease. The nephropathies caused by chronic exposure to the most abundant toxic metals—lead, cadmium, and mercury—are considered here in some detail; other nephropathies associated with heavy metal exposure are mentioned briefly. Acute tubular toxicity of heavy metals is discussed in Chapter 24.

### Lead Nephropathy

Lead exposure in the form of inhaled fumes and dust is an occupational illness for industrial workers (i.e., painters, printers, welders, foundry workers, and electric storage battery makers). In the form of dust and contaminating fluids and surfaces, it is still of some risk to the general population, in spite of banning lead as an additive in gasoline (392,393). Soil and paints containing lead are sources of lead exposure, particularly for children (394). Absorbed lead is widely distributed, but the principal sites of long-term storage are the bones, in which 94% of the lead in the body is found. This storage site constitutes a slow-exchange pool, and the biologic half-life of lead in bone is about

16 years (395). Another 4% is present in the blood, tissue fluids, and soft tissues, and these constitute a rapid-exchange pool. The remaining 2% is distributed between actively exchanging parts of the skeleton and soft tissues. Chronic lead intoxication has been widespread, and its history and effects on health are appreciated and well documented as a result of contamination of foods and as an occupational hazard of mining and smelting operation as early as 2500 BCE (396). An epidemic of childhood lead poisoning in Queensland, Australia, established lead nephropathy as a recognized clinical and pathologic entity (397).

## Clinical Presentation

The clinical diagnosis of lead nephropathy is based on history of exposure, evidence of renal dysfunction, and a positive calcium disodium edetate (EDTA) mobilization test. The test measures urinary excretion of lead after two 1-g doses of EDTA 12 hours apart (398). The test suggests lead nephropathy if excretion of lead is greater than 650 mg in 24 hours. Because the half-life of circulating lead is about 1 month, the test reflects only recent exposure (394), and the result can be normal for patients with chronic lead toxicity (394,398). The lead concentration can also be measured in tissues (primarily bone) by x-ray fluorescence and neutron activation analyses (395). In addition to its use as a diagnostic test, EDTA has also been advocated as a therapeutic agent (394,398). EDTA causes disruption of the lead inclusions and may contribute to their removal from tissues (399).

Many studies have confirmed a relationship between lead exposure and chronic renal disease (398,400–405). However, a well-controlled, prospective study comparing two groups of patients, one with high (more than 100 mg/dL) and the other with low (less than 40 mg/dL) lead concentrations in the blood failed to show significant differences in blood pressure and in various tests of renal function between these two groups 17 to 23 years after chelation therapy (406). On the other hand, a study from Taiwan recently examined the effect of environmental lead exposure on the progression of chronic renal disease and found that even low-level environmental lead exposure is associated with progressive renal insufficiency (402). One hundred and twenty one patients were included in the study with a baseline creatinine level between 1.5 and 3.9 mg/dL. Seventeen patients doubled their baseline serum creatinine volume within the follow-up period of 48 months. Blood lead levels and body lead burden at baseline were the most important risk factors to predict progression of renal insufficiency. None of the patients had a history of lead exposure, and all of them had blood lead levels and body lead burden above acceptable levels (402).

Staessen et al (407) investigated the effects of lead exposure in the general population and found that patients with decreased renal function had increased lead content in the blood and that the decrease in renal function was proportionate to increased lead concentration in the blood. Because of the nature of their study, they could not conclude whether lead exposure resulted in impaired renal function or whether impaired renal function caused increased concentration of lead in the blood. Chronic lead intoxication is manifested by proximal tubular defects, and decreased glucose reabsorptive capacity is an early indicator of tubular cell injury (408). Most patients have recurrent gout, hyperuricemia, and hypertension (409). Whether hypertension and hyperuricemia are caused by lead exposure, however, is controversial (394,396,403,404,410). Both increased uric acid levels and hypertension are more common in patients with renal insufficiency; therefore, it is difficult to decide whether these are secondary to the lead exposure itself or rather to the subsequent chronic renal injury. However, recent studies support the fact that lead can cause decreased renal uric acid excretion and uric acid deposition in the kidney, which may be one important factor in the development of chronic lead nephropathy (403,404,409). Also, long-term accumulation of lead in the body is probably an independent risk factor for the development of hypertension (403,405,409).

## Pathologic Findings

The kidneys are reduced in size, show a finely granular surface with reduction of the cortex, and may weigh one third of normal (397). There is variable multifocal tubular atrophy, tubular loss, and interstitial fibrosis (397,411). Nuclear inclusions seen in acute lead nephropathy (see Chapter 24) are not a common feature. Glomeruli are normal (411), and arteries and arterioles demonstrate medial thickening and luminal narrowing, probably related to hypertension. Urate, in the form of microtophi, may be seen in the medulla (397). Immunofluorescence studies are noncontributory or show only nonspecific findings. The glomeruli and vessels may be spared, except in patients with end-stage renal disease, whose kidneys may show features of nephrosclerosis because of the frequently severe hypertension in these patients.

## Etiology and Pathogenesis

The pathogenesis of lead nephropathy is not completely understood. Lead in fluids is bound to lead-binding proteins and is taken up by epithelial cells by membrane binding and possibly by passive transport; absorbed lead accumulates preferentially in proximal tubular cells (411,412). A cleavage product of $\alpha_2$-microglobulin is the principal component of complexed lead that makes $Pb^{2+}$ available to enzymes ($\Delta$-aminolevulinic acid dehydrase) and mediates intranuclear transport and chromatin binding, resulting in changes in gene expression. Lead interacts with renal membranes and enzymes; disrupts energy production, calcium metabolism, and glucose homeostasis; and interferes with ion transport. Oxidative stress most likely plays a significant role in the pathogenesis because serum levels of oxidative stress markers show a close correlation with lead exposure levels (412). It appears that urine level of alpha glutathione S-transferase, a marker of proximal tubular injury, may be an early marker of lead nephrotoxicity (412). The clinical usefulness of this marker needs further confirmation.

## Cadmium Nephropathy

Cadmium exposure from inhalation of cadmium oxide dust or cadmium fumes is an occupational illness (392) that occurs in the manufacture of pigments, plastics, electric storage batteries, and metal alloys. In the general population, exposure occurs by the oral route through contaminated water or food. Cigarette smoking is another potential source of exposure, because cadmium aerosol, produced during smoking, facilitates absorption of the metal (413). The kidney content of cadmium is greater in smokers than in nonsmokers (414). Cadmium has a biologic half-life of more than 30 years (399).

### Clinical Presentation

Cadmium toxicity is manifested by increased excretion of high– and low–molecular-weight proteins, such as $\beta_2$-microglobulin (415), kidney-derived antigens, enzymes, prostanoids, glycosaminoglycans, sialic acid (416), glucose, and amino acids (417) or the full complement of substances seen in the Fanconi syndrome (413,418). Subclinical changes in tubular function also occur in the general population above a threshold excretion of urinary cadmium of 2 mg in 24 hours (419). Once manifested, renal injury tends to be progressive, even if exposure is discontinued (420). In addition to irreversible dysfunction of proximal tubules, excess cadmium exposure is also known to cause hypercalciuria, nephrolithiasis, and osteomalacia. Nogawa (417) reported low-level prolonged environmental exposure to cadmium through contaminated water in the Kakehashi River basin in Japan. Patients in this area suffered from Itai-Itai disease (i.e., ouch-ouch disease), with bone pain from osteomalacia. Hypertension is present in patients with cadmium toxicity (421), but whether cadmium causes hypertension is controversial (414). A recent study from Sweden examined the effects of occupational and nonoccupational exposure to cadmium on the development of end-stage renal disease in a population working and/or living around a cadmium battery factory (415). They found a 2.3-fold increase in the ratio of end-stage renal disease in the population with occupational exposure and even a 1.4-fold increase in the patients with low expo-

sure living between 2 and 10 km away from the cadmium battery factory.

### Pathologic Findings

Very little is known about the pathologic findings in chronic cadmium nephrotoxicity. Yasuda et al (422) reported 15 cases of Itai-Itai disease. The kidneys were red-brown, had a granular surface described as sandpaperlike, were decreased in size, had a hard consistency, and weighed about 60 g each. Microscopically, there were extensive tubular atrophy and interstitial fibrosis involving preferentially the outer cortex. Inflammatory cells were present in small numbers. Some degree of glomerular sclerosis was present. However, five patients in the autopsy series of Smith et al (423), and three patients in the series of Kazantzis et al (424), including one autopsy case, showed no significant renal pathology. As judged by excessive mortality from chronic renal failure in areas of environmental cadmium pollution, tissue changes may be proportionate to the quantity of cadmium deposits, and accordingly, tissue changes may occur only in patients with substantial exposure (425).

### Etiology and Pathogenesis

The pathogenesis of chronic cadmium nephrotoxicity is poorly understood. Once absorbed, cadmium is initially deposited in the liver, where it is bound to metallothionein-forming complexes that are released in the circulation and are widely distributed. Filtered by the glomeruli, cadmium–metallothionein complexes are absorbed by proximal tubular epithelial cells and are degraded in lysosomes with release of $Cd^{2+}$ to the cytosol, where it is bound to metallothionein and to non–metallothionein-binding proteins. Cadmium complexed with non–metallothionein-binding proteins probably interferes with biogenesis of lysosomes, because it is this fraction that is temporally associated with cell injury and tubular dysfunction, as denoted by increased numbers of electron-dense lysosomes, decreased lysosomal protease activity, appearance of cellular vesiculation, increased excretion of low–molecular-weight protein, calciuria, and enzymuria (413,419,426,427). Renal excretion of cadmium occurs only after a threshold is exceeded (426). A pathogenetic role for heat shock protein (427) and oxidative stress has been raised (412).

## Mercury Nephropathy

Mercury exposure results from accidental or suicidal ingestion of inorganic mercurial compounds (e.g., mercuric chloride), from occupational activity (392) owing to inhalation of mercury vapors in the manufacture of scientific instruments and amalgam handling for dental fillings, from use of various products (e.g., topical ointments, cathartics, cosmetics, paints, pesticides), and from consumption of contaminated food. Mercury salts are methylated by bacteria in the environment, and the product, methyl mercury, finds its way into the food chain by accumulating in marine life, particularly in fish. Chronic mercury poisoning is becoming uncommon because of the elimination of mercury from most of these compounds. However, environmental pollution and the accumulation of mercury in fish still represent a slight risk. Mercury can be quantified in the kidneys by means of x-ray fluorescence analysis. In 20 exposed workers, excessive deposition of mercury was detected in the kidneys of 9 patients using this method of determination (428). Mercury can cause autoimmune disease in humans and in experimental animals (429).

Chronic mercury poisoning results in kidneys of normal or slightly decreased size. Initially interstitial edema, inflammatory infiltration with lymphocytes, and tubular cell changes such as necrosis, flattening of epithelium, and desquamation of epithelial cells are present (430–433). Later, there is progressive loss of tubules and interstitial fibrosis (431). Glomerular pathology is limited to membranous nephropathy (434,435).

Inorganic mercury affects proximal tubules and causes vesiculation and exfoliation of brush border membrane, followed by calcium influx and cell death. Mercury also inhibits water permeability in epithelia stimulated by vasopressin (436) and depolarizes mitochondria inner membrane, resulting in increased hydrogen peroxide production and oxidative tissue injury and in loss of respiratory function because of interference with the heme biosynthetic pathway in mitochondria.

### Miscellaneous Heavy Metal Nephropathy

Organic compounds containing *gold* are used in the treatment of rheumatoid arthritis. Gold salts cause various autoimmune diseases in humans (429). Patients chronically exposed to gold compounds develop proteinuria or the nephrotic syndrome (secondary to membranous glomerulonephritis), microscopic hematuria, tubular injury, and chronic tubulointerstitial nephritis with lymphocytic inflammatory infiltrate (437). Gold inclusions are often found in the cytoplasm of epithelial cells and free in the interstitium (437). The pathogenesis of gold nephropathy is unknown. Patients with HLA-DQA haplotype are more susceptible to develop gold nephropathy (see Chapter 6).

Exposure to *copper* and *iron* results in deposits of these metals in tubular cells. Iron may induce tubular cell necrosis and acute renal failure when ingested in large doses as sulfate salts (12). Copper also may cause tubulointerstitial nephritis. In the case reported by Hocher et al (438), tubulointerstitial nephritis, with diffuse inflammatory infiltration by lymphocytes and eosinophils and renal failure requiring dialysis, was induced by a copper-containing in-

trauterine device. Removal of the device was followed by near normalization of renal function.

Cis-platinum is a chemotherapeutic agent whose major toxicity is renal (439). Cis-platinum administration results in variable renal dysfunction and tubular cell injury, including flattening of epithelial cells, dilation of tubules, necrosis and desquamation of epithelial cells, and focal edema and interstitial fibrosis. Acute cis-platinum nephrotoxicity is discussed in Chapter 24. Cis-platinum has been associated with contracted kidneys (439). Studies in which platinum analogs were administered to rats suggest that nephrotoxicity is characterized by early inhibition of protein synthesis and late mitochondrial dysfunction (440).

Intoxication with *arsenic* is uncommon. Arsenic exposure can result in chronic renal injury (441) in the form of tubulointerstitial nephritis with interstitial fibrosis manifesting with the Fanconi syndrome and renal insufficiency (441). The source of arsenic was tentatively traced to consumption of "organic health foods" (442). Diagnosis rests on heavy metal screening.

The nephrotoxicity of *uranium* in humans is somewhat controversial, but it has been reported in uranium mill workers (443). There is now renewed interest in the toxicity of depleted uranium in soldiers exposed on battlefields. So far, there is no evidence that depleted uranium is associated with nephrotoxicity (444). Recent studies describing uranium nephrotoxicity are experimental (445).

## TUBULOINTERSTITIAL NEPHROPATHY ASSOCIATED WITH HEREDITARY DISEASES

The pathology of Alport's syndrome is discussed in Chapter 11. Tubulointerstitial diseases in renal developmental defects and cystic diseases, as well as familial metabolic renal diseases are discussed in Chapters 26 and 25, respectively. In this section, only two somewhat controversial entities will be addressed: familial tubulointerstitial nephritis with hypokalemia and familial tubulointerstitial nephritis secondary to mitochondrial DNA abnormalities.

### Familial Tubulointerstitial Nephritis With Hypokalemia

Patients with chronic tubulointerstitial nephritis and hypokalemia have been reported in three families (446–448). The interstitial inflammatory cells are predominantly lymphocytes, and there is associated interstitial fibrosis and variable tubular atrophy. In the report of Gullner et al (446) of three siblings, a characteristic tubular lesion was described wherein proximal tubular cells stained very darkly with methylene–basic fuchsin stain; TBMs were thickened; and the mitochondria showed dense, flocculent material

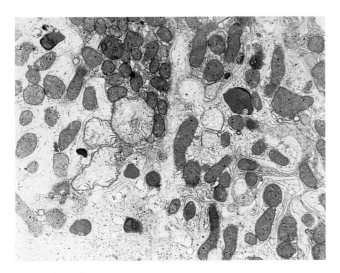

**Figure 23.24** Abnormally shaped and focally quite swollen mitochondria with flocculent electron-dense inclusions in the mitochondrial matrix in a biopsy from a 16-year-old patient with familial hypokalemic interstitial nephritis. (Uranyl acetate and lead citrate, ×20,000.)

and appeared enlarged. We have seen a kidney biopsy from a 16-year-old male with familial hyperkalemia who had mild interstitial nephritis and ultrastructural findings similar to those described by Gullner et al (446) (Fig. 23.24).

Familial tubulointerstitial nephritis with hypokalemia has an autosomal recessive mode of inheritance that is MHC linked, and one or more genes that control potassium reabsorption, present in the short arm of chromosome 6, appear to be involved (448). The pathogenesis is unknown. Although acquired hypokalemia owing to malnutrition or abuse of laxatives has been reported to result in chronic tubulointerstitial nephritis and chronic renal failure (449), this hypothesis is debated (450). Familial chronic tubulointerstitial nephritis with hypokalemia must be differentiated from nonfamilial chronic tubulointerstitial nephritis with secondary hypokalemia. This latter condition is possibly immune mediated, and the loss of potassium may be hormonally driven (451). Most affected patients are postpubertal females with systemic features of autoimmune disease (451). In one of the three families reported initially, renal failure developed in three siblings (448).

## Chronic Tubulointerstitial Nephritis Secondary to Mitochondrial Abnormalities

In 1994, Szabolcs et al (10) from Columbia University reported on an 8-year-old girl who had megaloblastic anemia, growth retardation, and progressive renal insufficiency. Renal biopsy revealed chronic tubulointerstitial disease with tubular atrophy and interstitial fibrosis. Ultrastructural examination showed extremely dysmorphic, bizarre mitochondria. Molecular analysis of the mitochon-

drial DNA detected a 2.7-kb mitochondrial DNA deletion. A year later, a group from France reported a young patient with progressive tubulointerstitial nephritis and leukodystrophy who had a 2.6-kb mitochondrial DNA deletion (32). Consequently, two groups described point mutations in mitochondrial DNA that was associated with progressive interstitial nephritis in three families (452,453). The patients of Zsurka et al (452), the patients had thoracolumbar scoliosis, muscle weakness, breathing difficulties, mitral prolapse, cardiac conduction defects, pigmented retinopathy, and psychiatric disorders. The patients of Tzen et al (453) had myopathy and central nervous system abnormalities. Some patients also had Fanconi's syndrome.

The morphologic findings in the kidney were dominated by chronic tubulointerstitial injury. The light microscopy and immunofluorescence obviously did not provide a diagnostic clue. Ultrastructurally, all patients had bizarre, sometimes curvilinear-appearing mitochondria (10,32,452). The mitochondrial also had abnormal cristae and inclusions. One has to keep in mind that dysmorphic, bizarre mitochondria are not necessarily diagnostic of mitochondrial DNA abnormality-associated renal diseases because abnormal mitochondria can occasionally be seen in various conditions, including drug toxicity (e.g., cyclosporine) (Fig. 23.25). Mitochondrial DNA abnormalities are associated not only with chronic progressive tubulointerstitial

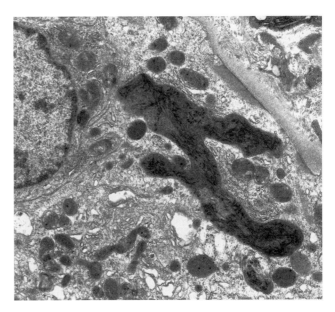

**Figure 23.25** A bizarre mitochondrion in a tubular epithelial cell in the renal biopsy from a patient with a history of hypertension, rheumatoid arthritis, and obesity. He developed acute renal insufficiency following contrast media administration and NSAID treatment. Light microscopy revealed acute tubular injury, mild to moderate interstitial fibrosis, and enlarged glomeruli. The patient was on many medications in addition to NSAID. Such bizarre mitochondria may occasionally occur in renal biopsies, and they most frequently probably represent toxic injury. (Uranyl acetate and lead citrate, ×7000.)

injury in the kidney, as cases of focal segmental glomerulosclerosis secondary to mitochondrial DNA abnormalities have now been reported (see Chapter 5).

The exact pathogenesis of mitochondrial DNA abnormality-related renal disease is unclear, but it is most likely related to disturbances in the mitochondrial respiratory chain. Renal disease is usually part of a multiorgan disease in these patients, which frequently involves the musculoskeletal system and the central nervous system. Interestingly, it appears that mutation of genes encoding mitochondrial proteins may also be associated with functional and morphologic mitochondrial abnormalities and renal disease, probably both in humans and in experimental animals (454,455).

## TUBULOINTERSTITIAL NEPHROPATHY ASSOCIATED WITH MISCELLANEOUS DISORDERS

### Systemic Karyomegaly

Mihatsch et al (456) in 1979 reported chronic tubulointerstitial nephritis concurrent with karyomegaly in three patients between 26 and 29 years of age, whose tubulointerstitial nephritis progressed to end-stage renal disease within 4 to 6 years. Spoendlin et al (457) reported four additional patients whose presentation in the third decade of life was asymptomatic but later experienced progressive renal failure associated with infections of the upper respiratory tract. Several additional cases have been reported (458–461), some of them in siblings. (459,461,462).

Renal changes include interstitial infiltration with mononuclear cells, tubular cell injury with focal loss of tubular cells, tubular atrophy, variable interstitial fibrosis, and nuclear changes in proximal and distal tubules. The nuclei are enlarged and measure up to 30 μm in diameter (Fig. 23.26). Enlarged nuclei are found in other cells such as those of bile duct, bronchi, smooth muscle, bowel, vessels, skeletal muscle, and connective tissue (456,458). The enlarged nuclei are polyploid (463). By immunofluorescence studies, no deposits of immunoreactants are found and electron microscopy is not helpful. No convincing viral particles have been found.

The pathogenesis is unknown. Mihatsch et al (456) reviewed the various causes of karyomegalic changes and suggested that chemical toxins or viral infections might be implicated. In the reports of Godin et al (459) and Hassen et al (461), high concentrations of ochratoxin, a mycotoxin that interferes with mitotic activity, was found in the blood of affected siblings. Spoendlin et al (457) studied Ki67 and proliferating cell nuclear antigen in tissues of four patients and concluded that there was inhibition of mitosis in karyomegalic cells. The hypothesis that the karyomegaly is secondary to a block in the G2 phase of the cell cycle has been

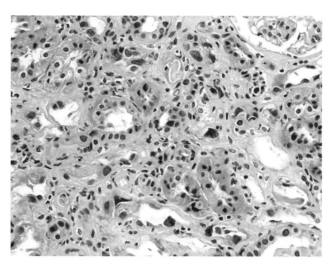

**Figure 23.26** Karyomegalic interstitial nephritis in the renal biopsy of a patient who underwent bone marrow transplantation and developed progressive renal insufficiency. Note the bizarre, large nuclei primarily in the tubular epithelial cells. Immunostaining for KI-67 was negative in the nuclei. (H&E, ×200.)

proposed (457,463). MHC typing revealed the A9/B35 haplotype, which suggested a genetic defect in chromosome 6 that was linked to the MHC locus. However, the study of Bhandari et al (463), based on their six patients, did not confirm clustering of A9 or B35.

### Balkan Endemic Nephropathy

Balkan endemic nephropathy is found in Croatia, Bosnia, Serbia, Bulgaria, and Romania. In villages where the disease is endemic, the prevalence varies between 2% and 10%. The disease occurs in families but is not hereditary, and most affected persons are farmers (464). The condition is geographically localized and occurs along major tributaries of the Danube river basin. It does not affect children and rarely is seen in patients younger than 20 years of age. Individuals who have lived for a short time in the endemic area do not develop the condition, but individuals from nonendemic areas who spend several years in villages where the condition is endemic may become ill (464).

### Clinical Presentation

Typical manifestations of the disease occur between 30 and 50 years of age, and the clinical presentation is insidious with weakness, anorexia, anemia, weight loss, copper-yellow skin, orange palms and soles, lumbar pain, mild proteinuria, and microscopic hematuria (465). Hypertension is relatively rare. Renal dysfunction, manifested by tubular proteinuria of usually less than 2 g/day with increased excretion of $\beta_2$-microglobulin, is an early sign of the nephropathy.

## Pathologic Findings

The kidneys are reduced in size and can weigh as little as 20 g each (466). The external surface is finely granular or smooth, and the cortex is thin. The predominant microscopic changes are in the tubules and interstitium. There are abundant interstitial fibrosis and variable amounts of interstitial inflammatory cells. Nephrons in the superficial cortex are predominantly involved, and there is extensive solidification of glomeruli (467). Based on a study of 50 kidney biopsies, Ferluga et al (468) described multifocal interstitial fibrosis spreading from the superficial to the deep cortex and tubular atrophy in most of their patients. Figures 23.27 and 23.28, which depict specimens from patients with Balkan endemic nephropathy, show prominent involvement of the superficial cortex with preservation of glomeruli in deeper cortex. By immunofluorescence, Ferluga et al (468) reported prominent glomerular capillary deposits of IgM in 16 of 50 patients. Papillary necrosis is uncommon, but benign and malignant tumors may be found in the pelvis and in the ureters (442,468,469). About 30% to 48% of Balkan nephropathy patients develop tumors of the upper urothelium, most frequently transitional

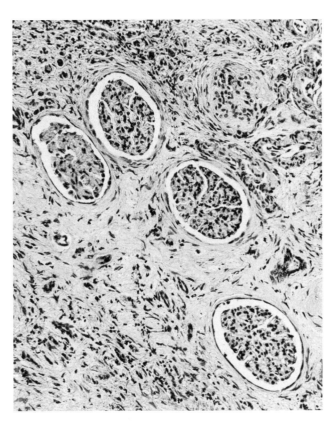

**Figure 23.28** Balkan endemic nephropathy. There is dense interstitial fibrosis in the deeper cortex with preservation of glomeruli. (H&E, ×70.) (Material courtesy of Dr. G. J. Dammin.)

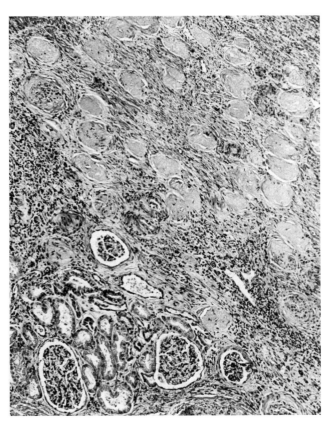

**Figure 23.27** Balkan endemic nephropathy. There is prominent involvement of the superficial cortex (*top*) by a process of solidification. In the deeper cortex (*bottom*), the glomeruli are little affected, and some tubules persist. (H&E, ×71.) (Material courtesy of Dr. G. J. Dammin.)

cell carcinoma. These tumors can be bilateral. Tumors other than transitional cell carcinoma have been reported, including papillomas and squamous cell carcinomas (470).

## Pathogenesis

The pathogenesis is unknown. A recent study indicated that Balkan endemic nephropathy is associated with the GSTM-1 allele of the glutathione S-transferase (471). However, the absence of association with these and other examined alleles has been reported by others (472). Similarly conflicting data have been published regarding viruses, including the possible role of coronavirus (473,474). Heavy metals (475), silica (476), low–molecular-weight proteins (477), and ochratoxin A (478,479) have been implicated but not substantiated. Pigs fed on barley contaminated with ochratoxin A, which is a fungal metabolite, develop tubular atrophy and interstitial fibrosis comparable to that seen in Balkan endemic nephropathy (480). The potential etiologic role of ochratoxin A or other mycotoxins as causative agents of Balkan endemic nephropathy is strengthened by the observation that 10% to 20% of cereals, pork meat, and bread from endemic regions are contaminated with ochratoxin A (481,482).

Another possibility, raised by the similarity of renal changes between Balkan endemic nephropathy and Chinese herbs nephropathy (483), implicates aristolochic acid, a nephrotoxin and carcinogenic agent present in *Aristolochia*, one of the Chinese herbs contaminating herbal preparations taken for weight reduction (484). Apparently, *Aristolochia clematis*, which contain aristolochic acid, is common in the endemic areas, and its seeds were found to be contaminants of wheat grains in endemic regions (485).

## Chinese Herb Nephropathy

During 1992 and 1993, an outbreak of rapidly progressive renal failure associated with a slimming regimen containing Chinese herbs occurred in Belgium (486). Withdrawal of the herbs did not prevent progression to chronic renal failure. A large body of subsequent literature appeared on herbal-induced nephropathies, initially mainly from Belgium (483–492). Subsequently, series of patients have been reported from Taiwan (493,494) and Japan (495,496). It became quickly evident that Chinese herb nephropathy is very similar to Balkan endemic nephropathy (487). There is some controversy about the name of the disease. Some investigators suggested that the term "Chinese herb nephropathy" should be abandoned because most of the cases occurred in Belgium and the term is prejudicial (496). They recommended using the term "aristolochic acid-associated nephropathy." Perhaps a more politically correct term would be simply "herbal nephropathy," but the name Chinese herb nephropathy remains the most widely accepted.

In a substantial proportion of patients, transitional cell carcinoma develops. The prevalence of carcinoma was 46% among patients with Chinese herb nephropathy who underwent nephrectomy (488). Because of this high prevalence rate in patients with end-stage renal disease secondary to Chinese herb nephropathy, bilateral nephrectomy may be an appropriate preventive measure (484).

## Clinical Presentation

Most patients present with rapidly progressive renal failure leading to end-stage renal disease typically within months. Proteinuria is mild and microscopic hematuria may be present. Hypokalemia or hyperkalemia may occur and Fanconi's syndrome is common in Japanese patients (495,496). Most patients in the Belgian studies are female, which may be related to gender differences in taking the diet aid. Males are frequently affected in far Eastern countries (495). Although many aspects of Chinese herb nephropathy are similar to Balkan endemic nephropathy, the clinical course is clearly different. Balkan endemic nephropathy leads to end-stage renal disease after many years (usually

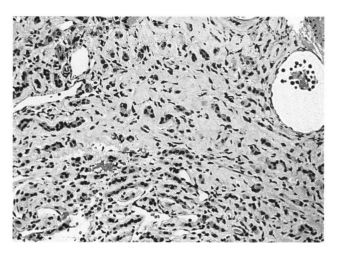

**Figure 23.29**    Prominent hypocellular interstitial fibrosis in the renal biopsy of a patient who developed rapidly progressive renal insufficiency following use of Chinese herbal medications. (H&E, ×100.)

20 years) whereas Chinese herb nephropathy is rapidly progressive.

## Pathologic Findings

Renal biopsy findings include extensive interstitial fibrosis with tubular atrophy and loss involving predominantly the outer cortex. Interlobular arteries frequently show fibromucoid intimal thickening. In the glomeruli, global sclerosis, collapse, and ischemic changes are common (485,486,487). The interstitial inflammatory cell infiltrate is usually sparse (Fig. 23.29). Immunofluorescence and ultrastructural studies are noncontributory. Scattered deposits of C3 may be present in the TBM and interstitium.

## Pathogenesis

There is now widespread agreement that Chinese herb nephropathy is primarily caused by aristolochic acid, which is the constituent of the Chinese herb *Stephania tetrandra* (489,490). Aristolochic acid can form premutagenic aristolochic acid—DNA adducts in the kidney and urothelium and aristolochic acid ; DNA adducts have been detected in a renal biopsy by Lo et al (497). Interestingly, the patient developed transitional cell carcinoma 5 months later. It appears that the cumulative dose of aristolochic acid and the progression rate of renal failure show a positive correlation (491). The nephrotoxicity of aristolochic acid was also proven in experimental animals (492,498). However, we would like to note that there are occasional case reports stating that Chinese herb nephropathy develops in the absence of aristolochic acid. In fact, we have encountered a case with typical historic and morphology of Chinese herb nephropathy, but we were unable to prove that the herbal medications the patient was taking contained aristolochic acid.

## Idiopathic Tubulointerstitial Nephritis

Idiopathic tubulointerstitial nephritis probably encompasses a group of diverse conditions. This diagnosis is applied only after known causes or etiologic agents of tubulointerstitial nephritis have been considered and excluded. To exclude every possibility, it is imperative to perform a full renal biopsy workup, including immunofluorescence and electron microscopy. Without immunofluorescence or electron microscopy, the possibility of underlying immune complex disease, anti-tubular basement membrane disease, monoclonal immunoglobulin deposition disease, mitochondrial abnormalities, and other forms of underlying diseases cannot be excluded. It is also very important to review the clinical history in detail and consider all possible pathogenetic factors to which the patient may have been exposed. The diagnosis of idiopathic tubulointerstitial nephritis reflects only that we are unable to identify the etiologic factor(s).

## REFERENCES

1. Councilman W. Acute interstitial nephritis. J Exp Med 1898;3: 393.
2. Pettersson E, von Bonsdorff M, Tornroth T, Lindholm H. Nephritis among young Finnish men. Clin Nephrol 1984;22:217.
3. Linton AL, Clark WF, Driedger AA, et al. Acute interstitial nephritis due to drugs: Review of the literature with a report of nine cases. Ann Intern Med 1980;93:735.
4. Wilson DM, Turner DR, Cameron JS, et al. Value of renal biopsy in acute intrinsic renal failure. Br Med J 1976;2:459.
5. Murray T, Goldberg M. Chronic interstitial nephritis: Etiologic factors. Ann Intern Med 1975;82:453.
6. Rostand SG, Kirk KA, Rutsky EA, Pate BA. Racial differences in the incidence of treatment for end-stage renal disease. N Engl J Med 1982;306:1276.
7. Laberke HG, Bohle A. Acute interstitial nephritis: Correlations between clinical and morphological findings. Clin Nephrol 1980;14:263.
8. Farrington K, Levison DA, Greenwood RN, et al. Renal biopsy in patients with unexplained renal impairment and normal kidney size. Q J Med 1989;70:221.
9. Fried T. Acute interstitial nephritis: Why do the kidneys suddenly fail? Postgrad Med 1993;93:105.
10. Szabolcs MJ, Seigle R, Shanske S, et al. Mitochondrial DNA deletion: A cause of chronic tubulointerstitial nephropathy. Kidney Int 1994;45:1388.
11. McCluskey R. Immunologically mediated tubulo-interstitial nephritis. Contemp Issues Nephrol 1983;10:121.
12. Churg J, Cotran R, Sinniah R, et al. Classification and atlas of tubulo-interstitial diseases. Tokyo, Igaku-Shoin, 1984.
13. Colvin R, Fang L. Interstitial nephritis. In: Tisher C, Brenner B, eds. Renal Pathology with Clinical and Functional Correlations, vol 1. Philadelphia: JB Lippincott, 1994:723.
14. Baker RJ, Pusey CD. The changing profile of acute tubulointerstitial nephritis. Nephrol Dial Transplant 2004;19:8.
15. Distler A, Keller F, Kunzendorf U, et al. The outcome of acute interstitial nephritis: Risk factors for the transition from acute to chronic interstitial nephritis. Clin Nephrol 2003;59:65.
16. Buysen JG, Houthoff HJ, Krediet RT, Arisz L. Acute interstitial nephritis: A clinical and morphological study in 27 patients. Nephrol Dial Transplant 1990;5:94.
17. Ruffing KA, Hoppes P, Blend D, et al. Eosinophils in urine revisited. Clin nephrol 1994;41:163.
18. Bender WL, Whelton A, Beschorner WE, et al. Interstitial nephritis, proteinuria, and renal failure caused by nonsteroidal anti-inflammatory drugs. Iimmunologic characterization of the inflammatory infiltrate. Am J Med 1984;76:1006.
19. Pamukcu R, Moorthy V, Singer JR, et al. Idiopathic acute interstitial nephritis: Characterization of the infiltrating cells in the renal interstitium as T helper lymphocytes. Am J Kidney Dis 1984;4:24.
20. Kobayashi Y, Honda M, Yoshikawa N, Ito H. Immunohistological study in sixteen children with acute tubulointerstitial nephritis. Clin Nephrol 1998;50:14.
21. D'Agati VD, Appel GB, Estes D, et al. Monoclonal antibody identification of infiltrating mononuclear leukocytes in lupus nephritis. Kidney Int 1986;30:573.
22. Hawkins EP, Berry PL, Silva FG. Acute tubulointerstitial nephritis in children: Clinical, morphologic, and lectin studies. A report of the southwest pediatric nephrology study group. Am J Kidney Dis 1989;14:466.
23. Ivanyi B, Marcussen N, Kemp E, Olsen TS. The distal nephron is preferentially infiltrated by inflammatory cells in acute interstitial nephritis. Virchows Arch A Pathol Anat Histopathol 1992;420:37.
24. Viero RM, Cavallo T. Granulomatous interstitial nephritis. Hum Pathol 1995;26:1347.
25. Nadasdy T, Laszik Z, Blick KE, et al. Tubular atrophy in the end-stage kidney: A lectin and immunohistochemical study. Hum Pathol 1994;25:22.
26. Pfaller W, Rittinger M. Quantitative morphology of the rat kidney. Int J Biochem 1980;12:17.
27. Knepper MA, Danielson RA, Saidel GM, Post RS. Quantitative analysis of renal medullary anatomy in rats and rabbits. Kidney Int 1977;12:313.
28. Muller GA, Rodemann HP. Characterization of human renal fibroblasts in health and disease. I. immunophenotyping of cultured tubular epithelial cells and fibroblasts derived from kidneys with histologically proven interstitial fibrosis. Am J Kidney Dis 1991;17:680.
29. Tang WW, Feng L, Xia Y, Wilson CB. Extracellular matrix accumulation in immune-mediated tubulointerstitial injury. Kidney Int 1994;45:1077.
30. Silva FG, Nadasdy T, Laszik Z. Immunohistochemical and lectin dissection of the human nephron in health and disease. Arch Pathol Lab Med 1993;117:1233.
31. Cogan M. Classification and patterns of renal dysfunction. Contemp Issues Nephrol 1983;10:35.
32. Rotig A, Goutieres F, Niaudet P, et al. Deletion of mitochondrial DNA in patient with chronic tubulointerstitial nephritis. J Pediatr 1995;126:597.
33. Isbel NM, Hill PA, Foti R, et al. Tubules are the major site of M-CSF production in experimental kidney disease: Correlation with local macrophage proliferation. Kidney Int 2001;60:614.
34. Rovin BH. Beyond a glomerulocentric view of inflammation. Kidney Int 2001;60:797.
35. Samuelson J, Von Lichtenberg F. Infectious diseases. In: Cotran R, Kumar V, Robbins S, eds. Robbins Pathologic Basis of Disease. Philadelphia: WB Saunders, 1994:305.
36. Rossert J. Drug-induced acute interstitial nephritis. Kidney Int 2001;60:804.
37. Clayman MD, Michaud L, Brentjens J, et al. Isolation of the target antigen of human anti-tubular basement membrane antibody-associated interstitial nephritis. J Clin Invest 1986;77:1143.
38. Crary GS, Katz A, Fish AJ, et al. Role of a basement membrane glycoprotein in anti-tubular basement membrane nephritis. Kidney Int 1993;43:140.
39. Yoshioka K, Morimoto Y, Iseki T, Maki S. Characterization of tubular basement membrane antigens in human kidney. J Immunol 1986;136:1654.
40. Kashtan C, Fish AJ, Kleppel M, et al. Nephritogenic antigen determinants in epidermal and renal basement membranes of kindreds with Alport-type familial nephritis. J Clin Invest 1986;78:1035.
41. Koffler D, Schur PH, Kunkel HG. Immunological studies concerning the nephritis of systemic lupus erythematosus. J Exp Med 1967;126:607.

42. Tax WJ, Kramers C, van Bruggen MC, Berden JH. Apoptosis, nucleosomes, and nephritis in systemic lupus erythematosus. Kidney Int 1995;48:666.

43. Hatanaka Y, Yuzawa Y, Nishikawa K, et al. Role of a rat membrane inhibitor of complement in anti-basement membrane antibody-induced renal injury. Kidney Int 1995;48:1728.

44. Kambham N, Markowitz GS, Tanji N, et al. Idiopathic hypocomplementemic interstitial nephritis with extensive tubulointerstitial deposits. Am J Kidney Dis 2001;37:388.

45. Kelly C, Tomaszewski J, Neilson E. Immunopathogenic mechanisms of tubulointerstitial injury. In: Tisher C, Brenner B, eds. Renal Pathology with Clinical and Functional Correlations, vol 1. Philadelphia: JB Lippincott, 1994:699.

46. Wada T, Furuichi K, Sakai N, et al. Eotaxin contributes to renal interstitial eosinophilia. Nephrol Dial Transplant 1999;14:76.

47. Sato M, Muragaki Y, Saika S, et al. Targeted disruption of TGF-beta1/Smad3 signaling protects against renal tubulointerstitial fibrosis induced by unilateral ureteral obstruction. J Clin Invest 2003;112:1486.

48. Bottinger EP, Bitzer M. TGF-beta signaling in renal disease. J Am Soc Nephrol 2002;13:2600.

49. August P, Suthanthiran M. Transforming growth factor beta and progression of renal disease. Kidney Int 2003;Nov(suppl):S99.

50. Okada H, Kikuta T, Kobayashi T, et al. Connective tissue growth factor expressed in tubular epithelium plays a pivotal role in renal fibrogenesis. J Am Soc Nephrol 2005;16:133.

51. Lan HY. Tubular epithelial-myofibroblast transdifferentiation mechanisms in proximal tubule cells. Curr Opin Nephrol Hypertens 2003;12:25.

52. Nadasdy T, Racusen L. Renal injury caused by therapeutic and diagnostic agents and abuse of analgesics and narcotics. In: Jennette J, Olson J, Schwartz M, Silva F, eds. Heptinstall's Pathology of the Kidney, 5th ed. Philadelphia: Lippincott-Raven, 1998:811.

53. Silva FG. Chemical-induced nephropathy: A review of the renal tubulointerstitial lesions in humans. Toxicol Pathol 2004;32(suppl 2):71.

54. Markowitz GS, Perazella MA. Drug-induced renal failure: A focus on tubulointerstitial disease. Clin Chim Acta 2005;351:31.

55. Cameron JS. Allergic interstitial nephritis: Clinical features and pathogenesis. Q J Med 1988;66:97.

56. Karras DJ. Severe low back pain secondary to acute interstitial nephritis following administration of ranitidine. Am J Emerg Med 1994;12:67.

57. Galpin JE, Shinaberger JH, Stanley TM, et al. Acute interstitial nephritis due to methicillin. Am J Med 1978;65:756.

58. Corwin HL, Korbet SM, Schwartz MM. Clinical correlates of eosinophiluria. Arch Intern Med 1985;145:1097.

59. Nolan CR 3rd, Anger MS, Kelleher SP. Eosinophiluria—a new method of detection and definition of the clinical spectrum. N Engl J Med 1986;315:1516.

60. Colvin RB, Burton JR, Hyslop NE Jr, et al. Letter: Penicillin-associated interstitial nephritis. Ann Intern Med 1974;81:404.

61. Parra E, Gota R, Gamen A, et al. Granulomatous interstitial nephritis secondary to allopurinol treatment. Clin Nephrol 1995;43:350.

62. Jennings M, Shortland JR, Maddocks JL. Interstitial nephritis associated with furosemide. J R Soc Med 1986;79:239.

63. Montseny JJ, Meyrier A. Immunoallergic granulomatous interstitial nephritis following treatment with omeprazole. Am J Nephrol 1998;18:243.

64. Fervenza FC, Kanakiriya S, Kunau RT, et al. Acute granulomatous interstitial nephritis and colitis in anticonvulsant hypersensitivity syndrome associated with lamotrigine treatment. Am J Kidney Dis 2000;36:1034.

65. Ramalakshmi S, Bastacky S, Johnson JP. Levofloxacin-induced granulomatous interstitial nephritis. Am J Kidney Dis 2003;41:E7.

66. Korzets Z, Elis A, Bernheim J, Bernheim J. Acute granulomatous interstitial nephritis due to nitrofurantoin. Nephrol Dial Transplant 1994;9:713.

67. Baldwin DS, Levine BB, McCluskey RT, Gallo GR. Renal failure and interstitial nephritis due to penicillin and methicillin. N Engl J Med 1968;279:1245.

68. Border WA, Lehman DH, Egan JD, et al. Antitubular basement-membrane antibodies in methicillin-associated interstitial nephritis. N Engl J Med 1974;291:381.

69. Olsen S, Asklund M. Interstitial nephritis with acute renal failure following cardiac surgery and treatment with methicillin. Acta Med Scand 1976;199:305.

70. Gabow PA, Lacher JW, Neff TA. Tubulointerstitial and glomerular nephritis associated with rifampin. report of a case. JAMA 1976;235:2517.

71. Minetti L, Barbiano di Belgioioso G, Busnach G. Immunohistological diagnosis of drug-induced hypersensitivity nephritis. Contrib Nephrol 1978;10:15.

72. Olsen TS, Wassef NF, Olsen HS, Hansen HE. Ultrastructure of the kidney in acute interstitial nephritis. Ultrastruct Pathol 1986;10:1.

73. Joh K, Aizawa S, Yamaguchi Y, et al. Drug-induced hypersensitivity nephritis: Lymphocyte stimulation testing and renal biopsy in 10 cases. Am J Nephrol 1990;10:222.

74. Shibasaki T, Ishimoto F, Sakai O, et al. Clinical characterization of drug-induced allergic nephritis. Am J Nephrol 1991;11:174.

75. Vlasveld LT, van de Wiel-van Kemenade E, de Boer AJ, et al. Possible role for cytotoxic lymphocytes in the pathogenesis of acute interstitial nephritis after recombinant interleukin-2 treatment for renal cell cancer. Cancer Immunol Immunother 1993;36:210.

76. Choi YJ, Chakraborty S, Nguyen V, et al. Peritubular capillary loss is associated with chronic tubulointerstitial injury in human kidney: Altered expression of vascular endothelial growth factor. Hum Pathol 2000;31:1491.

77. Schwarz A, Krause P, Kunzendorf U, et al. The outcome of acute interstitial nephritis: Risk factors for the transition from acute to chronic interstitial nephritis. Clin Nephrol 2003;59:65.

78. Benner EJ. Renal damage associated with prolonged administration of ampicillin, cephaloridine, and cephalothin. Antimicrobial Agents Chemother 1969;9:417.

79. Pickering MJ, Spooner GR, de Quesada A, Cade JR. Declining renal function associated with administration of cephalothin. South Med J 1970;63:426.

80. Foord RD. Cephaloridine, cephalothin and the kidney. J Antimicrob Chemother 1975;1:119.

81. Norrby R, Stenqvist K, Elgefors B. Interaction between cephaloridine and furosemide in man. Scand J Infect Dis 1976;8:209.

82. Fillastre JP, Kleinknecht D. Acute renal failure associated with cephalosporin therapy. Am Heart J 1975;89:809.

83. Burton JR, Lichtenstein NS, Colvin RB, Hyslop NE Jr. Acute renal failure during cephalothin therapy. JAMA 1974;229:679.

84. Engle JE, Drago J, Carlin B, Schoolwerth AC. Letter: Reversible acute renal failure after cephalothin. Ann Intern Med 1975;83:232.

85. Wade JC, Smith CR, Petty BG, et al. Cephalothin plus an aminoglycoside is more nephrotoxic than methicillin plus an aminoglycoside. Lancet 1978;2:604.

86. Dodds MG, Foord RD. Enhancement by potent diuretics of renal tubular necrosis induced by cephaloridine. Br J Pharmacol 1970;40:227.

87. Verma S, Kieff E. Cephalexin-related nephropathy. JAMA 1975;234:618.

88. Barza M. The nephrotoxicity of cephalosporins: An overview. J Infect Dis 1978;137(suppl):S60.

89. Mancini S, Iacovoni R, Fierimonte V, et al. Drug-induced interstitial nephritis. A case report. Minerva Pediatr 1994;46:557.

90. Goddard JK, Janning SW, Gass JS, Wilson RF. Cefuroxime-induced acute renal failure. Pharmacotherapy 1994;14:488.

91. Barrientos A, Bello I, Gutierrez-Millet V. Letter: Renal failure and cephalothin. Ann Intern Med 1976;84:612.

92. Perkins RL, Apicella MA, Lee IS, et al. Cephaloridine and cephalothin: Comparative studies of potential nephrotoxicity. J Lab Clin Med 1968;71:75.

93. Tune BM, Hsu CY. Toxicity of cephaloridine to carnitine transport and fatty acid metabolism in rabbit renal cortical

mitochondria: Structure-activity relationships. J Pharmacol Exp Ther 1994;270:873.

94. Lash LH, Tokarz JJ, Woods EB. Renal cell type specificity of cephalosporin-induced cytotoxicity in suspensions of isolated proximal tubular and distal tubular cells. Toxicology 1994;94:97.

95. Levine BB. Antigenicity and cross-reactivity of penicillins and cephalosporins. J Infect Dis 1973;128(suppl):S364.

96. Saxon A, Hassner A, Swabb EA, et al. Lack of cross-reactivity between aztreonam, a monobactam antibiotic, and penicillin in penicillin-allergic subjects. J Infect Dis 1984;149:16.

97. Hadimeri H, Almroth G, Cederbrant K, et al. Allergic nephropathy associated with norfloxacin and ciprofloxacin therapy. Report of two cases and review of the literature. Scand J Urol Nephrol 1997;31:481.

98. Okada H, Watanabe Y, Kotaki S, et al. An unusual form of crystal-forming chronic interstitial nephritis following long-term exposure to tosufloxacin tosilate. Am J Kidney Dis 2004; 44:902.

99. Allon M, Lopez EJ, Min KW. Acute renal failure due to ciprofloxacin. Arch Intern Med 1990;150:2187.

100. Helmink R, Benediktsson H. Ciprofloxacin-induced allergic interstitial nephritis. Nephron 1990;55:432.

101. Hootkins R, Fenves AZ, Stephens MK. Acute renal failure secondary to oral ciprofloxacin therapy: A presentation of three cases and a review of the literature. Clin Nephrol 1989;32:75.

102. Rastogi S, Atkinson JL, McCarthy JT. Allergic nephropathy associated with ciprofloxacin. Mayo Clin Proc 1990;65:987.

103. Shih DJ, Korbet SM, Rydel JJ, Schwartz MM. Renal vasculitis associated with ciprofloxacin. Am J Kidney Dis 1995;26:516.

104. Lo WK, Rolston KV, Rubenstein EB, Bodey GP. Ciprofloxacin-induced nephrotoxicity in patients with cancer. Arch Intern Med 1993;153:1258.

105. Lien YH, Hansen R, Kern WF, et al. Ciprofloxacin-induced granulomatous interstitial nephritis and localized elastolysis. Am J Kidney Dis 1993;22:598.

106. Garcia-Ortiz R, Espinoza RS, Silva GR, et al. Cloxacillin-induced acute tubulo interstitial nephritis. Ann Pharmacother 1992;26:1241.

107. Soto J, Bosch JM, Alsar Ortiz MJ, et al. Piperacillin-induced acute interstitial nephritis. Nephron 1993;65:154.

108. Pill MW, O'Neill CV, Chapman MM, Singh AK. Suspected acute interstitial nephritis induced by piperacillin-tazobactam. Pharmacotherapy 1997;17:166.

109. Gilbert DN, Gourley R, d'Agostino A, et al. Interstitial nephritis due to methicillin, penicillin and ampicillin. Ann Allergy 1970;28:378.

110. Ruley EJ, Lisi LM. Interstitial nephritis and renal failure due to ampicillin. J Pediatr 1974;84:878.

111. Tannenberg AM, Wicher KJ, Rose NR. Ampicillin nephropathy. JAMA 1971;218:449.

112. Woodroffe AJ, Weldon M, Meadows R, Lawrence JR. Acute interstitial nephritis following ampicillin hypersensitivity. Med J Aust 1975;1:65.

113. Ditlove J, Weidmann P, Bernstein M, Massry SG. Methicillin nephritis. Medicine (Baltimore) 1977;56:483.

114. Jensen HA, Halveg AB, Saunamaki KI. Permanent impairment of renal function after methicillin nephropathy. Br Med J 1971;4:406.

115. Appel GB, Neu HC. The nephrotoxicity of antimicrobial agents (first of three parts). N Engl J Med 1977;296:663.

116. Rennke HG, Roos PC, Wall SG. Drug-induced interstitial nephritis with heavy glomerular proteinuria. N Engl J Med 1980;302: 691.

117. Minetti L, di Belgiojoso GB, Civati G, et al. Drug induced hypersensitivity nephritis. Proc Eur Dial Transplant Assoc 1975; 11:526.

118. Mayaud C, Kanfer A, Kourilsky O, Sraer JD. Letter: Interstitial nephritis after methicillin. N Engl J Med 1975;292:1132.

119. Mery J, Morel-Maroger L. Acute interstitial nephritis: A hypersensitivity reaction to drugs. In: Giovannetti S, Bonomini V, D'Amico, eds. Proceedings of the Sixth International Congress of Nephrology. Basel: Karger, 1976:524.

120. Woodroffe AJ, Thomson NM, Meadows R, Lawrence JR. Nephropathy associated with methicillin administration. Aust N Z J Med 1974;4:256.

121. Hansen ES, Tauris P. Methicillin-induced nephropathy. A case with linear deposition of IgG and C3 on the tubular-basement-membrane. Acta Pathol Microbiol Scand (A) 1976;84:440.

122. Orfila C, Rakotoarivony J, Durand D, Suc JM. A correlative study of immunofluorescence, electron, and light microscopy in immunologically mediated renal tubular disease in man. Nephron 1979;23:14.

123. Pirani CL, Valeri A, D'Agati V, Appel GB. Renal toxicity of nonsteroidal anti-inflammatory drugs. Contrib Nephrol 1987;55: 159.

124. Flynn CT, Rainford DJ, Hope E. Acute renal failure and rifampicin: Danger of unsuspected intermittent dosage. Br Med J 1974;2:482.

125. Muthukumar T, Jayakumar M, Fernando EM, Muthusethupathi MA. Acute renal failure due to rifampicin: A study of 25 patients. Am J Kidney Dis 2002;40:690.

126. Campese VM, Marzullo F, Schena FP, Coratelli P. Acute renal failure during intermittent rifampicin therapy. Nephron 1973;10:256.

127. Cordonnier D, Muller JM. Acute renal failure after rifampicin. Lancet 1972;2:1364.

128. Ramgopal V, Leonard C, Bhathena D. Acute renal failure associated with rifampicin. Lancet 1973;1:1195.

129. Cochran M, Morrhead PJ, Platts M. Letter: Permanent renal damage with rifampicin. Lancet 1975;1:1428.

130. Quinn BP, Wall BM. Nephrogenic diabetes insipidus and tubulointerstitial nephritis during continuous therapy with rifampin. Am J Kidney Dis 1989;14:217.

131. Minetti L, Barbiano di Belgioioso G, et al. Nephritis caused by drug hypersensitivity (DHN). Clinico-histological observations in 15 cases [in Italian]. Minerva Nefrol 1974;21:197.

132. Poole G, Stradling P, Worlledge S. Potentially serious side effects of high-dose twice-weekly rifampicin. Br Med J 1971;3:343.

133. Tomonaga H. Detection of antibody specific to rifampicin metabolite by ELISA–mechanism of sensitization by rifampicin. Arerugi 1993;42:854.

134. French A. Hypersensitivity in the pathogenesis of the histopathologic changes associated with sulfonamide chemotherapy. Am J Pathol 1946;22:679.

135. More R, McMillan G, Duff G. The pathology of sulfonamide allergy in man. Am J Pathol 1946;22:703.

136. Dry J, Leynadier F, Herman D, Pradalier A. Letter: Sulfamethoxazole-trimethoprim combination (cotrimoxazole). Unusual immuno-allergic reaction [in French]. Nouv Presse Med 1975;4:36.

137. Robson M, Levi J, Dolberg L, Rosenfeld JB. Acute tubulo-interstitial nephritis following sulfadiazine therapy. Isr J Med Sci 1970;6:561.

138. Bailey RR, Little PJ. Deterioration in renal function in association with co-trimoxazole therapy. Med J Aust 1976;1:914–916.

139. Kalowski S, Nanra RS, Mathew TH, Kincaid-Smith P. Deterioration in renal function in association with co-trimoxazole therapy. Lancet 1973;1:394.

140. Farina LA, Palou Redorta J, Chechile Toniolo G. Reversible acute renal failure due to sulfonamide-induced lithiasis in an AIDS patient. Arch Esp Urol 1995;48:418.

141. Albala DM, Prien EL Jr, Galal HA. Urolithiasis as a hazard of sulfonamide therapy. J Endourol 1994;8:401.

142. Russinko PJ, Agarwal S, Choi MJ, Kelty PJ. Obstructive nephropathy secondary to sulfasalazine calculi. Urology 2003; 62:748.

143. Dowling H, Lepper M. Toxic reactions following therapy with sulfapyridine, sulfathiazole and sulfadiazine. JAMA 1943; 121:1190.

144. Cryst C, Hammar SP. Acute granulomatous interstitial nephritis due to co-trimoxazole. Am J Nephrol 1988;8:483.

145. Cimino MA, Rotstein C, Slaughter RL, Emrich LJ. Relationship of serum antibiotic concentrations to nephrotoxicity in cancer patients receiving concurrent aminoglycoside and vancomycin therapy. Am J Med 1987;83:1091.

146. Rybak MJ, Albrecht LM, Boike SC, Chandrasekar PH. Nephrotoxicity of vancomycin, alone and with an aminoglycoside. J Antimicrob Chemother 1990;25:679.

147. Nahata MC. Lack of nephrotoxicity in pediatric patients receiving concurrent vancomycin and aminoglycoside therapy. Chemotherapy 1987;33:302.

148. Codding CE, Ramseyer L, Allon M, et al. Tubulointerstitial nephritis due to vancomycin. Am J Kidney Dis 1989;14:512.

149. Wai AO, Lo AM, Abdo A, Marra F. Vancomycin-induced acute interstitial nephritis. Ann Pharmacother 1998;32:1160.

150. Hsu SI. Biopsy-proved acute tubulointerstitial nephritis and toxic epidermal necrolysis associated with vancomycin. Pharmacotherapy 2001;21:1233.

151. Yano Y, Hiraoka A, Oguma T. Enhancement of tobramycin binding to rat renal brush border membrane by vancomycin. J Pharmacol Exp Ther 1995;274:695.

152. Harris RC. Cyclooxygenase-2 in the kidney. J Am Soc Nephrol 2000;11:2387.

153. Galli G, Panzetta G. Do non-steroidal anti-inflammatory drugs and COX-2 selective inhibitors have different renal effects? J nephrol 2002;15:480.

154. Rocha JL, Fernandez-Alonso J. Acute tubulointerstitial nephritis associated with the selective COX-2 enzyme inhibitor, rofecoxib. Lancet 2001;357:1946.

155. Demke D, Zhao S, Arellano FM. Interstitial nephritis associated with celecoxib. Lancet 2001;358:1726.

156. Henao J, Hisamuddin I, Nzerue CM, et al. Celecoxib-induced acute interstitial nephritis. Am J Kidney Dis 2002;39:1313.

157. Alper AB Jr, Meleg-Smith S, Krane NK. Nephrotic syndrome and interstitial nephritis associated with celecoxib. Am J Kidney Dis 2002;40:1086.

158. Brewster UC, Perazella MA. Acute tubulointerstitial nephritis associated with celecoxib. Nephrol Dial Transplant 2004;19:1017.

159. Szalat A, Krasilnikov I, Bloch A, et al. Acute renal failure and interstitial nephritis in a patient treated with rofecoxib: Case report and review of the literature. Arthritis Rheum 2004;51:670.

160. Whelton A, Hamilton CW. Nonsteroidal anti-inflammatory drugs: Effects on kidney function. J Clin Pharmacol 1991;31:588.

161. Whelton A. Nephrotoxicity of nonsteroidal anti-inflammatory drugs: Physiologic foundations and clinical implications. Am J Med 1999;106:13S.

162. Murray MD, Brater DC. Adverse effects of nonsteroidal anti-inflammatory drugs on renal function. Ann Intern Med 1990;112:559.

163. Kleinknecht D, Landais P, Goldfarb B. Analgesic and nonsteroidal anti-inflammatory drug-associated acute renal failure: A prospective collaborative study. Clin Nephrol 1986;25:275.

164. Fox DA, Jick H. Nonsteroidal anti-inflammatory drugs and renal disease. JAMA 1984;251:1299.

165. Bonney SL, Northington RS, Hedrich DA, Walker BR. Renal safety of two analgesics used over the counter: Ibuprofen and aspirin. Clin Pharmacol Ther 1986;40:373.

166. Corwin HL, Bonventre JV. Renal insufficiency associated with nonsteroidal anti-inflammatory agents. Am J Kidney Dis 1984;4:147.

167. Clive DM, Stoff JS. Renal syndromes associated with nonsteroidal antiinflammatory drugs. N Engl J Med 1984;310:563.

168. Palmer BF, Henrich WL. Clinical acute renal failure with nonsteroidal anti-inflammatory drugs. Semin Nephrol 1995;15:214.

169. Marasco WA, Gikas PW, Azziz-Baumgartner R, et al. Ibuprofen-associated renal dysfunction. Pathophysiologic mechanisms of acute renal failure, hyperkalemia, tubular necrosis, and proteinuria. Arch Intern Med 1987;147:2107.

170. Whelton A, Stout RL, Spilman PS, Klassen DK. Renal effects of ibuprofen, piroxicam, and sulindac in patients with asymptomatic renal failure. A prospective, randomized, crossover comparison. Ann Intern Med 1990;112:568.

171. Calvo-Alen J, De Cos MA, Rodriguez-Valverde V, et al. Subclinical renal toxicity in rheumatic patients receiving longterm treatment with nonsteroidal antiinflammatory drugs. J Rheumatol 1994;21:1742.

172. Carmichael J, Shankel SW. Effects of nonsteroidal anti-inflammatory drugs on prostaglandins and renal function. Am J Med 1985;78:992.

173. Kleinknecht D. Interstitial nephritis, the nephrotic syndrome, and chronic renal failure secondary to nonsteroidal anti-inflammatory drugs. Semin Nephrol 1995;15:228.

174. Warren GV, Korbet SM, Schwartz MM, Lewis EJ. Minimal change glomerulopathy associated with nonsteroidal antiinflammatory drugs. Am J Kidney Dis 1989;13:127.

175. Lantz B, Cochat P, Bouchet JL, Fischbach M. Short-term niflumic-acid-induced acute renal failure in children. Nephrol Dial Transplant 1994;9:1234.

176. Kleinknecht D. Diseases of the kidney caused by nonsteroidal anti-inflammatory drugs. In: Stewart J, ed. Analgesic and NSAID-Induced Kidney Disease. Oxford: Oxford University Press, 1993: 160.

177. Kaplan BS, Restaino I, Raval DS, et al. Renal failure in the neonate associated with in utero exposure to non-steroidal anti-inflammatory agents. Pediatr Nephrol 1994;8:700.

178. van der Heijden BJ, Carlus C, Narcy F, et al. Persistent anuria, neonatal death, and renal microcystic lesions after prenatal exposure to indomethacin. Am J Obstet Gynecol 1994;171:617.

179. Voyer LE, Drut R, Mendez JH. Fetal renal maldevelopment with oligohydramnios following maternal use of piroxicam. Pediatr Nephrol 1994;8:592.

180. Ciabattoni G, Cinotti GA, Pierucci A, et al. Effects of sulindac and ibuprofen in patients with chronic glomerular disease. Evidence for the dependence of renal function on prostacyclin. N Engl J Med 1984;310:279.

181. Unsworth J, Sturman S, Lunec J, Blake DR. Renal impairment associated with non-steroidal anti-inflammatory drugs. Ann Rheum Dis 1987;46:233.

182. Gurwitz JH, Avorn J, Ross-Degnan D, Lipsitz LA. Nonsteroidal anti-inflammatory drug-associated azotemia in the very old. JAMA 1990;264:471.

183. Gentilini P. Cirrhosis, renal function and NSAIDs. J Hepatol 1993;19:200.

184. Baisac J, Henrich WL. Nephrotoxicity of nonsteroidal anti-inflammatory drugs. Miner Electrolyte Metab 1994;20:187.

185. Bjorck S. Paracetamol-induced renal tubular cell necrosis. In: Stewart J, ed. Analgesic and NSAID-Induced Kidney Disease. Oxford: Oxford University Press; 1993:174.

186. Blantz RC. Acetaminophen: Acute and chronic effects on renal function. Am J Kidney Dis 1996;28:S3.

187. D'Agati V. Does aspirin cause acute or chronic renal failure in experimental animals and in humans? Am J Kidney Dis 1996;28:S24.

188. Cheng HF, Nolasco F, Cameron JS, et al. HLA-DR display by renal tubular epithelium and phenotype of infiltrate in interstitial nephritis. Nephrol Dial Transplant 1989;4:205.

189. Schwarz A, Krause PH, Keller F, et al. Granulomatous interstitial nephritis after nonsteroidal anti-inflammatory drugs. Am J Nephrol 1988;8:410.

190. Feinfeld DA, Olesnicky L, Pirani CL, Appel GB. Nephrotic syndrome associated with use of the nonsteroidal anti-inflammatory drugs. Case report and review of the literature. Nephron 1984;37:174.

191. Maniglia R, Schwartz AB, Moriber-Katz S. Non-steroidal anti-inflammatory nephrotoxicity. Ann Clin Lab Sci 1988;18:240.

192. Schlondorff D. Renal prostaglandin synthesis. Sites of production and specific actions of prostaglandins. Am J Med 1986;81:1.

193. Anderson RJ, Berl T, McDonald KM, Schrier RW. Prostaglandins: Effects on blood pressure, renal blood flow, sodium and water excretion. Kidney Int 1976;10:205.

194. Zambraski EJ. The effects of nonsteroidal anti-inflammatory drugs on renal function: Experimental studies in animals. Semin Nephrol 1995;15:205.

195. Remuzzi A, Remuzzi G. The effects of nonsteroidal anti-inflammatory drugs on glomerular filtration of proteins and their therapeutic utility. Semin Nephrol 1995;15:236.

196. Spuhler O, Zollinger HU. Chronic interstitial nephritis. Z Klin Med 1953;151:1.

197. Elseviers MM, De Broe ME. A long-term prospective controlled study of analgesic abuse in Belgium. Kidney Int 1995;48:1912.
198. Elseviers MM, Waller I, Nenoy D, et al. Evaluation of diagnostic criteria for analgesic nephropathy in patients with end-stage renal failure: Results of the ANNE study. Analgesic Nephropathy Network of Europe. Nephrol Dial Transplant 1995;10:808.
199. Perneger TV, Whelton PK, Klag MJ. Risk of kidney failure associated with the use of acetaminophen, aspirin, and nonsteroidal antiinflammatory drugs. N Engl J Med 1994;331:1675.
200. Pommer W, Bronder E, Greiser E, et al. Regular analgesic intake and the risk of end-stage renal failure. Am J Nephrol 1989; 9:403.
201. Sandler DP, Smith JC, Weinberg CR, et al. Analgesic use and chronic renal disease. N Engl J Med 1989;320:1238.
202. Elseviers M, De Broe M. The implication of analgesic in human kidney disease. In: Stewart J, ed. Analgesic and NSAID-Induced Kidney Disease. Oxford: Oxford University Press, 1993:32.
203. Gault MH, Wilson DR. Analgesic nephropathy in Canada: Clinical syndrome, management, and outcome. Kidney Int 1978; 13:58.
204. Kincaid-Smith P. Analgesic nephropathy and the effect of nonsteroidal anti-inflammatory drugs on the kidney. In: Catto G, ed. Drugs and the Kidney. Dordrecht: Kluwer Academic, 1990:1.
205. Gonwa TA, Hamilton RW, Buckalew VM Jr. Chronic renal failure and end-stage renal disease in northwest North Carolina. Importance of analgesic-associated nephropathy. Arch Intern Med 1981;141:462.
206. Elseviers M, De Broe M. Epidemiology of analgesic nephropathy. J nephrol 1992;5:94.
207. Schwarz A, Preuschof L, Zellner D. Incidence of analgesic nephropathy in Berlin since 1983. Nephrol Dial Transplant 1999;14:109.
208. Michielsen P, de Schepper P. Trends of analgesic nephropathy in two high-endemic regions with different legislation. J Am Soc Nephrol 2001;12:550.
209. Feinstein AR, Heinemann LA, Curhan GC, et al. Relationship between nonphenacetin combined analgesics and nephropathy: A review. Ad Hoc Committee of the International Study Group on Analgesics and Nephropathy. Kidney Int 2000;58: 2259.
210. Kurth T, Glynn RJ, Walker AM, et al. Analgesic use and change in kidney function in apparently healthy men. Am J Kidney Dis 2003;42:234.
211. Schnuelle P, Van Der Woude FJ. Analgesics and renal disease in the postphenacetin era. Am J Kidney Dis 2003;42:385.
212. Nanra R. Functional defects in analgesic nephropathy. In: Stewart J, ed. Analgesic and NSAID-Induced Kidney Disease. Oxford: Oxford University Press, 1993: 102.
213. Griffin MD, Bergstralhn EJ, Larson TS. Renal papillary necrosis—a sixteen-year clinical experience. J Am Soc Nephrol 1995;6:248.
214. De Broe ME, Elseviers MM. Analgesic nephropathy. N Engl J Med 1998;338:446.
215. Burry A. Pathology of analgesic nephropathy: Australian experience. Kidney Int 1978;13:34.
216. Mihatsch M, Zollinger H. The pathology of analgesic nephropathy. In: Stewart J, ed. Analgesic and NSAID-Induced Kidney Disease. Oxford: Oxford University Press; 1993:67.
217. Berneis K, Korteweg E, Mihatsch MJ. Characterization of the brown pigment of the mucosa of the urinary tract. Virchows Arch A Pathol Anat Histopathol 1983;402:203.
218. Gloor F. Capillary sclerosis of the urinary tract caused by abuse of an analgesic agent (phenacetin) [in German]. Pathologe 1982;3:132.
219. Mihatsch MJ, Hofer HO, Gudat F, et al. Capillary sclerosis of the urinary tract and analgesic nephropathy. Clin Nephrol 1983;20:285.
220. Mihatsch MJ, Torhorst J, Steinmann E, et al. The morphologic diagnosis of analgesic (phenacetin) abuse. Pathol Res Pract 1979;164:68.
221. Burry A. The evolution of analgesic nephropathy. Nephron 1967;5:185.
222. Kincaid-Smith P. Pathogenesis of the renal lesion associated with the abuse of analgesics. Lancet 1967;1:859.
223. Zollinger H. Niere und albeitende Harnwege. Berlin: Springer Verlag, 1966.
224. Kincaid-Smith P, Saker BM, McKenzie IF, Muriden KD. Lesions in the blood supply of the papilla in experimental analgesic nephropathy. Med J Aust 1968;1:203.
225. Molland EA. Experimental renal papillary necrosis. Kidney Int 1978;13:5.
226. Lagergren C, Ljungqvist A. The intrarenal arterial pattern in renal papillary necrosis. A micro-angiographic and histologic study. Am J Pathol 1962;41:633.
227. Prescott LF. Analgesic nephropathy: A reassessment of the role of phenacetin and other analgesics. Drugs 1982;23:75.
228. Duggin GG. Mechanisms in the development of analgesic nephropathy. Kidney Int 1980;18:553.
229. Duggin GG. Combination analgesic-induced kidney disease: The Australian experience. Am J Kidney Dis 1996;28:S39.
230. Moeckel GW, Zhang L, Fogo AB, et al. COX2 activity promotes organic osmolyte accumulation and adaptation of renal medullary interstitial cells to hypertonic stress. J Biol Chem 2003;278:19352.
231. Li C, Liu J, Saavedra JE, et al. The nitric oxide donor, V-PYRRO/NO, protects against acetaminophen-induced nephrotoxicity in mice. Toxicology 2003;189:173.
232. Ahmed MH, Ashton N, Balment RJ. Renal function in a rat model of analgesic nephropathy: Effect of chloroquine. J Pharmacol Exp Ther 2003;305:123.
233. Goncalves AR, Fujihara CK, Mattar AL, et al. Renal expression of COX-2, ANG II, and AT1 receptor in remnant kidney: Strong renoprotection by therapy with losartan and a nonsteroidal anti-inflammatory. Am J Physiol Renal Physiol 2004;286: F945.
234. Schnellmann RG. Analgesic nephropathy in rodents. J Toxicol Environ Health B Crit Rev 1998;1:81.
235. Credie M. Analgesics as human carcinogens: Clinical and epidemiological evidence. In: Stewart J, ed. Analgesic and NSAID-Induced Kidney Disease. Oxford: Oxford University Press, 1993: 211.
236. Mihatsch MJ, Knusli C. Phenacetin abuse and malignant tumors. An autopsy study covering 25 years (1953–1977). Klin Wochenschr 1982;60:1339.
237. Taylor J. Carcinoma of the renal pelvis. In: Stewart J, ed. Analgesic and NSAID-Induced Kidney Disease. Oxford: Oxford University Press, 1993:211.
238. Chow WH, McLaughlin JK, Linet MS, et al. Use of analgesics and risk of renal cell cancer. Int J Cancer 1994;59:467.
239. Van Staa TP, Travis S, Leufkens HG, Logan RF. 5-Aminosalicylic acids and the risk of renal disease: A large British epidemiologic study. Gastroenterology 2004;126:1733.
240. Ransford RA, Langman MJ. Sulphasalazine and mesalazine: Serious adverse reactions re-evaluated on the basis of suspected adverse reaction reports to the committee on safety of medicines. Gut 2002;51:536.
241. Arend LJ, Springate JE. Interstitial nephritis from mesalazine: Case report and literature review. Pediatr Nephrol 2004;19: 550.
242. Agarwal BN, Cabebe FG, Hoffman BI. Diphenylhydantoin-induced acute renal failure. Nephron 1977;18:249.
243. Hyman LR, Ballow M, Knieser MR. Diphenylhydantoin interstitial nephritis. Roles of cellular and humoral immunologic injury. J Pediatr 1978;92:915.
244. Matson JR, Krous HF, Blackstock R. Diphenylhydantoin-induced hypersensitivity reaction with interstitial nephritis. Hum Pathol 1985;16:94.
245. Gaffey CM, Chun B, Harvey JC, Manz HJ. Phenytoin-induced systemic granulomatous vasculitis. Arch Pathol Lab Med 1986; 110:131.
246. Walker RG. Lithium nephrotoxicity. Kidney Int 1993;42(suppl): S93.
247. Presne C, Fakhouri F, Noel LH, et al. Lithium-induced nephropathy: Rate of progression and prognostic factors. Kidney Int 2003;64:585.

248. Bucht G, Wahlin A, Wentzel T, Winblad B. Renal function and morphology in long-term lithium and combined lithium-neuroleptic treatment. Acta Med Scand 1980;208:381.

249. Hestbech J, Hansen HE, Amdisen A, Olsen S. Chronic renal lesions following long-term treatment with lithium. Kidney Int 1977;12:205.

250. Cox M. Lithium in the kidney. Kidney Int 1981;19:379.

251. Jorkasky DK, Amsterdam JD, Oler J, et al. Lithium-induced renal disease: A prospective study. Clin Nephrol 1988;30:293.

252. Walker R, Edwards J. Lithium and the kidney: An update [editorial]. Psychol Med 1989;19:825.

253. Tam VK, Green J, Schwieger J, Cohen AH. Nephrotic syndrome and renal insufficiency associated with lithium therapy. Am J Kidney Dis 1996;27:715.

254. Markowitz GS, Radhakrishnan J, Kambham N, et al. Lithium nephrotoxicity: A progressive combined glomerular and tubulointerstitial nephropathy. J Am Soc Nephrol 2000;11:1439.

255. Dias N, Hocken AG. Oliguric renal failure complicating lithium carbonate therapy. Nephron 1973;10:246.

256. Lavender S, Brown JN, Berrill WT. Acute renal failure and lithium intoxication. Postgrad Med J 1973;49:277.

257. Aurell M, Svalander C, Wallin L, Alling C. Renal function and biopsy findings in patients on long-term lithium treatment. Kidney Int 1981;20:663.

258. Kincaid-Smith P, Burrows GD, Davies BM, et al. Renal-biopsy findings in lithium and prelithium patients. Lancet 1979;2:700.

259. Walker RG, Escott M, Birchall I, et al. Chronic progressive renal lesions induced by lithium. Kidney Int 1986;29:875.

260. Walker RG, Bennett WM, Davies BM, Kincaid-Smith P. Structural and functional effects of long-term lithium therapy. Kidney Int Suppl 1982;11:S13.

261. Santella RN, Rimmer JM, MacPherson BR. Focal segmental glomerulosclerosis in patients receiving lithium carbonate. Am J Med 1988;84:951.

262. Christensen BM, Marples D, Kim YH, et al. Changes in cellular composition of kidney collecting duct cells in rats with lithium-induced NDI. Am J Physiol Cell Physiol 2004;286:C952.

263. Myers RP, McLaughlin K, Hollomby DJ. Acute interstitial nephritis due to omeprazole. Am J Gastroenterol 2001;96:3428.

264. Delve P, Lau M, Yun K, Walker R. Omeprazole-induced acute interstitial nephritis. N Z Med J 2003;116:U332.

265. Moore I, Sayer JA, Nayar A, et al. Pantoprazole-induced acute interstitial nephritis. J Nephrol 2004;17:580.

266. Torpey N, Barker T, Ross C. Drug-induced tubulo-interstitial nephritis secondary to proton pump inhibitors: Experience from a single UK renal unit. Nephrol Dial Transplant 2004;19:1441.

267. Geevasinga N, Kairaitis L, Rangan GK, Coleman PL. Acute interstitial nephritis secondary to esomeprazole. Med J Aust 2005;182:235.

268. Sarcletti M, Petter A, Zangerle R. Indinavir and interstitial nephritis. Ann Intern Med 1998;128:320.

269. Olyaei AJ, deMattos AM, Bennett WM. Renal toxicity of protease inhibitors. Curr Opin Nephrol Hypertens 2000;9:473.

270. Jaradat M, Phillips C, Yum MN, et al. Acute tubulointerstitial nephritis attributable to indinavir therapy. Am J Kidney Dis 2000;35:E16.

271. Brewster UC, Perazella MA. Acute interstitial nephritis associated with atazanavir, a new protease inhibitor. Am J Kidney Dis 2004;44:e81.

272. Wuthrich RP, Sibalic V. Autoimmune tubulointerstitial nephritis: Insight from experimental models. Exp Nephrol 1998;6:288.

273. Miller K, Michael AF. Immunopathology of renal extracellular membranes in diabetes mellitus: Specificity of tubular basement-membrane immunofluorescence. Diabetes 1976;25:701.

274. Lehman DH, Wilson CB, Dixon FJ. Extraglomerular immunoglobulin deposits in human nephritis. Am J Med 1975;58:765.

275. Clayman MD, Martinez-Hernandez A, Michaud L, et al. Isolation and characterization of the nephritogenic antigen producing anti-tubular basement membrane disease. J Exp Med 1985;161:290.

276. Brentjens JR, Matsuo S, Fukatsu A, et al. Immunologic studies in two patients with antitubular basement membrane nephritis. Am J Med 1989;86:603.

277. Nelson TR, Charonis AS, McIvor RS, Butkowski RJ. Identification of a cDNA encoding tubulointerstitial nephritis antigen. J Biol Chem 1995;270:16265.

278. Bergstein J, Litman N. Interstitial nephritis with anti-tubular-basement-membrane antibody. N Engl J Med 1975;292:875.

279. Rakotoarivony J, Orfila C, Segonds A, et al. Human and experimental nephropathies associated with antibodies to tubular basement membrane. Adv Nephrol Necker Hosp 1981;10:187.

280. Freycon MT, Gilly J, Bouvier R, Braye A. Familial chronic tubulointerstitial nephritis with antibodies to the tubular basement membrane [in French]. Pediatrie 1982;37:371.

281. Helczynski L, Landing BH. Tubulointerstitial renal diseases of children: Pathologic features and pathogenetic mechanisms in Fanconi's familial nephronophthisis, antitubular basement membrane antibody disease, and medullary cyst disease. Pediatr Pathol 1984;2:1.

282. Kalluri R, Wilson CB, Weber M, et al. Identification of the alpha 3 chain of type IV collagen as the common autoantigen in antibasement membrane disease and Goodpasture syndrome. J Am Soc Nephrol 1995;6:1178.

283. Andres G, Brentjens J, Kohli R, et al. Histology of human tubulointerstitial nephritis associated with antibodies to renal basement membranes. Kidney Int 1978;13:480.

284. Biancone L, Andres G, Stamenkovic I. Autoimmune disease of the kidney: An update. Proc Soc Exp Biol Med 1996;212:225.

284a. Graindorge PP, Mahieu PR. Radioimmunologic method for detection of antitubular basement membrane antibodies. Kidney Int 1978;14:594.

285. Border WA, Baehler RW, Bhathena D, Glassock RJ. IgA antibasement membrane nephritis with pulmonary hemorrhage. Ann Intern Med 1979;91:21.

286. Merkel F, Kalluri R, Marx M, et al. Autoreactive T-cells in Goodpasture's syndrome recognize the N-terminal NC1 domain on alpha 3 type IV collagen. Kidney Int 1996;49:1127.

287. Levy M, Guesry P, Loirat C, et al. Immunologically mediated tubulo-interstitial nephritis in children. Contrib Nephrol 1979;16:132.

288. Katz A, Fish AJ, Santamaria P, et al. Role of antibodies to tubulointerstitial nephritis antigen in human anti-tubular basement membrane nephritis associated with membranous nephropathy. Am J Med 1992;93:691.

289. Makker S, Widstrom R, Huang J. Characterization of glomerular antigen of membranous nephropathy (MN) in the syndrome of MN, tubulointerstitial nephritis (TN) and Fanconi syndrome. J Am Soc Nephrol 1995;6:925.

290. Tay AH, Ren EC, Murugasu B, et al. Membranous nephropathy with anti-tubular basement membrane antibody may be X-linked. Pediatr Nephrol 2000;14:747.

291. Kerjaschki D, Farquhar MG. Immunocytochemical localization of the Heymann nephritis antigen (GP330) in glomerular epithelial cells of normal Lewis rats. J Exp Med 1983;157:667.

292. Ivanyi B, Haszon I, Endreffy E, et al. Childhood membranous nephropathy, circulating antibodies to the 58-kD TIN antigen, and anti-tubular basement membrane nephritis: An 11-year follow-up. Am J Kidney Dis 1998;32:1068.

293. Rotellar C, Noel LH, Droz D, et al. Role of antibodies directed against tubular basement membranes in human renal transplantation. Am J Kidney Dis 1986;7:157.

294. Klassen J, Kano K, Milgrom F, et al. Tubular lesions produced by autoantibodies to tubular basement membrane in human renal allografts. Int Arch Allergy Appl Immunol 1973;45:675.

295. Wilson CB, Lehman DH, McCoy RC, et al. Antitubular basement membrane antibodies after renal transplantation. Transplantation 1974;18:447.

296. Morel-Maroger L, Kourilsky O, Mignon F, Richet G. Antitubular basement membrane antibodies in rapidly progressive poststreptococcal glomerulonephritis: Report of a case. Clin Immunol Immunopathol 1974;2:185.

297. Makker SP. Tubular basement membrane antibody-induced interstitial nephritis in systemic lupus erythematosus. Am J Med 1980;69:949.

298. Dixit MP, Scott KM, Bracamonte E, et al. Kimura disease with advanced renal damage with anti-tubular basement membrane antibody. Pediatr Nephrol 2004;19:1404.

299. Hannigan NR, Jabs K, Perez-Atayde AR, Rosen S. Autoimmune interstitial nephritis and hepatitis in polyglandular autoimmune syndrome. Pediatr Nephrol 1996;10:511.

300. Yoshioka K, Hino S, Takemura T, et al. Isolation and characterization of the tubular basement membrane antigen associated with human tubulo-interstitial nephritis. Clin Exp Immunol 1992;90:319.

301. Butkowski RJ, Kleppel MM, Katz A, et al. Distribution of tubulointerstitial nephritis antigen and evidence for multiple forms. Kidney Int 1991;40:838.

302. Miyazato H, Yoshioka K, Hino S, et al. The target antigen of anti-tubular basement membrane antibody-mediated interstitial nephritis. Autoimmunity 1994;18:259.

303. Kalfa TA, Thull JD, Butkowski RJ, Charonis AS. Tubulointerstitial nephritis antigen interacts with laminin and type IV collagen and promotes cell adhesion. J Biol Chem 1994;269:1654.

304. Chen Y, Krishnamurti U, Wayner EA, et al. Receptors in proximal tubular epithelial cells for tubulointerstitial nephritis antigen. Kidney Int 1996;49:153.

305. Kanwar YS, Kumar A, Yang Q, et al. Tubulointerstitial nephritis antigen: An extracellular matrix protein that selectively regulates tubulogenesis vs. glomerulogenesis during mammalian renal development. Proc Natl Acad Sci U S A 1999;96:11323.

306. Yoshioka K, Takemura T, Hattori S. Tubulointerstitial nephritis antigen: Primary structure, expression and role in health and disease. Nephron 2002;90:1.

307. Yoshioka K, Kleppel M, Fish AJ. Analysis of nephritogenic antigens in human glomerular basement membrane by two-dimensional gel electrophoresis. J Immunol 1985;134:3831.

308. Tang WW, Feng L, Mathison JC, Wilson CB. Cytokine expression, upregulation of intercellular adhesion molecule-1, and leukocyte infiltration in experimental tubulointerstitial nephritis. Lab Invest 1994;70:631.

309. Neilson EG. Pathogenesis and therapy of interstitial nephritis. Kidney Int 1989;35:1257.

310. Ellis D, Fisher SE, Smith WI Jr, Jaffe R. Familial occurrence of renal and intestinal disease associated with tissue autoantibodies. Am J Dis Child 1982;136:323.

311. Hyun J, Galen MA. Acute interstitial nephritis. A case characterized by increase in serum IgG, IgM, and IgE concentrations. Eosinophilia, and IgE deposition in renal tubules. Arch Intern Med 1981;141:679.

312. Tokumoto M, Fukuda K, Shinozaki M, et al. Acute interstitial nephritis with immune complex deposition and MHC class II antigen presentation along the tubular basement membrane. Nephrol Dial Transplant 1999;14:2210.

313. Takeda S, Haratake J, Kasai T, et al. IgG4-associated idiopathic tubulointerstitial nephritis complicating autoimmune pancreatitis. Nephrol Dial Transplant 2004;19:474.

314. Markowitz GS, Fine PL, Kunis CL, et al. Polyclonal immunoglobulin G deposition diseas: A unique entity. Am J Kidney Dis 1998;32:328.

315. Brentjens JR, Sepulveda M, Baliah T, et al. Interstitial immune complex nephritis in patients with systemic lupus erythematosus. Kidney Int 1975;7:342.

316. Park MH, D'Agati V, Appel GB, Pirani CL. Tubulointerstitial disease in lupus nephritis: Relationship to immune deposits, interstitial inflammation, glomerular changes, renal function, and prognosis. Nephron 1986;44:309.

317. Schwartz MM, Fennell JS, Lewis EJ. Pathologic changes in the renal tubule in systemic lupus erythematosus. Hum Pathol 1982;13:534.

318. Biesecker G, Katz S, Koffler D. Renal localization of the membrane attack complex in systemic lupus erythematosus nephritis. J Exp Med 1981;154:1779.

319. Pijpe J, Vissink A, Van der Wal JE, Kallenberg CG. Interstitial nephritis with infiltration of IgG-kappa positive plasma cells in a patient with Sjögren's syndrome. Rheumatology (Oxford) 2004;43:108.

320. Tung K, Black W. Association of renal glomerular and tubular immune complex disease and antitubular basement membrane antibody. Lab Invest 1975;32:696.

321. Douglas MF, Rabideau DP, Schwartz MM, Lewis EJ. Evidence of autologous immune-complex nephritis. N Engl J Med 1981;305:1326.

322. Cavallo T. Membranous nephropathy. insights from Heymann nephritis. Am J Pathol 1994;144:651.

323. Markowitz GS, Kambham N, Maruyama S, et al. Membranous glomerulopathy with Bowman's capsular and tubular basement membrane deposits. Clin Nephrol 2000;54:478.

324. Ohsawa I, Ohi H, Fujita T, et al. Glomerular and extraglomerular immune complex deposits in a bone marrow transplant recipient. Am J Kidney Dis 2000;36:E3.

324a. Cornell LD, Chicano SL, Deshpande V, et al. IgGt immune complex tubulointerstitio nephritis associated with autoimmune pancreatitis. Lab Invest 2006;86:261A.

325. Adeyi OA, Sethi S, Rennke HG. Fibrillary glomerulonephritis: A report of 2 cases with extensive glomerular and tubular deposits. Hum Pathol 2001;32:660.

326. Kerjaschki D, Farquhar MG. The pathogenic antigen of Heymann nephritis is a membrane glycoprotein of the renal proximal tubule brush border. Proc Natl Acad Sci U S A 1982;79:5557.

327. Kerjaschki D. Molecular pathogenesis of membranous nephropathy. Kidney Int 1992;41:1090.

328. Nobel R, Andres G, Brentjens J. Passively transferred anti-brush border antibodies induce injury of proximal tubules in absence of complement. Clin Exp Immunol 1983;56:281.

329. Hoyer JR. Tubulointerstitial immune complex nephritis in rats immunized with Tamm-Horsfall protein. Kidney Int 1980;17:284.

330. Fasth A, Hoyer JR, Seiler MW. Renal tubular immune complex formation in mice immunized with Tamm-Horsfall protein. Am J Pathol 1986;125:555.

331. Seiler MW, Hoyer JR. Ultrastructural studies of tubulointerstitial immune complex nephritis in rats immunized with Tamm-Horsfall protein. Lab Invest 1981;45:321.

332. Fasth AL, Hoyer JR, Seiler MW. Extratubular Tamm-Horsfall protein deposits induced by ureteral obstruction in mice. Clin Immunol Immunopathol 1988;47:47.

333. Benkovic J, Jelakovic B, Cikes N. Antibodies to Tamm-Horsfall protein in patients with acute pyelonephritis. Eur J Clin Chem Clin Biochem 1994;32:337.

334. Fasth A, Ahlstedt S, Hanson LA, et al. Cross-reactions between the Tamm-Horsfall glycoprotein and Escherichia coli. Int Arch Allergy Appl Immunol 1980;63:303.

335. Faaber P, Rijke TP, van de Putte LB, et al. Cross-reactivity of human and murine anti-DNA antibodies with heparan sulfate. The major glycosaminoglycan in glomerular basement membranes. J Clin Invest 1986;77:1824.

336. Thomas DB, Davies M, Williams JD. Tamm-Horsfall protein: An aetiological agent in tubulointerstitial disease? Exp Nephrol 1993;1:281.

337. Nath KA, Hostetter MK, Hostetter TH. Pathophysiology of chronic tubulo-interstitial disease in rats. Interactions of dietary acid load, ammonia, and complement component C3. J Clin Invest 1985;76:667.

338. Dobrin RS, Vernier RL, Fish AL. Acute eosinophilic interstitial nephritis and renal failure with bone marrow-lymph node granulomas and anterior uveitis. A new syndrome. Am J Med 1975;59:325.

339. Spital A, Panner BJ, Sterns RH. Acute idiopathic tubulointerstitial nephritis: Report of two cases and review of the literature. Am J Kidney Dis 1987;9:71.

340. Ten RM, Torres VE, Milliner DS, et al. Acute interstitial nephritis: Immunologic and clinical aspects. Mayo Clin Proc 1988;63:921.

341. Takemura T, Okada M, Hino S, et al. Course and outcome of tubulointerstitial nephritis and uveitis syndrome. Am J Kidney Dis 1999;34:1016.

342. Wakaki H, Sakamoto H, Awazu M. Tubulointerstitial nephritis and uveitis syndrome with autoantibody directed to renal tubular cells. Pediatrics 2001;107:1443.

343. Howarth L, Gilbert RD, Bass P, Deshpande PV. Tubulointerstitial nephritis and uveitis in monozygotic twin boys. Pediatr Nephrol 2004;19:917.

344. Burnier M, Jaeger P, Campiche M, Wauters JP. Idiopathic acute interstitial nephritis and uveitis in the adult. report of 1 case and review of the literature. Am J Nephrol 1986;6:312.

345. Iida H, Terada Y, Nishino A, et al. Acute interstitial nephritis with bone marrow granulomas and uveitis. Nephron 1985;40:108.

346. Morino M, Inami K, Kobayashi T, et al. Acute tubulointerstitial nephritis in two siblings and concomitant uveitis in one. Acta Paediatr Jpn 1991;33:93.

347. Lessard M, Smith JD. Fanconi syndrome with uveitis in an adult woman. Am J Kidney Dis 1989;13:158.

348. Hirano K, Tomino Y, Mikami H, et al. A case of acute tubulointerstitial nephritis and uveitis syndrome with a dramatic response to corticosteroid therapy. Am J Nephrol 1989;9:499.

349. Itami N, Akutsu Y, Yasoshima K, et al. Acute tubulointerstitial nephritis with uveitis. Arch Intern Med 1990;150:688.

350. Yoshioka K, Takemura T, Kanasaki M, et al. Acute interstitial nephritis and uveitis syndrome: Activated immune cell infiltration in the kidney. Pediatr Nephrol 1991;5:232.

351. Van Acker KJ, Buyssens N, Neetens A, et al. Acute tubulo-interstitial nephritis with uveitis. Acta Paediatr Belg 1980;33:171.

352. Kikkawa Y, Sakurai M, Mano T, et al. Interstitial nephritis with concomitant uveitis. report of two cases. Contrib Nephrol 1975;4:1.

353. Gianviti A, Greco M, Barsotti P, Rizzoni G. Acute tubulointerstitial nephritis occurring with 1-year lapse in identical twins. Pediatr Nephrol 1994;8:427.

354. Hannedouche T, Grateau G, Noel LH, et al. Renal granulomatous sarcoidosis: Report of six cases. Nephrol Dial Transplant 1990;5:18.

355. Muther RS, McCarron DA, Bennett WM. Granulomatous sarcoid nephritis: A cause of multiple renal tubular abnormalities. Clin Nephrol 1980;14:190.

356. Ricker W, Clark M. Sarcoidosis: A clinicopathologic review of 300 cases including 22 autopsies. Am J Clin Pathol 1949;19:725.

357. Richmond JM, Chambers B, D'Apice AJ, et al. Renal disease and sarcoidosis. Med J Aust 1981;2:36.

358. Longcope WT, Freiman DG. A study of sarcoidosis; based on a combined investigation of 160 cases including 30 autopsies from the Johns Hopkins Hospital and Massachusetts General Hospital. Medicine (Baltimore) 1952;31:1.

359. Bergner R, Hoffmann M, Waldherr R, Uppenkamp M. Frequency of kidney disease in chronic sarcoidosis. Sarcoidosis Vasc Diffuse Lung Dis 2003;20:126.

360. Gobel U, Kettritz R, Schneider W, Luft F. The protean face of renal sarcoidosis. J Am Soc Nephrol 2001;12:616.

361. Brause M, Magnusson K, Degenhardt S, et al. Renal involvement in sarcoidosis—a report of 6 cases. Clin Nephrol 2002;57:142.

362. Ito Y, Suzuki T, Mizuno M, et al. A case of renal sarcoidosis showing central necrosis and abnormal expression of angiotensin converting enzyme in the granuloma. Clin Nephrol 1994;42:331.

363. Farge D, Liote F, Turner M, et al. Granulomatous nephritis and chronic renal failure in sarcoidosis. Long-term follow-up studies in two patients. Am J Nephrol 1986;6:21.

364. Mignon F, Mery JP, Mougenot B, et al. Granulomatous interstitial nephritis. Adv Nephrol Necker Hosp 1984;13:219.

365. Fauci AS, Wolff SM. Wegener's granulomatosis: Studies in eighteen patients and a review of the literature 1973. Medicine (Baltimore) 1994;73:315.

366. Caruana RJ, Carr AA, Rao RN. Idiopathic granulomatous nephritis in a patient with hypertension and an atrophic kidney. Nephron 1982;32:83.

367. Okada H, Konishi K, Suzuki H, et al. Steroid-responsive renal insufficiency due to idiopathic granulomatous tubulointerstitial nephritis. Am J Nephrol 1993;13:164.

368. O'Riordan E, Willert RP, Reeve R, et al. Isolated sarcoid granulomatous interstitial nephritis: Review of five cases at one center. Clin Nephrol 2001;55:297.

369. Robson MG, Banerjee D, Hopster D, Cairns HS. Seven cases of granulomatous interstitial nephritis in the absence of extrarenal sarcoid. Nephrol Dial Transplant 2003;18:280.

370. Thumfart J, Muller D, Rudolph B, et al. Isolated sarcoid granulomatous interstitial nephritis responding to infliximab therapy. Am J Kidney Dis 2005;45:411.

371. Pichler R, Giachelli C, Young B, et al. The pathogenesis of tubulointerstitial disease associated with glomerulonephritis: The glomerular cytokine theory. Miner Electrolyte Metab 1995;21:317.

372. Strutz F, Neilson EG. The role of lymphocytes in the progression of interstitial disease. Kidney Int 1994;45(suppl):S106.

373. Dodd S. The pathogenesis of tubulointerstitial disease and mechanisms of fibrosis. Curr Top Pathol 1995;88:51.

374. Roy-Chaudhury P, Wu B, King G, et al. Adhesion molecule interactions in human glomerulonephritis: Importance of the tubulointerstitium. Kidney Int 1996;49:127.

375. Kliem V, Johnson RJ, Alpers CE, et al. Mechanisms involved in the pathogenesis of tubulointerstitial fibrosis in 5/6-nephrectomized rats. Kidney Int 1996;49:666.

376. Boucher A, Droz D, Adafer E, Noel LH. Characterization of mononuclear cell subsets in renal cellular interstitial infiltrates. Kidney Int 1986;29:1043.

377. Husby G, Tung KS, Williams RC Jr. Characterization of renal tissue lymphocytes in patients with interstitial nephritis. Am J Med 1981;70:31.

378. Neilson EG. The nephritogenic T lymphocyte response in interstitial nephritis. Semin Nephrol 1993;13:496.

379. McCluskey RT, Bhan AK. Cell-mediated immunity in renal disease. Hum Pathol 1986;17:146.

380. Rubin-Kelley VE, Jevnikar AM. Antigen presentation by renal tubular epithelial cells. J Am Soc Nephrol 1991;2:13.

381. Haas C, Ryffel B, Aguet M, Le Hir M. MHC antigens in interferon gamma (IFN gamma) receptor deficient mice: IFN gamma-dependent up-regulation of MHC class II in renal tubules. Kidney Int 1995;48:1721.

382. Unanue ER, Allen PM. The basis for the immunoregulatory role of macrophages and other accessory cells. Science 1987;236:551.

383. Kelley VR, Singer GG. The antigen presentation function of renal tubular epithelial cells. Exp Nephrol 1993;1:102.

384. Shimokado K, Raines EW, Madtes DK, et al. A significant part of macrophage-derived growth factor consists of at least two forms of PDGF. Cell 1985;43:277.

385. Wahl SM, Hunt DA, Wakefield LM, et al. Transforming growth factor type beta induces monocyte chemotaxis and growth factor production. Proc Natl Acad Sci U S A 1987;84:5788.

386. Postlethwaite A, Seyer J, Kang A. Chemotactic attraction of human fibroblasts to type I, II, III collagens and collagen-derived peptides. Proc Natl Acad Sci 1978;75:871.

387. Roberts AB, Flanders KC, Kondaiah P, et al. Transforming growth factor beta: Biochemistry and roles in embryogenesis, tissue repair and remodeling, and carcinogenesis. Recent Prog Horm Res 1988;44:157.

388. Tang WW, Ulich TR, Lacey DL, et al. Platelet-derived growth factor-BB induces renal tubulointerstitial myofibroblast formation and tubulointerstitial fibrosis. Am J Pathol 1996;148:1169.

389. Bornstein P, Sage H. Regulation of collagen gene expression. Prog Nucleic Acid Res Mol Biol 1989;37:67.

390. Schmidt JA, Mizel SB, Cohen D, Green I. Interleukin 1, a potential regulator of fibroblast proliferation. J Immunol 1982;128:2177.

391. Vilcek J, Palombella VJ, Henriksen-DeStefano D, et al. Fibroblast growth enhancing activity of tumor necrosis factor and its relationship to other polypeptide growth factors. J Exp Med 1986;163:632.

392. Newman LS. Occupational illness. N Engl J Med 1995;333:1128.

393. Lockitch G. Perspectives on lead toxicity. Clin Biochem 1993;26:371.

394. Ibels LS, Pollock CA. Lead intoxication. Med Toxicol 1986;1:387.

395. Borjesson J, Mattsson S. Toxicology; in vivo x-ray fluorescence

for the assessment of heavy metal concentrations in man. Appl Radiat Isot 1995;46:571.

396. Bernard BP, Becker CE. Environmental lead exposure and the kidney. J Toxicol Clin Toxicol 1988;26:1.

397. Inglis JA, Henderson DA, Emmerson BT. The pathology and pathogenesis of chronic lead nephropathy occurring in Queensland. J Pathol 1978;124:65.

398. Wedeen RP, Malik DK, Batuman V. Detection and treatment of occupational lead nephropathy. Arch Intern Med 1979;139:53.

399. Goyer RA. Effect of toxic, chemical, and environmental factors on the kidney. Monogr Pathol 1979;20:202.

400. Bennett WM. Lead nephropathy. Kidney Int 1985;28:212.

401. Cooper WC. Deaths from chronic renal disease in U.S. battery and lead production workers. Environ Health Perspect 1988;78:61.

402. Yu CC, Lin JL, Lin-Tan DT. Environmental exposure to lead and progression of chronic renal diseases: A four-year prospective longitudinal study. J Am Soc Nephrol 2004;15:1016.

403. Perazella MA. Lead and the kidney: Nephropathy, hypertension, and gout. Conn Med 1996;60:521.

404. Weaver VM, Jaar BG, Schwartz BS, et al. Associations among lead dose biomarkers, uric acid, and renal function in Korean lead workers. Environ Health Perspect 2005;113:36.

405. Hu H, Aro A, Payton M, et al. The relationship of bone and blood lead to hypertension. The Normative Aging Study. JAMA 1996;275:1171.

406. Moel DI, Sachs HK. Renal function 17 to 23 years after chelation therapy for childhood plumbism. Kidney Int 1992;42:1226.

407. Staessen JA, Lauwerys RR, Buchet JP, et al. Impairment of renal function with increasing blood lead concentrations in the general population. The Cadmibel Study Group. N Engl J Med 1992;327:151.

408. Hong CD, Hanenson IB, Lerner S, et al. Occupational exposure to lead: Effects on renal function. Kidney Int 1980;18:489.

409. Batuman V. Lead nephropathy, gout, and hypertension. Am J Med Sci 1993;305:241.

410. Sharp DS, Becker CE, Smith AH. Chronic low-level lead exposure. Its role in the pathogenesis of hypertension. Med Toxicol 1987;2:210.

411. Cramer K, Goyer RA, Jagenburg R, Wilson MH. Renal ultrastructure, renal function, and parameters of lead toxicity in workers with different periods of lead exposure. Br J Ind Med 1974;31:113.

412. Garcon G, Leleu B, Zerimech F, et al. Biologic markers of oxidative stress and nephrotoxicity as studied in biomonitoring of adverse effects of occupational exposure to lead and cadmium. J Occup Environ Med 2004;46:1180.

413. Friberg L. Cadmium and the kidney. Environ Health Perspect 1984;54:1.

414. Scott R, Aughey E, Fell GS, Quinn MJ. Cadmium concentrations in human kidneys from the UK. Hum Toxicol 1987;6:111.

415. Hellstrom L, Elinder CG, Dahlberg B, et al. Cadmium exposure and end-stage renal disease. Am J Kidney Dis 2001;38:1001.

416. Roels H, Bernard AM, Cardenas A, et al. Markers of early renal changes induced by industrial pollutants. III. Application to workers exposed to cadmium. Br J Ind Med 1993;50:37.

417. Nogawa K. Biologic indicators of cadmium nephrotoxicity in persons with low-level cadmium exposure. Environ Health Perspect 1984;54:163.

418. Chan WY, Rennert OM. Cadmium nephropathy. Ann Clin Lab Sci 1981;11:229.

419. Bernard A, Roels H, Buchet JP, et al. Cadmium and health: The Belgian experience. IARC Sci Publ 1992;118:15.

420. Roels H, Lauwerys R, Buchet J, et al. Health significance of cadmium induced renal dysfunction: A five year follow up. Br J Ind Med 1989;46:755.

421. Geiger H, Bahner U, Anderes S, et al. Cadmium and renal hypertension. J Hum Hypertens 1989;3:23.

422. Yasuda M, Miwa A, Kitagawa M. Morphometric studies of renal lesions in Itai-Itai disease: Chronic cadmium nephropathy. Nephron 1995;69:14.

423. Smith J, Smith J, McCall A. Chronic poisoning from cadmium fume. J Pathol Bacteriol 1960;80:287.

424. Kazantzis G, Flynn FV, Spowage JS, Trott DG. Renal tubular malfunction and pulmonary emphysema in cadmium pigment workers. Q J Med 1963;32:165.

425. Lauwers R, De Wals P. Environmental pollution by cadmium and mortality from renal diseases. Lancet 1981;1:383.

426. Roels HA, Lauwerys RR, Buchet JP, et al. In vivo measurement of liver and kidney cadmium in workers exposed to this metal: Its significance with respect to cadmium in blood and urine. Environ Res 1981;26:217.

427. Weiss RA, Madaio MP, Tomaszewski JE, Kelly CJ. T cells reactive to an inducible heat shock protein induce disease in toxin-induced interstitial nephritis. J Exp Med 1994;180:2239.

428. Borjesson J, Barregard L, Sallsten G, et al. In vivo XRF analysis of mercury: The relation between concentrations in the kidney and the urine. Phys Med Biol 1995;40:413.

429. Bigazzi PE. Autoimmunity and heavy metals. Lupus 1994;3:449.

430. Burston J, Darmady EM, Stranack F. Nephrosis due to mercurial diuretics. Br Med J 1958;14:1277.

431. Joekes AM, Heptinstall RH, Porter KA. The nephrotic syndrome; a study of renal biopsies in 20 adult patients. Q J Med 1958;27:495.

432. Preedy JR, Russell DS. Acute salt depletion associated with the nephrotic syndrome developing during treatment with a mercurial diuretic. Lancet 1953;265:1181.

433. Riddle M, Gardner F, Beswick I, Filshie I. The nephrotic syndrome complicating mercurial diuretic therapy. Br Med J 1958;14:1274.

434. Mandema E, Arends A, Van Zeijst J, et al. Mercury and the kidney. Lancet 1963;1:1266.

435. Williams NE, Bridge HG. Nephrotic syndrome after the application of mercury ointment. Lancet 1958;2:602.

436. Grosso A, De Sousa RC. Mercury blockage of apical water channels in toad skin (bufo marinus). J Physiol 1993;468:741.

437. Cramer CR, Hagler HK, Silva FG, et al. Chronic interstitial nephritis associated with gold therapy. Arch Pathol Lab Med 1983;107:258.

438. Hocher B, Keller F, Krause PH, et al. Interstitial nephritis with reversible renal failure due to a copper-containing intrauterine contraceptive device. Nephron 1992;61:111.

439. Friedman AC, Lautin EM. Cis-platinum (II) diaminedichloride: Another cause of bilateral small kidneys. Urology 1980;16:584.

440. Leibbrandt ME, Wolfgang GH, Metz AL, et al. Critical subcellular targets of cisplatin and related platinum analogs in rat renal proximal tubule cells. Kidney Int 1995;48:761.

441. Prasad GV, Rossi NF. Arsenic intoxication associated with tubulointerstitial nephritis. Am J Kidney Dis 1995;26:373.

442. Petronic VJ, Bukurov NS, Djokic MR, et al. Balkan endemic nephropathy and papillary transitional cell tumors of the renal pelvis and ureters. Kidney Int Suppl 1991;34:S77.

443. Thun MJ, Baker DB, Steenland K, et al. Renal toxicity in uranium mill workers. Scand J Work Environ Health 1985;11:83.

444. Sztajnkrycer MD, Otten EJ. Chemical and radiological toxicity of depleted uranium. Mil Med 2004;169:212.

445. Tolson JK, Roberts SM, Jortner B, et al. Heat shock proteins and acquired resistance to uranium nephrotoxicity. Toxicology 2005;206:59.

446. Gullner HG, Gill JR Jr, Bartter FC, et al. A familial disorder with hypokalemic alkalosis, hyperreninemia, aldosteronism, high urinary prostaglandins and normal blood pressure that is not "Bartter's syndrome". Trans Assoc Am Physicians 1979;92:175.

447. Potter WZ, Trygstad CW, Helmer OM, et al. Familial hypokalemia associated with renal interstitial fibrosis. Am J Med 1974;57:971.

448. Wallace MR, Bruton D, North A, Wild DJ. End-stage renal failure due to familial hypokalaemic interstitial nephritis with identical HLA tissue types. N Z Med J 1985;98:5.

449. Cremer W, Bock KD. Symptoms and course of chronic hypokalemic nephropathy in man. Clin Nephrol 1977;7:112.

450. Lelamali K, Khunkitti W, Yenrudi S, et al. Potassium depletion in a healthy north-eastern Thai population: No association

with tubulo-interstitial injury. Nephrology (Carlton) 2003;8:28.

451. Wrong OM, Feest TG, MacIver AG. Immune-related potassium-losing interstitial nephritis: A comparison with distal renal tubular acidosis. Q J Med 1993;86:513.

452. Zsurka G, Ormos J, Ivanyi B, et al. Mitochondrial mutation as a probable causative factor in familial progressive tubulointerstitial nephritis. Hum Genet 1997;99:484.

453. Tzen CY, Tsai JD, Wu TY, et al. Tubulointerstitial nephritis associated with a novel mitochondrial point mutation. Kidney Int 2001;59:846.

454. Rotig A. Renal disease and mitochondrial genetics. J Nephrol 2003;16:286.

455. Peng M, Jarett L, Meade R, et al. Mutant prenyltransferase-like mitochondrial protein (PLMP) and mitochondrial abnormalities in kd/kd mice. Kidney Int 2004;66:20.

456. Mihatsch MJ, Gudat F, Zollinger HU, et al. Systemic karyomegaly associated with chronic interstitial nephritis: A new disease entity? Clin Nephrol 1979;12:54.

457. Spoendlin M, Moch H, Brunner F, et al. Karyomegalic interstitial nephritis: Further support for a distinct entity and evidence for a genetic defect. Am J Kidney Dis 1995;25:242.

458. Moch H, Spondlin M, Schmassmann A, Mihatsch MJ. Systemic karyomegaly with chronic interstitial nephritis: Discussion of the disease picture based on an autopsy case [in German]. Pathologe 1994;15:44.

459. Godin M, Francois A, Le Roy F, et al. Karyomegalic interstitial nephritis: Is ochratoxin A responsible? J Am Soc Nephrol 1995;6:997.

460. Vadiaka M, Sotsiou F, Koufos C. A case of systemic karyomegaly associated with interstitial nephritis. Ann Med Interne (Paris) 1998;149:291.

461. Hassen W, Abid-Essafi S, Achour A, et al. Karyomegaly of tubular kidney cells in human chronic interstitial nephropathy in Tunisia: Respective role of ochratoxin A and possible genetic predisposition. Hum Exp Toxicol 2004;23:339.

462. Rossini M, Coventry S, Duff DR, Fogo AB. Chronic renal failure and abnormal tubular cells in 2 siblings. Am J Kidney Dis 2005;46:982

463. Bhandari S, Kalowski S, Collett P, et al. Karyomegalic nephropathy: An uncommon cause of progressive renal failure. Nephrol Dial Transplant 2002;17:1914.

464. Ceovic S, Hrabar A, Saric M. Epidemiology of Balkan endemic nephropathy. Food Chem Toxicol 1992;30:183.

465. Radonic M, Radosevic Z. Clinical features of Balkan endemic nephropathy. Food Chem Toxicol 1992;30:189.

466. Vukelic M, Sostaric B, Fuchs R. Some pathomorphological features of Balkan endemic nephropathy in Croatia. IARC Sci Publ 1991;115:37.

467. Hall PW 3rd, Dammin GJ, Griggs RC, et al. Investigation of chronic endemic nephropathy in Yugoslavia. II. Renal pathology. Am J Med 1965;39:210.

468. Ferluga D, Hvala A, Vizjak A, et al. Renal function, protein excretion, and pathology of Balkan endemic nephropathy. III. Light and electron microscopic studies. Kidney Int Suppl 1991;34:S57.

469. Toncheva D, Galabov AS, Laich A, et al. Urinary neopterin concentrations in patients with Balkan endemic nephropathy (BEN). Kidney Int 2003;64:1817.

470. Sostaric B, Vukelic M. Characteristics of urinary tract tumours in the area of Balkan endemic nephropathy in Croatia. IARC Sci Publ 1991;115:29.

471. Andonova IE, Sarueva RB, Horvath AD, et al. Balkan endemic nephropathy and genetic variants of glutathione S-transferases. J Nephrol 2004;17:390.

472. Toncheva DI, Von Ahsen N, Atanasova SY, et al. Identification of NQO1 and GSTs genotype frequencies in Bulgarian patients with Balkan endemic nephropathy. J Nephrol 2004;17:384.

473. Uzelac-Keserovic B, Spasic P, Bojanic N, et al. Isolation of a coronavirus from kidney biopsies of endemic Balkan nephropathy patients. Nephron 1999;81:141.

474. Riquelme C, Escors D, Ortego J, et al. Nature of the virus associated with endemic Balkan nephropathy. Emerg Infect Dis 2002;8:869.

475. Wedeen RP. Environmental renal disease: Lead, cadmium and Balkan endemic nephropathy. Kidney Int Suppl 1991;34:S4.

476. Radovanovic Z, Markovic-Denic L, Marinkovic J, et al. Well water characteristics and the Balkan nephropathy. Nephron 1991;57:52.

477. Batuman V. Possible pathogenetic role of low-molecular-weight proteins in Balkan nephropathy. Kidney Int 1991;34(suppl): S89.

478. Bozic Z, Duancic V, Belicza M, et al. Balkan endemic nephropathy: Still a mysterious disease. Eur J Epidemiol 1995;11:235.

479. Vrabcheva T, Petkova-Bocharova T, Grosso F, et al. Analysis of ochratoxin A in foods consumed by inhabitants from an area with Balkan endemic nephropathy: A 1 month follow-up study. J Agric Food Chem 2004;52:2404.

480. Krogh P, Axelsen NH, Elling F, et al. Experimental porcine nephropathy. Changes of renal function and structure induced by ochratoxin A-contaminated feed. Acta Pathol Microbiol Scand (A) 1974;0:1.

481. Krogh P, Elling F. Letter: Fungal toxins and endemic (Balkan) nephropathy. Lancet 1976;2:40.

482. Pavlovic M, Plestina R, Krogh P. Ochratoxin A contamination of foodstuffs in an area with Balkan (endemic) nephropathy. Acta Pathol Microbiol Scand (B) 1979;87:243.

483. Vanherweghem JL. A new form of nephropathy secondary to the absorption of Chinese herbs [in French]. Bull Mem Acad R Med Belg 1994;149:128 discussion 135.

484. Cosyns JP, Jadoul M, Squifflet JP, et al. Urothelial lesions in Chinese-herb nephropathy. Am J Kidney Dis 1999;33:1011.

485. Depierreux M, Van Damme B, Vanden Houte K, Vanherweghem JL. Pathologic aspects of a newly described nephropathy related to the prolonged use of Chinese herbs. Am J Kidney Dis 1994;24:172.

486. Vanherweghem JL, Depierreux M, Tielemans C, et al. Rapidly progressive interstitial renal fibrosis in young women: Association with slimming regimen including Chinese herbs. Lancet 1993;341:387.

487. Cosyns JP, Jadoul M, Squifflet JP, et al. Chinese herbs nephropathy: A clue to Balkan endemic nephropathy? Kidney Int 1994;45:1680.

488. Nortier JL, Martinez MC, Schmeiser HH, et al. Urothelial carcinoma associated with the use of a Chinese herb (*Aristolochia fangchi*). N Engl J Med 2000;342:1686.

489. Vanhaelen M, Vanhaelen-Fastre R, But P, Vanherweghem JL. Identification of aristolochic acid in Chinese herbs. Lancet 1994;343:174.

490. Cosyns JP. Aristolochic acid and 'Chinese herbs nephropathy': A review of the evidence to date. Drug Saf 2003;26:33.

491. Martinez MC, Nortier J, Vereerstraeten P, Vanherweghem JL. Progression rate of Chinese herb nephropathy: Impact of *Aristolochia fangchi* ingested dose. Nephrol Dial Transplant 2002;17:408.

492. Cosyns JP, Dehoux JP, Guiot Y, et al. Chronic aristolochic acid toxicity in rabbits: A model of Chinese herbs nephropathy? Kidney Int 2001;59:2164.

493. Yang CS, Lin CH, Chang SH, Hsu HC. Rapidly progressive fibrosing interstitial nephritis associated with Chinese herbal drugs. Am J Kidney Dis 2000;35:313.

494. Chang C, Wang Y, Yang A, Chiang S. Rapidly progressive interstitial renal fibrosis associated with Chinese herbal drugs. Am J Nephrol 2001;21:441.

495. Tanaka A, Nishida R, Maeda K, et al. Chinese herb nephropathy in Japan presents adult-onset Fanconi syndrome: Could different components of aristolochic acids cause a different type of Chinese herb nephropathy? Clin Nephrol 2000;53:301.

496. Tanaka A, Nishida R, Yoshida T, et al. Outbreak of Chinese herb nephropathy in Japan: Are there any differences from Belgium? Intern Med 2001;40:296.

497. Lo SH, Wong KS, Arlt VM, et al. Detection of Herba Aristolochia Mollissemae in a patient with unexplained nephropathy. Am J Kidney Dis 2005;45:407.

498. Sato N, Takahashi D, Chen SM, et al. Acute nephrotoxicity of aristolochic acids in mice. J Pharm Pharmacol 2004;56: 221.

499. Nzerue C, Schlanger L, Jena M, et al. Granulomatous interstitial nephritis and uveitis presenting as salt-losing nephropathy. Am J Nephrol 1997;17:462.

500. Segal A, Dowling JP, Ireton HJ, et al. Granulomatous glomerulonephritis in intravenous drug users: A report of three cases in oxycodone addicts. Hum Pathol 1998;29: 1246.

501. Enriquez R, Cabezuelo JB, Gonzalez C, et al. Granuloma-

tous interstitial nephritis associated with hydrochlorothiazide/ amiloride. Am J Nephrol 1995;15:270.

502. Nast CC, Cohen AH. Renal cholesterol granulomas: Identification and morphological pattern of development. Histopathology 1985;9:1195.

503. Hegarty J, Picton M, Agarwal G, et al. Carbamazepine-induced acute granulomatous interstitial nephritis. Clin Nephrol 2002;57:310.

504. Pena de la Vega L, Fervenza FC, Lager D, et al. Acute granulomatous interstitial nephritis secondary to bisphosphonate alendronate sodium. Ren Fail 2005;27:485.

# Ischemic and Toxic Acute Tubular Injury and Other Ischemic Renal Injury

**24**

*Lorraine Racusen*     *Michael Kashgarian*

## ACUTE TUBULAR INJURY

Acute renal failure (ARF) is a clinical syndrome and not a distinct pathologic entity. It is characterized by rapid deterioration in renal function and glomerular filtration rate (GFR) over a relatively short period of time, ranging from hours to days. The result is a sudden inability to maintain normal fluid and electrolyte homeostasis. The acute reduction in renal function can be the result of the impairment of blood flow (so-called "prerenal failure"), obstruction of the urinary collecting system (so-called "postrenal failure"),

**TABLE 24.1**

**CLINICAL PHASES OF ACUTE KIDNEY INJURY**

1. Risk of renal dysfunction
   Increase in sCr by 1.5 times OR
   Decrease in GFR >25% for 6 hours OR
   Urine output <.5 mL/kg/hr for 6 hours

2. Renal injury
   Increase in sCr by 2 times OR
   Decrease in GFR >50% for 12 hours OR
   Urine output <.5 mL/kg/hr for 12 hours

3. Renal failure
   Increase in sCr by 3 times or >4 mg/dL OR
   Decrease in GFR by 75% for 24 hours OR
   Urine output <.3 mL/kg/hr for 24 hours OR
   Anuria for 12 hours

sCr, serum creatinine; GFR, glomerular filtration rate.
Modified from reference 7.

or a variety of intrinsic renal diseases ranging from glomerulonephritis to interstitial nephritis to acute tubular injury (ATI), which is the primary topic of discussion in this chapter. There has been a lack of uniformity in the definition of "acute renal failure," which is generally based on a rise in serum creatinine, making the literature in this area somewhat difficult to interpret. Based on the available literature, which uses somewhat variable definitions, ARF is commonly encountered in hospitalized patients (1–5). Its frequency ranges from 1% at admission to the hospital to as high as 31% in patients undergoing cardiopulmonary bypass or with other high-risk conditions.

Recently there has been an attempt to reach a consensus definition of acute renal dysfunction (6,7). The proposed classification system includes both GFR and urine output criteria (Table 24.1). The earliest phase, *risk of renal dysfunction*, is defined by an increase in serum creatinine (sCr) by 1.5 times, GFR decrease of more than 25%, or urine output below 0.5 mL/kg/hr for 6 hours. *Renal injury* is defined by sCr increase by 2 times, GFR decrease of more than 50%, or urine output less than 0.5 mL/kg/hr for 12 hours. *Renal failure* is defined as sCr increase by three times (or over 4 mg/dL), GFR decrease by 75%, urine output below 0.3 mL/kg/hr for 24 hours, or anuria for 12 hours. If accepted, this definition should lead to more uniformity in the literature related to acute renal dysfunction and should result in better recognition and enhanced understanding of the various stages of clinical renal dysfunction. However, even more refinement of definition could be possible. For example, differentiation of prerenal azotemia from intrinsic renal disease owing to tubular injury is enhanced by assessment of markers of tubular injury or function.

A consensus panel of the American Society of Nephrology recently discussed the nomenclature of the clinical term *acute renal failure* and decided that it was not a clear representation of the disease process to nonnephrologist clinicians, patients, and the general public. The term *acute kidney injury* was felt to reflect a recognition of the early stages of kidney injury. The term could be used to distinguish early from more advanced stages of kidney disease, in which there is more overt "failure" of clearance by the kidney. From a clinical point of view, use of this more general term would highlight the predictive value of acute or small changes in serum creatinine and facilitate recognition of renal injury and dysfunction at earlier stages of disease.

There is also lack of precision in the use of the term *acute tubular injury/necrosis*. The term should be reserved for the clinical pathologic entity of intrinsic renal failure that is the result of either an ischemic or toxic insult to the kidney, with evidence of tubular injury/dysfunction such as fractional excretion of sodium (8) and potentially other more specific biomarkers, when other causes have been excluded. As a result of the lack of uniformity in terminology, the percentage of cases of ARF that can be attributed to "acute tubular necrosis/injury" is difficult to accurately ascertain, but the condition is likely responsible for the majority of cases of ARF that require acute renal replacement therapy. The term *acute tubular necrosis* itself is a misnomer, since necrosis, while classically a feature of animal models, is only one morphologic manifestation of clinical ATI. It should also be noted that morphologic evidence of frank tubular necrosis is not a frequent feature in kidney biopsies obtained in the context of clinical ARF; morphologic changes of sublethal tubular injury are almost always present. The term *acute tubular injury* is more accurate and will be used throughout this chapter.

## Historical Background

A historical review of the clinical observations and experimental work relating to this entity over the past century gives some insight into the pathogenesis of ARF. It was not until World War I that acute renal dysfunction was recognized as a distinctive clinical and pathologic entity. Hackradt (9) described what he called "vasomotor nephrosis" following crushing injuries. In a review of autopsy material of war casualties, Minami (10) described the presence of pigment casts in medullary tubules associated with tubular changes and an interstitial infiltrate. On the basis of his morphologic observations, he suggested that myohemoglobinuria and subsequent precipitation in the tubules were factors involved in producing the observed anatomic and functional renal abnormalities.

Shortly thereafter, Baker and Dodds (11) studied a rabbit model of ARF that they believed to be caused by the precipitation of acid hematin in an acid urine of high sodium concentration; they emphasized tubular obstruction as important in the pathogenesis. Progress in the field was relatively dormant until the advent of World War II, when Bywaters and Beall (12) revived interest in ARF as a result of their study of London air casualties. Bywaters and Dible (13) and Dunn et al (14) described in detail the renal histopathologic features of the "crush syndrome or traumatic anuria" and emphasized the presence of intratubular hemoglobin and myoglobin casts associated with focal necrosis of tubules, interstitial edema, and mild interstitial inflammatory changes. Localization of these changes to specific portions of the nephron was noted. This finding led to the hypothesis that tubular obstruction by necrotic debris and precipitated pigment was the prime cause of the observed oliguria.

Bywaters and Dible (13), however, believed that obstruction alone could not explain all the clinical findings or the abnormal character of the urine that was produced by such patients. They reasoned that if obstruction were the sole explanation, the urine produced would be the product of remaining unobstructed and undamaged nephrons, which should produce urine of entirely normal composition. Because patients with ARF had urine that was quite abnormal and resembled an unaltered glomerular filtrate, and because there was a marked discrepancy between the degree of anatomic change and the severity of the oliguria, they postulated that other factors must play a part. Lucke (15) emphasized that the discrepancy between structure and function could be related to the observed localization of histologic changes to the distal nephrons, and he coined the term *lower nephron nephrosis*. His description in *Military Medicine* is classic, and the anatomic findings that he emphasized are still recognized today as hallmarks of ARF associated with crushing injuries and transfusion reactions.

Lucke's description includes pigment casts in the distal tubules and areas of tubular destruction and interstitial inflammatory reaction. His studies, however, did not directly address the dilemma of the lack of concordance between structure and function. It was this problem that led Oliver et al (16) to use nephron dissections to study cases of ARF, and they were able to show two distinct types of renal tubular injury. In the first, as a result of the direct cytotoxic effect of a specific nephrotoxin, there was segmental necrosis of the proximal tubular epithelium with denudation of the basement membrane, which remained intact. In the second type, which they termed the *tubulorrhexic lesion*, there was focal necrosis of tubular cells associated with rupture of the adjacent basement membrane, allowing communication of the tubular lumen with the interstitial tissue. This focal lesion could affect any portion of the nephron but was most commonly seen in the distal portions of the proximal tubule. It was believed that this lesion was most likely ischemic in origin. The focal and patchy nature of the necrosis, which was usually not associated with any interstitial reaction, was thought to be the reason that random histologic sections of such kidneys frequently did not demonstrate significant pathologic change. From these microdissection studies, Oliver et al suggested a mechanism of action whereby these lesions could lead to the leakage

of tubular fluid into the interstitial tissue, thus diminishing the amount of urine produced. At the same time, such leakage could cause a rise in intrarenal pressure, which could further potentiate oliguria by compression of thin afferent capillaries, resulting in diminished glomerular filtration.

While these investigators were concentrating on the tubular changes, Goormaghtigh (17,18) called attention to the renal arteriolar changes in kidneys of patients with the crush syndrome. He observed considerable hypertrophy and an increase in granularity of the juxtaglomerular cells in kidneys of patients with ARF. As early as 1940, he advanced the theory that these cells produced a vasoactive or prevasoactive substance that could act on the renal vasculature. He suggested that the anuria observed in the crush syndrome was the result of vasoconstriction, initially in the postglomerular arterioles and later in the glomerular tufts. He further postulated that vasoconstriction was followed by a period of paralytic dilatation and that glomerular hemodynamic changes would result in the diminution of glomerular filtration; he emphasized decreased glomerular function as a mechanism of oliguria.

Although Hackradt (9) had suggested a vasomotor basis for traumatic anuria as early as 1917, the physiologic aspects of this possibility were ignored until Trueta et al (19) proposed that the fundamental defect in the crush syndrome was a reduction of glomerular filtration as a result of the diversion of blood away from the outer cortical glomeruli through a juxtamedullary shunt. They arrived at this conclusion as a result of direct observation of the kidney as well as angiographic and morphologic studies of intrarenal vascular patterns. Brun et al (20,21) produced even more convincing evidence by measuring renal hemodynamics in vivo. Sheehan and Davis (22) also believed that ischemia was important, but they suggested that the mechanisms of action were related to vascular damage following an initial period of ischemia, which prevented adequate reperfusion once blood flow had been established. Sevitt (23) also commented on the poor correlation between the presence of tubular necrosis and the state of uremia, and felt that the diminution of glomerular filtration was a result of an abnormality of intrarenal blood flow.

Hollenberg et al (24,25) studied patients with ARF following a variety of initiating injuries and noted that it was impossible to see the cortical arteries in such patients; they also documented disappearance of the cortical flow component of xenon washout from the kidney. Munck (26) verified that such a decrease in blood flow was sufficient to result in renal hypoxia, once again calling attention to the intrarenal physiologic abnormalities associated with diminished blood flow and their relationship to glomerular filtration. These early studies suggested several physiologic mechanisms of action for the resultant oligoanuria, including tubular obstruction, back-leakage of tubular fluid, and changes in hemodynamics resulting in decreasing glomerular filtration.

The advent of micropuncture techniques led to the investigation of several animal models of ARF to identify the pathophysiologic mechanisms of action in greater detail. Oken et al (27) first applied the techniques of micropuncture to experimental mercury- or glycerol-induced ARF. Their work demonstrated that glomerular filtration progressively diminished as oliguria developed, leading these investigators to believe that suppressed filtration was the key pathophysiologic agency. Early work in our own laboratory (M.K.) studied two different models of ARF (28). In one, potassium dichromate was used to cause toxic cellular damage to the early ($S_{1-2}$) part of the proximal tubule, and in the other, purified human globin was administered to produce an intrarenal obstructive lesion of the distal nephron with minimal histologic evidence of proximal tubular damage. These models were studied in animals that had been made renin-rich and renin-poor by alterations of the salt content of their diet. The renal failure produced in both of these models was less severe in the salt-loaded, renin-poor animals.

The decrease in urine flow was accompanied by a diminution of the total and individual nephron GFR associated with a decrease in the tubular reabsorptive capacity for sodium, chloride, and water. There was evidence of mechanical tubular obstruction, reflected by an elevation of free-flow intratubular pressure. In addition, the glomerular filtration pressure appeared to be diminished, suggesting that the decreased glomerular blood flow and glomerular filtration were the result of preglomerular arteriolar constriction, which was mediated by activation of the local renin–angiotensin system. Studies of renal blood flow distribution demonstrated that a diminution of outer cortical flow correlated best with decreased glomerular filtration (29,30). These studies and those from several other laboratories (31–36) led to a proposal that tubular epithelial injury induced by either ischemia or by a toxin could be sublethal but had to be severe enough to result in decreased epithelial transport activity, which then would result in decreased tubular sodium reabsorption and local activation of the renin–angiotensin system. This, in turn, would alter glomerular hemodynamics and result in decreased glomerular filtration.

Decreased tubular urine flow associated with the shedding of cellular debris and the presence of Tamm-Horsfall protein would result in tubular obstruction when combined with focal areas of necrosis, as demonstrated by the micropuncture studies of Oliver. This situation could lead to a back-leakage of fluid, all of which contribute to the end result of oliguria. It is of interest that the term *acute renal success* was suggested by Thurau and Boylan (37), because they analyzed the pathophysiologic changes of decreased glomerular filtration as being thoroughly appropriate as a defense against loss of intravascular volume caused by the inability of the damaged tubules to reabsorb the glomerular filtrate. Although these studies primarily focused on pathophysiology and did not address the cellular pathologic characteristics of the oliguria of ARF, they did address the discrepancy between structure and function and emphasized the central role of renal tubular epithelial transport function and how this function is altered by ischemic or toxic injury.

This section of the chapter will focus on ATI caused by ischemia and/or nephrotoxins. Clinical features, pathology, and pathogenesis will be discussed for ischemia and toxic injury in general and for the major nephrotoxic agents.

## Clinical Presentation

Patients with injury to the tubular epithelium have clinical and laboratory evidence of tubular dysfunction that is sometimes quite subtle. Loss of normal resorptive function may lead to polyuria, glucosuria, phosphaturia, or aminoaciduria; Fanconi's syndrome has occasionally been reported. With more severe injury, intact and necrotic tubular cells appear in the urine sediment, individually or in cast form. Patients may become oliguric. In some cases, crystals, leukocyturia, and hematuria may also be detected on urinalysis.

Enzymuria is a useful marker for tubular cell injury; it is more sensitive than a rise in sCr and may be used to some extent to gauge the severity of cell injury. Elevated levels of $\beta_2$-microglobulin or enzymes may be detected in the urine and have been used in many clinical studies as markers of tubular toxicity (38,39). The presence in the urine of brush border enzymes, such as alkaline phosphatase and gamma-glutamyl transpeptidase, may reflect mild cellular injury. The appearance of lysosomal enzymes, such as N-acetyl glucosaminidase, and of cytoskeletal elements reflects more severe injury and cell loss from the tubular epithelium. Measurement of these enzymes has been used as a noninvasive marker of injury to the renal tubule (40–43). New unbiased genomic and proteomic techniques are leading to the discovery of many potential biomarkers that may be useful in detecting early tubular injury. Biomarkers proposed for early detection of acute kidney injury include proteins present in urine (Kidney Injury Molecule-$\alpha$ [KIM-1], cysteine rich-61 [cyr61], Na($+$) $-$ H($+$) antiporter isoform 3 [NHE3] membranes, lipocalin, actin) and serum (cystin C, tumor necrosis factor-a [TNFa] receptor) (44,45).

Acute tubular injury often results in reduction of GFR, with development of acute renal insufficiency and ARF. The acute reduction in renal function results in both biochemical and clinical abnormalities. They are related to the inability of the kidney to eliminate water, nitrogenous wastes, and acids and to regulate electrolyte balance. Oliguria is classically seen as an initial feature of many cases of ATI; the appearance of oliguria correlates with the extent of decline in GFR (46). Nonoliguric ARF is now commonly recognized as well (47,48), owing to the more critical observation and laboratory monitoring of seriously ill hospitalized patients.

In addition, the use of potentially nephrotoxic drugs such as aminoglycoside antibiotics or nonsteroidal antiinflammatory drugs, which can accentuate renal ischemia, may predispose seriously ill patients to develop overt ARF. It is of particular interest that patients with the nonoliguric form of disease tend to have less severe renal failure and fewer complications (49). Significant laboratory findings include elevations in blood urea nitrogen, serum creatinine, and serum potassium. Urinary sodium excretion is markedly amplified, consistent with a decreased resorptive capacity of the damaged tubules.

Between 5% and 10% of acute renal injury is caused, at least in part, by exposure to drugs (50). Patients with toxic injury to the tubular epithelium often show signs of renal failure. Hemoglobin and myoglobin are endogenous proteins that can function as nephrotoxins when they are present in large concentrations in the urine. Acute renal failure is associated with hemoglobinuria following acute hemolysis in patients with transfusion reactions and in patients with *Plasmodium falciparum* malaria. Whereas the toxicity of hemoglobin may contribute to the pathogenesis of ARF in these instances, ischemia and microcirculatory disturbances probably play a greater role in its development. Myoglobinuria stemming from rhabdomyolysis as a result of trauma, viral infection, or heat stress (51–54) produces a similar clinical picture. Rhabdomyolysis associated with cocaine abuse has also been demonstrated to result in ATI, as discussed in this chapter in the section on nephrotoxins.

A variety of exogenous agents can also cause ATI (Table 24.2). It must be noted that association of a particular drug or toxin with renal injury and dysfunction may be missed or may be difficult to establish as causative, especially in complex clinical settings. Repeated correlation of exposure and injury help to establish nephrotoxicity, and experimental models are often useful in defining the mechanism of injury.

Renal dysfunction may occur soon after exposure or after a predictable interval, as is seen with aminoglycosides, depending on the specific drug or toxin causing injury. Most patients experience a fall in GFR that is detectable on clearance studies, with only a minority proceeding to overt renal failure. A few tubular toxins cause injury only at high doses; with other agents, some level of injury can be detected at the usual therapeutic doses in most patients. Pigmented casts or crystals may appear in the urine, providing a clue to the diagnosis; in such cases, oliguria and even anuria may be the presenting feature. Hydration and maintenance of diuresis help prevent renal dysfunction or hasten recovery in cases with intratubular crystals or cast formation. Radiographic studies generally reveal normal-sized kidneys with increased echogenicity. Clinical features of major nephrotoxins are described in the text following; the focus of this chapter is on toxic effects of therapeutic agents. Toxic nephropathies caused by heavy metals and other environmental toxins have been reviewed recently (55).

## TABLE 24.2

### DRUGS THAT ARE INJURIOUS TO RENAL TUBULAR EPITHELIUM

Antiviral agents
    Nucleoside analogs
    Antiretroviral agents

Antibiotics
    Aminoglycosides
    Amphotericin B
    Cephalosporins
    Colistin/polymyxin B
    Rifampicin[a]
    Sulfonamides[a]

Immunomodulatory agents
    Calcineurin inhibitors
    Intravenous immunoglobulin
    Sirolimus

Antineoplastic agents
    Cis-platinum
    Other

Radiologic contrast media
Narcotics
Anesthetics
Herbal medications

[a]Discussed in Chapter 23.

New techniques have been developed to make the diagnosis of and to study ARF (56). Rapid and accurate measurement of GFR using radioactive and nonradioactive clearance techniques is now possible, even when GFR is not stable. New magnetic resonance imaging techniques may enhance the study of intrarenal perfusion and oxygenation.

## Clinical Features Associated with Specific Toxic Agents

### Antibiotics

*Antiviral Agents.* The nephrotoxicity of antiviral drugs has been recently reviewed (57). Early use of acyclovir, a nucleoside analog, was reported to be associated with renal dysfunction, and there is a significant incidence of renal dysfunction with newer agents as well. Tubular injury may lead to Fanconi-like syndrome (cidofovir, tenofovir, foscarnet), distal tubular acidosis (foscarnet), and nephrogenic diabetes insipidus (foscarnet). Adefovir has been reported to produce proximal tubulopathy in up to 50% of patients at high doses (58). A variety of these agents have been associated with renal failure, including acyclovir (59–63), foscarnet (64), ganciclovir (65), cidofovir (66–68), indinavir (69,70), tenofovir (71–73), and adefovir (58). Some agents are associated with crystalluria, and flank or abdominal pain may occur (acyclovir, ganciclovir, indinavir); crystals are needle-shaped and birefringent under polarized light and can be seen in voided urine. Proteinuria has also been described with cidofovir, more commonly than ARF (68).

Toxicity is dose-dependent, and volume depletion may predispose to toxicity. Renal failure often resolves rapidly when these drugs are discontinued, and the patient may be rechallenged with a lower dose of the drug without development of renal dysfunction. However, occasional cases of chronic renal failure have been reported in patients receiving cidofovir (74), indinavir (75), and tenofovir (72). Renal tubular functional defects may persist as well (76). Hydration to maintain diuresis may prevent renal toxicity (59,67). With acyclovir, toxicity has been frequently described with intravenous administration, but cases have been reported with oral administration as well (61). Older age and pre-existing renal failure are risk factors for ARF in patients receiving acyclovir (61). Renal impairment is also a risk factor for ARF induced by cidofovir, foscarnet, indinavir, interferon, and ritonavir, and dosage adjustment is required.

*Aminoglycosides.* Aminoglycoside antibiotics have long been recognized as nephrotoxic and ototoxic. They continue to be used, however, because of their efficacy in treating Gram-negative infections. The incidence of ARF in patients treated with gentamicin is about 20% (77). The nephrotoxicity of the various aminoglycosides is greatest in those with the largest number of free amino groups (78). Streptomycin, the least toxic, has two amino groups; those with intermediate toxicity, such as gentamicin, tobramycin, and kanamycin, have four to five groups; and neomycin, which is the most toxic, has six free amino groups. Changes in dosing to once-daily administration have evolved to avoid nephrotoxicity (79). Once-daily dosing with monitoring of trough levels may enable avoidance of significant renal toxicity, even in elderly patients (80). However, with prolonged treatment, differences between once-daily and twice-daily dosing diminish (81). The toxicity of aminoglycosides may be potentiated by ischemia or other drugs, including thalidomide (82).

Gentamicin is a broad-spectrum antibiotic that has intermediate nephrotoxicity. In humans, gentamicin alone may cause elevation of serum urea nitrogen (SUN) and serum creatinine, although the incidence is difficult to assess because of a variety of concomitant clinical variables, including advanced age, presence of pre-existing renal damage, or administration of other drugs that are potentially nephrotoxic. The frequency with which renal toxicity is reported varies from study to study, in part because of variable criteria for defining significant elevations in SUN and creatinine. Incidences ranging from 8% to 37% have been reported (83–86). Identified risk factors include advanced age, poor nutritional status, severe systemic illness, and ad-

ministration of other drugs, including amphotericin B, vancomycin, methicillin, or cephalosporins, which are themselves potentially nephrotoxic (87–90).

Onset of a detectable rise in serum creatinine is typically delayed for 8 to 10 days from initiation of therapy. Renal failure is usually mild, and most patients recover. Enzymuria may be detected in cases without elevations in serum creatinine, suggesting the presence of subclinical injury in many patients. Occasional cases have been reported in which proximal tubular dysfunction is severe enough to produce Fanconi's syndrome (91). In experimental studies, no functional abnormalities are present with doses comparable to those used therapeutically in humans. However, with large doses, there may be proteinuria, polyuria, and elevation of blood urea nitrogen (BUN) and serum creatinine levels (92–94). Oliguric renal failure has been described with very high doses in rats (93).

Kanamycin also has an intermediate potential for nephrotoxicity among the aminoglycosides. Winfield et al (95) have reported that after 6 to 31 days of treatment with kanamycin (mean total dose of 46.5 g), the creatinine clearances were lower in more than half of the patients, and para-amino hippurate (PAH) clearance declined in one third of patients. On urinalysis, microscopic hematuria was present in one third, but proteinuria was rare (95). Acute oliguric renal failure has been reported to occur in 10% of patients treated for several months with more modest doses (96). Tobramycin also is considered to have intermediate nephrotoxic potential. However, several large studies comparing gentamicin and tobramycin have shown that gentamicin induces nephrotoxicity more frequently than tobramycin (97,98). Nephrotoxicity was defined as a rise in the sCr level of 0.5 to 1.0 mg/mL (97) or by an elevation one third above the base level (98).

Neomycin is the most nephrotoxic of the aminoglycoside antibiotics. Because it is poorly absorbed from the gastrointestinal tract, it is used largely as a bowel-sterilizing drug. Neomycin also has been used parenterally and has caused deafness and renal damage. Acute renal failure, usually of an oliguric type, has been reported; recovery has been reported in most patients (99,100). Acute renal failure occurs most commonly after intravenous or intramuscular administration of the drug, although it has been recorded after oral administration as well (100).

*Amphotericin B.* Nephrotoxicity is the side effect that most commonly limits the use of this important antifungal agent. Renal insufficiency is usually observed, with a fall in the GFR and renal blood flow. In one large prospective series of patients being treated for cryptococcal meningitis, 26% had an increase in sCr level of more than 2 mg/dL (101). Such renal failure is usually reversible, but renal function may be permanently impaired in 40% of patients who receive more than 5 g of amphotericin (102). In addition, there is a defect in acid excretion by the tubules, resulting in renal tubular acidosis (103), which may precede a significant fall in the GFR and is generally reversible. A common side effect is an impaired ability to concentrate urine (104,105); this may be present without azotemia. Liposomal formulations may reduce nephrotoxicity.

*Cephalosporins.* The cephalosporin group of antibiotics comprises several "generations" of these useful agents, defined on the basis of antimicrobial activity. The first generation includes cefazolin, cephalothin, and cephalexin. Cefamandole, cefonicid, cefuroxime, cefaclor, cefoxitin, and cefotetan are second generation, while the third generation includes ceftazidime, cefotaxime, and ceftriaxone. Cefepime is a fourth-generation cephalosporin that is more resistant to β lactamase than the previous agents. These drugs may be nephrotoxic, especially at high doses or in patients with pre-existing renal insufficiency. Cephaloridine, the most toxic of the group, is no longer available in the United States but is used experimentally for toxicity studies.

The cephalosporins are most likely to produce renal failure in patients with pre-existing renal insufficiency (106,107), in those with drug overdose (108), and in those receiving other antibiotics (108). Patients simultaneously receiving furosemide (108) are also at increased risk, which is probably related to the ability of furosemide to prolong the half-life of the cephalosporins (109). Also, many of the patients reported to have nephrotoxicity owing to cephalosporins are acutely ill with severe infections, and many are old.

Cephalothin given alone (110–112) or with gentamicin, tobramycin (113,114), or other substances (115) can cause ARF in humans or can worsen pre-existing renal insufficiency (106,107). The ARF is usually reversible. Cephalexin (116) is less likely to cause nephrotoxicity, but acute renal dysfunction has been reported (116); clinical features suggest an immunologic basis. "Acute tubular necrosis" without hypersensitivity has also been reported with cephalexin (117). Acute renal failure with tubular proteinuria has been described with a combination of ceftriaxone and acyclovir (118), and cefodizime and vancomycin (119).

*Polymyxin B and Colistin.* Polymyxin B and colistin are older antibiotics that are re-emerging for treatment of multiple-drug–resistant Gram-negative bacteria. Polymyxin B is an antibiotic with well-recognized nephrotoxicity. At parenteral doses of 2.5 mg/kg, proteinuria, casts, and hematuria may be seen, and at doses above 3 mg/kg/day, renal failure occurs (120). When there is pre-existing impaired renal function, smaller doses can produce renal symptoms. Renal failure may occur with oliguria. Recovery is usual after withdrawal of the drug.

Colistin is an antibiotic closely related to polymyxin B. Nephrotoxicity, usually reversible, has been described with the use of this drug on several occasions and is more common in patients whose renal function is already impaired, probably owing to interference with the excretion of the drug (121). In a study of 288 patients treated with colistin, Koch-Weser et al found adverse renal reactions in 20%, with elevated BUN, hematuria, proteinuria, casts, or oliguria present in some patients (121). Acute tubular injury occurred in six patients, and five of them died. However, because few clinical details were given, it is impossible to assess the role of the original disease, or of other drugs administered concomitantly, in the pathogenesis of the renal damage.

Four cases of acute nonoliguric renal failure following colistin therapy were described by Adler and Segel (122); cephalothin was also used in three of these patients. In three of the cases, the renal failure was reversible. No description was given of the pathologic characteristics of the kidney in any of the cases. Intravenous therapy with colistin for nosocomial infections resulted in ARF in 27% of patients with initially normal renal function and worsening of renal dysfunction in 58% with abnormal baseline creatinine (123). Elwood et al (124) reported three deaths among their four patients who had acute oliguric renal failure following intramuscular administration of colistin.

## Immunosuppressive/Immunomodulatory Agents

*Cyclosporine.* Cyclosporine (CsA) is widely used in the prevention and treatment of transplant rejection and to treat autoimmune disease. The major side effect is nephrotoxicity, which is to some extent dose dependent. Both acute and chronic toxic effects have been described (125–130). In a large clinical study, Krupp et al (130) reported adverse effects in 3518 renal transplant recipients treated with CsA; clinical renal dysfunction occurred in 54%. With nephrotoxicity broadly defined to include an asymptomatic mild decline in the GFR, it is likely that many patients treated with immunosuppressive doses of CsA experience nephrotoxicity. Perico et al (131) observed a fall in the GFR and renal blood flow with daily dosing of CsA; these changes were transient and negatively correlated with peak CsA concentration (131). Renal transplant patients receiving cyclosporine have higher serum creatinine levels than those on other therapies, with reduction in sCr on conversion from CsA (132).

When more overt CsA-induced renal failure is superimposed on mild functional toxicity, it may manifest in the form of one or more different clinical syndromes: acute reversible renal functional impairment, delayed renal allograft function, tubular cell effects, acute vasculopathy (thrombotic microangiopathy), and chronic nephropathy with interstitial fibrosis.

The occurrence of *acute reversible renal failure*, while not absolutely related to circulating drug levels, is generally seen with serum levels rising above 200 ng/mL and is common at drug levels above 400 ng/mL. Other features may include hyperuricemia, hyperkalemia, hypomagnesemia, sodium retention, and concentrating defects (133,134). These relatively high levels are seen more commonly in heart and liver allograft patients than in patients with renal allografts. Acute renal failure may be severe, with polyuria or oliguria (and even rarely anuria). An important feature of acute reversible renal functional impairment is its rapid reversal when CsA dosing is reduced (132,135). This rapid return of function is evidence that there is no direct tubular toxicity, as is the low fractional excretion of sodium, which indicates intact tubular reabsorption mechanisms. In early phases, the underlying vasoconstriction can be reversed by dopamine (136). Cyclosporine can also produce significant injury to proximal tubule epithelium, potentially related to direct effects as well as ischemic injury owing to prolonged vasoconstriction. In this setting, renal dysfunction is not rapidly reversible on reducing dosage of the drug.

Cyclosporine also has a propensity for producing endothelial cell damage, which can lead to thrombotic microangiopathy. Glomerular thrombi and thromboembolic complications have been described in several series (137–140). A hemolytic uremic type of syndrome (HUS) has been reported, initially in bone marrow transplant recipients (138) and subsequently in other contexts as well. There may be ischemic tubulointerstitial changes downstream from involved vessels.

Myers et al (141) and others have drawn attention to the fact that chronic nephropathy with striped interstitial fibrosis may occur following long-term CsA therapy, particularly in cardiac allograft recipients. However, these changes develop in many other allograft patients, as well as in patients receiving chronic CsA for autoimmune disease (142). Proposed risk factors include episodes of clinical toxicity, high CsA trough levels, concurrent administration of other nephrotoxic drugs, unexplained episodes of dysfunction, acute rejection episodes and therapy, and high variability in CsA levels (143,144). The development of striped interstitial fibrosis has been described in these patients, probably as a consequence of the vascular effects of cyclosporine. Myers et al showed significant reductions in the GFR in cyclosporine-treated patients—to approximately 50% of that in azathioprine-treated patients (141,145). Patients may also have severe hypertension, mild proteinuria, and evidence of tubular dysfunction. A similar long-term reduction in the GFR has also been reported in liver allograft recipients (146), and comparable changes have been reported in the kidneys of pancreas transplant recipients as well (147). Even low-dose CsA therapy for psoriasis may effect long-term changes (148,149). Whereas persistent changes in the kidney in renal allografts may be caused by several factors, careful morphometric analysis has confirmed increased fibrosis in those on long-term CsA (150). This type of chronic cyclosporine toxicity may not be reversible (151). Risk factors for the development of chronic

cyclosporine nephrotoxicity have been evaluated in renal allograft recipients (141) and in patients treated for autoimmune disease (153). Previous episodes of ARF, high-dose treatment, and (for heart transplant patients) increasing age were found to be important risk factors.

*Tacrolimus.* Tacrolimus (FK506) produces a spectrum of nephrotoxicity very similar to that of CsA and is generally dose-dependent; toxic reactions are common at or above 20 ng/mL (154) but can occur even when trough levels have been in lower range (143). Reversible renal dysfunction has been reported with the use of FK506 for prevention of graft versus host disease in bone marrow transplantation (155) and in the context of pancreas (156), liver (157), and renal transplantation (158). The high incidence of renal functional impairment when FK506 and CsA are used together has led Fung et al (159) and others to suggest that combination therapy should be avoided. In addition to induction of posttransplant diabetes, patients may develop hypertension (160). Higher incidences of urinary tract infection, pyelonephritis (160), and of polyoma virus infection (161) have been reported as well, perhaps owing to the more potent immunosuppressive activity of the drug.

*Intravenous Immunoglobulin.* Intravenous immunoglobulin (IVIG) may produce ARF (162,163). Addition of sugar excipients, and especially sucrose, to IVIG formulations has reduced side effects of pain, fever, chills, and fatigue but may increase the frequency of ARF. Renal failure may be attenuated by slowing the rate of infusion. Renal function generally returns to normal with discontinuation of the drug. Switching to a D-sorbitol–stabilized formulation may prevent toxicity (163). Avoidance of sucrose-stabilized formulations is recommended in patients receiving other nephrotoxins, in the elderly, in those with pre-existing dysfunction, and in diabetics.

*Sirolimus.* Nephrotoxicity of sirolimus is an emerging problem in clinical medicine (164). The drug has been associated with higher mean sCr concentrations in CsA-treated patients (165), via mechanisms that are unclear; some pharmacokinetic potentiation of CsA was noted in sirolimus patients. In addition, delayed graft function was three times more common in one series in patients treated with FK506 and sirolimus compared to those without sirolimus (166); another study demonstrated that sirolimus-treated patients were half as likely to resolve delayed graft function (167). A few cases of acute oliguric renal allograft failure associated with combined use of FK506 and sirolimus have been described, apparently owing to ATI (168), and in one study of high-risk renal allograft recipients, FK506-treated patients on reduced sirolimus (5 to 10 ng/mL) had a significantly higher incidence of biopsy-proven FK506 toxicity (169). Occasional cases of acute renal dysfunction caused by sirolimus have been associated with thrombotic microangiopathy (170).

## Antineoplastic Agents

Several antineoplastic agents produce toxic effects in the kidney. Immunotherapeutic agents, discussed earlier, are among them. In addition, antineoplastic agents that lead to rapid tumor lysis may cause hyperuricemia, with precipitation of uric acid in renal tubules; this syndrome may be largely avoided by hydration and careful monitoring of the patient. Specific agents that are toxic to the kidney are discussed here.

*Cis-platinum.* Cis-platinum is a chemotherapeutic agent that frequently produces nephrotoxicity. Cis-platinum nephrotoxicity is dose related. It has been reported in 25% to 30% of patients on single-course therapy and 50% to 75% of patients on multiple courses (171,172). Patients show gradual signs of elevations in SUN and sCr. Polyuria is a prominent early clinical feature, but even oliguric ARF may be seen. Other presenting symptoms include proteinuria, hyperuricemia, enzymuria, glycosuria, and electrolyte disturbances reflecting tubular dysfunction (171,173–175). Aggressive hydration (176), administration of diuretics (177), or co-administration of thiosulfate or thiophosphate (178,179) reduce renal toxicity. Delay of dosing is recommended if renal toxicity occurs. Recovery of renal function following cessation of therapy is the rule, but it may be delayed and incomplete (170). Chronic renal dysfunction is best predicted by the cumulative dose administered. Newer platinum derivatives, including carboplatin, spiroplatin, and iproplatin, and liposome-entrapped platinum compounds appear to have limited nephrotoxicity. However, there is still a degree of nephrotoxicity, even with these formulations (180). Nephrotoxicity may be exacerbated by combination therapy with other agents such as Taxol (paclitaxel) (181).

*Other Chemotherapeutic Agents.* Nitrosoureas also produce nephrotoxicity. Streptozotocin, a nitrosourea compound, is toxic to pancreatic beta cells and is used to treat metastatic islet cell carcinoma, carcinoid tumors, and lymphoma. Up to 75% of patients experience some degree of nephrotoxicity with prolonged administration (182,183). The alkylating agent cyclophosphamide has only transient effects on water excretion, increasing urine osmolarity and decreasing plasma osmolarity (184). However, its analog, ifosfamide, has significant renal toxicity. Renal proximal tubular dysfunction is the most common effect, and features of Fanconi's syndrome, which may be severe, have been reported (185,186). Distal renal tubular acidosis occurs rarely. Mild drops in the GFR are common, but severe ARF may occur as well (184,187). Irreversible chronic renal failure has also been described (188). Use of thiophosphates may reduce toxicity (189).

## Radiologic Contrast Media

Renal failure is an important complication of contrast media administration; the reported incidence of radiocontrast nephrotoxicity (RN) varies between 2% and 70%, averaging 5% to 10% (190–193). In the United States and Europe, RN has been reported to be the cause of 10% of hospital-acquired ARF (194). Differences in reported incidence are primarily the result of problems with the definition of RN, optimally defined as "acute impairment in renal function following exposure to radiographic contrast materials." This impairment is measured by a rise in sCr by most investigators. However, the degree of change in sCr that is considered to be diagnostic of RN shows great variation. One criterion is a 20% to 50% increase from the baseline level, and another is an absolute increase, ranging from 0.3 mg/dL to 2.0 mg/dL within 24 to 120 hours after contrast media administration (190,191,195). Some prospective studies, which measured the sCr levels at regular intervals, have confirmed a diagnosis of RN even after relatively small increases. Thus, some of these studies may overestimate the incidence of clinically significant RN. The Iohexol Cooperative Study group (192) has defined RN as a 1.0 mg/dL rise in sCr within 48 to 72 hours of contrast exposure. Urinary levels of tubular cell enzymes and markers of oxidative stress rise in the urine of patients with RN (196,197).

Certain underlying conditions predispose to the development of RN; the most important of them is *pre-existing renal insufficiency* (192,198–200). Moore et al (198) demonstrated that the incidence of RN in patients with baseline sCr levels between 1.5 and 1.9 mg/dL was 4.7%; the incidence for those with sCr levels between 2.0 and 2.4 mg/dL was 14.3%, and for levels between 2.5 and 2.9 mg/dL, it was 20%. Analogous findings were reported in a recent large study, with incidence of RN (rise in sCr of more than 0.5 mg/dL) ranging from 2.4% with sCr of 0.1 to 1 mg/dL to 30.6% for sCr above 3 mg/dL (199). The Iohexol Cooperative Study group (192) found that patients with pre-existing renal insufficiency (baseline sCr over 1.5 mg/dL) had a 21.1 times greater risk of nephrotoxicity than patients with normal baseline renal function (sCr below 1.5 mg/dL). Dehydration is a risk factor for RN, which is not surprising because dehydration, and thus hypovolemia, may potentiate the development of renal failure owing to any insult. Effective prophylactic measures, such as rehydration, alleviate this problem (190,191). The efficacy of prophylactic hemodialysis and hemofiltration to reduce the incidence of RN in high risk groups is controversial (200).

*Diabetes* and *multiple myeloma* are also risk factors for RN. However, it appears that neither condition represents a higher risk if renal function is normal (192,201,202). Diabetes has a deleterious effect in patients with high baseline sCr levels, since patients with diabetes and pre-existing renal insufficiency are at higher risk compared with nondiabetic patients with renal insufficiency (192,202–205). The incidence of radiocontrast material–associated renal failure in people with advanced diabetes may be well over 50%. Patients with plasma cell dyscrasias may have a variety of renal pathologic patterns, such as myeloma cast nephropathy, amyloidosis, monoclonal immunoglobulin deposition disease, or interstitial nephritis. If there is pre-existing renal impairment because of these myeloma-associated renal diseases, contrast media administration will facilitate the development of ARF. However, the review of McCarthy and Becker (201) indicates a relatively low incidence of RN in myeloma patients (0.6% to 1.25%), and it appears that patients with normal renal function are not at higher risk.

Whether *dosage* and *route of administration* are independent risk factors is a matter of debate. Some studies found a significant correlation between the volume of administered contrast media and the degree of nephrotoxicity, particularly in patients with underlying renal disease, such as diabetes mellitus (204), and in the setting of reduced renal function (206). Other studies did not confirm this relationship (198). These differences probably reflect biases in selection of patients. Dose may not be a significant risk factor in patients with normal renal function, but dosage as an independent risk factor has not been investigated in most published studies. The incidence of RN appears to be somewhat higher following cardiac angiography than after other procedures (198). In such patients, atheroembolism and cardiac disease are also risk factors for renal failure, and many of these patients have pre-existing renal disease (207). Patients who develop RN reportedly have more frequent adverse events, including myocardial infarction, prolonged hospital stay, and higher 1-year mortality (208).

Following the introduction of nonionic (low-osmolality) contrast media, some studies suggested that they are less nephrotoxic than the conventional ionic (high-osmolality) contrast media (209,210). However, several prospective clinical studies comparing the nephrotoxic effect of low- and high-osmolality contrast media did not find differences in the incidence of nephrotoxicity (192,198,203,205). The randomized prospective multicenter Iohexol Cooperative Study group (192) found that in patients with normal renal function, the incidence rates of RN were not different between patients undergoing cardiac angiography using ionic (sodium diatrizoate) and nonionic (iohexol) contrast media. In contrast, patients with pre-existing renal impairment receiving ionic contrast material were 3.3 times more likely to develop RN than patients receiving nonionic contrast material. Thus, it appears that the considerably cheaper conventional ionic contrast media can be safely used in patients with normal renal function, but ionic contrast media should be used with caution in those with pre-existing renal insufficiency.

### Narcotics

Cocaine has been implicated in both acute and chronic renal failure (211). The clinical symptoms of myoglobinuric ARF associated with narcotic abuse are not different from myoglobinuric ARF of other origins. Patients show signs of ARF, with muscle pain and elevated serum levels of creatine phosphokinase, serum glutamic-oxaloacetic transaminase, serum glutamic-pyruvic transaminase, and lactate dehydrogenase. Hypotension, hypoxia, hypovolemia, and acidosis are common findings. Acute renal failure may be polyuric or oliguric and of varying severity and duration (212–214). Only about a third of patients with cocaine-induced rhabdomyolysis develop renal failure; risk factors for ARF include higher creatine phosphokinase levels, hyperthermia, and hypotension (212). With appropriate supportive therapy, the majority of patients recover, but the mortality rate in some cohorts approaches 15% (212). Renal infarction is a rare complication; patients present with flank pain, fever, leukocytosis, elevated lactate dehydrogenase, and hematuria.

### Anesthetics

Several cases of ARF, sometimes of the polyuric or high-output type, have been associated with the use of the anesthetic methoxyflurane (215,216).

### Angiotensin-Converting Enzyme Inhibitors

Angiotensin-converting enzyme (ACE) inhibitors have become widely used because of their proven beneficial effect on cardiovascular and renal disease. They decrease the GFR through reducing efferent arteriolar vascular tone by antagonizing the angiotensin II effect. There is ample evidence that by reducing glomerular transcapillary hydraulic pressure, ACE inhibitors slow the progression of chronic renal disease, particularly if it is attributable to glomerular hyperperfusion/hyperfiltration. However, data indicate that ACE inhibitors may induce ARF in some individuals (for review, see Textor [217]). Risk factors include pre-existing renal impairment, particularly if it is caused by compromise of the afferent arteriolar blood supply, such as renal artery stenosis. Another unwanted effect of ACE inhibitors is hyperkalemia. Fortunately, in the overwhelming majority of cases, renal failure is reversible, and the benefits of ACE inhibitors appear to far outweigh the risks. These agents may also produce interstitial nephritis and are discussed in detail in Chapter 23.

### Herbal Medications

The use of herbal therapies has increased over the past decade in the Western world, and much of the world depends on botanical medicines to treat a variety of health problems (218–221). A number of renal manifestations have been reported with these preparations. These include ARF, Fanconi's syndrome, and hypokalemia or hyperkalemia; the focus here will be on tubular injury in this context. Botanical/herbal preparations are inconsistent in composition and effect and in general poorly regulated (222). The use of traditional herbal remedies may underlie about 35% of all cases of ARF in Africa. Acute renal failure produced by herbal medications may be a result of direct tubular injury it but may also be part of a systemic reaction or owing to interstitial nephritis or urolithiasis. Herbs known to cause ATI/necrosis include *Securida longepedunculata, Euphoria matabelensis, Callilepsis laureola, Cape aloes, Taxus celebica,* and *Fakaout roumia.* Adulteration of herbal preparations by dichromate may underlie toxicity in some cases. Fanconi's syndrome has been described with Chinese herbs containing aristocholic acids or adulterated with cadmium (218). Urinary excretion of $\beta_2$-microglobulin and other low–molecular-weight proteins is increased, and proximal tubular enzymuria has been described with aristocholate exposure (223,224). Cases caused by *Fakaout roumia* (paraphenylenediamine) are often associated with rhabdomyolysis (225,226).

## Acute Renal Failure in Sepsis

The incidence of ARF is approximately 19% in moderate sepsis, 23% in severe sepsis, and 51% in septic shock with positive blood cultures (227,228). The combination of ARF and shock is associated with 70% mortality. Clinical definition of sepsis includes fever, high heart and respiratory rates, and elevation in white blood cells and/or immature white blood cell forms in the setting of infection. Severe sepsis is associated with lactic acidosis, and there may be altered mental status. In septic shock, hypotension persists despite adequate fluid replacement.

## Pathology of Acute Renal Failure

### Gross Pathology

At a gross level, as a result of extensive interstitial edema, the kidneys become enlarged and swollen. The combined weight of both kidneys is usually increased by about 25% to 30%. On cut section, the tissue bulges above the cut surface and has a flabby consistency. The cortex is widened and pale. The outer medulla may appear as a deep red band, in contrast to the more pale cortex and papillary tip, the result of congestion of the vasa recta. Glomeruli appear as distinct red dots in the pale cortex.

### Histopathology

#### Acute Tubular Injury
Our understanding of the pathology of human ARF is incomplete, since many cases occur without renal biopsy (229). Autopsy kidneys, even if optimally harvested and processed, often have major preservation artifacts, especially in tubules. Biopsy with rapid processing provides the best histologic preparation, although it has inherent sampling errors. However, while less than ideal, many useful

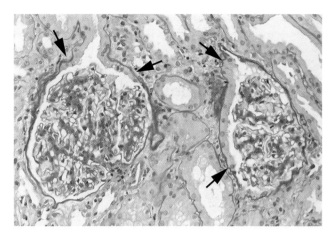

**Figure 24.1** "Tubularization" of parietal epithelial cells lining Bowman's capsule (*arrows*). Reactive changes in the proximal tubule extend from the tubular take-off to involve these epithelial cells, which have marked increase in cytoplasm compared to normal quiescent cells. (Hematoxylin & eosin [H&E]; ×640.)

observations have been made with available tissue from cases of ATI.

The lesions in both ischemic and toxic ATI primarily involve the tubules; the glomeruli are spared, as indicated by the nomenclature (230–232). Although no significant changes occur in the glomeruli, the parietal epithelium of Bowman's capsule is often prominent (Fig. 24.1), apparently reflecting reactive changes in the proximal tubule. Herniation of proximal tubular epithelium into Bowman's capsule is sometimes seen and may be the sole indicator of ATI when tubular epithelial changes are minimal. While these changes may be prominent, they are not specific. Glomeruli may show ischemic collapse, and Bowman's space may appear dilated.

Although "necrosis" has traditionally been included in the clinical term for ARF caused by tubular injury to distinguish this condition from other intrinsic causes of ARF (such as prerenal or postrenal failure or acute glomerular or interstitial nephritis), tubular epithelial cell death is often not evident by light microscopy (233,234). Acute tubular injury is generally divided into two subcategories: postischemic ATI and nephrotoxic ATI. Morphologic changes of cellular injury are usually more subtle in the ischemic type, and there are more obvious cytopathologic changes in the toxic form. In addition, the sites of tubular damage along the nephron differ between the two forms (Fig. 24.2). In the ischemic form, tubular damage is patchy, affecting relatively short lengths of the straight segments of the proximal tubule and focal areas of the ascending limbs of the loops of Henle. In the toxic form, the tubular epithelial damage is more extensive along segments of the proximal tubule, and the degree of involvement of the segments varies with the specific toxin. Although there is distal nephron damage, it is less extensive and more inconsistent in location than with ischemic ATI.

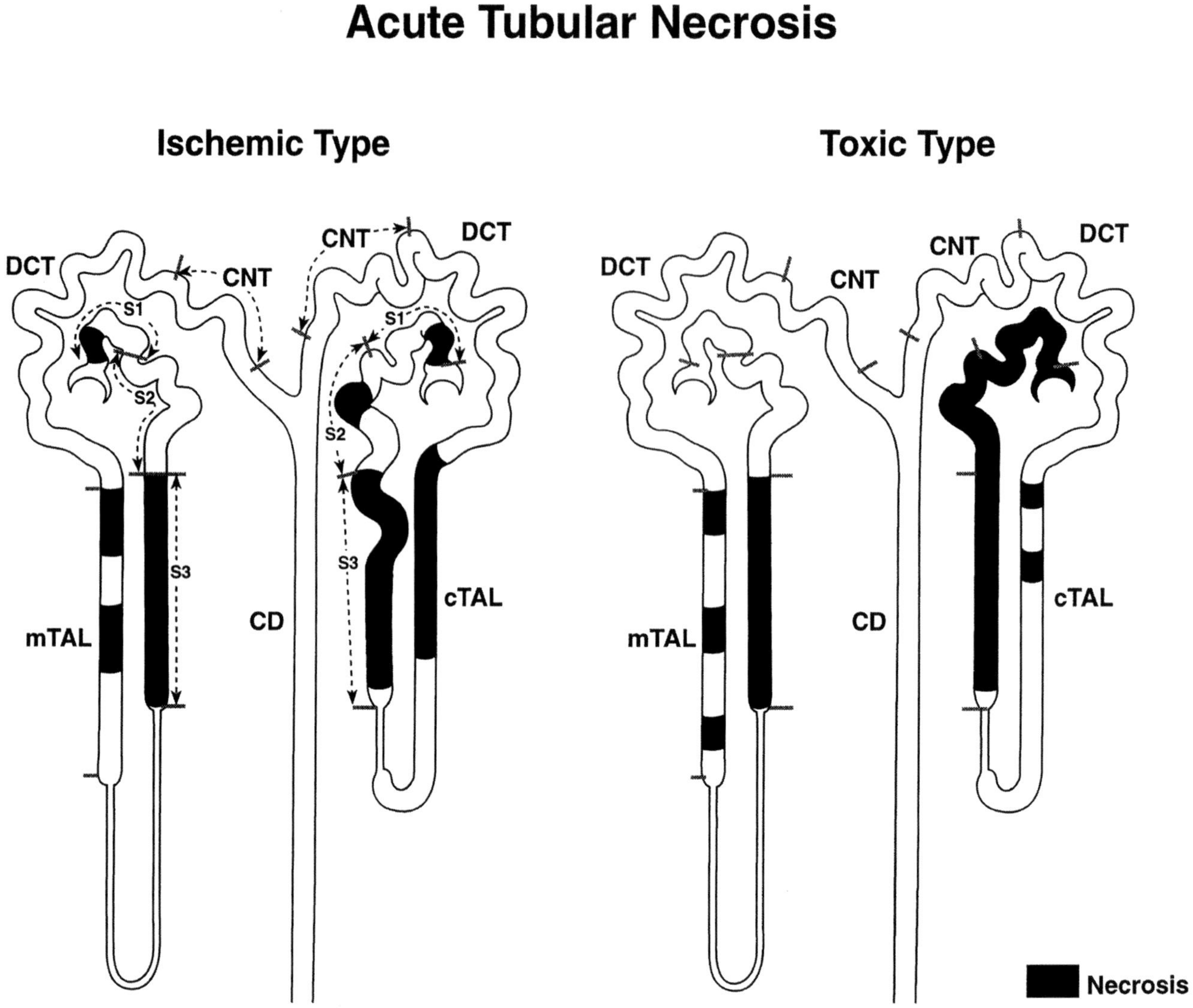

# Acute Tubular Necrosis

## Ischemic Type

## Toxic Type

**Figure 24.2**   Cartoon demonstrating the difference in the distribution of lesions between ischemic and classic nephrotoxic tubular injury. In addition to differences in localization along nephron segments, different degrees of damage are visible between cortical and juxtamedullary nephrons. In the ischemic form, the $S_3$ segments are most severely affected, along with focal areas of the ascending limbs of the loops of Henle. The cortical nephrons show more extensive damage than the juxtamedullary nephrons. In the toxic form, tubular epithelial damage is more extensive. Whereas mercury shows some predilection for the $S_3$ segment, other heavy metals and organic toxins often show more extensive involvement of all nephron segments, also with a greater predilection for cortical nephrons.

## Ischemic Acute Tubular Injury

The histologic picture varies with the severity of renal failure and the evolution of the lesion. Early in the course, cellular changes can range from minimal alterations to severe cell swelling (Fig. 24.3) to individual cell necrosis with denudation of the basement membrane (Fig. 24.4). With injury, there may be shedding of both viable (Fig. 24.5) and necrotic epithelial cells (Fig. 24.6) into the tubular lumen. Exfoliated epithelial cells, some viable, can be demonstrated in the urine (Fig. 24.7) (235).

In sections stained with periodic acid–Schiff (PAS), the brush border of proximal tubules is often thinned or ab-

sent. Blebs of apical membrane and intact cells shed from their basement membrane anchor are present in the lumen of the tubules (Fig. 24.8). Focal lesions of individual cell necrosis with disruption of the basement membrane also occur in the ascending limb of the loop of Henle. Hyaline, granular, cellular, and/or pigmented casts are seen in the distal portions of the nephron and are often particularly prominent in the collecting ducts (Fig. 24.9). These casts consist of Tamm-Horsfall protein, which stains positively with PAS mixed with cell debris (236). It is the relative prominence of these distal changes that gave rise to the term *lower nephron nephrosis*. In segments of the tubules

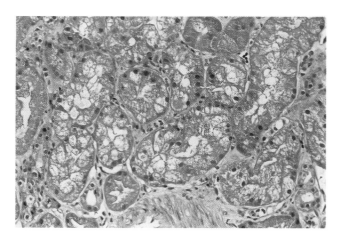

**Figure 24.3**   Tubular cells showing severe cell swelling, in some areas apparently obstructing the tubular lumen. (H&E; ×640.)

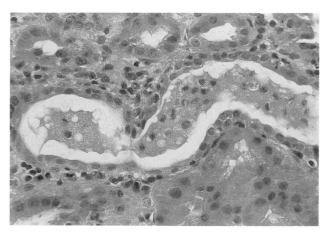

**Figure 24.5**   Intact exfoliated tubular cells in tubular lumen in a kidney with ischemic injury. (H&E; ×640.)

that do not show significant necrosis, the tubules are often dilated and lined by flattened epithelial cells—so-called "tubular simplification" (Fig. 24.10). The denuded basement membrane gaps are covered by spreading of adjacent viable epithelial cells.

The tubules are separated by sometimes markedly edematous interstitium. There may be evidence of transdifferentiation of tubular cells (237,238), which may express vimentin and other mesenchymal markers (Fig. 24.11). There is some evidence that transdifferentiated tubular cells may contribute to fibrogenesis in later stages (237,238).

As the lesion progresses after the initial injury, evidence of tubular regeneration can be seen. Histologic indicators of cellular proliferation, such as mitoses, hyperchromatic nuclei, and a high nuclear–cytoplasmic ratio, may be seen (Fig. 24.12). Immunostaining for transcription markers, such as

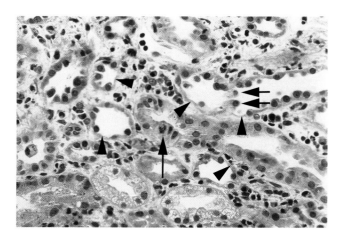

**Figure 24.4**   Areas of single tubular cell loss from a kidney with ischemic injury. Injured cells have detached, leaving areas of tubular basement membrane covered by a thin layer of cytoplasm from adjacent cells (*arrowheads*). A few detached cells can be seen in tubular lumina (*short arrows*). A mitotic figure can be seen in one tubular cell (*long arrow*). There is also interstitial edema and inflammatory cells largely marginating in capillaries. (H&E; ×400.)

proliferating cell nuclear antigen or Ki-67, reveal an elevated proliferative index (238) (Fig. 24.13).

The injured tubules are separated by sometimes markedly edematous interstitium. There may be a mild interstitial inflammatory infiltrate with small numbers of lymphocytes, macrophages, and neutrophils, or, occasionally, eosinophils (Fig. 24.4). The cellular infiltrate tends to be clustered around necrotic and ruptured segments of tubules or where Tamm-Horsfall protein has been extruded, forming small granulomata. It is in these late stages that distinctions have to be made between ischemic ATI and acute tubulointerstitial nephritis, but in general, the infiltrate is much less prominent in cases of ATI.

Tubular cell death during ischemia/reperfusion occurs via apoptosis as well as coagulative necrosis and has been documented in both animal models and in clinical renal disease (239–241). It is possible to detect the nuclear and cytoplasmic condensation of cells undergoing apoptosis by light microscopy. Apoptotic cells may appear triangular and may be extruded from the epithelium into the tubular lumen (Fig. 24.14). Apoptotic bodies, representing membrane-bound nuclear fragments, may also be detected in adjacent tubular cells, which have phagocytosed the cell remnants. However, the most reliable methods of detection are by nick-end labeling (TUNEL) of the chromatin that has been cleaved in a characteristic "ladder" pattern by the endonucleases, or by staining for apoptosis-associated markers. Coagulative necrosis is characterized by eosinophilic cytoplasm and pyknosis and eventual disappearance of nuclei (Fig. 24.15).

Acute tubular injury in renal allografts can show changes similar to those found in native kidneys, but more frank necrosis of tubular cross sections may be seen, and calcium oxalate deposits may be numerous in renal tubules (242) (Fig. 24.16). The cellular lesions are most prominent in the $S_3$ segment of the proximal tubule and tend to be more uniform in character. Apical blebbing may be the only finding

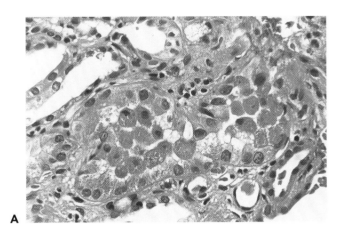
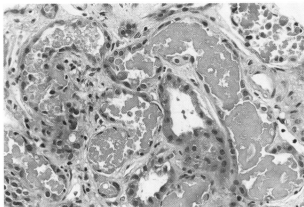

**Figure 24.6** **A:** Detached necrotic tubular cells, several with pyknotic nuclei, in lumen of proximal tubule. **B:** Granular casts with necrotic cell debris. Note flattened tubular epithelium in tubules containing necrotic debris. (H&E, ×640.)

in milder forms, whereas the more severe cases also show focal necrosis with rupture of the tubular basement membrane. It is interesting to note that one study has shown a correlation of loss of Na$^+$,K$^+$-adenosine triphosphatase (ATPase) polarity with delayed graft function (243).

Electron microscopy has been helpful in evaluating the tubular epithelial changes in ATI (230,244–248). In ischemic ATI, scattered epithelial cell changes show a variety of different cytopathic alterations (Fig. 24.17). These include loss of the apical brush border; blebbing of the apical membrane, with shedding of apical membrane blebs into the tubular lumina; high-amplitude swelling, with condensation of the cristae of the mitochondria; individual cell apoptosis, as demonstrated by cell shrinkage with nuclear fragmentation; and a variety of other cytopathic changes leading to necrosis (Fig. 24.18).

Interstitial inflammation is seen as a response to tubular injury. This inflammation is typically mononuclear and patchy. There is often associated interstitial edema, which may be severe (see Fig. 24.4).

A particularly interesting and useful finding in cases of ARF is the accumulation of nucleated cells in the vasa recta of the outer medulla (249–251). This is a very common feature, and in many cases it is the only histologic clue to the diagnosis of ATI (Fig. 24.19). The nature of the cell changes with progression of the ATI through its three different phases. Lymphocytes are predominant in the first 24 to 48 hours, followed later by immature cells of the myeloid series and eventually by nucleated red cells and red cell precursors. The accumulation of the larger nucleated cells in this location may be merely a reflection of the hemodynamic shifts that occur in ATI, with shifting of blood flow away from the superficial and midcortical glomeruli to the juxtamedullary glomeruli, resulting in a relative increase in blood flow to this nephron population, which gives rise to the vasa recta. The countercurrent nature of blood flow in the vasa recta would result in dilution of cellular elements as blood flows toward the hairpin turn, resulting in a concentration of cellular elements at the proximal end of the vasa

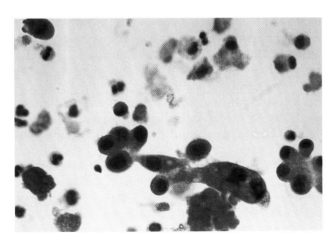

**Figure 24.7** Intact tubular cells in the urine from a patient with ischemic injury. (Papanicolaou; ×1000.)

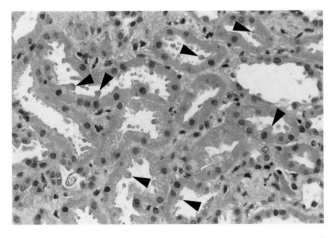

**Figure 24.8** Apical blebbing from the surface of injured proximal tubular cells (*arrowheads*). Apical cytoplasmic blebs can be seen in tubular lumina. (H&E; ×640.)

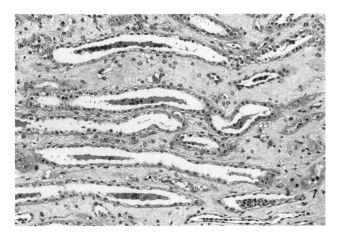

**Figure 24.9** Tubular cell casts in collecting ducts in papilla. Injured cells have detached from sites in proximal nephron, and aggregate into casts, often around a protein core. (H&E; ×400.)

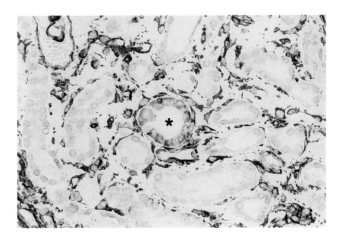

**Figure 24.11** Injured tubule with cells staining for vimentin (*center*). Adjacent tubules do not stain. Note bright background staining for vimentin in interstitial areas. (Immunoperoxidase; ×400.)

recta vasculature in the outer medulla. There is also some evidence that up-regulation of adhesion molecules on ischemic endothelium leads to accumulation of leukocytes in the microvasculature, which may contribute to stasis and lack of reflow in ischemia–reperfusion injury (see section "The Inflammatory Response in Ischemic Injury").

## Nephrotoxic Acute Tubular Injury

*Tubules.* Classically, toxic tubular injury may be associated with extensive epithelial necrosis, which tends to involve all nephrons more uniformly than in the ischemic form. However, a range of morphologic changes may be seen in the renal tubules as the result of toxic injury. The extent and severity of the changes will vary depending on the agent, the dose, and the timing of the morphologic assessment. Renal tubular cell changes detectable by light microscopy include the following:

- Alterations in the surface of the cells, including loss of brush border (detectable on PAS), loss of basolateral infoldings, and blebbing of apical cytoplasm
- Cytoplasmic swelling and vacuolation
- Intracellular inclusions
- Extensive tubular cell necrosis
- Loss of individual tubular cells, with gaps along the tubular basement membrane or tubular profiles with fewer and attenuated cells lining the tubule
- Intraluminal proteinaceous cellular debris, casts, or crystals
- Tubular dilatation with flattening of tubular epithelium
- Tubular rupture with urinary extravasation
- Regenerative changes, including flattening of epithelial cells, cytoplasmic basophilia, heterogeneity in cell size and shape, a higher nuclear-to-cytoplasmic ratio in individual cells, and cellular mitoses

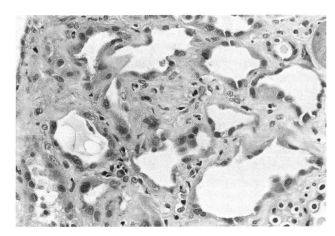

**Figure 24.10** Dilated tubules with flattened epithelium in the regenerative phase after tubular injury. Marginating inflammatory cells can be seen in capillaries. (H&E; ×640.)

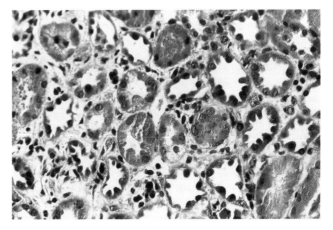

**Figure 24.12** Striking regenerative changes in tubular cells, with pleomorphic hyperchromatic nuclei, with relatively little cytoplasm. (H&E; ×640.)

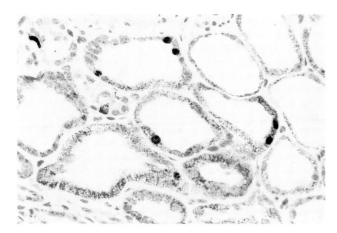

**Figure 24.13**    Immunostain for the transcription factor Ki-67. Note positive nuclear staining in several tubular cells. (Immunoperoxidase; ×640.)

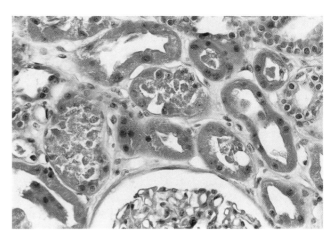

**Figure 24.15**    Coagulative necrosis of focal tubular epithelial cells, with cell debris in tubular lumina. (H&E; ×640.)

Swelling and vacuolation of proximal tubular cells may be seen; cells appear large and pale and may contain discrete vacuoles of varying size. Hypertonic solutions, including intravenous immunoglobulin preparations (252), have been reported to produce severe swelling and vacuolation of renal tubular cells.

Intracellular inclusions are occasionally seen in renal tubular cells exposed to drugs. Giant mitochondria, appearing as bright eosinophilic inclusions, have been described after the administration of relatively high doses of CsA to humans. In gold-induced nephropathy, gold can be demonstrated in tubular cells (253). Calcification of tubular cells has been described in cases of severe toxicity caused by amphotericin or bacitracin (254).

Extensive coagulative necrosis of tubular cells has been seen in cases of poisoning by heavy metals such as mercuric chloride, rarely seen today, or in cases of poisoning due to chemicals such as diethylene glycol (55). More often changes are more subtle, with individual tubular cell necrosis or loss, though there may be more obvious and

extensive necrosis than is seen in ischemic injury (255). Apoptosis has not been thoroughly studied in the context of toxic renal injury. However, apoptosis is a known toxic effect of agents in other cell systems and may be a central molecular mechanism in toxic injury at many sites (256). It is clear that both necrosis and apoptosis occur in toxic nephropathies in experimental models as well as in clinical tubular injury (240,257,258). In vitro studies have documented apoptosis in cell culture on exposure to nephrotoxins. For example, LLC-PK1 cells exposed to sublethal doses of mercuric chloride in vitro undergo apoptosis (259), and apoptosis can be induced in Lewis-lung cancer-porcine kidney-1 [LLC-PK1] cells by cisplatin as well via activation of caspases (260). Apoptosis has been described in clinical nephrotoxicity as well (261). This remains an area to be actively explored in both clinical and experimental models of toxic renal injury.

Tubular casts, which may include cells and cell debris, are frequently seen with toxic tubular injury. In addition, tubular crystalline deposits are found in cases of renal toxicity produced by nephrotoxins. Anesthetic agents, including methoxyflurane and halothane, and antiretroviral agents such as indinavir may produce tubular crystalline deposits. Mechanical obstruction may also result from deposition of intratubular crystals in patients treated with sulfonamides or acyclovir. In addition, radiocontrast agents are uricosuric and oxaluric, and casts and birefringent crystals have been identified following administration of these agents. Uric acid lithiasis with tubular obstruction has been reported with phenylbutazone (262). Finally, pigmented casts may result from hemolysis in rare cases of fulminant drug reactions and with the rhabdomyolysis caused by cocaine.

*Vessels.* Vessels usually show no remarkable features unless there is intercurrent disease. However, newer studies in experimental models have refocused attention on injury to the microvasculature, which may have been underappreciated in clinical specimens. Certainly, vascular congestion in the outer medulla with margination has been noted.

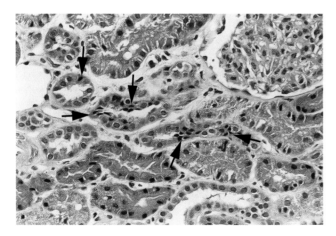

**Figure 24.14**    Focal tubular cell apoptosis, with condensed triangular cells in the epithelium (*arrows*), focally extruding from the epithelium. (H&E; ×640.)

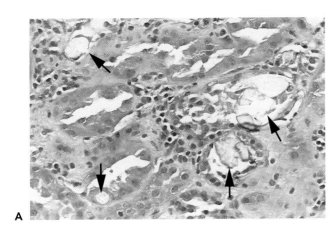 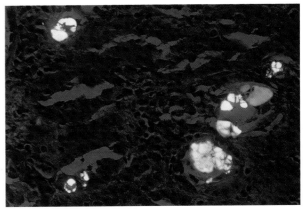

**Figure 24.16** A: Oxalate crystal precipitates (*arrows*) in acute tubular injury in an allograft kidney. B: Oxalate crystals in polarized light. (H&E; ×640.)

*Electron Microscopy.* Electron microscopy of injured tubules reveals loss of brush border microvilli and basolateral infoldings in the proximal tubules. Cells may show rarefaction of the cytoplasm, with intracellular vacuoles and swollen organelles. Degenerative changes in mitochondria, including swelling and loss of cristae, loss of endoplasmic reticulum, or alterations in lysosomes, are often visible. Within the cells, membrane-bound structures consisting of concentrically arranged whorls of membrane may form, especially with exposure to aminoglycosides; however, these so-called myeloid bodies do not necessarily indicate toxicity.

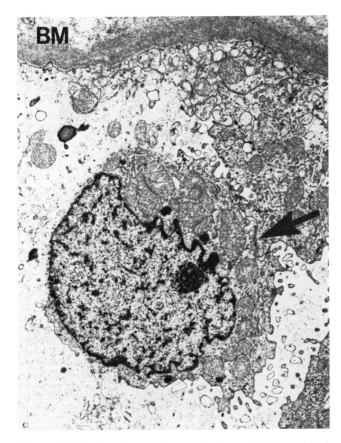

**Figure 24.17** An electron micrograph shows a tubular epithelial cell in the process of desquamation into the lumen. The cell has separated from the basement membrane (BM) but is still adherent to the adjacent epithelial cell through the cell-to-cell junction (*arrow*). (×10,230.) (From Olsen TS, Hansen HE. Ultrastructure of medullary tubules in ischemic acute tubular necrosis and acute interstitial nephritis in man. APMIS 1990;98:600.)

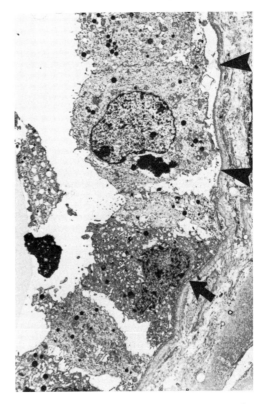

**Figure 24.18** An electron micrograph demonstrates loosening from the basement membrane (*arrowheads*) of an array of tubular epithelial cells. Most cells appear viable, but a cell undergoing apoptosis is also seen (*arrow*). (×3720.) (From Olsen TS, Hansen HE. Ultrastructure of medullary tubules in ischemic acute tubular necrosis and acute interstitial nephritis in man. APMIS 1990;98:600.)

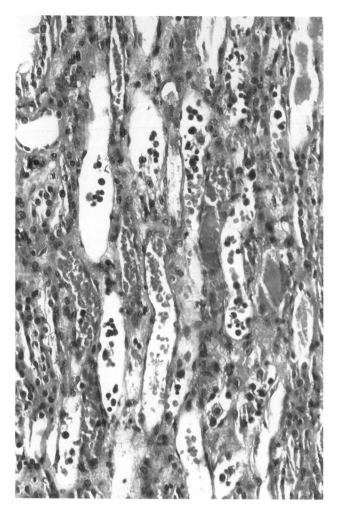

**Figure 24.19** Erythrocyte congestion and nucleated cells in dilated vasa recta in outer medulla of a kidney with ischemic injury. (H&E; ×400.)

## Pathology of Specific Nephrotoxins

As a preface to this discussion, it should be recognized that it is often difficult to establish a pathogenetic link between a pathologic lesion and a particular drug or toxin (263). Several factors contribute to this uncertainty, including concurrent factors that may produce renal injury, such as administration of other potentially nephrotoxic drugs; lack of or inadequacy of morphologic data in reported cases; and the fact that some drugs may have multiple effects. Moreover, experimental models of toxicity may not be relevant to a particular clinical context owing to interspecies variation and markedly different dosing of drug or toxin in these models. In general, we limit our discussion to those drugs for which toxicity has been well documented in humans by disappearance of toxic effects when the drug is withdrawn, recurrence of symptoms on rechallenge, or both.

A range of chemotherapeutic agents and other toxins may produce direct injury to the renal tubular epithelium. These agents are outlined in Table 24.2. The focus in this

discussion is on primary toxic tubular injury, recognizing that secondary injury to the renal tubule may also occur with other types of toxic renal injury, including tubulointerstitial nephritis, hemodynamic changes, and vascular disease.

### Antibiotics

There have been many reports of renal damage associated with antibiotic therapy. However, in many cases, there is an association, but the causative role of the antibiotic has not been firmly established. There are several reasons for this. First, the infection for which the drug is being used may damage the kidney directly or indirectly. Second, infections are frequently treated with several agents, making it difficult to implicate a particular drug. Finally, the paucity of renal biopsy studies makes it difficult to define the pathologic changes produced by individual drugs and the pathogenetic mechanisms involved in producing renal injury.

### Antiviral Agents

In experimental animal models and in humans receiving acyclovir, indinavir, or ganciclovir, renal histologic examination often shows drug crystals in tubules, especially collecting ducts, with dilatation of tubules reflecting obstruction (59,68–70,264–266) (Figs. 24.20 and 24.21). In other cases, there may be tubular dilatation and tubular cell injury without detectable crystals in the urine or kidney (62); crystals, of course, might be missed if relatively few collecting ducts are sampled. Patchy interstitial inflammation has been described without crystals (62,63), and, occasionally, granulomas have been described (63). Renal tubular cell apoptosis has been described in renal biopsy of a patient with irreversible cidofovir toxicity (261).

### Aminoglycosides

Pathologic changes in the kidney have not been well documented in most clinical cases of aminoglycoside-induced

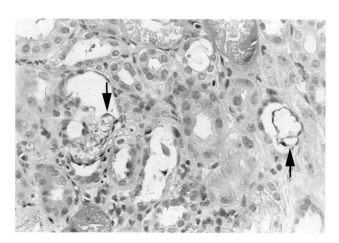

**Figure 24.20** Crystalline precipitates (*arrows*) in tubules in a patient treated with intravenous acyclovir. (H&E; ×640.)

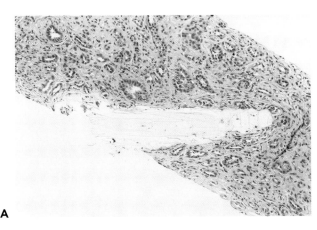
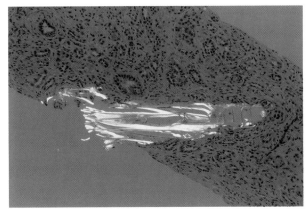

**Figure 24.21** **A:** Indinavir crystal in papilla of patient treated long-term with highly active antiretroviral therapy. The patient also had crystals in the urine. **B:** Indinavir crystal under polarized light. (H&E; ×200.)

nephrotoxicity. With gentamicin, ATI has been the lesion reported most often (267,268,269), although in some cases this lesion has been attributed to concomitant volume depletion and hypotension. Tubulointerstitial inflammation with tubular necrosis also has been reported; this pattern may be the most common in female patients (270). Houghton et al (271) observed that cytosegresomes are very common in the tubular epithelium of patients receiving gentamicin, but appeared to reflect exposure to the drug, since the presence of cytosegresomes did not correlate with a significant toxic effect of the drug.

Tubular necrosis in the kidney can be produced with high doses of gentamicin in rats and dogs. In rats, there are no detectable changes in the tubules with doses comparable to those used in humans (93). With high doses (40 to 100 mg/kg/day) there is necrosis of the $S_1$ and $S_2$ segments of the proximal convoluted tubules (92–94,272), the extent of which is dose-dependent. On electron microscopy, more subtle tubular cell changes are seen, including damage to the brush border, mitochondrial swelling with intramitochondrial densities, and accumulation within the cell of cytosegresomes with myeloid bodies (Fig. 24.22).

Zager (273) has shown experimentally that gentamicin in a dose that does not by itself cause renal failure will trigger severe renal failure when combined with 1 hour of moderate renal hypoperfusion, which also does not produce renal failure on its own. In those studies, there was tubular necrosis in the $S_3$ proximal tubule segment, a pattern of injury characteristic of renal ischemia rather than gentamicin toxicity; this suggests that in some instances gentamicin may worsen ischemic injury rather than causing injury to the $S_1$ and $S_2$ segments, which is more typical of toxic doses of gentamicin.

There are few descriptions of renal pathologic lesions in patients receiving kanamycin or tobramycin. In one patient with oliguria who received 21 g of kanamycin over a 2-week period (274), a renal biopsy was done 25 days after the on-set of oliguria (21 days after diuresis) and was reported to show some flattening of tubular epithelial cells. Whereas histologic findings have often not been documented in clinical cases of neomycin toxicity, one biopsy from a patient in the recovery phase revealed edema of the interstitium with flattening of tubular epithelial cells; some of the tubular cells showed vacuolation (102). It is worth noting that this patient also received kanamycin. Vacuolation of tubules has also been reported in two cases examined at autopsy (275).

In cases of ARF resulting from a combination of gentamicin and cephalothin, the pathologic features are those of ATI with normal glomeruli and vessels (89,90). Necrotic epithelial cells may be shed into the tubular lumen (90). However, experimental studies in the rat have found no potentiating effect of cephalosporins on gentamicin nephrotoxicity (276). Immunofluorescence studies have shown negative results, and Fillastre et al commented on the absence of antibodies to gentamicin and cephalothin (89).

### Amphotericin

In human autopsy or biopsy specimens from patients treated with amphotericin, extensive calcification in tubules, presumably developing in the context of severe tubular cell injury, has been reported frequently (103,277) (Fig. 24.23A). There may be vacuolation of smooth muscle cells in small arteries and arterioles (278) (Fig. 24.23B). This is likely a change that potentially reflects direct toxic effects on the arterial wall, some element of intrarenal vasospasm, or both, and it may be very striking.

### Cephalosporins

Renal biopsies have been obtained in relatively few cases of cephalosporin-induced renal injury, usually in those in which the older cephalosporins were given. In cases of cephaloridine-induced ARF, biopsies have shown a picture of interstitial edema with variable numbers of chronic

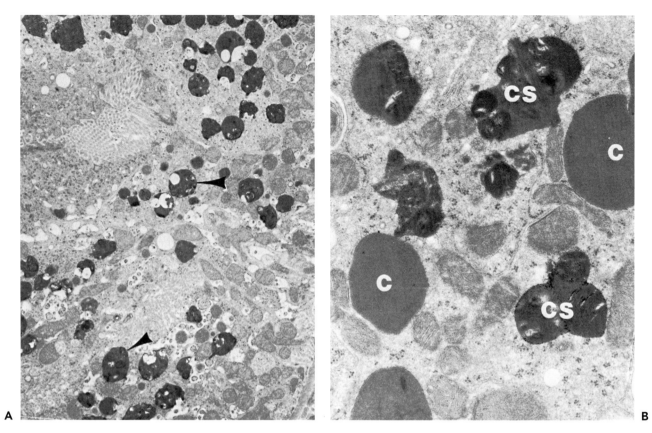

**Figure 24.22**    Electron micrographs of a rabbit killed 14 days after being given a high dose of gentamicin. **A:** Cytosegresomes (*arrowheads*) are scattered throughout the cytoplasm of the proximal convoluted tubule. The brush border can be seen at the top left (×5700). **B:** Numerous cytosomes (C) and cytosegresomes (CS) are visible at higher power (×2800) (lead citrate and uranyl acetate). (Courtesy of Dr. E. F. Cuppage.)

inflammatory cells accompanied by tubular dilatation or necroses (113). The renal histologic features in these cases showed what is described as ATI, with interstitial fibrosis or edema and infiltration by lymphocytes and mononuclear cells. Pathologic changes in cases induced by cephalothin

with or without other potential nephrotoxins consist of interstitial edema with variable numbers of lymphocytes and plasma cells; necrosis, swelling, and evidence of regeneration of tubular epithelium; and only trivial glomerular changes (110,279). Vacuolation of tubular cells has been

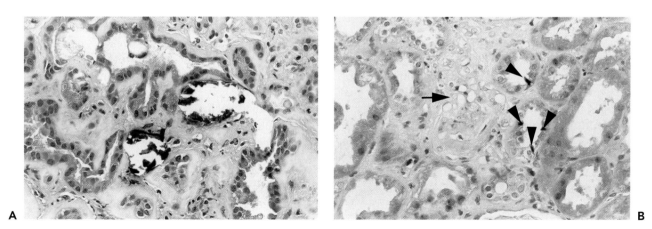

**Figure 24.23**    **A:** Calcification of tubular cells in a patient treated with amphotericin. **B:** Striking vacuolization of smooth muscle cells (*arrow*) in small vessels in the biopsy of a patient treated with amphotericin. Note apoptotic cells (*arrowheads*) in adjacent tubules. (H&E; ×640.)

evident on electron microscopy (279). A case of bilateral renal cortical necrosis associated with cefuroxime has been reported (280). Acute tubular injury has been described in patients treated with cephalexin (116,117).

## Polymyxin/Colistin

On biopsy of patients treated with polymyxin, there is interstitial edema with eosinophils, plasma cells, lymphocytes, and, occasionally, neutrophils (281). The cellular reaction may have granulomatous characteristics. Tubules show swelling of the epithelium with intramuscular administration of colistin; the lesion described was ATI (124).

## Immunosuppressive/Immunomodulatory Agents

*Cyclosporine.* Functional CsA nephrotoxicity can occur without any morphologic changes. The most common morphologic change observed in the kidneys of patients treated with CsA is isometric vacuolation of the proximal tubular cells (Fig. 24.24); this change is characteristic but not specific. Other changes include necrosis with or without calcification, inclusion bodies corresponding to giant mitochondria, and giant lysosomes (129,282). The megamitochondria and microcalcification in tubular cells of CsA-treated patients do not correlate with dysfunction (283). Strong staining for osteopontin protein and mRNA has been demonstrated in tubular epithelium in clinical CsA toxicity (284).

Vessels in CsA-induced acute renal dysfunction may show only vasospasm and vacuolation of smooth muscle cells—changes that often reflect vasoconstriction. The onset of hyaline arteriolar thickening, especially with nodular accumulation of hyaline in the periphery of the arteriolar wall, has been associated with CsA-induced renal dysfunction, although dysfunction can also exist without this change. The juxtaglomerular apparatus may be hyper-

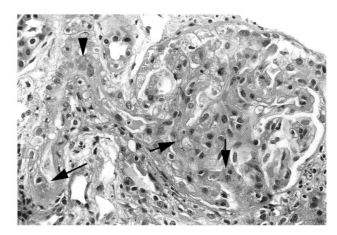

**Figure 24.25** Thrombotic microangiopathy in a patient on tacrolimus. Note arteriole with very focal intramural fibrin (*arrowhead*), focal erythrocyte extravasation into the intima (*long arrow*), and focal erythrocyte fragmentation in the glomerulus (*short arrows*). (H&E; ×640.)

plastic; this finding is significantly more prominent in renal transplant patients with CsA nephrotoxicity than in other posttransplant groups, probably indicating activation of the renin–angiotensin system (127). Thrombotic microangiopathy may be seen in particularly severe cases of toxicity.

Descriptions of the pathologic characteristics of both clinical and experimental long-term CsA toxicity have focused on interstitial fibrosis and tubular atrophy, which appears in a "striped" pattern reminiscent of ischemic injury, and hyaline arteriolar change, as described earlier. The fibrosis involves medulla and medullary rays in the cortex (281,285,286). Schieppati et al (287) have reported the renal biopsy changes observed in 10 cardiac allograft recipients with renal failure after they had received cyclosporine for 31 to 48 months. Obliterative arteriolopathy with ischemic glomerular changes was found. Serial reconstruction of the glomeruli showed the presence of populations of both abnormally small and abnormally large glomeruli. Sclerotic lesions were confined to the small glomeruli. Myers et al (288) and Remuzzi and Perico (289) have also emphasized sclerosing glomerular changes with long-term CsA therapy. The pathologic findings and the differential diagnosis of CsA nephrotoxicity in renal transplant recipients are discussed in detail in Chapter 28.

*Tacrolimus.* Pathologic changes owing to FK506 are very similar to those described for CsA. Changes include tubular cell vacuolization, calcification, myocyte vacuolization, necrotizing arteriolitis, thrombotic microangiopathy, arteriolar hyalinosis, and interstitial fibrosis. Morphologic changes with FK506 toxicity have been compared to those produced by CsA (290). Tubular cell vacuoles were small and focally confluent and involved proximal and distal tubules. Morizumi et al (291) have suggested that

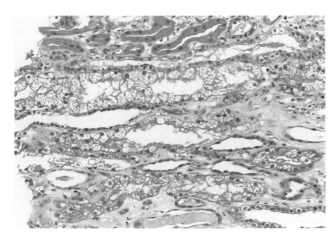

**Figure 24.24** "Isometric" vacuolization, with many small equalsized vacuoles in tubular cell cytoplasm, in a patient with high serum levels of calcineurin inhibitor. (H&E; ×400.)

FK506-related vacuoles are foamy and nonisometric and present in straight and convoluted portions of the proximal tubules. We have noted involvement of tubules in outer medulla as well (unpublished).

Glomerular capillary and arteriolar thrombi have been seen in renal allograft recipients (292) and a few kidney/liver allograft recipients (293). In several of these cases, other factors, including prior CsA therapy in three cases and fungal sepsis in a fourth case, may have contributed to the endothelial injury underlying thrombosis. A HUS-like syndrome with thrombotic microangiopathy may be seen (Fig. 24.25); the estimated incidence is approximately 1% (292), and cases are frequently associated with high serum levels of drug. Hyaline arteriolar change and interstitial fibrosis have been reported with long term therapy (158,281,282).

An increase in SUN and sCr has been documented in rats treated with FK506, with evidence of proximal tubular cell vacuolation and megamitochondria on histologic examination (294,295). Pathologic changes, including proximal tubular cell vacuolation and tubular regeneration similar to those reported with CsA therapy, also have been reported in dogs (296). Stillman et al developed a rat model of prolonged FK506 toxicity by combining FK506 with a low-salt diet for 6 weeks (297). In this model, sCr and plasma renin levels were elevated, and there was tubular atrophy and fibrosis in medullary rays and the inner stripe of the outer medulla. Tacrolimus alone produced increased juxtaglomerular apparatus granularity.

*Intravenous Immunoglobulin.* Intravenous administration of immunoglobulins has been associated with severe swelling of tubular epithelial cells (252) (Fig. 24.26). Of note, the brush border of the cells is generally well-preserved. Swelling may be severe enough to occlude the tubular lumen. In one series of transplant patients, isometric vacuolization appeared to precede the more severe cell swelling (298).

*Sirolimus.* Rats given sirolimus (3 mg/kg orally) for 2 weeks on a low-salt diet developed magnesium wasting and structural renal lesions consisting of tubular collapse, vacuolization, and nephrocalcinosis (299). Acute tubular injury has occasionally been described in patients (168). In one study of sirolimus-treated patients (also on FK506) there was a subset that developed striking intratubular cast formation, reminiscent of myeloma cast nephropathy (166). Vascular changes and glomerular disease have been reported with sirolimus; these are described in Chapter 28. Some reports have appeared that sirolimus may delay recovery from tubular injury, exacerbate acute FK506 tubular cell toxicity (168), or exacerbate chronic calcineurin inhibitor toxicity.

### Chemotherapeutic Agents

*Cis-platinum.* In the human kidney, focal necrosis of tubular cells is seen, primarily in the distal tubule and collecting ducts; cast formation and dilatation of proximal tubules may be observed (300,301). In animals, tubular changes are found in the proximal nephron, with or without accompanying distal changes (302). Dentino et al (300) found that many patients show continuing damage, and fail to regain pretherapy levels of renal function. Dobyan et al (303) studied the effects of chronic administration in animals and found cyst formation, interstitial fibrosis, and tubular atrophy.

*Other.* The pathologic picture produced by the alkylating agent ifosfamide is that of ATI or chronic tubulointerstitial changes (188,304). On pathologic examination of kidneys from patients with toxic injury caused by streptozotocin, there is ATI in the proximal tubules, with or without accompanying interstitial inflammation (183).

### Radiocontrast Agents

Because renal biopsies are not indicated in patients with transient renal failure after contrast media administration, human studies are scant. Patients who undergo biopsy are those who do not recover from renal failure, and in most of these cases the histologic picture reveals an underlying (and most likely pre-existing) renal disease. The majority of publications describing renal morphologic changes are based on experimental studies. The induction of renal failure in experimental animal models usually requires administration of additional agents (e.g., indomethacin, gentamicin, glycerol), ischemia, water or salt depletion, or a combination of these factors (305–309).

The overwhelming majority of both experimental and clinical studies report variable, transient proximal tubular

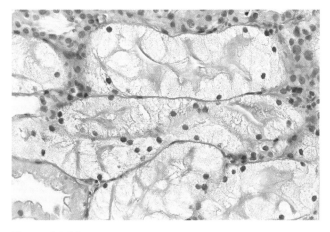

**Figure 24.26**  Severe cell swelling of tubular cells in the biopsy of a patient being treated with intravenous immunoglobulin. Note persistence of brush border. (H&E; ×640.)

vacuolation, which appears as soon as 30 minutes following administration, disappears within a few days (310,311), and seems to be dose dependent (312). One study emphasizes the selective injury of the thick ascending limb of Henle in the outer medulla after co-administration of indomethacin and iothalmate to unilaterally nephrectomized, salt-depleted rats (306). They describe mitochondrial swelling, pyknosis, cytoplasmic disruption, calcification, necrosis, and tubular collapse in the thick ascending limb of Henle in areas away from vascular bundles, suggesting hypoxic injury. They also report vacuolation of the proximal convoluted tubules.

Ultrastructural studies indicate that the vacuoles are membrane-bound, probably representing lysosomes (306,311). The fine structure of the mitochondria and the endoplasmic reticulum remains intact. Tervahartiala et al (311) believe that the vacuolation is caused by a nonspecific lysosomal injury and is not the consequence of osmotic diuresis. Autoradiographic and electron microscopic studies failed to demonstrate the presence of iodinated molecules within the vacuoles (306,313).

The most extensive studies in human beings come from the Necker Hospital in Paris, where radiocontrast examination of the kidney was routinely performed before renal biopsies in the 1970s (310,313). This group published the case studies of 211 patients who underwent biopsy within 10 days of urography or renal arteriography using ionic contrast media (310). Tubular vacuolation characteristic of "osmotic nephrosis" was found in 47 patients and was more severe in patients with pre-existing renal failure; however, they did not find a correlation between the extent of tubular vacuolation and the degree of renal functional impairment. The same group later described osmotic nephrosis in 14 of 33 patients who received low-osmolality contrast media before renal biopsy (313). They reported the case of one patient who had evidence of ATI on initial biopsy and showed signs of advanced tubular atrophy and interstitial fibrosis on a second biopsy. Other patients in the Necker Hospital also had evidence of ATI in the renal biopsy, but it appears that these patients had ARF as a pre-existing condition. They concluded that tubular vacuolation after radiocontrast administration probably does not represent true osmotic nephrosis and that it is not a reliable morphologic indicator of RN (310,313).

In 1970, two articles described hemorrhagic necrosis, primarily of the renal medulla, in six infants (314,315). Five of them underwent cardiac catheterization for heart problems, and one had excretory urography because of a flank mass. In these children, there were several confounding variables that might have contributed to the renal necrosis, such as seizures, cardiac developmental abnormalities, and sepsis. All six children died. Acute tubular injury has been reported only rarely (310,313,316), but the incidence of mild ATI may be underestimated in the absence of renal biopsy studies.

### Narcotics in Myoglobinuric Acute Renal Failure

The characteristic finding is the presence of pigmented casts, as in other forms of myoglobinuric ARF. Renal biopsy is rarely performed in affected patients, and for this reason pathologic reports are uncommon (317,318). The characteristic casts show mild brown pigmentation and usually have a granular appearance with irregular globules. These casts are frequently bright red as seen by trichrome stain. Immunohistochemistry is helpful in identifying myoglobin casts (Fig. 24.27). Hyalin and granular casts not containing detectable myoglobin may be present. Other features of ATI, such as tubular epithelial damage with exfoliation of tubular epithelial cells, thinning of the tubular epithelium, and tubular calcification, are usually noted. Immunofluorescence is typically not helpful. On ultrastructural examination, the myoglobin casts frequently consist of very electron-dense, finely granular globules that may have a somewhat less electron-dense rim (Fig. 24.28). In addition, electron microscopic signs of ATI are readily visible.

### Anesthetics

The renal lesion consists of interstitial edema with somewhat dilated tubules lined by flattened epithelium. In several cases, a striking degree of intratubular collection of oxalate crystals has been reported (215).

### Herbal Medications

There are relatively few reports of biopsy findings in ARF caused by herbal medications. Acute tubular injury has been described (reviewed by Isnard-Bagnis et al [218]). Pathology of the kidneys in patients with renal failure caused by *Aristocholia* species have shown hypocellular interstitial fibrosis and tubular loss, especially in the outer cortex, in lesions obtained later in the course of the injury (319).

## Etiology and Pathogenesis

Although the number of disease entities that have been associated with ATI is large, the basic etiologic factors are very similar (Table 24.3). Prolonged renal ischemia is the most common cause of ATI (2,320). Renal ischemia is frequently associated with major surgery, particularly when it involves the abdominal vasculature (321,322). Hemorrhage, burns, and crushing injuries associated with extensive trauma make up a second major group (12,14,323,324). A significant percentage can be attributed to conditions associated with obstetric accidents (325,326). In the hospital setting, severe congestive heart failure and septic shock are common predisposing conditions (327,328). The widespread use of nonsteroidal anti-inflammatory drugs (NSAIDs), which inhibit renal prostaglandins, is another potential mechanism through which renal ischemia can be initiated, and these drugs have been associated with the development

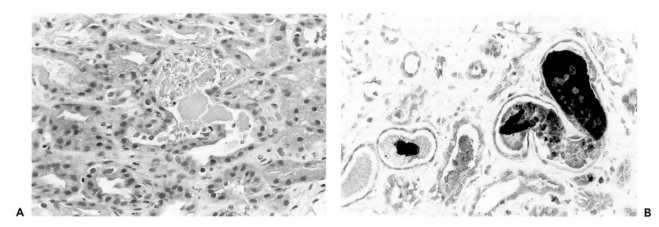

**Figure 24.27** Pigmented casts in tubular lumina of a biopsy from a patient with acute renal failure who had overdosed on cocaine. **A:** Light microscopy. (H&E; ×640). **B:** Immunostain for myoglobin. (Immunoperoxidase; ×640.)

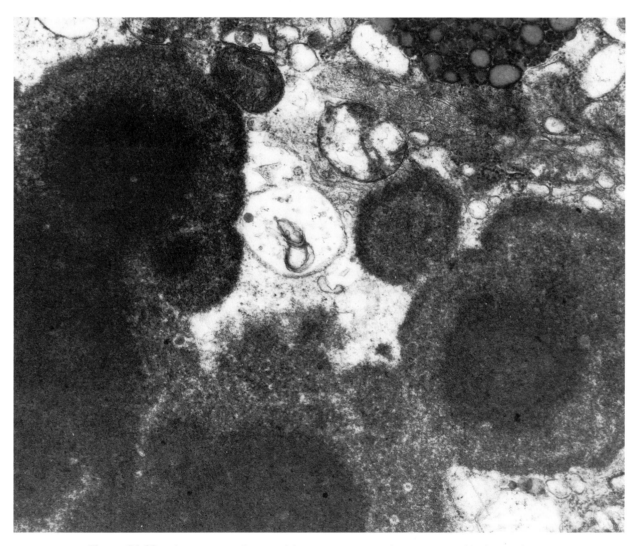

**Figure 24.28** Ultrastructure of a myoglobin-containing granular cast. Note the electron-lucent periphery relative to the dense core and rim. (Uranyl acetate and lead citrate; ×33,800.)

## TABLE 24.3

### CAUSES OF ACUTE RENAL FAILURE

| Causes | Examples |
|---|---|
| Prerenal azotemia (renal hypoperfusion)<br>Decreased cardiac output<br>Diminished intravascular volume | Cardiogenic shock, hemorrhage, gastrointestinal loss |
| Postrenal azotemia (obstructive uropathy)<br>Intraureteric obstruction<br>Extraureteric obstruction<br>Lower urinary tract obstruction | Stone, clot<br>Tumor, fibrosis<br>Urethral occlusion, prostatic disease |
| Renal causes of acute renal failure | |
| Glomerular/vascular disease | Glomerulonephritis, malignant hypertension, scleroderma, thrombotic purpura, emboli, arterial/venous occlusion |
| Interstitial disease | Drug-induced, hypercalcemia, hypokalemia, pyelonephritis, papillary necrosis |
| Intrarenal tubular occlusion | Crystal (uric acid, oxalic acid), protein (myeloma) deposition |
| Acute tubular injury<br>Ischemic injury | Severe trauma, aortic cross-clamping, hemorrhage |
| Nephrotoxic injury | Aminoglycosides, contrast material, heavy metals |
| Pigment-associated | Myoglobinuria, hemoglobinuria |

of ARF, particularly in patients who are volume depleted or dehydrated (329).

The second major category of etiologic agent is exposure to nephrotoxins. The kidney is uniquely susceptible to toxic injury, because it is the principal excretory organ of the body, with glomerular filtration of exposure of renal tubular epithelium to toxins. The route of exposure of the toxin is generally irrelevant—it can be through ingestion, inhalation, or cutaneous absorption. Some instances of severe nephrotoxic ATI are the result of industrial exposure or accidental or intentional ingestion of toxins, but numerous therapeutic agents may be associated with renal epithelial damage.

Drug exposure results in the most frequently encountered forms of nephrotoxicity. A problem that has been observed in developing countries is the contamination of commonly used drugs by nephrotoxins during their preparation under less-than-stringent conditions. Examples include the sudden occurrence of unexplained ARF in children in Pakistan and Haiti, where the cause was found to be contamination of the liquid vehicle of paracetamol with diethylene glycol (330–331). In many cases involving the use of diagnostic and therapeutic agents, the known risk of nephrotoxicity is outweighed by the clinical benefits of using the drug. While the range of injurious compounds is diverse, there are a limited number of patterns of injury produced in the kidney; the focus of this section will be on agents and specifically drugs that produce ATI.

Acute renal failure in the newborn may have a prenatal onset associated with maternal hypotension or in the setting of congenital diseases, such as renal dysplasia or polycystic kidney disease (322). In the postnatal period, hypoxic/ischemic injury and toxins are the most common etiologies. Toxic ARF is most commonly associated with administration of aminoglycoside antibiotics and NSAIDs given to close a patent ductus arteriosus. Decreased renal function can be documented in about 40% of premature infants receiving indomethacin; the decrease is usually reversible.

In hospitalized patients, ATI/ARF often occurs in the setting of both ischemic and toxic insults. Multiorgan failure, with or without sepsis, is a common scenario. Incidence of ARF is approximately 19% in moderate sepsis, 23% in severe sepsis, and 51% in septic shock with positive blood cultures (332–334). Clinical course and outcomes will be determined by multiple clinical factors and "cross-talk" between and among affected organs (335) (see following). Acute renal failure occurring in the critically ill has a significant impact on morbidity and mortality (336).

Much of our understanding of ATI and ARF has derived from experimental models, and extrapolation to human ARF may be problematic (337,338). This likely underlies the failure of various therapeutic agents defined in animal models to have clinical efficacy (339,340). Although they are imperfect, experimental models have provided important insights. New techniques, including imaging studies, may enable more precise definition of mechanisms of ARF in vivo (56). The rarity of renal biopsies in this setting has contributed to the difficulty of defining the pathobiology in humans (229). However, new techniques will likely make it possible to more precisely define mechanisms in clinical ARF in the future. Micro–magnetic resonance imaging techniques may ultimately be useful in assessing tubular cell function (341). Detection of renal inflammation may also be possible using these techniques (342). Imaging of subcellular processes, including apoptosis, enzyme markers, and cell pH and calcium, may ultimately be widely applicable in vivo (56).

## Ischemia

### Mechanisms of Injury and Cell Death

Alterations in cellular metabolism underlying ischemic cell injury in the kidney are analogous to those in ischemic injury in other organs and have been directly related to the severity of changes in renal cell structure and function regardless of the cause of ATI. Ischemia and reduced oxygen delivery to highly metabolically active tubular epithelial cells reduce oxidative metabolism and cell stores of high-energy phosphate compounds. Reperfusion with return of oxygen delivery enhances generation of oxygen free radicals, with resultant damage to cell components. An increase in intracellular calcium ion related to membrane injury enhances activation of injurious enzymes such as proteases and phospholipases. To some extent, these changes are reversible, but if severe or prolonged, they result in cell death. Definition of molecular mechanisms is a very active area of investigation; some major findings are outlined in the following sections.

A great deal of attention has focused on alterations in cellular polarity and cytoskeletal assembly that occur as a consequence of renal ischemia; these have been viewed as critical factors in the loss of normal renal epithelial structure and function. Several laboratories have verified that the polar distribution of $Na^+,K^+$-ATPase is directed to and maintained in its basolateral location by an interaction with the cortical cytoskeletal proteins ankyrin and fodrin (343–345). Other cellular components involved in the establishment and maintenance of cell polarity include proteins associated with organizing and maintaining cell-to-cell contact, such as E-cadherin, zonula occludens (ZO-1), β-catenin, and other novel proteins at the lateral membranes of the cell and integrins at the basal portions of the cell, where cell–matrix interactions occur (346,347). All of these components have been shown to have interactions with the actin-based cytoskeleton, which may coordinate interactions of the different membrane domains. Renal ischemia in vivo or intracellular ATP depletion in vitro induces disruption of this cytoskeletal complex with relocation of apical and basal lateral membrane–specific proteins and lipids into alternate membrane domains (348–352). After as little as 5 minutes of ATP depletion, there is loss of polarity, with internalization and blebbing of the apical brush border membranes. Shortly thereafter, basal lateral $Na^+,K^+$-ATPase has been shown to migrate from the basal lateral to the apical membrane. For $Na^+,K^+$-ATPase to be translocated to the apical domain, it must first be detached from its cytoskeletal tether. Renal ischemia in vivo results in increased solubility of $Na^+,K^+$-ATPase in rat renal proximal tubule cells, indicating disassembly from the cortical cytoskeleton. In humans, cadaveric transplant kidneys with ischemic injury and delayed graft function had significantly greater translocated cytoplasmic Na-K-ATPase and actin-binding proteins than kidneys that functioned well (353).

Re-establishment of normal cell organization comes about during recovery from renal ischemia at a rate dependent on the severity and duration of the insult; it is preceded by restoration of cellular ATP. Restoration of basal lateral $Na^+,K^+$-ATPase localization and of the brush border is a necessary prerequisite for restoration of tubular function (349–352). Restored localization of basolateral $Na^+,K^+$-ATPase is not caused by new synthesis of $Na^+,K^+$-ATPase

subunits, because the rate of transcription of each subunit decreases in parallel with diminished overall transcription, which occurs with ATP depletion (354). These findings suggest that recycling of misplaced $Na^+,K^+$-ATPase units, rather than increased biosynthesis, is the way in which renal tubule cells repolarize after an ischemic insult. Similar recycling of apical membrane proteins also occurs in the restoration of the brush border. The role of heat shock proteins can be invoked in this process, because they can serve as chaperones to protect the misfolded or misplaced proteins from degradation until ATP levels are restored and reorganization can take place (355).

Proper organization of the fodrin cytoskeleton is necessary to maintain $Na^+,K^+$-ATPase in its basolateral location. Fodrin is able to self-associate and bind actin (356), a process modulated by a unique regulatory cascade. Studies have demonstrated that this regulatory cascade appears to be involved in the disruption of the $Na^+,K^+$-ATPase ankyrin–fodrin complex following ischemia in hippocampal neurons as well as in the kidney (344). After 45 minutes of renal ischemia, the presence of fodrin cleavage products can be detected. Cleavage products increase during reperfusion, peaking at 6 hours; afterward there is a gradual return to a normal pattern, which corresponds to the repolarization of $Na^+,K^+$-ATPase to the basolateral membrane. This temporal pattern suggests that fodrin has a role in the loss and return of $Na^+,K^+$-ATPase polarity after ischemia and during recovery. Cleavage of the cytoskeleton and initiation of the stress response can also result from activation of the enzymes involved in the programed cell death pathway that leads to apoptosis (357–359).

The response of ankyrin to renal ischemia is similar to that of $Na^+,K^+$-ATPase. After ischemia there is a loss of the normal distribution of ankyrin, and ankyrin is immunodetected in the apical domain and in subapical vacuoles. During recovery, ankyrin co-distributes once again with $Na^+,K^+$-ATPase to the basolateral membrane. Examination of ankyrin turnover after renal ischemia has yielded interesting results that may help in analyzing its role in recovery. Kidney tissue that has been rendered completely ischemic displays a major time-dependent loss of ankyrin that is essentially complete after 2 hours of ischemia (360). This profound loss is not accompanied by the appearance of proteolytic degradation products and was not observed in ischemic brain or heart. These observations suggest that ischemia causes significant tissue-specific inhibition of ankyrin mRNA transcription, stability, or translation.

Studies of the biosynthetic response of ankyrin during recovery from renal ischemia have revealed that shortly after reperfusion, there is a significant loss of immunodetectable ankyrin associated with a concomitant loss of $Na^+,K^+$-ATPase polarization. However, after 6 hours of reflow, the amount of ankyrin increases to levels close to those of control kidney at a time when restitution of

Na$^+$,K$^+$-ATPase polarity has commenced. After 24 hours of reperfusion, immunodetectable ankyrin levels exceed control levels concomitant with the restitution of Na$^+$,K$^+$-ATPase polarity. These studies also suggest the potential role of the stress response (or the heat shock response) in ankyrin processing. This could occur by protecting the transcriptional apparatus for ankyrin so that its rapid synthesis can take place at a time when other protein synthesis is restricted. A second possibility is that the loss of ankyrin immunoreactivity is the result of interaction with heat shock protein 70, resulting in a pool of ankyrin available for recycling (354).

In intact proximal tubule epithelium, actin is primarily associated with the circumferential terminal web of the apical pole. In vivo renal ischemia results in redistribution of actin throughout the cytoplasm, with loss of its interactions with other cytoskeletal components and membrane domains. After intracellular ATP depletion in cultured cells, there is a disruption of the actin cytoskeleton and conversion of polymeric filamentous actin (F-actin) to monomeric G-actin with redistribution of residual F-actin from the membrane surface to a perinuclear and cytosolic location (361). These changes coincide with the rapid decrease in the amount of cytoskeletal-associated Na$^+$,K$^+$-ATPase, suggesting involvement of the actin cytoskeleton as well as the cortical cytoskeleton in maintaining Na$^+$,K$^+$-ATPase polarity. The possible role of actin disassembly in inducing apoptosis must also be considered (357).

Disruption of the cytoskeleton is associated not only with loss of cell polarity of transport proteins but also with relocation of basal integrins, tethered via the cytoskeleton and associated binding proteins in the basolateral domain. For example, nonlethal oxidative stress in cultured mouse tubular cells disrupts focal adhesion sites and is associated with redistribution of integrins to the apical domain (362,363). This results in disruption of the interaction of the cell with the underlying matrix, with loss of attachment of the epithelial cells from the basement membrane. Both cell–matrix and cell–cell adhesion may be disrupted with ATP depletion (364). Inhibition of cell–matrix adhesion in vitro by hydrogen peroxide has been shown to be reversible; recovery was associated with increased alpha-6 integrin expression (365). Inhibition of integrins during recovery can in turn lead to increase in cell apoptosis (366). Exfoliation of the epithelium into the tubular lumen can occur while the cells are still viable (235). Exfoliated cells and cell debris may interact with other epithelial cells, potentially with Tamm-Horsfall protein as a matrix. Aggregation of the exfoliated cells and adhesion to in situ cells can result in tubular obstruction. These exfoliated cells may interact with other cells via surface integrins (367,368). RGD peptides, which block these interactions, have been shown to ameliorate ARF in vivo (369). Gaps in the tubular epithelial barrier via cell loss or altered tight junctions could also be sites of backleak of glomerular filtrate. Clinical studies suggest that this is only a small component of fall in GFR, at least in native kidneys (370). Adhesion to the substratum is also necessary for cytoskeletal organization, and loss of adhesion has been shown to be an inducer of programmed cell death (359).

The alterations in cytoskeleton and Na$^+$,K$^+$-ATPase redistribution stemming from ATP depletion result in loss of Na$^+$,K$^+$-ATPase activity and the normal sodium and potassium gradients across the cell. The influx of sodium in conjunction with cytoskeletal disruption results in cell swelling, which has been proposed to also contribute to renal dysfunction—possibly by obstruction of the tubular lumina and vascular congestion of the outer medulla (371). This has led to clinical attempts to reduce cell swelling by the use of impermeable nonionic solutes such as mannitol. Although some clinical benefit has been identified, particularly in the prevention of ATI in patients undergoing cardiac bypass or aortic clamping, the protective effect of mannitol in ischemia most likely results from mechanisms independent of the effects on cell swelling, such as those related to osmotic diuresis, and potentially by the scavenging of oxygen radicals.

Reactive oxygen species (ROS) have been implicated as important effectors of cell injury in a variety of systems, including the kidney. Following ischemic injury, reactive oxygen species are formed when oxygen is restored to tissue during reperfusion. In ischemia, ATP is metabolized to adenosine and then to hypoxanthine. Calcium and calmodulin-dependent proteases convert xanthine dehydrogenase to xanthine oxidase, which then uses hypoxanthine as a substrate to generate superoxide formation. Superoxide dismutase (SOD) converts superoxide to hydrogen peroxide, which can then be converted to a highly reactive hydroxyl radical. Lecithinized SOD has been shown to ameliorate renal function and oxidative stress when administered to experimental animals. Reactive oxygen species may also come from infiltrating leukocytes as well as from the hypoxic renal epithelium (372).

Nitric oxide (NO) has also been implicated in ATI, but its effects are complex (373). Nitric oxide is generated by three separate nitric oxide synthase (NOS) enzyme systems, and effects depend on site of production, duration of effect, and concomitant levels of other ROS. Endothelial NOS (eNOS) results in transient high-level NO release, activating potentially protective heme-containing enzymes such as guanylate cyclase, mediating vasorelaxation, and triggering an anti-apoptotic phenotype. Treatment of mice with L-NAME, which is a nonspecific NOS inhibitor, has been reported to worsen ischemic renal injury (374). In contrast, generation of NO by inducible NOS (iNOS) results in sustained NO levels that may lead to lipid peroxidation, DNA damage, and apoptosis. In vitro, NOS inhibition prevents hypoxic damage in fresh proximal tubular preparations (375), and transfection of iNOS antisense oligodeoxynucleotide (AS-ODN) prevented nitrite accumulation and lethal cell injury in cultured green monkey kidney (BSC-1) cells (376). Proximal tubules isolated from mice with targeted deletion of iNOS were resistant to hypoxia (377). In vivo, S-ODN administration protected renal function and prevented tubular necrosis and decreased loss of brush border and cast formation (378). Effects of superoxide and NO may occur via formation of metabolites such as peroxynitrite and nitro-tyrosine that cause tubular damage during ischemia (379,380). α-Melanocyte–stimulating hormone protects against experimental ischemia/reperfusion injury via blockade of both iNOS induction and leukocyte infiltration (381).

Lethal injury to renal epithelial cells follows the same pathways and mechanisms that result in ischemic cell death in other cell types. Lethal injury can result in coagulative necrosis and/or apoptosis, depending on the nature of the agent and duration and severity of the insult. There is recent evidence that these two pathways may be parallel, may be activated by some of the same stimuli, and share common elements, including endonuclease activation, role of mitochondria, and caspase (382). In contrast to necrosis, apoptosis requires energy and is physiologically regulated. Apoptotic cells are rapidly removed from the environment, modulating the inflammatory responses to injury. It may also be important in the tissue remodeling that occurs after tubular epithelial injury. Recent studies have focused on the pathways that regulate cell death as potential targets for modulating recovery from acute renal injury (241).

As noted above, actin disassembly and altered adhesion of cells to the tubular basement membranes may trigger apoptosis (357,359). Central to the apoptotic process is activation of several members of a family of enzymes now referred to as caspases. They include interleukin-1–converting enzyme (ICE) and apopain (CPP 32). These enzymes have recently been shown to be able to use the cytoskeletal proteins fodrin and actin as substrates. It is interesting to note that their cleavage appears to have its peak at the same time as the peak of apoptosis during reperfusion after acute ischemia in experimental models, further suggesting the contribution of loss of polar distribution of $Na^+,K^+$-ATPase (and therefore disruption of its function) not only in the development of necrosis but also in apoptosis.

Cysteine proteases, including calpain and caspases, have been shown to be activated in experimental ischemic/hypoxic injury to tubules in vitro (383,384). Inhibition of calpain attenuated hypoxic injury, decreasing lactate dehydrogenase release (385). Calpastatin, an endogenous cellular inhibitor of calpain activation, is downregulated by caspases during hypoxia (384). Calcium activation of phospholipase A has also been shown to contribute to ischemic renal injury (386). Other mediators of apoptotic cell death include intracellular pH, calcium, free radicals, ceramide, and ATP depletion. Guanosine triphosphate depletion is an independent trigger of apoptosis via p53 (387). Guanosine triphosphate salvage with guanosine

or pifithrin-α inhibits apoptosis with a protective effect on experimental ischemic injury (388).

Over-activation of poly(ADP)-ribose polymerase (PARP), one of the molecules involved in necrotic cell death, has been demonstrated in renal ischemia (389). This leads to cellular depletion of substrate $NAD9^+$ and ATP, inducing cell injury. Expression of pro-inflammatory factors and adhesion molecules is also increased in ischemic kidney with PARP activation. Inhibitors of PARP-1 or gene ablation have been shown to reduce energy depletion and inflammation and improve renal function in ischemic kidney (390). There is evidence that the mitogen-activated protein kinase (MAPK) pathway also plays a role in oxidant injury to the kidney. Up-regulation of extracellular signal-regulated kinase (ERK) by previous ischemic pretreatment has been shown to provide protection against ischemia/reperfusion functional injury and c-Jun N-terminal kinase (JNK), p38, and MAPK activation (391). In an in vitro mouse proximal tubule preparation, inhibition of JNK activation of extracellular signal-regulates kinase (ERK) ameliorated oxidant-induced necrosis (392), an effect mediated by cyclic adenosine monophosphate (AMP)-response-element binding protein (393).

### Mechanisms of Cell Recovery

Heat shock proteins are molecular chaperones that play a key role in the adaptive response of cells to stress conditions. Both hsp72 and hsp25 increase in response to ischemia (394). In early time points after ischemia, hsp25 translocates transiently to the particulate cytoskeletal fraction (394). In vivo, increased hsp25 can be detected in renal epithelium, especially in proximal tubular cells (395). Renal ischemia in vivo rapidly induces the elaboration of hsp70 and hsp72 (354,396). The message for inducible hsp70 is found within minutes of an ischemic insult and peaks within the first 2 to 6 hours of reflow after 45 minutes of ischemia. The inducible protein appears shortly after the message and accumulates for the first few days after the injury, persisting for 5 days. The protein is found in membrane fractions as well as in cytosol, suggesting that it may be complexed with a variety of proteins that have been disassembled or denatured as a result of the ischemic insult.

Immunolocalization of hsp72 expression in proximal tubule cells after ischemia and reperfusion has provided additional information concerning the possible interactions between hsp72 and disrupted cytoskeletal or integral membrane proteins (355). After 15 minutes of reperfusion following 45 minutes of renal ischemia, hsp72 is found almost exclusively in the apical domain of the proximal tubule cells, where characteristic alterations of the brush border are seen, with breakdown of the apical cytoskeleton, loss of the brush border, and redistribution of $Na^+,K^+$-ATPase to the apical membrane. After 2 to 6 hours of reperfusion, hsp72 translocates to the cytoplasm in a granular pattern. Some of the granules also contain cathepsin and are presumed to be lysosomes in which irreversibly denatured proteins have been targeted by hsp72 to undergo proteolysis, but the majority of granules correspond to internalized membrane profiles that contain $Na^+, K^+$-ATPase and ankyrin. After 24 hours of reperfusion, hsp72 has migrated toward a more basolateral location coincident with the restitution of normal cell polarity. It is noteworthy that nuclear localization has not been identified during this time. Thus, induction of hsp72 corresponds with the initiation of ischemic damage, and its translocation through various cellular compartments correlates with the restitution of normal cellular structure, indicating a direct and important role for hsp72 in the repair process. Induction and altered localization of heat shock proteins have also been identified in rat kidneys with cisplatin-induced ARF, mercuric chloride nephrotoxicity, and cadmium-cystine toxicity (397–399).

A study of human biopsy material examined in situ expression of hsp72 in diseased and normal human kidneys (400). Although the pattern of expression varied, hsp72 was found in proximal tubules and collecting ducts of kidneys that had been subjected to an ischemic insult or that demonstrated ATI; hsp72 was not present in nondiseased human kidneys. The pattern of staining correlated with the severity of disease activity and the degree of the inflammatory response, suggesting that stress protein up-regulation represents cellular attempts at cytoprotection in ongoing sublethal injury.

The induction of hsp70 under stressful conditions has been found to occur rapidly through activation of the heat shock factor, by trimerization and binding to the heat shock element. While a variety of injurious agents result in such activation, the mechanisms of induction may differ. Adenosine triphosphate depletion, increases in intracellular calcium, decreases in intracellular pH, activation of phospholipases, and release of arachidonic acid metabolites have been shown to either initiate or modulate the heat shock response in a variety of cell systems.

Using gel retardation assays as an indication of heat shock activation, the role of ATP depletion was studied in an in vivo model of graded ATP depletion (354). Heat shock factor binding to the heat shock element is found as early as 15 minutes after total ischemia and is increased with prolongation of the ischemic interval. After 2 hours of reflow, heat shock factor binding begins to decline. Transcription and translation of hsp70 mRNA follows a similar pattern, resulting in the production of hsp72. This pattern is consistent with the concept that inducible hsp70 is negatively regulated at the transcriptional level. Reflow/perfusion injury is not necessary for initiation of the stress response, because activation of the transcription factor is present at both 15 and 45 minutes of maximal ATP depletion without reflow. Other signals identified as potential initiators of this response include the generation

of denatured unfolded or misfolded proteins, changes in intracellular calcium and intracellular pH, and the release of arachidonic acid.

The entire heat shock response appears to have an intimate and multifaceted relationship to cellular ATP. A phosphorylation step is required for activation of the heat shock factor, and heat shock proteins require ATP hydrolysis for their activity. The state of binding the heat shock proteins to denatured proteins depends on the presence or absence of ATP, and heat shock proteins appear to protect ATP synthesis in stressed cells. Using a model of graded vascular occlusion and continuous in vivo monitoring to achieve specific steady-state increments in cellular ATP, activation of heat shock factor in the renal cortex was evaluated after 45 minutes of energy depletion (354). When ATP levels were maintained above 60%, increased activation of heat shock factor could not be detected. Increased heat shock factor binding to the heat shock element consistently accompanied reductions in cortical ATP below 50% of pre-occlusion values, and further increases in hsp70 mRNA were found as more heat shock factor was activated, with reductions of cellular ATP by 20% to 25%. With higher ATP levels, less heat shock factor is present, and less heat shock protein mRNA accumulates. It is apparent that hsp72 has a multifaceted relationship with the metabolic state of stressed cells.

In ATP-depleted LLC-PK1 cells, inducible up-regulation of hsp70 protects against apoptosis (401). In vivo, up-regulation of hsp70 improves recovery from ischemia/reperfusion, associated with protection from apoptosis (402). The protection of cells from apoptosis by heat shock proteins depends on the subunit involved in refolding of damaged proteins and is apparently upstream from the mitochondria-dependent activation of apoptosis. Heat shock protein 70 also affects signaling pathways for onset of apoptosis. This heat shock factor interacts with protein complexes such as apoptosis signal–regulating kinase 1 (ASK1) and binds to the caspase activator recruitment domain of apoptosis protein–activating factor, preventing activation of caspases and apoptosis (reviewed by van de Water et al [403]).

Other protective mechanisms are also being defined. Caveolae are plasma membrane structures containing proteins. The caveolins are potential participants in protection and repair in both ischemic and toxic renal injury (404). Altered caveolin-1 expression and localization may affect renal cell survival following oxidative stress. Up-regulation of caveolin-1 has been demonstrated in ATI (405,406). More studies are required to determine whether this up-regulation contributes to cell survival or is an epiphenomenon. Lipoxins are lipoxygenase-derived lipid mediators with anti-inflammatory and pro-repair properties. There is some experimental evidence that these compounds have therapeutic potential in ARF. Bioactivity of lipoxins is mediated through receptor cross-talk (407). Kidney injury molecule 1 appears in the urine early during acute kidney injury and is potentially a reliable and early biomarker of renal damage (see previous). The protein contains a novel immunoglobulin-like domain and a mucin domain and is up-regulated in renal injury in dedifferentiated cells undergoing replication (408,409). It is proposed that shedding of this molecule allows the tubular epithelial cells to move and reconstitute the tubular epithelial barrier (410).

The interesting interrelationships among alterations of cellular metabolic processes, the integrity of cellular structure and function, and those systems that may serve to protect or repair the injured epithelium will doubtless provide insights into the type of fundamental biologic processes that may be modified therapeutically to modulate the severity of injury and enhance recovery.

### Gene Expression and Growth Factors in Tubular Epithelial Injury and Recovery

While cells that have suffered anoxia-induced sublethal injury can be remodeled, those cells that are lethally injured must be replaced. Renal epithelial cells are stable cells that do not normally divide but must be stimulated by growth factors to undergo mitosis. The growth factors that are important during renal development are good candidates to become involved in a reparative process; they include insulin-like growth factor type 1 (IGF-1), hepatocyte growth factor (HGF), and the epidermal growth factor (EGF)-like peptide, transforming growth factor α (TGFα). Epidermal growth factor and IGF-1 bind to specific receptors in the proximal tubule and not only act as mitogens but also regulate a variety of transport processes (411–414).

The kidney constitutively expresses high levels of EGF mRNA, which suggests that it is an abundant source of the peptide. It is of interest that levels of mature EGF peptide in the kidney have been reported to be higher following acute renal ischemic injury, and that EGF immunoreactivity is detected in injured proximal tubules. Because EGF amplifies DNA synthesis after tubular injury, it may be an important factor in regulating the regenerative process (412,415–417). The beneficial effects of postischemic infusion of thyroxin may also derive from this mechanism, because thyroxin raises EGF mRNA and EGF levels in the kidney (418).

In addition to EGF, a number of growth factors are activated in sublethally injured cells following anoxia; they include HGF and IGF-1. Research has shown that IGF-1 administered after acute ischemic injury accelerates recovery of normal renal function and regeneration of damaged epithelium (411,414,419,420–421). Although several different mechanisms of action have been proposed, including changes in the GFR, the effect of IGF-1 on enhanced DNA synthesis and its action as an anabolic agent seem most likely to be important in the beneficial effects that are achieved. Similar results have been obtained with HGF administration, but whereas IGF-1 has a definite anabolic effect, HGF appears to exert its salutary outcome primarily by enhancing DNA synthesis. It seems likely, therefore, that

each of these growth factors contributes in different ways to the recovery process and that they act synergistically to achieve resolution of the injury (413).

The commitment to DNA synthesis and regeneration involves the immediate induction of early genes that encode for transcription factors that have been associated with the induction of mitogenesis, such as c-*fos*, c-*jun*, *myc*, and early growth response gene (*EGR 1*) (416,422,423). This induction is associated with specific initial down-regulation of the expression of genes, such as kinase induced by depolarization (*KID 1*), that are associated with differentiation during development. In addition, a number of other genes that encode for small secreted peptides are activated. These proteins have cytokine-like activity that may play a part in the recruitment and activation of the inflammatory response that accompanies the renal response to ischemia. It has been suggested that the inflammatory response that takes place during reperfusion contributes to the amplification of the ischemic injury by activation of oxygen radicals in the brain and liver.

Restoration of structure and function following ATI is dependent on the replacement of necrotic or exfoliated tubular epithelial cells by viable epithelium. Several possible mechanisms have been suggested to participate in the resolution of tubular epithelial structure. Wound healing may occur by extension of adjacent viable epithelial cells to close gaps along the basement membrane with dedifferentiation of existing tubular epithelial cells into a proliferative phenotype, with stimulation of proliferation by growth factors (424). There is evidence from studies of ischemic injury in chimeric mice that restoration of epithelial integrity resulted from intrinsic tubular cell proliferation and not from circulating bone marrow–derived cells (425). However, studies of transplanted kidneys of male patients who received an allograft from a female donor have demonstrated a potential role for recipient-derived cells in reconstituting epithelial damage (426). Other studies have suggested that circulating recipient cells (presumably circulating pluripotential cells) play a role in renal remodeling after injury (427–429). Recent studies have suggested that stem cells either derived from the kidney or circulating bone marrow–derived cells may play a role in tubular repair. Experimental studies from several different groups have demonstrated that hematopoietic stem cells are capable of protecting the kidney from ischemic injury and assisting in repair and recovery from ischemia/reperfusion and toxin-induced injury (427,428,430–432). In a recent study, mobilization of bone marrow cells by granulocyte colony-stimulating factor rescued mice from cisplatin-induced renal failure, an effect enhanced by macrophage colony stimulating factor (M-CSF) (433). While all groups concluded that the majority of tubular repair occurred via proliferation of endogenous renal cells, the exact mechanism by which renotropic stem cells participate in this repair was unclear. Some studies found that some bone marrow–derived cells did appear to differentiate and be incorporated into the tubular epithelium, whereas other studies found that the protection did not act by direct incorporation into the repaired tubular segments. The findings of these experimental studies taken in context of findings in transplanted kidneys suggest that some form of cell therapy may improve the prognosis of patients with ATI.

### The Inflammatory Response in Ischemic Injury

The inflammatory response to ischemia has been invoked as an amplifier of ischemic injury during the reperfusion period in a variety of organ systems and has been the focus of recent investigation in ARF (for reviews, see 434–436). The importance of this response in the pathogenesis of ATI has been investigated (437–439). In one study, administration of a monoclonal antibody to intercellular adhesion molecule type 1 (ICAM-1) protected the kidney from perfusion injury both functionally and histologically when administered at the time of bilateral renal ischemia. Furthermore, anti–ICAM-1 protected the kidney when administered 0.5 to 2 hours after restoration of blood flow but not after 8 hours. The protection corresponded with the degree of neutrophilic infiltration and suggested that leukocyte endothelial adhesion and migration do contribute to reperfusion injury in the kidney, as they do in other organs (438). In a complementary study, inhibition of leukocyte adhesion using antibodies to the leukocyte adhesion molecules CD11/CD18 also resulted in a significant protective response (439). The agency by which inhibition of the initial steps of the inflammatory response limits the severity of ischemic damage is likely to be complex and not related just to the additive effect of the release of leukocyte enzymes or oxidative damage. Production of cytokines, such as interleukin-1β, may have direct effects on cell viability and the induction of apoptosis. Activation of ICE (caspase-1) not only activates interleukin-1 but also induces initiation of the apoptotic pathway (440–442).

Several recent studies have implicated T cells and B cells in the etiology of ischemic ARF. Marked depletion of T cells using anti–T-cell antibodies in thymectomized mice conferred protection of renal function and structure after ischemia/reperfusion (443). B-cell–deficient mice were also partially protected, with ischemic phenotype restored by serum transfer, but not B-cell transfers (444). However, T- and B-cell–deficient mice (RAG-1 deficient) were not protected from ischemia/reperfusion injury; adoptive transfer of B cells or T cells into these mice, however, afforded partial protection, indicating complex interactions between T cells and B cells in this setting (445).

### Renal Vasculature in Ischemic Injury

As noted, early experimental studies demonstrated that injury and dysfunction of the tubular epithelium lead to renal vasoconstriction via activation of tubuloglomerular feedback mechanisms (31–36). Renin-angiotensin was identified early as a potential mediator. More recent studies have documented roles for altered prostaglandin and NO at the macula densa in altering blood flow in response to intraluminal salt concentrations (446,447). It was recognized early that tubuloglomerular feedback served a protective function, preventing loss of intravascular volume with loss of tubular resorptive capacity (37), but the mechanism is pathogenic if prolonged.

Endothelial cell swelling with luminal narrowing in the setting of renal ischemia was noted decades ago (448), potentially contributing to reduced flow in ischemic injury. Altered renal vascular resistance with failure of normal relaxation has been shown in animal models of ARF (449), and ischemic injury in rats results in lack of response to endothelium-dependent vasodilators (450). Production of the major endothelium-derived relaxing factor, NO, is suppressed in ischemic kidneys (378). Endothelial injury and dysfunction clearly play a role in initiation and especially the maintenance/extension phase of ischemic tubular injury (451). Imbalance in iNOS and eNOS, oxidant stress, and generation of peroxynitrite have roles in the pathophysiology (373). Infusion of endothelial cells or surrogates containing NO have been efficacious in experimental models (452), opening up an exciting new avenue for therapeutic intervention.

Outer medullary congestion is a vascular hallmark of acute renal ischemia, and it has been proposed that this may worsen hypoxic injury to the S3 segments and medullary thick ascending limb, which traverse this area of the kidney (453). This congestion and stasis could be the result of altered hemodynamics, increased viscosity, compression by interstitial edema and/or swollen tubular cells, and up-regulation of cell adhesion molecules with stasis of leukocytes. Some toxic agents exert toxic effects on the kidney via reduction of renal blood flow. These agents include ACE inhibitors, angiotensin-2 receptor blockers, and NSAIDs. These mechanisms are discussed in the following section, which covers specific nephrotoxins.

## Nephrotoxins

In vivo and in vitro experimental models have been widely used to define the pathogenesis of renal tubular injury produced by the various types of drugs. Heavy metal exposure, especially to mercury, was the basis of early models of toxicity; these will not be discussed in detail here. Aminoglycoside antibiotics and cis-platinum have been the most widely studied nephrotoxic drugs; pathogenesis of injury owing to these and other agents are discussed in detail later in this chapter. Some drugs and toxins are injurious in their native form. In other cases, metabolic by-products are the actual injurious agents. Drug catabolism may take place in the liver, at other systemic sites, or in the renal epithelium (see Rankin and Valentovic [454] for review). In the case of many drugs and toxins, injury to the nephron may be zonal, depending on the site of uptake or catabolism. A few agents specifically injure segments of the proximal tubule (e.g., aminoglycosides), whereas others produce effects distally (e.g., lithium). Endocytosis, discussed in detail for aminoglycoside toxicity, plays a role in the pathogenesis of nephrotoxicity of a number of nephrotoxins (see Sundin and Molitoris [455] for review).

Toxic agents may interfere with normal mitochondrial function and oxidative metabolism, leading to depletion of cellular high-energy phosphate compounds and failure of energy-requiring enzymes and active transport mechanisms. Some alter lysosomes, causing leakage of digestive enzymes and membrane injury, or disrupt protein synthesis. Free radical compounds may be produced by systemic or local metabolism of a drug or by drug effects on cell metabolism. Free radicals, in turn, can interact with lipids to produce membrane damage and with proteins to alter cellular enzyme activity. Membrane damage results in loss of critical cell compartmentation, leading to loss of the normal cellular distribution of ions and the gradients that drive critical cell processes. Concentrations of intracellular ionic calcium rise, with resulting secondary effects on cell enzymes and cytoskeletal elements, causing loss of the normal cell substructure.

While apoptotic mechanisms play an obvious and important role in ischemia reperfusion injury, their contribution to toxic nephropathies may be even more complex. Toxins may initiate apoptosis not only through the mitochondrial pathways discussed above, but also by directly initiating the signaling pathway for tumor necrosis factor signaling pathway or through p53 via genotoxic stress. Paracetamol toxicity has been linked to the direct activation of Bcl-xL in mouse proximal tubular cells in culture (456). The antiviral drug cidofovir has been shown to induce apoptotic epithelial injury in renal biopsy and human renal tubular cells in culture, via direct effects on epithelial cell membranes (261).

Some nephrotoxic agents interfere with renal function by altering renal hemodynamics. In some cases, the effects are prerenal, but tubular epithelial cell injury may ensue if vasoconstriction/hypoperfusion persists. In addition, inflammatory cells may play a role in some forms of toxic injury; this is an area that requires further exploration (see previous). Finally, mechanisms of recovery are likely analogous to those described for ischemic injury. Removal of the offending agent or significant reduction in dose may be necessary to allow recovery.

There is currently a focus on prediction of nephrotoxic action by identification of toxicity-related biomarkers (457,458). Profiling of gene expression microarray in rats exposed to a range of nephrotoxins revealed clustering based on similarities in severity and type of pathology. A set of potential biomarkers showing time- and dose-response related to progression of proximal tubular toxicity included several transporters: kidney injury molecule 1 (Kim-1), IGF bp-1, osteopontin, α fibrinogen and glutathione transferase (Gst α). Other potential biomarkers include c-*myc*, multidrug resistance gene (MDR-1), clusterin, vimentin, and hepatitis A virus cell receptor (HAVcr-1) (459). Similar studies in cynomolgus monkeys using gentamicin and everninomycin as nephrotoxins confirmed modulation of genes identified in rodent models, including *waf-1*, matrix metalloproteinase-9, and vimentin. Three early gene biomarkers predictive of drug-induced nephrotoxicity included clusterin, osteopontin, and HAV cr-1 (460).

## Antibiotics

*Antiviral Agents.* Mechanisms of injury involved in antiviral agent-induced renal tubular cell injury and renal failure are currently being defined (57). There is experimental evidence that acyclovir has direct effects on tubular function (461). In vitro studies have shown that acyclovir blocks the swelling-dependent chloride current in fibroblasts and human T-cell lymphoma (H9) cells and the cyclic adenosine monophosphate-dependent chloride current in CaCo cells—effects that were blocked by thymidine diphosphate or uridine (462). These studies provide a potential molecular mechanism of action for direct toxic effects of this drug and related nucleoside analogs. Increased influx of drug via organic ion transporters, or decreased efflux via the multidrug resistance protein, may enhance cytotoxicity (463,464).

Programmed cell death and effects on mitochondrial function have been invoked as potential mechanisms of renal toxicity of antiviral agents (57). Stimulated by tubular cell apoptosis in a renal biopsy of a patient with irreversible ARF caused by cidofovir, Ortiz and Justo (261) studied induction of apoptosis in primary cultures and a cell line (HK2) of human proximal tubular cells with time and dose parallel to clinical toxicity. Apoptosis was prevented by probenecid and by an inhibitor of caspase-3. Insulin-like growth factor type 1 and HGF were protective as well.

Several of these agents induce nephrogenic diabetes insipidus, potentially by down-regulation of the water channel aquaporin-2 or inhibition of vasopressin responsiveness. The proteinuria seen in patients treated with cidofovir is likely caused by tubular injury and failure of normal resorption. Deposition of crystals in the kidney is seen with a variety of these agents, including acyclovir and indinavir (59,60,465,466). Several of these agents have relatively low solubility in urine; rapid infusion, volume depletion, and underlying renal insufficiency are important risk factors for crystal formation.

*Aminoglycosides.* Molecular mechanisms in aminoglycoside toxicity have been reviewed (467–470). Aminoglycosides are freely filtered by the glomerulus and are not metabolized in the body. About 10% of intravenously administered drugs accumulate in the kidney, with little uptake in other tissues. At the brush border of proximal tubular cells, polyanionic inositol phospholipids serve as the binding site. Megalin, a giant endocytic receptor expressed at the apical membrane, plays a major role in binding and endocytosis of these drugs (reviewed by Nagai and Takano [469]). Studies in megalin–knock-out mice demonstrated almost no renal accumulation of $H^3$-gentamicin, compared to 10.6% of the total dose accumulated in the kidney in control animals (471). Other megalin ligands also have been shown to reduce gentamicin accumulation and nephrotoxicity (472). There is some evidence that gentamicin is trafficked retrogradely through the secretory pathway and is released into the cytosol via the endoplasmic reticulum (473).

Clinical pathologic findings and experimental studies support the direct toxic effects of aminoglycosides on renal tubules. The amino side chains are associated with membrane binding, and avidity of binding correlates with nephrotoxicity (474). These drugs induce formation of myeloid bodies containing phospholipids and proteins, apparently related to proximate cationic side chains and an apolar ring structure, resulting in a high affinity for the phospholipid components, and especially the acidic phospholipids, of cell membranes. Via binding, aminoglycosides also inhibit lysosomal phospholipases, leading to accumulation of phospholipid myelin figures in the lysosomes. The interaction of the drugs and the membranes leads to lamellar aggregates and lysosomal drug accumulation (475). Membrane aggregation correlates with the toxic potential of aminoglycosides and may contribute to its toxicity (476). Aminoglycosides have been shown to traffic rapidly to the Golgi complex in cell culture. Cells previously depleted of nucleotides accumulated significantly more gentamicin within a dispersed Golgi complex (477). Polyamino acids such as polyaspartic acid reduce aminoglycoside nephrotoxicity in vivo, despite increases in renal gentamicin and amikacin accumulation, suggesting that the site of action of polyaspartic acid may be in preventing interactions of aminoglycoside with acidic phospholipases in the lysosomes (478,479).

Destabilization of lysosomal membranes allows escape of enzymes, which cause further cell injury. In addition, aminoglycoside in the cell cytoplasm interacts with mitochondrial membranes and microsomes. There has been evidence for some time that gentamicin inhibits mitochondrial respiration and cellular protein synthesis (480–482). Aminoglycosides affect protein synthesis as well as protein–protein interactions involving protein disulfide isomerase (PDI). Gentamicin and ribostamycin have been shown to bind to PDI, an enzyme that stabilizes some proteins and participates in mechanisms degrading misfolded proteins in the cell, inhibiting its chaperone activity (483,484). Gentamicin binds to a number of kidney microsomal proteins, including calreticulin, a chaperone protein, and has selective effects on chaperone activity of this molecule in vitro (485).

Gentamicin also enhances the generation of reactive oxygen metabolites in renal cortical mitochondria, and many studies suggest that oxygen and hydroxyl radicals have an important role in gentamicin-induced ARF (486–489). Iron plays a role in stimulating oxidative stress. Gentamicin has been shown to cause release of iron from mitochondria and to complex with ferrous ion, forming a high-spin complex (490,491). Chelators and antioxidants depress aminoglycoside-induced oxidant stress (492–494). Gentamicin-induced ROS are inhibited by $N^G$-nitro-L-arginine methyl ester (L-NAME), consistent with a role for endothelin receptor β/NO pathway in toxicity (495). Aminoglycosides stimulate endothelin-1 and subsequently NO in proximal tubules (496) and mesangial cells (497), effects that are blocked by L-NAME. Aminoglycosides also increase intracellular calcium levels and ERK activity in proximal tubular cell lines, correlating with cell injury (498). At sublethal concentrations, aminoglycosides, when administered to the basolateral solution in cell culture, disrupted electrogenic transport in human renal tubular cells (499). The effects of different aminoglycosides followed the pattern of known in vivo toxicity. These changes, and lethal cell injury, presumably result from the mechanisms of action described earlier.

The renin–angiotensin system also appears to play a role in the adverse effects of gentamicin (500). Baylis et al (501) have documented a decline in the glomerular capillary ultrafiltration coefficient with gentamicin. At doses of 4 mg/kg per day, there was no decline in other determinants of glomerular ultrafiltration. However, at doses of 40 mg/kg per day, there were decreases in plasma flow rate, transglomerular hydraulic pressure difference, and GFR (501).

The N-methyl-D-aspartate (NMDA) receptor plays a major role in gentamicin-induced ototoxicity, and expression of NMDA receptor has recently been shown to be increased in gentamicin-induced renal toxicity in rats. Endothelin B receptor expression and urinary nitrite concentration were also significantly increased, with increases in blood pressure, urine pH, and creatinine; an NMDA receptor antagonist ameliorated these effects (502). Calpain isoforms were unaltered by the short-term regimen used.

Mechanisms of fibrosis and progression following gentamicin exposure have recently been explored. In one study, rats treated with gentamicin were sacrificed at 5 and 30 days after drug injections. Fibronectin, α-smooth muscle actin (myofibroblast marker), ED-1 (monocyte marker), endothelin, angiotensin II, and TGFβ were all increased in renal cortex compared with controls. At 30 days, treated rats also had fibrosis and increased TGFβ content in cortex, despite normalization of creatinine (503).

*Amphotericin.* Amphotericin B has been shown to bind to sterol-containing membranes, causing changes in their permeability via formation of intramembranous pores (504–506). This property, which underlies its antifungal efficacy, may also cause the vascular or tubular toxicity produced by the drug. Studies in rats have shown potentiation of tubular toxicity, as measured by fractional excretion of sodium, with potassium depletion (507). Amphotericin also affects water and urea transport in the inner medullary collecting duct. While amphotericin B causes hypokalemia, which may itself produce a concentrating defect, the defect may be seen with normal serum potassium as well (508). It may also come about in part as the result of the fall in the GFR that can develop in these patients.

In dogs and rats, vasoconstriction has been documented after infusion of amphotericin into the renal artery (508,509). Experimental studies in the rat have suggested that the vasoconstriction brought about by amphotericin B is in part thromboxane-mediated (510) and involves activation of the tubuloglomerular feedback response (511). It appears, however, that the vasoconstriction brought about by amphotericin may also be the result of a direct effect on renal vessels (505).

### Cephalosporins

Cephalosporins appear to be capable of producing direct toxic injury to tubular cells. Tune and Hsu (512) have shown that cephalosporins interfere with mitochondrial function in the renal tubule via inhibition of substrate transport across the mitochondrial inner membrane. Cephaloridine has structural homology to carnitine, and it has toxic effects on carnitine transport and fatty acid metabolism in rabbit renal cortical mitochondria in vivo; in vitro effects on pyruvate metabolism were seen, although only at very high concentrations (512). Cephaloridine also produces lipid peroxidation and acylation and inactivation of some tubular cell proteins. Other cephalosporins, which lack cephaloridine's side group constituents, largely affect tubular cell proteins and especially mitochondrial anionic substrate transporters. In vitro, proximal tubular cells show evidence of cytotoxicity on exposure to cephaloridine (greatest injury), cephalexin, and cephalothin, while distal tubules do not; these studies provide evidence of the role of oxidative stress, cytochrome P450 activation, and mitochondrial dysfunction in tubular cell toxicity (513). Cytochrome C oxidase has been shown to be a target in LLC-PK1 cells (514).

Cephaloridine, ceftazidime, and cefotaxime have also been shown to produce dose-dependent disruption of LLC-PK1 monolayers in vitro, as measured by transepithelial potentials, morphologic changes, and enzyme release (515); cephaloridine was the most toxic and cefotaxime the least toxic, dose for dose. Proximal localization of injury is apparently the result of concentration of drug within these cells; the drug readily enters the cell via the organic anion transporters, but it is a poor substrate for efflux porters at the brush border membrane, leading to accumulation in the cell. Despite these experimental findings, clinically significant cases of renal tubular toxicity are rare at the recommended doses of these agents, and newer agents have even less toxic potential.

In addition, cephalosporins are known to cause hypersensitivity reactions. In some cases, there has been resolution with drug withdrawal and, in a few cases, recurrence on rechallenge (119). The cephalosporins are structurally similar to the penicillins, which produce similar reactions, and cross-reactivity may occur in 1% to 20% of patients. No specific cephalosporin is more likely than others to cause such a reaction (covered further in Chapter 23).

### Immunosuppressive/Immunomodulatory Agents

*Cyclosporine.* Cyclosporine is very lipophilic, circulating in plasma and erythrocytes and accumulating in liver and adipose tissue. It is extensively metabolized in the liver; its metabolites are minimally nephrotoxic. Most excretion is in the bile. It interacts with many other drugs through the hepatic cytochrome P450-3A system. Cyclosporine binds in cells to cyclophilin, which interacts with calcineurin to inhibit the enzyme, affecting a wide variety of downstream genes via its substrate, nuclear factor of activated T cells (NFAT). The latter in turn regulates transcription of interleukin 2 (IL-2), TNF-$\alpha$, and granulocyte-macrophage colony-stimulating factor. Calcineurin also regulates transcription of IL-2 receptor, NO synthase, TGF$\beta$, endothelin-1, collagen types I and II, and Bcl-2 protein (133,135,516).

Intrarenal vasoconstriction appears to be the central pathogenetic mechanism for most types of CsA nephrotoxicity (134,135,517,518). This vasoconstriction can result from: a direct vasoconstrictive effect (517), endothelin mediation (518–520), increased local production of angiotensin in renal vessels without the usual compensatory release of vasodilatory prostaglandins (521–523), activation of the sympathetic nervous system (524), selective impairment of endothelium-dependent relaxation related to prostaglandins or NO release (525–527), or increased thromboxane production (528–530).

Several lines of evidence implicate the role of endothelin in the vascular effects of CsA. Endothelin plasma and urine levels have been shown to be elevated in CsA-treated patients, and in vitro, CsA causes cultured vascular cells to release endothelin (531–533). Anti-endothelin antibody or receptor blockade prevents a CsA-induced fall in the GFR in rats (519,520,533). Cyclosporine also up-regulates endothelin receptors in the kidney of rats (534). Thromboxane receptor blockade or modulation of thromboxane metabolism has been shown to reduce CsA toxicity in experimental animal models (529,530). In addition, inhibition of thromboxane synthetase has been demonstrated to improve renal allograft function in patients taking CsA (528). Platelet-derived growth factor, another vasoconstrictor substance, has been found to be increased in arterioles of CsA-treated rats (535). Another intriguing finding is markedly enhanced immunostaining for vascular clusterin after 4 and 6 weeks of CsA treatment in the rat (536);

clusterin has a variety of effects, including chemotactic effects, in injured and regenerating tissue.

The nephrotoxic effect of CsA appears to be tightly linked to its immunosuppressive effects (283). The mechanisms of action of CsA as an immunosuppressive drug involve binding to cyclophilin, a 17-kD basic cytosolic polypeptide with peptidyl-prolyl cis-trans isomerase activity. This enzyme is involved in protein folding, an activity that is inhibited by immunosuppressive concentrations of CsA. Kidney androgen-regulated protein (KAP) specifically interacts with cyclophilin B; KAP levels are decreased in CsA-treated rats. Overexpression of KAP in proximal tubular cells significantly decreased toxic effects of CsA, a protective stress response (537). The intracellular target of cyclophilin A-CsA is calcineurin, a protein phosphatase required for signaling via the T-cell receptor (reviewed by Ryffel et al [538]). Calcineurin regulates both baseline and receptor-activated Na/K-ATPase activity (539). There is evidence that CsA also decreases cell levels of the calcium binding protein calbindin D (540,541), which increases urinary calcium excretion, promoting intratubular calcifications that can be seen with CsA toxicity.

A variety of factors may act together to injure the endothelium and cause a HUS-like syndrome, especially in patients with renal allografts; these factors include drugs, inflammation, and hypertension. It has been shown experimentally that at high doses, CsA exhibits direct endothelial toxicity in vitro (542). At lower doses, it may inhibit endothelial repair (543). Increased platelet aggregation and thromboxane release have been documented in patients and volunteers receiving CsA (544).

The hyaline arteriolar lesions observed in humans have been difficult to reproduce in experimental animal models, with the exception of the spontaneously hypertensive rat. However, Young et al reported such a model in persistently salt-depleted rats (545). The lesions, first detected at day 10, began with granular eosinophilic transformation of smooth muscle cells in afferent arterioles, followed by vacuolation of smooth muscle cells and discrete hyaline deposits in vessel walls. Immunocytochemistry and electron microscopy revealed accumulation of renin granules in the smooth muscle cells. It is possible that the lesion is more likely to develop clinically if the arterioles are abnormal before CsA treatment. Indeed, CsA nephrotoxicity appears to be much more severe in patients with pre-existing kidney disease, and age has been identified as an additional risk factor (153).

Tubular injury may be enhanced by the antiproliferative effects of CsA on renal tubular cells, an effect which may be explained, in part, by stimulation of TGFβ expression in renal tubular cells (546). In vivo, CsA significantly inhibits $H^3$-thymidine incorporation in a time- and dose-dependent manner; p53 levels increased coincident with cell-cycle arrest (547). Oxidants may play a role in tubular cell injury in CsA toxicity. Renal lipid peroxidation has been

shown in vivo and in vitro. Atrial natriuretic factor reduces toxicity in renal cells via cyclic guanine monophosphate and heme oxygenase (548). Melatonin is also protective in isolated perfused rat kidney (549). In vitro exposure of LLC-PK1 cells to CsA increased glucose consumption and pyruvate production, consistent with a shift to glycolysis; interruption of glucose influx and glycolysis increased lactate dehydrogenase release, whereas the *Glut-1* gene was protective (550). In primary cultures of rat renal epithelial cells, CsA-induced increases in mitochondrial $Ca^{2+}$, reduction in mitochondrial membrane potential, and reduction in ATP have been detected; all these changes may play an important role in CsA-related cell cytotoxicity (551). However, while direct treatment of cells in vitro inhibits mitochondrial respiration, cells isolated from CsA-treated rats showed mitochondrial inhibition only at high dose (75 mg/kg/day), not at immunosuppressive doses (552). Cyclosporine-induced apoptosis has been described in a murine cell line in vitro at relatively low doses. However, despite increased expression of apoptosis stimulating fragment (Fas) and evidence of endoplasmic reticulum (ER) stress, the pathway of apoptosis did not involve apoptosis stimulating fragment ligand (FasL)-induced mechanisms of caspase-12, but instead involved *Bax* translocation to the mitochondria and activation of caspases 2, 3, and 9 (553).

Charuk et al (554) found that CsA has a high affinity for human renal P-glycoprotein and also described enhanced cell accumulation of the drug and other agents transported by P-glycoprotein. The authors postulated that this binding may competitively inhibit excretion of an endogenous P-glycoprotein substrate (554).

Rosen et al (555,556) described a model of chronic CsA-induced nephropathy in which CsA (12.5 mg/kg) was injected daily into sodium-depleted rats. Histologic assessment revealed focal atrophy of the thick ascending limb and fibroblast proliferation. Structural lesions and renal functional impairment were less severe in animals who had been fed a normal sodium diet. Based on this model, Heyman et al proposed a role for medullary ischemia in CsA-induced lesions (557).

Young et al used this model (558) to study the pathogenesis of interstitial fibrosis. Proliferation of tubular and interstitial cells was documented in the medulla by day 5. By day 35, proliferation was maximal, and there was increased cortical tubular staining for osteopontin, a macrophage adhesion protein. A significant influx of macrophages was detected by day 35, which was associated with maximal cortical interstitial fibrosis. These changes correlated with functional abnormalities, and the authors concluded that these cellular events may be important in the pathogenesis of chronic CsA nephrotoxicity. Studies in rats have implicated angiotensin II in effecting fibrosis with prolonged CsA administration (519). Transforming growth factor β also likely plays a role in induction of fibrosis in chronic CsA nephropathy (559). In a rat model of chronic CsA toxicity, administration of anti-TGFβ antibodies reversed most of the CsA-induced renal lesions (560). There is evidence that CsA may bind to the promotor for collagen type III, stimulating collagen expression in renal cells (561). Loss of peritubular capillaries has been demonstrated in chronic CsA toxicity; in an experimental model, vascular endothelial growth factor ameliorated the chronic nephropathy (562). Inappropriate apoptosis and the vascular effects described above leading to chronic vasoconstriction also likely contribute to chronic effects of CsA.

*FK506 (Tacrolimus).* Tacrolimus appears to have a mechanism of action similar to that of CsA (563). Like CsA, FK506 binds to an intracellular binding protein, FKBP12; this complex targets calcineurin within the cell (reviewed by Dumont [564]). Studies have shown inhibition of renal calcineurin in rats treated with FK506, suggesting that renal toxicity is mediated in part by inhibition of the phosphatase activity of calcineurin (565). Tacrolimus also binds to FKBP59, a heat shock protein associated with the nucleus, cytoskeleton, and mitotic apparatus (566). Like cyclosporine, FK506 is bound to proteins and erythrocytes in the blood. Like CsA, FK506 is metabolized by the hepatic cytochrome P450 3A4 system, and there is potential for drug interactions (567). Metabolites are generally inactive, and excretion is largely via the biliary tract.

Studies in mesangial cells cultured in vitro have shown that FK506 induces release of endothelin-1, an effect that may be mediated by FKBP (568). Clinically, endothelin levels in the urine have been shown to rise with FK506 immunosuppression after liver transplantation, whereas 6-keto-PG1-α levels fell; the changes in levels of these vasoactive substances persisted for 2 years, over a period when the GFR dropped and renal vascular resistance rose (569). In an experimental rat model, 2 weeks of treatment with FK506 produced a rise in SUN and sCr levels, luminal narrowing of arterioles, increases in plasma renin and urine thromboxane, and a decline in urinary 6-keto-PG1-α; the effects were reversible (570). The drug also induces TGFβ in experimental FK506 toxicity (571), suggesting that the drug may induce renal fibrosis by mechanisms analogous to CsA.

*Sirolimus.* Sirolimus has been shown to impair recovery from experimental ARF. A role for cell-cycle arrest and apoptosis of tubular cells has been demonstrated (572). This compound has also been studied in a rat model of CsA toxicity (573). The drug potentiated the renal toxicity of low-dose (5 mg/kg/day) CsA. Sirolimus alone increased TGFβ expression by 44%. In the setting of a combination of sirolimus and low-dose CsA, TGFβ mRNA and protein were increased by 121% and 176%. Lieberthal et al (572) found that rapamycin inhibits growth factor-induced proliferation of cultured proximal tubular cells and fosters apoptosis by blocking survival effects of the growth factors. The drug also impaired recovery from experimental ARF caused

by renal artery occlusion via increased apoptosis and inhibition of regeneration; these effects were attributable to the inhibition of p70 S6 kinase.

*Intravenous Immunoglobulin.* The toxicity of IVIG appears to be osmotic. Highly osmotic, sucrose-stabilized formulations have a disproportionately high rate of ARF compared to non–sucrose-stabilized products (163). Rate of infusion may be an important risk factor for renal tubular injury.

## Chemotherapeutic Agents

*Cis-platinum.* Cis-platinum is a tubular toxin that accumulates in the kidney, especially at the corticomedullary junction. There is evidence that renal damage is not caused by the heavy metal platinum moiety in this compound; cis-platinum toxicity is delayed in onset, renal failure is not prevented by chelators (574,575), and trans-platinum is not toxic (576). An aquated cationic form of cisplatin forms in the cell and binds to essential macromolecules, forming cisplatin adducts that are highly toxic (577). In vitro, inhibition of mitochondrial respiration is early and dose-dependent (578). Oxidative mechanisms play a role in mitochondrial toxicity (579). Indeed, there is considerable evidence that reactive oxygen metabolites play a role in cis-platinum toxicity. Cisplatin induces hydrogen peroxide generation by proximal tubular cells (580); catalase was protective. There is evidence that catalytic iron derived via cytochrome P450 and capable of catalyzing free radical reactions is increased in renal cells on exposure to cisplatin both in vitro and in vivo (581,582). In vitro studies have documented nucleolar disruption and inhibition of lysosomal function and protein synthesis, leading to mitochondrial dysfunction (583,584).

Cisplatin produces both necrotic and apoptotic cell death (585), the former at very high doses. Antioxidants could ameliorate low-dose effects but not high-dose effects. In vitro studies have documented a role for mitochondrial caspase pathway in cis-platinum–induced apoptosis (586–588), as well as a separate P53-dependent mechanism (587).

An intrarenal inflammatory response may contribute to cis-platinum–induced ARF (589). Cisplatin has been reported to increase chemokine and cytokine production in an experimental cisplatin toxicity model, an effect mediated by TNFα; inhibition of TNF ameliorated the nephrotoxicity (590). Anti-CD54 antibody blockade of leukocyte adhesion is also protective (591). Interleukin-10, an anti-inflammatory cytokine, also inhibits cis-platinum nephrotoxicity (592).

*Nitrosureas.* The mechanism of injury appears to be direct renal tubular toxicity. Metabolites of the drug ifosfamide may be responsible for the tubular injury induced by that agent (593). Methotrexate also causes direct toxic injury to the proximal tubule. In addition, precipitation of the drug in renal tubules, with resultant obstruction, has been reported (594).

### Radiocontrast Agents

Based on the existing clinical and experimental studies, it appears that the tubules and the vasculature of the kidney are the key targets in the development of radiocontrast nephrotoxicity (RN). Increased tubular protein and enzyme excretion have been detected in the urine of patients undergoing radiocontrast studies (199,200,309,595,596), suggesting a direct tubular toxic effect of contrast media. Rise in urinary levels of markers of oxidative stress have been documented (200). The pattern of amplified enzyme and protein excretion (e.g., more urinary brush border enzymes, folate-binding protein) was suggestive of a primarily proximal tubular injury. Mechanisms have been recently reviewed (597).

In general, it is difficult to induce ARF with contrast media in most animal species, and contrast media alone are not sufficient to cause renal injury in animal models. The combination of unilateral nephrectomy, salt depletion, and administration of indomethacin and other injurious agents is necessary to cause renal injury in animals after contrast media exposure. In this model, apoptosis of medullary tubular cells has been noted, ascribed to hypoxia (598). Some experimental studies describe proximal tubular vacuolation (309,595). Other investigators have emphasized the selective injury of the thick ascending limb of Henle in a rat experimental model for RN (306,599). However, this thick ascending limb injury appears to have been the consequence of hypoxia rather than direct toxic damage in this model. The thick ascending limb of Henle is the site where Tamm-Horsfall protein is produced, and some data indicate that contrast media may increase the urinary excretion of Tamm-Horsfall protein, an important cast-forming protein (600). Contrast media may also facilitate the urinary excretion of oxalate and urate (601,602), but there is no evidence that urinary obstruction by any form of cast plays a role in RN.

There is both human and experimental evidence that vasoconstriction and subsequent ischemic injury may play an important role in RN (305,600,603–605). The injection of contrast media causes a biphasic response in the renal blood flow. There is an initial short phase of increased flow followed by a long phase of reduced flow caused by intrarenal vasoconstriction (603,606). Some experimental studies suggest that high endothelin levels, low NO levels, or both are key mediators of this intrarenal vasoconstriction (599,604,605). However, early results with endothelin receptor blockade in clinical trials have not shown benefit (606). Other factors, such as increased adenosine release and decreased prostanoid levels (e.g., owing to the concomitant administration of indomethacin or other prostaglandin synthase inhibitors) may also play a part in pathogenesis (599,600).

More recently developed iso-osmolar contrast media are dimers, while the widely used nonionic, low-osmolar contrast media are monomers. The viscosity of these dimers is higher than that of blood, potentially interfering with flow within the kidney. Experimental studies suggest greater perturbation in renal function with the dimers, although clinical trials have yielded conflicting results (607).

Whereas vascular effects are important, in vitro studies demonstrate toxic effects of contrast media on cultured renal epithelial cells (608). Iodinated radiocontrast agents produce cytotoxic effects in glomerular mesangial cells as well as tubular epithelial cells in vitro. Exposure of cultured tubular cells to ionic contrast media induces opening of intercellular junctions and redistribution of surface proteins (609,610). More severe injury is usually characterized by cell shrinkage and nuclear fragmentation, consistent with apoptosis (611–614). Most studies utilize the madin darby kidney cells (MDCK) cell line (predominantly distal phenotype), but changes occur in LLCPK-1 cells (proximal phenotype) as well. There is loss of cellular energy stores, disruption of calcium homeostasis, and disturbance of cell polarity. All agents appear to variably affect mitochondrial function (611). Some experimental evidence has accrued that oxidative stress is an underlying mechanism (615). In vitro cell injury is variably correlated with osmolality of the contrast media (613,615).

### Narcotics: Myoglobinuric Acute Renal Failure

Rhabdomyolysis in drug addicts is associated primarily with the use of opiates and cocaine (212,213,616). The pathogenesis of muscle damage following substance abuse is obscure. Cocaine and opiates may have a toxic effect on the skeletal muscle, but seizures, muscle injury, hyperthermia, and coma-induced ischemic or pressure injury of the muscle may also be important factors (214,317,616). Once rhabdomyolysis evolves, three major mechanisms are thought to be involved in the development of ARF: direct tubulotoxicity of myoglobin, renal tubular obstructive cast formation, and vasoconstriction/hypoperfusion (for a review, see Zager [214]). Several factors have been implicated in renal infarction, including intense renal vasoconstriction from adrenergic stimulation, endothelial injury, and platelet activation (617). Cocaine-induced endothelial injury has also been implicated in the few cases of microangiopathy associated with cocaine use (618).

### Anesthetics

The toxicity of methoxyflurane may be related to the fluoride ion, but other fluoride-containing anesthetics are not associated with renal failure (619,620).

### Herbal Medications

Poisoning caused by these formulations may be a result of the presence of undisclosed drugs or heavy metals, interaction with conventional medications, or misidentified herbal species (218). Mechanisms of tubular injury have not been well-studied.

## Acute Renal Failure in Sepsis

Acute renal failure is one manifestation of acute organ dysfunction occurring in severe sepsis (332). Patients with severe sepsis frequently develop prerenal failure as a result of septic shock (621). Renal vasoconstriction plays a role in sepsis-induced prerenal failure (622). Arterial vasodilatation in sepsis is a predisposition to ARF and is caused by cytokine-mediated induction of NO synthesis (623). Acidosis and decrease in vascular smooth muscle ATP lead to alteration in $K^+$ channels and resistance to vasopressin (624). Knock-out of eNOS in mice makes the animals very vulnerable to ARF when treated with endotoxin, consistent with a role for endothelial injury in sepsis (625). In a rat model, a specific iNOS inhibitor, L-NIL, protected against ARF (626). The inflammatory cytokine TNF has been implicated in sepsis by studies showing preservation from renal injury in experimental endotoxemia in mice with TNF receptor blockade (627), although clinical trials with anti-TNF antibody have not shown improved patient survival in these complex patients (627,628). Other experimental studies have implicated ROS. In animal studies, oxygen radical scavengers, including superoxide dismutase, have been shown to protect against endotoxemia-induced acute renal injury (629). Caspase-1 knock-out mice are resistant to ARF induced by endotoxemia (630), implicating this protease in sepsis-associated ARF. A possible role for complement has been proposed in studies documenting the protective effect of blockade of complement component C5a in sepsis (631).

## Acute Renal Failure and Multiple Organ Failure

Acute renal failure often occurs in the setting of other acute organ dysfunction. Potential "cross-talk" between affected organs is emerging as an area of interest for nephrology and critical care medicine (see Bonventre [335] and Kielar et al [632] for review). For example, mechanical ventilation may initiate or aggravate ARF. Three mechanisms have been invoked: permissive hypercapnia or hypoxemia with compromise of renal blood flow, effects on cardiac output, and barotrauma with pulmonary inflammation and release of inflammatory mediators (633). Conversely, ARF may potentiate acute lung injury. Acute renal failure leads to macrophage-mediated increase in pulmonary vascular permeability (634). Acute renal failure also leads to dysregulation of lung salt and water channels in bilateral ischemic injury or bilateral nephrectomy, though not in unilateral ischemic injury, suggesting a role for "uremic toxins" (635). Mechanisms underlying combined ARF and acute lung injury in the intensive care unit have been reviewed (636).

## Differential Diagnosis

As indicated previously, the causes of ARF are varied, although a significant portion of cases can be attributed to ATI. A similar clinical syndrome is seen in a variety of primary renal diseases, including rapidly progressive glomerulonephritis and thrombotic microangiopathies, and "secondary" ATI may occur in these settings owing to ischemia, inflammation, and potentially other mechanisms. Clinical differentiation between ischemic and toxic injury may be difficult in some settings, especially in hospitalized patients. Morphologically, toxic injury is more strongly associated with frank cellular necrosis. There are features, as discussed above, that may make it possible to identify the mechanism and even occasionally a specific agent.

There may be an inflammatory response in ATI. The single most distinguishing feature between ATI and acute interstitial nephritis is the severity and nature of the interstitial infiltrate. Although eosinophils can be present during the recovery phase of some cases of ATI, they are usually low in number and found only in a scattered distribution. The changes associated with postrenal failure owing to obstruction may lead to tubular dilatation and interstitial edema, but the characteristic focal areas of necrosis and sublethal cell injury generally absent.

## Clinical Course

The clinical course of ATI is usually divided into three phases: the initiation phase, the maintenance phase, and the recovery phase. The *initiation phase*, which usually comprises the initial oliguric symptoms, consists of a rapid decline in renal function followed by stabilization to the maintenance phase, with GFR at a relatively low 5 to 10 mL per minute. As noted above, the extent of decrease in GFR correlates with the appearance of oliguria. The *maintenance phase* typically lasts 1 to 2 weeks, but it may be prolonged for several months in individual patients with complications. During the *recovery phase*, patients gradually recover renal function, with normalization of urine output and a fall in sCr. Patients may experience polyuria with significant diuresis, which occasionally can be excessive and require careful management of fluid and electrolyte balance.

The period of renal insufficiency varies from patient to patient, ranging from a few days to as long as several weeks (637–639). The morbidity of ATI is largely the result of the multiple possible accompanying complications and the clinical setting in which it occurs (Table 24.4). The severity of these complications correlates with mortality (2,3,327,637,640,641). The overall mortality rate for ATI approximates 50% and has changed little since the advent of renal replacement therapy. A variety of pharmacologic agents have been tried in attempts to ameliorate the severity of the failure and to hasten recovery, but none have been

## TABLE 24.4
## COMPLICATIONS OF ACUTE RENAL FAILURE

**Metabolic**
  Hyperkalemia
  Metabolic acidosis
  Hyponatremia
  Hypocalcemia
  Hyperphosphatemia
  Hypermagnesemia
  Hyperuricemia

**Cardiovascular**
  Pulmonary edema
  Arrhythmias
  Pericarditis
  Pericardial effusion
  Hypertension
  Myocardial infarction
  Pulmonary embolism
  Pneumonitis

**Gastrointestinal**
  Nausea
  Vomiting
  Malnutrition
  Gastritis
  Gastrointestinal ulcers
  Gastrointestinal bleeding
  Stomatitis or gingivitis
  Parotitis or pancreatitis

**Neuromuscular irritability**
  Asterixis
  Seizures
  Mental status changes
  Somnolence
  Coma

**Hematologic**
  Anemia
  Bleeding

**Infectious**
  Pneumonia
  Wound infections
  Intravenous line infections
  Septicemia
  Urinary tract infection

**Other**
  Hiccups
  Decreased insulin catabolism
  Mild insulin resistance
  Elevated parathyroid hormone
  Reduced 1,25-dihydroxy- and 25-hydroxyvitamin D
  Low total triiodothyronine and thyroxine
  Normal free thyroxine

shown to be consistently of value. The mortality rates do differ, however, depending on the initiating cause of ARF; trauma and major surgery are associated with the highest mortality rate, and ARF in pregnancy has the lowest rate. In addition, mortality rates are higher in older debilitated peo-

ple and those with multiple organ disease. Death is almost inevitable if ARF is associated with failure of more than three other organ systems (642,643). Acute renal failure in itself may play an important role in multiple organ dysfunction (638). In the critically ill, assessment of epidemiology and natural history of ARF has been complicated by the absence of a universally accepted definition of ARF and of measurable end points (643,645,646).

### Prognosis

Patients who survive an episode of ARF generally recover sufficient renal function and do not usually suffer from overt progressive chronic renal deterioration. Patients with the greatest impairment of renal hemodynamics have the lowest potential for recovery of renal function long-term (646), and an accurate estimate of GFR may be of prognostic significance. Toxic tubular injury will continue as long as there is exposure to the offending agent. Discontinuation of the drug or adjustment of the dosage will allow recovery of tubular cells and of renal function, although permanent damage has been seen with some toxins, and some drugs such as calcineurin inhibitors, lithium, and herb medications routinely cause fibrosis (74,75,141,142,170). Recovery is the rule, although recovery may be incomplete, with persistent decrease in creatinine clearance and urine concentrating ability in 35% to 71% of patients (647,648), with some evidence of progression of dysfunction after 1 to 5 years in one follow-up study (648). Persistent renal dysfunction has been reported in adults and children (649,650). In the newborn, prognosis and recovery are also dependent upon the underlying etiology. Hypoxic/ ischemic and nephrotoxic injury to the developing kidney in the perinatal period can result in a reduced number of nephrons, and monitoring for the late developments of chronic renal insufficiency is recommended. Early ischemic injury in the renal allograft has persistently been shown to predispose to later graft injury and loss (see Chapter 28).

Chronic renal failure and fibrosis have been described in animal models when these animals have been followed long term, and although the renal insults in these models are not completely analogous to those in clinical ARF, these studies provide some insights into mechanisms of progression. Both ischemic injury (651) and cisplatin toxicity (652) have been reported to result in concentrating defects in rats. In the ischemic model, chronic renal insufficiency develops after several months, following recovery of function and morphologic tubular injury and has been associated with progressive proteinuria (653–655). Early increases in macrophages and myofibroblasts have been documented in early experimental ischemic injury (656) and gentamicin toxicity (503).

Early postischemia there are significant alterations in renal blood flow, with reduced and chaotic cortical flow demonstrable by videomicroscopy (657). Increased capillary leakiness has been documented following ischemia/reperfusion injury by tracking diffusion of fluorescent high–molecular-weight dextrans by 2-photon confocal microscopy (658), associated with disorganization of F-actin in endothelial and vascular smooth muscle cells and loss of E-cadherin–positive tight junction. Late microvascular damage and loss of peritubular capillaries have been documented in animal models with ischemic injury. These changes persist even as tubules recover from the acute insult. In a study using microfil injection, a 30% to 50% reduction in vascular density was demonstrated at 4, 8, and 40 weeks following ischemia/reperfusion injury in the rat (653). It has been hypothesized that rarefaction of peritubular capillaries permanently alters renal function and predisposes to chronic renal insufficiency (654). Other possible mechanisms for progressive decline in renal function include inability of some nephrons to regenerate following ischemic injury (654). Inhibition of B7 costimulatory factor in experimental ischemic injury attenuates the development of progressive renal failure (659), suggesting a role for inflammation, which may be a factor in both ischemic and some types of toxic injury. A possible role for endothelin has also been implicated (655). All of these factors could be interrelated. The hypoxia marker 2-pimonidizole has been used to demonstrate persistent hypoxia in the outer medulla at 5 weeks following experimental ischemia/reperfusion injury, when function and renal tubular structure have recovered. Treatment with L-arginine increased blood flow and attenuated the hypoxia and later interstitial fibrosis (660).

### Therapy

Therapy for ARF includes prevention and interventions during or after the insult. Any inciting agents or factors should be removed or corrected. Depending on the toxic agent and severity of injury, recovery may be rapid or prolonged. Careful management of fluid, electrolytes, and acid-base status is critical, especially if renal insufficiency is severe. Renal replacement therapy, including dialysis or other forms of hemofiltration, may be required (331,661–664). Intermittent hemodialysis is the most common modality. Peritoneal dialysis is not widely used in adults, and use of this modality is decreasing in pediatric patients, except for neonates and very small infants (331). Hemofiltration is increasingly common in the pediatric population (331,665). A number of therapeutic agents and strategies have been efficacious in experimental models to prevent or ameliorate ARF, although many have been generally disappointing in clinical trials.

Prevention of ARF is a goal, and some strategies have been developed, including perioperative hydration, maintenance of perfusion pressure, and avoidance of nephrotoxins or minimization of toxic effects of potential nephrotoxins, to lessen occurrence of ARF (666). Many experimental models have focused on therapies administered before the onset of ARF. However, the efficacy of these approaches is limited to scenarios in which development of ATI can be anticipated, including preoperatively, following myocardial infarction, prior to use of potential nephrotoxic agents, and in renal transplantation. In humans, some of the best results in prevention of ARF have been seen with RN (200,667); isotonic sodium bicarbonate infusion, N-acetylcysteine combined with hydration (197,668), and ascorbic acid (669) have been used to prevent RN. However, results have been heterogeneous, and caution is advised in adopting this as standard of care (670).

More generally useful therapies are those that are effective when given during or after the onset of injury and dysfunction. A variety of agents, including growth factors, have some efficacy in experimental models. In humans, ANP has proven efficacious in nonoliguric renal failure (671); however, use of atrial natriuretic peptide (ANP) to prevent RN has had variable efficacy, although perhaps with some utility in diabetic patients (200). Treatment with insulin-like growth factor had no measurable benefit in a randomized clinical trial in ARF patients (672). However, clinical trials using single agents based on findings in experimental models have not identified significant efficacy. Combination therapies, for example, use of a vasodilator such as ANP combined with mannitol to maintain tubular flow, could be an optimal approach; this combination has been shown to be effective in experimental animals (673). ANP and dopamine in combination have also been effective in a rat model of ischemic ARF (674).

The bioartificial kidney, which combines hemofiltration and a device containing human tubular cells in hopes of replacing some of the metabolic and endocrine functions of the renal tubules, has been in development for some years (675). This device is currently in clinical trials. More recently, based on experimental evidence that extrarenal cells, including bone marrow-derived cells, may have efficacy in recovery and repair following renal tubular injury, there has been a focus on how endothelial cells or stem cells might be used to accelerate recovery from ATI. Future strategies in the treatment of ARF include use of growth factors or stem cells and other novel therapies (676,677).

## RENAL CORTICAL NECROSIS

Bilateral renal cortical necrosis is a rare and dramatically unique cause of ARF. The clinical course is similar to that of ATI, except that it almost always presents with anuria or profound oliguria. It most commonly is seen in association with obstetric accidents, such as abruptio placentae, but it is also seen in instances of severe trauma, systemic sepsis, postoperative shock, and some specific poisonings, including snake venom, diethylene glycol, and arsenic (678–681).

Hemorrhage associated with abruptio placentae, abortion, or placenta previa is reported as being responsible for 50% to 60% of all cases of acute bilateral renal cortical necrosis (678). Twin–twin or twin–maternal transfusions with resultant activation of the complement cascade can also lead to cortical necrosis. In infants and children, the precipitating event is often gastroenteritis with severe vomiting, diarrhea, and dehydration. Overwhelming infection with bacterial sepsis is the other major cause in adults.

The pathogenesis of cortical necrosis remains unknown. There are several major theories, and they are not mutually exclusive. On the basis of examination of the kidneys from patients who died after abruptio placentae, Sheehan and Davis (22) proposed that vasospasm is the primary event causing cortical necrosis. Alternatively, it has been suggested that acute cortical necrosis may be a severe form of thrombotic microangiopathy, resulting from acute vascular injury followed by activation of coagulation and thrombosis (680,682–684). To support the vasospasm hypothesis, Sheehan and Davis (22) developed an experimental model in which prolonged clamping of the renal pedicle produced a lesion similar to that seen in humans. Several other investigators found that it was possible to experimentally induce the Shwartzman reaction in pregnant rabbits with only a single injection of bacterial endotoxin, which resulted in a lesion that resembled cortical necrosis in humans. A third hypothesis suggests that acute cortical necrosis may be the consequence of an immunologic mechanism akin to hyperacute rejection of renal allografts. All of these hypotheses have some supporting evidence, but there is no convincing proof that any one of them fully explains the sequence of events that occurs in human patients.

The clinical course of acute cortical necrosis depends on the extent of involvement. If necrosis is extensive, death occurs within the first few days unless dialysis is undertaken. With timely renal replacement therapy, renal function may recover sufficiently to allow patients to become dialysis independent after a period of 1 to 3 months, and renal function may continue to improve over a period of 1 to 2 years. No specific therapeutic approaches have been successful, although anticoagulants, beta blockers, cytotoxic drugs, and mannitol have all been tried.

## Gross Pathology

Bilateral cortical necrosis in its diffuse form is a condition in which there is widespread destruction of the renal cortex, except for a narrow rim of cortical tissue just underneath the capsule and with relative preservation of the medulla and the adjacent juxtamedullary cortex. This is the most severe form and can be detected on imaging studies (Fig. 24.29A). It is generally recognized on gross examination as large, swollen kidneys in which the necrotic portion of the cortex is pale or yellowish white, with congestion of the adjacent, relatively well-preserved tissue (Fig. 24.29B).

Patchy and focal forms affect smaller amounts of cortex and appear grossly similar to areas of infarction, except that they are surrounded on all sides by viable tissue and do not have the characteristic wedge-shaped pattern of the classic infarct.

## Histopathology

By light microscopy, the findings are very similar to those seen with ischemic infarcts. There is coagulation of the central necrotic areas with relative preservation of the architecture of the tubules and the glomeruli but loss of normal cytologic features (Fig. 24.30). The arteries and arterioles are also necrotic and dilated and frequently contain thrombi. Glomeruli and vessels in the border zones may show evidence of capillary and vascular thrombosis (Fig. 24.31). As the lesion progresses toward healing, leukocytic infiltration, organization, scarring, calcification, and even ossification may take place as the necrotic tissue is gradually replaced by scarring (Fig. 24.32).

# INFARCTION OF THE KIDNEY

Infarction of the kidney results from complete obstruction of major branches of the renal arteries or renal veins, and when it is extensive, it may appear as ARF. Arterial occlusion, however, is more frequently seen as a cause of renal infarction than venous occlusion. It can result from embolism, thrombosis, or vessel wall damage such as accompanies malignant hypertension or systemic vasculitis. Renal infarction caused by arterial occlusion is not uncommon, largely because there is little collateral circulation available and because complete occlusion of an arterial branch results in absolute ischemia of the distal parenchyma. The majority of infarcts in adults are often clinically silent and are frequently caused by sudden and complete arterial blockage by emboli. They can originate as ventricular thrombi or from vegetations on heart valves with verrucous or infective endocarditis. Less commonly, arterial obstruction is produced by thrombosis owing to changes in the wall of the vessel associated with atherosclerosis, systemic sclerosis, malignant hypertension, polyarteritis, or aneurysm formation as a result of dysplastic disease of the renal artery. Renal infarction has also rarely been described as a result of cocaine use (685,686). Renal infarction frequently goes undetected, particularly if the area of infarction is small. Large infarcts can be associated with loin pain followed by hematuria and transient proteinuria.

## Gross Pathology

The gross appearance of a renal infarct depends on the age of the lesion, the size of the vessel obstructed, and the presence or absence of infection. Initially, the infarct is red and

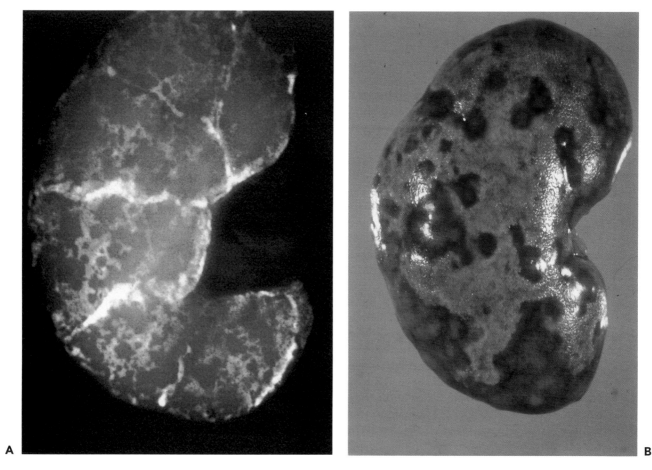

**Figure 24.29** A: Radiograph with contrast of a kidney with cortical necrosis showing hypoperfusion and areas of hemorrhage. B: Gross specimen of kidney with extensive areas of pallor representing necrotic cortex with intervening areas of congested nonnecrotic parenchyma.

pyramidal in shape, with the apex toward the obstructed artery. Within hours it becomes gray, with a narrow red rim of adjacent congested parenchyma; as intralesional coagulation occurs, the infarcted area develops a yellow coloration (Fig. 24.33). As necrotic tissue is removed and re- placed by collagenous tissue, the area of infarct shrinks and eventually becomes a V-shaped scar. The medulla is generally spared in renal infarction, and the lesions are confined to the cortex. Infarcts resulting from septic embolization are associated with the presence of liquefactive necrosis

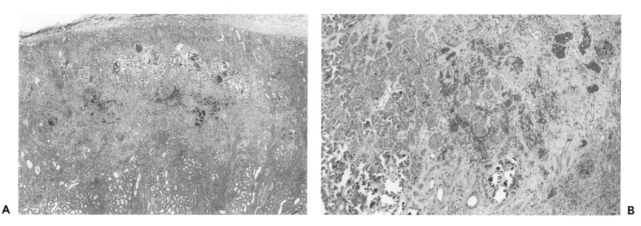

**Figure 24.30** A: Cortical necrosis, with sparing of subcapsular cortex and medulla. (H&E; ×64.) B: Cortical necrosis with coagulative necrosis with focal hemorrhage. (H&E; ×200.)

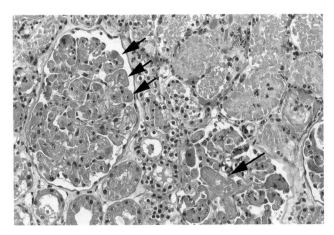

**Figure 24.31** Cortical necrosis, with thromboses *(arrows)* in glomeruli adjacent to necrotic area. (H&E; ×640.)

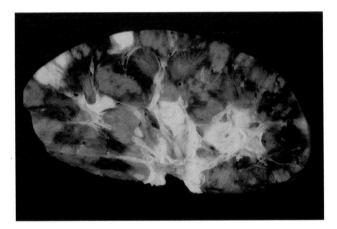

**Figure 24.33** Kidney with focal pale wedge-shaped cortical infarcts. Note congestion at the corticomedullary junction.

and abscess formation as a result of digestion by leukocytic enzymes.

## Histopathology

Histologically, sterile infarcts show the findings of classic coagulative necrosis. Initially, there is marked congestion, followed by cytoplasmic and nuclear changes, where the tubular and glomerular architecture is preserved but gradual loss of viable cytologic structure occurs. The cytoplasm becomes homogeneous and eosinophilic, and the nuclei demonstrate condensation and karyorrhexis (Fig. 24.34). Peripheral to the central area of necrosis is a marginal zone in which there is a gradual transition from frank necrotic changes to sublethal injury in which glomerular and tubular changes are less striking and are similar to those seen in ATI (Fig. 24.35). As the lesion develops, it is in this zone that polymorphonuclear leukocytic infiltration becomes prominent. As the lesion progresses, the central necrotic area becomes smaller, and organization and regeneration

center around the periphery, with eventual collapse of the central necrotic area and replacement by collagenous scarring. As mentioned previously, the lesions are generally confined to the cortical tissue, and the medulla is spared. This picture helps distinguish scars resulting from infarction from those caused by reflux or pyelonephritis, in which medullary involvement is prominent.

## Venous Infarction

Venous obstruction as a cause of infarction is much less common than arterial obstruction. It is seen in infancy as a complication of severe dehydration stemming from diarrheal diseases. Thrombosis of intrarenal veins and, occasionally, of the main renal vein produces an infarct of the hemorrhagic type (Fig. 24.36), as opposed to the relatively bland ischemic infarction that follows arterial occlusion. Whether infarction occurs in the kidney as a result of venous thrombosis depends on the completeness of the occlusion and the speed at which thrombosis and

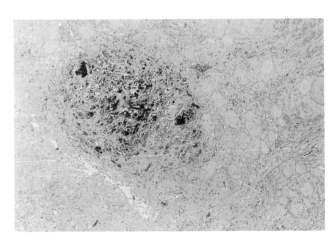

**Figure 24.32** Chronic cortical necrosis with calcification. (H&E; ×80.)

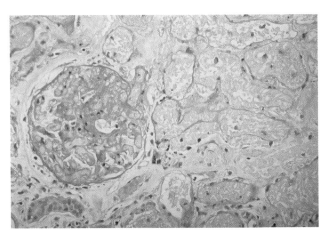

**Figure 24.34** Renal infarct, with coagulative necrosis of all cellular elements. (H&E; ×400.)

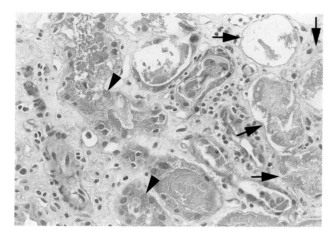

**Figure 24.35** Transition zone at the edge of a cortical infarct. Note completely necrotic tubules (*arrows*) and relatively intact tubules with individual cell necrosis (*arrowheads*) containing necrotic debris. (H&E; ×640.)

occlusion take place. Sudden, complete occlusions can be associated with infarction in adults, although this is rare; in most instances, thrombosis of the renal vein does not lead to infarction after infancy.

## LOIN PAIN HEMATURIA SYNDROME

The loin pain hematuria syndrome is an ill-defined clinical syndrome characterized by recurrent episodes of loin pain accompanied by hematuria (687). It was first described by Little et al in 1967 (688) and is essentially a diagnosis of exclusion. Renal colic associated with hematuria can be seen in patients with ureteric stones, urinary tract infections, and known causes of glomerular hematuria, such as acute glomerulonephritis or IgA nephropathy (689). Loin pain with hematuria is also occasionally seen in patients with thin basement membrane disease (690). This syndrome

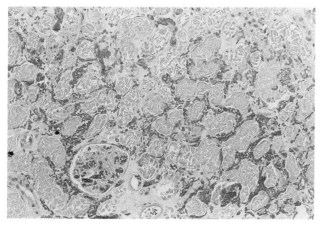

**Figure 24.36** Hemorrhagic infarct with severe congestion of microvessels. (H&E; ×400.)

of loin pain hematuria should therefore be invoked only when the other causes of hematuria have been excluded. Thus, the clinical definition of a patient with this syndrome is a person with intermittent or persistent loin pain and intermittent or persistent hematuria (either gross but more usually microscopic) in the context of a normal collecting system, as confirmed by radiography. If it is performed, a renal biopsy should not show any form of primary or secondary glomerular lesion.

The majority of patients are women between the ages of 20 and 40, but the syndrome has also been reported in older children. Its incidence appears to be higher in Great Britain than in the United States (687,691). Many patients show psychologic or psychopathologic features (692,693), and this finding has inspired considerable skepticism about the validity of the diagnosis, particularly since many of these patients demand long-term narcotic analgesic therapy. The pain can be so severe that narcotic analgesics are administered on a long-term basis, and this long-term administration has engendered attempts to alleviate pain by other means, including autotransplantation (694,695). Clinical evaluation shows nothing unusual, except for the presence of pain and hematuria. Blood pressure and renal function are normal, and evidence of proteinuria is generally absent. Radiologic findings have been variable, but several investigators have described tortuosity, beading, and obliteration of medium-size intrarenal vessels (696,697). Areas of underperfusion have also been described, and it has been thought by some researchers that these findings can be explained by reversible intrarenal arteriolar spasm (698). Most commonly, however, arteriography results are completely normal.

### Microscopic Findings

When biopsy is performed, renal histology generally shows only minor abnormalities (696,699). One study has described mild mesangial hypertrophy and patchy interstitial fibrosis with tubular atrophy. If there are any abnormal findings, they generally involve the renal vessels. Arterial and arteriolar hyalinosis has been described, and immunofluorescence studies have reported prominent deposition of C3 in affected vessels (700). Immunoglobulin deposits have never been recorded. The radiologic and histologic findings suggest that the syndrome may result from diseases affecting the intrarenal vessels, but this theory has not been confirmed.

An interesting hypothesis has been advanced by Boyd et al based on the observation that the majority of these patients are women and that a significant number of young women had been taking estrogen-containing oral contraceptives (701). Estrogens are known to produce an increase in platelet factor 3, and some studies have suggested that levels of platelet factor 3 are higher in patients with loin pain hematuria. These findings have suggested that platelet activation and fibrin deposition may play a role (698). The possibility of a defect in prostacyclin production has also been put forward (702). Despite the dramatic nature of the clinical features, the prognosis from a renal point of view is excellent. There have been no reports of progressive renal injury or evolution to chronic disease.

## ATHEROEMBOLIC DISEASE OF THE KIDNEY

Embolization of the kidney by fragments of atheromatous plaques is extremely common and is found in nearly 5% of autopsies of men over the age of 50 and 3% of women in the same age group (703–706). Although emboli do appear spontaneously, they more commonly follow invasive arterial procedures, including arteriography, coronary angiography, coronary artery bypass, and repair of aortic aneurysms; they are found in as many as 25% of patients who have undergone such procedures (707). The emboli are usually derived from atheromatous lesions of the abdominal aorta that become impacted in intralobular or smaller arcuate vessels (Fig. 24.37). Arteriolar and glomerular embolization can also occur (Fig. 24.38). When obstruction is complete, distal areas of infarction and necrosis are evident. Often the obstruction is incomplete, and the distal parenchyma demonstrates only ischemic atrophy (Fig. 24.39).

Cholesterol emboli are identified by the characteristic needle-shaped clefts that remain after the lipid has been dissolved during histologic processing. In early stage lesions, the crystals are surrounded by fibrin, whereas with older embolic lesions, organization is evident, and the crystals are surrounded by fibrous tissue. Renal atheroemboli are frequently part of more generalized atheroembolic disease, resulting from multiple showers of cholesterol-containing microemboli in many organs, including the

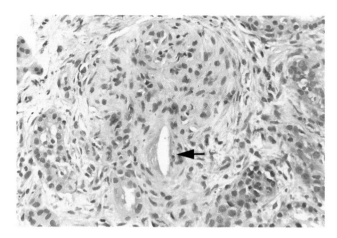

**Figure 24.38**   Atheroembolus in an arteriole. The glomerulus appears ischemic. (H&E; ×400.)

retina, brain, pancreas, and, in particular, the muscles and skin of the legs in addition to the kidney. Multisystem involvement often mimics systemic vasculitides, such as microscopic polyarteritis. In some instances, showers of emboli may be so extensive as to result in the clinical syndrome of ARF, mimicking the findings of rapidly progressive glomerulonephritis. The presence of eosinophilia, hypocomplementemia, and sometimes eosinophiluria further complicates the clinical recognition of this disease.

## THE HEPATORENAL SYNDROME

The term *hepatorenal syndrome* (HRS) is not a definable histopathologic entity of intrinsic renal disease. It describes a clinical syndrome of ARF that may complicate advanced liver disease (708). Two types have been defined: type 1, with rapid reduction of renal function; and type 2, with slowly progressive decline in renal function. The five criteria

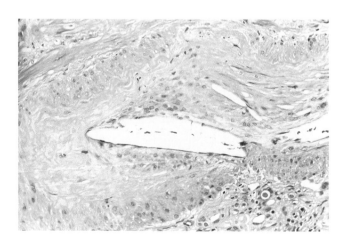

**Figure 24.37**   Atheroembolus in an artery, with cleft-like spaces surrounded by fibrotic reaction. (H&E; ×400.)

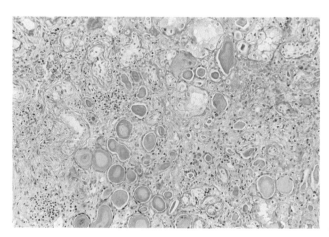

**Figure 24.39**   Ischemic atrophy downstream from chronic arterial atheroembolus. (H&E; ×200.)

for HRS, as defined by the International Ascites Club, include: severe cirrhosis, glomerular hypofiltration, lack of other functional or organic cause, failure of plasma expansion to improve renal function, and absence of proteinuria. The syndrome is thought to be common, but the incidence is not known. In a recent multivariate retrospective study of 355 patients with cirrhosis and ARF, 58% had prerenal failure (71 of 206 with type 1, the remainder type 2). Forty-two percent had "acute tubular necrosis." No cases of ARF owing to acute glomerulonephritis were identified (709). This study confirms that the vast majority of cases of ARF in cirrhosis are caused by hypoperfusion.

This syndrome is characterized physiologically by intense intrarenal vasoconstriction and hypoperfusion, resulting in a primary decrease in the GFR, and is a variant of prerenal failure, because it is accompanied by diminished effective systemic circulatory volume. Urinalysis will usually reveal a benign urinary sediment and concentrated urine; in contrast to the chemical composition of the urine in ATI caused by ischemia or nephrotoxins, the sodium concentration is usually low. This finding could be a useful addition to the five criteria for hepatorenal syndrome outlined above. The pathogenetic mechanisms of action of the dramatic hemodynamic alterations accompanying severe hepatic disease are incompletely understood. The presence of ascites and other shifts in total body fluid volume are major contributors. Gastrointestinal bleeding may underlie the ARF in some of these patients (710). Other risk factors in this setting include vomiting, diarrhea, diuretic therapy, or treatment with NSAIDs, ACE inhibitors, or angiotensin II receptor blockers. However, a significant number of cases occur without these antecedents. The renin–angiotensin–aldosterone system, vasoactive intestinal peptides, endothelin, NO, prostaglandins, and the kallikrein–kinin system have all been implicated as possibly playing a role. Patients with type 1 HRS have improved renal function after therapy with vasoconstrictors such as terlipressin (709). This response could also serve as an additional diagnostic criterion for HRS (708).

Because the pathogenesis appears to be primarily hemodynamic, the morphologic changes associated with this syndrome are nonspecific and not distinctive. Although bile-stained casts and crystals can be seen within tubular lumina, the cytologic changes visible in patients with ATI are not consistently present. Relatively few renal biopsy studies have been performed, because the biopsy procedure is often contraindicated in the clinical context of end-stage liver disease; the findings of postmortem studies must be evaluated with consideration of the changes caused by autolysis and other comorbid features. Nevertheless, some authors have emphasized particular histologic findings, including "tubularization" of Bowman's capsular epithelium, tubular dilatation, interstitial edema, bile-stained intratubular casts, leucine crystals in the tubules and interstitium, and sometimes an interstitial leukocytic infiltrate.

# REFERENCES

1. Chertow GM, Levy EM, Hammermeister KM, et al. Independent association between acute renal failure and mortality following cardiac surgery. Am J Med 1998;104:343.
2. de Mendonca A, Vincent JL, Suter PM, et al. Acute renal failure in the ICU: Risk factors and outcome evaluated by the SOFA score. Intensive Care Med 2000;26:915.
3. Vivino G, Antonelli M, Moro M, et al. Risk factors for acute renal failure in trauma patients. Intensive Care Med 1998;24:808.
4. Pascual J, Liano F, Ortuno J. The elderly patient with acute renal failure. J Am Soc Nephrol 1995;6:144.
5. Zanardo G, Michielon P, Paccagnella A, et al. Acute renal failure in the patient undergoing cardiac operation: Prevalence, mortality rate, and main risk factors. J Thorac Cardiovasc Surg 1994;107:1489.
6. Schrier RW, Wang W, Poole B, Mitra A. Acute renal failure: Definitions, diagnosis, pathogenesis, and therapy [Erratum appears in J Clin Invest 2004;114:598]. J Clin Invest 2004;114(1):5.
7. Bellomo R. Defining, quantifying, and classifying acute renal failure. Crit Care Clin 2005;21:223.
8. Carvounis CP, Nisar S, Guro-Razuman S. Significance of the fractional excretion of urea in the differential diagnosis of acute renal failure. Kidney Int 2002;62:2223.
9. Hackradt A. Vasomotorische Nephrosen nach Verschuttung. Munich: Wagner, 1917.
10. Minami S. Ueber Nierenveranderungen nach Verschuttung. Virchows Arch (Pathol Anat) 1923;246:246.
11. Baker SL, Dodds EC. Obstruction of the renal tubules during the excretion of haemoglobin. Br J Exp Pathol 1925;6:247.
12. Bywaters EGL, Beall D. Crush injuries with impairment of renal function. Br Med J 1941;1:427.
13. Bywaters EGL, Dible JH. The renal lesion in traumatic anuria. J Pathol Bacteriol 1942;54:111.
14. Dunn JS, Gillespie M, Niven JSF. Renal lesions in two cases of crush syndrome. Lancet 1941;2:549.
15. Lucke B. Lower nephron nephrosis: The renal lesions of the crush syndrome, of burns, transfusions and other conditions affecting the lower segments of the nephrons. Mil Surgeon 1946;99:371.
16. Oliver J, MacDowell M, Tracy A. The pathogenesis of acute renal failure associated with traumatic and toxic injury: Renal ischemia, nephrotoxic damage and the ischemic episode. J Clin Invest 1951;30:1307.
17. Goormaghtigh N. Vascular and circulatory changes in renal cortex in the anuric crush-syndrome. Proc Soc Exp Biol Med 1945;59:303.
18. Goormaghtigh N. The renal arteriolar changes in the anuric crush syndrome. Am J Pathol 1947;23:513.
19. Trueta J, Barclay AE, Daniel PM, et al. Studies of the Renal Circulation. Springfield, IL: Charles C. Thomas, 1947.
20. Brun C. Acute Anuria: A Study Based on Renal Function Tests and Aspiration Biopsy of the Kidney. Copenhagen: E Munksgaard, 1965.
21. Brun C, Crone C, Davidsen HG, et al. Renal interstitial pressure in normal and in anuric man: Based on wedged renal vein pressure. Proc Soc Exp Biol Med 1956;91:199.
22. Sheehan HL, Davis JC. Renal ischaemia with failed reflow. J Pathol Bacteriol 1959;78:105.
23. Sevitt S. Pathogenesis of traumatic uraemia: A revised concept. Lancet 1959;2:135.
24. Hollenberg NK, Adams DF, Oken DE, et al. Acute renal failure due to nephrotoxins: Renal hemodynamic and angiographic studies in man. N Engl J Med 1970;282:1329.
25. Hollenberg NK, Epstein M, Rosen SM, et al. Acute oliguric renal failure in man: Evidence for preferential renal cortical ischemia. Medicine (Baltimore) 1968;47:455.
26. Munck O. Renal Circulation in Acute Renal Failure. Oxford: Blackwell, 1958.
27. Oken DE, Acre ML, Wilson DR. Glycerol-induced hemoglobinuric acute renal failure in the rat. I. Micropuncture study of the development of oliguria. J Clin Invest 1966;45:724.

28. Henry LN, Lane CE, Kashgarian M. Micropuncture studies of the pathophysiology of acute renal failure in the rat. Lab Invest 1968;19:309.
29. Kashgarian M, Siegel NJ, Ries AL, et al. Hemodynamic aspects in development and recovery phases of experimental postischemic acute renal failure. Kidney Int 1976;6:S160.
30. Siegel NJ, Gunstream SK, Handler RI, Kashgarian M. Renal function and cortical blood flow during the recovery phase of acute renal failure. Kidney Int 1977;12:199.
31. Arendshorst WJ, Finn WF, Gottschalk CW. Pathogenesis of acute renal failure following temporary renal ischemia in the rat. Circ Res 1975;37:558.
32. Bank N, Mutz BF, Aynedjian HS. The role of "leakage" of tubular fluid in anuria due to mercury poisoning. J Clin Invest 1967;46:695.
33. Beeuwkes R, Bonventre JV. Tubular organization and vascular-tubular relations in the dog kidney. Am J Physiol 1975;229:695.
34. Biber TUL, Mylle M, Baines AD, et al. A study by micropuncture and microdissection of acute renal damage in rats. Am J Med 1968;44:664.
35. Brown JJ, Gleadle RI, Lawson DH, et al. Renin and acute renal failure: Studies in man. Br Med J 1970;1:253.
36. Flamenbaum W, McDonald FD, Dibona GF, Oken DE. Micropuncture study of renal tubular factors in low dose mercury poisoning. Nephron 1971;8:221.
37. Thurau K, Boylan JW. Acute renal success. Am J Med 1976;1:308.
38. Tolkoff-Rubin NE, Rubin RH, Bonventre JV. Noninvasive renal diagnostic studies. Clin Lab Med 1988;8:507.
39. Mutti A, Lucertini S, Valcavi P, et al. Urinary excretion of brush-border antigen revealed by monoclonal antibody: Early indicator of toxic nephropathy. Lancet 1985;2:914.
40. Scherberich JE, Wolf G, Schoeppe WL. Shedding and repair of renal cell membranes following drug-induced nephrotoxicity in humans. Eur J Clin Pharmacol 1993;44(suppl 1):S33.
41. Herget-Rosenthal S, Poppen D, Husing J, et al. Prognostic value of tubular proteinuria and enzymuria to nonoliguric acute tubular necrosis. Clin Chem 2004;50:552.
42. Stonard MD, Gore CW, Oliver GJ, et al. Urinary enzymes and protein patterns as indicators of injury in different regions of the kidney. Fundam Appl Toxicol 1987;9:339.
43. Westhuyzen J, Endre ZH, Reece G, et al. Measurement of tubular enzymuria facilitates early detection of acute renal impairment in the intensive care unit. Nephrol Dial Transplant 2003;18:543.
44. Hewitt SM, Dear J, Star RA. Discovery of protein biomarkers for renal diseases. J Am Soc Nephrol 2004;15:1677.
45. Han WK, Bonventre JV. Biologic markers for the early detection of acute kidney injury. Curr Opin Crit Care 2004;10:476.
46. Allgren RL, Marbury TC, Rahman SN, et al. Anaritide in acute tubular necrosis. Auriculin Anaritide Acute Renal Failure Study Group. New Engl J Med 1997;336:828.
47. Abreo K, Moorthy AV, Osborne M. Changing patterns and outcome of acute renal failure requiring hemodialysis. Arch Intern Med 1986;146:1338.
48. Brady H, Brenner B, Lieberthal W. Acute Renal Failure. Philadelphia: WB Saunders, 1996.
49. Meyers C, Roxe D, Hano J. The clinical course of nonoliguric acute renal failure. Cardiovasc Med 1977;2:699.
50. Porter GA, Palmer BF, Henrich WL. Clinical relevance. In: De-broe ME, Porter GA, Bennett WM, Verpooten GA, eds. Clinical Nephrotoxins: Renal Injury by Drugs and Chemicals. Dordrecht, The Netherlands, Kluwer Academic Publishers, 2003:3.
51. Planas M, Wachtel T, Frank H, Henderson LW. Characterization of acute renal failure in the burned patient. Arch Intern Med 1982;142:2087.
52. Polderman KH. Acute renal failure and rhabdomyolysis. Int J Artif Organs 2004;27:1030.
53. Holt SG, Moore KP. Pathogenesis and treatment of renal dysfunction in rhabdomyolysis. Intensive Care Med 2001;27:803.
54. Vanholder R, Sever MS, Erek E, Lameire N. Rhabdomyolysis. J Am Soc Nephrol 2000;11:1553.
55. van Vleet TR, Schnellman RG. Toxic nephropathy: Environmental chemicals. Semin Nephrol 2003;23:500.
56. Dagher PC, Herget-Rosenthal S, Ruehm SG, et al. Newly developed techniques to study and diagnose acute renal failure. J Am Soc Nephrol 2003;14:2188.
57. Izzedine H, Launay-Vacher V, Deray G. Antiviral drug-induced nephrotoxicity. Am J Kidney Dis 2005;45:804.
58. Fisher EJ, Chaloner K, Cohn DL, et al. The safety and efficacy of adefovir dipivoxil in patients with advanced HIV disease: A randomized placebo-controlled trial. AIDS 2001;15:1695.
59. Sawyer MH, Webb DE, Balow JE, Straus SE. Acyclovir-induced renal failure. Am J Med 1988;84:1067.
60. Spiegal DM, Lau K. Acute renal failure and coma secondary to acyclovir therapy. JAMA 1986;255:1882.
61. Johnson GL, Limon L, Trikha G, Wall H. Acute renal failure and neurotoxicity following oral acyclovir. Ann Pharmacother 1994;28:460.
62. Becker BN, Fall P, Hall C, et al. Rapidly progressive acute renal failure due to acyclovir: Case report and review of the literature. Am J Kidney Dis 1993;22:611.
63. Perazella MA. Crystal-induced acute renal failure. Am J Med 1999;106:459.
64. Jacobson MA, O'Donnell JJ, Mills J. Foscarnet treatment of cytomegalovirus retinitis in patients with the acquired immunodeficiency syndrome. Antimicrob Agents Chemother 1989;33:736.
65. Winston DJ, Wirin D, Shaked A, Busuttil RW. Randomised comparison of ganciclovir and high-dose acyclovir for long-term cytomegalovirus prophylaxis in liver-transplant recipients. Lancet 1995;346:69.
66. Lalezari JP, Stagg RJ, Jaffe HS, et al. A preclinical and clinical overview of the nucleotide-based antiviral agent cidofovir (HPMPC). Adv Exp Med Biol 1996;394:105.
67. Polis MA, Spooner KM, Baird BF, et al. Anticytomegaloviral activity and safety of cidofovir in patients with human immunodeficiency virus infection and cytomegalovirus viruria. Antimicrob Agents Chemother 1995;39:882.
68. Lalezari JP, Holland GN, Kramer F, et al. Randomized controlled study of the safety and efficacy of intravenous cidofovir for the treatment of relapsing cytomegalovirus retinitis in patients with AIDS. J Acquir Immune Defic Syndr Hum Retrovirol 1998;17:339.
69. Tashima KT, Horowitz JD, Rosen S. Indinavir nephropathy. N Engl J Med 1997;336:138.
70. Kopp JB, Miller KD, Mican JA, et al. Crystalluria and urinary tract abnormalities associated with indinavir. Ann Intern Med 1997;127:119.
71. Chugh S, Bird R, Alexander EA. Ritonavir and renal failure. N Engl J Med 1997;336:138.
72. Zimmermann AE, Pizzoferrato T, Bedford J, et al. Tenofovir-associated acute and chronic kidney disease: A case of multiple drug interactions. Clin Infect Dis 2006;42:283.
73. Izzedine H, Isnard-Bagnis C, Hulot JS, et al. Renal safety of tenofovir in HIV treatment-experienced patients. AIDS 2004;18:1074.
74. Vandercam B, Moreau M, Goffin E, et al. Cidofovir-induced end-stage renal failure. Clin Infect Dis 1999;29:948.
75. Hanabusa H, Tagami H, Hataya H. Renal atrophy associated with long-term treatment with indinavir. New Engl J Med 1999;340:392.
76. Noble S, Goa KL. Adefovir dipivoxil. Drugs 1999;58:479.
77. Cronin RE, Henrich WL. Toxic nephropathies. In: Brenner BM, ed. The Kidney, 6th ed. Philadelphia: WB Saunders, 2000:563.
78. Cronin RE. Aminoglycoside nephrotoxicity: Pathogenesis and prevention. Clin Nephrol 1979;11:251.
79. Hitt CM, Klepser ME, Nightengale CH, et al. Pharmacoeconomic impact of once-daily aminoglycoside administration. Pharmacotherapy 1997;17:810.
80. Raveh D, Kopyt M, Hite Y, et al. Risk factors for nephrotoxicity in elderly patients receiving once-daily aminoglycosides. QJM 2002;95:291.
81. Rougier F, Ducher M, Maurin M, et al. Aminoglycoside dosages and nephrotoxicity: Quantitative relationships. Clin Pharmacokinet 2003;42:493.
82. Montagut C, Bosch F, Villela L, et al. Aminoglycoside-associated severe renal failure in patients with multiple myeloma treated with thalidomide. Leuk Lymphoma 2004;45:1711.

83. Appel GB, Neu HC. The nephrotoxicity of antimicrobial agents. I, II, III. N Engl J Med 1977;296:663,722,784.

84. Mingeot-Leclercq MP, Tulkens PM. Aminoglycosides: Nephrotoxicity. Antimicrob Agents Chemo Ther 1999;43:1003.

85. Swan SK. Aminoglycoside nephrotoxicity. Semin Nephrol 1997; 17:27.

86. Humes HD. Aminoglycoside nephrotoxicity. Kidney Int 1988;33:900.

87. Bertino JS Jr, Booker LA, Franck PA, et al. Incidence of and significant risk factors for aminoglycoside-associated nephrotoxicity in patients dosed by using individualized pharmacokinetic monitoring. J Infect Dis 1993;167:173.

88. Chow AW, Azar RM. Glycopeptides and nephrotoxicity. Intensive Care Med 1994;20:S23.

89. Fillastre JP, Laumonier R, Humbert G, et al. Acute renal failure associated with combined gentamicin and cephalothin therapy. Br Med J 1973;2:396.

90. Kleinknecht D, Ganeval D, Droz D. Acute renal failure after high doses of gentamicin and cephalothin. Lancet 1973;1:1129.

91. Melnick JZ, Baum M, Thompson JR. Aminoglycoside-induced Fanconi's syndrome. Am J Kidney Dis 1994;23:118.

92. Houghton DC, Hartness M, Campbell-Boswell M, et al. A light and electron microscopic analysis of gentamicin nephrotoxicity in rats. Am J Pathol 1976;81:589.

93. Kosek JC, Mazze RI, Cousins MJ. Nephrotoxicity of gentamicin. Lab Invest 1974;30:48.

94. Luft FC, Patel V, Yum MN, et al. Experimental aminoglycoside nephrotoxicity. J Lab Clin Med 1975;86:213.

95. Winfield M, Crist GO, Maxwell MH, Kleeman DR. Nephrotoxic effects of kanamycin: A preliminary report. Ann N Y Acad Sci 1958;76:140.

96. Kuntz E. Klinische Untersuchungen zur Nephrotoxicität von Kanamycin. Klin Wochenschr 1962;40:830.

97. Kumin GD. Clinical nephrotoxicity of tobramycin and gentamicin. JAMA 1980;244:1808.

98. Smith CR, Lipsky JJ, Laskin OL, et al. Double-blind comparison of the nephrotoxicity and auditory toxicity of gentamicin and Tobramycin. N Engl J Med 1980;302:1106.

99. De Beukelaer MD, Travis LB, Dodge WF, Guerra FA. Deafness and acute tubular necrosis following parenteral administration of neomycin. Am J Dis Child 1971;121:250.

100. Greenberg LH, Momary H. Audiotoxicity and nephrotoxicity due to orally administered neomycin. JAMA 1965;194:827.

101. Stamm AM, Diasio RB, Dismukes WE, et al. Toxicity of amphotericin B plus flucytosine in 194 patients with cryptococcal meningitis. Am J Med 1987;83:236.

102. Mery JP, Morel-Maroger L. Acute interstitial nephritis: A hypersensitivity reaction to drugs. In: Giovannetti S, Bonomini V, D'Amico, eds. Proceedings of the Sixth International Congress of Nephrology. Basel: Karger, 1976:524.

103. McCurdy DK, Frederic M, Elkinton JR. Renal tubular acidosis due to amphotericin B. N Engl J Med 1968;278:124.

104. Douglas JB, Healy JK. Nephrotoxic effects of amphotericin B, including renal tubular acidosis. Am J Med 1969;46:154.

105. Yano Y, Monteiro JL, Seguro AC. Effect of amphotericin B on water and urea transport in the inner medullary collecting duct. J Am Soc Nephrol 1994;5:68.

106. Benner EJ. Renal damage associated with prolonged administration of ampicillin, cephaloridine, and cephalothin. Antimicrob Agents Chemother 1969;9:417.

107. Pickering MJ, Spooner GR, de Quesada A, Cade JR. Declining renal function associated with administration of cephalothin. South Med J 1970;63:426.

108. Foord RD. Cephaloridine, cephalothin and the kidney. J Antimicrob Chemother 1975;1:119.

109. Norrby R, Stenqvist K, Elgefors B. Interaction between cephaloridine and furosemide in man. Scand J Infect Dis 1976;8:209.

110. Barrientos A, Bello I, Gutierrez-Millett V, et al. Renal failure and cephalothin. Ann Intern Med 1976;84:612.

111. Burton JR, Lichtenstein NS, Colvin RB, Hyslop NE Jr. Acute renal failure during cephalothin therapy. JAMA 1974;229:679.

112. Engle JE, Drago J, Calin B, Schoolwerth AC. Reversible acute renal failure after cephalothin. Ann Intern Med 1975;1:232.

113. Fillastre JP, Kleinknecht D. Acute renal failure associated with cephalosporin therapy. Am Heart J 1975;1:809.

114. Wade JC, Smith CR, Petty BG, et al. Cephalothin plus an aminoglycoside is more nephrotoxic than methicillin plus an aminoglycoside. Lancet 1978;1:604.

115. Dodds MG, Foord RD. Enhancement by potent diuretics of renal tubular necrosis induced by cephaloridine. Br J Pharmacol 1970;1:227.

116. Moran H, Beattie TJ. Acute tubular necrosis associated with cephalexin therapy. Clin Nephrol 1985;24:212.

117. Longstreth KL, Robbins SD, Smavatkul C, Doe NS. Cephalexin-induced acute tubular necrosis. Pharmacotherapy 2004;24:808.

118. Vomiero G, Carpenter B, Robb I, Filler G. Combination of ceftriaxone and acyclovir: An underestimated nephrotoxic potential? Pediatr Nephrol 2002;17:633.

119. Fiaccadori E, Maggiore U. Arisi A, et al. Outbreak of acute renal failure due to cefodizime-vancomycin associated in a heart surgery unit. Intensive Care Med 2001;27:1819.

120. Jawetz E. Polymyxin, colistin, and bacitracin. Pediatr Clin North Am 1961;8:1057.

121. Koch-Weser J, Sidel VW, Federman EB, et al. Adverse effects of sodium colistimethate: Manifestations and specific reaction rates during 317 courses of therapy. Ann Intern Med 1970;72:857.

122. Adler S, Segel DP. Nonoliguric renal failure secondary to sodium colistimethate: A report of four cases. Am J Med Sci 1971;262:107.

123. Levin AS, Barone AA, Penco J, et al. Intravenous colistin as therapy for nosocomial infections caused by multidrug-resistant *Pseudomonas aeruginosa and Actinobacter baumannii*. Clin Infect Dis 1999;28:1008.

124. Elwood CM, Lucas GD, Muehrcke RC. Acute renal failure associated with sodium colistimethate treatment. Arch Intern Med 1966;118:326.

125. Andoh TF, Burdmann EA, Bennett WM. Nephrotoxicity of immunosuppressive drugs: Experimental and clinical observations. Semin Nephrol 1997;17:34.

126. Kopp J, Klotman PE. Cellular and molecular mechanisms of cyclosporin nephrotoxicity. J Am Soc Nephrol 1990;1:162.

127. Remuzzi G, Perico N. Cyclosporine-induced renal dysfunction in experimental animals and humans. Kidney Int 1995;48 (suppl 52):S70.

128. Solez K, Racusen LC, Mihatsch M. Nephrotoxicity of cyclosporine and newer immunosuppressive agents. In: Solez K, Racusen L, Billingham M, eds. Solid Organ Allograft Rejection. New York: Marcel Dekker, 1996:587.

129. Charney D, Solez K, Racusen L. Nephrotoxicity of cyclosporine and other immunosuppressive and immunotherapeutic agents. In: Tarloff JB, Lash LH, eds. Toxicology of the Kidney, 3rd ed. New York: CRC Press, 2005:687.

130. Krupp P, Gulich A, Timoren P. Side effects and safety of Sandimmune in long-term treatment of renal transplant. Transplant Proc 1986;18:991.

131. Perico N, Ruggenenti P, Gaspari F, et al. Daily renal hypoperfusion induced by cyclosporine in patients with renal transplantation. Transplantation 1992;54:56.

132. Ader JL, Rostaing L. Cyclosporin nephrotoxicity: Pathophysiology and comparison with FK506. Curr Opin Nephrol Hypertens 1998;7:539.

133. Mihatsch MJ, Kyo M, Morozumi K, et al. The side-effects of ciclosporine-A and tacrolimus. Clin Nephrol 1998;49:356.

134. Rodicio JL. Calcium antagonists and renal protection from cyclosporine nephrotoxicity: Long-term trial in renal transplantation patients. J Cardiovasc Pharmacol 2000;35(suppl 1):S7.

135. Campistol JM, Sacks SH. Mechanisms of nephrotoxicity. Transplantation 2000;69:SS5.

136. Conte G, Dal Canton A, Sabbatini M, et al. Acute cyclosporine renal dysfunction reversed by dopamine infusion in healthy subjects. Kidney Int 1989;36:1086.

137. Neild G, Reuben R, Hartley RB, Cameron JS. Glomerular thrombi in renal allografts associated with cyclosporine therapy. J Clin Pathol 1985;38:253.

138. Shulman H, Striker G, Deeg HJ, et al. Nephrotoxicity of cyclosporin A after allogeneic marrow transplantation: Glomerular thromboses and tubular injury. N Engl J Med 1981;305:1392.

139. Vanrenterghem Y, Roels L, Lerut T, et al. Thromboembolic complications and haemostatic changes in cyclosporin-treated cadaveric kidney allograft recipients. Lancet 1985;1:999.

140. Young BA, Marsh CL, Alpers CE, Davis CL. Cyclosporine-associated thrombotic microangiopathy/hemolytic uremic syndrome following kidney and kidney–pancreas transplantation. Am J Kidney Dis 1996;28:561.

141. Myers BD, Ross J, Newton L, et al. Cyclosporine-associated chronic nephropathy. N Engl J Med 1984;311:699.

142. Zachariae H. Renal toxicity of long-term cyclosporin. Scand J Rheumatol 1999;28:65.

143. de Mattos AM, Olyaei AJ, Bennett WM. Nephrotoxicity of immunosuppressive drugs: Long-term consequences and challenges for the future. Am J Kidney Dis 2000;35:333.

144. Levy G, Thervet E, Lake J, Uchida K. Patient management by Neoral C2 monitoring: An international consensus statement. Transplantation 2002;73(9 Suppl):S12.

145. Myers BD. Cyclosporine nephrotoxicity [Review]. Kidney Int 1986;30:964.

146. McCauley J, Van Thiel DH, Starzl TE, Puschett JB. Acute and chronic renal failure in liver transplantation. Nephron 1990;55:121.

147. Fioretto P, Steffes MW, Mihatsch MJ, et al. Cyclosporine associated lesions in native kidneys of diabetic pancreas transplant recipients. Kidney Int 1995;48:489.

148. Messana JM, Johnson KJ, Mihatsch MJ. Renal structure and function effects after low dose cyclosporine in psoriasis patients: A preliminary report. Clin Nephrol 1995;43:150.

149. Zachariae H, Olsen TS. Efficacy of cyclosporin A in psoriasis: An overview of dose response, indications, contraindications and side-effects. Clin Nephrol 1995;43:154.

150. Ruiz P, Kolbeck PC, Scroggs MW, Sanfilippo F. Associations between cyclosporine therapy and interstitial fibrosis in renal allograft biopsies. Transplantation 1988;45:91.

151. Rao KV, Crosson JT, Kjellstrand CM. Chronic irreversible nephrotoxicity from cyclosporin A. Nephron 1985;41:75.

152. Mihatsch MJ, Steiner K, Abeywickrama KH, et al. Risk factors for the development of chronic cyclosporine nephrotoxicity. Clin Nephrol 1988;29:165.

153. Feutren G, Mihatsch MJ. Risk factors associated with cyclosporine A nephropathy in patients treated for autoimmune diseases. N Engl J Med 1992;326:654.

154. McMaster P, Mirza DF, Ismail T, et al. Therapeutic drug monitoring of tacrolimus in clinical transplantation. Ther Drug Monit 1995;17:602.

155. Fay JW, Wingard JR, Antin JH, et al. FK506 (Tacrolimus) monotherapy for prevention of graft-versus-host disease after histocompatible sibling allogenic bone marrow transplantation. Blood 1996;87:3514.

156. Gruessner RW, Burke GW, Stratta R, et al. A multicenter analysis of the first experience with FK506 for induction and rescue therapy after pancreas transplantation. Transplantation 1996;61:261.

157. Neuhaus P, Blumhardt G, Bechstein WO, et al. Comparison of FK506- and cyclosporine-based immunosuppression in primary orthotopic liver transplantation: A single center experience. Transplantation 1995;59:31.

158. Randhawa PS, Shapiro R, Jordan ML, et al. The histopathological changes associated with allograft rejection and drug toxicity in renal transplant recipients maintained on FK506. Am J Surg Pathol 1993;17:60.

159. Fung JJ, Todo S, Jain A, et al. Conversion from cyclosporine to FK506 in liver allograft recipients with cyclosporine-related complications. Transplant Proc 1990;22:6.

160. Radermacher J, Meiners M, Bramlage C, et al. Pronounced renal vasoconstriction and systemic hypertension in renal transplant patients treated with cyclosporin A versus FK506. Transplant Int 1998;11:3.

161. Ramos E, Drachenberg CB, Papadimitriou JC, et al. Clinical course of polyoma virus nephropathy in 67 renal transplant patients. J Am Soc Nephrol 2002;13:2145.

162. Itkin YM, Trujillo TC. Intravenous immunoglobulin-associated acute renal failure: Case series and literature review. Pharmacotherapy 2005;25:886.

163. Chapman SA, Gilkerson KL, Davin TD, Pritzker MR. Acute renal failure and intravenous immune globulin: Occurs with sucrose-stabilized, but not with D-sorbitol-stabilized, formulation. Ann Pharmacother 2004;38:2059.

164. Marti H-P, Frey FJ. Nephrotoxicity of rapamycin: An emerging problem in clinical medicine. Nephrol Dial Transplant 2005;20:13.

165. Kahan BD. Two-year results of multicenter phase III trials on the effect of the addition of sirolimus to cyclosporine-based immunosuppressive regimens in renal transplantation. Transplant Proc 2003;35(Suppl 3):37S.

166. Smith KD, Wrenshall LE, Nicosia RF, et al. Delayed graft function and cast nephropathy associated with tacrolimus plus rapamycin use. J Am Soc Nephrol 2003;14:1037.

167. McTaggart RA, Gottlieb D, Brooks J, et al. Sirolimus prolongs recovery from delayed graft function after cadaveric renal transplantation. Am J Transplant 2003;3:416.

168. Lawsin L, Light JA. Severe acute renal failure after exposure to sirolimus-tacrolimus in two living donor kidney recipients. Transplantation 2003;75:157.

169. Lo A, Egidi MF, Gaber LW, et al. Observations regarding the use of sirolimus and tacrolimus in high-risk cadaveric renal transplantation. Clin Transplant 2004;18:53.

170. Sartelet H, Toupance O, Lorenzato M, et al. Sirolimus-induced thrombotic microangiopathy is associated with decreased expression of vascular endothelial growth factor in kidneys. Am J Transplant 2005;5:2441.

171. Madias NE, Harrington JT. Platinum nephrotoxicity. Am J Med 1978;65:307.

172. Lippman AJ, Helson C, Helson L, Krakoff IH. Clinical trials with cis-diamminedichloro platinum. Cancer Chemother Rep 1975;57:191.

173. Ries F, Klastersky J. Nephrotoxicity induced by cancer chemotherapy with special emphasis on cisplatin toxicity. Am J Kidney Dis 1986;8:368.

174. Von Hoff DD, Schilsky R, Reichert CM, et al. Toxic effects of cis-dichlorodiamine-platinum (II) in man. Cancer Treat Rep 1979;63:1527.

175. Heyman SN, Lieberthal W, Rogiers P, Bonventre JV. Animal models of acute tubular necrosis. Curr Opin Crit Care 2002;8:526.

176. Ozols RF, Corden BJ, Jacob J, et al. High-dose cisplatin in hypertonic saline. Ann Intern Med 1984;100:19.

177. Hayes DM, Cvitkovic E, Golbey RB, et al. High dose cis-platinum diamine dichloride amelioration of renal toxicity by mannitol diuresis. Cancer 1977;39:1372.

178. Nagai N, Hotta K, Yamamura H, Ogata H. Effects of sodium thiosulfate on the pharmacokinetics of unchanged cisplatin and on the distribution of platinum species in rat kidney: Protective mechanism against cisplatin nephrotoxicity. Cancer Chemother Pharmacol 1995;36:404.

179. Schuchter LM, Hensley ML, Meropol NJ, Winer EP. 2002 update of recommendations for the use of chemotherapy and radiotherapy protectants. J Clin Oncol 2002;20:2895.

180. McDonald BR, Kirmani S, Vasquez M, Mehta RL. Acute renal failure associated with the use of intraperitoneal carboplatin: A report of two cases and review of the literature. Am J Med 1991;90:386.

181. Merouani A, Davidson SA, Schrier RW. Increased nephrotoxicity of combination taxol and cisplatin chemotherapy in gynecologic cancers as compared to cisplatin alone. Am J Nephrol 1997;17:53.

182. Moertel CG, Lefkopoulo M, Lipsitz S, et al. Streptozocin-doxorubicin, streptozocin-fluorouracil or chlorozotocin in the treatment of advanced islet-cell carcinoma. N Engl J Med 1992;326:519.

183. Weiss RB. Streptozocin: A review of its pharmacology, efficacy, and toxicity. Cancer Treat Rep 1982;66:427.

184. DeFronzo RA, Braine H, Colvin M, Davis PJ. Water intoxication in man after cyclophosphamide therapy. Ann Intern Med 1973;78:861.

185. Pratt CB, Meyer WH, Jenkins JJ, et al. Ifosamide, Fanconi's syndrome and rickets. J Clin Oncol 1991;9:1495.

186. Skinner R, Sharkey IM, Pearson AD, Craft AW. Ifosamide, mesna, and nephrotoxicity in children. J Clin Oncol 1993;11:173.

187. Elias AD, Eder JP, Shea T, et al. High-dose ifosamide with mesna uroprotection: A phase I study. J Clin Oncol 1990;8:170.

188. Berns JS, Haghighat A, Staddon A, et al. Severe irreversible renal failure after ifosamide treatment: A clinicopathologic report of two patients. Cancer 1995;76:497.

189. Hartmann JT, Knop S, Fels LM, et al. The use of reduced doses of amifostine to ameliorate nephrotoxicity of cisplatin/ifosamide-based chemotherapy in patients with solid tumors. Anticancer Drugs 2000;11:1.

190. Barrett BJ. Contrast nephrotoxicity. J Am Soc Nephrol 1994;5:125.

191. Rudnick MR, Berns JS, Cohen RM, Goldfarb S. Nephrotoxic risks of renal angiography: Contrast media–associated nephrotoxicity and atheroembolism. A critical review. Am J Kidney Dis 1994;24:713.

192. Rudnick MR, Goldfarb S, Wexler L, et al. Nephrotoxicity of ionic and nonionic contrast media in 1196 patients: A randomized study. Kidney Int 1995;47:254.

193. Meyrier A. Nephrotoxicity of iodine contrast media. Ann Radiol (Paris) 1994;37:286.

194. Briguori C, Tavano D, Colombo A. Contrast agent-associated nephrotoxicity. Prog Cardiovasc Dis 2003;45:493.

195. Porter GA. Experimental contrast-associated nephropathy and its clinical implications. Am J Cardiol 1990;66:18F.

196. Erley CM, Duda SH, Rehfuss D, et al. Prevention of radiocontrast-media-induced nephropathy in patients with pre-existing renal insufficiency by hydration in combination with the adenosine antagonist theophylline. Nephrol Dial Transplant 1999;14:1146.

197. Drager LF, Andrade L, Barros de Toledo JF, et al. Renal effects of N-acetyl cysteine in patients at risk for contrast nephropathy: Decrease in oxidant stress-mediated renal tubular injury. Nephrol Dial Transplant 2004;19:1803.

198. Moore RD, Steinberg EP, Powe NR, et al. Nephrotoxicity of high-osmolality versus low-osmolality contrast media. Radiology 1992;182:649.

199. Rihal CS, Textor SC, Grill DE, et al. Incidence and prognostic importance of acute renal failure after percutaneous coronary intervention. Circulation 2002;105:2259.

200. Itoh Y, Yano T, Sendo T, Oishi R. Clinical and experimental evidence for prevention of acute renal failure induced by radiographic contrast media. J Pharmacol Sci 2005;97:473.

201. McCarthy CS, Becker JA. Multiple myeloma and contrast media. Radiology 1992;183:519.

202. Parfrey PS, Griffiths SM, Barrett BJ, et al. Contrast material–induced renal failure in patients with diabetes mellitus, renal insufficiency, or both. N Engl J Med 1989;320:143.

203. Harris KG, Smith TP, Cragg AH, Lemke JH. Nephrotoxicity from contrast material in renal insufficiency: Ionic versus nonionic agents. Radiology 1991;179:849.

204. Manske CL, Sprafka JM, Strony JT, Wang Y. Contrast nephropathy in azotemic diabetic patients undergoing coronary angiography. Am J Med 1990;89:615.

205. Taliercio CP, Vlietstra RE, Ilstrup DM, et al. A randomized comparison of the nephrotoxicity of iopamidol and diatrizoate in high risk patients undergoing cardiac angiography. J Am Coll Cardiol 1991;17:384.

206. Cigarroa RG, Lange RA, Williams RH, Hillis LD. Dosing of contrast material to prevent contrast nephropathy in patients with renal disease. Am J Med 1989;86:649.

207. Lajoie G, Laszik Z, Nadasdy T, Silva FG. The renal-cardiac connection: Renal parenchymal alterations in patients with heart disease. Semin Nephrol 1994;14:441.

208. Dangas G, Iakovou I, Nikolsky E, et al. Contrast-induced nephropathy after percutaneous coronary interventions in relation to chronic kidney disease and hemodynamic variables. Am J Cardiol 2005;95:13.

209. McClennan BL. Low-osmolality contrast media: Premises and promises. Radiology 1987;162:1.

210. Spataro RF. Newer contrast agents for angiography. Radiol Clin North Am 1984;22:365.

211. Gitman MD, Singhal PC. Cocaine-induced renal disease. Expert Opin Drug Saf 2004;3:441.

212. Roth D, Alarcon FJ, Fernandez JA, et al. Acute rhabdomyolysis associated with cocaine intoxication. N Engl J Med 1988;319:673.

213. Singhal P, Horowitz B, Quinones MC, et al. Acute renal failure following cocaine abuse. Nephron 1989;52:76.

214. Zager RA. Rhabdomyolysis and myohemoglobinuric acute renal failure. Kidney Int 1996;49:314.

215. Frascino JA, Vanamee P, Rosen PQ. Renal oxalosis and azotemia after methoxyflurane anesthesia. N Engl J Med 1970;283:676.

216. Hollenberg NK, McDonald FD, Cotran R, et al. Irreversible acute oliguric renal failure: A complication of methoxyflurane anesthesia. N Engl J Med 1972;286:877.

217. Textor SC. Renal failure related to angiotensin-converting enzyme inhibitors. Semin Nephrol 1997;17:67.

218. Isnard-Bagnis C, Deray G, Baumelou A, et al. Herbs and the kidney. Am J Kidney Dis 2004;44:1.

219. De Smet PA. Herbal remedies. N Engl J Med 2002;347:2046.

220. Jha V, Chugh K. Nephropathy associated with animal, plant and chemical toxins in the tropics. Semin Nephrol 2003;23:49.

221. Depierreux M, Van Damme B, Vanden Houte K, Vanherweghem JL. Pathologic aspects of a newly described nephropathy related to the prolonged use of Chinese herbs. Am J Kidney Dis 1994;24:172.

222. Marcus D, Grollman A. Botanical medicines: The need for new regulations. N Engl J Med 2002;347:2073.

223. Kabanda A, Jadoul M, Lauwerys R, et al. Low molecular weight proteinuria in Chinese herbs nephropathy. Kidney Int 1995;48:1571.

224. Nortier JL, Deschodt-Lanckman MM, Simon S, et al. Proximal tubular injury in Chinese herbs nephropathy: Monitoring by neutral endopeptidase enzymuria. Kidney Int 1997;51:288.

225. Sir Hashim M, Hamza YO, Yahia B, et al. Poisoning from henna dye and para-phenylenediamine mixtures in children in Khartoum. Ann Trop Paediatr 1992;12:3.

226. Shemesh IY, Mishal Y, Baruchin AM, et al. Rhabdomyolysis in paraphenylenediamine intoxication. Vet Hum Toxicol 1995;31:244.

227. Riedemann NC, Guo RF, Ward PA. The enigma of sepsis. J Clin Invest 2003;112:460.

228. Rangel-Frausto MS, Pittet D, Costigan M, et al. The natural history of the systemic inflammatory response syndrome (SIRS): A prospective study. JAMA 1995;273:117.

229. Solez K, Racusen LC. Role of the renal biopsy in acute renal failure. Contrib Nephrol 2001;132:68.

230. Dalgaard O. An electron microscopic study on glomeruli in renal biopsies taken from human shock kidney. Lab Invest 1960;9:364.

231. Olsen S, Skjoldborg H. The fine structure of the renal glomerulus in acute anuria. Acta Pathol Microbiol Scand 1967;70:205.

232. Waugh D, Schlieter W, James A. Infraglomerular epithelial reflux: An early lesion of acute renal failure. Arch Pathol 1964;77:93.

233. Racusen LC. The morphologic basis of acute renal failure. In: Molitoris BA, Finn WF, eds. Acute Renal Failure: A Companion to Brenner and Rector's The Kidney, 1st ed. Philadelphia: WB Saunders, 2001:1.

234. Bohle A, Jahnecke J, Meyer D, Schubert GE. Morphology of acute renal failure: Comparative data from biopsy and autopsy. Kidney Int 1976;6:S9.

235. Racusen LC, Fivush BA, Li Y-L, et al. Dissociation of tubular cell detachment and tubular cell death in clinical and experimental "acute tubular necrosis." Lab Invest 1991;64:546.

236. Hoyer J, Seiler M. Pathophysiology of Tamm-Horsfall protein. Kidney Int 1979;16:279.

237. Vongwiwatana A, Tasanarong A, Rayner DC, et al. Epithelial to mesenchymal transition during late deterioration of human

kidney transplants: The role of tubular cells in fibrogenesis. Am J Transplant 2005;5:1367.

238. Nadasdy T, Laszik Z, Blick KE, et al. Human acute tubular necrosis: A lectin and immunohistochemical study. Hum Pathol 1995;26:230.

239. Castaneda MP, Swiatecka-Urban A, Mitsnefes MM, et al. Activation of mitochondrial apoptotic pathways in human renal allografts after ischemia reperfusion injury. Transplantation 2003;76:50.

240. Gobe GC, Endre ZH. Cell death in toxic nephropathies. Semin Nephrol 2003;23:416.

241. Ortiz A, Justo P, Sanz A, et al. Targeting apoptosis in acute tubular injury. Biochem Pharmacol 2003;66:1589.

242. Solez K, Racusen LC, Marcussen N, et al. Morphology of ischemic acute renal failure, normal function, and cyclosporine toxicity in cyclosporine-treated renal allograft recipients. Kidney Int 1993;43:1058.

243. Alejandro VS, Nelson WJ, Huie P, et al. Postischemic injury, delayed function and Na$^+$/K$(+)$-ATPase distribution in the transplanted kidney. Kidney Int 1995;48:1308.

244. Jones D. Ultrastructure of human acute renal failure. Lab Invest 1982;46:254.

245. Olsen S. Ultrastructure of the renal tubules in acute renal insufficiency. Acta Pathol Microbiol Scand 1967;71:203.

246. Olsen T, Hansen H. Ultrastructure of medullary tubules in ischemic acute tubular necrosis and acute interstitial nephritis in man. APMIS 1990;98:1139.

247. Olsen T, Hansen H, Olsen H. Tubular ultrastructure in acute renal failure: Alterations of cellular surfaces (brush-border and basolateral infoldings). Virchows Arch 1985;406:91.

248. Olsen T, Olsen H, Hansen H. Tubular ultrastructure in acute renal failure in man: Epithelial necrosis and regeneration. Virchows Arch 1985;406:75.

249. Solez K, Morel-Maroger L, Sraer J. The morphology of "acute tubular necrosis" in man: Analysis of 57 renal biopsies and a comparison with the glycerol model. Medicine (Baltimore) 1979;58:362.

250. Baker SBD. Intravascular haemopoiesis in the renal medulla in shock. J Pathol Bacteriol 1958;75:421.

251. Solez K, Kramer E, Fox J, Heptinstall R. Medullary plasma flow and intravascular leukocyte accumulation in acute renal failure. Kidney Int 1974;6:24.

252. Cantu TG, Hoehn-Saric EW, Burgess KM, et al. Acute renal failure associated with immunoglobulin therapy. Am J Kidney Dis 1995;25:228.

253. Viol GW, Minielly JA, Bistricki T. Gold nephropathy. Arch Pathol Lab Med 1977;101:635.

254. Genkins G, Bryer MS. Bacitracin nephropathy: Report of a case of acute renal failure and death. JAMA 1954;155:894.

255. Abuelo J. Renal failure caused by chemicals, foods, plants, animal venoms, and misuse of drugs. An overview. Arch Int Med 1990;150:505.

256. Corcoran GB, Fix L, Jones DP, et al. Apoptosis: Molecular control point in toxicity. Toxicol Appl Pharmacol 1994;128:169.

257. Nagothu KK, Bhatt R, Kaushal GP, Portilla D. Fibrate prevents cisplatin-induced proximal tubule cell death. Kidney Int 2005;68:2680.

258. Bonegio R, Lieberthal W. Role of apoptosis in the pathogenesis of acute renal failure. Curr Opin Nephrol Hypertens 2002;11:301.

259. Duncan-Achanzar KB, Jones JT, Burke MF, et al. Inorganic mercury chloride-induced apoptosis in the cultured porcine renal cell line LLC-PK1. J Pharmacol Exp Ther 1996;277:1726.

260. Kaushal GP, Kaushal V, Hong X, Shah SV. Role and regulation of activation of caspases in cisplatin-induced injury to renal tubular epithelial cells. Kidney Int 2001;60:1726.

261. Ortiz A, Justo P, Sanz A, et al. Tubular cell apoptosis and cidofovir-induced acute renal failure. Antivir Ther 2005;10:185.

262. Weisman JI, Bloom B. Anuria following phenylbutazone therapy. N Engl J Med 1955;252:1086.

263. Heptinstall RH. Renal complications of therapeutic and diagnostic agents, analgesic abuse, and addiction to narcotics. In: Hep-

tinstall RH, ed. Pathology of the Kidney, 3rd ed. Boston: Little Brown, 1983:1149.

264. Brigden D, Rosling AE, Woods NC. Renal function after acyclovir intravenous injection. Am J Med 1982;73:182.

265. Lacy CH. Gancyclovir: Drug information. UpToDate 2000;8:1.

266. Tucker WE. Preclinical toxicology profile of acyclovir: An overview. Am J Med 1982;73:27.

267. Pisoni R, Ruggenenti P, Remuzzi G. Drug-induced thrombotic microangiopathy: Incidence, prevention, and management. Drug Saf 2001;24:491.

268. Bennett WM, Gilbert DN, Houghton D, Porter GA. Gentamicin nephrotoxicity: Morphologic and pharmacologic features. West J Med 1977;126:65.

269. Wilfert JN, Burke JP, Bloomer HA, Smith CB. Renal insufficiency associated with gentamicin therapy. J Infect Dis 1971;124(suppl):S148.

270. Kourilsky O, Solez K, Morel-Maroger L, et al. The pathology of acute renal failure due to interstitial nephritis in man with comments on the role of interstitial inflammation and sex in gentamicin nephrotoxicity. Medicine (Baltimore) 1982;61:258.

271. Houghton DC, Campbell-Boswell MV, Bennett WM, et al. Myeloid bodies in the renal tubules of humans: Relationship to gentamicin therapy. Clin Nephrol 1978;10:140.

272. Cuppage FE, Setter K, Sullivan P, et al. Gentamicin nephrotoxicity. II. Physiological, biochemical and morphological effects of prolonged administration to rats. Virchows Arch B Cell Pathol 1977;24:121.

273. Zager RA. Gentamicin nephrotoxicity in the setting of acute renal hypoperfusion. Am J Physiol 1988;254:F574.

274. Berman LB, Katz S. Kanamycin nephrotoxicity. Ann N Y Acad Sci 1958;76:149.

275. Einspruch BC, Gonzalez VV. Clinical and experimental nephropathy resulting from use of neomycin sulfate. JAMA 1960;173:809.

276. Harrison WO, Silverblatt FJ, Turck M. Gentamicin nephrotoxicity: Failure of three cephalosporins to potentiate injury in rats. Antimicrob Agents Chemother 1975;8:209.

277. Westlake PT, Burlter WT, Hill GJ, Utz JP. Nephrotoxic tubular damage and calcium deposition following amphotericin B therapy. Am J Pathol 1963;43:449.

278. Bullock WE, Luke RG, Nuttall CE, Bhathena D. Can mannitol reduce amphotericin B nephrotoxicity? Double-blind study and description of a new vascular lesion in kidneys. Antimicrob Agents Chemother 1976;10:555.

279. Perkins RL, Apicella MA, Lee IS, et al. Cephaloridine and cephalothin: Comparative studies of potential nephrotoxicity. J Lab Clin Med 1968;71:75.

280. Manley HJ, Bailie GR, Eisele G. Bilateral renal cortical necrosis associated with cefuroxime axetil. Clin Nephrol 1998;49:268.

281. Beirne GJ, Hansing CE, Octaviano GN, Burns RO. Acute renal failure caused by hypersensitivity to polymyxin B sulfate. JAMA 1967;202:156.

282. Davies DR, Bittmann I, Pardo J. Histopathology of calcineurin inhibitor-induced nephrotoxicity. Transplantation 2000;69 (Suppl 12):SS11.

283. Foxwell BMJ, Ryffel B. The mechanisms of action of cyclosporine. Cardiol Clin 1990;8:107.

284. Hudkins KL, Le QC, Segerer S, et al. Osteopontin expression in human cyclosporine toxicity. Kidney Int 2001;60:635.

285. Andoh TF, Bennett WM. Chronic cyclosporine nephrotoxicity. Curr Opin Nephrol Hypertens 1998;7:265.

286. Ader JL, Rostaing L. Cyclosporin nephrotoxicity: Pathophysiology and comparison with FK506. Curr Opin Nephrol Hypertens 1998;7:539.

287. Bertani T, Ferrazzi P, Schieppati A, et al. Nature and extent of glomerular injury induced by cyclosporine A in heart transplant patients. Kidney Int 1991;40:243.

288. Myers BD, Newton L, Boshkos C, et al. Chronic injury of human renal microvessels with low-dose cyclosporine therapy. Transplantation 1988;46:694.

289. Remuzzi G, Perico N. Cyclosporine-induced renal dysfunction in experimental animals and humans. Kidney Int 1995;52(Suppl):S70.

290. Randhawa PS, Shapiro R, Jordan ML, et al. The histopathological changes associated with allograft rejection and drug toxicity in renal transplant recipients maintained on FK506. Clinical significance and comparison with cyclosporine. Am J Surg Pathol 1993;17:60.

291. Morozumi K, Sugito K, Oda A, et al. A comparative study of morphological characteristics of renal injuries of tacrolimus (FK506) and cyclosporin (CyA) in renal allografts. Transplant Proc 1996;28:1076.

292. Randhawa PS, Tsamandas AC, Magnone M, et al. Microvascular changes in renal allografts associated with FK506 (Tacrolimus) therapy. Am J Surg Pathol 1996;20:306.

293. Demetris AJ, Fung JJ, Todo S, et al. Pathologic observations in human allograft recipients treated with FK506. Transplant Proc 1990;22:25.

294. Nalesnik MA, Lai HS, Murase N, et al. The effect of FK506 and CyA on the Lewis rat renal ischemia model. Transplant Proc 1990;22:87.

295. Stephen M, Woo J, Hasan NU, Whiting PH, Thomson AW. Immunosuppressive activity, lymphocyte subset analysis, and acute toxicity of FK506 in the rat. Transplantation 1989;47:60.

296. Todo S, Ueda Y, Demetris JA, et al. Immunosuppression of canine, monkey, and baboon allografts by FK506: With special reference to synergism with other drugs and to tolerance induction. Surgery 1988;104:239.

297. Stillman IE, Andoh TF, Burdmann EA, et al. FK506 nephrotoxicity: Morphologic and physiologic characterization of a rat model. Lab Invest 1995;73:794.

298. Haas M, Sonnenday CJ, Cicone JS, et al. Isometric tubular epithelial vacuolization in renal allograft biopsy specimens of patients receiving low-dose intravenous immunoglobulin for a positive crossmatch. Transplantation 2004;78:549.

299. Andoh TF, Burdmann EA, Fransechini N, et al. Comparison of acute rapamycin nephrotoxicity with cyclosporine and FK506. Kidney Int 1996;50:1110.

300. Dentino M, Luft FC, Yum MN, et al. Long-term effect of cis-diamminedichloride platinum (CDDP) on renal function and structure in man. Cancer 1978;41:1274.

301. Gonzalez-Vitale JC, Hayes DM, Cvitkovic E, Sternberg SS. The renal pathology in clinical trials of cis-platinum. II. Diamminedichloride. Cancer 1977;39:1362.

302. Dobyan DC, Levi J, Jacobs C, et al. Mechanisms of cis-platinum nephrotoxicity. II. Morphologic observations. J Pharmacol Exp Ther 1980;213:551.

303. Dobyan DC, Hill D, Lewis T, Bulger RE. Cyst formation in rat kidney induced by cis-platinum administration. Lab Invest 1981;45:260.

304. Rossi R, Helmchen U, Schellong G. Tubular function and histologic findings in ifosfamide-induced renal Fanconi syndrome: A report of two cases. Eur J Pediatr 1992;151:384.

305. Deray G, Martinez F, Cacoub P, et al. A role for adenosine, calcium and ischemia in radiocontrast-induced intrarenal vasoconstriction. Am J Nephrol 1990;10:316.

306. Heyman SN, Brezis M, Reubinoff CA, et al. Acute renal failure with selective medullary injury in the rat. J Clin Invest 1988;82:401.

307. Thomsen HS, Golman K, Larsen S, et al. Urine profiles and kidney histology following intravenous diatrizoate and iohexol in the degeneration phase of gentamicin nephropathy in rats. Invest Radiol 1991;26:951.

308. Thomsen HS, Larsen S, Hemmingsen L, et al. Nephropathy induced by intramuscularly administered glycerol and contrast media in rats: A comparison between diatrizoate, iohexol and ioxilan. Acta Radiol 1989;30:217.

309. Yoshioka T, Fogo A, Beckman JK. Reduced activity of antioxidant enzymes underlies contrast media–induced renal injury in volume depletion. Kidney Int 1992;41:1008.

310. Moreau J-F, Droz D, Sabto J, et al. Osmotic nephrosis induced by water-soluble triiodinated contrast media in man: A retrospective study of 47 cases. Radiology 1975;115:329.

311. Tervahartiala P, Kivisaari L, Kivisaari R, et al. Contrast media–induced renal tubular vacuolization: A light and electron microscopic study on rat kidneys. Invest Radiol 1991;26:882.

312. Hofmeister R, Bhargava AS, Günzel P. The use of urinary N-acetyl-b-D-glucosaminidase (NAG) for the detection of contrast-media-induced "osmotic nephrosis" in rats. Toxicol Lett 1990;50:9.

313. Moreau JF, Droz D, Noel LH, et al. Tubular nephrotoxicity of water-soluble iodinated contrast media. Invest Radiol 1980;15:S54.

314. Gilbert EF, Khoury GH, Hogan GR, Jones B. Hemorrhagic renal necrosis in infancy: Relationship to radiopaque compounds. J Pediatr 1970;76:49.

315. Gruskin AB, Oetliker OH, Wolfish NM, et al. Effects of angiography on renal function and histology in infants and piglets. J Pediatr 1970;76:41.

316. Whalley DW, Ibels LS, Eckstein RP, et al. Acute tubular necrosis complicating bilateral retrograde pyelography. Aust N Z J Med 1987;17:536.

317. Herrera GA. Myoglobin and the kidney: An overview. Ultrastruct Pathol 1994;18:113.

318. Turbat-Herrera EA. Myoglobinuric acute renal failure associated with cocaine use. Ultrastruct Pathol 1994;18:127.

319. Cosyns JP, Jadoul M, Squifflet JP, et al. Chinese herbs nephropathy: A clue to Balkan endemic nephropathy? Kidney Int 1994;45:1680.

320. Myers B, Moran S. Hemodynamically mediated acute renal failure. N Engl J Med 1986;314:97.

321. Gornick C, Kjellstrand C. Acute renal failure complicating aortic aneurysm surgery. Nephron 1983;35:145.

322. Andreoli SP. Acute renal failure in the newborn. Semin Perinatol 2004;28:112.

323. Clarkson P, Cameron J. Disturbances of renal function in burned patients. Proc R Soc Med 1969;62:49.

324. Lordon R, Burton J. Post-traumatic renal failure in military personnel in Southeast Asia. Am J Med 1972;53:137.

325. Hayslett J. Postpartum renal failure. N Engl J Med 1985;312:1556.

326. Lindheimer M, Katz A, Ganeval D, Grunfeld J. Acute Renal Failure. New York: Churchill Livingstone, 1993.

327. Maher ER, Robinson KN, Scoble JE, et al. Prognosis of critically-ill patients with acute renal failure: APACHE II score and other predictive factors. Q J Med 1989;72:857.

328. Hou SH, Bushinsky DA, Wish J, et al. Hospital acquired renal insufficiency: A prospective study. Am J Med 1983;74:243.

329. Kleinknecht C, Broyer M, Gubler M, Palcoux J. Irreversible renal failure after indomethacin in steroid resistant nephrosis. N Engl J Med 1980;302:691.

330. Hanif M, Mobarak M, Ronan A, et al. Fatal renal failure caused by diethylene glycol in paracetamol elixir: The Bangladesh experience. Br Med J 1995;311:88.

331. McKenzie K. Epidemic of acute renal failure in Haiti. Br Med J 1996;313:70.

332. Schrier RW, Wang W. Acute renal failure and sepsis. New Engl J Med 2004;351:159.

333. Riedemann NC, Guo RF, Ward PA. The enigma of sepsis. J Clin Invest 2003;112:460.

334. Rangel-Frausto MS, Pittet D, Costigan M, et al. The natural history of the systemic inflammatory response syndrome (SIRS): A prospective study. JAMA 1995;273:117.

335. Bonventre JV. Pathophysiology of ischemic acute renal failure. Inflammation, lung-kidney cross-talk, and biomarkers. Contrib Nephrol 2004;144:19.

336. Hoste EA, Kellum JA. Acute renal failure in the critically ill: Impact on morbidity and mortality. Contrib Nephrol 2004;144:1.

337. Lieberthal W, Nigam SK. Acute renal failure II. Experimental models of acute renal failure: Imperfect but indispensable. Am J Physiol Renal Physiol 2000;278:F1.

338. Rosen S, Heyman SN. Difficulties in understanding human "acute tubular necrosis." Limited data and flawed animal models. Kidney Int 2001;60:1220.

339. Kelly KJ, Molitoris BA. Acute renal failure in the new millennium: Time to consider combination therapy. Semin Nephrol 2000;20:4.

340. Star RA. Treatment of acute renal failure. Kidney Int 1998;54:1817.

341. Zhou H, Miyaji T, Kato A, et al. Attenuation of cisplatin-induced acute renal failure is associated with less apoptotic cell death. J Lab Clin Med 1999;134:649.

342. Hauger O, Delalande C, Deminiere C, et al. Nephrotoxic nephritis and obstructive nephropathy: Evaluation with MR imaging enhanced with ultrasmall superparamagnetic iron oxide-preliminary findings in a rat model. Radiology 2000;217:819.

343. Kashgarian M, Morrow JS, Foellmer HG, et al. Na,K-ATPase co-distributes with ankyrin and spectrin in renal tubular epithelial cells. Prog Clin Biol Res 1988;268B:245.

344. Morrow JS, Cianci CD, Ardito T, et al. Ankyrin links fodrin to the alpha subunit of Na,K-ATPase in Madin-Darby canine kidney cells and in intact renal tubule cells. J Cell Biol 1989;108:455.

345. Rodriguez-Boulan E, Nelson WJ. Morphogenesis of the polarized epithelial cell phenotype [Review]. Science 1989;245:718.

346. Hinck L, Nathke IS, Papkoff J, Nelson WJ. Dynamics of cadherin/catenin complex formation: Novel protein interactions and pathways of complex assembly. J Cell Biol 1994;125:1327.

347. Nelson WJ, Shore EM, Wang AZ, Hammerton RW. Identification of a membrane-cytoskeletal complex containing the cell adhesion molecule uvomorulin (E-cadherin), ankyrin, and fodrin in Madin-Darby canine kidney epithelial cells. J Cell Biol 1990;110:349.

348. Canfield PE, Geerdes AM, Molitoris BA. Effect of reversible ATP depletion on tight-junction integrity in LLC-PK1 cells. Am J Physiol,. 1991;261:F1038.

349. Molitoris BA, Dahl R, Geerdes A. Cytoskeleton disruption and apical redistribution of proximal tubule Na(+)-K(+)-ATPase during ischemia. Am J Physiol 1992;263:F488.

350. Molitoris BA, Falk SA, Dahl RH. Ischemia-induced loss of epithelial polarity: Role of the tight junction. J Clin Invest 1989;84:1334.

351. Molitoris BA, Wilson PD, Schrier RW, Simon FR. Ischemia induces partial loss of surface membrane polarity and accumulation of putative calcium ionophores. J Clin Invest 1985;76:2097.

352. Spiegel DM, Wilson PD, Molitoris BA. Epithelial polarity following ischemia: A requirement for normal cell function. Am J Physiol 1989;256:F430.

353. Alejandro VS, Nelson WJ, Huie P, et al. Post-ischemic injury, delayed function and Na/K-ATPase distribution in the transplanted kidney. Kidney Int 1995;48:1308.

354. Van Why SK, Mann AS, Ardito T, et al. Expression and molecular regulation of Na(+)-K(+)-ATPase after renal ischemia. Am J Physiol 1994;267:F75.

355. Van Why SK, Hildebrandt F, Ardito T, et al. Induction and intracellular localization of HSP-72 after renal ischemia. Am J Physiol 1992;263:F769.

356. Harris AS, Croall DE, Morrow JS. Calmodulin regulates fodrin susceptibility to cleavage by calcium-dependent protease I. J Biol Chem 1989;264:17401.

357. Chen Z, Naito M, Mashima T, Tsuruo T. Activation of actin-cleavable interleukin 1beta-converting enzyme (ICE) family protease CPP-32 during chemotherapeutic agent–induced apoptosis in ovarian carcinoma cells. Cancer Res 1996;56:5224.

358. Cryns VL, Bergeron L, Zhu H, et al. Specific cleavage of alpha-fodrin during Fas- and tumor necrosis factor—induced apoptosis is mediated by an interleukin-1beta-converting enzyme/Ced-3 protease distinct from the poly(ADP-ribose) polymerase protease. J Biol Chem 1996;271:31277.

359. Stanger BZ. Looking beneath the surface: The cell death pathway of Fas/APO-1 (CD95). Mol Med 1996;2:7.

360. Doctor RB, Bennett V, Mandel LJ. Degradation of spectrin and ankyrin in the ischemic rat kidney. Am J Physiol 1993;264:C1003.

361. Molitoris BA, Geerdes A, McIntosh JR. Dissociation and redistribution of Na (+)-K(+)-ATPase from its surface membrane actin cytoskeletal complex during cellular ATP depletion. J Clin Invest 1991;88:462.

362. Gailit J, Colflesh D, Rabiner I, et al. Redistribution and dysfunction of integrins in cultured renal epithelial cells exposed to oxidative stress. Am J Physiol 1993;264:F149.

363. Lieberthal W, McKenney JB, Kiefer CR, et al. Beta integrin-mediated adhesion between renal tubular cells after anoxic injury. J Am Soc Nephrol 1997;8:175.

364. Kroshian VM, Sheridan AM, Lieberthal W. Functional and cytoskeletal changes induced by sublethal injury in proximal tubular epithelial cells. Am J Physiol 1994;266:F21.

365. Nigam S, Weston CE, Liu CH, Simon EE. The actin cytoskeleton and integrin expression in the recovery of cell adhesion after oxidant stress to a proximal tubule cell line (JRC-12). J Am Soc Nephrol 1998;9:1787.

366. Wijesekera DS, Zarama MJ, Paller MS. Effects of integrins on proliferation and apoptosis of renal epithelial cells after acute injury. Kidney Int 1997;52:1511.

367. Goligorsky MS, DiBona GF. Pathogenetic role of Arg-Gly-Asp-recognizing integrins in acute renal failure. Proc Natl Acad Sci USA 1993;90:5700.

368. Goligorsky MS, Lieberthal W, Racusen L, Simon EE. Integrin receptors in renal tubular epithelium: New insights into pathophysiology of acute renal failure. Am J Physiol 1993;264:F1.

369. Noiri E, Gailit J, Sheth D, et al. Cyclic RGD peptides ameliorate ischemic acute renal failure in rats. Kidney Int 1994;46:1050.

370. Myers BD, Chui F, Hilberman M, Michaels A. Transtubular leakage of glomerular filtrate in human acute renal failure. Am Physiol 1979;237:F319.

371. Mason J, Joeris B, Welsch J, Kriz W. Vascular congestion in ischemic renal failure: The role of cell swelling. Miner Electrolyte Metab 1989;15:114.

372. Noiri E, Nakao A, Uchida K, et al. Oxidative and nitrosative stress in acute renal ischemia. Am J Physiol Renal Physiol 2001;281:F948.

373. Goligorsky MS, Brodsky SV, Noiri E. NO bioavailability, endothelial dysfunction, and acute renal failure: New insights into pathophysiology. Semin Nephrol 2004;24:316.

374. Atanasova I, Burke TJ, McMurtry IF, Schrier RW. Nitric oxide synthase inhibition and acute renal ischemia: Effect on systemic hemodynamics and mortality. Ren Fail 1995;17:389.

375. Yu L, Gengaro P, Niederberger M, et al. Nitric oxide: A mediator in rat tubular hypoxia/reoxygenation injury. Proc Natl Acad Sci 1994;91:1691.

376. Peresleni T, Noiri E, Bahou WF, Goligorsky M. Antisense oligodeoxynucleotides to inducible NO synthase rescue epithelial cells from oxidative stress injury. Am J Physiol 1996;270:F971.

377. Ling H, Gengaro PE, Edelstein CL, et al. Effect of hypoxia on proximal tubules isolated from nitric oxide synthase knockout mice. Kidney Int 1998;53:1642.

378. Noiri E, Peresleni T, Miller F, Goligorsky M. In vivo targeting of inducible NO synthase with oligodeoxynucleotides protects rat kidney against ischemia. J Clin Invest 1996;97:2377.

379. Xia Y, Dawson VL, Dawson TM, et al. Nitric oxide synthase generates superoxide and nitric oxide in arginine-depleted cells leading to peroxynitrite-mediated cellular injury. Proc Natl Acad Sci USA 1996;93:6770.

380. Wangsiripaisan A, Gengaro PE, Nemenoff RA, et al. Effect of nitric oxide donors on renal tubular epithelial cell-matrix adhesion. Kidney Int 1999;55:2281.

381. Chiao H, Kohda Y, McLeroy P, et al. Alpha-melanocyte stimulating hormone protects against renal injury after ischemia in mice and rats. J Clin Invest 1997;99:1165.

382. Kaushal GP, Basnakian AB, Shah SV. Apoptotic pathways in ischemic acute renal failure. Kidney Int 2004;66:500.

383. Edelstein CL, Wieder ED, Yaqoob MM, et al. The role of cysteine proteases in hypoxic-induced rat renal proximal tubular injury. Proc Natl. Acad Sci USA 1995;92:7662.

384. Shi Y, Melnikov VY, Schrier RW, Edelstein CL. Downregulation of the calpain inhibitor protein calpastatin by caspases during renal ischemia-reperfusion. Am J Physiol Renal Physiol 2000;279:F509.

385. Edelstein CL, Ling H, Gengaro PE, et al. Effect of glycine on prelethal and postlethal increases in calpain activity in rat renal proximal tubules. Kidney Int 1997;52:1271.

386. Choi KH, Edelstein CL, Gengaro P, et al. Hypoxia induces changes in phospholipase A2 in rat proximal tubules: Evidence for multiple forms. Am J Physiol 1995;269:F846.

387. Dagher PC. Apoptosis in ischemic renal injury: Roles of GTP depletion and p53. Kidney Int 2004;66:506.

388. Kelly KJ, Plotkin Z, Dagher PC. Guanosine supplementation reduces apoptosis and protects renal function in the setting of ischemic injury. J Clin Invest 2001;108:1291.

389. Devalaraja-Narashimha K, Singaravelu K, Padanilam BJ. Poly (ADP-ribose) polymerase-mediated cell injury in acute renal failure. Pharmacol Res 2005;52:44.

390. Zheng J, Devalaraja-Narashimha K, Singaravelu K, Padanilam BJ. Poly (ADP-ribose) polymerase-1 gene ablation protects mice from ischemic renal injury. Am J Physiol Renal Physiol 2005; 288:F387.

391. Park KM, Chen A, Bonventre JV. Prevention of kidney ischemia/reperfusion-induced functional injury and JNK, p38, and MAPK kinase activation by remote ischemic pretreatment. J Biol Chem 2001;276:11870.

392. Arany I, Megyesi JK, Kaneto H, et al. Activation of ERK or inhibition of JNK ameliorates $H_2O_2$ cytotoxicity in mouse renal proximal tubule cells. Kidney Int 2004;65:1231.

393. Arany I, Megyesi JK, Reusch JE, Safirstein RL. CREB mediates ERK-induced survival of mouse renal tubular cells after oxidant stress. Kidney Int 2005;68:1573.

394. Schober A, Muller E, Thurau K, Beck FX. The response of heat shock protein 25 and 72 to ischaemia in different kidney zones. Pflugers Arch 1997;434:292.

395. Park KM, Chen A, Bonventre JV. Prevention of kidney ischemia/reperfusion induced functional injury and JNK, p38, and MAP kinase activation by remote ischemic pretreatment. J Biol Chem 2001;276:11870.

396. Emami A, Schwartz JH, Borkan SC. Transient ischemia or heat stress induces a cytoprotectant protein in rat kidney. Am J Physiol 1991;260:F479.

397. Goering PL, Fisher BR, Chaudhary PP, Dick CA. Relationship between stress protein induction in rat kidney by mercuric chloride and nephrotoxicity. Toxicol Appl Pharmacol 1992;113:184.

398. Goering PL, Kish CL, Fisher BR. Stress protein synthesis induced by cadmium-cysteine in rat kidney. Toxicology 1993;85:25.

399. Lovis C, Mach F, Donati YR, et al. Heat shock proteins and the kidney [Review]. Ren Fail 1994;16:179.

400. Dodd SM, Martin JE, Swash M, Mather K. Expression of heat shock protein epitopes in renal disease. Clin Nephrol 1993;39:239.

401. Wang YH, Knowlton AA, Li FH, Borkan SC. Hsp 72 expression enhances survival in adenosine triphosphate-depleted renal epithelial cells. Cell Stress Chaperones 2002;7:137.

402. Yang CW, Kim BS, Kim J, et al. Preconditioning with sodium arsenite inhibits apoptotic cell death in rat kidney with ischemia/reperfusion or cyclosporine-induced injuries: The possible role of heat shock protein 70 as a mediator of ischemic tolerance. Exp Nephrol 2001;9:284.

403. van de Water B, Imamdi R, de Graauw M. Signal transduction in renal repair and regeneration. In: Torloff JB, Lash LH, eds. Toxicology of the Kidney, 3rd ed. New York: CRC Press, 2005: 299.

404. Percy C, Waters MJ, Gobe G. Caveolins in the repair phase of acute renal failure after oxidative stress. Nephrology 2004;9: 374.

405. Zager RA, Johnson A, Hanson S, dela Rosa V. Altered cholesterol localization and caveolin expression during the evolution of acute renal failure. Kidney Int 2002;61:1674.

406. Mahmoudi M, Willgoss D, Cuttle L, et al. In vivo and in vitro models demonstrate a role for caveolin-1 in the pathogenesis of ischaemic acute renal failure. J Pathol 2003;200:396.

407. Kieran NE, Maderna P, Godson C. Lipoxins: Potential anti-inflammatory, proresolution, and antifibrotic mediators in renal disease. Kidney Int 2004;65:1145.

408. Han WK, Bailly V, Abichandani R, et al. Kidney Injury molecule-1 (KIM-1): A novel biomarker for human renal proximal tubule injury. Kidney Int 2002;62:237.

409. Ichimura T, Bonventre JV, Bailly V, et al. Kidney injury molecule-1 (KIM-1), a putative epithelial cell adhesion molecule containing a novel immunoglobulin domain, is up-regulated in renal cells after injury. J Biol Chem 1998;273:4135.

410. Bailly V, Zhang Z, Meier W, et al. Shedding of kidney injury molecule-1, a putative adhesion protein involved in renal regeneration. J Biol Chem 2002;277:39739.

411. Humes HD, Beals TF, Cieslinski DA, et al. Effects of transforming growth factor-beta, transforming growth factor-alpha, and other growth factors on renal proximal tubule cells. Lab Invest 1991;64:538.

412. Humes HD, Cieslinski DA, Coimbra TM, et al. Epidermal growth factor enhances renal tubule cell regeneration and repair and accelerates the recovery of renal function in postischemic acute renal failure. J Clin Invest 1989;84:1757.

413. Kawaida K, Matsumoto K, Shimazu H, Nakamura T. Hepatocyte growth factor prevents acute renal failure and accelerates renal regeneration in mice. Proc Natl Acad Sci U S A 1994;91: 4357.

414. Martin AA, Gillespie CM, Moore L, et al. Effects of insulin-like growth factor-I peptides in rats with acute renal failure. J Endocrinol 1994;140:23.

415. Coimbra TM, Cieslinski DA, Humes HD. Epidermal growth factor accelerates renal repair in mercuric chloride nephrotoxicity. Am J Physiol 1990;259:F438.

416. Safirstein R. Gene expression in nephrotoxic and ischemic acute renal failure [Editorial]. J Am Soc Nephrol 1994;4:1387.

417. Schaudies RP, Nonclercq D, Nelson L, et al. Endogenous EGF as a potential renotrophic factor in ischemia-induced acute renal failure. Am J Physiol 1993;265:F425.

418. Humes HD, Cieslinski DA, Johnson LB, Sanchez IO. Triiodothyronine enhances renal tubule cell replication by stimulating EGF receptor gene expression. Am J Physiol 1992;262:F540.

419. Ding H, Kopple JD, Cohen A, Hirschberg R. Recombinant human insulin-like growth factor-I accelerates recovery and reduces catabolism in rats with ischemic acute renal failure. J Clin Invest 1993;91:2281.

420. Miller SB, Martin DR, Kissane J, Hammerman MR. Rat models for clinical use of insulin-like growth factor I in acute renal failure. Am J Physiol 1994;266:F949.

421. Noguchi S, Kashihara Y, Ikegami Y, et al. Insulin-like growth factor-1 ameliorates transient ischemia-induced acute renal failure in rats. J Pharmacol Exp Ther 1993;267:919.

422. Goes N, Urmson J, Ramassar V, Halloran PF. Ischemic acute tubular necrosis induces an extensive local cytokine response: Evidence for induction of interferon-gamma, transforming growth factor-beta 1, granulocyte-macrophage colony-stimulating factor, interleukin-2, and interleukin-10. Transplantation 1995;59:565.

423. Verstrepen WA, Nouwen EJ, De Broe ME. Renal epidermal growth factor and insulin-like growth factor I in acute renal failure. Nephrol Dial Transplant 1994;9:57.

424. Price PM, Megyesi J, Safirstein RL. Cell cycle regulation: Repair and regeneration in acute renal failure. Kidney Int 2004;23:499.

425. Duffield JS, Park KM, Hsiao LL, et al. Restoration of tubular epithelial cells during repair of the postischemic kidney occurs independently of bone marrow-derived stem cells. J Clin Invest 2005;115:1743.

426. Gupta S, Verfaillie C, Chmielewski D, et al. A role for extrarenal cells in the regeneration following acute renal failure. Kidney Int 2002;62:1285.

427. Herrera MB, Bussolati B, Bruno S, et al. Mesenchymal stem cells contribute to the renal repair of acute tubular epithelial injury. Int J Mol Med 2004;14:1035.

428. Morigi M, Imberti B, Zoja C, et al. Mesenchymal stem cells are renotropic, helping to repair the kidney and improve function in acute renal failure. J Am Soc Nephrol 2004;15:1794.

429. de Groot K, Bahlmann CH, Bahlmann E, et al. Kidney graft function determines endothelial progenitor cell number in renal transplant recipients. Transplantation 2005;79:941.

430. Kale S, Karihaloo A, Clark PR, et al. Bone marrow stem cells contribute to repair of the ischemically injured renal tubule. J Clin Invest 2003;112:42.

431. Stokman G, Leemans JC, Claessen N, et al. Hematopoietic stem cell mobilization therapy accelerates recovery of renal function independent of stem cell contribution. J Am Soc Nephrol 2005;16:1684.

432. Lin F, Cordes K, Li L, et al. Hematopoietic stem cells contribute to the regeneration of renal tubules after ischemia-reperfusion injury in mice. J Am Soc Nephrol 2003;14:1188.

433. Iwasaki M, Adachi Y, Minamino K, et al. Mobilization of bone marrow cells by G-CSF rescues mice from cisplatin-induced renal failure and M-CSF enhances the effects of G-CSF. J Am Soc Nephrol 2005;16:658.

434. Bonventre JV, Zuk A. Ischemic acute renal failure: An inflammatory disease? Kidney Int 2004;66:480.

435. Friedewald JJ, Rabb H. Inflammatory cells in ischemic acute renal failure. Kidney Int 2004;66:486.

436. Ysebaert DK, DeGreef KE, DeBeuf A, et al. T cells as mediators in renal ischemia/reperfusion injury. Kidney Int 2004;66:491.

437. Gibbs P, Berkley LM, Bolton EM, et al. Adhesion molecule expression (ICAM-1, VCAM-1, E-selectin and PECAM) in human kidney allografts. Transpl Immunol 1993;1:109.

438. Kelly KJ, Williams WW Jr, Colvin RB, Bonventre JV. Antibody to intercellular adhesion molecule 1 protects the kidney against ischemic injury. Proc Natl Acad Sci U S A 1994;91:812.

439. Rabb H, Mendiola CC, Saba SR, et al. Antibodies to ICAM-1 protect kidneys in severe ischemic reperfusion injury. Biochem Biophys Res Commun 1995;211:67.

440. Bhat RV, DiRocco R, Marcy VR, et al. Increased expression of IL-1beta converting enzyme in hippocampus after ischemia: Selective localization in microglia. J Neurosci 1996;16:4146.

441. Chinnaiyan AM, Hanna WL, Orth K, et al. Cytotoxic T-cell-derived granzyme B activates the apoptotic protease ICE-LAP3. Curr Biol 1996;6:897.

442. Kuida K, Zheng TS, Na S, et al. Decreased apoptosis in the brain and premature lethality in CPP32-deficient mice. Nature 1996;384:368.

443. Yokota N, Daniels F, Crosson J, Rabb H. Protective effect of T cell depletion in murine renal ischemia-reperfusion injury. Transplantation 2002;74:759.

444. Burne-Taney MJ, Ascon DB, Daniels F, et al. B cell deficiency confers protection from renal ischemia reperfusion injury. J Immunol 2003;171:3210.

445. Burne-Taney MJ, Yokota-Ikeda N, Rabb H. Effects of combined T- and B-cell deficiency on murine ischemia reperfusion injury. Am J Transplant 2005;5:1186.

446. Komlosi P, Fintha A, Bell PD. Current mechanisms of macula densa cell signalling. Acta Physiol Scand 2004;181:463.

447. Wilcox CS. Redox regulation of the afferent arteriole and tubuloglomerular feedback. Acta Physiol Scand 2003;179:217.

448. Conger JD, Robinette J, Guggenheim S. Effect of acetylcholine on the early phase of norepinephrine-induced acute renal failure. Kidney Int 1981;19:399.

449. Flores J, DiBona D, Beck CH, Leaf A. The role of cell swelling in ischemic renal damage and the protective effect of hypertonic solute. J Clin Invest 1972;51:118.

450. Conger J, Robinette J, Villar A, et al. Increased nitric oxide synthase activity despite lack of response to endothelium-dependent vasodilators in postischemic acute renal failure in rats. J Clin Invest 1995;96:631.

451. Molitoris BA, Sutton TA. Endothelial injury and dysfunction: Role in the extension phase of acute renal failure. Kidney Int 2004;66:496.

452. Brodsky SV, Yamamoto T, Tada T, et al. Endothelial dysfunction in ischemic acute renal failure: Rescue by transplanted endothelial cells. Am J Physiol 2002;282:F1140.

453. Mason J, Torhorst J, Welsch J. Role of the medullary perfusion defect in the pathogenesis of ischemic renal failure. Kidney Int 1984;26:283.

454. Rankin GO, Valentovic MA. Role of xenobiotic metabolism. In: Tarloff JB, Lash LH, eds. Toxicology of the Kidney, 3rd ed. New York: CRC Press, 2005;375.

455. Sundin DP, Molitoris BA. The role of endocytosis in nephrotoxicity. In: Tarloff JB, Lash LH, eds. Toxicology of the Kidney, 3rd ed. New York: CRC Press, 2005;375.

456. Lorz C, Justo P, Sanz AB, et al. Role of Bcl-xL in paracetamol-induced tubular epithelial cell death. Kidney Int 2005;67:592.

457. Huang Q, Dunn RT, Jayadev S, et al. Assessment of cisplatin-induced nephrotoxicity by microarray technology. Toxicol Sci 2001;63:196.

458. Goodsaid FM. Genomic biomarkers of toxicity. Curr Opin Drug Discov Devel 2003;6:41.

459. Thukral SK, Nordone PJ, Hu R, et al. Prediction of nephrotoxicant action and identification of candidate toxicity-related biomarkers. Toxicol Pathol 2005;33:343.

460. Davis JW, Goodsaid FM, Bral CM, et al. Quantitative gene expression analysis in a nonhuman primate model of antibiotic-induced nephrotoxicity. Toxicol Appl Pharmacol 2004;200:16.

461. Campos SB, Seguro AC, Cesar KR, Rocha AS. Effects of acyclovir on renal function. Nephron 1992;62:74.

462. Gschwentner M, Susanna A, Woll E, et al. Antiviral drugs from the nucleoside analog family block volume-activated chloride channels. Mol Med 1995;1:407.

463. Ho ES, Lin DC, Mendel DB, Cihlar T. Cytotoxicity of antiviral nucleotides adefovir and cidofovir is induced by the expression of human renal organic anion transporter 1. J Am Soc Nephrol 2000;11:383.

464. Wijnholds J, Mol CA, VanDeemter L, et al. Multiple drug resistance protein 5 is a multispecific organic anion transporter able to transport nucleotide analogs. Proc Natl Acad Sci USA 2000;97:7476.

465. Berns JS, Cohen RM, Stumacher RJ, Rudnick MR. Renal aspects of therapy for human immunodeficiency virus and associated opportunistic infections. J Am Soc Nephrol 1991;1:1061.

466. Perazella MA. Drug-induced renal failure: Update on new medications and unique mechanisms of nephrotoxicity. Am J Med Sci 2003;325:349.

467. Kaloyanides GJ. Drug-phospholipid interactions: Role in aminoglycoside nephrotoxicity. Renal Fail 1992;14:351.

468. Mingeot-Leclercq MP, Brasseur R, Schanck A. Molecular parameters involved in aminoglycoside nephrotoxicity. J Toxicol Environ Health 1995;44:263.

469. Nagai J, Takano M. Molecular aspects of renal handling of aminoglycosides and strategies for preventing the nephrotoxicity. Drug Metab Pharmacokinet 2004;19:159.

470. Mingeot-Leclercq MP, Tulkens PM. Aminoglycosides: Nephrotoxicity. Antimicrob Agents Chemother 1999;43:1003.

471. Schmitz C, Hilpert J, Jacobsen C, et al. Megalin deficiency offers protection from renal aminoglycoside accumulation. J Biol Chem 2002;277:618.

472. Watanabe A, Nagai J, Adachi Y, et al. Targeted prevention of renal accumulation and toxicity of gentamicin by aminoglycoside binding receptor antagonists. J Control Release 2004;95:423.

473. Sandoval RM, Molitoris BA. Gentamicin traffics retrograde through the secretory pathway and is released in the cytosol via the endoplasmic reticulum. Am J Physiol Renal Physiol 2004;286:F617.

474. Williams PD, Bennett DB, Gleason CR, Hottendorf GH. Correlation between renal membrane binding and nephrotoxicity of aminoglycosides. Antimicrob Agents Chemother 1987;31:570.

475. Laurent G, Kishore BK, Tulkens PM. Aminoglycoside-induced renal phospholipidosis and nephrotoxicity. Biochem Pharmacol 1990;40:2383.

476. Van Bambeke F, Tulkens PM, Brasseur R, Mingeot-Leclercq MP. Aminoglycoside antibiotics induce aggregation but not fusion of negatively charged liposomes. Eur J Pharmacol 1995;289:321.

477. Sandoval RM, Bacallao RL, Dunn KW, et al. Nucleotide depletion increases trafficking of gentamicin to the Golgi complex in LLC-PK1 cells. Am J Physiol Renal Physiol 2002;283:F1422.

478. Ramsammy LS, Josepovitz C, Lane BP, Kaloyanides GJ. Polyaspartic acid protects against gentamicin nephrotoxicity in the rat. J Pharmacol Exp Ther 1989;250:149.

479. Kishore BK, Ibrahim S, Lambricht P, et al. Comparative assessment of poly-L-aspartic and poly-L-glutamic acids as protectants against gentamicin-induced renal lysosomal phospholipidosis, phospholipiduria, and cell proliferation in rats. J Pharmacol Exp Ther 1992;262:424.

480. Sundin DP, Sandoval R, Molitoris BA. Gentamicin inhibits renal protein and phospholipid metabolism in the rat: Implications involving intracellular trafficking. J Am Soc Nephrol 2001;12:114.

481. Okuda M, Takano A, Yasuhara M, Hori R. Inhibition of apical membrane enzyme activities and protein synthesis by gentamicin in a kidney epithelial cell line LLC-PK1. Chem Pharm Bull (Tokyo) 1992;40:3307.

482. Takano M, Okuda M, Yasuhara M, Hori R. Cellular toxicity of aminoglycoside antibiotics in G418-sensitive and -resistant LLC-PK1 cells. Pharmacol Res 1994;11:609.

483. Horibe T, Nagai H, Sakakibara K, et al. Ribostamycin inhibits the chaperone activity of protein disulfide isomerase. Biochem Biophys Res Commun 2001;289:967.

484. Horibe T, Nagai H, Matsui H, et al. Aminoglycoside antibiotics bind to protein disulfide isomerase and inhibit its chaperone activity. J Antibiot 2002;55:528.

485. Horibe T, Matsui H, Tanaka M, et al. Gentamicin binds to the lectin site of calreticulin and inhibits its chaperone activity. Biochem Biophys Res Commun 2004;323:281.

486. Walker PD, Shah SV. Evidence suggesting a role for hydroxyl radical in gentamicin-induced acute renal failure in rats. J Clin Invest 1988;81:334.

487. Guidet BR, Shah SV. In vivo generation of hydrogen peroxide by rat kidney cortex and glomeruli. Am J Physiol 1989;256:F158.

488. Cuzzocrea S, Mazzon E, Dugo L, et al. A role for superoxide in gentamicin-mediated nephropathy in rats. Eur J Pharmacol 2002;450:67.

489. Walker PD, Barri Y, Shah SV. Oxidant mechanisms in gentamicin nephrotoxicity. Renal Fail 1999;21:433.

490. Ueda N, Guidet B, Shah SV. Gentamicin-induced mobilization of iron from renal cortical mitochondria. Am J Physiol (Renal Fluid Elect Physiol) 1993;265:F435.

491. Priuska EM, Clark-Baldwin K, Pecorato VL, Schacht J. NMR studies of iron-gentamicin complexes and the implication for aminoglycoside toxicity. Inorg Chim Acta 1998;273:85.

492. Peddraza-Chaverri J, Maldonado PD, Medina-Campos ON, et al. Garlic ameliorates gentamicin nephrotoxicity: Relation to antioxidant enzymes. Free Radical Biol Med 2000;29:602.

493. Maldonado PD, Barrera D, Rivero I, et al. Anti-oxidant S-allylcysteine prevents gentamicin-induced oxidative stress and renal damage. Free Rad Biol Med 2003;35:317.

494. Abdel-Naim AB, Abdel-Wahab MH, Attia FF. Protective effect of vitamin E and probucol against gentamicin-induced nephrotoxicity in rats. Pharmacol Res 1999;40:183.

495. Martinez-Salgado C, Eleno N, Tavares P, et al. Involvement of reactive oxygen species on gentamicin-induced mesangial cell activation. Kidney Int 2002;62:1682.

496. Notenboom S, Miller DS, Smits P, et al. Role of NO in endothelin-regulated drug transport in the renal proximal tubule. Am J Physiol Renal Physiol 2002;282:F458.

497. Rivas-Cabanero L, Rodriguez-Lopez AM, Martinez-Salgado C, et al. Gentamicin treatment increases mesangial cell nitric oxide production. Exp Nephrol 1997;5:23.

498. Ward DT, McLarnon SJ, Riccardi D. Aminoglycosides increase intracellular calcium levels and ERK activity in proximal tubular OK cells expressing the extracellular calcium-sensing receptor. J Am Soc Nephrol 2002;13:1481.

499. Todd JH, Sens DA, Hazen-Martin DJ, et al. Aminoglycoside antibiotics alter the electrogenic transport properties of cultured human proximal tubule cells. Toxicol Pathol 1992;20:608.

500. Bennett WM, Hartnett MN, Gilbert D, et al. Effects of sodium intake on gentamicin nephrotoxicity in the rat. Proc Soc Exp Biol Med 1976;151:736.

501. Baylis C, Rennke HR, Brenner BM. Mechanisms of the defect in glomerular ultrafiltration associated with gentamicin administration. Kidney Int 1977;12:344.

502. Leung JC, Marphis T, Craver RD, Silverstein DM. Altered NMDA receptor expression in renal toxicity: Protection with a receptor antagonist. Kidney Int 2004;66:167.

503. Geleilete TJ, Melo GC, Costa RS, et al. Role of myofibroblasts, macrophages, transforming growth factor-beta, endothelin, angiotensin II and fibronectin in the progression of tubulointerstitial nephritis induced by gentamicin. J Nephrol 2002;15:633.

504. Hsuchen CC, Feingold DS. Selective membrane toxicity of the polyene antibiotics. Antimicrob Agents Chemother 1973;4:316.

505. Sawaya BP, Briggs JP, Schnermann J. Amphotericin B nephrotoxicity: The adverse consequences of altered membrane properties. J Am Soc Nephrol 1995;6:154.

506. Weissmann G. A common mechanism for the fungicidal and nephrotoxic effects of amphotericin B. J Clin Invest 1966;45: 1084.

507. Bernardo JF, Murakami S, Branch RA, Sabra R. Potassium depletion potentiates amphotericin-B-induced toxicity to renal tubules. Nephron 1995;70:235.

508. Sawaya BP, Weihprecht H, Campbell WR, et al. Direct vasoconstriction as a possible cause for amphotericin B–induced nephrotoxicity in rats. J Clin Invest 1991;87:2097.

509. Tolins JP, Raij L. Adverse effect of amphotericin B administration on renal hemodynamics in the rat: Neurohumoral mechanisms and influence of calcium channel blockade. J Pharmacol Exp Ther 1988;245:594.

510. Hardie WD, Ebert J, Frazer M, et al. The effect of thromboxane A2 receptor antagonism on amphotericin B-induced renal vasoconstriction in the rat. Prostaglandins 1993;45:47.

511. Sabra R, Takahashi K, Branch RA, Badr KF. Mechanism of amphotericin B–induced reduction of the glomerular filtration rate: A micropuncture study. J Pharmacol Exp Ther 1990;253:34.

512. Tune BM, Hsu CY. Toxicity of cephaloridine to carnitine transport and fatty acid metabolism in rabbit renal cortical mitochondria: Structure-activity relationships. J Pharmacol Exp Ther 1994;270:873.

513. Lash LH, Tokarz JJ, Woods EB. Renal cell type specificity of cephalosporine-induced cytotoxicity in suspensions of isolated proximal tubular and distal tubular cells. Toxicology 1994;94:97.

514. Kiyomiya K, Matsushita N, Matsuo S, Kurebe M. Cephaloridine-induced inhibition of cytochrome c oxidase activity in the mitochondria of cultured renal epithelial cells (LLC-PK1) as a possible mechanism of its nephrotoxicity. Toxicol Appl Pharmacol 2000;167:151.

515. Steinmassl D, Pfaller W, Gstraunthaler G, Hoffmann W. LLC-PK1 epithelia as a model for in vitro assessment of proximal tubular nephrotoxicity. In Vitro cell Dev Biol Anim 1995;31:94.

516. Dunn CJ, Wagstaff AJ, Perry CM, et al. Cyclosporin: An updated review of the pharmacokinetic properties, clinical efficacy and tolerability of a micro-emulsion-based formulation (Neoral) 1 in organ transplantation. Drugs 2001;61:1957.

517. English J, Evan A, Houghton DC, Bennett WM. Cyclosporine-induced acute renal dysfunction in the rat: Evidence of arteriolar vasoconstriction with preservation of tubular function. Transplantation 1987;44:135.

518. Hunley TE, Fogo A, Iwasaki S, Kon V. Endothelin A receptor mediates functional but not structural damage in chronic cyclosporine nephrotoxicity. J Am Soc Nephrol 1995;5:1718.

519. Kon V, Hunley TE, Fogo A. Combined antagonism of endothelin A/B receptors links endothelin to vasoconstriction whereas angiotensin II effects fibrosis: Studies in chronic cyclosporine nephrotoxicity in rats. Transplantation 1995;60:89.

520. Kon V, Sugiura M, Inagami T, et al. Role of endothelin in cyclosporine-induced glomerular dysfunction. Kidney Int 1990;37:1487.

521. Edwards BD, Daley-Yates PT, Maiza A, et al. Cyclosporin toxicity: Haemodynamics, tubular dysfunction and abrogation in the normal human kidney. J Am Soc Nephrol 1990;1:610.

522. Lassila M. Interaction of cyclosporine A and the renin-angiotensin system: New perspectives. Curr Drug Metab 2002;3: 61.

523. Lee DB. Cyclosporine and the renin-angiotensin axis. Kidney Int 1997;52:248.

524. Moss NG, Powell SL, Falk RJ. Intravenous cyclosporine activates afferent and efferent renal nerves and causes sodium retention in innervated kidneys in rats. Proc Natl Acad Sci U S A 1985;82: 8222.

525. Bloom IT, Bentley FR, Spain DA, Garrison RN. An experimental study of altered nitric oxide metabolism as a mechanism of cyclosporin-induced renal vasoconstriction. Br J Surg 1995;82:195.

526. Gaston RS, Schlessinger SD, Sanders PW, et al. Cyclosporine inhibits the renal response to L-arginine in human kidney transplant recipients. J Am Soc Nephrol 1995;5:1426.

527. Stephan D, Billing A, Krieger JP, et al. Endothelium-dependent relaxation in the isolated rat kidney: Impairment by cyclosporine A. J Cardiovasc Pharmacol 1995;26:859.

528. Coffman T, Carr DR, Yarger WE, Klotman PE. Evidence that renal prostaglandin and thromboxane production is stimulated in chronic cyclosporine nephrotoxicity. Transplantation 1987;43:282.

529. Rossini M, Belloni A, Remuzzi G, Perico N. Thromboxane receptor blockade attenuates the toxic effect of cyclosporine in experimental renal transplantation. Circulation 1990;81:I61.

530. Spruney RF, Mayros SD, Collins D, et al. Thromboxane receptor blockade improves cyclosporine nephrotoxicity in rats. Prostaglandins 1989;1:135.

531. Bunchman TE, Brookshire CA. Cyclosporine-induced synthesis of endothelin by cultured human endothelial cells. J Clin Invest 1991;88:310.

532. Haug C, Duell I, Voisard R, et al. Cyclosporine A stimulates endothelin release. J Cardiovasc Pharmacol 1995;26(suppl. 3): S239.

533. Perico N, Dadan J, Remuzzi G. Endothelin mediates the renal vasoconstriction induced by cyclosporine in the rat. J Am Soc Nephrol 1990;1:76.

534. Nambi P, Pullen M, Contino LC, Brooks DP. Upregulation of renal endothelin receptors in rats with cyclosporine A–induced nephrotoxicity. Eur J Pharmacol 1990;187:113.

535. Shehata M, El Nahas AM, Barkworth E, et al. Increased platelet-derived growth factor in the kidneys of cyclosporin-treated rats. Kidney Int 1994;46:726.

536. Darby IA, Hewitson T, Jones C, et al. Vascular expression of clusterin in experimental cyclosporine nephrotoxicity. Exp Nephrol 1995;3:234.

537. Cebrian C, Areste C, Nicolas A, et al. Kidney androgen-related protein interacts with cyclophilin b and reduces cyclosporine A-mediated toxicity in proximal tubule cells. J Biol Chem 2001;276:29410.

538. Ryffel B, Su Q, Eugster H-P, Car BD. New immunosuppressive agents. In: Solez K, Racusen L, Billingham M, eds. Solid Organ Allograft Rejection. New York: Marcel Dekker, 1996:561.

539. Ader JL, Rostaing L. Cyclosporin nephrotoxicity: Pathophysiology and comparison with FK506. Curr Opin Nephrol Hypertens 1998;7:539.

540. Steiner S, Aicher L, Raymackers J, et al. Cyclosporine A decreases the protein level of the calcium-binding protein calbindin-D 28kDa in rat kidney. Biochem Pharmacol 1996;51:253.

541. Aicher L, Meier G, Norcross AJ, et al. Decrease in kidney calbindin-D 28 kDa as a possible mechanism mediating cyclosporine A- and FK506-induced calciuria and tubular mineralization. Biochem Pharmacol 1997;53:723.

542. Zoja C, Furci L, Ghiladri F, et al. Cyclosporin-induced endothelial cell injury. Lab Invest 1986;55:455.

543. Lau DC, Wong K-L, Hwang WS. Cyclosporine toxicity on cultured rat microvascular endothelial cells. Kidney Int 1989;35:604.

544. Grace AA, Barradas MA, Mikhailidis DP, et al. Cyclosporine A enhances platelet aggregation. Kidney Int 1987;32:889.

545. Young BA, Burdmann EA, Johnson RJ, et al. Cyclosporine A–induced arteriolopathy in a rat model of chronic cyclosporine nephropathy. Kidney Int 1995;48:431.

546. Wolf G, Thaiss F, Stahl RA. Cyclosporine stimulates expression of transforming growth factor-beta in renal cells: Possible mechanism of cyclosporine's antiproliferative effects. Transplantation 1995;60:237.

547. Lally C, Healy E, Ryan MP. Cyclosporine A-induced cell cycle arrest and cell death in renal epithelial cells. Kidney Int 1999;56:1254.

548. Polte T, Hemmerle A, Berndt G, et al. Atrial natriuretic peptide reduces cyclosporin toxicity in renal cells: Role of cGMP and heme oxygenase-1. Free Rad Biol Med 2002;32:56.

549. Longoni B, Migliori M, Ferretti A, et al. Melatonin prevents cyclosporine-induced nephrotoxicity in isolated and perfused rat kidney. Free Rad Res 2002;36:357.

550. Dominguez JH, Soleimani M, Batiuk T. Studies of renal injury IV. The Glut-1 gene protects renal cells from cyclosporine A toxicity. Kidney Int 2002;62:127.

551. Jiang T, Acosta D Jr. Mitochondrial Ca2$^+$ overload in primary cultures of rat renal cortical epithelial cells by cytotoxic concentrations of cyclosporine: A digitized fluorescence imaging study. Toxicology 1995;1:155.

552. Strzelecki T, Kumar S, Khauli R, Menon M. Impairment by cyclosporine of membrane-mediated functions in kidney mitochondria. Kidney Int 1988;34:234.

553. Justo P, Lorz C, Sanz A, et al. Intracellular mechanisms of cyclosporin-induced tubular cell apoptosis. J Am Soc Nephrol 2003;14:3072.

554. Charuk JH, Wong PY, Reithmeier RA. Differential interactions of human renal P-glycoprotein with various metabolites and analogues of cyclosporin A. Am J Physiol 1995;269:F31.

555. Rosen S, Brezis M, Stillman I. The pathology of nephrotoxic injury: A reappraisal. Miner Electrolyte Metab 1994;20:174.

556. Rosen S, Greenfeld Z, Brezis M. Chronic cyclosporine-induced nephropathy in the rat. Transplantation 1990;49:445.

557. Heyman SN, Fuchs S, Brezis M. The role of medullary ischemia in acute renal failure. New Horiz 1995;3:597.

558. Young BA, Burdmann EA, Johnson RJ, et al. Cellular proliferation and macrophage influx precede interstitial fibrosis in cyclosporine nephrotoxicity. Kidney Int 1995;48:439.

559. Shihab FS, Andoh TF, Tanner AM, et al. Role of transforming growth-factor beta-1 in experimental chronic cyclosporine nephropathy. Kidney Int 1996;49:1141.

560. Islam M, Burke JF Jr, McGowan TA, et al. Effect of anti-transforming growth factor-beta antibodies in cyclosporine-induced renal dysfunction. Kidney Int 2001;59:498.

561. Oleggini R, Musante L, Menoni S, et al. Characterization of a DNA binding site that mediates the stimulatory effect of cyclosporin A on type III collagen expression in renal cells. Nephrol Dial Transplant 2000;15:778.

562. Kang DH, Kim YG, Andoh TF, et al. Post-cyclosporine-mediated hypertension and nephropathy: Amelioration by vascular endothelial growth factor. Am J Physiol Renal Physiol 2001;280:F727.

563. Suzuki N, Sakane T, Tsunematsu T. Effects of a novel immunosuppressive agent, FK506, on human B-cell activation. Clin Exp Immunol 1990;79:240.

564. Dumont FJ. FK506, an immunosuppressant targeting calcineurin function. Curr Med Chem 2000;7:731.

565. Su Q, Weber L, Le Hir M, et al. Nephrotoxicity of cyclosporine A and FK506: Inhibition of calcineurin phosphatase. Renal Physiol Biochem 1995;18:128.

566. Perrot-Applanat M, Cibert C, Geraud G, et al. The 59 kDa FK506-binding protein, a 90 kDa heat shock protein binding immunophilin (FKBP59-HBI), is associated with the nucleus, the cytoskeleton and mitotic apparatus. J Cell Sci 1995;108:2037.

567. Christians U, Jacobsen W, Benet LZ, Lampen A. Mechanisms of clinically relevant drug interactions associated with tacrolimus. Clin Pharmacokinet 2002;41:813.

568. Goodall T, Kind CN, Hammond TG. FK506-induced endothelin release by cultured rat mesangial cells. J Cardiovasc Pharmacol 1995;26(suppl 3):S482.

569. Textor SC, Burnett JC Jr, Romero JC, et al. Urinary endothelin and renal vasoconstriction with cyclosporine or FK506 after liver transplantation. Kidney Int 1995;47:1426.

570. Mitamura T, Yamada A, Ishida H, et al. Tacrolimus (FK506)-induced nephrotoxicity in spontaneous hypertensive rats. J Toxicol Sci 1994;19:219.

571. Shihab FS, Bennett WM, Tanner AM, Andoh TF. Mechanisms of fibrosis in experimental tacrolimus toxicity. Transplantation 1997;64:1829.

572. Shihab FS, Bennett WM, Yi H, et al. Sirolimus increases transforming growth factor-beta 1 expression and potentiates chronic cyclosporine nephrotoxicity. Kidney Int 2004;65:1262.

573. Lieberthal W, Fuhro R, Andry CC, et al. Rapamycin impairs recovery from acute renal failure; role of cell-cycle arrest and apoptosis in tubular cells. Am J Physiol Renal Physiol 2001;281:F693.

574. Graziano J, Jones B, Pisciotto P. The effect of heavy metal chelators on the renal accumulation of platinum after cis-dichlorodiammine platinum II administration to the rat. Br J Pharmacol 1981;73:649.

575. Safirstein R, Miller P, Dikman S, et al. Cis-platinum nephrotoxicity in rats: Defect in papillary hypertonicity. Am J Physiol 1981;241:F175.

576. Van den Berg EK Jr, Brazy PC, Huang AT, Dennis VW. Cisplatinum-induced changes in sodium, chloride, and urea transport by the frog skin. Kidney Int 1981;19:8.

577. Jordan P, Carmo-Fonseca M. Molecular mechanisms involved in cisplatin cytotoxicity. Cell Mol Life Sci 2000;57:1229.

578. Brady HR, Kone BC, Stromski ME, et al. Mitochondrial injury: An early event in cisplatin toxicity in renal proximal tubules. Am J Physiol 1990;258:F1181.

579. Zhang JG, Lindup WE. Cisplatin nephrotoxicity: Decreases in mitochondrial protein sulfhydryl concentration and calcium uptake by mitochondria from rat renal cortical slices. Biochem Pharmacol 1994;47:1127.

580. Tsutsumishita Y, Onda T, Okada K, et al. Involvement of $H_2O_2$ production in cisplatin-induced nephrotoxicity. Biochem Biophys Res Commun 1998;242:310.

581. Baliga R, Zhang Z, Baliga M, et al. Role of cytochrome P450 as a source of catalytic iron in cisplatin-induced nephrotoxicity. Kidney Int 1998;54:1562.

582. Baliga R, Ueda N, Walker PD, Shah SV. Oxidant mechanisms in toxic acute renal failure. Drug Metab Rev 1999;31:971.

583. Leibbrandt MEI, Wolfgang GH, Metz AL, et al. Critical subcellular targets of cisplatin and related platinum analogs in rat renal proximal tubule cells. Kidney Int 1995;48:761.

584. Tay LK, Bregman CL, Masters BA, William PD. Effects of cis-diamminedichlorplatinum (II) in rabbit kidney in vivo and rabbit renal proximal tubule cells in culture. Cancer Res 1988;48:2538.

585. Lieberthal W, Triaca V, Levine J. Mechanisms of death induced by cisplatin in proximal tubular epithelial cells: Apoptosis vs necrosis. Am J Physiol 1996;270:F700.

586. Park MS, De Leon M, Devarajan P. Cisplatin induces apoptosis in LLC-PK1 cells via activation of mitochondrial pathways. J Am Soc Nephrol 2002;13:858.

587. Cummings BS, Schnellmann RG. Cisplatin-induced renal cell apoptosis. Caspase 3-dependent and independent pathways. J Pharmacol Exp Therap 2002;302:8.

588. Bonegio R, Lieberthal W. Role of apoptosis in the pathogenesis of acute renal failure. Curr Opin Nephrol Hypertens 2002;11:301.

589. Schrier RW. Cancer therapy and renal injury. J Clin Invest 2002;110:743.

590. Ramesh G, Reeves WB. TNF-alpha mediates chemokine and cytokine expression and renal injury in cisplatin nephrotoxicity. J Clin Invest 2002;110:835.

591. Kelly KJ, Meehan SM, Colvin RB, et al. Protection from toxicant-mediated renal injury in the rat with anti-CD54 antibody. Kidney Int 1999;56:922.

592. Deng J, Kohda Y, Chiao H, et al. Interleukin-10 inhibits ischemic and cisplatin-induced acute renal injury. Kidney Int 2001;60:2118.

593. Rossi R, Helmchen U, Schellong G. Tubular function and histologic findings in ifosfamide-induced renal Fanconi syndrome: A report of two cases. Eur J Pediatr 1992;151:384.

594. Rieselbach RE, Garnick MB. Renal disease induced by antineoplastic agents. In: Schrier RW, Gottschalk CW, eds. Diseases of the Kidney, 4th ed. Boston: Little, Brown, 1988:1275.

595. Ludwin D, Luxton GC. Renal urinary antigens and the diagnosis of acute renal failure. In: Solez K, Racusen LC, eds. Acute Renal Failure: Diagnosis, Treatment, and Prevention. New York: Marcel Dekker, 1991:139.

596. Nicot GS, Merle LJ, Charmes JP, et al. Transient glomerular proteinuria, enzymuria, and nephrotoxic reaction induced by radiocontrast media. JAMA 1984;252:2432.

597. Persson PB, Hansell P, Liss P. Pathophysiology of contrast medium-induced nephropathy. Kidney Int 2005;68:14.

598. Beeri R, Symon Z, Brezis M, et al. Rapid DNA fragmentation from hypoxia along the thick ascending limb of rat kidneys. Kidney Int 1995;47:1806.

599. Agmon Y, Peleg H, Greenfeld Z, et al. Nitric oxide and prostanoids protect the renal outer medulla from radiocontrast toxicity in the rat. J Clin Invest 1994;94:1069.

600. Bakris GL, Gaber AO, Jones JD. Oxygen free radicals involvement in urinary Tamm-Horsfall protein excretion after intrarenal injection of contrast medium. Radiology 1990;175:57.

601. Gelman ML, Ropwe JW, Coggins CH, Athanasoulis C. Effects of an angiographic contrast agent on renal function. Cardiovasc Med 1979;1:313.

602. Postlethwaite AE, Kelley WN. Uricosuric effect of radiocontrast agents: A study in man of four commonly used preparations. Ann Intern Med 1971;74:845.

603. Lantz B, Cochat P, Bouchet JL, Fischbach M. Short-term niflumic-acid-induced acute renal failure in children. Nephrol Dial Transplant 1994;9:1234.

604. Oldroyd SD, Haylor JL, Morcos SK. Bosentan, an orally active endothelin antagonist: Effect on the renal response to contrast media. Radiology 1995;196:661.

605. Schwartz D, Blum M, Peer G, et al. Role of nitric oxide (EDRF) in radiocontrast acute renal failure in rats. Am J Physiol 1994;267:F374.

606. Wang A, Holcslaw T, Bashore TM, et al. Exacerbation of radiocontrast nephrotoxicity by endothelin receptor antagonism. Kidney Int 2000;57:1675.

607. Persson PB, Hansell P, Liss P. Pathophysiology of contrast medium-induced nephropathy. Kidney Int 2005;68:14.

608. Andersen KJ, Christensen EI, Vik H. Effects of iodinated x-ray contrast media on renal epithelial cells in culture. Invest Radiol 1994;29:955.

609. Haller C, Schick CS, Zorn M, Kubler W. Cytotoxicity of radiocontrast agents in polarized renal epithelial cell monolayers. Cardiovasc Res 1997;33:655.

610. Schick CS, Haller C. Comparative cytotoxicity of ionic and nonionic radiocontrast agents on MDCK cell monolayers in vitro. Nephrol Dial Transplant 1999;14:342.

611. Hardiek K, Katholi RE, Ramkumar V, Dietrick C. Proximal tubule cell response to radiographic contrast media. Am J Physiol Renal Physiol 2001;280:F61.

612. Hizoh I, Haller C. Radiocontrast-induced renal tubular cell apoptosis: Hypertonic versus oxidative stress. Invest Radiol 2002;37:428.

613. Yano T, Itoh Y, Sendo T, et al. Cyclic AMP reverses radiocontrast media-induced apoptosis in LLC-PK1 cells by activating A kinase/P13 kinase. Kidney Int 2003;64:2052.

614. Zager RA, Johnson AC, Hanson S. Radiographic contrast media-induced tubular injury: Evaluation of oxidant stress and plasma membrane integrity. Kidney Int 2003;64:128.

615. Haller C, Hizoh I. The cytotoxicity of iodinated radiocontrast agents on renal cells in vitro. Invest Radiol 2004;39:149.

616. Krohn KD, Slowman-Kovacs S, Leapman SB. Cocaine and rhabdomyolysis. Ann Intern Med 1988;108:639.

617. Heng MC, Haberfeld G. Thrombotic phenomenon associated with intravenous cocaine. J Am Acad Dermatol 1987;16:462.

618. Keung YK, Morgan D, Cobos E. Cocaine-induced microangiopathies, hemolytic anemia, and thrombocytopenia simulating thrombotic thrombocytopenic purpura. Ann Hematol 1996;72:155.

619. Burchardi H, Kaczmarczyk G. The effect of anaesthesia on renal function. Eur J Anaesthesiol 1994;11:163.

620. Munday IT, Stoddart PA, Jones RM, et al. Serum fluoride concentration and urine osmolality after enflurane and sevoflurane anesthesia in male volunteers. Anesth Analg 1995;81:353.

621. American College of Chest Physicians-Society of Critical Care Medicine Consensus conference: Definitions for sepsis and organ failure and guidelines for the use of innovative therapies in sepsis. Crit Care Med 1992;20:864.

622. Thadhani R, Pascual M, Bonventre JV. Acute renal failure. N Engl J Med 1996;334:1448.

623. Landry DW, Oliver JA. The pathogenesis of vasodilatory shock. N Engl J Med 2001;345:588.

624. Keung EC, Li Q. Lactate activates ATP-sensitive potassium channels in guinea pig ventricular myocytes. J Clin Invest 1991;88:1772.

625. Wang W, Mitra A, Poole B, et al. Endothelial nitric oxide synthase deficient mice exhibit increased susceptibility to endotoxin-induced acute renal failure. Am J Physiol 2004;287:F1044.

626. Schwartz D, Mendonca M, Schwartz I, et al. Inhibition of constitutive nitric oxide synthase (NOS) by nitric oxide generated by inducible NOS after lipopolysaccharide administration provokes renal dysfunction in rats. J Clin Invest 1997;100: 439.

627. Knotek M, Rogachev B, Wang W, et al. Endotoxemic renal failure in mice: Role of tumor necrosis factor independent of inducible nitric oxide synthase. Kidney Int 2001;59:2243.

628. Gallagher J, Fisher C, Sherman B, et al. A multi-center, open-label, prospective, randomized, dose-ranging pharmacokinetic study of the anti-TNF-alpha antibody afelimomab in patients with sepsis syndrome. Intensive Care Med 2001;27:1169.

629. Wang W, Jittikanont S, Falk SA, et al. Interaction among nitric oxide, reactive oxygen species, and antioxidants during endotoxemia-related acute renal failure. Am J Physiol Renal Physiol 2003;284:F532.

630. Wang W, Faubel S, Ljubanovic D, et al. Endotoxemic acute renal failure is attenuated in caspase-1-deficient mice. Am J Physiol Renal Physiol 2005;288:F997.

631. Czermak BJ, Sarma V, Pierson CL, et al. Protective effects of C5a blockade in sepsis. Nat Med 1999;5:788.

632. Kielar ML, Rohan Jeyarajah D, Lu CY. The regulation of ischemic acute renal failure by extrarenal organs. Curr Opin Nephrol Hypertens 2002;11:451.

633. Kuiper JW, Groeneveld AB, Slutsky AS, Plotz FB. Mechanical ventilation and acute renal failure. Crit Care Med 2005;33:1408.

634. Kramer AA, Postler G, Salhab KF, et al. Renal ischemia/ reperfusion leads to macrophage-mediated increase in pulmonary vascular permeability. Kidney Int 1999;55:2362.

635. Rabb H, Wang Z, Nemoto T, et al. Acute renal failure leads to dysregulation of lung salt and water channels. Kidney Int 2003;63:600.

636. Chien CC, King LS, Rabb H. Mechanisms underlying combined acute renal failure and acute lung injury in the intensive care unit. Contrib Nephrol 2004;144:53.

637. Anderson R, Schrier R. Clinical spectrum of oliguric and non-oliguric acute renal failure. In: Brenner BM, Stein J, eds. Acute Renal Failure. Contemporary Issues in Nephrology. New York: Churchill Livingstone, 1980.

638. Hall J, Johnson W, Maher F, Hunt J. Immediate and long-term prognosis in acute renal failure. Ann Intern Med 1970;73:515.

639. Minuth A, Terrell J, Suki W. Acute renal failure: A study of the course and prognosis of 104 patients and of the role of furosemide. Am J Med Sci 1976;271:317.

640. Chertow GM, Christiansen CL, Cleary PD, et al. Prognostic stratification in critically ill patients with acute renal failure requiring dialysis. Arch Intern Med 1995;155:1505.

641. Lima EQ, Dirce MT, Castro I, Yu L. Mortality risk factors and validation of severity scoring systems in critically ill patients with acute renal failure. Ren Fail 2005;27:547.

642. Woodrow G, Turney JH. Cause of death in acute renal failure. Nephrol Dial Transplant 1992;7:230.

643. Liano F, Gallego A, Pascual J, et al. Prognosis of acute tubular necrosis: An extended prospectively contrasted study. Nephron 1993;63:21.

644. Hoste EA, DeWaele JJ. Physiologic consequences of acute renal failure on the critically ill. Crit Care Clin 2005;21:251.

645. Joannidis M, Metnitz PG. Epidemiology and natural history of acute renal failure in the ICU. Crit Care Clin 2005;21:239.

646. Ilic S, Rajic M, Vlajkovic M, et al. The predictive value of 131I: hippurate clearance in the prognosis of acute renal failure. Ren Fail 2000;22:581.

647. Lewers D, Mathew TH, Maher JF, Schreiner G. Long-term follow-up of renal function and histology after acute tubular necrosis. Ann Intern Med 1970;73:523.

648. Bonomini V, Stefoni S, Vangelista A. Long-term patient and renal prognosis in acute renal failure. Nephron 1984;36:169.

649. Finn WF. Recovery from acute renal failure. In: Molitoris BA, Finn WF, eds. Acute Renal Failure: A Companion to Brenner & Rector's The Kidney. Philadelphia: W. B. Saunders, 2001:425.

650. Alon US. Neonatal acute renal failure: The need for long-term follow-up. Clin Pediatr (Phila) 1998;37:387.

651. Anderson R, Gordon J, Kim J, et al. Renal concentration defect following non-oliguric acute renal failure in the rat. Kidney Int 1982;21:583.

652. Safirstein R, Miller P, Dikman S, et al. Cisplatin nephrotoxicity in rats: Defect in papillary hypertonicity. Am J Physiol 1981;241:F175.

653. Basile DP, Donohoe D, Roethe K, Osborn J. Renal ischemic injury results in permanent damage to peritubular capillaries and influences long-term function. Am J Physiol 2001;281:F887.

654. Basile DP. Rarefaction of peritubular capillaries following ischemic acute renal failure: A potential factor predisposing to progressive nephropathy. Curr Opin Nephrol Hypertens 2004; 13:1.

655. Gueler F, Gwinner W, Schwarz A, Haller H. Long-term effects of acute ischemia and reperfusion injury. Kidney Int 2004;66:523.

656. Forbes JM, Hewitson TD, Becker GJ, Jones CL. Ischemic acute renal failure: Long-term histology of cell and matrix changes in the rat. Kidney Int 2000;57:2375.

657. Yamamoto T, Tada T, Brodsky SV, et al. Intravital videomicroscopy of peritubular capillaries in renal ischemia. Am J Physiol Renal Physiol 2002;282:F1150.

658. Sutton TA, Mang H, Campos SB, et al. Injury of the renal microvascular endothelium alters barrier function after ischemia. Am J Physiol Renal Physiol 2003;285:F191.

659. Chandraker A, Takada M, Nadeau KC, et al. CD28-b7 blockade in organ dysfunction secondary to cold ischemia/reperfusion injury. Kidney Int 1997;52:1678.

660. Basile D, Donohoe DL, Roethe K, Mattson DL. Chronic renal hypoxia following ischemia/reperfusion injury: Effects of L-arginine on hypoxia and secondary damage. Am J Physiol Renal Physiol 2003;284:F338.

661. Quan A, Quigley R. Renal replacement therapy and acute renal failure. Curr Opin Pediatr 2005;17:205.

662. Palevsky PM. Renal replacement therapy I. Indications and timing. Crit Care Clin 2005;21:347.

663. Ricci Z, Ronco C. Renal replacement II. Dialysis dose. Crit Care Clin 2005;21:357.

664. O'Reilly P. Tolwani A. Renal replacement III. IHD, CRRT, SLED. Crit Care Clin 2005;21:367.

665. Barletta GM, Bunchman TE. Acute renal failure in children and infants. Curr Opin Crit Care 2004;10:499.

666. Venkataraman R. Prevention of acute renal failure. Crit Care Clin 2005;21:281.

667. Lin J, Bonventre JV. Prevention of radiocontrast nephropathy. Curr Opin Nephrol Hypertens 2005;14:105.

668. Pannu N, Manns B, Lee H, Tonelli M. Systematic review of the impact of N-acetylcysteine on contrast nephropathy. Kidney Int 2004;65:1366.

669. Spargias K, Alexopoulos E, Kyrzopoulos S, et al. Ascorbic acid prevents contrast-mediated nephropathy in patients with renal dysfunction undergoing coronary angiography or intervention. Circulation 2004;110:2837.

670. Goldenberg I, Matetzky S. Nephropathy induced by contrast media: Pathogenesis, risk factors and preventive strategies. CMAJ 2005;172:1461.

671. Rahman SN, Kim GE, Mathew AS, et al. Effects of atrial natriuretic peptide in clinical acute renal failure. Kidney Int 1994;45:1731.

672. Hirschberg R, Kopple J, Lipsett P, et al. Multicenter clinical trial of recombinant human insulin-like growth factor I in patients with acute renal failure. Kidney Int 1999;55:2423.

673. Lieberthal W, Sheridan AM, Valeri CR. Protective effect of atrial natriuretic factor and mannitol following renal ischemia. Am J Physiol 1990;258:F1266.

674. Conger JD, Falk SA, Yuan BH, Schrier RW. Atrial natriuretic peptide and dopamine in a rat model of ischemic acute renal failure. Kidney Int 1989;35:1126.

675. Tiranathanagul K, Eiam-Ong S, Humes HD. The future of renal support: High-flux dialysis to bioartificial kidneys. Crit Care Med 2005;21:379.

676. Bates CM, Lin F. Future strategies in the treatment of acute renal failure: Growth factors, stem cells, and other novel therapies. Curr Opin Pediatr 2005;17:215.

677. Ricardo SD, Deane JA. Adult stem cells in renal injury and repair. Nephrology (Carlton) 2005;10:276.

678. Alwall N, Erlanson P, Tornberg A, et al. Two cases of gross renal cortical necrosis in pregnancy with severe oliguria and anuria for 116 and 79 days respectively: Clinical course, roentgenological studies of the kidneys (size, outlines and calcifications) and post-mortem findings. Acta Med Scand 1958;161:93.

679. Geiling E, Cannon P. Pathologic effects of elixir of sulfanilamide (diethylene glycol) poisoning: A clinical and experimental correlation. Final report. JAMA 1938;111:9191.

680. Mckay D, Jewett J, Reid D. Endotoxin shock and the generalized Shwartzman reaction in pregnancy. Am J Obstet Gynecol 1959;78:546.

681. Robboy S, Major MC, Colman R, Minna J. Pathology of disseminated intravascular coagulation (DIC): Analysis of 26 cases. Hum Pathol 1972;3:327.

682. Raij L, Keane W, Michael A. Unilateral Shwartzman reaction: Cortical necrosis in one kidney following in vivo perfusion with endotoxin. Kidney Int 1977;2:91.

683. Marcussen H, Asnaes S. Renal cortical necrosis: An evaluation of the possible relation to the Shwartzman reaction. Acta Pathol Microbiol Scand (A) 1972;80:351.

684. McKay D. Disseminated Intravascular Coagulation: An Intermediary Mechanism of Disease. New York: Harper & Row, 1965.

685. Goodman PE, Rennie WP. Renal infarction secondary to nasal insufflation of cocaine. Am J Emerg Med 1995;13:421.

686. Kramer RK, Turner RC. Renal infarction associated with cocaine use and latent protein C deficiency. South Med J 1993;86:1436.

687. Burke JR, Hardie IR. Loin pain haematuria syndrome. Pediatr Nephrol 1996;10:216.

688. Little PJ, Sloper JS, de Wardener HE. A syndrome of loin pain and haematuria associated with disease of peripheral renal arteries. Q J Med 1967;36:253.

689. Higgins PM, Aber GM. Renal pain and haematuria. Br J Urol 1974;46:601.

690. Hebert LA, Betts JA, Sedmak DD, et al. Loin pain-hematuria syndrome associated with thin glomerular basement membrane disease and hemorrhage into renal tubules. Kidney Int 1996;49:168.

691. Weisberg LS, Bloom PB, Simmons RL, Viner ED. Loin pain hematuria syndrome [Editorial]. Am J Nephrol 1993;13:229.

692. Lucas PA, Leaker BR, Murphy M, Neild GH. Loin pain and haematuria syndrome: A somatoform disorder. Q J Med 1995;88:703.

693. Lucas PA, Leaker BR, Neild GH. Psychiatric aspects of loin pain/haematuria syndrome. Lancet 1992;340:1038.

694. Karvelas JP, Ramsey EW. Renal autotransplantation in patients with loin pain-hematuria syndrome. Can J Surg 1996;39:121.

695. Parnham AP, Low A, Finch P, Perlman D, Thomas MA. Recurrent graft pain following renal autotransplantation for loin pain haematuria syndrome. Br J Urol 1996;78:25.

696. Burden RP, Booth LJ, Ockenden BG, et al. Intrarenal vascular changes in adult patients with recurrent haematuria and loin pain: A clinical, histological and angiographic study. Q J Med 1975;44:433.

697. Miller F, Lane BP, Kirsch M, et al. Loin pain-hematuria syndrome with a distinctive vascular lesion and alternative pathway complement activation. Arch Pathol Lab Med 1994;118:1016.

698. Leaker BR, Gordge MP, Patel A, Neild GH. Haemostatic changes in the loin pain and haematuria syndrome: Secondary to renal vasospasm? Q J Med 1990;76:969.

699. Fletcher P, Al-Khader AA, Parsons V, Aber GM. The pathology of intrarenal vascular lesions associated with the loin pain-haematuria syndrome. Nephron 1979;24:150.

700. Naish PF, Aber GM, Boyd WN. C3 deposition in renal arterioles in the loin pain and haematuria syndrome. Br Med J 1975;3:746.

701. Boyd WN, Burdern RP, Aber GM. Intrarenal vascular changes in patients receiving oestrogen-containing compounds: A clinical, histological and angiographic study. Q J Med 1975;44:415.

702. Siegler RL, Brewer ED, Hammond E. Platelet activation and prostacyclin supporting capacity in the loin pain hematuria syndrome. Am J Kidney Dis 1988;12:156.

703. Modi KS, Rao VK. Atheroembolic renal disease. Am Soc Nephrol 2001;12:1781.

704. Cosio F, Zager R, Sharma H. Atheroembolic renal disease causes hypocomplementamia. Lancet 1985;2:118.

705. Kasinath B, Lewis E. Eosinophilia as a clue to the diagnosis of atheroembolic renal disease. Arch Intern Med 1987;147:1384.

706. Saleem S, Lakkis FG, Martinez-Maldonado M. Atheroembolic renal disease. Semin Nephrol 1996;16:309.

707. Thurlbeck W, Castleman B. Atheromatous emboli to the kidneys after aortic surgery. N Engl J Med 1957;257:442.

708. Moreau R, Lebrec D. Review article: Hepatorenal syndrome–Definitions and diagnosis. Aliment Pharmacol Ther 2004;20 (Suppl 3):24.

709. Moreau R, Durand F, Poynar T, et al. Terlipressin in patients with cirrhosis and type I hepatorenal syndrome: A retrospective multicenter study. Gastroenterology 2002;122:923.

710. Gardenas A, Gines P, Uriz J, et al. Renal failure after upper gastrointestinal bleeding in cirrhosis: Incidence, clinical course, predictive factors, and short-term prognosis. Hepatology 2001;34:671.

# Renal Disease Caused by Familial Metabolic and Hematologic Diseases

25

*Laura S. Finn    Jay Bernstein*

This chapter covers familial metabolic defects in the kidney, along with more systemic metabolic and hematologic defects that affect the kidney secondarily. Renal involvement in the first group includes several lysosomal storage diseases caused by deficiencies of lysosomal enzymes in renal tissues, for example, as in Fabry's disease. Not all lysosomal storage diseases primarily affect the kidney, however; renal involvement in Gaucher's disease, for example, results from the entrapment in the kidney of circulating macrophages engorged with glucosyl ceramide. Clearly, secondary renal involvement follows the hyperlipidemia of familial lecithin–cholesterol acyl transferase (LCAT) deficiency, hyperoxaluria of hepatic peroxisomal alanine–glyoxylate aminotransferase deficiency, and the microcirculatory abnormality of hemoglobinopathies. The defect of tubular transport in inherited Fanconi syndrome is intrinsic to the proximal convoluted tubule, although an identical transport abnormality is much more commonly secondary to the renal accumulation of cystine, as the re-

sult of a generalized primary defect in lysosomal membrane transport. Therefore, simple categorization of these disorders into primary and secondary groups serves little purpose. The diseases are grouped into broad categories, with descriptions of the functional abnormalities and the renal consequences.

## LIPID DISORDERS

### Familial Lecithin–Cholesterol Acyl Transferase Deficiency

Familial LCAT deficiency is an uncommon autosomal recessive disorder resulting from a heritable defect in the esterification of plasma cholesterol. Increased plasma concentrations of unesterified cholesterol, triglycerides, and phosphatidylcholine result in lipid deposition in tissues. The enzyme LCAT is carried by high-density lipoprotein with apolipoprotein (Apo) AI as a cofactor, and it catalyzes the esterification of free cholesterol bound to lipoproteins. Mutations in the LCAT gene, localized to chromosome 16q21-q22, cause classic familial LCAT deficiency (FLD) and fish eye disease (FED) (1). More than 36 mutations have been described that produce a variety of defects, including normal secretion of LCAT with low activity, reduced secretion of a fully or partially active LCAT, secretion of an unstable or rapidly catabolized enzyme, and complete degradation of the enzyme at its site of synthesis (2). All result in greatly reduced concentrations of high-density lipoprotein (HDL). The residual plasma HDL is characterized on electron microscopy by an accumulation of disk-shaped pre-β HDL that may form rouleaux. Other lipid phenotypes include morphologically abnormal low-density lipoprotein (LDL) and very–low-density lipoprotein (VLDL) particles and the formation of free cholesterol- and phospholipid-rich, triglyceride-poor vesicles known as lipoprotein X (LpX) (3).

Homozygous patients often have a complete deficiency of LCAT catalytic activity; heterozygotes lack clinical symptoms, although they may have partial deficiency. Classic LCAT deficiency comprises deficits in the activities of both α-LCAT and β-LCAT. The disease, originally described in Norway (4), appears to be widely distributed. Clinical manifestations of FLD include corneal opacities, hemolytic anemia, accelerated peripheral atherosclerosis, and proteinuria with renal insufficiency. Lipid deposits also occur in liver, spleen, and bone marrow, in which foam cells (sea-blue histiocytes) are present (5). In contrast to FLD, FED patients have no major clinical manifestations except corneal opacity.

Renal involvement, the major cause of morbidity and mortality, commonly begins with proteinuria during childhood, sometimes in the neonatal period (6), and it culminates after several decades of renal insufficiency. The

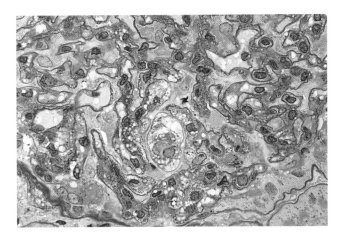

**Figure 25.1** Glomerulus from a patient with LCAT deficiency. It shows mesangial and focal capillary wall thickening with prominent bubbly lipid interposed between what appear to be two layers of basement membrane (double contours). (Periodic acid-Schiff [PAS]; ×400.)

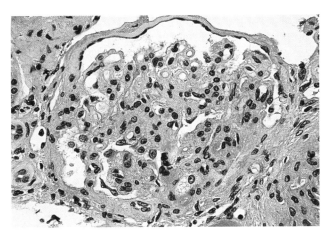

**Figure 25.2** Glomerulus in LCAT deficiency showing thickened basement membranes and mesangial foam cells (*bottom*) entrapped within increased eosinophilic matrix. (Hematoxylin & eosin [H&E]; ×200.)

progression of renal disease is variable; some patients show severe proteinuria and others experience little. Hypertension may appear early in the course or as a late complication of renal insufficiency. Urinalysis usually shows mild hematuria, leukocyturia, and cylindruria. Renal insufficiency is not invariable (7); when present, it usually develops by the fourth decade.

## Pathologic Changes

The glomeruli are the principal site of renal injury, undergoing mesangial expansion and a characteristic capillary wall thickening. Foamy lipid is most obvious in thickened capillary walls, which have a bubbly, vacuolated, or honeycomb appearance that is accentuated when stained with toluidine blue (Fig. 25.1). Silver-stained sections show craters in and vacuolization of the glomerular basement membrane, resembling late-stage membranous glomerulonephritis; double contours are often noted (8–10). Mesangial cellularity is normal to mildly increased, and the mesangium is often expanded, with the same vacuolated appearance as the capillary walls. Collections of endocapillary foam cells are an occasional feature. The mesangium also contains acellular, eosinophilic matrix that accumulates in areas of segmental sclerosis and eventual global sclerosis (Fig. 25.2). Interstitial foam cells may be present, and lipid deposition has been noted in arterial walls. The tubules are generally normal until atrophy accompanies interstitial fibrosis. Immunofluorescence is usually negative for immunoglobulin and complement components, occasionally showing mild, nonspecific changes. The deposits have been shown by immunostaining to contain large amounts of ApoB and ApoE (10).

Electron microscopy has shown a mixture of glomerular epimembranous, intramembranous, subendothelial, and

mesangial lipid deposits (Fig. 25.3). One study of sequential biopsy specimens showed early subepithelial and intramembranous deposition, followed by predominantly subendothelial and mesangial deposits (11). The lipid deposits are partly lucent and partly deeply osmiophilic, the latter including cross-striated curvilinear serpiginous fibrils, rounded lamellar densities, and granular densities (12). Densely osmiophilic basement membrane deposits have resembled the glomerular alterations of dense-deposit disease (13). The lamellar and serpiginous densities are predominantly in epimembranous and intramembranous deposits. The intramembranous lipid deposits may increase basement membrane fragility because focal disruptions are identifiable. The granular densities are predominantly in subendothelial deposits. The mesangial deposits tend to be large and dense, comprising increased matrix and hyalin. Foam cells may be present in the mesangium, as shown by

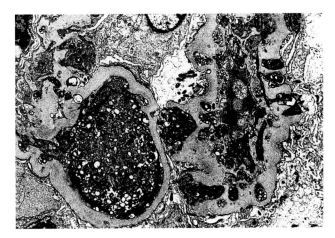

**Figure 25.3** Electron microscopy in LCAT deficiency shows glomerular epimembranous, intramembranous, subendothelial, and mesangial accumulations of extracellular lipid material with membranous profiles and granules. (×9000.)

light microscopy; they rarely seem to be endocapillary. Arteriolar endothelial and medial cells may also contain lipid deposits. Tubular atrophy and interstitial fibrosis progress variably.

Mesangial lipid deposits recur rapidly in renal allografts (14), sometimes within weeks (Figs. 25.4 and 25.5). The deposits do not necessarily impair renal function, because long-term graft survival has been described (15–17). Renal transplantation has no effect on the systemic metabolic disorder (14).

The renal abnormality, although easily recognizable, is not exactly specific, because similar lipid deposits occur in kidneys of patients with chronic liver disease, for example, Alagille's syndrome and cirrhosis of various etiologies, who also have elevated serum lipoprotein (18–20).

## Pathogenesis

The cause of renal injury, despite lipid accumulation, has not been completely elucidated. A role for LpX has been supported by animal studies. In vitro experiments

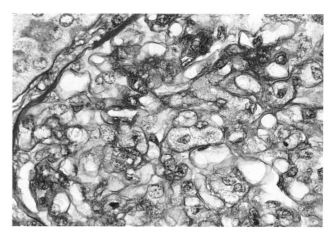

**Figure 25.4** Glomerulus from renal allograft in a patient with LCAT deficiency, 7 weeks after transplantation, with recurrence of foamy mesangial cells. (PAS; ×400.)

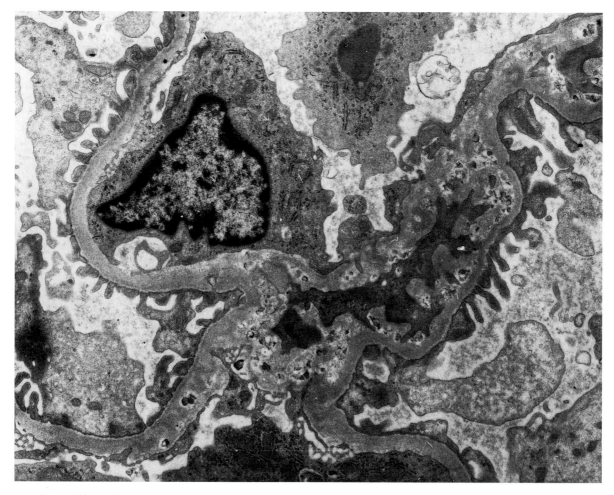

**Figure 25.5** Electron microscopy shows recurrence of mesangial and subendothelial lipid deposits in renal allograft at 7 weeks after renal transplantation in a patient with LCAT deficiency. (×10,400.)

have shown up-regulation of monocyte chemoattractant protein-1 mRNA expression and protein levels and increased nuclear activities of nuclear factor κB in rat mesangial cells, suggesting that LpX may induce a proinflammatory response (21). In the LCAT knock-out mouse, high-fat diets produced LpX accumulation, with the development of proteinuria and glomerulosclerosis in a subset (22). A more recent analysis circumvented the potentially confounding contribution of coexisting hyperlipidemia in the prior study by generating a novel murine model in which circulating lipoproteins were predominantly LpX. These mice spontaneously developed progressive glomerular lesions that had light and electron microscopic abnormalities similar to those seen in human LCAT deficiency (23).

## Lipoprotein Glomerulopathy

Lipoprotein glomerulopathy (LPG) is a rare disorder with an autosomal recessive pattern of inheritance that is associated with severe proteinuria and progression to renal failure. The condition was initially described in the review of renal lipidoses by Faraggiana and Churg (24), with the above appellation later coined by Saito (25). The glomerular lesion takes the form of lipoprotein thrombi in ectatic capillary lumina. Patients are typically of Asian ancestry, mostly Japanese, and of approximately 40 reported cases, only 2 were Caucasian in origin (26–29). The disease may present in childhood, and males outnumber females two to one (30,31). Subjects have a characteristic plasma lipoprotein profile, usually with elevation of β-lipoprotein and pre-β-lipoprotein, that resembles type III hyperlipoproteinemia; ApoE is elevated twofold to threefold (31). Unlike type III hyperlipoproteinemia, systemic manifestations of hyperlipidemia, corneal arcus, cutaneous xanthomas, and atherosclerosis are very uncommon in LPG, and the presence of ApoE isoforms E2/3, E3/3, E2/4, and E4/4 helps to differentiate the diseases. One European patient, however, was homozygous for ApoE3, the most common phenotype in Whites (26).

Clinical onset is usually marked by proteinuria and steroid-resistant nephrotic syndrome. The disease may undergo spontaneous amelioration, but slow progression to renal failure has been observed in half of patients (32). Various treatments, including immunosuppressive agents, anticoagulants, plasmapheresis, and LDL apheresis, are ineffective, though intensive lipid-lowering therapy induced resolution of symptoms and pathology in a few subjects (31,33). Recurrence of the lesion in renal allografts has also been described (28,34,35).

## Pathologic Changes

The glomeruli are large and contain capillaries distended with lipoprotein thrombi (Fig. 25.6). The capillary ecta-

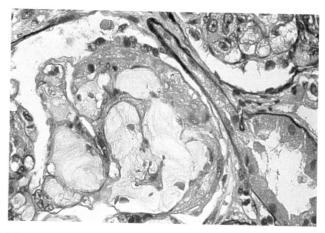

**Figure 25.6** The glomerulus from a patient with lipoprotein glomerulopathy. The capillaries are distended by pale lipoprotein thrombi that have a vague laminated appearance. Dilation of the capillary is associated with mesangiolysis. (PAS-silver methenamine; ×200.)

sia is accompanied by mesangiolysis. Capillary walls may be at first attenuated, but they often become thickened, with double contour, as in other types of mesangiolysis. The thrombi are weakly periodic acid-Schiff (PAS)-positive, periodic acid/silver methenamine-positive, and pale blue with Masson trichrome, in contrast to the typical fuchsinophilia of fibrin thrombi, with which they might be confused. The lack of congophilia excludes amyloid. The material has a moderately vacuolated and laminated structure under high magnification and is also strongly positive with oil red O and variably sudanophilic in frozen section. Increasing mesangial cellularity and matrix, segmental sclerosis, and hyalinosis progress to global sclerosis (Fig. 25.7). Tubulointerstitial changes are secondary,

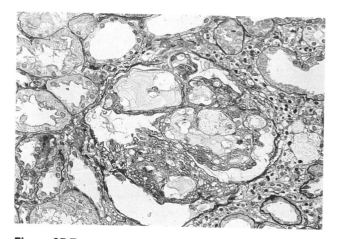

**Figure 25.7** Capillaries in the glomerulus with lipoprotein glomerulopathy are distended with lipoprotein thrombi. The lobule at bottom has increased mesangial cellularity and matrix. There are multiple adhesions to Bowman's capsule, which will progress with sclerosis and hyalinosis. (PAS; ×100.)

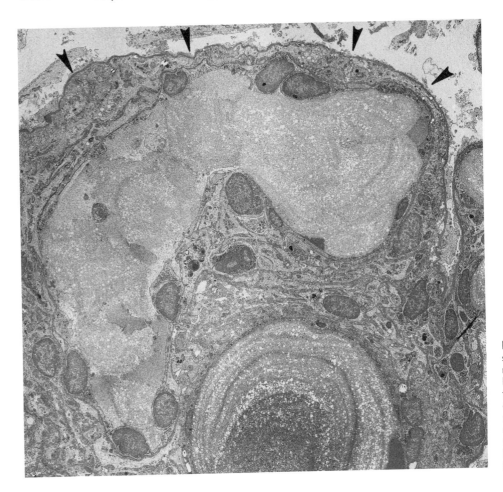

**Figure 25.8** Electron micrograph shows the glomerular capillary lumina to be filled with partially lamellated, finely vacuolated lipoprotein thrombi. The mesangium is thickened by cell processes and increased matrix. The capillary wall is also thickened, with mesangial interposition and duplication of the glomerular basement membrane (*arrowheads*). (×1900.)

although interstitial foam cells may appear early in the course. Lipoprotein glomerulopathy can coexist with other glomerular diseases.

Immunofluorescence shows that the glomerular thrombi contain β-lipoprotein, ApoB, and ApoE. Immunoglobulin M, C1q, and fibrinogen often surround the thrombi.

Electron microscopy shows the thrombi to be finely, almost concentrically lamellated, with numerous small lipid vacuoles (Fig. 25.8). In milder cases, lipid deposits may localize to the mesangium and then extend into the subendothelial space. Endothelial hypertrophy may be present in unobstructed capillary segments. Mesangial hypercellularity is associated with segmental interposition and double contour. Changes in foot processes correlate with proteinuria.

## Pathogenesis

Apolipoprotein E plays a major role in lipid and lipoprotein metabolism by functioning as the ligand for receptor-mediated catabolism of chylomicrons, VLDLs, and some HDLs. The *ApoE* gene, located on chromosome 19q13.2, has three common alleles—$\epsilon2$, $\epsilon3$, and $\epsilon4$—that code the three main isoforms: E2, E3, and E4 (36). Six common polymorphisms are *ApoE2/2*, *ApoE3/3*, *ApoE4/4*, *ApoE3/2*, *ApoE4/2*, and *ApoE4/3*. *ApoE* and its polymorphisms are also instrumental in the pathogenesis of renal disease; they are implicated in the development and progression of diabetic nephropathy and influence the serum lipid profile in end-stage renal disease (ESRD)—and thus the risk of atherosclerotic vascular disease. Novel missense mutations and deletions in the *ApoE* gene are thought to be pathogenic in LPG. Several rare mutant isoforms—*ApoE2* Sendai, *ApoE* Kyoto, *ApoE* Tokyo, and *ApoE* Maebashi—have been associated with LPG, and the development of LPG in *ApoE2* Sendai–infected mice suggests an etiologic role for these atypical isoforms (37–42). However, not all family members with mutant isoforms develop LPG, and the glomerular lesion has been described in those with nonmutated *ApoE2* (43). Moreover, LPG-like lesions may develop spontaneously in ApoE-deficient mice in the absence of *ApoE2* Sendai (44). Rare normolipidemic individuals have developed LPG, excluding a direct effect of hyperlipidemia (45). The exact mechanism remains to be defined, but a lack of systemic manifestations suggests abnormal intraglomerular lipid trafficking; the development of LPG in Fc receptor γ–deficient mice supports a role for the interference of lipoprotein uptake by mononuclear cells (46). A possible disturbance in LDL receptor binding is theorized, given that several *ApoE* mutations occur within

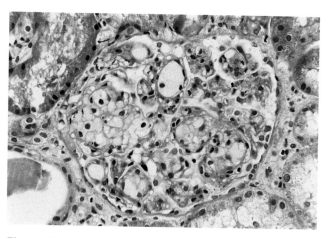

**Figure 25.9** Glomerulus from a child with type III hyperlipoproteinemia that shows groups of foam cells in the mesangium and distending the capillary lumens. (Masson's trichrome; ×400.)

the LDL receptor binding domain (47). Other genetic and environmental factors are feasibly influential in this ever more heterogenous disorder.

## Type III Hyperlipoproteinemia (Familial Dysbetalipoproteinemia)

Type III hyperlipoproteinemia with characteristic xanthomas develops in approximately 1% of patients who are homozygous for *ApoE2/2*, where it is associated with combined and often severe mixed hyperlipidemia caused by the accumulation of β-VLDL, which leads to accelerated atherosclerosis (36). Uncommonly, these patients develop glomerular lipidosis, manifest as proteinuria. Renal biopsies have shown large numbers of foam cells in the glomerular mesangium and distending glomerular capillaries (Fig. 25.9). Interstitial foam cells have been noted. Lipid vacuoles focally admixed with lamellated electron-dense material and occasional cholesterol clefts have been detected by electron microscopy in the cytoplasm of capillary foam cells, as well as in mesangial, endothelial, and tubular lining cells. Podocyte foot processes may be fused. Renal lipid deposits have cleared with plasmapheresis and lipid-lowering agents (48–50). Lipoprotein glomerulopathy has also been described in a few patients with type III hyperlipoproteinemia, including one Japanese woman with glomerular IgA deposits and two siblings with nonmutated *ApoE2* whose glomerular lipoprotein thrombi lacked the typical lamellated striae by electron microscopy (43,51).

## LYSOSOMAL STORAGE DISEASES

Several dozen diseases are caused by the pathologic accumulation of naturally occurring molecules inside lysosomes. Taxonomic classification is based on the stored material, which allows organization but does not necessarily reflect a common clinical manifestation. Many lysosomal storage diseases present in infancy or early childhood, although milder adult variants are known. Diagnosis is ascertained by combining the clinical phenotype with biochemical parameters, pathology, and possibly genetic confirmation. Fabry's disease is the classic example of a lysosomal disorder with primary kidney impairment, and in a few settings, the diagnosis is made by kidney biopsy. Most lysosomal storage diseases, however, demonstrate only morphologic involvement without clinical renal manifestations; it is unlikely that a renal biopsy in those disorders will lead to the unsuspected diagnosis. More often these become evident by disturbances of the central nervous and skeletal systems, hepatosplenomegaly, and/or dysmorphic features. In rare cases, clinical renal disease has been described, for example, nephrotic syndrome in two children with Hurler's syndrome and proximal tubular dysfunction in I-cell disease (52,53). Several observations about the kidney and lysosomal storage disease are worth noting. Renal involvement in Gaucher's disease, the most common lysosomal storage disease, only becomes symptomatic after splenectomy, a therapeutic procedure in type 1 nonneuropathic disease (54–60). Its characteristic "wrinkled paper" appearance allows the diagnosis of Gaucher's disease by light microscopy, whereas the pathology of the majority of lysosomal disorders is not distinct. Rather, storage cells are typified by clear and sometimes foamy cytoplasm, the consequence of storage material dissolving with processing. Special histochemical staining, especially on frozen sections where water and alcohol soluble substances are preserved, may help to characterize the stored material, but is frequently nonspecific. Electron microscopy can usually define the disorder further. In most instances, the diagnosis will already be known from the history, laboratory data, and enzyme analysis.

The lysosomal storage diseases that primarily involve the kidney or cause symptoms are briefly discussed below, whereas those that only secondarily involve the kidney appear in Table 25.1. Representative features of I-cell disease and neuronal ceroid lipofuscinosis are illustrated in Figures 25.10 to 25.14. Cystinosis, a lysosomal membrane transport defect, is discussed in the section with Fanconi's syndrome.

## Fabry's Disease (Angiokeratoma Corporis Diffusum Universale)

This condition, described by both Fabry (61) and Anderson (62) in 1898, is a rare metabolic disorder arising from a deficiency of a lysosomal exoglycohydrolase, ceramidetrihexosidase, commonly referred to as α-galactosidase A (63). The enzyme catalyzes the cleavage of glycosphingolipids, especially globotriaosylceramide, which is present in most

## TABLE 25.1
### RENAL INVOLVEMENT BY LYSOSOMAL STORAGE DISORDERS (WITHOUT SIGNIFICANT FUNCTIONAL IMPAIRMENT)

| Disease | Stored Material | Enzyme Defect | Storage Location | Light Microscopy | Electron Microscopy | Other |
|---|---|---|---|---|---|---|
| **Sphingolipidoses** | | | | | | |
| Gaucher's disease | Glycosyl ceramide | β-Glucosidase | MC, MI; rare, BM | Gaucher macrophage with "wrinkled" cytoplasm | 50-nm tubular bilayers | Renal involvement follows splenectomy |
| Niemann pick (types A and B) | Sphingomyelin | Sphingomyelinase | P, E, MI, PT, DT | Small, uniform cytoplasmic vacuoles | Myelin-like lamellae | Involved in >50% of cases; red birefringence with polarization |
| Metachromatic leukodystrophy | Galactocerebroside sulfate | Arylsulfatase A | H, DT, CT, rare PT | 15- to 20-μm cytoplasmic spheroids | 6- to 8-nm "stacked disks"; honeycomb pattern opposite plane | Kidney is major site of pathology in fetus; green birefringence with polarization |
| Neuronal ceroid lipofuscinosis | Ceroid (lipofuscin); subunit c of mitochondrial ATP synthase, Saposin A and D | Palmitoyl-protein thioesterase 1; tripeptidyl peptidase 1 | E, DT, PT, P | Tan, waxy lipid globules | Granular osmiophilic bodies, curvilinear profiles, fingerprints, rectilinear complexes | Yellow-green autofluorescence |
| Gangliosidosis | Ganglioside ($G_{M1}$) | β-Galactosidase | P, H, M | Clear cytoplasmic vacuoles | Finely granular material with some lipid lamellae | |
| Sandhoff's disease | Ganglioside ($G_{M2}$) and other sphingolipid | Hexosaminidase A and B | H | Clear cytoplasmic vacuoles | Finely granular material with some lipid lamellae | |
| **Mucolipidosis** | | | | | | |
| I-cell | Sialyl oligosaccharides | N-acetylglucosamine-phosphotransferase deficiency | P, rare PT, fibroblasts | Ballooning of cells with clear cytoplasmic vacuoles | Fibrillogranular | Light microscopy resembles $G_{M1}$; defect in multiple enzyme transport |
| **Mucopolysaccharidosis** | | | | | | |
| Hurler's disease (I) | Heparan sulfate, dermatan sulfate | A-L-iduronidase | P, rare PT | Clear cytoplasmic vacuoles | Sparse fibrillogranular | Reported with nephrotic syndrome |
| **Glycoproteinoses** | | | | | | |
| Fucosidosis | Fucosyl oligos | A-fucosidase | P | Clear cytoplasmic vacuoles | Sparse fibrillogranular and lamellar | |
| Mannosidosis | Mannosyl oligos | A-mannosidase, β-mannosidase | P | Clear cytoplasmic vacuoles | Sparse fibrillogranular | |
| Aspartyl glucosaminuria | Aspartyl glucosamine | Aspartyl glucosaminidase | P | Clear cytoplasmic vacuoles | Sparse fibrillogranular | |

PAS, periodic acid–Schiff; SB, Sudan black; AB, Alcian blue; P, podocyte; E, glomerular capillary endothelium; M, mesangial cells; BM, basement membrane; PT, proximal tubular cells; DT, distal tubular cells; H, loop of Henle cells; CT, collecting tubular cells; A, arterial endothelium; MI, interstitial macrophage; MC, circulating and entrapped macrophage; oligos, oligosaccharides.

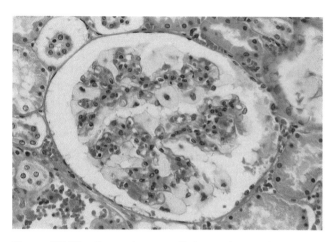

**Figure 25.10**    Glomerulus in I-cell disease has profoundly enlarged, finely vacuolated podocytes. (H&E; ×400.)

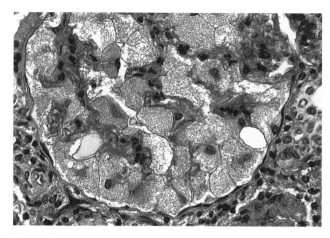

**Figure 25.11**    The vacuolated podocytes in I-cell disease contain abundant glycolipids and acidic glycosaminoglycans. (Hale colloidal iron; ×400.)

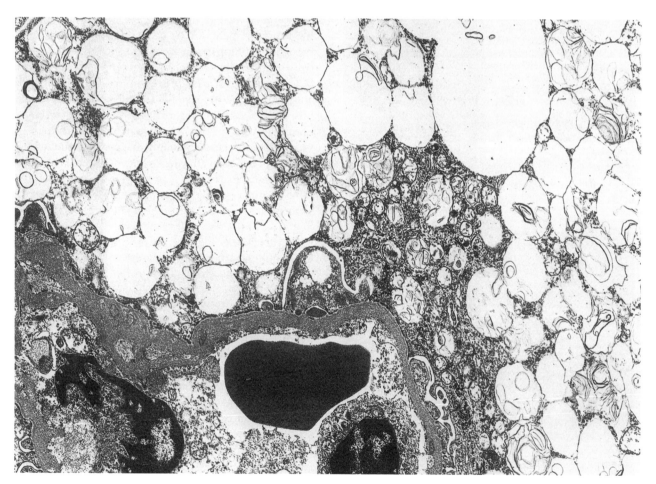

**Figure 25.12**    Electron micrograph of a podocyte in I-cell disease shows that the vacuoles contain a few membranous and lamellated inclusions. The material in the largely "empty" vacuoles may have been dissolved during processing. (×9215.)

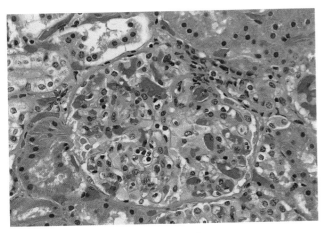

**Figure 25.13** Glomerulus from a 13-year-old boy with neuronal ceroid lipofuscinosis. The child had severe cerebral atrophy and neurologic impairment but normal renal function. The visceral podocytes are distended with granular ceroid material. (H&E; ×200.)

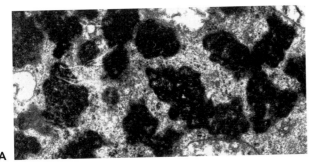

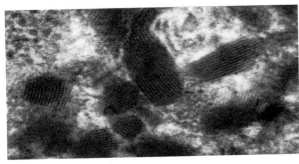

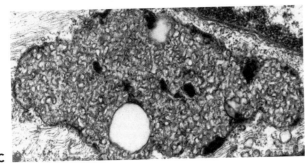

**Figure 25.14** Electron microscopy of storage material in neuronal ceroid lipofuscinosis showing characteristic granular osmiophilic bodies (**A**) and fingerprint (**B**) and curvilinear (**C**) profiles. (×31,500.)

cell membranes. Deficient enzyme activity results in the systemic accumulation of neutral glycosphingolipids with terminal α-linked galactosyl moieties, primarily globotriaosylceramide (Gb3), in plasma and particularly lysosomes of vascular endothelia of the kidneys, heart, brain, and skin.

The disease is uncommon, although it is the second most prevalent inherited lysosomal storage disorder after Gaucher's disease. Recent estimates of the frequency range from 1 in 40,000 to 1 in 117,000 births; however, Fabry's disease may be more prevalent because of a lack of recognition in patients with isolated renal or cardiac involvement. About 5% of the cases are sporadic. More than 300 mutations of the α-galactosidase gene at Xq22.1 have been described, and most are family-specific (64,65). The X-linked disease is completely expressed in hemizygous males, and heterozygous females commonly have intermediate levels of α-galactosidase A activity, occasionally with renal insufficiency (64,66). The random lyonization of the abnormal X chromosome in females leads, in fact, to highly variable levels of enzyme activity and, therefore, a broader range of clinical symptoms. Most females, contrary to historical accounts, are affected; notably, 12% of the Fabry's patients on dialysis are women (67–69). Although renal biopsy may be diagnostic (70,71), the specificity of intracellular myeloid bodies has been questioned (72); similar structures are present in silicon nephropathy and chloroquine-induced lipidosis (73–75). An aid to diagnosis may be immunofluorescence with a monoclonal anticeramide trihexoside (76). Affected males with classic and variant phenotypes are reliably diagnosed by the demonstration of deficient enzyme activity in plasma, leukocytes, or cultured cells (66). By contrast, female carriers can exhibit normal α-galactosidase A levels, such that exclusion of a carrier status can only be done by mutational analysis of the α-galactosidase A gene. Prenatal diagnosis is possible by amniocentesis at about 14 weeks and by chorionic villus sampling earlier (77). Diagnosis by molecular probes is typically limited to patients with a positive family history and known mutation; DNA sequencing has proven to be the most reliable strategy for mutation detection. A faster and more economical approach using denaturing high-performance liquid chromatography was recently reported (78).

Manifestations in hemizygous males include lesions in the skin, heart, central nervous system, blood vessels, lymph nodes, and kidneys. The skin lesions—angiokeratomas—cluster on the lower trunk and thighs as reddish-purple dark spots or papules with dilatation of superficial capillaries and variable hyperkeratosis. Vacuolization occurs in myocardiocytes, brain neurons, vascular endothelial and muscle cells, and renal glomerular and tubular epithelial cells. In addition to the classical phenotype, there are milder variants with residual α-galactosidase A activity that lack the classic features. "Cardiac" and "renal" variants present with late-onset manifestations primarily limited to heart and kidney, respectively (79,80).

Clinical features in hemizygotes commonly begin before puberty, often in infancy (81), and include, in addition to the cutaneous eruption and corneal opacities, fever, anhidrosis or hypohidrosis, acroparesthesia, and proteinuria (82). Clinical evolution to renal insufficiency and hypertension is variable over several decades and correlates with residual α-galactosidase activity (83). Progressive renal impairment is reflected in increasing proteinuria and decreasing glomerular filtration rate. Loss of urine-concentrating ability leads to polyuria, resembling diabetes insipidus, and polydipsia. Altered tubular functions have also been identified, such as impaired glucose resorption, to a greater degree than can be accounted for by reduced glomerular filtration (84,85). The urine sediment contains lipid globules showing Maltese crosses on polarization and desquamated cells containing myeloid bodies (86–88). Patients have early and extensive atherosclerosis, with an increased risk of myocardial infarction and stroke. Heterozygous females may develop corneal opacities and renal insufficiency, often without acroparesthesia.

## Pathologic Changes

Gross descriptions of the kidney in Fabry's disease are limited, but the kidneys may be enlarged by the accumulation of storage material. Renal cortical or parapelvic cysts have been demonstrated by ultrasound, magnetic resonance imaging, and computed tomographic imaging in up to 50% of patients studied, which includes classically affected hemizygous males, female carriers, and cardiac variants. The prevalence of the cysts increases with age, but their presence does not correlate with residual enzyme activity, mutation type, proteinuria, or kidney function (89,90). The nature and pathogenesis of the cysts remain undetermined.

Light microscopic changes are remarkable and can easily yield a diagnosis. The glomerular tuft contains strikingly enlarged and vacuolated glomerular cells, especially podocytes (Fig. 25.15). Similar changes are present in endothelial and mesangial cells, and occasionally in the parietal epithelial cells lining Bowman's capsule. They appear empty in paraffin sections because the accumulated glycosides are removed during clearing and paraffin embedding of the tissue. The material is preserved by prior osmification and is easily demonstrated in semithin sections of tissue embedded in epoxy resin (Fig. 25.16) (91). The material in frozen sections, whether fresh or formalin fixed, is birefringent, autofluorescent, sudanophilic, and positive to oil red O and PAS. It may also be demonstrated in frozen sections by lectin binding (92). A similar vacuolated appearance, variable in quantity but sometimes considerable, is present in tubules, particularly distal tubules and the loop of Henle (Figs. 25.15 and 25.17). Small

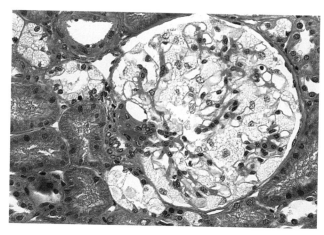

**Figure 25.15** The glomerular podocytes are swollen and finely vacuolated in a patient with Fabry's disease. Epithelial cells of distal tubules are also vacuolated. (Mallory's trichrome; ×200.)

arteries and arterioles show vacuolation of the endothelial cells and finely vacuolated areas in the smooth muscle (Fig. 25.18). Interstitial foam cells can be seen. Progression of the disease leads to glomerular mesangial sclerosis (Fig. 25.19) and capillary wall thickening, tubular atrophy, interstitial fibrosis, and arterial and arteriolar sclerosis. Immunofluorescence is negative or nonspecific. Storage of myeloid bodies has been shown also in liver and spleen (93). Hemizygotes have more severe lipid storage than do heterozygotes (94).

Electron microscopy shows enlarged secondary lysosomes filled with osmiophilic, granular to lamellated membrane structures (zebra bodies) (Fig. 25.20) (71,94). The inclusions are present especially in podocytes, Bowman's epithelium, distal tubular epithelium, and vascular myocytes, although a few inclusions may be present in virtually all renal cells (95). The periodicity of the

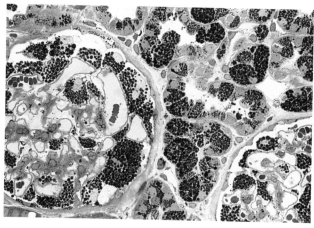

**Figure 25.16** The intracellular lipid inclusions in Fabry's disease are preserved in osmicated, epoxy-embedded tissue. The enlarged podocytes and tubular epithelial cells contain lamellated inclusion bodies (same patient as in Fig. 25.15). (Methylene blue; ×250.)

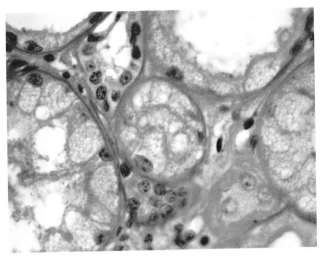

**Figure 25.17** Fine, foamy vacuolation of tubular cells from a patient with Fabry's disease. (PAS; ×400.)

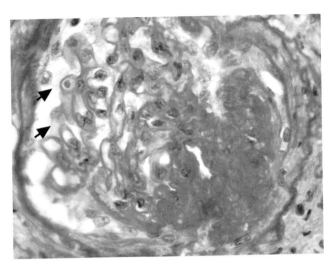

**Figure 25.19** Glomerulus in Fabry's disease shows thickened capillary walls and partial solidification. Fine vacuolation is still evident in a few podocytes (*arrows*) over an intact portion of the tuft. (PAS; ×400.)

lamellated structures, when measured in plastic thin sections, varies between 3.5 and 5.0 nm but is estimated at 14 to 15 nm when studied by freeze-fracture electron microscopy (96,97).

## Pathogenesis

The accumulation of lipid in endothelial cells is believed to promote leukocyte activation and thrombosis, leading to microvascular obstruction and ischemia (98). Endothelial deposits may be pathogenic in renal disease, as they are absent in the Fabry's knock-out mouse model that does not develop renal failure (99). Interestingly, deposits are also unapparent in endothelial cells from Fabry's car-

diac variants (64). A prothrombotic, age-dependent phenotype nonetheless exists in the α-galactosidase A knock-out, where there is progressive accumulation of Gb3 in arterial walls (100). Gubler et al (94) proposed that renal injury in human beings was ischemic, secondary to Gb3-induced fibrinoid degenerative changes in arterial walls, resulting in vascular compromise.

## Treatment

Kidney transplantation successfully corrects renal failure in Fabry's disease, yielding good graft function and patient survival (101,102). Normal renal allografts contain α-galactosidase but do not provide sufficient enzyme for systemic correction of the disorder (103,104). Myeloid bodies can appear in the allograft and are usually limited to arteriolar endothelial cells, tubular epithelial cells, and infiltrating monocytes but do not contribute significantly to graft loss or mortality (105–108). Asymptomatic living related donors must be screened carefully for heterozygosity (109,110).

Enzyme replacement therapy with recombinant human α-galactosidase (rhα-GAL) has proven to be safe and effective in hemizygous male and heterozygous female patients (111–114). Clinical trials have shown an improvement in pain, reduction in left ventricular mass, and a decline in blood and urine Gb3 levels, despite the development of antibodies to rhα-GAL. Interestingly, antibodies are not detected in women treated with rhα-GAL, likely a consequence of residual native enzyme activity (114,115). Although a trend toward stabilizing kidney functional decline has been shown, a consistent effect on proteinuria or renal function remains to be proven. These studies, however, were

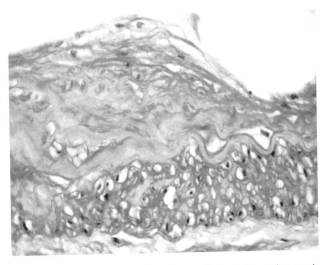

**Figure 25.18** Renal artery in end-stage Fabry's disease has moderate intimal fibroplasia, cleared endothelial cells (*top*), and empty spaces in the media (*bottom*). (PAS; ×400.)

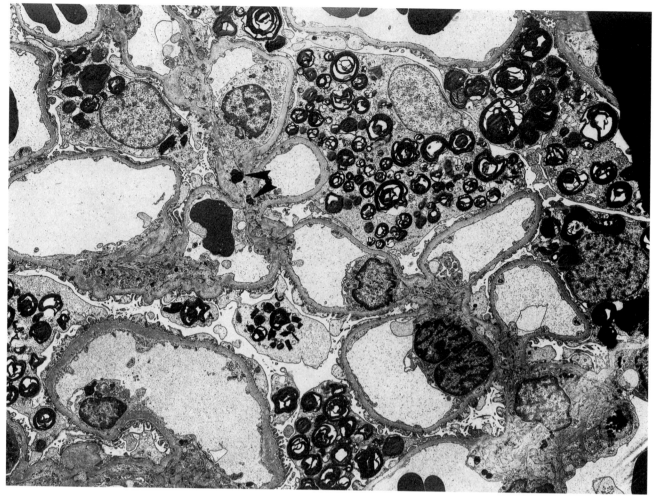

**Figure 25.20** Electron micrograph of glomerulus in Fabry's disease shows lamellated lipid inclusions ("myeloid bodies") in podocytes. A few mesangial inclusions are also present (*arrowheads*, just above center). (×3000.)

all of short duration, and extended therapy may produce significant stabilization or improvement of renal function (116). Preliminary experience with enzyme replacement therapy in kidney transplant patients with Fabry's disease also appears to be safe and often effective against extrarenal involvement (117,118).

Examination of tissues from rhα-GAL–treated patients showed clearing of deposits from endomyocardium, skin, liver, and kidney. The percentage of glomeruli without mesangial widening or sclerosis increased on therapy (112). Detailed analysis of sequential kidney biopsies from patients on enzyme replacement therapy showed lipid clearance from mesangial and interstitial cells and endothelium of peritubular capillaries, glomeruli, and arteries (111,113). Only moderate clearance was seen in tubular epithelial cells and vascular smooth muscle; podocytes were most resistant to clearance. The persistence of Gb3 in podocytes is possibly related to their low turnover and limited access to enzyme.

## Nephrosialidosis and Variants

### Sialidosis

Sialidosis is an autosomal recessive disorder affecting the degradation of glycoprotein. A deficiency of α-neuroaminidase leads to the accumulation of several sialyl oligosaccharides and glycoproteins, which are excreted in the urine and are useful in diagnosis. Type 1 sialidosis, the milder form, usually presents in the second decade with visual impairment, generalized myoclonus, ataxia, and epilepsy. Sialidosis type 2 is divided into at least two subgroups, congenital and infantile, and is distinguished by its earlier onset and mucopolysaccharide-like phenotype with abnormal facies, dysostosis multiplex, hepatosplenomegaly, and psychomotor retardation (119). Early infantile sialidosis severely affecting the kidney and causing symptomatic renal disease has been termed *nephrosialidosis* (120,121). These patients may sometimes present with congenital ascites (122). Macular cherry-red spots, myoclonus, and delayed neurodevelopment soon become manifest. Proteinuria, developing in infancy, progresses to nephrotic syndrome and to early renal insufficiency (123–126).

## Galactosialidosis

Galactosialidosis is closely related to sialidosis and results from a combined deficiency of neuraminidase and β-galactosidase owing to a defect in another lysosomal protein, the protective protein/cathepsin A, with which they are complexed (119,127). Patients have coarse facies, cherry-red spots, skeletal anomalies, and foam cells in the bone marrow. A juvenile/adult form is characterized by myoclonus, ataxia, and neurologic deterioration and is found predominantly in consanguineous Japanese families, whereas the late infantile form has hepatosplenomegaly, growth retardation, and cardiac valvular disease (126,128,129). In addition to hydrops, visceromegaly, and skeletal dysplasia, the kidneys are affected in the early infantile form of galactosialidosis, with histopathologic features and progression to renal insufficiency matching that of nephrosialidosis.

## Free Sialic Acid Storage Disorders (Salla and Infantile Sialic Acid Storage Diseases)

Sialic acid storage disorders are characterized by the lysosomal accumulation of free sialic acid as a result of defects in sialin, a carrier-mediated lysosomal membrane transport protein (130). The disorder is divided into two phenotypes: the milder Salla disease, nearly unique to the Finnish population, which shows reduced but residual function; and the severe infantile sialic acid storage disease, which is associated with complete loss of sialin activity. Patients store in their tissues and excrete in their urine approximately 10 to 100 times the normal amounts of sialic acid. The infantile form can present at birth with hepatosplenomegaly, failure to thrive, severe mental and motor retardation, coarse facies, and dysostosis multiplex; those with Salla disease are normal at birth but develop psychomotor delay and ataxia during infancy. They, too, are histopathologically similar to nephrosialidosis, and have been associated with steroid-resistant nephrotic syndrome (131–134).

## Pathologic Changes in Nephrosialidosis and Variants

The glomerular podocytes are enlarged by abundant foamy and vesicular cytoplasm (Fig. 25.21) (125,129,133,134). Similar histopathologic abnormalities in the podocytes occur in asymptomatic sialidosis. The vesicles in paraffin sections are clear, although they stain lightly with colloidal

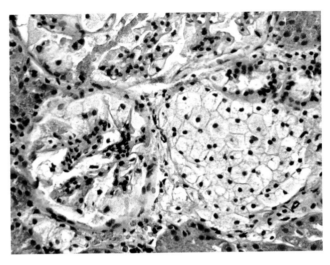

**Figure 25.21** The glomerulus in nephrosialidosis contains vacuolated podocytes that fill Bowman's space. The adjacent interstitium and tubules contain vacuolated storage cells. (H&E; ×200.)

iron, indicating partial preservation of the material during processing. Periodic acid-Schiff staining shows only a fine granularity. Tubular cells, especially in proximal tubules, and interstitial cells are also vacuolated. Cytoplasmic vacuoles have also been found in endothelial cells of renal vessels (135).

Immunofluorescence may show small, nonspecific glomerular deposits of IgM and C3, reflecting hyalinosis. In sialidosis, some podocyte vacuoles in frozen sections bind concanavalin A and wheat germ agglutinin, demonstrating mannose and sialic acid residues within the stored oligosaccharides (18).

Electron microscopy shows the vacuoles to be membrane bound and almost empty (Fig. 25.22). Some vacuoles contain granules and membranous profiles of electron-dense material. Similar vacuoles are present in tubules and occasionally in mesangial cells (132). Podocyte changes relate to proteinuria, and renal insufficiency is associated with glomerular collapse and sclerosis.

No specific treatment exists for this rare group of lysosomal storage disorders. A few attempts at bone marrow transplantation have met with limited success (136).

## VITAMIN DISORDERS

### Cobalamin C Deficiency

Cobalamin C (cblC) is required for conversion of dietary vitamin $B_{12}$ to its reduced and methylated forms, which function as coenzymes. Deficiency of cblC, inherited as an autosomal recessive trait, leads to impaired activities of methylmalonyl CoA mutase and methionine synthase, resulting in methylmalonic aciduria and homocystinuria. Major clinical problems in cblC-deficient patients typically

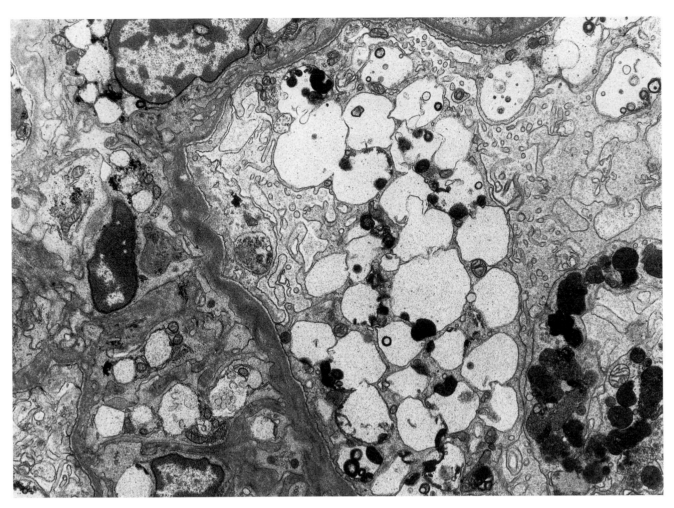

**Figure 25.22** Electron microscopy of a glomerulus in nephrosialidosis shows vacuolated podocytes and mesangial cells. The vacuoles are partially filled with electron-dense bodies and also contain lucent and finely granular material. (×10,400.) (Courtesy of Drs. C. E. Kashtan and Z. Posalaky.)

become apparent in the first few months as failure to thrive, neurologic and ophthalmologic abnormalities, and hematologic disturbances (especially megaloblastic anemia); a few present in early childhood and adolescence (137). Several patients have had proteinuria and features of hemolytic-uremic syndrome, rarely as the sole manifestation of late-onset disease (138). Diagnosis is made by finding the combination of methylmalonic aciduria and homocystinuria with normal serum vitamin $B_{12}$ and transcobalamin II concentrations.

Renal pathology in this group of patients has been that of thrombotic microangiopathy (139–142). The glomeruli have shown mild mesangial and endothelial proliferation, capillary dilatation, and basement membrane splitting (Fig. 25.23). Intracapillary fibrin or platelet thrombi are unusual. Foot process fusion with endothelial cell detachment and expansion of the subendothelial space by granular, fibrillary material has been noted by electron microscopy (Fig. 25.24). Immunofluorescence is typically negative or nonspecific, but peripheral membrane and

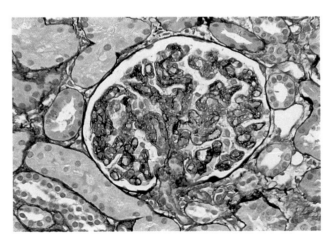

**Figure 25.23** Mildly hypercellular glomerulus from a 5-year-old boy with cobalamin C deficiency. Chronic microangiopathic changes include thickened and duplicated basement membranes without capillary thrombi. (PAS-silver methenamine; ×400.)

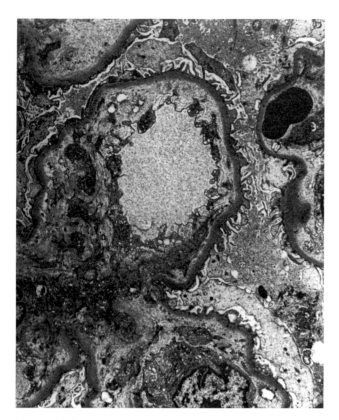

**Figure 25.24**   Electron microscopy in cobalamin C deficiency showing narrowing of the capillary lumen by subendothelial granular and fibrillar material and focal mesangial cell interposition. Foot process fusion is only focal. (×2500.)

primarily mesangial C3, C1q, and IgM were found in a single case, which also had widespread electron-dense deposits (142).

The precise locations of defects and the responsible genes have not yet been identified. Presumed mechanisms for the renal pathology include endothelial dysfunction, with contributions from homocysteine. Successful management requires large amounts of hydroxocobalamin and betaine. Many patients die from severe hemolytic anemia despite intensive therapy, although delayed presentation is associated with improved outcomes.

## ORGANIC ACID DISORDERS

### Methylmalonic Acidemia

Isolated methylmalonic acidemia is an autosomal recessive disorder of branched chain amino acid metabolism that presents with recurrent vomiting, lethargy, dehydration, failure to thrive, hypotonia, and metabolic ketoacidosis. It is caused by a deficiency of the enzyme methylmalonyl–CoA mutase (MCM); defects in cobalamin metabolism (cblA, cblB) also yield methylmalonic acidemia. Children with MCM deficiency are cobalamin nonresponsive and

typically develop renal tubular dysfunction that often progresses to ESRD by early adolescence (143). Analyses of nonvolatile organic acid patterns and acylcarnitine profiles are useful for diagnosis. Treatment is centered on dietary control and carnitine supplementation, with emergency support during times of illness.

Chronic organ damage ensues despite improved outcome of the acute metabolic crisis. Impaired renal function occurs in the majority of patients, and kidney pathology has shown tubulointerstitial nephritis with interstitial fibrosis, tubular atrophy, and mononuclear cell infiltrates (144–146). Chronic renal failure usually develops in the first or second decade and can be treated with dialysis. Liver transplantation provides enzyme to effectively avoid systemic metabolic derangement, but combined kidney/liver transplantation is required for replacement of localized kidney enzyme. The effectiveness of combination transplantation as a therapeutic option remains to be proven (147,148).

## CARBOHYDRATE DISORDERS

### Glycogen Storage Disease

The glycogen storage diseases are genetic defects that result in the storage of abnormal amounts and/or abnormal forms of glycogen. Some affect several tissues, whereas others may affect only one, most commonly the liver or muscle because of their abundant quantities of glycogen.

Glycogen storage disease type I (GSD-I) is a group of autosomal recessive disorders with an incidence of 1 in 100,000. It includes two major subtypes: GSD-Ia (von Gierke disease), caused by a deficiency of glucose-6-phosphatase (G6Pase), which accounts for about 80% of cases; and GSD-Ib, caused by a deficiency in the glucose-6-phosphate transporter (G6PT) (149). Glucose-6 translocates glucose-6-phosphate from the cytoplasm into the lumen of the endoplasmic reticulum, where G6Pase hydrolyses it into glucose and phosphate; together these enzymes maintain glucose homeostasis, and their deficiency results in an accumulation of glycogen, as conversion of glucose-6-phosphate to glucose in both glycogenolysis and gluconeogenesis is impaired. Glucose-6-phosphatase is expressed in high levels in the gluconeogenetic liver and kidney, whereas G6PT is ubiquitous.

Patients with GSD-I commonly become symptomatic in early infancy, presenting with hepatorenomegaly. They are hypoglycemic, with large abdomens and rounded faces, and some present with seizures. Hyperlipidemia, paralleling that in type IV hyperlipidemia, causes xanthomas; hyperuricemia may cause symptoms of gout in older children. The diagnosis, based on clinical and biochemical findings, is confirmed by measurement of G6Pase activity in fresh liver biopsy samples. More recent recommendations for diagnosis combine clinical and biochemical abnormalities with mutational analysis, the latter of which can also be used for carrier testing of at-risk families and prenatal diagnosis (150).

Renal enlargement begins early, and functional impairment is a late complication (151). Effective renal plasma flow and glomerular filtration are increased at first, and proteinuria and hypertension develop later (152–154). Increased prostaglandin production secondary to renal tubulopathy may be responsible for glomerular hyperperfusion and hyperfiltration (155). The degree of hyperfiltration correlates with renal size (156). Patients have an incomplete form of distal tubular acidosis, and they are prone to nephrocalcinosis and stone disease, which can be demonstrated within the first year of life (157–160). A form of Fanconi's syndrome, originally thought to be associated with GSD-I, is now attributed to Fanconi-Bickel's syndrome (see section later in this chapter).

## Pathologic Changes

Renal enlargement and glomerular hyperperfusion are associated with twofold to threefold glomerular hypertrophy. The glomeruli may be mildly hypercellular, and they contain large amounts of mesangial lipid. Tubules are lined with large vacuolated cells engorged with glycogen (Fig. 25.25). Progressive renal damage leads to focal segmental and, eventually, complete glomerular sclerosis (Fig. 25.26), the latter with arteriolar sclerosis, tubular atrophy, and interstitial fibrosis (161). Immunofluorescence is often positive for immunoglobulin and complement components; it may be positive for ApoAI (162).

Electron microscopy shows twofold thickening of the glomerular basement membrane, sometimes diffusely.

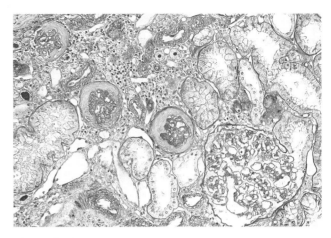

**Figure 25.26** Nephrectomy kidney from a child with GSD-I shows an enlarged glomerulus and extensive global glomerulosclerosis. Atrophic tubules are associated with interstitial inflammation, fibrosis, and thickened arteries. (PAS; ×50.)

Lamellation and irregular contour, reminiscent of the abnormality in Alport's syndrome, occur in areas of severe thickening (Fig. 25.27) (163,164). Glycogen granules are present among the basement membrane lamellae and focally within mesangial, epithelial, and endothelial cells. Widening of foot processes relates to proteinuria. Mesangial widening and segmental sclerosis are also present. The glomerular abnormality partially resembles that of diabetic nephropathy. Glycogen is present both diffusely and in membrane-bound vesicles in tubular epithelial cells.

## Pathogenesis and Treatment

The *G6PC* gene for G6Pase is located on chromosome 17q21, and 84 mutations in the catalytic subunit have been identified in patients with GSD-Ia; a stringent genotype–phenotype correlation does not exist (150,165–167). More than 70 mutations in the *SLC37A4* gene on chromosome 11q23, which encodes G6PT, are responsible for GSD-Ib (non-Ia) (168). Both conditions result in multiorgan system impairment, but dietary control may ameliorate dysfunction with early intervention (151,169). Captopril reduced microalbuminuria in some patients, but ESRD and complications of liver adenomas contribute to increased morbidity and mortality (169,170). Kidney transplantation has been used for those who develop ESRD, although glucose metabolism will not be improved. Combined liver/kidney transplantation may be indicated, but posttransplant complications have been noted (171).

Kidney involvement in other GSD subtypes is limited. Renal tubules in GSD-II (acid maltase deficiency) accumulate glycogen without functional impairment. Acute tubular necrosis secondary to rhabdomyolysis has been reported in McArdle's disease (GSD-V) (172,173).

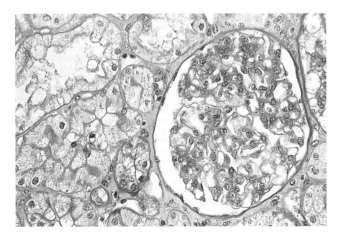

**Figure 25.25** A glomerulus in a patient with GSD-I is hypertrophied and has mildly increased numbers of prominent mesangial cells. Adjacent tubules show intense vacuolation of epithelial cells. (PAS; ×100.)

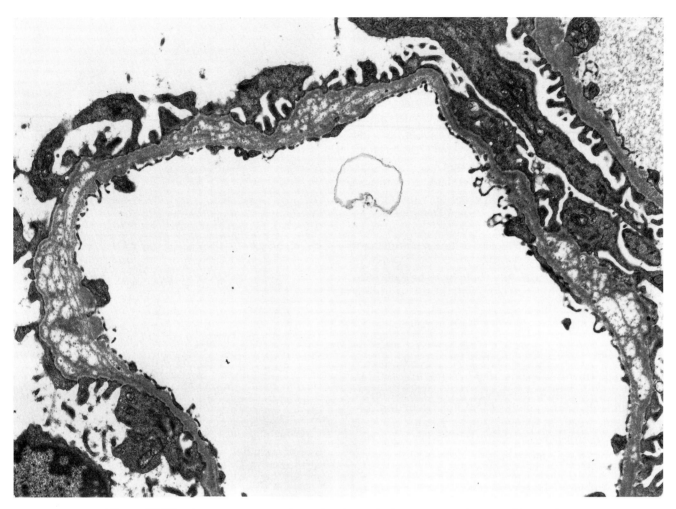

**Figure 25.27**    Electron microscopy shows the glomerular basement membrane in GSD-I to be frequently lamellated, incorporating irregular lucencies and fine granules. (×12,000.) (Courtesy of Dr. R. Verani.)

## PEROXISOMAL DISORDERS

Peroxisomes are single membrane–bound organelles that are found in nearly all cells and participate in β- and α-oxidation of fatty acids; the synthesis of bile acids, cholesterol, and plasmalogens; as well as amino acid and purine metabolism. Disorders are grouped as those that affect single peroxisomal enzymes and as biogenesis disorders (assembly deficiencies) in which the organelle fails to form normally, resulting in defects that involve multiple peroxisomal functions (174). Defects in peroxisomes cause multiorgan disease that often involves the nervous system. Those discussed here include renal abnormalities.

### Zellweger's Syndrome

Zellweger's syndrome (cerebrohepatorenal syndrome) is caused by defective biogenesis of peroxisomes owing to various mutations in at least 12 different *PEX* genes that encode peroxins, which are proteins required for peroxi-

some assembly. Peroxisomal enzymes, synthesized in the cytosol, fail to be incorporated into peroxisomes, resulting in a complete dearth of functional peroxisomes and all peroxisomal functions (175). Peroxisomes are markedly reduced and sometimes absent in the kidney, liver, and other organs (176). Infants are affected at birth and show severe hypotonia, feeding disability, and elevated very long-chain fatty acids in blood and tissues. They have abnormal facies, with high forehead and hypertelorism. Histopathologic studies of the brain have shown abnormal neuronal migration and abnormal cortical convolutions. Cerebral white matter is poorly myelinated, and it contains abundant sudanophilic lipid. Hepatocellular hemosiderosis is characteristic, and cell damage and death progress to cirrhosis. Stippled epiphyses are often demonstrated radiographically. More than 90% of patients have renal cortical cysts, often of glomerular origin, that may develop in utero and vary from microscopic dimensions to several centimeters in size (Figs. 25.28 and 25.29) (174,177). Most patients die within the first year of life.

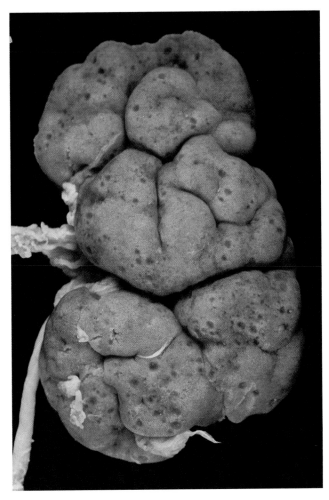

**Figure 25.28**  Autopsy kidney from infant with Zellweger's syndrome shows prominent fetal lobulation and numerous small, thin-walled cysts in the peripheral cortex and subcapsular area.

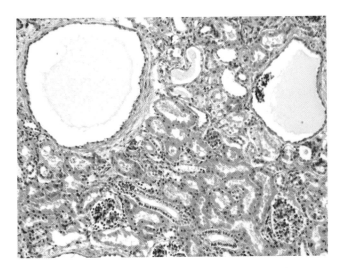

**Figure 25.29**  Microcysts of both tubular and glomerular origin are evident in the cortex of a Zellweger's kidney without significant functional implication. (H&E; ×100.)

Although the renal cysts are usually asymptomatic and renal function is usually normal, occasional instances of albuminuria, aminoaciduria, and mild azotemia have been described. In addition, several babies with the Zellweger phenotype were reported to have severe renal cystic dysplasia and early-onset renal failure, although their diagnoses may be arguable because these reports predate the current classification of peroxisomal disorders (178,179). The hypotonia, hepatic dysfunction, facial dysmorphism, and renal cysts of Zellweger could theoretically evoke a diagnosis of glutaric aciduria type 2 (multiple acyl CoA dehydrogenase deficiency), a mitochondrial electron transfer disorder, but a characteristic organic acid pattern in the urine establishes the latter diagnosis. Renal anomalies in glutaric aciduria type 2 may be dramatic and include extensive cortical and medullary cyst formation, sometimes with dysplastic changes (180–183).

## Adult Refsum's Disease

Adult (classic) Refsum's disease (heredopathia atactica polyneuritiformis), a rare autosomal recessive disorder, results from an abnormal accumulation of phytanic acid owing to a defect in phytanoyl-CoA hydroxylase (PhyH). Most patients harbor mutations in the *PHYH* gene, although in a subset, mutations have been found in *PEX7*, which encodes the peroxisomal targeting signal receptor that is required for the import of PhyH into peroxisomes (184). Heterozygotes, with approximately 50% enzyme activity, do not accumulate phytanic acid.

Phytanic acid is a 20-carbon, branched-chain fatty acid derived from phytol, a component of chlorophyll. The human source of phytol and phytanic acid is entirely dietary, from dairy products and animal fats. Phytanic acid is stored in plasma and tissues, mostly adipose tissue, liver, kidney, muscle, and nerve, predominantly in triglycerides, and to a lesser extent in phospholipids and cholesterol esters (185).

Clinical symptoms usually present in late childhood as anosmia and night blindness, caused by retinitis pigmentosa. Peripheral neuropathy, cerebellar ataxia, nerve deafness, cardiac arrhythmias, and ichthyosis often occur in the following decades (186). About 35% of patients have bone abnormalities, especially in the hands and feet, that are present at birth but typically are not recognized until other disease manifestations become evident (187). High concentrations of protein are present in spinal fluid. Full expression of the disease occurs during the fourth or fifth decade, but it can manifest in childhood.

Renal involvement is demonstrated by proteinuria, mild renal insufficiency, glycosuria, and lipiduria. Elevated plasma phytanic acid esters are demonstrated by gas chromatography, but these elevations are not specific to Refsum's disease since they are seen in peroxisome biogenesis disorders. The condition is treated by dietary restriction.

Treatment of acute exacerbations by plasmapheresis may allow a less restrictive diet (188).

## Pathologic Changes

Renal tubular epithelial cells, both proximal and distal, are filled with fine sudanophilic vacuoles. Glomeruli are initially minimally affected, with only mild podocyte vacuolization. Glomerular sclerosis and interstitial fibrosis correlate with renal insufficiency. Electron microscopy shows perinuclear cytoplasmic vacuoles and membrane-bound vesicles in glomerular and tubular epithelial cells. Lancet-shaped inclusions of microtubular material are present within cells of the distal tubules and loop of Henle (189); they are visible in semithin plastic sections. The inclusions resemble mitochondrial paracrystalline structures, but they are not membrane bound. They contain quadrangular microtubular arrays, shown in cross section to have geometric patterns (Fig. 25.30) (190). Their origin and composition are unknown, although they may be lipid organized into lamellae (191).

## Primary Hyperoxaluria

Primary hyperoxaluria (PH) exists in two autosomal recessive forms. In type 1 (PH1), which is more common, continuing renal deposition of calcium oxalate leads to nephrocalcinosis, recurrent nephrolithiasis, and chronic renal insufficiency. The disease is caused by a deficiency of the liver-specific peroxisomal alanine–glyoxylate amino-transferase (AGT), which transaminates glyoxylate to glycine (192). Glyoxylate thus accumulates and is instead oxidized to oxalate and reduced to glycolate. Oxalate is not metabolized further and is eliminated from the body in the urine. Crystallization occurs from highly concentrated solutions, causing renal tubulointerstitial damage and progressive renal functional impairment. Type 2 hyperoxaluria (PH2), which produces oxalate urolithiasis without renal failure, is caused by defective cytosolic D-glycerate dehydrogenase-glyoxylate reductase (193).

Primary hyperoxaluria type 1 is characterized by hyperoxaluria and hyperglycolic aciduria. Renal colic and hematuria, secondary to urolithiasis, often commence in

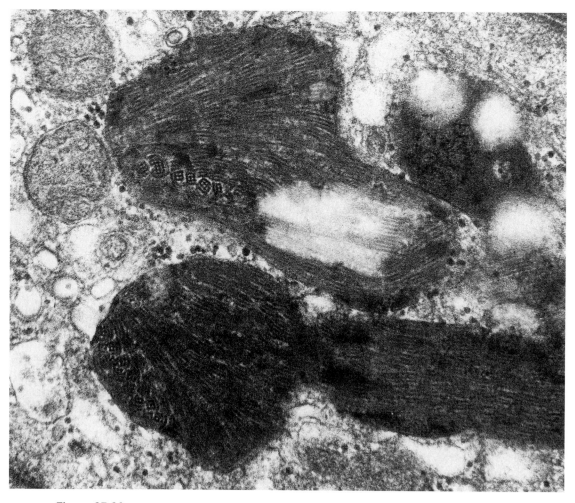

**Figure 25.30** The tubular epithelial cells in adult Refsum's disease contain crystalloid inclusions, with geometric structures. (×77,000.) (Courtesy of Dr. B. Panner.)

childhood, although there is marked heterogeneity in the onset and severity. Approximately 10% of patients have severe disease, with early infantile onset manifesting as failure to thrive, severe metabolic acidosis, anemia, and rapid progression to renal failure, whereas another 10% may not become symptomatic before the fourth or fifth decades (194). Progressive parenchymal deposition of calcium oxalate impairs renal function, which ultimately leads to systemic oxalosis. Complications include severe deforming osteopathy, arthropathy, cardiomyopathy, retinopathy, neuropathy, and pancytopenia. The kidneys are often small and may feel gritty on cut section (Fig. 25.31). Small, polyhedral or rhomboid, doubly refractile crystals are recognized histologically and accumulate in tubules, where they compress and destroy epithelium. The crystals can extend into the interstitium and induce fibrosis (Fig. 25.32). End-stage kidneys show extensive

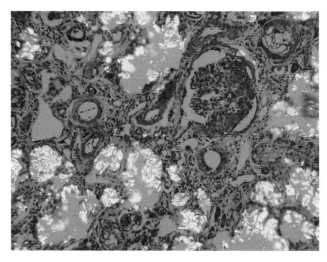

**Figure 25.32** Renal tubules in primary hyperoxaluria are filled with rhomboid and polyhedral refractile oxalate crystals. A glomerulus is collapsed and segmentally sclerotic (same kidney as Fig. 25.31). (H&E, partial polarization; ×200.)

glomerulosclerosis and widespread interstitial fibrosis that encases abundant crystals (Fig. 25.33).

The combination of renal failure and urolithiasis should prompt clinical suspicion of PH; however, none of the symptoms is unique. Markedly elevated levels of urinary oxalate in the absence of any likely causes of secondary hyperoxaluria usually indicate PH. Histologic demonstration of calcium oxalate deposition in the kidney has been used for diagnosis, but, again, it is not specific for primary disease. Definitive diagnosis of PH1 is achieved by determining the AGT activity in a liver biopsy sample.

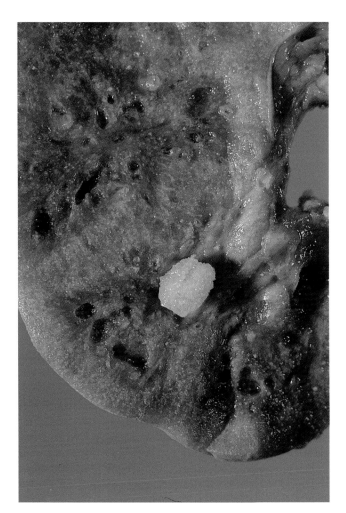

**Figure 25.31** Autopsy kidney of 5-year-old boy with primary hyperoxaluria who presented at 5 months with seizures and failure to thrive. The kidneys were one third the expected weight and had a gritty consistency caused by yellow-tan oxalate crystals. A 0.3-cm calculus occupies a calix. (Courtesy of J. Siebert, Ph.D., Children's Hospital and Regional Medical Center, University of Washington.)

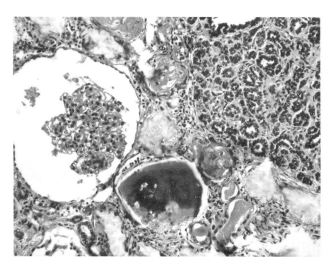

**Figure 25.33** The end-stage kidney in primary hyperoxaluria has interstitial fibrosis and inflammation that separate crystal-filled tubules. This unique case had marked embryonal hyperplasia characterized by nodular proliferations of small basophilic tubules peppering the cortex; the patient was not dialyzed. Osseous metaplasia is present adjacent to the glomerulus. (H&E; ×250.)

More than 50 mutations have been identified in the *AGXT* gene, which resides on chromosome 2q37.3 (195). Mutations result in peroxisome-to-mitochondrion targeting defects, intraperoxisomal AGT aggregation, absence of AGT catalytic activity, and absence of both catalytic activity and immunoreactivity. The clinical heterogeneity may relate to great variability in enzymatic activity among patients but is clearly influenced by potential modifier genes, environmental factors, and genetic background, as the genotype/phenotype correlation is limited (196,197).

Type 2 PH is rare and can be distinguished from PH1 by finding elevated glycolate and L-glycerate in addition to high oxalate levels. Clinical manifestations are less severe and consist primarily of urolithiasis, although ESRD has been documented (198–200). Liver enzyme analysis confirms the diagnosis. At least 14 mutations in the *GRHPR* gene on chromosome 9 are responsible for PH2 (201).

Generous fluid intake and drugs that increase the urinary solubility product are important therapeutic measures (202). Pyridoxine (vitamin $B_6$), which affects AGT expression or activity, lowers urinary oxalate in only about one third of patients (202). Pyridoxamine, by scavenging carbonyl intermediates in the glyoxylate pathway, inhibits oxalate biosynthesis, has been shown to decrease crystal formation in hyperoxaluric animal models, and may offer therapeutic hope for the treatment of PH (203). Combined liver/kidney transplantation, which results in enzyme replacement, has been met with better outcomes than the disappointing early results from isolated kidney transplantation, in which oxalate deposits constantly recurred in the graft (204,205). Preemptive liver transplantation may be considered in some settings.

# MEMBRANE TRANSPORT DISORDERS

Functional tubular abnormalities take the form of both specific defects in solute resorption and generalized disorders of proximal tubular transport. Most specific transport defects are heritable and are not associated with structural abnormalities.

Fanconi's syndrome is a heterogeneous disorder of proximal tubular transport, by definition comprising aminoaciduria, glucosuria, and phosphaturia. Children develop hypophosphatemic, vitamin D-resistant rickets; adults develop osteomalacia. The disorder commonly includes proximal tubular acidosis, impaired urine concentration, and impaired resorption of potassium, urate, and citrate. Fanconi's syndrome occurs as a primary idiopathic disease (Lignac-de Toni-Debré-Fanconi's syndrome), a heritable tubular defect, or a secondary manifestation of a recognized heritable metabolic disease. Acquired Fanconi's syndrome is the result of a variety of toxic and immunologic renal tubular injuries. The renal manifestations are largely the same in all forms. So-called incomplete

Fanconi's syndromes with, for example, only renal glycosuria and aminoaciduria may be caused by the same basic tubular disturbances as occur in the complete syndrome.

Fanconi's syndrome seems to be the final common manifestation of assorted cellular perturbations that interfere with tubular epithelial function by affecting solute uptake and/or excretion. Diverse etiologies can all affect the delicate balance that maintains tubular function; these include (a) altered energy production, for example, mitochondrial dysfunction that inhibits $Na^+$, $K^+$-ATPase and thereby impedes $Na^+$-dependent transport; (b) abnormal apical or basolateral membrane transport molecules, for example, mutations in *SLC6A19* or *GLUT2*; and (c) interference with membrane trafficking and recycling, for example, *CLCN5* mutations that interrupt the activities of megalin and cubilin. As new discoveries are made, so-called idiopathic Fanconi's syndrome may cease to exist.

## Inherited Fanconi's Syndrome

### Idiopathic Fanconi's Syndrome

Primary Fanconi's syndrome occurs in both adults and children as familial traits that appear to be predominantly autosomal dominant (206). Sporadic cases without identifiable nephrotoxicity are not necessarily genetic. Although a defined genetic defect is currently unknown, this form of the syndrome can only be diagnosed when no underlying metabolic disease exists and all possible acquired causes have been excluded. The demonstrated absence or partial loss of proximal tubular brush border is common to all forms of Fanconi's syndrome. The occurrence of heavy glycogen deposition (Armanni-Ebstein's lesion), similar to that in diabetes mellitus, has been described in the pars recta of some patients with Fanconi's syndrome (207). Clinical manifestations in children include failure to thrive, growth retardation, polydipsia, polyuria, rickets, and unexplained fever. Adults have weakness and bone pain, with polydipsia and polyuria.

### Cystinosis

Cystinosis, a rare autosomal recessively inherited lysosomal transport disorder, is the most common identifiable cause of Fanconi's syndrome in children. It has an estimated incidence of 1 in 100,000 to 200,000 live births, although higher incidences are reported in some regions of France, Germany, Quebec, and the United Kingdom (208). More than 85 mutations have been identified in the responsible gene, *CTNS*, which resides on chromosome 17p13 and encodes cystinosin, a lysosomal transmembrane protein (209,210). It differs thereby from other lysosomal storage diseases, which are caused by deficiencies in lysosomal acid hydrolases.

## Clinical Presentation

Cystinosis is clinically classified into three forms. Infantile cystinosis is nephropathic, with early onset of Fanconi's syndrome and progression to ESRD usually within the first decade of life. Less severe variants probably form a continuum, but two distinct subtypes include (a) intermediate cystinosis ("juvenile" or "late-onset"), which causes a mild nephropathy with slow progression of renal impairment, without Fanconi's syndrome; and (b) ocular or nonnephropathic cystinosis ("benign" or "adult"), which is characterized by ocular findings but no renal involvement.

Free cystine, from lysosomal protein hydrolysis, increases in cells to concentrations between 10 and 1000 times normal. Cystine accumulation and crystal formation vary considerably among tissues and may be related to different rates of protein degradation and cell turnover. The diagnosis can be made by demonstrating increased concentrations of cystine in peripheral leukocytes and other cells or by demonstrating cystine crystals in the cornea by slit-lamp examination and in bone marrow macrophages, conjunctiva, intestinal mucosa, and kidney by polarization microscopy. In contrast to cystinuria, urinary cystine levels are not elevated. Diagnosis of fetal disease can be made by measurement of cystine in amniotic fluid, amniocytes, or chorionic villi. The crystals, easily dissolved from the tissues in aqueous solutions during tissue processing, are preserved in alcoholic solutions. They have a hexagonal, rhombohedral, or polymorphous configuration; are birefringent; and, even when sparse, are demonstrable by polarization microscopy in frozen sections.

Children with infantile nephropathic cystinosis develop polyuria, polydipsia, dehydration, and febrile episodes within the first year of life. Features of Bartter's syndrome and nephrogenic diabetes insipidus have preceded the development of Fanconi's syndrome in occasional patients (211,212). Proximal tubular dysfunction, with aminoaciduria, glycosuria, phosphaturia, and renal tubular acidosis, leads to vitamin D-refractory rickets and growth retardation. Patients may develop muscle weakness as a consequence of myopathy. Glomerular impairment leads to end-stage renal failure by 10 years of age. With renal replacement therapy, widespread end-organ damage may develop from cystine deposition in eyes, liver, endocrine glands, and the muscular and central nervous systems. Photophobia and abnormal retinal pigmentation are not uncommon. Caucasian children have noticeably less skin and hair pigmentation than their unaffected siblings as a consequence of defective melanin synthesis; the skin and hair of patients from darkly pigmented ethnic groups appear normally pigmented.

## Pathologic Changes

The ultimate histopathologic abnormality in all forms of Fanconi's syndrome is tubular atrophy with interstitial fibrosis, variable inflammation, and progressive glomerular

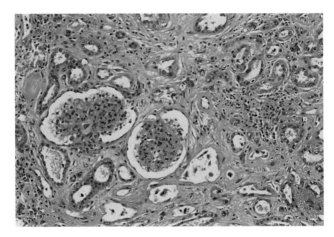

**Figure 25.34** Renal cortex from an 8-year-old boy with cystinosis showing considerable atrophy of the tubules, interstitial fibrosis, and glomerular solidification. (H&E; ×200.)

sclerosis (Fig. 25.34). Morphologic complications include the occasional development of nephrocalcinosis.

The tubular atrophy has been shown by microdissection to be particularly pronounced in the first part of the proximal tubule, in which a shortened and narrow postglomerular segment has been described as the "swan-neck deformity" (Fig. 25.35) (213). This abnormality probably represents a moderately severe degree of secondary tubular atrophy and is neither specific to Fanconi's syndrome nor a likely explanation of its functional derangements. Among the earlier tubular changes, loss of brush border accompanies cell shortening, and the generalized absence of brush border mentioned in the description of idiopathic Fanconi's syndrome may well be a secondary phenomenon. Other secondary changes include cellular vacuolization and basement membrane calcification, the latter perhaps a consequence of renal insufficiency and secondary hyperparathyroidism.

Cystinosis is distinguished by the deposition of cystine crystals, predominantly in the interstitium (Fig. 25.36). Large extracellular collections of crystals lie among the tubules in the cortical labyrinth. A few crystals may be present in tubular and glomerular epithelial cells, and clefts are identified by electron microscopy in podocytes and mesangial cells (Fig. 25.37) (214,215).

Glomerular podocytes in cystinosis are sometimes opaque on light microscopic examination of semithin sections of osmicated, plastic-embedded tissue; transmission electron microscopy confirms the observation, showing the dark cells to be filled with electron-dense granular material (215). Dark cells are present rarely in tubules and occasionally in the interstitium. The phenomenon is probably caused by a reaction between osmium and intracellular cystine; electron-probe analysis shows that the dark cells contain sulfide, a constituent of cystine. Early and distinctive abnormalities in cystinosis are multinucleated

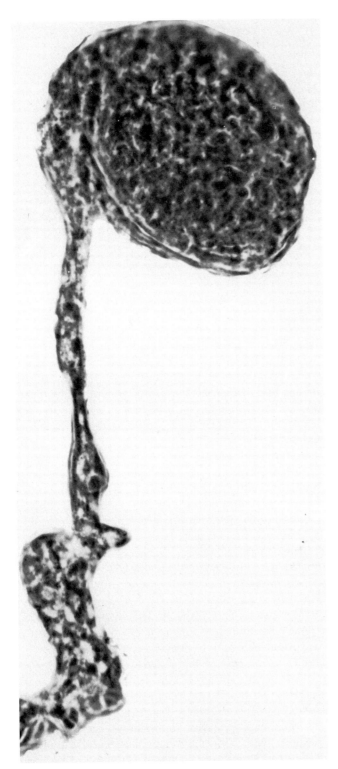

**Figure 25.35**   "Swan neck" appearance of a dissected proximal convoluted tubule. The thinned early part of the proximal convoluted segment is apparent (glomerulus at top). (Courtesy of Dr. E. M. Darmady.)

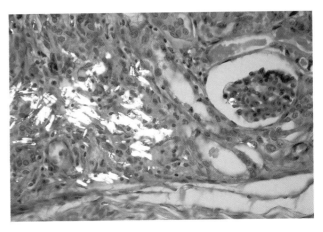

**Figure 25.36**   Alcohol-fixed kidney section from a child with cystinosis showing interstitial deposition of rectangular refractile cystine crystals. A rare crystal is also evident in the glomerulus. (H&E, partial polarization; ×100.)

podocytes (Fig. 25.38) and occasionally, tubular cells, a finding not unique to cystinosis but helpful in diagnosis (214,216). Similar cells occur in noncystinotic Fanconi's syndrome and few other conditions.

Intermediate, or juvenile, cystinosis causes predominantly glomerular disease, with mesangial hypercellularity,

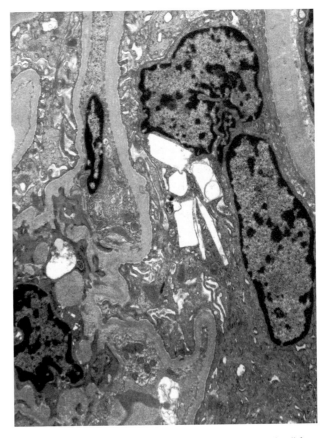

**Figure 25.37**   Electron micrograph shows an epithelial cell from a glomerular tuft that contains rectangular and spindle-shaped clear areas, presumably once occupied by cystine. (×4000.)

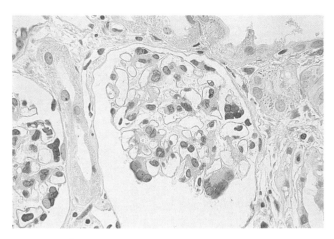

**Figure 25.38** Glomeruli from a child with cystinosis showing multinucleated visceral epithelial cells. (H&E; ×160.)

increased matrix, capillary wall thickening, and segmental and global glomerular sclerosis (217,218). Crystal deposition may only be detected by electron microscopy.

### Pathogenesis and Treatment

Cystinosin, a seven transmembrane domain protein, is a highly specific $H^+$-driven cystine transporter (219). Mutations usually associated with infantile cystinosis cause premature termination of cystinosin and tend to abolish transport of cystine, whereas those associated with milder clinical phenotypes tend to reduce transport (220). The most common mutation is a 57-kilobase deletion found typically in people of northern European descent (210). The etiology of Fanconi's syndrome in cystinosis is not understood, but in vitro studies using cystine-loaded cells have shown a decrease in cellular adenosine triphosphate (ATP) concentration and an inhibition of $Na^+$-dependent transporters, which could potentially account for urinary losses of amino acids, $HCO_3^-$, and phosphate (221,222). Cystinotic cells undergo apoptosis at two- to fourfold higher rates than controls, and renal proximal tubular cells are especially vulnerable, leading to speculation that lysosomal cystine promotes inappropriate cell death and decreased cell numbers in many tissues (223). Curiously, the *ctns* –/– mouse shows no proximal tubulopathy, although the kidney contains a high level of cystine and focal crystal deposits are within proximal tubular cells (224). These observations suggest alternative pathways in the mice that rescue these cells from ATP depletion and apoptosis.

Treatment with oral cysteamine can prevent or significantly delay the complications of cystinosis, allowing survival into adulthood and making early diagnosis and proper treatment critical (208). Kidney transplantation improves survival in cystinosis, although extrarenal deposition of cystine continues. Cystine deposits can recur in allografts. Interstitial dark cells, probably macrophages, are often present without an obvious relation to crystal

deposition (225), and glomerular mesangial crystals also occur in host-derived macrophages (226). Nonetheless, renal allograft survival has been good, allowing patients to develop other serious cystinotic complications, including vision impairment, peripheral myopathy, and diabetes mellitus (227–229).

## Dent's Disease

Dysfunction of renal proximal tubules with low–molecular-weight proteinuria, hypercalciuria, nephrocalcinosis, nephrolithiasis, and rickets characterizes Dent's disease (230). Renal function may begin to decline in the teenage years, and renal failure eventually develops in about two thirds of patients (231). Proximal tubular dysfunction is variable but may become evident in the neonatal period. Hypercalciuria, the hallmark of Dent's disease, can be detected in the first year of life, but stone formation may not be present in pediatric patients. Hypophosphatemic rickets is not universal but can be one of the first clinical presentations. The disease occurs at equal rates in the two sexes, but males are affected more severely (232,233). There is no cure, but thiazide diuretics have been helpful in reducing urinary calcium excretion (234). Recurrent stone formation has not occurred in renal allografts (235). Carrier detection can be difficult on clinical grounds and may require molecular analysis. Different clinical features predominated in the original descriptions, but it is now recognized that Dent's disease and its "variants"—X-linked recessive hypophosphatemic rickets and X-linked recessive nephrolithiasis—are a single disease caused by inactivating mutations in the *CLCN5* gene, located on chromosome Xp11.22 (231,236,237). Additional genes, potentially involving proteins necessary for endosomal function, likely harbor mutations, as normal *CLCN5* has been found in several patients with Dent's disease (238). Interestingly, mutations in *OCRL1*, the gene responsible for Lowe's syndrome (see following), have recently been identified in 5 of 13 families with a classic Dent's disease phenotype who lacked mutations in *CLCN5* (239).

### Pathologic Changes

Light microscopic findings are progressive but nonspecific (233,240,241). Normal glomeruli and well-preserved tubules are typical in childhood. Pathologic changes in older individuals of both sexes include hyaline casts, tubular epithelial degeneration, tubulointerstitial calcium deposition, mild interstitial fibrosis with tubular atrophy, and occasionally, glomerular hypercellularity with progressive hyalinosis. Electron microscopy fails to show ultrastructural abnormalities in proximal tubular cells (241).

### Pathogenesis

The voltage-gated chloride channel CLCN5 is predominantly expressed in the kidney, where it is found in subapical endosomes of cells of the proximal tubule and thick ascending limb of Henle's loop and intercalated cells of the collecting ducts (242). Megalin and cubilin are major receptors in the endocytotic reabsorption of polypeptides that are freely filtered by the glomerulus (243,244). CLCN5 is believed to provide the chloride conductance necessary for the endosomal acidification by electrogenic vacuolar $H^+$-ATPase. Defects in CLCN5 interrupt megalin recycling to the membrane brush border and abolish megalin-mediated endocytosis of proteins, causing low–molecular-weight proteinuria (245). Abnormalities in membrane recycling could explain other defects, such as phosphaturia, aminoaciduria, and glycosuria. A loss of CLCN5 in the thick ascending limb, a major site of calcium reabsorption, may account for the hypercalciuria. Alternatively, disturbances in renal phosphate and calcium handling might be secondary to symptoms of impaired renal endocytosis and metabolism of calciotropic hormones (246). Disruption of the interaction between CLCN5 and $H^+$-ATPase appears to alter its polarity or expression in proximal tubular and intercalated cells and may be implicated in urinary acidification deficits in Dent's disease (241).

## Mitochondrial Disorders

Oxidative phosphorylation is a ubiquitous metabolic pathway that supplies energy to most tissues. Genetic defects in oxidative phosphorylation, therefore, produce a variety of clinical symptoms involving multiple organ systems, most typically the neuromuscular system. Renal involvement is noted in 5% of patients with respiratory chain deficiency, with the first symptoms developing in the neonatal period or before age 2 (247). The most common kidney presentation in a mitochondrial disorder is a proximal tubulopathy with Fanconi's syndrome, although other disorders, including glomerular disease and chronic tubulointerstitial nephritis, have been reported (248–257).

Effects on active transport in the nephron are not surprising, given the prominence of mitochondria in proximal tubules. Mitochondrial defects result in deficient ATP to drive the sodium-potassium-ATPase pump that maintains the sodium gradient across the proximal tubular epithelium and is responsible for all proximal tubular cell activities. Fanconi's syndrome in mitochondrial disease is usually part of a multisystem disorder with extrarenal neuropathic, myopathic, endocrine, or cardiac symptoms but can be the initial presentation (249,258,259). It is occasionally seen with specific syndromes of respiratory chain deficiency, including Leigh's, Kearns-Sayre's, and Pearson's syndromes (258,260–262).

## Pathologic Changes

The renal biopsy shows generally intact glomeruli with nonspecific tubular changes, including dilation, cast formation, and epithelial atrophy (263). Giant or abnormal

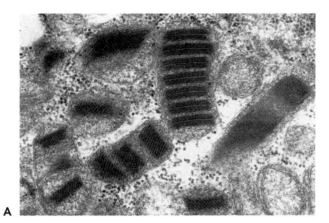

**A**

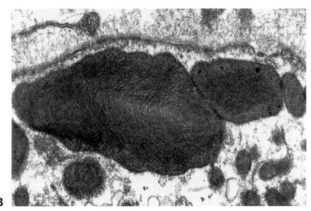

**B**

**Figure 25.39**  Tubular epithelial cells in this patient with myopathy and Fanconi's syndrome contain enlarged, irregular mitochondria with paracrystalline arrays (**A**) and dense circular cristae (**B**). (×16,000.)

mitochondria with paracrystalline arrays, or deficient, circular, or otherwise aberrant cristae are often evident with ultrastructural examination; however, their absence does not exclude the diagnosis (Fig. 25.39). Moreover, similar mitochondria can be observed in the presence of certain drugs and toxins, including antiepileptics, antimicrobials, and alcohol, as well as systemic illnesses such as diabetes and Wilson's disease, and can be induced by hypoxic injury and hypertonic fixatives.

## Diagnosis

The diagnosis is suspected in any patient with a complex association of symptoms involving unrelated organs. Renal symptoms appear to be more common in children than in adults. Proximal tubulopathy is often moderate, and isolated hyperaminoaciduria has been reported (263). Respiratory chain defects lead to a rise in blood lactate, pyruvate, and ketone bodies. Impaired proximal tubule reabsorption may lower blood lactate to normal levels; urinary lactate is increased in Fanconi's syndrome, where the lactate/creatinine ratio is higher than in healthy individuals or those with other renal disease (264). Therefore, a normal plasma lactate concentration does not rule out a mitochondrial disorder. Other methods of evaluation include polarographic and spectrophotometric studies that evaluate isolated mitochondrial oxygen consumption and enzyme activities. Respiratory chain disorders are genetically heterogeneous, owing to the multitude of genes involved in polypeptide synthesis and assembly, which are located in mitochondrial and nuclear DNA. Mitochondrial DNA defects undergo maternal transmission, and nuclear mutations are of autosomal recessive, autosomal dominant, and X-linked inheritance; sporadic cases exist. Disease-causing mutations have been identified for only a minority of patients. Nuclear gene mutations are becoming more recognized and may be responsible for the majority of respiratory chain deficiencies (247).

## Lowe's Syndrome

Lowe's oculocerebrorenal syndrome (265) comprises congenital ocular abnormalities, severe cerebral dysfunction, and renal tubular dysfunction similar to that of Fanconi's syndrome (266). The ocular abnormalities include microphthalmos, congenital cataracts, glaucoma, and buphthalmos. Cerebral dysfunction results in mental retardation, muscular hypotonia and hyporeflexia, and behavior disorders. The renal findings include tubular acidosis, aminoaciduria, tubular proteinuria, and phosphaturia. Glycosuria is usually slight. The renal tubular dysfunction is not severe, although the affected children are rachitic and have growth retardation. Proteinuria may dominate, however, and Lowe's syndrome is one of the causes of congenital and early infantile nephrotic syndrome. Although the onset is commonly in infancy, slowly progressive disease may lead to renal failure after several decades.

### Pathologic Changes

Renal morphologic features may be normal or minimally altered at first, with tubular dilation and loss of brush border (267,268). Mitochondrial swelling in proximal tubules has been described (269). The lesion progresses to tubular atrophy and interstitial fibrosis (270). Glomerular involvement develops early, with basement membrane thickening and splitting, widening of the foot process, and progressive glomerular sclerosis. The changes are secondary and nonspecific.

### Pathogenesis

The majority of cases in this rare X-linked recessive disorder are boys. Female carriers may have lenticular abnormalities that are detected by slit-lamp exam; full expression in females has been related to a balanced X:autosome translocation (266). At least 75 mutations have been identified in the gene responsible for Lowe's syndrome, *OCRL1*, located in the Xq25-26 region (271). Laboratory diagnosis is made by detecting a deficiency of the encoded enzyme, phos-

phatidylinositol (4,5) bisphosphate 5-phosphatase (272). Primarily localized in the Golgi network, mutations result in accumulation of the phosphatase in cells. The role of the enzyme deficiency in the Lowe's phenotype has not been completely deciphered, but it appears to be involved in membrane ruffling upon which cells depend for migration and cell–cell contact (273). Its importance in vesicle trafficking is also supported by the finding of markedly decreased megalin in urine of patients with Lowe's syndrome (274).

## Fanconi-Bickel's Syndrome

Originally described in 1949 and long considered a type of glycogen storage disease, interest in this rare autosomal recessive disorder has been re-energized by the discovery of mutations in the genes for facilitative glucose transporter membrane proteins (275,276). The detection of a genetic defect in the glucose transporter 2 gene (*GLUT2*) helps to disprove the postulated link to an inherited deficiency in phosphoglucomutase and will necessitate redefining "glycogen storage disease type XI." Patients typically present at 3 to 10 months and have stunted growth, hepatomegaly secondary to glycogen accumulation, glucose and galactose intolerance, fasting hypoglycemia, and severe Fanconi's syndrome, with disproportionate glucosuria. Fever, vomiting, and failure to thrive with chronic diarrhea may be evident at a younger age (277). Unusual features have included the absence of hepatomegaly, intestinal malabsorption, and glomerular disease (278,279). Older patients typically develop a protuberant abdomen, moon facies, and fat deposits on their shoulders and abdomen. Growth and puberty are severely retarded, and hypophosphatemic rickets is frequent. There is no specific treatment, although symptomatic replacement therapy consisting of supplemental water, electrolytes, and vitamin D; restriction of galactose; and administration of uncooked cornstarch has improved growth.

### Pathologic Changes

Renomegaly has been documented by imaging. The kidney may appear normal by light microscopy; however, glycogen accumulation and megamitochondria are evident in proximal tubular epithelial cells by electron microscopy (277).

### Pathogenesis

At least 34 mutations in *GLUT2 (SLC2A2)*, localized to chromosome 3q26.1-q26.3, have been reported, although other genes are potentially involved in Fanconi-Bickel's syndrome (279–281). No "hot spots" have emerged, making the molecular diagnosis laborious. Affected individuals have either homozygous or compound heterozygous mutations. The significance of *GLUT2* heterozygosity remains to be established, although isolated renal glucosuria has been observed; a link to diabetes mellitus remains to be proven (282,283).

Glucose transporter 2 is primarily involved in glucose homeostasis through its role in glucose uptake from the intestine, reabsorption by the kidney, sensing in the pancreatic β cells, and uptake and release by the liver (284). Glucose, reabsorbed by energy-dependent transport at the apical membrane of a proximal tubule cell, is passively released into the circulation via GLUT2 located in the basolateral membrane. Mutations in *GLUT2* are predicted to yield defective proteins with impaired function and/or localization. Interference with glucose transport out of the cell might cause tubular dysfunction by inducing an osmotic destruction of the cell, altering driving forces of other substances, or by producing an unspecified energy problem, the latter suggested by the finding of abnormal mitochondria in tubular cells. A genotype-phenotype correlation has not yet been shown (282).

### Other

Fanconi's syndrome secondary to other primary diseases, is much more common than idiopathic Fanconi's syndrome. Additional inborn errors of metabolism that can induce Fanconi's syndrome include tyrosinemia, galactosemia, hereditary fructose intolerance, and Wilson's disease. In these settings, Fanconi's syndrome is reversible with restriction of the offending substrate—respectively, tyrosine or phenylalanine, galactose or lactose, fructose, and copper with chelation.

### Acquired Fanconi's Syndrome

Acquired causes of Fanconi's syndrome include a variety of toxic and immunologic renal tubular injuries that impair net proximal tubular reabsorption. In contrast to those seen with heritable diseases, acquired Fanconi's syndrome is primarily an adult disease. These include drug-induced nephropathy, particularly anticancer agents, anticonvulsants, and antimicrobials (antibiotics and antiretrovirals); heavy metal intoxication; nephrotic syndrome; dysproteinemias or multiple myeloma; and membranous nephropathy with antitubular basement membrane antibodies (285). A reversible Fanconi's syndrome has followed renal transplantation and been associated with various malignancies, including nonossifying fibroma and lymphomas (206). Mitochondrial derangement, the generation of reactive oxygen species, and induction of apoptosis have been suggested mechanisms of cellular injury in these acquired settings (286–288).

### Specialized Heritable Tubular Defects

Heritable defects in specific tubular epithelial cell transporter systems can lead to aminoaciduria, renal tubular acidosis, or phosphaturia, largely without demonstrable morphologic abnormalities. They may, however, be accompanied by secondary morphologic changes. Nephrocalcinosis, with tubulointerstitial damage, occurs early in primary distal tubular acidosis, but it is prevented by therapy to reduce acidemia and hypercalciuria. Stone disease, the common clinical manifestation of classic cystinuria, is ameliorated by bicarbonate therapy to alkalinize the urine and by high fluid intake to maintain high urine volume. Chronic interstitial disease can eventually ensue in some instances. The clinical features range from asymptomatic to life threatening. The major conditions are listed in Table 25.2 (289–298).

## PURINE METABOLISM AND HANDLING DISORDERS

Uric acid is the end product of purine metabolism in humans. Purine nucleotides—specifically adenine and guanine—are synthesized from salvaged purines, from dietary purines, or de novo. Endogenous production of purines proceeds by stepwise addition of small molecules on to 5-phosphoribosyl pyrophosphate (PP-ribose-P), which is formed from a sugar derivative, D-ribose-5-phosphate, in a process catalyzed by the enzyme PP-ribose-P synthetase. Another enzyme, PP-ribose-P aminotransferase, initiates a series of reactions that lead to inosinic acid, a hypoxanthine nucleotide and the parent compound of purines (299,300). It can be converted by the so-called interconversion or salvage pathway to adenylic or to guanylic acid nucleotides, as a step in the synthesis of nucleic acids. Hypoxanthine–guanine phosphoribosyl transferase (HPRT) is a critical enzyme in the interconversion, and its absence leads to the loss or marked decrease of the ability to salvage purine bases. If not utilized in the body, the bases xanthine and hypoxanthine are degraded to uric acid by xanthine oxidase.

Hyperuricemia, defined as a concentration of uric acid in blood plasma above 7 mg/dL, may be caused by overproduction, underexcretion, or both. Known causes of hyperproduction include uncommon enzymatic defects such as complete absence or decrease of HPRT, raised activity of PP-ribose-P synthetase (301,302), hereditary fructose intolerance (303), and deficiency of G6Pase as in GSD-I (149), various drugs, ethanol- and protein-rich diets, and diverse disease states such as certain malignancies or obesity. Decreased excretion because of decreased tubular secretion or increased reabsorption occurs in many situations, such as chronic lead intoxication (saturnine gout), certain drugs (thiazide diuretics, cyclosporine), dehydration, malnutrition, preeclampsia, polycystic kidney disease, chronic renal insufficiency, hypertension, and hyperinsulinemia. Excretion is influenced by age, gender, and race (304). With few exceptions, however, these stimuli seldom result in

## TABLE 25.2

### HERITABLE INTRINSIC DISORDERS OF RENAL TUBULAR MEMBRANE TRANSPORT

| Disease | Inheritance | Gene | Mechanism | Clinical Effects |
|---|---|---|---|---|
| Cystinuria<br>Type I (type A)<br>Non–type I (type B, type AB) | AR<br>AD | SLC3A1<br>SLC7A9 | Impaired reabsorption of cystine and dibasic amino acids (lysine, arginine, ornithine) owing to defective shared b$^{0,+}$AT-rBAT system | Urolithiasis secondary to precipitation of highly insoluble cystine |
| Lysinuric protein intolerance | AR | SLC7A7 | Impaired reabsorption of cationic amino acids, especially lysine, owing to defect in y+LAT1 subunit of cationic amino acid transporter | Aminoaciduria and poor intestinal absorption lead to hyperammonemia, nausea, vomiting, protein malnutrition with hepatosplenomegaly, hypotonia, osteoporosis, occasional mental retardation, respiratory compromise, immunodeficiency |
| Dicarboxylic aminoaciduria | AR | SLC1A1 | Impaired reabsorption of anionic amino acids (glutamic and aspartic acids) owing to defective EAAT3 transport system | Asymptomatic aminoaciduria |
| Hartnup's disease | AR | SLC6A19 | Impaired reabsorption of neutral amino acids owing to defective B$^0$AT1 transport system | Reduced renal and intestinal absorption of tryptophan, leading to nicotinamide deficiency with pellagra-like rash, ataxia, mental retardation |
| Iminoglycinuria | AR | ?SLC36A1,<br>?SLC6A20 | Impaired reabsorption of proline and glycine owing to defective shared transport system IMINO | Asymptomatic aminoaciduria |
| Glycosuria | AR | SLC5A2 | Impaired reabsorption of glucose owing to defect in low-affinity, glucose-specific SGLT2 transporter | Asymptomatic glycosuria |
| Hypophosphatemic rickets (phosphaturia) | X-linked<br>AD | PHEX<br>FGF23 | Impaired phosphate reabsorption owing to defective phosphate homeostasis and renal vitamin D metabolism | Hypophosphatemia and normocalcemia, growth retardation, rickets, osteomalacia |
| Primary distal tubular acidosis | AD<br>AR<br>AR | SLC4A1<br>ATP6V0A4<br>ATP6V1B1 | Defective membrane transporters owing to dysfunction of anion exchanger AE1 or proton pump vacuolar H$^+$-ATPase | Hyperchloremic, hypokalemic metabolic acidosis, hypercalciuria, nephrocalcinosis and lithiasis, rickets or osteomalacia, +/− deafness |
| Primary proximal tubular acidosis | AR<br>AR<br>AD | SLC4A4<br>CA2<br>Unknown | Impaired bicarbonate reabsorption owing to dysfunction of NBC1 and carbonic anhydrase II | Hyperchloremic metabolic acidosis, with ocular abnormalities or osteopetrosis |

AD, autosomal dominant; AR, autosomal recessive; b$^0$AT1, b$^{0,+}$ amino acid transport; rBAT, related to b$^{0,+}$ transportor; y + LAT1, y$^+$L isoform 1 amino acid transport; EAAT3, excitatony amino acid transporter 3; IMINO, imino acid transporter; NBC1, Na$^+$, Na$^+$/HCO$_3^-$ cotransporter.

clinically significant disease. Gout, the best known manifestation of hyperuricemia, is caused mainly by decreased renal excretion (300). For any given level of plasma uric acid, subjects with gout excrete less uric acid than normal (305). The possible role of overproduction in the common form of gout in adults has not been defined.

## Uric Acid and the Kidney

About two thirds of the daily elimination of uric acid or urate takes place in the kidney, and one third occurs in the gastrointestinal tract (306). Uric acid is freely filtered by the glomerulus and is almost completely absorbed in the S1 segment of the proximal tubule, after which it is then secreted and again is partly reabsorbed in the S3 segment of the proximal tubule (307–313). A voltage-sensitive urate transporter and a urate/anion exchanger are two mechanisms for urate transport within the kidney (314,315). The final amount in the urine is 10% to 12% of the original quantity filtered. When uric acid or urate reaches the collecting ducts, it precipitates out because of the decreased solubility in the acid medium. The clinical presentation depends on the concentration and the speed of precipitation, which will lead either to ARF, with tubular obstruction mainly by uric acid, or to chronic renal disease and gouty nephropathy, with formation of granulomas (microtophi) in the tubules and interstitium around the crystals of urate.

## Hereditary Disorders

### Enzyme Defects

#### Hypoxanthine–Guanine Phosphoribosyltransferase Deficiency

Hypoxanthine–guanine phosphoribosyltransferase (HPRT) deficiency is an X-linked defect that causes high purine turnover and overproduction of uric acid; hypoxanthine cannot be reutilized without adequate HPRT and is therefore degraded to uric acid (316). Clinical manifestations relate to the degree of enzyme deficiency and have been described in women, likely because of skewed lyonization (317). Male hemizygotes with a defective gene show a broad spectrum of presentation. Mutational analysis of the *HPRT1* gene has shown a correlation between the predicted functional consequences of the amino acid substitution on enzyme activity and the phenotype (318). Complete deficiency of HPRT (Lesch-Nyhan's syndrome), a condition of late infancy and early childhood, comprises hyperuricemia, choreoathetoid movement, spasticity, mental retardation, and compulsive self-mutilation (319,320). Partial deficiency of HPRT causes less severe nervous system manifestations, although a significant proportion of these patients exhibit spasticity, cerebellar ataxia, and mild mental retardation; they also have a greater tendency to develop gouty arthritis, which

is rare in the Lesch-Nyhan's syndrome (320). Patients with greater than 8% enzyme activity have hyperuricemia without neurologic symptoms (321).

Those with total or partial HPRT deficiency can present in infancy with crystalluria, stone formation, or acute renal failure (ARF) (320,322,323). Xanthine stones may form in addition to uric acid stones (324). Gross kidney findings at autopsy have included diffuse atrophy and stones. The microscopic changes are a combination of intratubular crystalline deposition and interstitial microtophi. Biopsies in patients with HPRT deficiency have shown intratubular and interstitial amorphous or needle-like crystalline deposition with surrounding giant cells; interstitial fibrosis and tubular atrophy may be present along with an inflammatory response induced by uric acid crystals (325,326). Electron microscopy reveals occasional stacks of needle-like crystals in tubular lumina but not in tubular epithelial cells. Intratubular deposition may lead to tubular obstruction, decline in renal function, and further increase in serum uric acid levels (327). The diagnosis is made by demonstrating hyperuricemia, elevated uric acid:creatinine ratio, decreased HPRT enzyme activity in peripheral blood cells, and increased purine metabolites in urine (328).

### 5-Phosphoribosyl Pyrophosphate Synthase Superactivity

5-Phosphoribosyl pyrophosphate synthetase hyperactivity, caused by mutations at two distinct loci (PRS1 and PRS2) in the *PRPS* gene located on chromosome X, leads to an uncontrolled increase in PP-ribose-P, thus enhancing de novo synthesis of purines (329). As with HPRT deficiencies, the clinical spectrum varies from childhood presentation with severe neurologic deficits to isolated hyperuricemia, gouty arthritis, and renal stone formation that becomes apparent in adolescence or early childhood (301,302).

### Glucose-6-Phosphatase Deficiency

Glucose-6-phosphatase deficiency, an autosomal recessive trait that is typically found in GSD-I, may cause hyperuricemia and gout. Mechanisms include both an increased rate of purine catabolism and a decreased renal clearance of urate secondary to lactic academia and ketonemia (149). The hyperuricemia begins in infancy, and gouty arthritis may occur by the second decade (330). Hyperuricemia may also be encountered in type III glycogenosis, with clinical myopathy, as well as types V and VII, although these patients do not have gout (323).

### Tubular Defects

#### Familial Juvenile Hyperuricemic Nephropathy (Familial Nephropathy with Gout)

In 1960, Duncan and Dixon described a 19-year-old man with gouty arthritis, hyperuricemia, hypertension, severe renal failure, and bilateral small kidneys (331). Since that time several families with a similar constellation of findings have been described, and most have been grouped under the clinical rubric of familial juvenile hyperuricemic nephropathy (FJHN) (317).

Hyperuricemia is detected in childhood or adolescence, both sexes are involved, and gout and renal failure develop over the ensuing years, although gout is an inconsistent feature (322). The condition is inherited as an autosomal dominant trait, and HPRT and PP-ribose-P synthetase activities have been normal (300). Biochemical hallmarks include hyperuricemia that is out of proportion to renal dysfunction and extreme hypoexcretion of urate.

Renal biopsies show focal and segmental or global glomerular sclerosis, sometimes with glomerular collapse, thickening of Bowman's capsule, and patchy loss and atrophy of tubules associated with interstitial fibrosis. Thickening and reduplication of the basement membranes of distal tubules and collecting ducts have been observed, as well as intimal thickening of intrarenal arterioles and arteries (332–334). Electron microscopy has been unrevealing, and immunofluorescence studies have been indeterminate (335). Uric acid crystals are almost invariably described as absent (317). Treatment includes pharmaceutical control of hyperuricemia that sustains renal function if initiated before renal damage exists (336). High renal allograft failure rates have been reported (317).

Genetic heterogeneity clearly exists. Mutations in the gene encoding hepatocyte nuclear factor-1β have been demonstrated in rare families with features of FJHN (337). Mutations in the *UMOD* gene, on 16p12.3, leading to the synthesis of mutant forms of uromodulin (Tamm-Horsfall protein) have been found in about 50% of the cases of FJHN, after its initial cloning in three families with FJHN and one with autosomal dominant medullary cystic kidney disease (338). The pathogenesis of the condition is not clear. Postulated mechanisms include the extratubular deposition of mutant uromodulin, which has proinflammatory capabilities, with ensuing tubulointerstitial nephritis accompanied by a subtle defect in tubular excretion of urate, or the interference by mutant uromodulin with sorting of the Na-K-2 Cl co-transporter, resulting in fewer molecules at the luminal epithelial surface of the thick ascending loop of Henle, and subsequent depletion of the extracellular volume, diminished glomerular filtration rate, and increased reabsorption of urate in the proximal tubule (338,339).

### Idiopathic Renal Hypouricemia

The urate–anion exchanger in the human kidney has recently been identified as URAT1 and localized to proximal tubules. Homozygous inactivating mutations in its gene, *SLC22A12*, have been found in Japanese and Korean patients with idiopathic renal hypouricemia and serum uric acid levels well below 2 mg/dL (340–343). These indi-

viduals have presented with exercise-induced ARF, associated with nausea and vomiting several hours after exercise. The kidney shows acute tubular necrosis and possible subcapsular infarcts and, despite the need for dialysis, the short-term prognosis seems good. After recovery, most patients had normal creatinine levels, although decreased concentrating abilities were evident. Urolithiasis has been noted in few patients (343–346). Despite a favorable outcome, some have demonstrated progressive interstitial fibrosis, tubular atrophy, and chronic renal dysfunction (347).

### Acute Uric Acid Nephropathy

In contrast to enzymatic defects causing excessive purine and urate biosynthesis, this form of renal injury, caused by uric acid overproduction, typically results from massive tissue destruction, as seen in patients with rhabdomyolysis syndromes or acute tumor lysis syndrome associated with certain hematologic or solid malignancies (348,349). The onset is usually one of ARF related to the commencement of cytotoxic therapy, which releases large amounts of nucleoproteins and may lead to high levels of plasma uric acid (20 to 50 mg/dL) that is filtered into the renal tubules and precipitates in the collecting ducts and deep cortical and medullary vessels (350,351). Deposits of inorganic and organic phosphates, released with tumor cell death, along with calcium, produce nephrocalcinosis and contribute to ARF. Xanthine or other purine metabolites are rarely involved. Obstructions that cause oliguria can often be cleared with diuretics and alkalinization of urine. The great increase in uric acid output during therapy of leukemias and lymphomas has been recognized for many years, and the dangers of actual stone formation have been stressed (352). Standard preventative measures using vigorous hydration and allopurinol have decreased the incidence of acute hyperuricemic renal failure. Recombinant urate oxidase may prove to be an effective alternative (349,353).

### Pathologic Changes

The kidneys contain linear yellow striations in the medulla and papillae, corresponding to the distribution of the collecting ducts in which precipitation has taken place (Fig. 25.40). The collecting tubules contain large amounts of uric acid. This may take the form of amorphous masses or, when frozen sections are examined, of doubly refractile, radially disposed crystals. Some acicular crystals of monosodium urate are present, and these may be seen penetrating the tubular wall, inciting a giant cell reaction and uncommonly in the interstitium. Electron microscopic studies have shown crystals in the epithelium of collecting tubules, accompanied by an increase in lysosomal bodies (354). Dilatation of the glomerular

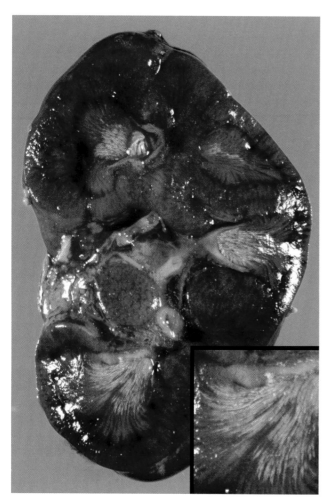

**Figure 25.40** Gross picture of a kidney from a 3-year-old boy with tumor lysis syndrome and acute urate nephropathy. The papilla (*inset*) has pale yellow linear streaking that corresponds to the presence of uric acid and urates in the collecting ducts. (Courtesy of J. Siebert, Ph.D., Children's Hospital and Regional Medical Center, University of Washington.)

space and the tubular system proximal to the obstruction plus edema of the cortical interstitium are sometimes present.

## Uric Acid Infarcts

Deposits of uric acid crystals may be seen in the kidneys of newborns who die within the first few weeks of life and appear macroscopically as yellow striations along the collecting ducts in the inner medulla, identical in appearance to Figure 25.40. This finding has become less common with better neonatal fluid management but seems to represent a normal physiologic state without functional disturbances; it is possibly related to cellular destruction associated with the remodeling of fetal tissues. Histologically, the streaks are amorphous, eosinophilic sediment (355).

## Chronic Uric Acid Nephropathy

Uric acid in human extracellular fluids exists almost exclusively as a salt, monosodium urate monohydrate. Both uric acid and sodium urate are poorly soluble and cannot exceed the concentration of about 7 mg/dL without forming a supersaturated solution that promotes deposition of urates in the tissue (i.e., tophi) (356). Not all persons with high serum levels of urate develop gout (300). Nephropathy in gout results from the precipitation of sodium urate in the renal tissues, with tubular damage and interstitial granulomatous inflammation (microtophi). Uric acid stones are common. These manifestations of chronic gout were once common but have declined substantially as a result of more effective therapy, particularly uricosurics (probenecid and sulfinpyrazone) and allopurinol (304,357).

The prognosis of gouty nephropathy has changed over the years. Data from the older literature indicate that impairment of renal function and renal failure were frequent, affecting at least 40% of cases, and 10% of patients died with uremia (358–360). Studies conducted since the introduction of effective treatment of gout with uricosuric agents and allopurinol have found considerable reduction in the incidence and severity of gouty nephropathy (357,361–363). In fact, the mild and uncomplicated renal disease, if present at all, gives rise to few symptoms and only infrequently leads to renal failure, although some reduction of renal function and asymptomatic hypertension might be seen (364,365).

The involvement of lead in renal damage and gout has long been debated. Lead may inhibit urate excretion both directly and indirectly by causing proximal tubular dysfunction and reducing renal blood flow through its influence on the renin-angiotensin system (366–368). More mobilizable lead has been found in gouty patients with renal impairment than in those with normal kidney function, and lead chelation has been shown to improve urate excretion and renal function in the general population and in nondiabetic, nongout patients with chronic renal insufficiency, respectively (369–371). Other investigations, however, do not support these findings (372,373). Comorbid states and medication, for example, hyperlipidemia, ischemic heart disease, and anti-inflammatory drugs, likely contribute to any decline in renal function in patients with gout (374,375).

## Pathologic Changes

The kidneys are affected equally, unless they are asymmetrically obstructed by stones; they are usually reduced in size. Granularity of the subcapsular surface may be accompanied by some coarser scars; the cortex is often reduced in width. The medulla contains small white specks and occasional radiating pale-yellow urate deposits. The pelvis may be dilated and contain small uric acid stones; the papillae in these cases are often blunted. In certain cases, the presence of acute infection is apparent grossly. The kidneys occasionally appear normal or even enlarged.

The glomeruli in most cases contain no abnormalities other than those attributable to aging, ischemia, and the effects of obstruction. However, in the early stages a distinctive, uniform fibrillary thickening of the glomerular basement membrane (GBM) with increased numbers of nuclei in capillary loops may be observed (376,377). The glomeruli are slightly enlarged, the mesangial areas are moderately expanded by matrix and some cells, and the capillary walls are thickened, occasionally showing "double outlines." On electron microscopy, the capillary basement membranes often measure 700 to 800 nm, which is twice their normal size, and the endothelium is focally separated from the basement membranes in a manner reminiscent of hemolytic uremic syndrome or radiation nephropathy (Fig. 25.41). Hyalinization of glomeruli can occur in the course of the disease, and glomerular deposits of amyloid have been seen (360).

The tubules may be atrophic as the result of ischemia, obstruction, or conceivably chronic infection. Dilatation of tubules occurs with extensive urate deposition in medullary tubules, rarely in the cortical tubules, or when uric acid stones in the pelvis or ureter cause obstruction (378). Degeneration and pigmentation of the loops of Henle have been described (376). Neutrophils are frequent in tubules, stimulated by the crystals or by an acute infective process (379,380).

The collecting tubules in the medulla often contain crystals of monosodium urate that are elongated (Fig. 25.42), rectangular, or so fragmented as to be amorphous. The doubly refractile crystals are best seen in alcohol-fixed material but are often surprisingly well preserved with formalin fixation. Some of the crystalline masses in hematoxylin and eosin sections are deep blue, perhaps because of concomitant calcium deposition, and they may be refractile under polarized light. In many deposits, the crystalline appearance and birefringence are partially lost, and a pale blue, faintly staining, amorphous substance is seen (Fig. 25.43).

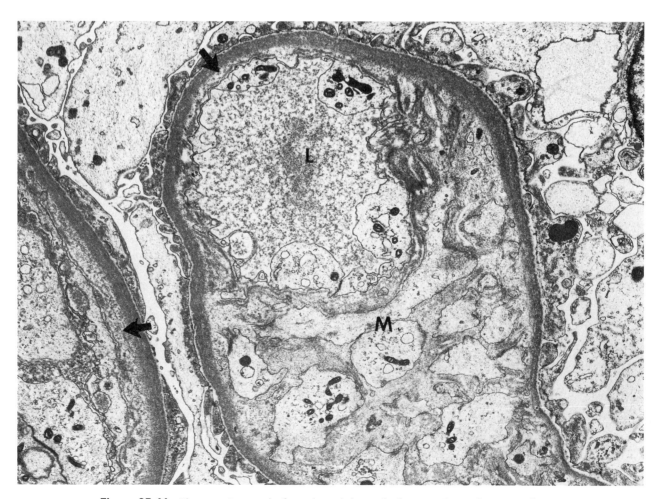

**Figure 25.41** Electron micrograph of an enlarged glomerulus from a patient with gouty nephropathy. Capillary walls show segmental separation of the endothelium from the basement membranes (*arrow*). The resulting space is filled with granular material similar to that in the capillary lumen. L, capillary lumen; M, mesangium. (×7125.)

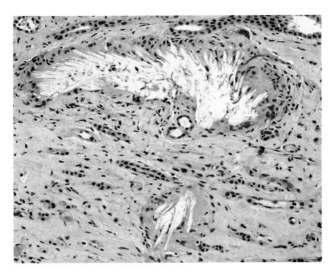

**Figure 25.42** Collection of elongated urate crystals with a giant cell reaction at the periphery. This collection probably originated in a collecting tubule, the walls of which are no longer apparent. Considerable loss of tubules has occurred. (Formalin fixation; H&E; ×400.) (Specimen courtesy of Dr. K. Smith, University of Washington.)

The walls of the tubules are frequently deficient, and the crystalline deposits appear to be in the interstitium, outlined by giant cells and other mononuclear cells, beyond which a layer of loose connective tissue may be seen, replacing almost all the local tubules. Microcalculi have been described in the lumen of tubules (381). Cortical tubular or interstitial urate deposits may also occur, but this change is inconstant.

The interstitium may be scarred and contains urate collections with giant cells and acute inflammatory cells (Fig. 25.44). Interstitial deposition of calcium, iron, and phosphate has been seen (382). In general, interstitial

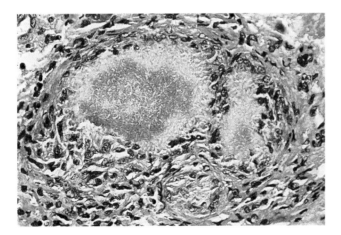

**Figure 25.43** Urate deposits (microtophus) of amorphous, faintly crystalline material in the medulla with an adjacent narrow zone of inflammatory cells and fibrosis at periphery. (Formalin fixation, Masson's trichrome; ×200.)

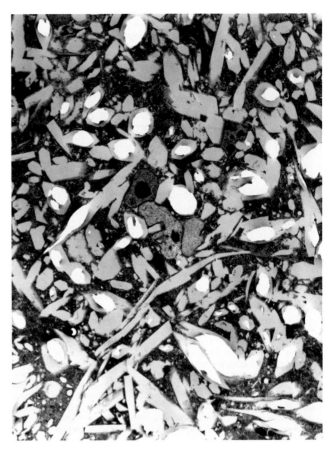

**Figure 25.44** Electron micrograph of substantial angular and irregularly shaped interstitial urate deposits admixed with inflammatory cells. (×16,000.) (Specimen courtesy of Dr. K. Smith, University of Washington.)

changes have been regarded as secondary to tubular damage. Blood vessels show arterial and arteriolar sclerosis, which is sometimes severe and may contribute to tubular atrophy. The correlation between the two is not good, however, and other factors, such as obstruction, are clearly at work (359).

## Urolithiasis

Uric acid stones occur in 10% to 25% of patients with gout (300). In a United States population-based analysis, the frequency of kidney stones in subjects with gout was almost three times greater than that in the general population (383). Stones are more likely to form in acidic urine (384); they occur after the administration of uricosuric drugs (385). The stones are characteristically radiolucent, but they become radiopaque if covered by calcium salt. Mixed uric acid and calcium oxalate stones may also be found (386). Uric acid or monosodium urate crystals are thought to serve as a nidus for stone formation, and heparin sulfate and aspartic and glutamic acids comprise the matrix (385).

Xanthine stone formation has been described in Lesch-Nyhan's syndrome after treatment with allopurinol (324). Stones composed of 2,8-dihydroxyadenine occur in homozygotes with adenine phosphoribosyl transferase deficiency, a purine salvage enzyme companion to HPRT (384).

# SICKLING DISORDERS

Sickled cells were first reported in the literature by Dr. James Herrick; however, the deadly disease hallmarked by painful episodes was known in Africa for centuries (387,388). A single nucleotide change, from GAG to GTG in the sixth codon of the β-globin gene on chromosome 11p15.5, results in the single amino acid substitution of valine for glutamic acid in the hemoglobin peptide (389–391). Although the sickle gene has a genetic advantage of protecting heterozygous carriers from endemic *Plasmodium falciparum* malaria infection, carriers of two gene defects are well known to suffer vaso-occlusive pain crises, acute chest syndromes, splenic sequestration, aplastic crises, cerebrovascular accidents, priapism, and chronic organ dysfunction, including effects on the kidney (392,393).

Sickle cell disease denotes all genotypes that contain at least one sickle gene. In addition to the homozygous HbSS disease (sickle cell anemia [SCA]) and sickle cell trait (HbAS), other major compound heterozygous genotypes, listed in order of clinical severity, include HbS/β⁰ thalassemia, HbS/HbC disease, HbS/β⁺ thalassemia, HbS/HPFH (hereditary persistence of fetal Hb), HbS/HbE syndrome, and additional rare combinations (HbS/Hb β$^{D-Punjab}$, HbS/Hb β$^{O-Arab}$, HbS/Hb β$^{D-Lepore}$). In the United States, 9% of African Americans have AS, and 1 in 600 has SS (394).

Sickle cell disease manifests in the kidney with both tubular and glomerular effects that culminate as ESRD. Renal involvement is most significant and well characterized in sickle cell anemia, which is the main focus of this section. In one large series of 310 patients followed in sickle cell clinics, 71% had HbSS, 17% had HbSC, 11% had HbS/β⁺ thalassemia or HbS = β⁰ thalassemia, and 1% had hemoglobin S-other (395). Reference below to HbS heterozygotes implies HbS/β thalassemia and HbS/HbC.

## Clinical Presentation

Sickle cell nephropathy (SCN) includes hematuria, papillary necrosis, urinary concentrating defect, impaired renal acidification and potassium excretion, supranormal proximal tubular function, proteinuria, and renal failure (reviewed by several authors [393,396–399]). Renal manifestations of sickling disorders are presented in chronologic order of onset.

## Hyposthenuria

The inability to concentrate urine maximally is the most frequent renal abnormality in sickle cell disease patients and the earliest evidence of a renal abnormality (400,401). An impaired capacity to concentrate urine can be demonstrated in patients with sickle cell anemia as early as 6 months of age. Patients under 10 years of age cannot concentrate their urine greater than 600 to 800 mOsm/kg H₂O. In young children, maximum urine osmolality can be increased with blood transfusions. However, this capability is lost with progressive ischemic damage to the renal medulla, and the defect is irreversible by age 15 (402). A maximum urinary osmolality of 400 to 450 mOsm/kg H₂O is typically seen under water deprivation in adults with sickle cell anemia. By contrast, urine osmolalities on water loading reach significantly lower values in sickle cell patients than in normal subjects, confirming the preservation of the capacity to maximally dilute the urine (403).

In HbS heterozygotes, HbSC, HbS-β thalassemia and HbAS, the defects can be as significant, though typically milder, with more gradual onset that usually becomes apparent later in life (404–406). In sickle cell trait, the severity of hyposthenuria is heterogeneous and dependent on the percentage of HbS, which is modulated by the α-globin genotype (407,408).

Hyposthenuria can produce polyuria, thereby increasing the risk of dehydration. High urine volumes may contribute to nocturnal enuresis, a relatively common disorder in children and young adults, with any form of sickle cell disease (409,410). The intensity of enuresis has been linked to the severity of sickle cell disease, with a higher incidence in those with anemia and painful crisis and low concentrations of fetal hemoglobin (409,411).

Although intranasal desmopressin has yielded complete or partial resolution of nocturnal enuresis in sickle cell disease, the condition is considered multifactorial (410,412).

## Altered Glomerular Function

Children with sickle cell disease have supranormal renal hemodynamics, with elevated glomerular filtration rate (GFR) and renal plasma flow (RPF). The GFR is usually normal in sickle cell trait, but, like sickle cell anemia, the filtration fraction is decreased, owing to a small increase in RPF (413). Both GFR and RPF normalize during adolescence but are frequently subnormal after the age of 40 (400,414–416).

Proteinuria is an early manifestation of SCN and develops in as many as 20% to 30% of adults with sickle cell trait and 12% of older children, where it increases with age (395,416–419). Proteinuria is more commonly associated with sickle cell anemia than other hemoglobinopathies (420). A 10-year prospective analysis of 442 pediatric patients found proteinuria, defined as greater than 1+ protein on urinalysis for at least 6 months, in no children younger than 6 years. Proteinuria was associated with lower hemoglobin concentrations, and children with HbS/β thalassemia were similarly affected (416). Lonsdorfer et al found proteinuria in approximately 18% of 52 patients over 16 with sickle cell trait (421).

Microalbuminuria is a sensitive marker of preclinical glomerular damage and has been detected in 39% (16 of 41) of teenagers or adults with HbSS, 25% (1 of 4) with HbS/β thalassemia, and 9% (1 of 11) with HbSC disease (422). Although it has been documented in children less than 4 years old, the overall incidence of microalbuminuria in HbSS children is 19% to 27% and is usually detectable around 7 years of age (423–425). The prevalence of microalbuminuria increases with age, reaching adult incidence in the second decade, but does not correlate with clinical severity of disease (i.e., painful crises, transfusion requirements). Microalbuminuria can also be demonstrated among patients with sickle cell trait, although at a lower frequency (426).

## Hyperfunctioning Proximal Tubules

Patients with sickle cell disease have lower than normal serum creatinine levels and supranormal proximal tubular function generating increased secretion of uric acid and creatinine (427). The latter can lead to significant overestimation of GFR by creatinine clearance. A discrepancy of 30% was found between creatinine and inulin clearance in a group of patients with sickle cell disease with normal GFR (CrCl, $2.57 \pm 0.12$ mL/s, versus inulin clearance, $1.98 \pm 0.8$ mL/s) (403). Homozygous SS patients may actually have a significant deterioration in renal function long before it is detected by traditional measurements of creatinine clearance. Herrera et al (428), however, recently challenged the notion of increased secretion of creatinine, finding lower baseline tubular secretion of creatinine and impaired response to an intravenous creatinine load in 16 sickle cell anemia patients versus controls. They argued that a difference in conclusions regarding creatinine secretion between their study and that of de Jong (427) was the result of differences in values between control subjects (428).

Abnormalities of proximal tubular reabsorption include increased reabsorption of phosphate and $\beta_2$-microglobulin, which can lead to elevated serum phosphate (429,430). However, the opposite has been found in children with sickle cell anemia, who have lower mean serum phosphate and lower maximal tubular phosphate reabsorption values compared to controls, possibly owing to higher parathyroid hormone levels in this age group (431,432).

## Incomplete Renal Tubular Acidosis

In addition to urinary concentrating defects, those with sickle cell disease often have impaired distal tubular handling of potassium and hydrogen. Under normal conditions, neither defect of acidification nor potassium secretion is clinically apparent, but either may become so with renal insufficiency or dehydration (433). During acid loading, HbSS patients were unable to lower their urine pH below 5, but normal renal acidification has been observed in HbAS (413,434). Results similar to those seen in HbSS have been reported for HbS/β thalassemia (405,406).

Homozygous SS patients usually have normal serum potassium concentrations that remain so, even with potassium loading. The defect in potassium excretion is independent of aldosterone deficiency but may be related to a shift of potassium from the extracellular to intracellular compartment (435). The fractional excretion of potassium is also lower in HbSS children, but normal potassium excretion is observed in patients of all ages with sickle cell trait (432,436).

## Hematuria

Asymptomatic hematuria is one of the most prevalent features of the disease. Although usually self limited, it may be dramatic and prolonged, rarely resulting in the passage of clots and severe anemia. Hematuria is often seen with papillary necrosis and is associated with sloughing of the renal papillae, which can produce obstruction to urine outflow and ARF—an outcome that is, however, uncommon, as papillary necrosis is usually a focal disease (401,437,438). Ultrasonography can identify renal papillary necrosis, which can evolve to calcification of the medullary pyramids and may be an incidental finding in the asymptomatic patient. Other variable presentations of papillary necrosis range from renal colic to symptoms of urinary tract infection or sepsis (439).

Hematuria occurs at any age in HbSS, HbSC or HbS-β thalassemia and most commonly presents in HbAS patients in the third or fourth decade. It should be cautioned that renal medullary carcinoma in sickle cell trait often presents with hematuria (see following).

## Hypotension

Individuals with sickle cell disease have significantly lower blood pressure than the general population. The Cooperative Study of Sickle Cell Disease showed that the prevalence of hypertension in sickle cell anemia is less common than in the Black population as a whole and than in control populations at all ages (440). In a more recent large study of approximately 4000 patients older than 2 years, blood pressure was measured annually for 15 years and was found to be significantly lower in sickle cell anemia than published norms for age, race, and sex; the difference was noted to increase with age. HbSC patients deviated from normal but to a lesser degree than HbSS patients. Therefore, those with sickle cell disease should have their blood pressure monitored, but values obtained must be assessed relative to lower values expected for patients with sickle disease (441).

## Acute Renal Failure

Acute renal failure is not common in sickle cell disease but becomes more probable during periods of acidosis and hypoxia. Acute renal failure has been described as part of the multiorgan failure syndrome (dysfunction of at least two major organ systems) that complicates a severe sickle pain episode (442). Acute renal failure in sickle cell disease may be related to rhabdomyolysis, sepsis, or general anesthesia, which often accompanies it, but patients generally have good survival and recovery of function without progression to ESRD (443). It has rarely been described in patients with sickle trait (444).

## Pathologic Changes

### Gross Pathology

The kidney in patients with sickle cell anemia who die of nonrenal causes is grossly no different from other patients. Progressive renal impairment is more common with advancing age and autopsy studies have shown a negative correlation of kidney weight with age (445). Kidneys typically show papillary changes ranging from blunting to obvious necrosis and scarring, with the more severe changes occurring in those who died of renal failure. An extensive review by Vaamonde (437) showed that renal papillary necrosis is a frequent complication of SCN in HbSS, as well as in heterozygotes, and has an incidence ranging from 15% to 36%. The acute lesion of papillary necrosis is pale infarction of the papillary tip, sometimes accompanied by sloughing (420). Loss of caliceal cupping, irregular renal outline, and cystic extension from the calix have been demonstrated by intravenous urography and correlate with chronic injury (Fig. 25.45) (446). Renal cortical infarction with subsequent cortical scarring has been observed, and many kidneys show coarsely irregular subcapsular surfaces, which are worse with evidence of uremia, though not to the degree that is common in pyelonephritis (397,445). Generalized cortical thinning is associated with reduced renal weight, and diminished numbers of glomeruli are enlarged and easily visualized on gross examination.

Renal enlargement, however, is apparent in childhood. Annual ultrasound evaluation of renal length in 237 subjects between the ages of 6 and 20 years with HbSS showed a significantly greater mean length with age, compared to 147 subjects with HbSC disease and 78 age-matched controls with normal (HbAA) hemoglobin (447). Renal length correlated negatively with hemoglobin levels and correlated positively with reticulocyte counts.

Most of the 21 patients with hematuria in the report of Mostofi et al were thought to have sickle cell trait (448). Unilateral nephrectomy specimens showed medullary or

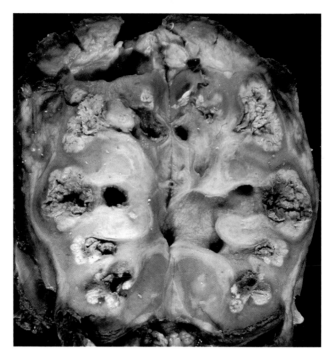

**Figure 25.45** Bisected kidney from a patient with sickle cell anemia (SS) showing papillary necrosis and destruction with cystically dilated calices. Multifocal pyelonephritis is evident. (Courtesy of Dr. R. Peel, University of Pittsburgh.)

cortical hemorrhages as well as necrotic papillae. Renal papillary necrosis usually presents later in HbAS than HbSS, but it may occur in up to 50% of patients with sickle cell trait who present for evaluation of hematuria. Papillary necrosis has been observed radiographically in patients with both HbS-thalassemia and HbSC (439,449).

Microradiographic studies revealed gross lesions of the vessels of the renal medulla with almost complete absence of vasa recta in sickle cell anemia; those that remained were spiraled, dilated, and ended blindly (450). Vasa recta in sickle cell trait and HbSC disease were shown to be reduced in number and to have lost the normal bundle architecture.

## Microscopic Pathology

### Vascular Abnormalities

Large blood vessels are usually unremarkable except for sickled erythrocytes. Arterioles and capillaries are dilated and congested with aggregates of erythrocytes without fibrin thrombi (451,452). Only rarely are afferent arterioles or cortical capillaries hyalinized (445,452).

### Tubulointerstitial Abnormalities

The most frequently reported cortical tubular change is hemosiderin deposition, primarily in proximal tubular epithelial cells (Fig. 25.46) (395,452,453). Early descriptions in children include tubular epithelial necrosis, regeneration, and pigmentation of tubular casts (451,454). Tubular atrophy and interstitial scarring with mononuclear cell

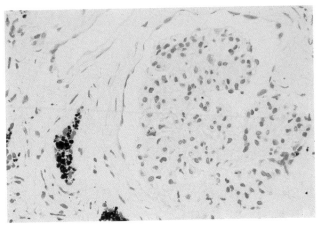

**Figure 25.46** Tubular epithelial cells in sickle cell anemia kidney contain abundant cytoplasmic iron. Rare granules are evident in glomerular visceral podocytes. (Perls Prussian blue; ×400.) (Specimen courtesy of Dr. A. Chang, University of Chicago.)

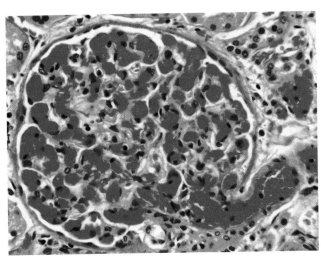

**Figure 25.48** A glomerulus in a patient with sickle cell anemia has its arteriole and capillaries distended by sickled erythrocytes. (H&E; ×400.) (Specimen courtesy of Dr. E. Manci, University of South Alabama.)

infiltrates have also been noted in the cortex of patients with renal failure (445).

Medullary lesions are more prominent, with early changes consisting of edema and telangiectasia (451). Destruction of the vasa recta results in multiple, small infarcts of the papilla that progress to focal scars. Eventually, tubular atrophy and dropout leave only a few surviving collecting ducts within broad areas of inflamed fibrous tissue (Fig. 25.47) (437,455,456).

### Glomerular Abnormalities

*Hypertrophy.* Structural changes were first described by Sydenstricker et al in 1923 as prominent glomeruli distended with blood, though without thrombi (454). Afferent and efferent arterioles can be dilated and congested with sickled red cells (Fig. 25.48) (451). Nonsclerotic glomeruli are often enlarged, with an increase in the total number of cross-sectioned capillary lumens accompanied by an increase in epithelial, endothelial, and mesangial cells (Fig. 25.49) (451,452,457). Iron deposition is limited and can occasionally be demonstrated in parietal epithelial cells with a lesser amount in visceral epithelial cells (Fig. 25.46) (451,452,458). Glomerular enlargement, particularly in a juxtamedullary location, to as much as 30% more than normal has been demonstrated in children as young as 2 years of age whose renal function was unknown; glomeruli in even younger children were normal except for variable degrees of congestion (451,452). In adults, glomerular hypertrophy of approximately the same degree has been documented at all cortical levels and

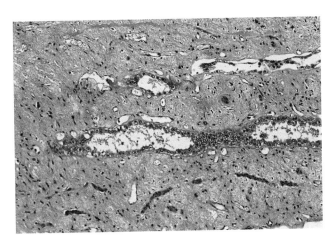

**Figure 25.47** Sclerotic area of papilla with loss of vasculature and tubular atrophy in an autopsy kidney from a patient with sickle cell disease. (H&E; ×200.) (Specimen courtesy of Dr. E. Manci, University of South Alabama.)

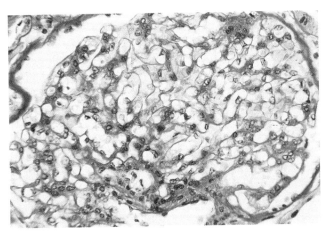

**Figure 25.49** An enlarged glomerulus from a sickle cell patient has an increased number of capillary lumen cross sections and mild mesangial hypercellularity. (PAS; ×400.) (Specimen courtesy of Dr. A. Chang, University of Chicago.)

exists before evidence of proteinuria. The mean glomerular area increases over a wide age range and has been measured to be more than double that of normal controls (395,445,453,457). No significant difference in glomerular size or densities per unit area of cortex was found in adults with HbAS and controls, as the glomeruli in sickle cell trait can appear virtually normal (457).

*Focal Segmental Glomerulosclerosis.* Glomerular abnormalities can be seen in sickle cell disease, with or without proteinuria. The fundamental pathologies in sickle cell glomerulopathy are hypertrophy and focal segmental glomerulosclerosis, sometimes accompanied by global sclerosis (395,453). Tejani et al (459) described similar lesions in children. The focal segmental glomerulosclerosis is often perihilar in location and typically adherent to Bowman's capsule (Fig. 25.50). Solidification of glomerular tuft segments is associated with hyalinosis, lipid vacuolation, and foam cells, with loss of its capillary bed (395). Bhathena and Sondheimer recognized two patterns, collapsing and expansive; the former was dominated by mesangial atrophy and wrinkling collapse of the capillaries, whereas the obliterated tuft in the latter was characterized by mesangial matrix expansion (453). Glomerular ischemia and sclerosis are more frequent in HbSS than HbAS.

Immunofluorescent microscopy has shown irregular immunostaining for IgM, C3, and C1q in areas of sclerosis, whereas nonsclerotic segments are either negative or contain trace amounts of IgM, IgG, and C3. Electron microscopy shows focal effacement of visceral epithelial foot processes, no or only rare electron-dense deposits, residual bodies in mesangial cells, and limited mesangial interposition (395,453). Falk et al (395) noted focal electron-lucent expansion of the subendothelial zone, suggestive of early lesions that could evolve to those

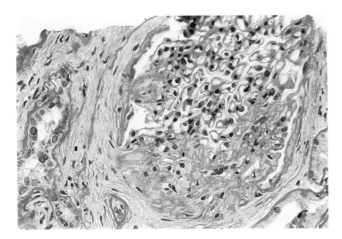

**Figure 25.50** The enlarged glomerulus has developed segmental sclerosis. The surrounding interstitium is fibrotic, and iron is visible in tubular epithelial cells. (PAS; ×400.) (Specimen courtesy of Dr. A. Chang, University of Chicago.)

in advanced SCN that resemble membranoproliferative glomerulonephritis.

*Membranoproliferative Pattern.* Nine of 12 proteinuric patients studied by Bakir et al (417) had glomerular lesions that resembled membranoproliferative glomerulonephritis, although the lobular pattern was not as striking. The hypercellular glomeruli had circumferential mesangial expansion, often associated with duplication of the GBM, causing characteristic "tram-tracking" (417). Similar changes have been described by others (445,457,460–462). Basement membrane duplication may only be focal, and variable degrees of segmental or global glomerulosclerosis can often accompany this lesion.

Immunofluorescent microscopy is usually negative but can show occasional nonspecific mesangial or capillary loop positivity for C3, IgM, IgG, or even IgA, although staining has typically been very faint (417,457,462). Electron microscopy does not show electron-dense deposits but increased mesangial matrix and mesangial cells. Podocyte foot process fusion is variable. Endothelial cells can be separated from the GBM by electron-lucent material in the subendothelial region (Fig. 25.51). There is often scalloping of the subendothelial aspect of the basement membrane and interposition of mesangial cells between the outer original basement membrane and the new inner basement membrane-like material (460,462). Small siderosomes can be seen in endothelial and mesangial cells. Similar subendothelial zone expansion has been described in a patient with HbSC (463).

*Other.* Only a few instances of potential immune complex–mediated glomerular lesions have been characterized in the literature. Pardo et al (464) maintained the existence of a normocomplementemic autologous immune complex–mediated process in seven individuals with sickle cell anemia and proteinuria or nephrotic syndrome. Biopsies from these patients showed glomeruli with increased mesangial matrix and cellularity, splitting of the basement membranes, and glomerular enlargement with evolution to sclerosis and complete obliteration. Immunofluorescent microscopy demonstrated granular IgG and C3 in the mesangium and GBM in addition to IgM, C2, and C4 in several cases. Antibodies against renal tubular antigen decorated glomeruli in the same pattern in two subjects. Electron microscopy showed electron-dense deposits on the inner aspect of the lamina densa in four patients in addition to mesangial and visceral epithelial siderosomes. Mesangial interposition and basement membrane duplication were noted. Antibody to renal tubular epithelial antigen was detected in the serum of two subjects. Ozawa et al described similar findings in a patient with sickle cell trait (465).

Renal biopsy is of value in patients with sickle cell disorders to differentiate the lesions associated with

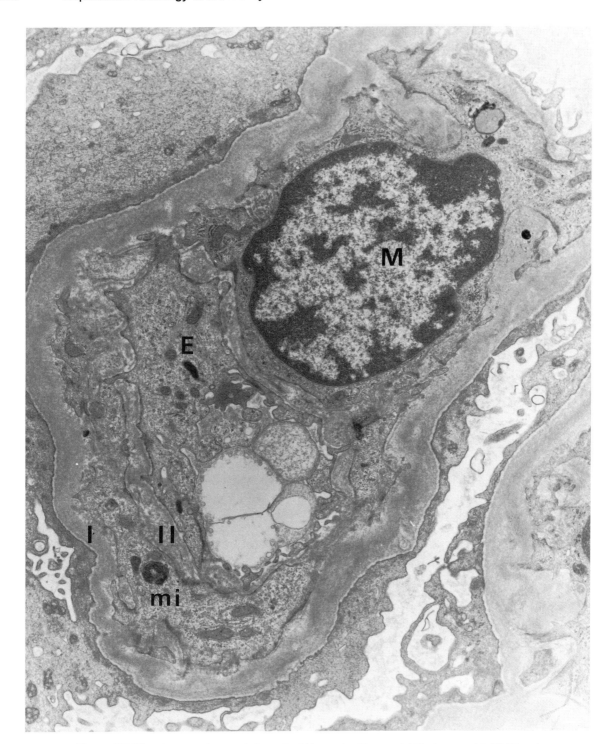

**Figure 25.51** Electron micrograph from the kidney of a 31-year-old Black man with HbSS and nephrotic syndrome (proteinuria 3.1 g/24 hr) showing glomerular capillary surrounded by podocytes with effaced foot processes. The capillary is double contoured (I and II) with mesangial interposition (mi). M, mesangial cell nucleus; E, capillary endothelium. (×13,120.)

hemoglobinopathies from other acute diseases that may overlap clinically. Coincident diagnoses, including lupus nephritis in a patient with HbS-thalassemia (466), immunotactoid glomerulopathy in a boy with HbSS (467), and amyloidosis in a patient with sickle cell anemia and Familial Mediterranean fever (468), have been demonstrated. Amyloid has also been seen in SS patients without a familial predisposition, presumably secondary to frequent sickle cell crises that may provoke recurrent acute inflammation and the development of amyloid protein (469).

Not surprisingly, coexistent immune complex-mediated diseases such as acute poststreptococcal glomerulonephritis can occur (470). Unusual to patients with sickle cell disease and acute poststreptococcal glomerulonephritis is a normal complement level, suggested to be secondary to an abnormality of the alternative pathway of complement activation (471). Proliferative segmental glomerulonephritis with immune complexes or microscopic vasculitis has been described in patients with sickle cell disease following Parvovirus-induced aplastic crises (472–474).

## Malignancies

The incidence of malignancy and sickle cell disease deserves further analysis as changes in management offer longer life expectancies with exposure to more medications. A cancer incidence rate of 1.04 cases per 1,000 patient years was calculated from a single institution review of 696 patients, results comparable to the Surveillance, Epidemiology, and End Results (SEER) data for age-specific cancer incidence in African Americans (475). Based on genotypic frequencies, however, Baron et al reported a surprising 16.7-fold excess of HbSS patients and an expected incidence of HbAS patients among those at their institution with renal cell carcinoma (476). Those with sickle cell trait, it turns out, may have had a tumor other than renal cell carcinoma.

Davis et al described a rare, highly aggressive neoplasm, which they termed *renal medullary carcinoma* (RMC), that is almost unique to African Americans with sickle cell trait (477). Rare cases have been documented in Caucasians and Brazilians (478). The tumor occurs in children and young adults and has a slight male predominance. Presenting symptoms most commonly include gross hematuria, abdominal or flank pain, and a palpable mass. Typically, the tumor is widely metastatic at diagnosis to regional lymph nodes and lungs, with spread to liver, adrenals, and bone reported. The response to therapy including radical surgery and combination chemotherapy has been poor, with most deaths occurring within months of diagnosis (479).

Nearly all patients described to date have HbAS, with rare documented exceptions of HbSS and HbSC (477,478). One White female patient in Davis's original report had no evidence of a sickling disorder, implying that the tumor is not restricted to those with hemoglobinopathies (477). However, this supposition was based on the absence of sickled erythrocytes, and without hemoglobin analysis, it remains unproven.

## Pathologic Change

These bulky tumors are poorly circumscribed, occupy the renal medulla and adjacent soft tissue, and spread to the cortex as multiple satellite nodules. Tumor size has ranged from 2 cm to 18 cm (mean, 7 cm), with hemorrhage and necrosis common. The light microscopic appear-

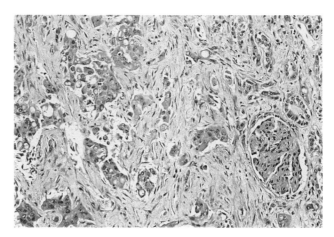

**Figure 25.52** Renal medullary carcinoma from a 16-year-old African American boy with sickle cell trait. The kidney tumor has glandular structures comprised of pleomorphic and mitotically active cells with occasional cytoplasmic lumina. The desmoplastic stroma surrounds tumor cell islands and encases a single sclerotic glomerulus. (H&E; ×200.)

ance is variable but most commonly includes a cribriform architecture with tumor cell aggregates forming uneven glandular spaces sometimes surrounded by a hypocellular desmoplastic reaction with inflammation (Fig. 25.52). The low-power view is sometimes reminiscent of a yolk sac (endodermal sinus) tumor. Other growth patterns—microcystic with micropapillations, solid, or sarcomatoid—may be present as well as solid sheets of poorly differentiated areas. The tumor cells have large vesicular nuclei with prominent nucleoli and abundant eosinophilic cytoplasm, with cytoplasmic lumina in some cases. Cytoplasmic inclusions resembling rhabdoid tumor are not uncommon (Fig. 25.53). Mitotic activity is highly variable but lymphatic or vascular invasion is the rule, which occasionally extends into the main renal vein. Tumors coexpress cytokeratin (CAM 5.2 and AE1/AE3) and vimentin (477,478).

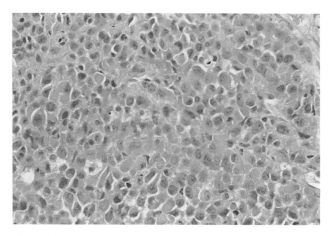

**Figure 25.53** Renal medullary carcinoma (same patient as Fig. 25.52) with rhabdoid cellular features, including prominent nucleoli and perinuclear cytoplasmic inclusions. (H&E; ×400.)

Cytogenetic studies have been limited, but two cases showed triploidy with numerous structural abnormalities, while in a third, a karyotype of 46,XX,inv(2)(p23q11.2) was found (478–480). The analysis of nine RMCs by comparative genomic hybridization demonstrated no genetic gains or losses in eight cases and loss of chromosome 22 in one case (478).

## Differential Diagnosis

Renal medullary carcinomas are classified as a subtype of collecting duct carcinoma (CDC) in most texts, despite their clinical and pathologic differences. Collecting duct carcinoma is a rare neoplasm that arises from the medullary collecting ducts and characteristically expresses cytokeratin 34β E12 and Ulex europeus agglutinin 1 lectin by immunohistochemical analysis. Renal medullary carcinoma has been shown to lack the former and demonstrate only focal staining of Ulex europeus in only a minority of cases, supporting the distinctiveness of RMC from CDC (478). Gene expression profiling of two RMCs, however, revealed close clustering with transitional cell carcinoma, perhaps supporting an origin from urothelium of the renal pelvis (481). The perception that CDC is commonly found in young adults is mostly because of its lack of distinction in many references from RMC. Collecting duct carcinoma may in fact be rare in adolescents, once the diagnosis of RMC is excluded. A single case report of CDC in a patient with sickle cell trait was reported in a 61-year-old Black woman (482).

## Etiology and Pathogenesis

### Sickling Cells

The polymerization of HbS is the required event in the molecular pathogenesis of sickle cell disease and is enhanced by deoxygenation, low pH, increased intracellular HbS, and decreased intracellular concentration of protective hemoglobins such as HbF and HbA2 (483). The polymer, a ropelike fiber, bundles with others to distort the erythrocyte into a rigid sickled shape, interfering with its usual deformability. The kinetics of polymerization, including a delay time followed by exponential polymerization, is usually longer than the transit time of microcirculation, so that most cells fail to undergo HbS polymerization. Prolongation of erythrocyte transit time is caused by enhanced erythrocyte adhesion to endothelium, cell dehydration, and abnormal vasomotor tone that favors vasoconstriction (393). Microcirculatory obstruction, originally thought to result from impaired capillary transit of sickled cells, is probably caused by trapping of deformed erythrocytes in the slow-flowing venular side and their aggregation with leukocytes, resulting in obstruction, local hypoxia, increased HbS polymerization, and propagation of the occlusion to adjacent vasculature (484).

## Renal Medullary Alterations

Hemoglobin S aggregation and polymerization are the seminal events in the erythrocytes of individuals with the various sickle syndromes and the primary pathophysiologic factor in renal injury. The hyperosmolar environment of the renal medulla, with its low $O_2$ tension and pH, increases the risk of sickling within vessels of the vasa recta (485). Congestion and sickling produce severe stasis, which leads to peritubular hemorrhage and ischemic necrosis in the medullary pyramids. The resultant hematuria is usually unilateral and more frequently involves the left kidney, perhaps because of the increased venous pressure owing to the greater length of the left renal vein (448).

Impaired local blood flow through the vasa recta decreases the oxygen supply to the tubular cells in the medullary loop of Henle, reducing the ability to absorb sodium from the tubular lumen and resulting in a decrease in the medullary interstitial osmolality (450). The functional defect in the maximal ability of the collecting duct to concentrate urine becomes irreversible with advancing age because sustained ischemia, which produces repeated sludging with thrombosis and progressive infarction of papillae and inner medulla, leads to scarring and permanent anatomic alterations. The intact ability to maximally dilute urine is explained by unimpaired solute reabsorption from the ascending limb of Henle. These are restricted to the outer medullary zone in approximately 85% of nephrons and receive blood via intact patent peritubular capillaries.

Oxidative stress has been implicated in sickle cell disease and originates from multiple sources, including increased levels of tumor necrosis factor-α and interleukin 6, repetitive ischemia-reperfusion, and the generation of oxidants by endothelial cells stimulated by erythrocytes, leukocytes, or the sickled erythrocytes themselves (486). The role for oxidative stress in mediating renal tubular damage has been demonstrated. Transgenic mouse models of sickle cell exposed to hypoxic conditions have vaso-occlusion of medullary vessels by sickled erythrocytes and a marked increase in nitric oxide (NO) synthases (487). More recent data suggest that NO and/or peroxynitrite, an extremely destructive reactive oxygen species, initiate cell damage that leads to apoptosis of epithelial cells and that inhibition of NO-mediated oxidant stress ameliorates renal cellular injury (488).

## Renal Cortical Alterations

Supranormal proximal tubular function may be prostaglandin mediated (403). Ischemia in the medullary region results in altered renal production of prostaglandins, the net effect of which can also lead to vasodilation of afferent glomerular arterioles and to glomerular hypertension (427,456,489). Sickle cell glomerulopathy appears to be the consequence of focal and segmental glomerular sclerosis superimposed on maximally hypertrophied glomeruli.

Glomerular hypertrophy in sickle cell anemia is not likely the consequence of anemia, as hypertrophied juxtamedullary glomeruli were not observed in children with other severe chronic anemias (451). Hypoxemia may be a stimulus for glomerular hypertension and hypertrophy, as similar lesions have been noted in children with cyanotic heart disease, who share the chronic hypoxia and elevated blood viscosity of HbSS children (490). The deleterious effect of increased viscosity has been suggested by its worsening the glomerulopathy in partially nephrectomized rats (491).

Rodent studies have correlated increased glomerular pressure and flow with glomerular hypertrophy (492). Falk et al (420) reasoned that focal glomerulosclerosis developing in the hypertrophied glomeruli of SS is analogous to the focal segmental glomerulosclerosis that develops in the renal remnant after subtotal nephrectomy, where glomerular injury occurs from glomerular hypertension (493). In this model, increased glomerular capillary pressure and resulting glomerular destruction is attenuated with angiotensin-converting enzyme that decreases glomerular hypertension (494).

Hyperfiltration-mediated sclerosis of the glomerular capillaries can lead to progressive renal insufficiency (495). Guasch et al (496) and Schmitt et al (497) have suggested that hyperfiltration in sickle patients is associated not only with enhanced renal perfusion but also with an alteration in glomerular permeability. Both researchers showed a loss of permselectivity with significantly elevated fractional clearance of neutral dextrans. The ultrafiltration coefficient was found to be increased in proteinuria and decreased in association with renal insufficiency in patients with sickle cell anemia. Enhanced transglomerular trafficking of macromolecules associated with loss of restrictive membrane pores because of podocyte stretch lesions (defects) induced by glomerular hypertrophy was proposed as the basis for this form of focal segmental glomerulosclerosis (497,498).

Glomerular lesions in sickle cell sometimes resemble those of thrombotic microangiopathy. The increased viscosity and enhanced adhesion of sickled erythrocytes to endothelium support the proposal of primary endothelial injury with mesangial interposition and secondary GBM production (462). Other mechanisms have been advanced over the years for the pathogenesis of glomerular injury. McCoy endorsed iron overload in the glomerulus, analogous to intravenously administered saccharated iron oxide that caused nephrotic syndrome in rabbits (460). That iron is generally deposited in the interstitium and along the lower nephron rather than glomeruli argues against the theory. Moreover, glomerular lesions of sickle cell anemia are not seen in other iron overload states such as hemochromatosis or with excessive blood transfusions. Strauss et al (499) and Pardo et al (464) postulated the glomerular deposition of immune complexes of antibodies targeted to renal tubular epithelial antigen and argued a mechanism that included an undue susceptibility to infection, inadequate host defense and sensitization, and production of antibodies to tubular antigens released from proximal tubules damaged by ischemia. The case for immune complex disease is lessened by the absence of immune deposits in biopsies of patients with early disease.

Oxidative stress may also contribute to glomerular damage. The instability of HbS allows degradation to its heme and globin moieties, and increased amounts of heme have been found in the transgenic sickle mouse kidney (500,501). Heme, as an extremely active oxidant of LDLs, may play a role in glomerular injury (502). Interestingly, up-regulation of heme oxygenase-1 (HO-1), an antioxidant involved in the degradation of heme, has been demonstrated in the kidney vasculature, interstitium, and tubular epithelial cells, as well as circulating endothelial cells in sickle cell patients (501). Increased glomerular nitric oxide synthase has also been demonstrated in a rodent model of sickle cell, suggesting that nitric oxide may play a role in the glomerular hyperfiltration by its vasodilatory effect (487).

## Clinical Course and Prognosis

Individuals with sickle cell disease have a decreased life expectancy, with mortality in children contributing significantly to this shortened survival. Neonatal screening and the introduction of prophylactic penicillin in early childhood has reduced mortality to less than 2% by 10 years of age (503,504). The average life span in the United States for men and women with HbSS has increased to 42 and 48 years, respectively, compared with ages of 60 and 68 years in those with HbSC disease (505). Improved life expectancy has shifted the focus of clinical problems in developed countries to chronic organ dysfunction. Where optimal medical care is unavailable, for example, in most parts of Africa, life expectancy for affected individuals with sickle cell disease is less than 30 years, and it remains the third leading cause of mortality in children receiving hospital care (506).

## Multifactorial/Pleiotropic Genes

There is marked variation in clinical severity of sickle cell anemia, owing in part to environmental, psychosocial, cultural, and even socioeconomic influences. Despite sickle cell anemia being the first monogenetic disease ever described, numerous other genes modify the phenotype. Genetic modification of the expression was originally suspected by notable geographic differences in clinical severity. The HbS gene is found on a genetic background of four major β-globin–like gene cluster haplotypes. Identified by various restriction endonucleases and assigned the name of the geographic area in which they are most frequent, they include the principal African haplotypes—Benin, Central African Republic (CAR or Bantu), and Senegal—in addition to the major Indo-European sickle mutation, Arab-India (507). The CAR haplotype has been associated with the highest incidence of organ damage and renal failure and the poorest HbF response to hydroxyurea (508–510). Other multigenic influences on clinical presentations include: copresence of β thalassemia or α thalassemia and possibly G6Pase deficiency, pyruvate kinase deficiency, and hereditary spherocytosis; regulators of HbF production such as female sex, XmnI-Gγ polymorphism and growth factor levels (erythropoietin, transforming growth factor-β); modulators of erythrocyte-endothelial adhesion and leukocyte numbers; and even human leukocyte antigen alleles (511–513). That renal failure occurs in a minority of sickle patients underscores the influence of genetically determined non-sickle cell disease genes.

## Chronic Renal Failure

Increased lifespan in sickle cell anemia patients increases the probability of developing chronic renal failure (419,456). Ineffective erythropoiesis with increasingly severe anemia, hypertension, proteinuria, nephrotic syndrome, and microscopic hematuria were shown by Powars (514) to be pre-azotemic predictors of chronic renal failure. A low hematocrit serves as a protective mechanism in sickle cell disease by reducing blood viscosity and thus decreasing vaso-occlusive crises; however, an increased number of pain crises does not lead to an increased risk for renal failure (508,515). Severe anemia appears to have an indirect adverse effect on the kidney, as hemoglobin levels have strongly correlated with creatinine clearance, especially in patients over 40 years of age (446,516). Hyposthenuria, unlike glomerular injury, does not correlate with subsequent renal impairment (421).

Compared to other African Americans, patients with sickle cell disease have a decrease in life expectancy of 25 to 30 years and a mortality rate that rose from 18% overall to 40% in those with glomerulopathy leading to end-stage renal failure (505). Morphologic evidence of the cause of death in 306 autopsies of sickle cell disease (including HbSS, HbSC, HbS-β thalassemia) accrued between 1929 and 1996 as part of the National Institutes of Health Centralized Pathology Unit for Sickle Cell Disease found infection to be most common for all ages (33% to 48%). Renal failure was implicated as the cause of death in 4.9% of cases, although additional evidence of chronic renal injury was noted as papillary necrosis (14.5%) and renal infarc-

tion and atrophy (23.4%) (517). Renal failure contributed to mortality in nearly 9% of 241 Jamaican patients with sickle cell disease (518). The prospective, 25-year longitudinal demographic and clinical cohort study by Powers et al showed that 4.2% of patients with sickle cell anemia (HbSS) and 2.4% with HbSC disease developed renal failure. Once renal failure develops, there is a substantially increased risk for early death. The survival of patients with sickle cell anemia was 4 years after the onset of ESRD, with a median age at the time of death of 27 years (508). A retrospective analysis of the 1999 United States Renal Data System database revealed a mean age of end-stage renal failure of 40.68 ± 14 years (519).

Renal insufficiency is not typical before age 40, but approximately 30% of patients who survive beyond that age are affected (418,420). Therapeutic advances may be responsible for even fewer patients showing the onset of renal insufficiency in their 20s as compared to earlier studies (516). Proteinuria is the hallmark of glomerular injury in patients with sickle cell disease and the antecedent to renal insufficiency and failure. In several large series, proteinuria was documented in approximately 20% of adults and 5% of children (395,416,418). Forty percent to more than 60% of sickle cell patients with ESRD had nephrotic range proteinuria (395,417,508,514).

It is apparent that renal involvement begins in childhood, and microalbuminuria will likely be a helpful predictor of end-organ damage in sickle cell disease, as it is in diabetes and hypertension. Microalbuminuria, as a preclinical marker of glomerular injury, has been documented in about 20% of children under 20 years of age (423–425). Early detection may theoretically allow therapeutic intervention to prevent progressive renal insufficiency.

## Therapy

Management of sickle cell disease requires a concerted team effort addressing pain management, preventative care including prophylactic penicillin, nutritional services, and specialist interventions around pulmonary, ophthalmologic, neurologic, orthopedic, prenatal, and renal issues. Treatment is directed toward prevention of vaso-occlusive crises and control of infections that can worsen renal function.

## Treatment of Hematuria

Usually bed rest is sufficient for spontaneous resolution of most episodes of gross hematuria. Intravenous hypotonic solutions to decrease medullary tonicity, sodium bicarbonate to alkalinize HbS, plus hyperbaric oxygen and diuretics, can eliminate clots from the bladder, reduce sickling, and potentially prevent papillary necrosis (396). The use of aminocaproic acid for fibrinolysis and irrigation of the pyelocaliceal system may be necessary. Qunibi reported "autotransplantation" in a 22-year-old woman with sickle cell trait whose gross hematuria was unresponsive to conservative therapy or silver nitrate instillation (520). Rarely is nephrectomy required.

## Drug Therapy

### Nonsteroidal Anti-inflammatory Agents

The use of nonsteroidal anti-inflammatory agents (NSAIDs) as pain management for sickle cell crises carries untoward consequences on renal function. Nonsteroidal anti-inflammatory agents can produce significant declines in creatinine clearance and the rates of glomerular filtration and renal blood flow, owing to the maintenance of GFR by the prostaglandin system (427). Because NSAIDs have a demonstrated antinatriuretic effect and can increase the rate of progression to ESRD, these agents should be avoided in those sickle cell disease patients with evidence of SCN (403).

### Angiotensin-Converting Enzyme Inhibitors

Careful attention to blood pressure control is important as effective treatment of hypertension has been reported to delay the progression to ESRD in sickle cell patients (521). However, diuretics should be used with caution because of impaired potassium excretion (435).

Urinary protein excretion was shown to decrease with angiotensin-converting enzyme (ACE) inhibitors, presumably through dilation of the efferent arterioles. Ten selected patients with mild renal insufficiency and biopsy-documented prevalence of glomerular enlargement and perihilar focal segmental glomerulosclerosis had a 57% mean decrease in the proteinuria below baseline ($P < .001$) after a short course of enalapril (395). However, 2 to 3 weeks after discontinuation of enalapril, protein excretion was 75% of the baseline value ($P <.168$). The fall in proteinuria was not a consequence of a drop in mean systemic pressure or a decreased GFR; neither effective renal plasma flow nor filtration fraction was significantly altered at any time. Six of eight additional patients with albuminuria who received a 6-month course of enalapril showed a reduction to normal; one additional patient experienced a reduction of 70% (522). Urinary albumin concentration increased relative to pretreatment levels in two of these individuals, returned to pretreatment levels in two patients, and remained below 30 mg/L in two subjects at 2 years after treatment was discontinued. A more recent 6-month controlled trial evaluating microalbuminuria in 22 normotensive patients documented a mean decrease from baseline of 37% ($P <.01$) compared to a gain in the placebo group (523). Enalapril therapy has also been shown to reduce urinary protein excretion and normalize serum albumin in children (524). The sustained benefit on protein excretion and prevention of renal insufficiency

from long-term ACE inhibitor therapy is anticipated but unproven.

### Hydroxyurea

In vivo evidence of mild disease in individuals with sickle cell disease with high concentrations of HbF, led to the use of hydroxyurea, an S-phase cytologic drug that increases HbF in vivo. Other benefits of hydroxyurea include modulation of sickle erythrocytes' adhesive properties and enhanced NO production. A multicenter study of hydroxyurea in sickle cell anemia, with a 9-year follow-up, showed reduced incidence of painful crises and a 40% reduction in mortality (525). The long-term hematologic efficacy of hydroxyurea at maximal tolerated dose in children with sickle cell disease has been demonstrated in 122 pediatric patients, which included 106 with HbSS, 7 with HbSC, 7 with HbS/β-thalassemia, and 2 with HbS/Hb$^{O-Arab}$ over a study period longer than 8 years without adverse effects on growth, increased numbers of acquired DNA mutations, or renal toxicity. These encouraging results support the use of hydroxyurea in all eligible patients with sickle cell disease at escalated doses to achieve maximal hematologic effects (526). Early intervention with hydroxyurea may be considered for the prevention of proteinuria and renal disease, because microalbuminuria appears to be associated with a decreased hemoglobin level (424). The addition of hydroxyurea to enalapril therapy in children with proteinuria may further normalize the urine protein/creatinine ratio than enalapril alone (524).

### Renal Replacement Therapy: Dialysis and Renal Transplantation

Like others with ESRD, the treatment options available to sickle cell patients include dialysis and renal transplantation. Renal replacement therapy in the form of hemodialysis remains the standard management for end-stage SCN, although little is known about the long-term outcome of this group. An early report on survival of patients on hemodialysis showed a 30-month survival of 59%, equivalent to other nondiabetic ESRD patients (527). A retrospective cohort study of Saudi Arabian patients revealed a higher mortality and significantly younger age and shorter dialytic age in comparison with ESRD patients without sickle cell disease who were receiving long-term hemodialysis (528). That group suffered an earlier onset of ESRD, a higher prevalence of hepatitis B and C infections, and a significantly elevated incidence of vascular access-related septicemia. Poor survival rates were largely related to the bacterial and viral infections in the asplenic sickle cell population. There was a trend toward improved survival in African American transplant recipients compared to their dialysis-treated (wait-listed) counterparts (relative risk = 0.14, $P = .056$) (529). Information from the year 2000 U.S. Renal Data System files A was used to compare 153 transplanted sickle cell disease patients with those who received no transplant and showed a far better survival curve—56% versus 14% at 10 years—even in comparison to those 133 sickle cell disease patients who were placed on the transplant waiting list but never received a transplant (399). Renal transplantation has certainly become a viable alternative to chronic dialysis. These superior survival rates of renal transplant recipients compared with patients who are receiving hemodialysis suggest that transplantation is a better option for sickle cell disease patients with renal failure and that patients should be encouraged to undergo renal transplantation at an earlier stage.

The conclusions from two sequential national surveys of U.S. transplant centers conducted by Chatterjee were that renal transplantation in patients with sickle cell hemoglobinopathies achieved results comparable to that of other ESRD populations (530,531). The initial study in 1980 found 34 transplants, including 9 HbSS and the remainder HbAS, that resulted in a 1-year graft and patient survival of 67% and 87%, respectively. The second survey of 45 transplants included 13 HbSS patients with 5 repeat transplants and showed 1-year graft and patient survival rates of 88% and 67%, respectively. However, many of these transplants predated the use of cyclosporine, and the patients were predominantly those who developed ESRD with HbAS, implying other etiologies for ESRD, an extremely rare sequela of sickle cell trait (401).

The study by Ojo et al (529) consisted of 22,647 African American end-stage SCN patients who were identified through the U.S. Renal Data System and the United Network of Organ Sharing; 82 (81 HbSS and 1 HbSC) of them received kidney transplantation between 1984 and 1996. There was no difference in the 1-year cadaveric graft survival (SCN 78% versus other ESRD 77%) and the multivariable adjusted 1-year risk for graft loss indicated no significant effect of SCN (relative risk = 1.39, $P = .149$). However, the 3-year cadaveric graft survival tended to be lower in the SCN group (48% versus 60%, $P = .055$), and their adjusted 3-year risk of graft loss was significantly greater (relative risk = 1.60, $P = .003$). Patient survival in SCN was significantly lower than that of others at 1 year (78% versus 90%) and 3 years (59% versus 81%). On average, transplants performed between 1990 and 1996 had a 35% lower risk of 3-year graft loss compared to transplants performed between 1984 and 1989 (relative risk = 0.65, $P = .0001$), perhaps influenced by improved immunosuppression and posttransplant patient care, as the adjusted mortality risk declined by 62% in patients who received their transplants after 1990.

Sickle cell disease is a rare cause of ESRD in pediatric patients, accounting for only 0.5% and 0.2% of patients registered in dialysis and transplant arms of the North American Pediatric Renal Transplant Cooperative Study. In this series, 10 transplants in 9 patients (7 HbSS, 1 HbS-thalassemia, 1 HbSC) had a 2-year graft and patient survival of 71% and

89%, respectively, suggesting that renal transplantation is also a viable option for adolescent patients (532).

An important rationale for not offering renal transplantation to those with end-stage SCN is the risk of infections from immunosuppressive therapy in patients who have already undergone splenic involution. Other considerations include the poorer survival owing to the systemic nature of the disease, increased frequency of painful crises in association with improved posttransplant hematocrit, avascular osteonecrosis related to steroid therapy, and disease recurrence in the allograft (530,531,533,534).

In summary, results of renal transplantation in patients with ESRD caused by SCN are comparable to those of age- and race-matched recipients with ESRD from other causes. Although the long-term patient and allograft survival are still lagging behind those of other ESRD patients, there is a trend toward better patient survival relative to maintenance dialysis. Some argue that the higher death rates in SCN transplant recipients result from the underlying disease itself rather than an adverse impact of renal transplantation.

### Bone Marrow Transplantation

Bone marrow transplantation is the only available potentially curative therapy for sickle cell disease, and more than 200 patients treated with myeloablative hematopoietic stem cell transplantation from genotypically identical siblings have been described in the literature with an 85% disease-free survival, a 7% transplant-related mortality, and a 9% graft failure rate with autologous recovery and return to sickle cell anemia; slightly improved results are noted for thalassemia (535,536).

New developments that hold promise include non-myeloablative conditioning that leads to stable mixed chimerism, novel targeted posttransplantation treatments, and alternative donor sources, including umbilical cord blood and unrelated stem cell donors (537–539). Whether bone marrow transplantation in the early stage of the disease can reverse or halt the progression of established SCN is currently not known. Gene therapy is regarded with cautious optimism after successful results in the sickle transgenic mouse (540).

### Mouse Models of Sickle Cell Disease

Mouse models of sickle cell anemia have been helpful in understanding the pathophysiology of the disease and the development of antisickling drugs (541,542). Initial models expressing variable degrees of severity include the SAD-1 mouse, which provided information about glomerular abnormalities and the protective effect of human γ globulin; the Costantini-Fabry-Nagel (NYC1) model, in which it was concluded that increased glomerular filtration rate was not causally related to anemia and that nitric oxide and nitric oxide synthase participate in the pathogenesis of renal abnormalities; and the S+S− Antilles model, where in vivo adhesion of sickle cells to endothelium was first observed. Transgenic models with exclusively human globin chains have been widely used for the past decade and offer more realistic models because they are anemic and have abundant irreversibly sickled cells, although they tend to have low mean cell hemoglobin concentrations (MCHCs). These mice are particularly desirable for testing antisickling hemoglobins proposed for use in gene therapy.

## REFERENCES

1. McLean J, Wion K, Drayna D, et al. Human lecithin-cholesterol acyltransferase gene: Complete gene sequence and sites of expression. Nucleic Acids Res 1986;14:9397.
2. Kuivenhoven JA, Pritchard H, Hill J, et al. The molecular pathology of lecithin:cholesterol acyltransferase (LCAT) deficiency syndromes. J Lipid Res 1997;38:191.
3. Glomset JA, Mitchell CD, King WC, et al. In vitro effects of lecithin:cholesterol acyltransferase on apolipoprotein distribution in familial lecithin:cholesterol acyltransferase deficiency. Ann N Y Acad Sci 1980;348:224.
4. Gjone E, Norum KR. Familial serum cholesterol ester deficiency: Clinical study of a patient with a new syndrome. Acta Med Scand 1968;183:107.
5. Hovig T, Gjone E. Familial plasma lecithin:cholesterol acyltransferase (LCAT) deficiency. Ultrastructural aspects of a new syndrome with particular reference to lesions in the kidneys and the spleen. Acta Pathol Microbiol Scand [A] 1973;81:681.
6. Hiramatsu M, Karashima S, Hattori S, et al. A case of congenital nephrotic syndrome associated with partial deficiency of lecithin cholesterol acyltransferase (LCAT) and hypothyroidism. Int J Pediatr Nephrol 1984;5:183.
7. Borysiewicz LK, Soutar AK, Evans DJ, et al. Renal failure in familial lecithin:cholesterol acyltransferase deficiency. Q J Med 1982;51:411.
8. Imbasciati E, Paties C, Scarpioni L, Mihatsch MJ. Renal lesions in familial lecithin-cholesterol acyltransferase deficiency: Ultrastructural heterogeneity of glomerular changes. Am J Nephrol 1986;6:66.
9. Magil A, Chase W, Frohlich J. Unusual renal biopsy findings in a patient with familial lecithin:cholesterol acyltransferase deficiency. Hum Pathol 1982;13:283.
10. Ohta Y, Yamamoto S, Tsuchida H, et al. Nephropathy of familial lecithin-cholesterol acyltransferase deficiency: Report of a case. Am J Kidney Dis 1986;7:41.
11. Lager DJ, Rosenberg BF, Shapiro H, Bernstein J. Lecithin cholesterol acyltransferase deficiency: Ultrastructural examination of sequential renal biopsies. Mod Pathol 1991;4:331.
12. Hovig T, Gjone E. Familial lecithin:cholesterol acyltransferase deficiency: Ultrastructural studies on lipid deposition and tissue reactions. Scand J Clin Lab Invest 1974;137(suppl):135.
13. Sessa A, Battini G, Meroni M, et al. Hypocomplementemic type II membranoproliferative glomerulonephritis in a male patient with familial lecithin-cholesterol acyltransferase deficiency due to two different allelic mutations. Nephron 2001;88:268.
14. Gjone E. Familial lecithin:cholesterol acyltransferase deficiency: A new metabolic disease with renal involvement. Adv Nephrol Necker Hosp 1981;10:167.
15. Horina JH, Wirnsberger G, Horn S, et al. Long-term follow-up of a patient with lecithin cholesterol acyltransferase deficiency syndrome after kidney transplantation. Transplantation 1993;56:233.
16. Flatmark AL, Hovig T, Myhre E, Gjone E. Renal transplantation in patients with familial lecithin: Cholesterol-acetyltransferase deficiency. Transplant Proc 1977;9:1665.
17. Panescu V, Grignon Y, Hestin D, et al. Recurrence of lecithin cholesterol acyltransferase deficiency after kidney transplantation. Nephrol Dial Transplant 1997;12:2430.
18. Chung-Park M, Petrelli M, Tavill AS, et al. Renal lipidosis associated with arteriohepatic dysplasia (Alagille's syndrome). Clin Nephrol 1982;18:314.
19. Habib R, Dommergues JP, Gubler MC, et al. Glomerular mesangiolipidosis in Alagille syndrome (arteriohepatic dysplasia). Pediatr Nephrol 1987;1:455.
20. Russo PA, Ellis D, Hashida Y. Renal histopathology in Alagille's syndrome. Pediatr Pathol 1987;7:557.
21. Lynn EG, Siow YL, Frohlich J, et al. Lipoprotein-X stimulates monocyte chemoattractant protein-1 expression in mesangial cells via nuclear factor-kappa B. Kidney Int 2001;60:520.
22. Lambert G, Sakai N, Vaisman BL, et al. Analysis of glomerulosclerosis and atherosclerosis in lecithin cholesterol acyltransferase−deficient mice. J Biol Chem 2001;276:15090.
23. Zhu X, Herzenberg AM, Eskandarian M, et al. A novel in vivo lecithin-cholesterol acyltransferase (LCAT)−deficient mouse expressing predominantly LpX is associated with spontaneous glomerulopathy. Am J Pathol 2004;165:1269.
24. Faraggiana T, Churg J. Renal lipidoses: A review. Hum Pathol 1987;18:661.
25. Saito T, Sato H, Kudo K, et al. Lipoprotein glomerulopathy: Glomerular lipoprotein thrombi in a patient with hyperlipoproteinemia. Am J Kidney Dis 1989;13:148.
26. Meyrier A, Dairou F, Callard P, Mougenot B. Lipoprotein glomerulopathy: First case in a white European. Nephrol Dial Transplant 1995;10:546.
27. Mourad G, Cristol JP, Turc-Baron C, Djamali A. Lipoprotein glomerulopathy: A new apolipoprotein-E−related disease that recurs after renal transplantation. Transplant Proc 1997;29:2376.
28. Saito T, Oikawa S, Sato H, Sasaki J. Lipoprotein glomerulopathy: Renal lipidosis induced by novel apolipoprotein E variants. Nephron 1999;83:193.
29. Zhang B, Liu ZH, Zeng CH, et al. Plasma level and genetic variation of apolipoprotein E in patients with lipoprotein glomerulopathy. Chin Med J (Engl) 2005;118:555.
30. Koitabashi Y, Ikoma M, Miyahira T, et al. Long-term follow-up of a paediatric case of lipoprotein glomerulopathy. Pediatr Nephrol 1990;4:122.
31. Liberopoulos E, Siamopoulos K, Elisaf M. Apolipoprotein E and renal disease. Am J Kidney Dis 2004;43:223.
32. Saito T, Ishigaki Y, Oikawa S, Yamamoto TT. Etiological significance of apolipoprotein E mutations in lipoprotein glomerulopathy. Trends Cardiovasc Med 2002;12:67.
33. Ieiri N, Hotta O, Taguma Y. Resolution of typical lipoprotein glomerulopathy by intensive lipid-lowering therapy. Am J Kidney Dis 2003;41:244.
34. Mourad G, Djamali A, Turc-Baron C, Cristol JP. Lipoprotein glomerulopathy: A new cause of nephrotic syndrome after renal transplantation. Nephrol Dial Transplant 1998;13:1292.
35. Miyata T, Sugiyama S, Nangaku M, et al. Apolipoprotein E2/E5 variants in lipoprotein glomerulopathy recurred in transplanted kidney. J Am Soc Nephrol 1999;10:1590.
36. Utermann G. Apolipoprotein E polymorphism in health and disease. Am Heart J 1987;113(2 Pt 2):433.
37. Oikawa S, Matsunaga A, Saito T, et al. Apolipoprotein E Sendai (arginine 145→ proline): A new variant associated with lipoprotein glomerulopathy. J Am Soc Nephrol 1997;8:820.
38. Ando M, Sasaki J, Hua H, et al. A novel 18-amino acid deletion in apolipoprotein E associated with lipoprotein glomerulopathy. Kidney Int 1999;56:1317.
39. Konishi K, Saruta T, Kuramochi S, et al. Association of a novel 3-amino acid deletion mutation of apolipoprotein E (Apo E Tokyo) with lipoprotein glomerulopathy. Nephron 1999;83:214.
40. Matsunaga A, Sasaki J, Komatsu T, et al. A novel apolipoprotein E mutation, E2 (Arg25Cys), in lipoprotein glomerulopathy. Kidney Int 1999;56:421.
41. Ogawa T, Maruyama K, Hattori H, et al. A new variant of apolipoprotein E (apo E Maebashi) in lipoprotein glomerulopathy. Pediatr Nephrol 2000;14:149.

42. Ishigaki Y, Oikawa S, Suzuki T, et al. Virus-mediated transduction of apolipoprotein E (ApoE)-sendai develops lipoprotein glomerulopathy in ApoE-deficient mice. J Biol Chem 2000; 275:31269.

43. Sakatsume M, Kadomura M, Sakata I, et al. Novel glomerular lipoprotein deposits associated with apolipoprotein E2 homozygosity. Kidney Int 2001;59:1911.

44. Wen M, Segerer S, Dantas M, et al. Renal injury in apolipoprotein E-deficient mice. Lab Invest 2002;82:999.

45. Saito T, Sato H, Oikawa S, et al. Lipoprotein glomerulopathy: Report of a normolipidemic case and review of the literature. Am J Nephrol 1993;13:64.

46. Kanamaru Y, Nakao A, Shirato I, et al. Chronic graft-versus-host autoimmune disease in Fc receptor gamma chain-deficient mice results in lipoprotein glomerulopathy. J Am Soc Nephrol 2002;13:1527.

47. Hoffmann M, Scharnagl H, Panagiotou E, et al. Diminished LDL receptor and high heparin binding of apolipoprotein E2 Sendai associated with lipoprotein glomerulopathy. J Am Soc Nephrol 2001;12:524.

48. Suzaki K, Kobori S, Ueno S, et al. Effects of plasmapheresis on familial type III hyperlipoproteinemia associated with glomerular lipidosis, nephrotic syndrome and diabetes mellitus. Atherosclerosis 1990;80:181.

49. Ellis D, Orchard TJ, Lombardozzi S, et al. Atypical hyperlipidemia and nephropathy associated with apolipoprotein E homozygosity. J Am Soc Nephrol 1995;6:1170.

50. Balson KR, Niall JF, Best JD. Glomerular lipid deposition and proteinuria in a patient with familial dysbetalipoproteinaemia. J Intern Med 1996;240:157.

51. Amenomori M, Haneda M, Morikawa J, et al. A case of lipoprotein glomerulopathy successfully treated with probucol. Nephron 1994;67:109.

52. Taylor J, Thorner P, Geary DF, et al. Nephrotic syndrome and hypertension in two children with Hurler syndrome. J Pediatr 1986;108(Pt 1):726.

53. Bocca G, Monnens LA. Defective proximal tubular function in a patient with I-cell disease. Pediatr Nephrol 2003;18:830.

54. de Brito T, Gomes dos Reis V, Penna DO, Camargo ME. Glomerular involvement in Gaucher's disease: A light, immunofluorescent, and ultrastructural study based on kidney biopsy specimens. Arch Pathol 1973;95:1.

55. Rosenmann E, Aviram A. Glomerular involvement in storage diseases. J Pathol 1973;111:61.

56. Smith RL, Hutchins GM, Sack GH Jr, Ridolfi RL. Unusual cardiac, renal and pulmonary involvement in Gaucher's disease: Interstitial glucocerebroside accumulation, pulmonary hypertension and fatal bone marrow embolization. Am J Med 1978;65: 352.

57. Chander PN, Nurse HM, Pirani CL. Renal involvement in adult Gaucher's disease after splenectomy. Arch Pathol Lab Med 1979;103:440.

58. Siegal A, Gutman A, Shapiro MS, Griffel B. Renal involvement in Gaucher's disease. Postgrad Med J 1981;57:398.

59. Morimura Y, Hojo H, Abe M, Wakasa H. Gaucher's disease, type I (adult type), with massive involvement of the kidneys and lungs. Virchows Arch 1994;425:537.

60. Santoro D, Rosenbloom BE, Cohen AH. Gaucher disease with nephrotic syndrome: Response to enzyme replacement therapy. Am J Kidney Dis 2002;40:E4.

61. Fabry J. Ein Beitrag zur Kenntniss der Purpura haemorrhagica nodularis (Purpura papulosa haemorrhagica Hebrae). Arch Dermatol Syphilol 1898;43:187.

62. Anderson W. A case of "angiokeratoma." Br J Dermatol 1898; 10:113.

63. Desnick RJ, Astrin KH, Bishop DF. Fabry disease: Molecular genetics of the inherited nephropathy. Adv Nephrol Necker Hosp 1989;18:113.

64. Desnick RJ, Ioannou YA, Eng CM. Fabry disease. In: Sciver CR, Beaudet AL, Sly WS, Valle D, eds. The Metabolic and Molecular Bases of Inherited Disease, 8th ed. New York: McGraw-Hill, 2001:3733.

65. Stenson PD, Ball EV, Mort M, et al. Human Gene Mutation Database (HGMD): 2003 update. Hum Mutat 2003;21: 577.

66. Desnick RJ, Allen KY, Desnick SJ, et al. Fabry's disease: Enzymatic diagnosis of hemizygotes and heterozygotes: Alpha-galactosidase activities in plasma, serum, urine, and leukocytes. J Lab Clin Med 1973;81:157.

67. Whybra C, Kampmann C, Willers I, et al. Anderson-Fabry disease: Clinical manifestations of disease in female heterozygotes. J Inherit Metab Dis 2001;24:715.

68. MacDermot KD, Holmes A, Miners AH. Anderson-Fabry disease: Clinical manifestations and impact of disease in a cohort of 60 obligate carrier females. J Med Genet 2001;38:769.

69. Thadhani R, Wolf M, West ML, et al. Patients with Fabry disease on dialysis in the United States. Kidney Int 2002;61:249.

70. Farge D, Nadler S, Wolfe LS, et al. Diagnostic value of kidney biopsy in heterozygous Fabry's disease. Arch Pathol Lab Med 1985;109:85.

71. Schatzki PF, Kipreos B, Payne J. Fabry's disease: Primary diagnosis by electron microscopy. Am J Surg Pathol 1979;3:211.

72. McNamara TE, Goodloe S, Butkus DE. Myeloid bodies in patients without clinical Fabry's disease. Arch Pathol Lab Med 1980;104:14.

73. Banks DE, Milutinovic J, Desnick RJ, et al. Silicon nephropathy mimicking Fabry's disease. Am J Nephrol 1983;3:279.

74. Muller-Hocker J, Schmid H, Weiss M, et al. Chloroquine-induced phospholipidosis of the kidney mimicking Fabry's disease: Case report and review of the literature. Hum Pathol 2003;34: 285.

75. Albay D, Adler SG, Philipose J, et al. Chloroquine-induced lipidosis mimicking Fabry disease. Mod Pathol 2005;18:733.

76. Fukushima M, Tsuchiyama Y, Nakato T, et al. A female heterozygous patient with Fabry's disease with renal accumulation of trihexosylceramide detected with a monoclonal antibody. Am J Kidney Dis 1995;26:952.

77. Kleijer WJ, Hussaarts-Odijk LM, Sachs ES, et al. Prenatal diagnosis of Fabry's disease by direct analysis of chorionic villi. Prenat Diagn 1987;7:283.

78. Shabbeer J, Robinson M, Desnick RJ. Detection of alpha-galactosidase A mutations causing Fabry disease by denaturing high performance liquid chromatography. Hum Mutat 2005;25:299.

79. Nakao S, Takenaka T, Maeda M, et al. An atypical variant of Fabry's disease in men with left ventricular hypertrophy. N Engl J Med 1995;333:288.

80. Nakao S, Kodama C, Takenaka T, et al. Fabry disease: Detection of undiagnosed hemodialysis patients and identification of a "renal variant" phenotype. Kidney Int 2003;64:801.

81. Desbois J-C, Maziere J-C, Gubler M-C, et al. La maladie de Fabry chez l'enfent. Ann Pediatr 1977;24:575.

82. Desnick RJ, Brady RO. Fabry disease in childhood. J Pediatr 2004;144(Suppl):S20.

83. Branton MH, Schiffmann R, Sabnis SG, et al. Natural history of Fabry renal disease: Influence of alpha-galactosidase A activity and genetic mutations on clinical course. Medicine (Baltimore) 2002;81:122.

84. Pabico RC, Atancio BC, McKenna BA, et al. Renal pathologic lesions and functional alterations in a man with Fabry's disease. Am J Med 1973;55:415.

85. Burkholder PM, Updike SJ, Ware RA, Reese OG. Clinicopathologic, enzymatic, and genetic features in a case of Fabry's disease. Arch Pathol Lab Med 1980;104:17.

86. Chatterjee S, Gupta P, Pyeritz RE, Kwiterovich PO Jr. Immunohistochemical localization of glycosphingolipid in urinary renal tubular cells in Fabry's disease. Am J Clin Pathol 1984;82:24.

87. Katz SM, Lyons PJ. Urinary ultrastructural findings in Fabry disease. JAMA 1977;237:1121.

88. Wenk RE, Bhagavan BS, Francis E. Myelin bodies in urine sediment in hemizygotes with Anderson-Fabry disease. Ultrastruct Pathol 1983;5:123.

89. Glass RB, Astrin KH, Norton KI, et al. Fabry disease: Renal sonographic and magnetic resonance imaging findings in affected males and carrier females with the classic and cardiac variant phenotypes. J Comput Assist Tomogr 2004;28:158.

90. Ries M, Bettis KE, Choyke P, et al. Parapelvic kidney cysts: A distinguishing feature with high prevalence in Fabry disease. Kidney Int 2004;66:978.

91. Savi M, Olivetti G, Neri TM, Curtoni C. Clinical, histopathological, and biochemical findings in Fabry's disease: A case report and family study. Arch Pathol Lab Med 1977;101:536.

92. Alroy J, Sabnis S, Kopp JB. Renal pathology in Fabry disease. J Am Soc Nephrol 2002;13 Suppl 2:S134.

93. Tondeur M, Resibois A. Fabry's disease in children: An electron microscopic study. Virchows Arch B Cell Pathol 1969;2:239.

94. Gubler MC, Lenoir G, Grunfeld JP, et al. Early renal changes in hemizygous and heterozygous patients with Fabry's disease. Kidney Int 1978;13:223.

95. Sessa A, Toson A, Nebuloni M, et al. Renal ultrastructural findings in Anderson-Fabry disease. J Nephrol 2002;15:109.

96. Simon M, Frey H, Gruler H, Bultmann B. Glycolipid storage material in Fabry's disease: A study by electron microscopy, freeze-fracture, and digital image analysis. J Struct Biol 1990;103:40.

97. Sessa A, Meroni M, Battini G, et al. Renal pathological changes in Fabry disease. J Inherit Metab Dis 2001;24(suppl 2):66.

98. DeGraba T, Azhar S, Dignat-George F, et al. Profile of endothelial and leukocyte activation in Fabry patients. Ann Neurol 2000;47:229.

99. Takahashi H, Hirai Y, Migita M, et al. Long-term systemic therapy of Fabry disease in a knockout mouse by adeno-associated virus-mediated muscle-directed gene transfer. Proc Natl Acad Sci U S A 2002;99:13777.

100. Eitzman DT, Bodary PF, Shen Y, et al. Fabry disease in mice is associated with age-dependent susceptibility to vascular thrombosis. J Am Soc Nephrol 2003;14:298.

101. Ojo A, Meier-Kriesche HU, Friedman G, et al. Excellent outcome of renal transplantation in patients with Fabry's disease. Transplantation 2000;69:2337.

102. Mignani R, Gerra D, Maldini L, et al. Long-term survival of patients with renal transplantation in Fabry's disease. Contrib Nephrol 2001;229.

103. Spence MW, MacKinnon KE, Burgess JK, et al. Failure to correct the metabolic defect by renal allotransplantion in Fabry's disease. Ann Intern Med 1976;84:13.

104. Kramer W, Thormann J, Mueller K, Frenzel H. Progressive cardiac involvement by Fabry's disease despite successful renal allotransplantation. Int J Cardiol 1985;7:72.

105. Faraggiana T, Churg J, Grishman E, et al. Light- and electron-microscopic histochemistry of Fabry's disease. Am J Pathol 1981;103:247.

106. Friedlaender MM, Kopolovic J, Rubinger D, et al. Renal biopsy in Fabry's disease eight years after successful renal transplantation. Clin Nephrol 1987;27:206.

107. Mosnier JF, Degott C, Bedrossian J, et al. Recurrence of Fabry's disease in a renal allograft eleven years after successful renal transplantation. Transplantation 1991;51:759.

108. Gantenbein H, Bruder E, Burger HR, et al. Recurrence of Fabry's disease in a renal allograft 14 years after transplantation. Nephrol Dial Transplant 1995;10:287.

109. Popli S, Molnar ZV, Leehey DJ, et al. Involvement of renal allograft by Fabry's disease. Am J Nephrol 1987;7:316.

110. Puliyanda DP, Wilcox WR, Bunnapradist S, et al. Fabry disease in a renal allograft. Am J Transplant 2003;3:1030.

111. Eng CM, Guffon N, Wilcox WR, et al. Safety and efficacy of recombinant human alpha-galactosidase A-replacement therapy in Fabry's disease. N Engl J Med 2001;345:9.

112. Schiffmann R, Kopp JB, Austin HA III, et al. Enzyme replacement therapy in Fabry disease: A randomized controlled trial. JAMA 2001;285:2743.

113. Thurberg BL, Rennke H, Colvin RB, et al. Globotriaosylceramide accumulation in the Fabry kidney is cleared from multiple cell types after enzyme replacement therapy. Kidney Int 2002;62:1933.

114. Baehner F, Kampmann C, Whybra C, et al. Enzyme replacement therapy in heterozygous females with Fabry disease: Results of a phase IIIB study. J Inherit Metab Dis 2003;26:617.

115. Linthorst GE, Hollak CE, Donker-Koopman WE, et al. Enzyme therapy for Fabry disease: Neutralizing antibodies toward agalsidase alpha and beta. Kidney Int 2004;66:1589.

116. De Schoenmakere G, Chauveau D, Grunfeld JP. Enzyme replacement therapy in Anderson-Fabry's disease: Beneficial clinical effect on vital organ function. Nephrol Dial Transplant 2003;18:33.

117. Mignani R, Cagnoli L. Enzyme replacement therapy in Fabry's disease: Recent advances and clinical applications. J Nephrol 2004;17:354.

118. Mignani R, Panichi V, Giudicissi A, et al. Enzyme replacement therapy with agalsidase beta in kidney transplant patients with Fabry disease: A pilot study. Kidney Int 2004;65:1381.

119. Thomas GH. Disorders of glycoprotein degradation: α-mannosidosis, β-mannosidosis, fucosidosis, and sialidosis. In: Sciver CR, Beaudet AL, Valle D, Sly WS, eds. The Metabolic and Molecular Bases of Inherited Disease, 8th ed. New York: McGraw-Hill, 2001:3507.

120. LeSec G, Stanescu R, Lyon G. Un nouveau type de sialidose avec atteinte renale: La nephrosialidose. Arch Fr Pediatr 1978;35:830.

121. Maroteaux P, Humbel R, Strecker G, et al. Un nouveau type de sialidose avec atteinte renale: La nephrosialidose. Arch Fr Pediatr 1978;35:819.

122. Burin MG, Scholz AP, Gus R, et al. Investigation of lysosomal storage diseases in nonimmune hydrops fetalis. Prenat Diagn 2004;24:653.

123. Aylsworth AS, Thomas GH, Hood JL, et al. A severe infantile sialidosis: Clinical, biochemical, and microscopic features. J Pediatr 1980;96:662.

124. Roth KS, Chan JC, Ghatak NR, et al. Acid alpha-neuraminidase deficiency: A nephropathic phenotype? Clin Genet 1988;34:185.

125. Kashtan CE, Nevins TE, Posalaky Z, et al. Proteinuria in a child with sialidosis: Case report and histological studies. Pediatr Nephrol 1989;3:166.

126. Strehle EM. Sialic acid storage disease and related disorders. Genet Test 2003;7:113.

127. Galjart NJ, Morreau H, Willemsen R, et al. Human lysosomal protective protein has cathepsin A-like activity distinct from its protective function. J Biol Chem 1991;266:14754.

128. Sewell AC, Pontz BF, Weitzel D, Humburg C. Clinical heterogeneity in infantile galactosialidosis. Eur J Pediatr 1987;146:528.

129. d'Azzo A, Andria G, Strisciuglio P, Galjaard H. Galactosialidosis. In: Sciver CR, Beaudet AL, Valle D, Sly WS, eds. The Metabolic and Molecular Bases of Inherited Disease, 8th ed. New York: McGraw-Hill, 2001:3811.

130. Wreden CC, Wlizla M, Reimer RJ. Varied mechanisms underlie the free sialic acid storage disorders. J Biol Chem 2005;280:1408.

131. Hale LP, van de Ven CJ, Wenger DA, et al. Infantile sialic acid storage disease: A rare cause of cytoplasmic vacuolation in pediatric patients. Pediatr Pathol Lab Med 1995;15:443.

132. Sperl W, Gruber W, Quatacker J, et al. Nephrosis in two siblings with infantile sialic acid storage disease. Eur J Pediatr 1990;149:477.

133. Lemyre E, Russo P, Melancon SB, et al. Clinical spectrum of infantile free sialic acid storage disease. Am J Med Genet 1999;82:385.

134. Ishiwari K, Kotani M, Suzuki M, et al. Clinical, biochemical, and cytochemical studies on a Japanese Salla disease case associated with a renal disorder. J Hum Genet 2004;49:656.

135. Yamano T, Shimada M, Sugino H, et al. Ultrastructural study on a severe infantile sialidosis (beta-galactosidase-alpha-neuraminidase deficiency). Neuropediatrics 1985;16:109.

136. Krivan G, Timar L, Goda V, et al. Bone marrow transplantation in non-malignant disorders. Bone Marrow Transplant 1998;22(suppl 4):S80.

137. Rosenblatt DS, Fenton WA. Inherited disorders of folate and cobalamin transport and metabolism. In: Sciver CR, Beaudet AL, Valle D, Sly WS, eds. The Metabolic and Molecular Bases of Inherited Disease, 8th ed. New York: McGraw-Hill, 2001:3897.

138. Van Hove JL, Van Damme-Lombaerts R, Grunewald S, et al. Cobalamin disorder Cbl-C presenting with late-onset

thrombotic microangiopathy. Am J Med Genet 2002;111:195.

139. Baumgartner ER, Wick H, Linnell JC, et al. Congenital defect in intracellular cobalamin metabolism resulting in homocystinuria and methylmalonic aciduria. II. Biochemical investigations. Helv Paediatr Acta 1979;34:483.

140. Geraghty MT, Perlman EJ, Martin LS, et al. Cobalamin C defect associated with hemolytic-uremic syndrome. J Pediatr 1992;120:934.

141. Russo P, Doyon J, Sonsino E, et al. A congenital anomaly of vitamin B12 metabolism: A study of three cases. Hum Pathol 1992;23:504.

142. Brunelli SM, Meyers KE, Guttenberg M, et al. Cobalamin C deficiency complicated by an atypical glomerulopathy. Pediatr Nephrol 2002;17:800.

143. Baumgarter ER, Viardot C. Long-term follow-up of 77 patients with isolated methylmalonic acidaemia. J Inherit Metab Dis 1995;18:138.

144. D'Angio CT, Dillon MJ, Leonard JV. Renal tubular dysfunction in methylmalonic acidaemia. Eur J Pediatr 1991;150:259.

145. Molteni KH, Oberley TD, Wolff JA, Friedman AL. Progressive renal insufficiency in methylmalonic acidemia. Pediatr Nephrol 1991;5:323.

146. Rutledge SL, Geraghty M, Mroczek E, et al. Tubulointerstitial nephritis in methylmalonic acidemia. Pediatr Nephrol 1993;7:81.

147. van 't Hoff WG, Dixon M, Taylor J, et al. Combined liver-kidney transplantation in methylmalonic acidemia. J Pediatr 1998;132:1043.

148. Nagarajan S, Enns GM, Millan MT, et al. Management of methylmalonic acidaemia by combined liver-kidney transplantation. J Inherit Metab Dis 2005;28:517.

149. Chen Y-T. Glycogen storage disease. In: Sciver CR, Beaudet AL, Valle D, Sly WS, eds. The Metabolic and Molecular Bases of Inherited Disease, 8th ed. New York: McGraw-Hill, 2001:1521.

150. Chou JY, Matern D, Mansfield BC, Chen YT. Type I glycogen storage diseases: Disorders of the glucose-6-phosphatase complex. Curr Mol Med 2002;2:121.

151. Chen YT, Scheinman JI, Park HK, et al. Amelioration of proximal renal tubular dysfunction in type I glycogen storage disease with dietary therapy. N Engl J Med 1990;323:590.

152. Baker L, Dahlem S, Goldfarb S, et al. Hyperfiltration and renal disease in glycogen storage disease, type I. Kidney Int 1989;35:1345.

153. Chen YT, Coleman RA, Scheinman JI, et al. Renal disease in type I glycogen storage disease. N Engl J Med 1988;318:7.

154. Chen YT. Type I glycogen storage disease: Kidney involvement, pathogenesis and its treatment. Pediatr Nephrol 1991;5:71.

155. Lee PJ, Dalton RN, Shah V, et al. Glomerular and tubular function in glycogen storage disease. Pediatr Nephrol 1995;9:705.

156. Reitsma-Bierens WC, Smit GP, Troelstra JA. Renal function and kidney size in glycogen storage disease type I. Pediatr Nephrol 1992;6:236.

157. Fick JJ, Beek FJ. Echogenic kidneys and medullary calcium deposition in a young child with glycogen storage disease type 1a. Pediatr Radiol 1992;22:72.

158. Restaino I, Kaplan BS, Stanley C, Baker L. Nephrolithiasis, hypocitraturia, and a distal renal tubular acidification defect in type 1 glycogen storage disease. J Pediatr 1993;122:392.

159. Talente GM, Coleman RA, Alter C, et al. Glycogen storage disease in adults. Ann Intern Med 1994;120:218.

160. Lin CC, Tsai JD, Lin SP, Lee HC. Renal sonographic findings of type I glycogen storage disease in infancy and early childhood. Pediatr Radiol 2005;35:786.

161. Obara K, Saito T, Sato H, et al. Renal histology in two adult patients with type I glycogen storage disease. Clin Nephrol 1993;39:59.

162. Yokoyama K, Hayashi H, Hinoshita F, et al. Renal lesion of type Ia glycogen storage disease: The glomerular size and renal localization of apolipoprotein. Nephron 1995;70:348.

163. Jonas AJ, Verani RR, Howell RR, Conley SB. Hypertension in a child with type IA glycogen storage disease. Am J Kidney Dis 1988;11:264.

164. Verani R, Bernstein J. Renal glomerular and tubular abnormalities in glycogen storage disease type I. Arch Pathol Lab Med 1988;112:271.

165. Lei KJ, Shelly LL, Pan CJ, et al. Mutations in the glucose-6-phosphatase gene that cause glycogen storage disease type 1a. Science 1993;262:580.

166. Janecke AR, Mayatepek E, Utermann G. Molecular genetics of type 1 glycogen storage disease. Mol Genet Metab 2001;73:117.

167. Matern D, Seydewitz HH, Bali D, et al. Glycogen storage disease type I: Diagnosis and phenotype/genotype correlation. Eur J Pediatr 2002;161(suppl 1):S10.

168. Gerin I, Veiga-da-Cunha M, Achouri Y, et al. Sequence of a putative glucose 6-phosphate translocase, mutated in glycogen storage disease type Ib. FEBS Lett 1997;419:235.

169. Rake JP, Visser G, Labrune P, et al. Glycogen storage disease type I: Diagnosis, management, clinical course and outcome. Results of the European Study on Glycogen Storage Disease Type I (ESGSD I). Eur J Pediatr 2002;161(suppl 1):S20.

170. Ozen H, Ciliv G, Kocak N, et al. Short-term effect of captopril on microalbuminuria in children with glycogen storage disease type Ia. J Inherit Metab Dis 2000;23:459.

171. Labrune P. Glycogen storage disease type I: Indications for liver and/or kidney transplantation. Eur J Pediatr 2002;161(suppl 1):S53.

172. Mittal SK, Dash SC, Mittal R, et al. McArdle's disease presenting as acute renal failure. Nephron 1995;71:109.

173. Walker AR, Tschetter K, Matsuo F, Flanigan KM. McArdle's disease presenting as recurrent cryptogenic renal failure due to occult seizures. Muscle Nerve 2003;28:640.

174. Moser HW. Molecular genetics of peroxisomal disorders. Front Biosci 2000;5:D298.

175. Gould SJ, Raymond GV, Valle D. The peroxisome biogenesis disorders. In: Sciver CR, Beaudet AL, Sly WS, Valle D, eds. The Metabolic and Molecular Bases of Inherited Disease, 8th ed. New York: McGraw-Hill, 2001:3181.

176. Depreter M, Espeel M, Roels F. Human peroxisomal disorders. Microsc Res Tech 2003;61:203.

177. Powers JM, Moser HW, Moser AB, et al. Fetal cerebrohepatorenal (Zellweger) syndrome: Dysmorphic, radiologic, biochemical, and pathologic findings in four affected fetuses. Hum Pathol 1985;16:610.

178. Bernstein J, Brough AJ, McAdams AJ. The renal lesion in syndromes of multiple congenital malformations. Cerebrohepatorenal syndrome; Jeune asphyxiating thoracic dystrophy; tuberous sclerosis; Meckel syndrome. Birth Defects 1974;10:35.

179. Gilchrist KW, Gilbert EF, Goldfarb S, et al. Studies of malformation syndromes of man XIB: The cerebro-hepato-renal syndrome of Zellweger: Comparative pathology. Eur J Pediatr 1976;121:99.

180. Harkin JC, Gill WL, Shapira E. Glutaric acidemia type II. Phenotypic findings and ultrastructural studies of brain and kidney. Arch Pathol Lab Med 1986;110:399.

181. Wilson GN, de Chadarevian JP, Kaplan P, et al. Glutaric aciduria type II: Review of the phenotype and report of an unusual glomerulopathy. Am J Med Genet 1989;32:395.

182. Whitfield J, Hurst D, Bennett MJ, et al. Fetal polycystic kidney disease associated with glutaric aciduria type II: An inborn error of energy metabolism. Am J Perinatol 1996;13:131.

183. Kjaergaard S, Graem N, Larsen T, Skovby F. Recurrent fetal polycystic kidneys associated with glutaric aciduria type II. APMIS 1998;106:1188.

184. van den Brink DM, Brites P, Haasjes J, et al. Identification of PEX7 as the second gene involved in Refsum disease. Am J Hum Genet 2003;72:471.

185. Jansen GA, Waterham HR, Wanders RJ. Molecular basis of Refsum disease: Sequence variations in phytanoyl-CoA hydroxylase (PHYH) and the PTS2 receptor (PEX7). Hum Mutat 2004;23:209.

186. Wierzbicki AS, Lloyd MD, Schofield CJ, et al. Refsum's disease: A peroxisomal disorder affecting phytanic acid alpha-oxidation. J Neurochem 2002;80:727.

187. Plant GR, Hansell DM, Gibberd FB, Sidey MC. Skeletal abnormalities in Refsum's disease (heredopathia atactica polyneuritiformis). Br J Radiol 1990;63:537.

188. Weinstein R. Phytanic acid storage disease (Refsum's disease): Clinical characteristics, pathophysiology and the role of therapeutic apheresis in its management. J Clin Apheresis 1999; 14:181.

189. Pabico RC, Gruebel BJ, McKenna BA, et al. Renal involvement in Refsum's disease. Am J Med 1981;70:1136.

190. D'Agrosa MC, Deteix P, Fonck Y, et al. [The kidney in Refsum's disease. Clinical, histologic and ultrastructural study of a case.] Nephrologie 1988;9:269.

191. Hughes JL, Poulos A, Robertson E, et al. Pathology of hepatic peroxisomes and mitochondria in patients with peroxisomal disorders. Virchows Arch A Pathol Anat Histopathol 1990;416: 255.

192. Danpure CJ, Jennings PR. Peroxisomal alanine: glyoxylate aminotransferase deficiency in primary hyperoxaluria type I. FEBS Lett 1986;201:20.

193. Danpure CJ. Primary Hyperoxaluria. In: Sciver CR, Beaudet AL, Valle D, Sly WS, eds. The Metabolic and Molecular Bases of Inherited Disease, 8th ed. New York: McGraw Hill, 2001: 3323.

194. Coulter-Mackie MB, Rumsby G. Genetic heterogeneity in primary hyperoxaluria type 1: Impact on diagnosis. Mol Genet Metab 2004;83:38.

195. Danpure CJ. Molecular aetiology of primary hyperoxaluria type 1. Nephron Exp Nephrol 2004;98:e39.

196. Pirulli D, Marangella M, Amoroso A. Primary hyperoxaluria: Genotype-phenotype correlation. J Nephrol 2003;16:297.

197. Leumann E, Hoppe B. Primary hyperoxaluria type 1: Is genotyping clinically helpful? Pediatr Nephrol 2005;20:555.

198. Marangella M, Petrarulo M, Cosseddu D. End-stage renal failure in primary hyperoxaluria type 2. N Engl J Med 1994;330: 1690.

199. Milliner DS, Wilson DM, Smith LH. Phenotypic expression of primary hyperoxaluria: Comparative features of types I and II. Kidney Int 2001;59:31.

200. Johnson SA, Rumsby G, Cregeen D, Hulton SA. Primary hyperoxaluria type 2 in children. Pediatr Nephrol 2002;17:597.

201. Webster KE, Ferree PM, Holmes RP, Cramer SD. Identification of missense, nonsense, and deletion mutations in the GRHPR gene in patients with primary hyperoxaluria type II (PH2). Hum Genet 2000;107:176.

202. Leumann E, Hoppe B. The primary hyperoxalurias. J Am Soc Nephrol 2001;12:1986.

203. Chetyrkin SV, Kim D, Belmont JM, et al. Pyridoxamine lowers kidney crystals in experimental hyperoxaluria: A potential therapy for primary hyperoxaluria. Kidney Int 2005;67:53.

204. Gagnadoux MF, Lacaille F, Niaudet P, et al. Long term results of liver-kidney transplantation in children with primary hyperoxaluria. Pediatr Nephrol 2001;16:946.

205. Cibrik DM, Kaplan B, Arndorfer JA, Meier-Kriesche HU. Renal allograft survival in patients with oxalosis. Transplantation 2002;74:707.

206. Bergeron M, Gougoux A, Noel J, Parent L. The renal Fanconi syndrome. In: Sciver CR, Beaudet AL, Sly WS, Valle D, eds. The Metabolic and Molecular Bases of Inherited Disease, 8th ed. New York: McGraw-Hill, 2001:5023.

207. Bendon RW, Hug G. Glycogen accumulation in the pars recta of the proximal tubule in Fanconi syndrome. Pediatr Pathol 1986;6:411.

208. Gahl WA, Thoene JG, Schneider JA. Cystinosis. N Engl J Med 2002;347:111.

209. Linkage of the gene for cystinosis to markers on the short arm of chromosome 17. The Cystinosis Collaborative Research Group. Nat Genet 1995;10:246.

210. Town M, Jean G, Cherqui S, et al. A novel gene encoding an integral membrane protein is mutated in nephropathic cystinosis. Nat Genet 1998;18:319.

211. Lemire J, Kaplan BS. The various renal manifestations of the nephropathic form of cystinosis. Am J Nephrol 1984;4:81.

212. Pennesi M, Marchetti F, Crovella S, et al. A new mutation in

213. Clay RD, Darmady EM, Hawkins M. The nature of the renal lesion in the Fanconi syndrome. J Pathol Bacteriol 1953;65: 551.

214. Jackson JD, Smith FG, Litman NN, et al. The Fanconi syndrome with cystinosis. Electron microscopy of renal biopsy specimens from five patients. Am J Med 1962;33:893.

215. Spear GS, Slusser RJ, Tousimis AJ, et al. Cystinosis. An ultrastructural and electron-probe study of the kidney with unusual findings. Arch Pathol 1971;91:206.

216. Spear GS, Slusser RJ, Schulman JD, Alexander F. Polykaryocytosis of the visceral glomerular epithelium in cystinosis with description of an unusual clinical variant. Johns Hopkins Med J 1971;129:83.

217. Manz F, Harms E, Lutz P, et al. Adolescent cystinosis: Renal function and morphology. Eur J Pediatr 1982;138:354.

218. Hory B, Billerey C, Royer J, Saint Hillier Y. Glomerular lesions in juvenile cystinosis: Report of 2 cases. Clin Nephrol 1994;42: 327.

219. Kalatzis V, Cherqui S, Antignac C, Gasnier B. Cystinosin, the protein defective in cystinosis, is a H(+)-driven lysosomal cystine transporter. Embo J 2001;20:5940.

220. Kalatzis V, Nevo N, Cherqui S, et al. Molecular pathogenesis of cystinosis: Effect of CTNS mutations on the transport activity and subcellular localization of cystinosin. Hum Mol Genet 2004;13:1361.

221. Coor C, Salmon RF, Quigley R, et al. Role of adenosine triphosphate (ATP) and NaK ATPase in the inhibition of proximal tubule transport with intracellular cystine loading. J Clin Invest 1991;87:955.

222. Cetinkaya I, Schlatter E, Hirsch JR, et al. Inhibition of Na(+)-dependent transporters in cystine-loaded human renal cells: Electrophysiological studies on the Fanconi syndrome of cystinosis. J Am Soc Nephrol 2002;13:2085.

223. Park M, Helip-Wooley A, Thoene J. Lysosomal cystine storage augments apoptosis in cultured human fibroblasts and renal tubular epithelial cells. J Am Soc Nephrol 2002;13:2878.

224. Cherqui S, Sevin C, Hamard G, et al. Intralysosomal cystine accumulation in mice lacking cystinosin, the protein defective in cystinosis. Mol Cell Biol 2002;22:7622.

225. Spear GS, Gubler MC, Habib R, Broyer M. Dark cells of cystinosis: Occurrence in renal allografts. Hum Pathol 1989;20:472.

226. Spear GS, Gubler MC, Habib R, Broyer M. Renal allografts in cystinosis and mesangial demography. Clin Nephrol 1989; 32:256.

227. Theodoropoulos DS, Krasnewich D, Kaiser-Kupfer MI, Gahl WA. Classic nephropathic cystinosis as an adult disease. JAMA 1993;270:2200.

228. Kashtan CE, McEnery PT, Tejani A, Stablein DM. Renal allograft survival according to primary diagnosis: A report of the North American Pediatric Renal Transplant Cooperative Study. Pediatr Nephrol 1995;9:679.

229. Robert JJ, Tete MJ, Guest G, et al. Diabetes mellitus in patients with infantile cystinosis after renal transplantation. Pediatr Nephrol 1999;13:524.

230. Scheinman SJ, Pook MA, Wooding C, et al. Mapping the gene causing X-linked recessive nephrolithiasis to Xp11.22 by linkage studies. J Clin Invest 1993;91:2351.

231. Knohl SJ, Scheinman SJ. Inherited hypercalciuric syndromes: Dent's disease (CLC-5) and familial hypomagnesemia with hypercalciuria (paracellin-1). Semin Nephrol 2004;24: 55.

232. Wrong OM, Norden AG, Feest TG. Dent's disease; a familial proximal renal tubular syndrome with low-molecular-weight proteinuria, hypercalciuria, nephrocalcinosis, metabolic bone disease, progressive renal failure and a marked male predominance. QJM 1994;87:473.

233. Langlois V, Bernard C, Scheinman SJ, et al. Clinical features of X-linked nephrolithiasis in childhood. Pediatr Nephrol 1998;12:625.

234. Burgess HK, Jayawardene SA, Velasco N. Dent's disease: Can we slow its progression? Nephrol Dial Transplant 2001;16:1512.

two siblings with cystinosis presenting with Bartter syndrome. Pediatr Nephrol 2005;20:217.

235. Pearce SH. Straightening out the renal tubule: Advances in the molecular basis of the inherited tubulopathies. QJM 1998; 91:5.

236. Lloyd SE, Pearce SH, Fisher SE, et al. A common molecular basis for three inherited kidney stone diseases. Nature 1996;379: 445.

237. Scheinman SJ. X-linked hypercalciuric nephrolithiasis: Clinical syndromes and chloride channel mutations. Kidney Int 1998; 53:3.

238. Hoopes RR Jr, Raja KM, Koich A, et al. Evidence for genetic heterogeneity in Dent's disease. Kidney Int 2004;65:1615.

239. Hoopes RR Jr, Shrimpton AE, Knohl SJ, et al. Dent Disease with mutations in OCRL1. Am J Hum Genet 2005;76:260.

240. Frymoyer PA, Scheinman SJ, Dunham PB, et al. X-linked recessive nephrolithiasis with renal failure. N Engl J Med 1991;325: 681.

241. Moulin P, Igarashi T, Van der Smissen P, et al. Altered polarity and expression of H+-ATPase without ultrastructural changes in kidneys of Dent's disease patients. Kidney Int 2003;63: 1285.

242. Devuyst O, Christie PT, Courtoy PJ, et al. Intra-renal and subcellular distribution of the human chloride channel, CLC-5, reveals a pathophysiological basis for Dent's disease. Hum Mol Genet 1999;8:247.

243. Christensen EI, Birn H. Megalin and cubilin: Multifunctional endocytic receptors. Nat Rev Mol Cell Biol 2002;3:256.

244. Christensen EI, Gburek J. Protein reabsorption in renal proximal tubule-function and dysfunction in kidney pathophysiology. Pediatr Nephrol 2004;19:714.

245. Christensen EI, Devuyst O, Dom G, et al. Loss of chloride channel ClC-5 impairs endocytosis by defective trafficking of megalin and cubilin in kidney proximal tubules. Proc Natl Acad Sci U S A 2003;100:8472.

246. Gunther W, Piwon N, Jentsch TJ. The ClC-5 chloride channel knock-out mouse—an animal model for Dent's disease. Pflugers Arch 2003;445:456.

247. Rotig A, Munnich A. Genetic features of mitochondrial respiratory chain disorders. J Am Soc Nephrol 2003;14:2995.

248. Szabolcs MJ, Seigle R, Shanske S, et al. Mitochondrial DNA deletion: A cause of chronic tubulointerstitial nephropathy. Kidney Int 1994;45:1388.

249. Mochizuki H, Joh K, Kawame H, et al. Mitochondrial encephalomyopathies preceded by de-Toni-Debre-Fanconi syndrome or focal segmental glomerulosclerosis. Clin Nephrol 1996;46:347.

250. Ormos J, Zsurka G, Turi S, Ivanyi B. Familial mitochondrial tubulointerstitial nephropathy. Nephrol Dial Transplant 1999; 14:785.

251. Tzen CY, Tsai JD, Wu TY, et al. Tubulointerstitial nephritis associated with a novel mitochondrial point mutation. Kidney Int 2001;59:846.

252. de Lonlay P, Valnot I, Barrientos A, et al. A mutant mitochondrial respiratory chain assembly protein causes complex III deficiency in patients with tubulopathy, encephalopathy and liver failure. Nat Genet 2001;29:57.

253. Hotta O, Inoue CN, Miyabayashi S, et al. Clinical and pathologic features of focal segmental glomerulosclerosis with mitochondrial tRNALeu(UUR) gene mutation. Kidney Int 2001;59: 1236.

254. Yamagata K, Muro K, Usui J, et al. Mitochondrial DNA mutations in focal segmental glomerulosclerosis lesions. J Am Soc Nephrol 2002;13:1816.

255. Guery B, Choukroun G, Noel LH, et al. The spectrum of systemic involvement in adults presenting with renal lesion and mitochondrial tRNA(Leu) gene mutation. J Am Soc Nephrol 2003;14:2099.

256. Dinour D, Mini S, Polak-Charcon S, et al. Progressive nephropathy associated with mitochondrial tRNA gene mutation. Clin Nephrol 2004;62:149.

257. Rotig A. Renal disease and mitochondrial genetics. J Nephrol 2003;16:286.

258. Eviatar L, Shanske S, Gauthier B, et al. Kearns-Sayre syndrome presenting as renal tubular acidosis. Neurology 1990;40:1761.

259. Kuwertz-Broking E, Koch HG, Marquardt T, et al. Renal Fanconi syndrome: First sign of partial respiratory chain complex IV deficiency. Pediatr Nephrol 2000;14:495.

260. Ogier H, Lombes A, Scholte HR, et al. de Toni-Fanconi-Debre syndrome with Leigh syndrome revealing severe muscle cytochrome c oxidase deficiency. J Pediatr 1988;112:734.

261. Niaudet P, Heidet L, Munnich A, et al. Deletion of the mitochondrial DNA in a case of de Toni-Debre-Fanconi syndrome and Pearson syndrome. Pediatr Nephrol 1994;8:164.

262. Smith OP, Hann IM, Woodward CE, Brockington M. Pearson's marrow/pancreas syndrome: Haematological features associated with deletion and duplication of mitochondrial DNA. Br J Haematol 1995;90:469.

263. Niaudet P. Mitochondrial disorders and the kidney. Arch Dis Child 1998;78:387.

264. Thirumurugan A, Thewles A, Gilbert RD, et al. Urinary L-lactate excretion is increased in renal Fanconi syndrome. Nephrol Dial Transplant 2004;19:1767.

265. Lowe CU, Terrey M, Mac Lachlan EA. Organic-aciduria, decreased renal ammonia production, hydrophthalmos, and mental retardation; A clinical entity. Am J Dis Child 1952;83:164.

266. Nussbaum RL, Suchy SF. The oculocerebrorenal syndrome of Lowe (Lowe Syndrome). In: Sciver CR, Beaudet AL, Sly WS, Valle D, eds. The Metabolic and Molecular Bases of Inherited Disease, 8th ed. New York: McGraw-Hill, 2001:6257.

267. Van Acker KJ, Roels H, Beelaerts W, et al. The histologic lesions of the kidney in the oculo-cerebro-renal syndrome of Lowe. Nephron 1967;4:193.

268. Witzleben CL, Schoen EJ, Tu WH, McDonald LW. Progressive morphologic renal changes in the oculo-cerebro-renal syndrome of Lowe. Am J Med 1968;44:319.

269. Ores RO. Renal changes in oculo-cerebro-renal syndrome of Lowe. Electron microscopic study. Arch Pathol 1970;89:221.

270. Hayashi Y, Hanioka K, Kanomata N, et al. Clinicopathologic and molecular-pathologic approaches to Lowe's syndrome. Pediatr Pathol Lab Med 1995;15:389.

271. Leahey AM, Charnas LR, Nussbaum RL. Nonsense mutations in the OCRL-1 gene in patients with the oculocerebrorenal syndrome of Lowe. Hum Mol Genet 1993;2:461.

272. Zhang X, Jefferson AB, Auethavekiat V, Majerus PW. The protein deficient in Lowe syndrome is a phosphatidylinositol-4,5-bisphosphate 5-phosphatase. Proc Natl Acad Sci U S A 1995; 92:4853.

273. Faucherre A, Desbois P, Nagano F, et al. Lowe syndrome protein Ocrl1 is translocated to membrane ruffles upon Rac GTPase activation: A new perspective on Lowe syndrome pathophysiology. Hum Mol Genet 2005;14:1441.

274. Norden AG, Lapsley M, Igarashi T, et al. Urinary megalin deficiency implicates abnormal tubular endocytic function in Fanconi syndrome. J Am Soc Nephrol 2002;13:125.

275. Fanconi G, Bickel H. Die chronische aminoacidurie (aminosaurediabetes oder nephrotisch-glukosurischer zwergwuchs) bei der Glykogenose und der cystinkrankheit. Helv Paediatr Acta 1949;4:359.

276. Santer R, Schneppenheim R, Dombrowski A, et al. Mutations in GLUT2, the gene for the liver-type glucose transporter, in patients with Fanconi-Bickel syndrome. Nat Genet 1997;17:324.

277. Manz F, Bickel H, Brodehl J, et al. Fanconi-Bickel syndrome. Pediatr Nephrol 1987;1:509.

278. Berry GT, Baker L, Kaplan FS, Witzleben CL. Diabetes-like renal glomerular disease in Fanconi-Bickel syndrome. Pediatr Nephrol 1995;9:287.

279. Santer R, Groth S, Kinner M, et al. The mutation spectrum of the facilitative glucose transporter gene SLC2A2 (GLUT2) in patients with Fanconi-Bickel syndrome. Hum Genet 2002;110: 21.

280. Fukumoto H, Seino S, Imura H, et al. Sequence, tissue distribution, and chromosomal localization of mRNA encoding a human glucose transporter-like protein. Proc Natl Acad Sci U S A 1988;85:5434.

281. Ozer EA, Aksu N, Uclar E, et al. No mutation in the SLC2A2 (GLUT2) gene in a Turkish infant with Fanconi-Bickel syndrome. Pediatr Nephrol 2003;18:397.

282. Santer R, Steinmann B, Schaub J. Fanconi-Bickel syndrome-A congenital defect of facilitative glucose transport. Curr Mol Med 2002;2:213.

283. Barroso I, Luan J, Middelberg RP, et al. Candidate gene association study in type 2 diabetes indicates a role for genes involved in beta-cell function as well as insulin action [erratum appears in PLoS Biol 2003 Dec;1(3):445]. PLoS Biol 2003 Oct;1(1): E20.

284. Brown GK. Glucose transporters: Structure, function and consequences of deficiency. J Inherit Metab Dis 2000;23:237.

285. Izzedine H, Launay-Vacher V, Isnard-Bagnis C, Deray G. Drug-induced Fanconi's syndrome. Am J Kidney Dis 2003;41:292.

286. Hawkins E, Brewer E. Renal toxicity induced by valproic acid (Depakene). Pediatr Pathol 1993;13:863.

287. Tanji N, Tanji K, Kambham N, et al. Adefovir nephrotoxicity: Possible role of mitochondrial DNA depletion. Hum Pathol 2001;32:734.

288. Thevenod F. Nephrotoxicity and the proximal tubule. Insights from cadmium. Nephron Physiol 2003;93:87.

289. Dello Strologo L, Pras E, Pontesilli C, et al. Comparison between SLC3A1 and SLC7A9 cystinuria patients and carriers: A need for a new classification. J Am Soc Nephrol 2002;13:2547.

290. Font-Llitjos M, Jimenez-Vidal M, Bisceglia L, et al. New insights into cystinuria: 40 new mutations, genotype-phenotype correlation, and digenic inheritance causing partial phenotype. J Med Genet 2005;42:58.

291. Santer R, Kinner M, Lassen CL, et al. Molecular analysis of the *SGLT2* gene in patients with renal glucosuria. J Am Soc Nephrol 2003;14:2873.

292. Magen D, Sprecher E, Zelikovic I, Skorecki K. A novel missense mutation in SLC5A2 encoding SGLT2 underlies autosomal-recessive renal glucosuria and aminoaciduria. Kidney Int 2005; 67:34.

293. Wright EM, Loo DD, Hirayama BA, Turk E. Surprising versatility of Na+-glucose cotransporters: SLC5. Physiology (Bethesda) 2004;19:370.

294. Palacin M, Bertran J, Chillaron J, et al. Lysinuric protein intolerance: Mechanisms of pathophysiology. Mol Genet Metab 2004;81 Suppl 1:S27.

295. Verrey F, Ristic Z, Romeo E, et al. Novel renal amino acid transporters. Annu Rev Physiol 2005;67:557.

296. Laing CM, Toye AM, Capasso G, Unwin RJ. Renal tubular acidosis: Developments in our understanding of the molecular basis. Int J Biochem Cell Biol 2005;37:1151.

297. Yu X, White KE. FGF23 and disorders of phosphate homeostasis. Cytokine Growth Factor Rev 2005;16:221.

298. Takanaga H, Mackenzie B, Suzuki Y, Hediger MA. Identification of mammalian proline transporter SIT1 (SLC6A20) with characteristics of classical system imino. J Biol Chem 2005;280: 8974.

299. Wyngaarden JB, Kelley WN. Gout and Hyperuricemia. New York: Grune and Stratton, 1976.

300. Becker MA. Hyperuricemia and gout. In: Sciver CR, Beaudet AL, Valle D, Sly WS, eds. The Metabolic and Molecular Bases of Inherited Disease, 8th ed. New York: McGraw-Hill, 2001:2513.

301. Becker MA, Meyer LJ, Seegmiller JE. Gout with purine overproduction due to increased phosphoribosylpyrophosphate synthetase activity. Am J Med 1973;55:232.

302. Sperling O, Eilam G, Persky-Brosh S, De Vries A. Accelerated erythrocyte 5-phosphoribosyl-1-pyrophosphate synthesis. A familial abnormality associated with excessive uric acid production and gout. Biochem Med 1972;6:310.

303. Seegmiller JE, Dixon RM, Kemp GJ, et al. Fructose-induced aberration of metabolism in familial gout identified by 31P magnetic resonance spectroscopy. Proc Natl Acad Sci U S A 1990;87: 8326.

304. Bieber JD, Terkeltaub RA. Gout: On the brink of novel therapeutic options for an ancient disease. Arthritis Rheum 2004; 50:2400.

305. Simkin PA. Urate excretion in normal and gouty men. Adv Exp Med Biol 1977;76B:41.

306. Dykman D, Simon EE. Hyperuricemia and uric acid nephropathy. Arch Intern Med 1987;147:1341.

307. Bordley J, Richards AN. Quantitative studies of acute gout. Hosp. Pract. 6: Studies of the composition of glomerular urine. J Biol Chem 1933;101:193.

308. Roch-Ramel F, Weiner IM. Excretion of urate by the kidneys of Cebus monkeys: A micropuncture study. Am J Physiol 1973;224:1369.

309. Diamond HS, Paolino JS. Evidence for a postsecretory reabsorptive site for uric acid in man. J Clin Invest 1973;52:1491.

310. Abramson RG, Levitt MF. Micropuncture study of uric acid transport in rat kidney. Am J Physiol 1975;228:1597.

311. Abramson RG, Levitt MF. Use of pyrazinamide to assess renal uric acid transport in the rat: A micropuncture study. Am J Physiol 1976;230:1276.

312. Weinman EJ, Steplock D, Suki WN, Eknoyan G. Urate reabsorption in proximal convoluted tubule of the rat kidney. Am J Physiol 1976;231:509.

313. Levinson DJ, Sorensen LB. Renal handling of uric acid in normal and gouty subjects: Evidence for a four-component system. Ann Rheum Dis 1980;39:173.

314. Kahn AM, Shelat H, Weinman EJ. Urate and p-aminohippurate transport in rat renal basolateral vesicles. Am J Physiol 1985; 249(5 Pt 2):F654.

315. Roch-Ramel F, Werner D, Guisan B. Urate transport in brush-border membrane of human kidney. Am J Physiol 1994;266 (5 Pt 2):F797.

316. Seegmiller JE, Rosenbloom FM, Kelley WN. Enzyme defect associated with a sex-linked human neurological disorder and excessive purine synthesis. Science 1967;155:1682.

317. Cameron JS, Simmonds HA. Hereditary hyperuricemia and renal disease. Semin Nephrol 2005;25:9.

318. Duan J, Nilsson L, Lambert B. Structural and functional analysis of mutations at the human hypoxanthine phosphoribosyl transferase (HPRT1) locus. Hum Mutat 2004;23:599.

319. Lesch M, Nyhan WL. A familial disorder of uric acid metabolism and central nervous system function. Am J Med 1964;36: 561.

320. Jinnah HA, Friedmann T. Lesch-Nyhan disease and its variants. In: Sciver CR, Beaudet AL, Valle D, Sly WS, eds. The Metabolic and Molecular Bases of Inherited Disease, 8th ed. New York: McGraw-Hill, 2001:2537.

321. Nyhan WL. The recognition of Lesch-Nyhan syndrome as an inborn error of purine metabolism. J Inherit Metab Dis 1997;20:171.

322. Cameron JS, Moro F, Simmonds HA. Gout, uric acid and purine metabolism in paediatric nephrology. Pediatr Nephrol 1993;7: 105.

323. Nyhan WL. Inherited hyperuricemic disorders. Contrib Nephrol 2005;147:22.

324. Ogawa A, Watanabe K, Minejima N. Renal xanthine stone in Lesch-Nyhan syndrome treated with allopurinol. Urology 1985; 26:56.

325. Holland PC, Dillon MJ, Pincott J, et al. Hypoxanthine guanine phosphoribosyl transferase deficiency presenting with gout and renal failure in infancy. Arch Dis Child 1983;58:831.

326. Lorentz WB Jr, Burton BK, Trillo A, Browning MC. Failure to thrive, hyperuricemia, and renal insufficiency in early infancy secondary to partial hypoxanthine-guanine phosphoribosyl transferase deficiency. J Pediatr 1984;104: 94.

327. Marangella M. Uric acid elimination in the urine. Pathophysiological implications. Contrib Nephrol 2005;147:132.

328. Ohdoi C, Nyhan WL, Kuhara T. Chemical diagnosis of Lesch-Nyhan syndrome using gas chromatography-mass spectrometry detection. J Chromatogr B Analyt Technol Biomed Life Sci 2003;792:123.

329. Ishizuka T, Iizasa T, Taira M, et al. Promoter regions of the human X-linked housekeeping genes PRPS1 and PRPS2 encoding phosphoribosylpyrophosphate synthetase subunit I and II isoforms. Biochim Biophys Acta 1992;1130:139.

330. Chen YT, Van Hove JL. Renal involvement in type I glycogen storage disease. Adv Nephrol Necker Hosp 1995;24:357.

331. Duncan H, Dixon AS. Gout, familial hypericaemia, and renal disease. QJM 1960;29:127.

332. Richmond JM, Kincaid-Smith P, Whitworth JA, Becker GJ. Familial urate nephropathy. Clin Nephrol 1981;16:163.
333. McBride MB, Rigden S, Haycock GB, et al. Presymptomatic detection of familial juvenile hyperuricaemic nephropathy in children. Pediatr Nephrol 1998;12:357.
334. Dahan K, Fuchshuber A, Adamis S, et al. Familial juvenile hyperuricemic nephropathy and autosomal dominant medullary cystic kidney disease type 2: Two facets of the same disease? J Am Soc Nephrol 2001;12:2348.
335. Massari PU, Hsu CH, Barnes RV, et al. Familial hyperuricemia and renal disease. Arch Intern Med 1980;140:680.
336. Fairbanks LD, Cameron JS, Venkat-Raman G, et al. Early treatment with allopurinol in familial juvenile hyperuricaemic nephropathy (FJHN) ameliorates the long-term progression of renal disease. QJM 2002;95:597.
337. Bingham C, Ellard S, van't Hoff WG, et al. Atypical familial juvenile hyperuricemic nephropathy associated with a hepatocyte nuclear factor-1beta gene mutation. Kidney Int 2003;63:1645.
338. Hart TC, Gorry MC, Hart PS, et al. Mutations of the *UMOD* gene are responsible for medullary cystic kidney disease 2 and familial juvenile hyperuricaemic nephropathy. J Med Genet 2002;39:882.
339. Kudo E, Kamatani N, Tezuka O, Taniguchi A, Yamanaka H, Yabe S, et al. Familial juvenile hyperuricemic nephropathy: Detection of mutations in the uromodulin gene in five Japanese families. Kidney Int 2004;65:1589.
340. Enomoto A, Kimura H, Chairoungdua A, et al. Molecular identification of a renal urate anion exchanger that regulates blood urate levels. Nature 2002;417:447.
341. Iwai N, Mino Y, Hosoyamada M, et al. A high prevalence of renal hypouricemia caused by inactive SLC22A12 in Japanese. Kidney Int 2004;66:935.
342. Takahashi T, Tsuchida S, Oyamada T, et al. Recurrent *URAT1* gene mutations and prevalence of renal hypouricemia in Japanese. Pediatr Nephrol 2005;20:576.
343. Cheong HI, Kang JH, Lee JH, et al. Mutational analysis of idiopathic renal hypouricemia in Korea. Pediatr Nephrol 2005;20:886.
344. Hisatome I, Tanaka Y, Kotake H, et al. Renal hypouricemia due to enhanced tubular secretion of urate associated with urolithiasis: Successful treatment of urolithiasis by alkalization of urine K+, Na(+)-citrate. Nephron 1993;65:578.
345. Yeun JY, Hasbargen JA. Renal hypouricemia: Prevention of exercise-induced acute renal failure and a review of the literature. Am J Kidney Dis 1995;25:937.
346. Hirasaki S, Koide N, Fujita K, et al. Two cases of renal hypouricemia with nephrolithiasis. Intern Med 1997;36:201.
347. Kikuchi Y, Koga H, Yasutomo Y, et al. Patients with renal hypouricemia with exercise-induced acute renal failure and chronic renal dysfunction. Clin Nephrol 2000;53:467.
348. Steele TH. Hyperuricemic nephropathies. Nephron 1999;81 Suppl 1:45.
349. Davidson MB, Thakkar S, Hix JK, et al. Pathophysiology, clinical consequences, and treatment of tumor lysis syndrome. Am J Med 2004;116:546.
350. Kjellstrand CM, Cambell DC II, von Hartitzsch B, Buselmeier TJ. Hyperuricemic acute renal failure. Arch Intern Med 1974;133:349.
351. Hsu HH, Chan YL, Huang CC. Acute spontaneous tumor lysis presenting with hyperuricemic acute renal failure: Clinical features and therapeutic approach. J Nephrol 2004;17:50.
352. McCrea LE. Formation of uric acid calculi during chemotherapy for leukemia. J Urol 1955;73:29.
353. Jeha S, Pui CH. Recombinant urate oxidase (rasburicase) in the prophylaxis and treatment of tumor lysis syndrome. Contrib Nephrol 2005;147:69.
354. Kanwar YS, Manaligod JR. Leukemic urate nephropathy. Arch Pathol 1975;99:467.
355. Manzke H, Eigster G, Harms D, et al. Uric acid infarctions in the kidneys of newborn infants. A study on the changing incidence and on oxypurine ratios. Eur J Pediatr 1977;126:29.
356. Gutman AB. Significance of uric acid as a nitrogenous waste in vertebrate evolution. Arthritis Rheum 1965;8:614.
357. Terkeltaub RA. Clinical practice. Gout. N Engl J Med 2003;349:1647.
358. Schnitker MA, Richter AB. Nephritis in gout. Am J Med Sci 1936;192:241.
359. Barlow KA, Beilin LJ. Renal disease in primary gout. QJM 1968;37:79.
360. Talbott JH, Terplan KL. The kidney in gout. Medicine (Baltimore) 1960;39:405.
361. Berger L, Yu TF. Renal function in gout. IV. An analysis of 524 gouty subjects including long-term follow-up studies. Am J Med 1975;59:605.
362. Yu TF, Berger L, Dorph DJ, Smith H. Renal function in gout. V. Factors influencing the renal hemodynamics. Am J Med 1979;67:766.
363. Fessel WJ. Renal outcomes of gout and hyperuricemia. Am J Med 1979;67:74.
364. Gibson T, Highton J, Potter C, Simmonds HA. Renal impairment and gout. Ann Rheum Dis 1980;39:417.
365. Klinenberg JR, Gonick HC, Dornfeld L. Renal function abnormalities in patients with asymptomatic hyperuricemia. Arthritis Rheum 1975;18(6 suppl):725.
366. Hollenberg NK, Borucki LJ, Adams DF. The renal vasculature in early essential hypertension: Evidence for a pathogenetic role. Medicine (Baltimore) 1978;57:167.
367. Lin JL, Tan DT, Hsu KH, Yu CC. Environmental lead exposure and progressive renal insufficiency. Arch Intern Med 2001;161:264.
368. Lin JL, Yu CC, Lin-Tan DT, Ho HH. Lead chelation therapy and urate excretion in patients with chronic renal diseases and gout. Kidney Int 2001;60:266.
369. Batuman V, Maesaka JK, Haddad B, et al. The role of lead in gout nephropathy. N Engl J Med 1981;304:520.
370. Lin JL, Tan DT, Ho HH, Yu CC. Environmental lead exposure and urate excretion in the general population. Am J Med 2002;113:563.
371. Lin JL, Lin-Tan DT, Hsu KH, Yu CC. Environmental lead exposure and progression of chronic renal diseases in patients without diabetes. N Engl J Med 2003;348:277.
372. Reynolds PP, Knapp MJ, Baraf HS, Holmes EW. Moonshine and lead. Relationship to the pathogenesis of hyperuricemia in gout. Arthritis Rheum 1983;26:1057.
373. Miranda-Carus E, Mateos FA, Sanz AG, et al. Purine metabolism in patients with gout: The role of lead. Nephron 1997;75:327.
374. Reif MC, Constantiner A, Levitt MF. Chronic gouty nephropathy: A vanishing syndrome? N Engl J Med 1981;304:535.
375. Beck LH. Requiem for gouty nephropathy. Kidney Int 1986;30:280.
376. Gonick HC, Rubini ME, Gleason IO, Sommers SC. The renal lesion in gout. Ann Intern Med 1965;62:667.
377. Bernstein J, Churg J. Heritable metabolic diseases. In: Jennette JC, Olson JL, Schwartz MM, Silva FG, eds. Heptinstall's Pathology of the Kidney, 5th ed. Philadelphia: Lippincott-Raven, 1998:1287.
378. Sommers SC, Churg J. Kidney pathology in hyperuricemia and gout. In: Yu T, Berger L, eds. The Kidney in Gout and Hyperuricemia. New York: Futura, 1982:95.
379. Brown J, Mallory GK. Renal changes in gout. N Engl J Med 1950;243:325.
380. Robinson RR, Yarger WE. Acute uric acid nephropathy. Arch Intern Med 1977;137:839.
381. Bluestone R, Waisman J, Klinenberg JR. The gouty kidney. Semin Arthritis Rheum 1977;7:97.
382. Pardo V, Perez-Stable E, Fisher ER. Ultrastructural studies in hypertension. III. Gouty nephropathy. Lab Invest 1968;18:143.
383. Kramer HM, Curhan G. The association between gout and nephrolithiasis: The National Health and Nutrition Examination Survey III, 1988–1994. Am J Kidney Dis 2002;40:37.
384. Cameron JS, Simmonds HA. Uric acid, gout and the kidney. J Clin Pathol 1981;34:1245.

385. Shekarriz B, Stoller ML. Uric acid nephrolithiasis: Current concepts and controversies. J Urol 2002;168(4 Pt 1):1307.
386. Khatchadourian J, Preminger GM, Whitson PA, et al. Clinical and biochemical presentation of gouty diathesis: Comparison of uric acid versus pure calcium stone formation. J Urol 1995;154:1665.
387. Herrick JB. Peculiar elongated and sickle-shaped red blood corpuscles in a case of severe anemia. Arch Intern Med 1910;6:517.
388. Onwubalili JK. Sickle-cell anaemia: An explanation for the ancient myth of reincarnation in Nigeria. Lancet 1983;322:503.
389. Ingram VM. Gene mutations in human haemoglobin: The chemical difference between normal and sickle cell haemoglobin. Nature 1957;180:326.
390. Hunt JA, Ingram VM. A terminal peptide sequence of human haemoglobin? Nature 1959;184:640.
391. Marrotta CA, Wilson JT, Forget BJ, Weissmann SM. Human β-globin messenger RNA. III. Nucleotide sequences derived from complementary DNA. J Biol Chem 1977;252:5040.
392. Kwiatkowski D. Genetic susceptibility to malaria getting complex. Curr Opin Genet Dev 2000;10:320.
393. Stuart MJ, Nagel RL. Sickle-cell disease. Lancet 2004;364:1343.
394. Steinberg MH. Management of sickle cell disease. N Engl J Med 1999;340:1021.
395. Falk RJ, Scheinman J, Phillips G, et al. Prevalence and pathologic features of sickle cell nephropathy and response to inhibition of angiotensin-converting enzyme. N Engl J Med 1992;326:910.
396. Saborio P, Scheinman JI. Sickle cell nephropathy. J Am Soc Nephrol 1999;10:187.
397. Pham PT, Pham PC, Wilkinson AH, Lew SQ. Renal abnormalities in sickle cell disease. Kidney Int 2000;57:1.
398. Ataga KI, Orringer EP. Renal abnormalities in sickle cell disease. Am J Hematol 2000;63:205.
399. Scheinman JI. Sickle cell disease and the kidney. Semin Nephrol 2003;23:66.
400. Hatch FE Jr, Azar SH, Ainsworth TE, et al. Renal circulatory studies in young adults with sickle cell anemia. J Lab Clin Med 1970;76:632.
401. Allon M. Renal abnormalities in sickle cell disease. Arch Intern Med 1990;150:501.
402. Statius van Eps LW, Schouten H, La Porte-Wijsman LW, Struyker Boudier AM. The influence of red blood cell transfusions on the hyposthenuria and renal hemodynamics of sickle cell anemia. Clin Chim Acta 1967;17:449.
403. Allon M, Lawson L, Eckman JR, et al. Effects of nonsteroidal antiinflammatory drugs on renal function in sickle cell anemia. Kidney Int 1988;34:500.
404. Statius van Eps LW, Schouten H, Haar Romeny-Wachter CC, La Porte-Wijsman LW. The relation between age and renal concentrating capacity in sickle cell disease and hemoglobin C disease. Clin Chim Acta 1970;27:501.
405. Kontessis P, Mayopoulou-Symvoulidis D, Symvoulidis A, Kontopoulou-Griva I. Renal involvement in sickle cell-beta thalassemia. Nephron 1992;61:10.
406. Katopodis KP, Elisaf MS, Pappas HA, et al. Renal abnormalities in patients with sickle cell-beta thalassemia. J Nephrol 1997;10:163.
407. Gupta AK, Kirchner KA, Nicholson R, et al. Effects of alpha-thalassemia and sickle polymerization tendency on the urine-concentrating defect of individuals with sickle cell trait. J Clin Invest 1991;88:1963.
408. Guasch A, Zayas CF, Eckman JR, et al. Evidence that microdeletions in the alpha globin gene protect against the development of sickle cell glomerulopathy in humans. J Am Soc Nephrol 1999;10:1014.
409. Readett DR, Morris JS, Serjeant GR. Nocturnal enuresis in sickle cell haemoglobinopathies. Arch Dis Child 1990;65:290.
410. Figueroa TE, Benaim E, Griggs ST, Hvizdala EV. Enuresis in sickle cell disease. J Urol 1995;153:1987.
411. Mabiala Babela JR, Loumingou R, Pemba-Loufoua A, et al.

Enuresis in children with sickle cell disease. Arch Pediatr 2004;11:1168.
412. Readett DR, Morris J, Serjeant GR. Determinants of nocturnal enuresis in homozygous sickle cell disease. Arch Dis Child 1990;65:615.
413. Oster JR, Lespier LE, Lee SM, et al. Renal acidification in sickle-cell disease. J Lab Clin Med 1976;88:389.
414. Etteldorf JN, Tuttle AW, Clayton GW. Renal function studies in pediatrics. 1. Renal hemodynamics in children with sickle cell anemia. AMA Am J Dis Child 1952;83:185.
415. Etteldorf JN, Smith JD, Tuttle AH, Diggs LW. Renal hemodynamic studies in adults with sickle cell anemia. Am J Med 1955;18:243.
416. Wigfall DR, Ware RE, Burchinal MR, et al. Prevalence and clinical correlates of glomerulopathy in children with sickle cell disease. J Pediatr 2000;136:749.
417. Bakir AA, Hathiwala SC, Ainis H, et al. Prognosis of the nephrotic syndrome in sickle glomerulopathy. A retrospective study. Am J Nephrol 1987;7:110.
418. Sklar AH, Campbell H, Caruana RJ, et al. A population study of renal function in sickle cell anemia. Int J Artif Organs 1990;13:231.
419. Serjeant GR. Sickle-cell disease. Lancet 1997;350:725.
420. Falk RJ, Jennette JC. Sickle cell nephropathy. Adv Nephrol Necker Hosp 1994;23:133.
421. Lonsdorfer A, Comoe L, Yapo AE, Lonsdorfer J. Proteinuria in sickle cell trait and disease: An electrophoretic analysis. Clin Chim Acta 1989;181:239.
422. Aoki RY, Saad ST. Microalbuminuria in sickle cell disease. Braz J Med Biol Res 1990;23:1103.
423. Dharnidharka VR, Dabbagh S, Atiyeh B, et al. Prevalence of microalbuminuria in children with sickle cell disease. Pediatr Nephrol 1998;12:475.
424. McBurney PG, Hanevold CD, Hernandez CM, et al. Risk factors for microalbuminuria in children with sickle cell anemia. J Pediatr Hematol Oncol 2002;24:473.
425. Datta V, Ayengar JR, Karpate S, Chaturvedi P. Microalbuminuria as a predictor of early glomerular injury in children with sickle cell disease. Indian J Pediatr 2003;70:307.
426. Sesso R, Almeida MA, Figueiredo MS, Bordin JO. Renal dysfunction in patients with sickle cell anemia or sickle cell trait. Braz J Med Biol Res 1998;31:1257.
427. de Jong PE, de Jong-Van Den Berg TW, Sewrajsingh GS, et al. The influence of indomethacin on renal haemodynamics in sickle cell anaemia. Clin Sci 1980;59:245.
428. Herrera J, Avila E, Marin C, Rodriguez-Iturbe B. Impaired creatinine secretion after an intravenous creatinine load is an early characteristic of the nephropathy of sickle cell anaemia. Nephrol Dial Transplant 2002;17:602.
429. de Jong PE, de Jong-Van Den Berg LTW, Statius van Eps LW. The tubular reabsorption of phosphate in sickle-cell nephropathy. Clin Sci Mol Med 1978;55:429.
430. de Jong PE, de Jong-van den Berg LTW, Sewrajsingh GS, et al. Beta-2-microglobulin in sickle cell anaemia. Nephron 1981;29:138.
431. Al-Harbi N, Annobil SH, Abbag F, et al. Renal reabsorption of phosphate in children with sickle cell anemia. Am J Nephrol 1999;19:552.
432. Bayazit AK, Noyan A, Aldudak B, et al. Renal function in children with sickle cell anemia. Clin Nephrol 2002;57:127.
433. Batlle D, Itsarayoungyuen K, Arruda JA, Kurtzman NA. Hyperkalemic hyperchloremic metabolic acidosis in sickle cell hemoglobinopathies. Am J Med 1982;72:188.
434. Oster JR, Lee SM, Lespier LE, et al. Renal acidification in sickle cell trait. Arch Intern Med 1976;136:30.
435. DeFronzo RA, Taufield PA, Black H, et al. Impaired renal tubular potassium secretion in sickle cell disease. Ann Intern Med 1979;90:310.
436. Oster JR, Lanier DC Jr, Vaamonde CA. Renal response to potassium loading in sickle cell trait. Arch Intern Med 1980;140:534.
437. Vaamonde CA. Renal papillary necrosis in sickle cell hemoglobinopathies. Semin Nephrol 1984;4:48.

438. Chauhan PM, Kondlapoodi P, Natta CL. Pathology of sickle cell disorders. Pathol Annu 1983;18:253.

439. Zadeii G, Lohr JW. Renal papillary necrosis in a patient with sickle cell trait. J Am Soc Nephrol 1997;8:1034.

440. Johnson CS, Giorgio AJ. Arterial blood pressure in adults with sickle cell disease. Arch Intern Med 1981;141:891.

441. Pegelow CH, Colangelo L, Steinberg M, et al. Natural history of blood pressure in sickle cell disease: Risks for stroke and death associated with relative hypertension in sickle cell anemia. Am J Med 1997;102:171.

442. Hassell KL, Eckman JR, Lane PA. Acute multiorgan failure syndrome: A potentially catastrophic complication of severe sickle cell pain episodes. Am J Med 1994;96:155.

443. Sklar AH, Perez JC, Harp RJ, Caruana RJ. Acute renal failure in sickle cell anemia. Int J Artif Organs 1990;13:347.

444. Helzlsouer KJ, Hayden FG, Rogol AD. Severe metabolic complications in a cross-country runner with sickle cell trait. JAMA 1983;249:777.

445. Morgan AG, Shah DJ, Williams W. Renal pathology in adults over 40 with sickle-cell disease. West Indian Med J 1987;36:241.

446. Morgan AG, Serjeant GR. Renal function in patients over 40 with homozygous sickle-cell disease. Br Med J (Clin Res Ed) 1981;282:1181.

447. Walker TM, Beardsall K, Thomas PW, Serjeant GR. Renal length in sickle cell disease: Observations from a cohort study. Clin Nephrol 1996;46:384.

448. Mostofi FK, Vorder Bruegge CF, Diggs LW. Lesions in kidneys removed for unilateral hematuria in sickle-cell disease. Arch Pathol 1957;63:336.

449. Pandya KK, Koshy M, Brown N, Presman D. Renal papillary necrosis in sickle cell hemoglobinopathies. J Urol 1976;115:497.

450. Statius van Eps LW, Pinedo-Veels C, de Vries GH, de Koning J. Nature of concentrating defect in sickle-cell nephropathy. Microradioangiographic studies. Lancet 1970;1:450.

451. Bernstein J, Whitten CF. A histologic appraisal of the kidney in sickle cell anemia. Arch Pathol 1960;70:407.

452. Pitcock JA, Muirhead EE, Hatch FE, et al. Early renal changes in sickle cell anemia. Arch Pathol 1970;90:403.

453. Bhathena DB, Sondheimer JH. The glomerulopathy of homozygous sickle hemoglobin (SS) disease: Morphology and pathogenesis. J Am Soc Nephrol 1991;1:1241.

454. Sydenstricker VP, Mulherin WA, Houseal RW. Sickle cell anemia: Report of two cases in children with necropsy in one case. Am J Dis Child 1923;26:132.

455. Alleyne GA. The kidney in sickle cell anemia. Kidney Int 1975;7:371.

456. de Jong PE, Statius van Eps LW. Sickle cell nephropathy: New insights into its pathophysiology. Kidney Int 1985;27:711.

457. Elfenbein IB, Patchefsky A, Schwartz W, Weinstein AG. Pathology of the glomerulus in sickle cell anemia with and without nephrotic syndrome. Am J Pathol 1974;77:357.

458. Buckalew VM Jr, Someren A. Renal manifestations of sickle cell disease. Arch Intern Med 1974;133:660.

459. Tejani A, Phadke K, Adamson O, et al. Renal lesions in sickle cell nephropathy in children. Nephron 1985;39:352.

460. McCoy RC. Ultrastructural alterations in kidney of patients with sickle cell disease and the nephrotic syndrome. Lab Invest 1969;21:85.

461. Arakawa M, Kimmelstiel P. Circumferential mesangial interposition. Lab Invest 1969;21:276.

462. Vogler C, Wood E, Lane P, et al. Microangiopathic glomerulopathy in children with sickle cell anemia. Pediatr Pathol Lab Med 1996;16:275.

463. Freedman BI, Burkart JM, Iskandar SS. Chronic mesangiolytic glomerulopathy in a patient with SC hemoglobinopathy. Am J Kidney Dis 1990;14:361.

464. Pardo V, Strauss J, Kramer H, et al. Nephropathy associated with sickle cell anemia: An autologous immune complex nephritis. II. Clinicopathologic study of seven patients. Am J Med 1975;59:650.

465. Ozawa T, Mass MF, Guggenheim S, et al. Autologous immune complex nephritis associated with sickle cell trait: Diagnosis of the haemoglobinopathy after renal structural and immunologic studies. Br Med J 1976;1:369.

466. Flanagan G, Packham DK, Kincaid-Smith P. Sickle cell disease and the kidney. Am J Kidney Dis 1993;21:325.

467. Aviles DH, Craver R, Warrier RP. Immunotactoid glomerulopathy in sickle cell anemia. Pediatr Nephrol 2001;16:82.

468. Akar H, Keven K, Nergizoglu G, et al. Renal amyloidosis in a patient with homozygous sickle cell anemia and M694V/M694V mutation. Nephron 2000;86:383.

469. Win N, Brozovic M, Gabriel R. Secondary amyloidosis accompanying multiple sickle cell crises. Trop Doct 1993;23:45.

470. Assar R, Pitel PA, Lammert NL, Tolaymat A. Acute poststreptococcal glomerulonephritis and sickle cell disease. Child Nephrol Urol 1988–89;9:176.

471. Johnston RP, Newton SL, Struth AG. An abnormality of the alternate pathway of complement activation in sickle-cell disease. N Engl J Med 1973;288:803.

472. Iskandar SS, Morgann RG, Browning MC, Lorentz WB. Membranoproliferative glomerulonephritis associated with sickle cell disease in two siblings. Clin Nephrol 1991;35:47.

473. Wierenga KJJ, Pattison JR, Brink N, et al. Glomerulonephritis after human parvovirus infection in homozygous sickle-cell disease. Lancet 1995;346:475.

474. Tolaymat A, Al Mousily F, MacWilliam K, et al. Parvovirus glomerulonephritis in a patient with sickle cell disease. Pediatr Nephrol 1999;13:340.

475. Dawkins FW, Kim KS, Squires RS, et al. Cancer incidence rate and mortality rate in sickle cell disease patients at Howard University Hospital: 1986–1995. Am J Hematol 1997;55:188.

476. Baron BW, Mick R, Baron JM. Hematuria in sickle cell anemia—not always benign: Evidence for excess frequency of sickle cell anemia in African Americans with renal cell carcinoma. Acta Haematol 1994;92:119.

477. Davis CJ Jr, Mostofi FK, Sesterhenn IA. Renal medullary carcinoma. The seventh sickle cell nephropathy. Am J Surg Pathol 1995;19:1.

478. Swartz MA, Karth J, Schneider DT, et al. Renal medullary carcinoma: Clinical, pathologic, immunohistochemical, and genetic analysis with pathogenetic implications. Urology 2002;60:1083.

479. Avery RA, Harris JE, Davis CJ Jr, et al. Renal medullary carcinoma: Clinical and therapeutic aspects of a newly described tumor. Cancer 1996;78:128.

480. Stahlschmidt J, Cullinane C, Roberts P, Picton SV. Renal medullary carcinoma: Prolonged remission with chemotherapy, immunohistochemical characterisation and evidence of bcr/abl rearrangement. Med Pediatr Oncol 1999;33:551.

481. Yang XJ, Sugimura J, Tretiakova MS, et al. Gene expression profiling of renal medullary carcinoma: Potential clinical relevance. Cancer 2004;100:976.

482. Yip D, Steer C, al-Nawab M, et al. Collecting duct carcinoma of the kidney associated with the sickle cell trait. Int J Clin Pract 2001;55:415.

483. Noguchi CT, Schechter AN, Rodgers GP. Sickle cell disease pathophysiology. Baillieres Clin Haematol 1993;6:57.

484. Kaul DK, Fabry ME, Nagel RL. Microvascular sites and characteristics of sickle cell adhesion to vascular endothelium in shear flow conditions: Pathophysiological implications. Proc Natl Acad Sci U S A 1989;86:3356.

485. Eaton WA, Hofrichter J. Hemoglobin S gelation and sickle cell disease. Blood 1987;70:1245.

486. Kaul DK, Hebbel RP. Hypoxia/reoxygenation causes inflammatory response in transgenic sickle mice but not in normal mice. J Clin Invest 2000;106:411.

487. Bank N, Aynedjian HS, Qiu JH, et al. Renal nitric oxide synthases in transgenic sickle cell mice. Kidney Int 1996;50:184.

488. Bank N, Kiroycheva M, Singhal PC, et al. Inhibition of nitric oxide synthase ameliorates cellular injury in sickle cell mouse kidneys. Kidney Int 2000;58:82.

489. de Jong PE, Saleh AW, de Zeeuw D, et al. Urinary prostaglandins in sickle cell nephropathy: A defect in 9-ketoreductase activity? Clin Nephrol 1984;22:212.

490. Bauer WC, Rosenberg BF. A quantitative study of glomerular enlargement in children with tetralogy of Fallot. A condition of glomerular enlargement without an increase in renal mass. Am J Pathol 1960;37:695.

491. Garcia DL, Anderson S, Rennke HG, Brenner BM. Anemia lessens and its prevention with recombinant human erythropoietin worsens glomerular injury and hypertension in rats with reduced renal mass. Proc Natl Acad Sci U S A 1988;85:6142.

492. Yoshida Y, Fogo A, Ichikawa I. Glomerular hemodynamic changes vs. hypertrophy in experimental glomerular sclerosis. Kidney Int 1989;35:654.

493. Hostetter TH, Olson JL, Rennke HG, et al. Hyperfiltration in remnant nephrons: A potentially adverse response to renal ablation. Am J Physiol 1981;241:F85.

494. Anderson S, Meyer TW, Rennke HG, Brenner BM. Control of glomerular hypertension limits glomerular injury in rats with reduced renal mass. J Clin Invest 1985;76:612.

495. Brenner BM, Meyer TW, Hostetter TH. Dietary protein intake and the progressive nature of kidney disease: The role of hemodynamically mediated glomerular injury in the pathogenesis of progressive glomerular sclerosis in aging, renal ablation, and intrinsic renal disease. N Engl J Med 1982;307:652.

496. Guasch A, Cua M, Mitch WE. Early detection and the course of glomerular injury in patients with sickle cell anemia. Kidney Int 1996;49:786.

497. Schmitt F, Martinez F, Brillet G, et al. Early glomerular dysfunction in patients with sickle cell anemia. Am J Kidney Dis 1998;32:208.

498. Guasch A, Cua M, You W, Mitch WE. Sickle cell anemia causes a distinct pattern of glomerular dysfunction. Kidney Int 1997;51:826.

499. Strauss J, Pardo V, Koss MN, et al. Nephropathology associated with sickle cell anemia: An autologous immune complex nephritis. I. Studies of nature of glomerular-bound antibody and antigen identification in a patient with sickle cell disease and immune deposit glomerulonephritis. Am J Med 1975;58:382.

500. Hebbel RP. The sickle erythrocyte in double jeopardy: Autoxidation and iron decompartmentalization. Semin Hematol 1990;27:51.

501. Nath KA, Grande JP, Haggard JJ, et al. Oxidative stress and induction of heme oxygenase-1 in the kidney in sickle cell disease. Am J Pathol 2001;158:893.

502. Lee HS, Kim YS. Identification of oxidized low density lipoprotein in human renal biopsies. Kidney Int 1998;54:848.

503. Cunningham G, Lorey F, Kling S, et al. Mortality among children with SCD identified by newborn screening during 1990–1994 in California, Illinois and New York. MMWR Morb Mortal Wkly Rep 1998;47:169.

504. Quinn CT, Rogers ZR, Buchanan GR. Survival of children with sickle cell disease. Blood 2004;103:4023.

505. Platt OS, Brambilla DJ, Rosse WF, et al. Mortality in sickle cell disease. Life expectancy and risk factors for early death. N Engl J Med 1994;330:1639.

506. Diallo D, Tchernia G. Sickle cell disease in Africa. Curr Opin Hematol 2002;9:111.

507. Powars DR. BetaS-gene-cluster haplotypes in sickle cell anemia. Hematol Oncol Clin North Am 1991;5:475.

508. Powars DR, Elliott-Mills DD, Chan L, et al. Chronic renal failure in sickle cell disease: Risk factors, clinical course, and mortality. Ann Intern Med 1991;115:614.

509. Steinberg MH, Lu ZH, Barton FB, et al. Fetal hemoglobin in sickle cell anemia: Determinants of response to hydroxyurea. Multicenter Study of Hydroxyurea. Blood 1997;89:1078.

510. Bakanay SM, Dainer E, Clair B, et al. Mortality in sickle cell patients on hydroxyurea therapy. Blood 2005;105:545.

511. Chui DH, Dover GJ. Sickle cell disease: No longer a single gene disorder. Curr Opin Pediatr 2001;13:22.

512. Nagel RL. Pleiotropic and epistatic effects in sickle cell anemia. Curr Opin Hematol 2001;8:105.

513. Steinberg MH. Predicting clinical severity in sickle cell anaemia. Br J Haematol 2005;129:465.

514. Powars DR. Sickle cell anemia and major organ failure. Hemoglobin 1990;14:573.

515. Faulkner M, Turner EA, Deus J, et al. Severe anemia: A risk factor for glomerular injury in sickle cell disease. J Natl Med Assoc 1995;209.

516. McKerrell TDH, Cohen HW, Billett HH. The older sickle cell patient. Am J Hematol 2004;76:101.

517. Manci EA, Culberson DE, Yang YM, et al. Causes of death in sickle cell disease: An autopsy study. Br J Haematol 2003;123:359.

518. Thomas AN, Pattison C, Serjeant GR. Causes of death in sickle-cell disease in Jamaica. Br Med J (Clin Res Ed) 1982;285:633.

519. Abbott KC, Hypolite IO, Agodoa LY. Sickle cell nephropathy at end-stage renal disease in the United States: Patient characteristics and survival. Clin Nephrol 2002;58:9.

520. Qunibi WY. Renal autotransplantation for severe sickle cell haematuria. Lancet 1988;331:236.

521. Wong WY, Elliott-Mills D, Powars D. Renal failure in sickle cell anemia. Hematol Oncol Clin North Am 1996;10:1321.

522. Aoki RY, Saad ST. Enalapril reduces the albuminuria of patients with sickle cell disease. Am J Med 1995;98:432.

523. Foucan L, Bourhis V, Bangou J, et al. A randomized trial of captopril for microalbuminuria in normotensive adults with sickle cell anemia. Am J Med 1998;104:339.

524. Fitzhugh CD, Wigfall DR, Ware RE. Enalapril and hydroxyurea therapy for children with sickle nephropathy. Pediatr Blood Cancer 2005;45(7):982.

525. Steinberg MH, Barton F, Castro O, et al. Effect of hydroxyurea on mortality and morbidity in adult sickle cell anemia: Risks and benefits up to 9 years of treatment. JAMA 2003;289:1645.

526. Zimmerman SA, Schultz WH, Davis JS, et al. Sustained long-term hematologic efficacy of hydroxyurea at maximum tolerated dose in children with sickle cell disease. Blood 2004;103:2039.

527. Nissenson AR, Port FK. Outcome of end-stage renal disease in patients with rare causes of renal failure. I. Inherited and metabolic disorders. QJM 1989;73:1055.

528. Saxena AK, Panhotra BR, Al-Ghamdi AM. Should early renal transplantation be deemed necessary among patients with end-stage sickle cell nephropathy who are receiving hemodialytic therapy? Transplantation 2004;77:955.

529. Ojo AO, Govaerts TC, Schmouder RL, et al. Renal transplantation in end-stage sickle cell nephropathy. Transplantation 1999;67:291.

530. Chatterjee SN. National study on natural history of renal allografts in sickle cell disease or trait. Nephron 1980;25:199.

531. Chatterjee SN. National study in natural history of renal allografts in sickle cell disease or trait: A second report. Transplant Proc 1987;19(2 suppl 2):33.

532. Warady BA, Sullivan EK. Renal transplantation in children with sickle cell disease: A report of the North American Pediatric Renal Transplant Cooperative Study (NAPRTCS). Pediatr Transplant 1998;2:130.

533. Miner DJ, Jorkasky DK, Perloff LJ, et al. Recurrent sickle cell nephropathy in a transplanted kidney. Am J Kidney Dis 1987;10:306.

534. Montgomery R, Zibari G, Hill GS, Ratner LE. Renal transplantation in patients with sickle cell nephropathy. Transplantation 1994;58:618.

535. Iannone R, Ohene-Frempong K, Fuchs EJ, et al. Bone marrow transplantation for sickle cell anemia: Progress and prospects. Pediatr Blood Cancer 2005;44:436.

536. Krishnamurti L, Abel S, Maiers M, Flesch S. Availability of unrelated donors for hematopoietic stem cell transplantation for hemoglobinopathies. Bone Marrow Transplant 2003;31:547.

537. Krishnamurti L, Blazar BR, Wagner JE. Bone marrow transplantation without myeloablation for sickle cell disease. N Engl J Med 2001;344:68.

538. Vermylen C. Hematopoietic stem cell transplantation in sickle cell disease. Blood Rev 2003;17:163.

539. Iannone R, Casella JF, Fuchs EJ, et al. Results of minimally toxic nonmyeloablative transplantation in patients with sickle cell

anemia and beta-thalassemia. Biol Blood Marrow Transplant 2003;9:519.
540. Pawliuk R, Westerman KA, Fabry ME, et al. Correction of sickle cell disease in transgenic mouse models by gene therapy. Science 2001;294:2368.
541. Blouin MJ, Beauchemin H, Wright A, et al. Genetic correction of sickle cell disease: Insights using transgenic mouse models. Nature Med 2000;6:177.
542. Nagel RL, Fabry ME. The panoply of animal models for sickle cell anaemia. Br J Haematol 2001;112:19.

# Cystic Diseases and Developmental Kidney Defects

26

*Helen Liapis*  *Paul Winyard*

## CYSTIC KIDNEY DISEASES

Cystic diseases of the kidney are a heterogeneous group of genetic, acquired, and sporadic disorders characterized by multiple renal cysts. Early classification was based on morphologic characteristics (1) but in recent decades clinical, radiologic, and genetic criteria were incorporated (2,3).

These modifications replace old terms with new that reflect mechanisms and etiology, but there is no universally accepted classification and it appears likely that cystic diseases of the kidney will be repeatedly reclassified with future insights into their pathogenesis. We base our classification on the most recently updated criteria, and the text is set in the same sequence as in Table 26.1.

Multiple bilateral renal cysts are the most frequent finding in familial disease in contrast to isolated, unilateral cysts that are most frequently acquired. The term *polycystic* is conventionally reserved for hereditary autosomal dominant (ADPKD) and autosomal recessive kidney disease (ARPKD) characterized by multiple cortical and medullary cysts. *Multicystic* is a term favored for a subcategory of renal dysplasia characterized by diffuse cysts that may mimic ADPKD in early childhood, but it is usually unilateral and readily distinguished by the presence of dysplasia. Glomerulocystic kidney disease (GCKD) describes cystic dilatation of the Bowman's space generically, but it is a prominent feature in childhood ADPKD and in distinct hereditary forms characterized by renal hypoplasia. These include familial GCKD associated with mutations in hepatocyte nuclear factor (HNF)-1β and early-onset diabetes (4,5) and a separate familial renal hypoplasia associated with glomerular cysts that has not been linked to HNF-1β mutations (6).

Medullary cystic disease is a recently revised category that includes two disorders that have corticomedullary cysts and similar clinical features but different modes of inheritance. It encompasses the nephronophthisis-medullary cystic kidney disease complex (NPH-MCKD). Both entities present with end stage renal disease (ESRD). NPH is the juvenile form inherited as an autosomal recessive trait, previously known as familial juvenile nephronophthisis and MCKD is an autosomal dominant disorder that presents in adults, previously called medullary cystic disease (7).

Medullary sponge kidney (MSK) is characterized by cysts that originate in the collecting ducts and is primarily a disease of adults. Cysts are often discovered incidentally by excretory urography in patients investigated for urinary tract infections or stones. The classic picture is of dilated collecting ducts filled with calcified deposits that appear as filling defects (8).

Cystic lesions in the kidney may on occasion be neoplastic (9). Classic examples are renal cysts associated with hereditary cancer syndromes such as von Hippel-Lindau disease and tuberous sclerosis. These are typically multiple and bilateral.

Multilocular renal cysts are a distinct entity seen predominantly in children with cystic neoplasms unrelated to other kidney tumors (10). Other names are multilocular cystic nephroma, polycystic nephroblastoma, and cystic differentiated nephroblastoma, because of the presence of blastema cells in some cases that mimic Wilms' tumor. An intermediate form is known as cystic partially differentiated nephroblastoma. Multilocular cystic nephroma is typically a unilateral lesion, and bilateral presentation is exceptionally rare (11).

Simple cortical cysts, extrarenal cysts (parapelvic lymphangiectasis and perinephric pseudocysts), and hemodialysis-induced cysts have distinct pathogenesis and are discussed as separate entities (Table 26.1).

---

## TABLE 26.1

## CLASSIFICATION OF CYSTIC KIDNEY DISEASES

**A. Polycystic kidney disease**
1. Autosomal dominant (ADPKD)
   Classic ADPKD
   Early-onset ADPKD in children
2. Autosomal recessive (ARPKD)
   Classic ARPKD in neonates and infants
   Medullary duct ectasia in older children with hepatic fibrosis
3. Glomerulocystic kidney disease (GCKD)
   Familial GCKD
     Renal hypoplasia and UROM mutations
     Associated with HNFβ1 mutations
   Hereditary GCKD
     Associated with ADPKD/ARPKD/TSC
   Syndromic nonhereditary GCKD
   Sporadic GCKD
   Acquired GCKD

**B. Renal medullary cysts**
1. Nephronophthisis (NPH)
   Nephronophthisis, autosomal recessive
   Juvenile nephronophthisis
   NPH1, NPH4
   NPH1, NPH5 associated with Senior-Loken syndrome
   Infantile NPH2
   Adolescent NPH3
2. Medullary cystic kidney disease (MCKD)
   Autosomal dominant MCKD
   MCKD associated with hyperuricemia
3. Medullary sponge kidney

**C. Cysts in hereditary cancer syndromes**
1. von Hippel-Lindau disease
2. Tuberous sclerosis

**D. Multilocular renal cyst**

**E. Localized cystic disease**

**F. Simple cortical cysts**

**G. Acquired (dialysis-induced) cysts**

**H. Miscellaneous**
1. Pyelocaliceal diverticula
2. Perinephric pseudocysts
3. Hygroma renalis

Multiple cysts also may occur with renal dysplasia, but are not considered cystic disease in this context.

## Polycystic Kidney Disease

### Autosomal Dominant Polycystic Kidney Disease (ADPKD)

#### Incidence, Clinical Presentation, and Genetics

Autosomal dominant polycystic kidney disease (ADPKD) is the most common inherited kidney disease, affecting 1:1000 individuals accounting for about 5% to 10% of patients in dialysis or with a renal transplant in the United States (12–14). Both males and females are affected with no significant racial preference. Women have a less severe disease compared with men. Children are rarely affected. Ninety percent of affected individuals have a parent with the disease, and their children have a 50% chance of inheriting the condition. ADPKD is a systemic disease, and patients experience multiple renal and extrarenal complications. Renal complications include stones, infections, flank pain, and gross hematuria. Hypertension and gross hematuria are often diagnosed before the age of 30 years. Renal cysts develop progressively over many decades, but kidneys are typically enlarged and palpable in individuals older than 30 years of age. This is the cutoff for ultrasound diagnosis—more than 95% of patients will have renal cysts by this age. All patients develop cysts in both kidneys eventually, but early appearances may be asymmetric. The cysts vary in size over the long course of the disease, but invariably they enlarge with time. The liver is palpable in many cases because of liver cysts, which affect more than 75% of patients. Pancreatic cysts are rare (present in only about 10% of patients), a distinguishing feature from other multiorgan hereditary cysts such as von Hippel-Lindau disease (15). Other extrarenal manifestations include intracranial (arachnoid cysts) and extracranial aneurysms (5% to 10%), colon diverticula, and mitral valve prolapse (25%). Systemic hypertension is very common, affecting 50% to 75% of patients before the onset of renal insufficiency, and is thought to accelerate progression to end-stage renal disease (ESRD). The relative frequency of renal and extrarenal cysts and the most frequent clinical manifestations and age of onset in patients with ADPKD are shown in Table 26.2.

Mutations have been found in two genes, PKD1 and PKD2. Two hundred PKD1 and more than 50 PKD2 mutations are described, most of which are private (12–14). A third gene (PKD3) is suspected based on reported isolated cases, but is not yet confirmed. PKD1 mutations are found in 80% to 85% of patients, and PKD2 mutations in the remaining 10% to 15%. Patients with PKD1 have earlier onset of symptoms, in contrast to patients carrying PKD2 mutations who tend to have delayed cyst formation, hypertension, and ESRD, by 10 to 20 years. In a study of 315 PKD1 patients, women had a later onset of hypertension and tended to have more liver cysts; however, there was no gender difference when it came to the onset of ESRD

#### TABLE 26.2

**RELATIVE FREQUENCY OF CLINICAL MANIFESTATIONS IN ADPKD AND AGE AT ONSET**

| Clinical Manifestations | Frequency (%) | Mean Age (Years) |
|---|---|---|
| Kidney cysts | 100 | 15–29 |
| Liver cysts | 75 >60 years | 45 |
| Pancreatic cysts | 10 | 47 |
| Intracranial aneurysms | 5–10 | 37 |
| Hypertension | 50–75 | 31 |
| Cardiac valve defects, | 25 | Later in life |

Modified from Chatha RK, Johnson AM, Rothberg PG, et al. Von Hippel-Lindau disease masquerading as autosomal dominant polycystic kidney disease. Am J Kidney Dis 2001;37:852.

(16). Median age at reaching ESRD was 61 years in younger cohorts and 56 years in older relatives, demonstrating improved clinical management in recent decades. Both PKD1 and PKD2 genes exhibit extensive allelic heterogeneity that correlates with variability in clinical manifestations (12–14). For example, mutations in PKD1 are more common in the 3′ half of the gene. These are associated with a somewhat later ESRD, with onset at 56 years on average, compared with 53 years in patients with PKD1 5′ mutations; therefore, phenotypic variability may in part be explained by molecular genetics (14). In addition, 18% to 59% of the phenotypic differences in PKD1 are attributed to inherited background genes and perhaps environmental factors that modify disease expression (16). Phenotypic heterogeneity in patients with ADPKD has been documented in recent studies without any significant difference in life expectancy (16–21).

The PKD1 gene is located on chromosome 16p13.3 and consists of a large 53 kb genomic DNA with 46 exons. It encodes a 460-kDa protein, polycystin 1. PKD2 maps to chromosome 4q13-q23 and consists of a smaller DNA sequence of 5.4 kb with 15 exons that encodes polycystin 2. The precise role of mutated polycystins in cyst formation is still under investigation, although it has been proposed that a second somatic mutation is required (the second hit hypothesis). Activated normal polycystin 1 is thought to be an epithelial cell membrane receptor sensing cues in the extracellular environment required for renal tubular epithelial cell division and differentiation. Mutated polycystin 1 is detected only in cytoplasmic pools in cystic cells, suggesting a pathologic role in cyst formation. Polycystin 2 is a smaller molecule localized in plasma membrane and the endoplasmic reticulum and has structural similarities with a family of sodium/calcium channels, thus thought to modulate intracellular levels of $Ca2+$. Polycystin 1 and

2 have similar cellular distribution, providing a biochemical basis for the identical phenotypes caused by PKD1 and PKD2 mutations. However, other factors such as altered responsiveness to c-AMP may be more important inducers of cysts (19) and there may be an important role for effects on primary cilia (22,23).

Genetic testing is possible by linkage analysis in large families with several affected members but not in small families with a single individual affected. Mutation analysis is particularly difficult in ADPKD because of marked allelic heterozygosity. Loss of heterozygosity (LOH), a loss of one of the two alleles in a specific location, has also been observed in PKD1 (17). Direct nucleotide sequencing gives a 60% to 70% detection rate, but is extremely time consuming. Genetic analysis has dramatically improved the understanding of ADPKD and is rapidly progressing to preimplantation diagnosis. For example, a twin pregnancy of selected oocytes resulted in the birth of two healthy babies by in vitro fertilization (24). However, in affected patients, molecular genetic testing is not yet useful in predicting rate of progression, onset, and type of symptoms. Ultrasound, computed tomography (CT), and magnetic resonance imaging (MRI) scans are more useful for diagnosis and follow-up, along with regular assessment of blood pressure and urinalysis so that therapy for hypertension can be started as soon as possible.

### Radiologic Evaluation

Ultrasonography is an effective imaging technique for diagnosis of ADPKD. The following diagnostic criteria have been established (25). Patients with at least two cysts in one or both kidneys age 30 years and younger, two cysts in each kidney between 30 to 60 years, or four cysts in each kidney in patients older than 60 years are considered to be at high risk for ADPKD. The test is 100% sensitive in identifying patients with PKD1 mutations and 67% for those with PKD2 (25). Conversely, if at-risk patients do not have cysts by the time they are 30 years old, they are unlikely to have ADPKD. Characteristic imaging findings of classic ADPKD are bilaterally enlarged kidneys with multiple cysts that have varying signal intensity: most cysts have low signal intensity, but hemorrhage, tumors within a cyst, or infection generates a high-intensity signal on CT or MRI. Concurrent liver cysts are a frequent finding (Fig. 26.1). Early in the disease, there is a sizable amount of renal parenchyma between the cysts (3). As cysts grow, however, renal parenchyma is replaced and may not be identified. Renal parenchyma and cyst volume are inversely related and correlate directly with urinary albumin secretion and presence of hypertension (25). Diagnosis is not problematic in classic ADPKD, but phenotypic variability in early stages may hamper recognition and management of patients with only a few cysts, even when family history of ADPKD is known. This is frequently the case in infantile- and childhood-onset ADPKD (25–28). Most fetuses screened by ultrasound will show

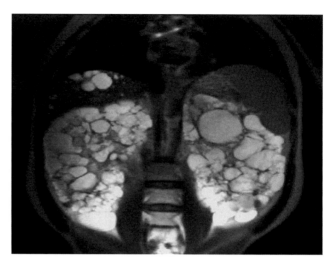

**Figure 26.1**   Coronal T2-weighted image that allows for bright appearance of cysts demonstrates innumerable cysts replacing both kidneys and liver of a 54-year-old man with ADPKD. (Courtesy Dr. Cary Lynn Siegel, Mallinckrodt Institute of Radiology, Washington University, St. Louis, MO.)

no apparent renal or extrarenal cysts, and children may be both asymptomatic and not develop cysts for 10 to 20 years after birth. In one study of 55 children with known ADPKD pedigree, diagnosis was made by fetal ultrasound in only 18%. In the first year of life, 9% of affected children were diagnosed; between 10 and 18 years of age, 38%. In adolescent children, bilateral disease was present in 78%. Of those with unilateral disease (22%), cysts more frequently affected the right kidney. None of these patients had liver cysts, a much more frequent finding in older adults. Diagnostic radiologic criteria for children were recently modified by defining one cyst as the threshold for positive identification (25–28). None the less, a 19% to 38% false-negative rate is reported in age-specific radiologic analysis of patients with known ADPKD genotype (25). This does not include the small proportion (5% to 10%) of children with no apparent history of ADPKD at the time of first presentation with a presumed new mutation. Overall, ultrasonography has improved significantly the rate of early detection and provides the added benefit of close follow-up and genetic counseling, but it should be stressed that normal ultrasound examination does not exclude ADPKD in young individuals. Linkage analysis should be considered if there is a strong clinical suspicion.

### Pathology of Classic ADPKD

ADPKD kidneys are not resected unless there are severe complications such as recurrent severe back pain, bleeding, and infection, or before renal transplantation. Resected kidneys in classic ADPKD weigh on average 2.5 kg each and appear enormous compared with normal kidneys (mean weight 0.150 kg). The reniform appearance is lost, and the external surface is distorted by multiple cysts that

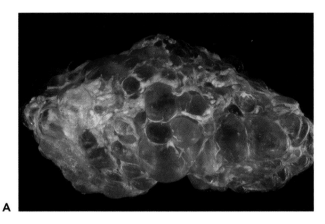

A

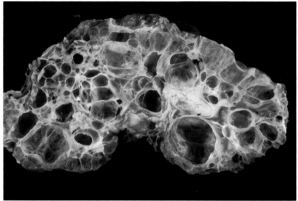

B

**Figure 26.2** Left kidney of a 39-year-old man with ADPKD: external and sagittal section view. Massively enlarged kidney (weight 3900 g) demonstrates numerous large and small cysts filled with clear or slightly turbid fluid. Remnant kidney parenchyma is barely visible.

may contain clear, turbid, gelatinous, or hemorrhagic fluid (Fig. 26.2). Cysts vary in size from millimeters to several centimeters and are randomly distributed. On sagittal sections cysts are typically unilocular, oval or spherical. The renal pelvis and calyces may be impossible to identify, but there is great variability in the extent of renal parenchyma replacement and cyst size. Younger patients tend to have fewer and smaller cysts and more residual renal parenchyma (Fig. 26.3), which correlates with better functional renal mass. Residual renal parenchyma is compressed by the enlarging cysts and eventually becomes atrophic. Interstitial fibrosis abounds in most specimens (Fig. 26.4). However, even at end stage there is significant amount of residual renal parenchyma that has raised questions over how cyst formation from only a small proportion of nephrons causes ESRD in ADPKD (see below).

Cysts are tubular in origin, arising from all parts of the excretory nephron as demonstrated by lectin staining.

Cysts may stain with both proximal and distal tubule markers, tetragonolobus and arachis hypogaea (peanut lectin), respectively (29). Immunohistochemistry with polycystin antibodies reveals positive staining in most renal cysts that express and may even overexpress polycystin 1 (30). It is unclear whether the detected signal represents mutated polycystin or presence of polycystin encoded by the "normal" allele. Glomerular cysts in the form of dilated Bowman's space are frequently present, especially in disease that manifests in childhood (Fig. 26.4). Tubular cysts are denuded of epithelium or lined by flat epithelium. Epithelial cell proliferations in the form of hyperplastic papillae vary in number, but they are a characteristic feature of ADPKD (Fig. 26.4). Micropolyps are present in as many as 90% of

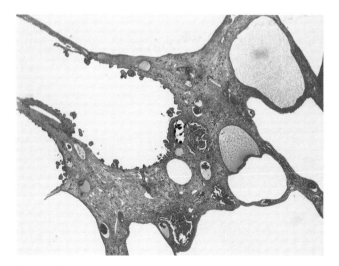

**Figure 26.4** ADPKD cysts are devoid of epithelial lining, filled with eosinophilic fluid; some cysts contain micropapillae. Glomeruli show capillary tuft retraction, tubules are atrophic; the interstitium is fibrotic and contains microcalcifications. (×40.)

**Figure 26.3** Right kidney from a 15-year-old boy with marked enlargement (weight 1500 g) and 80% replacement of parenchyma by cysts. Residual renal parenchyma is present.

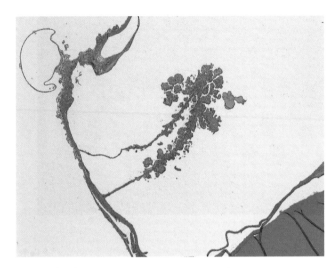

**Figure 26.5**   Intracystic papillary microadenoma in ADPKD. (×100.)

patients with ADPKD (31). They may be small with broad base or flowerlike microadenomas (Fig. 26.5). Epithelial cells lining the cysts studied with electron microscopy show hypertrophy of cytoplasmic organelles, thickened or lamellated basement membrane, and absence of differentiating features between proximal and distal tubules (3,32). Increased cytoplasmic volume, numerous membrane-bound lysosomes, and invariably loss of proximal tubule microvilli are present. These features are characteristic of cellular hyperplasia and concomitant degeneration (Fig. 26.6). ADPKD cysts in the early stages may also demonstrate abnormal mitochondria and spherical extrusion (apoptotic)

bodies. In later stages, features of cytoplasmic fragmentation predominate (3,32). Furthermore, tubular epithelial cells in human ADPKD are actively proliferating (33). In the process, they lose cell polarity and show characteristic mispolarization of proteins such as NaK-ATPase (34). Grantham et al (35) have demonstrated that cysts arise in a small fraction (1% to 2%) of proximal and distal tubules early in childhood, and new cysts are unlikely to develop over a patient's lifetime. Cyst development follows gradual luminal dilation by tubular epithelial cell proliferation, apoptosis, and fluid accumulation. Eventually cysts separate from the parent tubules and become a saclike structure while their lining epithelial cells continue autonomous proliferation. Cell proliferation is accompanied by secretion of high amounts of electrolyte transport proteins that result in excessive secretion of solute and fluid into the cysts. These phenomena are consistent with a neoplasticlike phenotype in epithelia with ADPKD, perhaps because the mutated polycystins are unable to maintain the normal state of differentiation/maturation of these epithelia (see under molecular biology of ADPKD). Other factors such as epidermal growth factor may also mediate cell proliferation and fluid secretion within the cysts (36). The observation that cyst formation involves a fraction and not all nephrons has immediate clinical implications and has prompted intense research in designing methods for early intervention to control cyst size, but these have been relatively unsuccessful (26) (see under Clinical Management).

The relation between kidney size and progression to renal failure is still debated. In patients who develop renal failure, there is loss of noncystic parenchyma in association

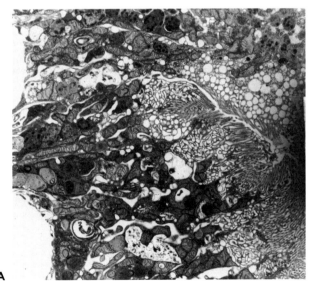
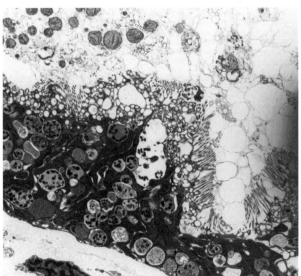

**Figure 26.6**   Electron microscopy of ADPKD cystic tubules. **A.** The cytoplasm contains increased number of mitochondria, some of which are degenerating. **B.** Proximal tubules show cytoplasmic and brush border fragmentation. The tubular basement membrane is thickened.

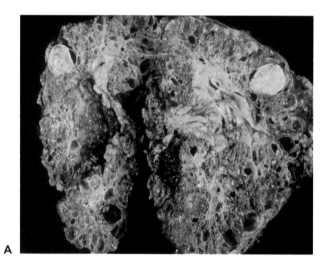
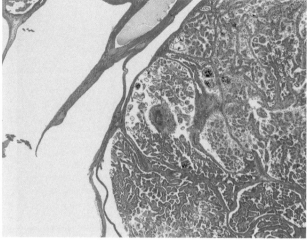

**Figure 26.7**   ADPKD with intracystic renal cell adenocarcinoma (RCC). **A:** A distinct solid yellow tumor mass fills one of the cysts. **B:** The tumor consists of typical papillary RCC with focal microcalcifications.

with mass replacement by interstitial fibrosis; the latter appears likely to be the most important pathogenic factor rather than mechanical displacement of renal parenchyma by enlarging cysts. Concurrent with progressive ADPKD there is increased expression of proto-oncogenes (fos, myc, ras, erb), growth factors (epidermal, EGF; hepatic, HGF; acid and basic fibroblast, FGF), chemokines (MCP-1. osteopontin), metalloproteinases, apoptotic markers, collagen type I and IV, laminin, fibronectin, and macrophages, all of which are known to participate in extracellular matrix remodeling (36).

## Malignancy in ADPKD

There are numerous case reports of renal cell carcinoma developing in cysts of ADPKD kidneys and small patient series that show more than 10-fold increase of malignancy compared with the general population (31). However, others find no significantly increased risk. In the last 10 years, we have seen 6 cases of renal cell carcinoma (RCC) in 22 resected ADPKD kidneys (that is equal to about 27% of resected ADPKD kidneys), but this number certainly represents a selection bias. Intracystic renal cell carcinomas usually range from 1 to 4 cm and can be unilateral or bilateral. Histologically, tumors are typically renal cell carcinomas, clear cell, papillary, or chromophobe type (Fig. 26.7). The predominant histologic type appears to be papillary RCC (Fig. 26.7). Tumors are diagnosed on routine radiologic follow-up screening. Multifocal and bilateral renal cell carcinoma was reported by Jay Bernstein et al (31) in as many as 20% of ADPKD kidneys, enforcing the view that epithelial cells lining ADPKD cysts have neoplastic properties. Beyond RCC, other kidney malignancies, for example, transitional cell carcinoma, may also be found incidentally. (Fig. 26.8).

## Early-Onset ADPKD

ADPKD in infants and young children is rare, and it may present diagnostic difficulties to radiologists and pathologists alike. ADPKD cysts that develop in utero are minuscule compared with those in the adult, and by sonography they may resemble an infiltrative instead of a cystic process. Currently refined sonographic criteria for prenatal diagnosis and lower thresholds for cyst number in children has improved sensitivity for diagnosis, but distinguishing ADPKD from other cystic kidney diseases of childhood may not be easy or always successful as discussed earlier. Renal biopsy

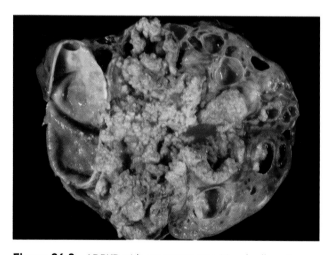

**Figure 26.8**   ADPKD with concurrent transitional cell carcinoma. Left nephrectomy from a 44-year-old woman. The kidney is enlarged (weight 2300 g) and contains a tumor centered in the renal pelvis. Multiple oval cysts are appreciated in the cortex. The tumor has a micropapillary gross appearance and infiltrates around the cysts. Microscopically, the tumor was transitional cell carcinoma arising in the renal pelvis. It involved the calyces and the ureter, but did not extend into the cysts.

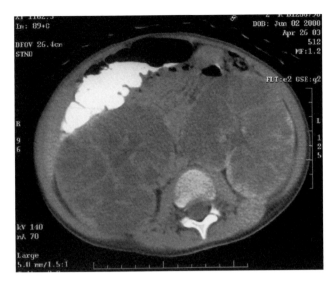

**Figure 26.9** Early-onset ADPKD. CT shows bilaterally enlarged kidneys interpreted as diffuse nephroblastomatosis. There are no visible cysts. The patient, a 4½-year-old boy who presented with acute renal failure, hypertension, and acute pyelonephritis.

is sometimes performed to elucidate the diagnosis when there is no family history/sonographic evidence of ADPKD or when presentation is atypical. For example, a 4½-year-old boy presented with acute renal failure, fever, and acute pyelonephritis. CT showed bilateral and diffuse kidney enlargement interpreted initially as bilateral nephroblastomatosis (Fig. 26.9). Renal biopsy revealed focal tubular dilation and glomerulocystic changes, and no evidence of blastema (Fig. 26.10). There were neither papillary proliferations nor well-developed tubular cysts. Tubular atrophy

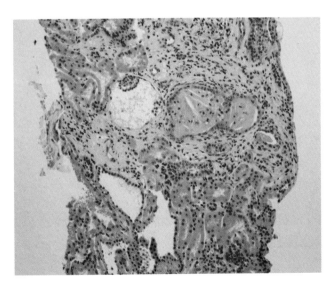

**Figure 26.10** Light microscopy in childhood-onset ADPKD. Renal biopsy shows mild ectasia of collecting ducts and focal glomerular capillary tuft collapse consistent with glomerulocystic kidney disease. (×40.)

and chronic interstitial inflammation was minimal. Acute inflammatory cells were present in some tubules consistent with recent history of acute pyelonephritis. Features such as in this biopsy may be interpreted as nonspecific, but one must raise the question of polycystic kidney disease whenever glomerular cysts are present in a renal biopsy from young individuals with bilaterally enlarged kidneys. Early-onset ADPKD with glomerular cysts raises a complex differential diagnosis that includes glomerulocystic kidney disease (see below). In a study of nine children with diffuse cystic kidney disease and no ADPKD family history at the time, two patients were proven by renal biopsy to have early-onset ADPKD (one confirmed by genetics as PKD2), three had ARPKD, three had GCKD, and one child had multicystic dysplasia (37). The diagnosis of unilateral cystic disease in children may be problematic not only in ultrasound but also pathologically. For example, as shown in Fig. 26.11, a 19-year-old man with family history of ADPKD in the mother had renal biopsy performed because of asymmetric cysts on CT. Renal biopsy revealed dilation of collecting ducts, microscopic tubular cysts, and interstitial fibrosis, but no glomerular cysts. Other patients may have a few large cysts. Intracystic epithelial micropolyps are a helpful diagnostic hint when present. The cases shown in Figures 26.10 and 26.11 demonstrate that findings on renal biopsy are frequently vague. Medullary duct ectasia may be the only remarkable change. To confirm a presumptive histopathologic diagnosis of early ADPKD, it is important to know whether kidneys are bilaterally enlarged, or in cases of unilateral disease, whether there is relevant family history. Genetic analysis may be necessary in ambiguous cases.

Pathogenesis of cysts in fetal and infantile ADPKD is difficult to explain with the two-hit hypothesis that presupposes a time interval for the second hit. Alternatively, such early manifestation of the disease may not be due solely to mutation type (PKD1 versus PKD2) but to modifier genes that accentuate the disease phenotype without a second hit.

*Differential Diagnosis of Early-Onset ADPKD.* The differential diagnosis of early-onset ADPKD is primarily from classic ARPKD and secondly from other cystic diseases of childhood such as tuberous sclerosis, bilateral Wilms' tumor, or lymphoma, and malformation syndromes including cystic dysplasia (38). Moreover, a rare but very intriguing entity, the so-called contiguous TSC2/PKD1 gene syndrome, is now described as characterized by concurrent ADPKD and tuberous sclerosis complex (TSC) (39). The TSC2 gene locus is adjacent to PKD1 on chromosome 16p. Kidneys contain multiple cysts lined by flattered epithelium next to typical TSC lesions such as angiomyolipomas or intraglomerular hamartomas (see under Tuberous Sclerosis). In contrast to polycystic kidneys, multicystic dysplastic kidneys are usually smaller or normal in size and tend to regress in early childhood rather than get larger, a

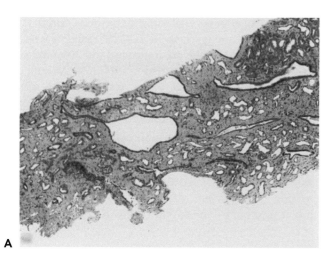
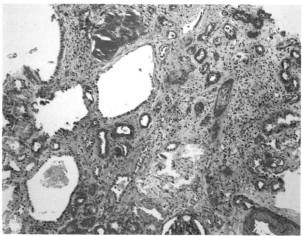

**Figure 26.11**   Early onset ADPKD. **A:** Renal biopsy reveals a. medullary duct ectasia. (H&E, ×20.) **B:** Focal cyst formation in the cortex. (PAS, ×40.) Cysts are lined by cuboidal epithelium; some contain PAS-positive fluid. The biopsy is from a 19-year-old man whose mother was known to have ADPKD. Renal ultrasound showed slightly enlarged kidneys and small asymmetric cortical cysts. (×200.)

feature that is distinctly helpful in the clinical differential diagnosis of cystic kidney disease of childhood (40).

## Molecular Biology of ADPKD

Several cell biology defects were identified in ADPKD prior to the identification of the genes mutated in this condition. Many of these are remarkably similar to ARPKD (discussed later) and include deregulation of proliferation and apoptosis of cystic epithelia and surrounding tissues, altered polarity of cyst epithelia with mislocalization of receptor and transporter proteins leading to increased fluid secretion into cysts (33,34,40–43), and abnormal cell–cell and cell–matrix interactions (43). Evidence also implicates altered structure or function of the primary cilium in PKD, and it may transpire that many of these defects arise secondary to ciliary dysfunction (44,45).

A logical approach to understanding any form of cystogenesis is to consider how processes involved in forming and maintaining normal structures go wrong to generate cysts. One paradigm of de novo tubule formation and subsequent cystogenesis involves three steps: (i) cell aggregation, (ii) lumen formation by vesicle exocytosis and apoptotic clearance of central cells, and (iii) cyst expansion with deregulation of proliferation/apoptosis and vectorial fluid/solute shift (45). Initial kidney development is normal in heterozygous ADPKD patients, which suggests that the third mechanism (deregulated apoptosis/proliferation/secretion) may be most important; this contrasts markedly with the severely disturbed initial tubulogenetic process in dysplastic kidneys described later. There is ample evidence for aberrant proliferation in ADPKD. Normal postnatal renal tubules have a relatively low proliferative index, but this is significantly increased in PKD (33,46). Aberrant expression of proteins associated

with proliferation occur within polycystic epithelia, such as the oncogene C-MYC (47), and renal cyst expansion is promoted in mice with up-regulated epithelial proliferation (33,35,48). Similarly, increased apoptosis occurs in AD and ARPKD (48,49), particularly in areas around the epithelia, which leads to loss of normal surrounding functional renal tissues. This may be one of the mechanisms, along with interstitial fibrosis, by which cyst formation in less than 10% of nephrons has such a profound effect on global kidney function. Intriguingly, mice with mutations in bcl-2, a prototypical antiapoptotic molecule, also develop cystic kidney disease (50).

In addition to deregulation of the balance between proliferation and apoptosis, there is also altered polarity of cells within ADPKD epithelia. Examples of mislocalized proteins include $Na^+/K^+$-ATPase, EGF receptors, E-cadherin, and matrix metalloproteinase 2, which immunolocalize to the apical surface (rather than the basolateral membrane in mature tubular epithelia) (34). This apical pattern reiterates embryonic distribution for some of these proteins; hence, the term embryonic dedifferentiation has been applied. One effect of the mislocalization is vectorial fluid secretion into the tubular and (eventually) cystic lumen, particularly via the sodium pump. Another is increased activation of receptors in their novel location. The classical example is the EGF receptor, which normally homodimerizes in its basal location, but forms heterodimers with erb-b2 and has increased activity apically. Several murine PKD studies have demonstrated that EGFR inhibition reduces cyst formation (51–54), which has led to phase 1 and 2 clinical trials of anti-EGFR therapy (53). Finally, mislocalization potentially exposes receptors to higher concentrations of their ligands within cyst fluid; there is increased adenosine triphosphate (ATP) and cyclic adenosine monophosphate (cAMP) in cyst fluid, for example, and activated purinergic signaling appears important in at least one mouse model of PKD (55).

Many of these cellular defects might stem from defects in primary cilia within renal epithelia. Primary cilia (one per cell) project from the apical cell surface and are thought to function as flow-sensitive mechanoreceptors that stimulate calcium influx via several channels (including polycystin-2) (Fig. 26.12). This leads to activation of intracellular signaling cascades and stabilization of epithelial maturation (23,56). Cilia are nucleated from the basal body, a modified centriole from the centrosome. Virtually all the well-established PKD proteins are expressed in

cilia or centrosomes including polycystins, fibrocystin, cystin, polaris, and inversin (the oral-facial-digital [OFD]-1 protein) (56,57). Some are important for structure, such as polaris. Cilia are malformed in orpk mice lacking this molecule, and molecular rescue restores their normal length and abrogates cystogenesis (57–59). Others affect function: cells lacking functional polycystin-1, for example, have cilia but fail to increase intracellular calcium levels in response to physiologic fluid flow, whereas polycystin-2 blocking antibodies also perturb the flow response of wild-type cells (60). Polycystins are not expressed just in cilia, however, and defects in other subcellular sites might also contribute to PKD pathogenesis, particularly

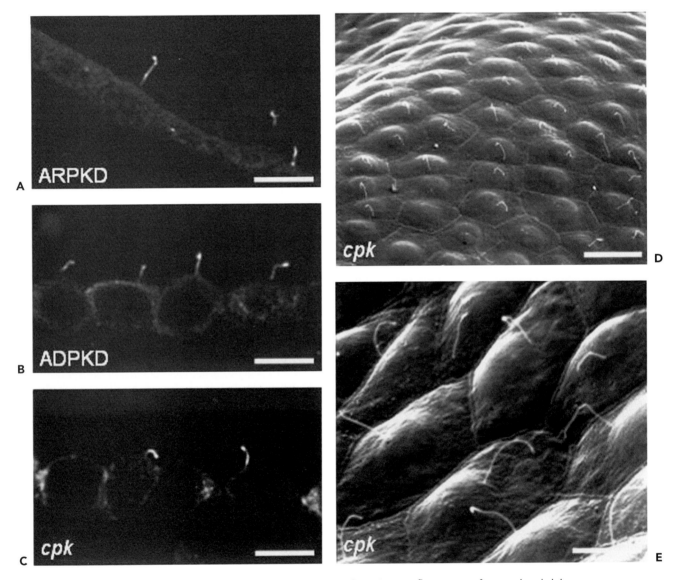

**Figure 26.12**   Cilia in human and murine PKD. **A–C:** are immunofluorescence for acetylated alpha tubulin on paraffin-embedded sections of human ARPKD **(A)**, ADPKD **(B)**. and the cpk mouse model of ARPKD **(C)**. Apical cilia are clearly seen in all of these PKD samples; length and gross structure were indistinguishable from tubules from normal samples. **D–E:** scanning electron micrographs of cpk cystic kidneys. Cilia are clearly visualized on more than 95% of epithelial cells. Scale bars correspond to 10 μm in **(D)** and 5 μm in all other sections.

in adherens junctions in lateral cell membranes and focal adhesion complexes involved in cell–matrix contacts (43). Interestingly, although strong residual immunostaining for both polycystin-1 and -2 is observed within cystic epithelia, this is predominantly cytoplasmic and no longer in the above locations, and may reflect increased inactivated protein rather than normal functioning polycystin (61,62).

Further in the molecular pathogenesis of ADPKD, abnormal interplay between epithelial cells and the extracellular matrix is thought to be crucial (63–65). Most of the evidence has come from localization studies that show up-regulation of matrix metalloproteinases (MMPs) in cyst-lining epithelia. MMP-14, MMP7, and TGF-β, a cytokine known to regulate the MMP expression, are increased. Treatment with metalloproteinase inhibitors (batimastat) in animals results in significant reduction of cyst number, suggesting that MMP inhibitors may represent a new therapeutic tool for ADPKD (63,64). Novel genetically engineered mouse models focused on the interaction of polycystins with extracellular matrix and demonstrated that defects in extracellular matrix can independently cause polycystic kidney. For example, in a mouse carrying an insertional mutation of laminin α5, homozygote mice exhibit polycystic kidneys at birth and die from renal failure at 4 weeks of age (65). These and other studies underscore the importance of cell–matrix interactions in ADPKD pathogenesis.

## Autosomal Recessive Polycystic Kidney Disease (ARPKD)

### Incidence, Clinical Presentation, and Genetics

ARPKD is much less common than ADPKD with an incidence of 1:20,000 live births (66–70). Historically, this disease was known as Potter cystic kidney type I. it classically presents antenatally or in the neonatal period and is usually associated with hepatic fibrosis. Later presentations do occur, however, in infancy or in adulthood. Neonates and infants with the classic phenotype have characteristic Potter's sequence, bilateral massive kidney enlargement and hepatic fibrosis. About 30% die of respiratory failure because of lung hypoplasia or sepsis. ARPKD in older children may present primarily with liver symptoms that range from acute cholangitis to cirrhosis. A database with clinical information of patients surviving infancy is available that has accumulated data from 34 centers in America (66). More than 200 patients are enrolled and were categorized in two groups; 79.4% were born before 1990 and 20.35% after 1990. Overall survival for patients for whom data were available was as follows: 85% were alive at 1 month, 78% at 1 year, and 75% at 5 years. Respiratory and chronic renal insufficiency was a significant predictor for mortality. Hypertension and liver disease did not affect survival. The most frequent complications were chronic

lung disease, growth retardation, hyponatremia, and urinary tract infections. Hypertension was common but not seen in all patients. Sonographic evaluation among 191 of the patients in the database reported echogenic kidneys without cysts (because there are masses of tiny cysts that increase echogenicity, but each individual cyst is below the limits of resolution of current ultrasound) in about 50% and the remaining had small cortical cysts. Liver imaging was normal in about 50% of patients; 16% had liver cysts consistent with Caroli's disease and of those, three (13%) had episodes of acute cholangitis. These data show that patients who survive infancy do much better than previously reported, with a mean life expectancy of 27 years (range, 18 to 55). Parallel studies from the United Kingdom suggest actuarial renal survival of 86% at 1 year and 67% at 15 years for those patients who survive the first month (67). Systemic and liver hypertension is a common complication in older patients. A few patients will not go into ESRD, but most will have dialysis or transplantation. Complications may arise in women during pregnancy, such as acute decline of renal function and preeclampsia (71).

In ARPKD, neither parent has the disease; each child of parents who are both carriers has a 1:4 chance of inheriting the disease and 1:2 chance of being a carrier. All patients with ARPKD have mutations in a single gene called the polycystic kidney and hepatic disease 1 gene (PKHD1), which is located on chromosome 6p21 and encodes a protein named fibrocystin/polyductin. There have been no new genes identified to explain infantile versus juvenile onset. Screens of PKHD1 revealed 119 different mutations of various types spread throughout the gene. Most patients are compound heterozygotes. Mutations are private, usually heterozygous, and vary widely (no hot spots). About 45% of a total of 29 mutations were truncating mutations (64–66). Haplotype-based diagnostic tests for at risk-pregnancies are available with a mutation detection rate of about 60% to 80% for those with kidney cysts and about 30% for those with liver cysts but no renal cysts.

Fibrocystin appears to be a transmembrane receptor that plays a role in collecting duct and biliary differentiation. The major site of fibrocystin expression in the kidney is the primary cilium of renal epithelial cells. During development, fibrocystin is also localized to the branching ureteric bud and collecting ducts in the kidney and in biliary ducts. It is often absent in ARPKD cysts.

### Radiology

Neonatal ARPKD is diagnosed by fetal ultrasound as early as 17 weeks of gestation. Kidneys are bilaterally enlarged and hyperechogenic, attributed to innumerous 1- to 2-mm cystic dilatation of the collecting ducts that increases acoustic interface frequencies. MRI can be used for evaluation of fetuses that have equivocal second trimester ultrasound. In older children, liver findings range from bile duct dilatation to portal hypertension and esophageal varices. Combined

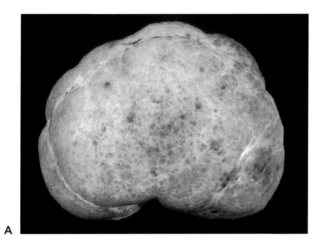
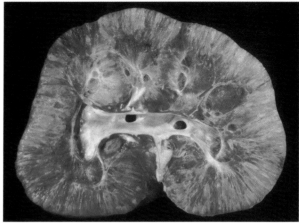

**Figure 26.13**   Gross pathology of neonatal ARPKD. Left nephrectomy from a 10-week-old baby girl. **A:** The kidney is markedly enlarged (weight 745 g). Multiple small cysts are seen through the capsule. Lines of fetal kidney lobulation are apparent. **B:** The renal parenchyma is uniformly cystic, replaced by fusiform cysts that occupy the entire cortex and the medulla. (Courtesy Dr. Ashley Hill, Department of Pathology and Immunology, Washington University, St. Louis, MO.)

use of radionuclide renal and liver scans is also reported to show diagnostic abnormalities in ARPKD.

### Kidney Pathology

In classic ARPKD, kidneys are massively enlarged with diffuse replacement of renal parenchyma by thousands of microcysts, although the reniform outline of the kidney is generally maintained (Fig. 26.13A). Sagittal sectioning reveals extensive distortion of the renal parenchyma by fusiform cysts that run perpendicular to the cortex (Fig. 26.13B). Microscopically, cysts are tubular involving predominantly the collecting ducts (Fig. 26.14). There is no increased interstitial tissue. Glomerular cysts may be present, but are

much less conspicuous than with ADPKD (37). The cylindrical cyst pattern is classic and should not be mistaken for any other cystic disease in the kidney. However, in fetal or neonatal ARPKD, cysts occasionally have a branching, not diffusely cylindrical pattern (Fig. 26.15). Cylindrical profiles may be very focal. This ARPKD variant can be misleading, but examination of the liver for portal, interlobular fibrosis and or multifocal dilation of the biliary tree will help distinguish ARPKD from infantile ADPKD. On occasion, renal biopsy will be submitted from older children with clinically unexpected juvenile ARPKD. The findings on biopsy can be very subtle. For example, mild medullary duct ectasia instead of the classic cylindrical cysts may be the

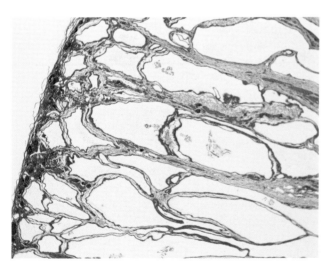

**Figure 26.14**   Light microscopy of ARPKD. Renal cysts are cylindrical, arising predominantly in collecting ducts and distal tubules (×200).

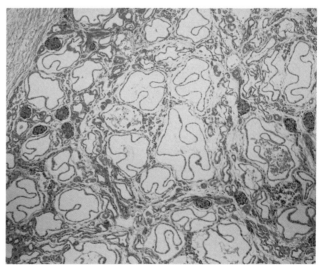

**Figure 26.15**   Light microscopy of ARPKD variant. Cysts have an angulated, branching pattern throughout. (H&E, ×40.)

sole finding, and the differential diagnosis from ADPKD may be very difficult based on histology only (37).

Entities to be considered in the differential diagnosis other than early-onset ADPKD include bilateral cystic dysplasia, sporadic or syndromic, including Meckel's syndrome. Meckel's syndrome is an autosomal recessive disease characterized by cystic kidneys associated with hepatic fibrosis, polydactyly, and central nervous system abnormalities such as encephaloceles (72). Immunohistochemistry using peanut lectin and antibodies to Na-K-ATPase that tags principal cells in the collecting duct may be helpful when morphology is inconclusive. ARPKD cysts are positive with both peanut lectin and antibodies to Na-K-ATPase, but Meckel kidney cysts are negative for Na-K-ATPase, suggesting that principal cells may be involved in the pathogenesis of the latter (73).

## Polycystic Liver Disease and Hepatic Fibrosis

Intrahepatic liver disease occurs in both ADPKD and ARPKD and should not be a point of confusion. Hepatic fibrosis is an obligatory finding in ARPKD. Liver cysts are invariably present but often asymptomatic in ADPKD (74–78). Cysts may be few in number (intrahepatic or perihilar) or grossly replace the entire liver (Figs. 26.16 and 26.17). Microscopically, cysts have the appearance of bile duct microhamartomas composed of dilated bile ducts embedded in a fibrous stroma (known as von Meyenburg complex) and appear disconnected from the biliary tree (Fig. 26.18). Conflicting data have been reported on correlations between renal and liver disease in ARPKD, with some early reports suggesting that severity of periportal fibrosis increases with prolonged survival of children with renal disease at the milder end of the spectrum, but this inverse relationship was not confirmed in a large U.S.-based study (66). Nevertheless, in individual cases hepatic involvement can be minimal in neonates who present with severe renal insufficiency, whereas hepatosplenomegaly and liver

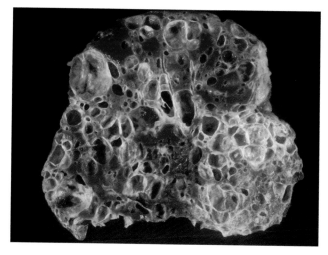

**Figure 26.17** Polycystic liver disease in a 41-year-old man with ADPKD and concurrent kidney cysts.

failure may predominate in older patients who have late-onset ESRD. The liver may be grossly cirrhotic (Fig. 26.19A). Microscopically, there is typical florid proliferation of bile ductules and liver cirrhosis (Fig. 26.19B). The hepatic portal tracts contain abnormally elongated and tortuous bile ducts. These are thought to derive from abnormal ductal plate formation in utero, justifying the term biliary dysgenesis. Hepatic precursor cells normally migrate from the foregut and form a double layer around portal veins, which is called the *ductal plate*. The ductal plate remodels into bile ducts and portal tracts over several weeks during embryonal development. The rest of the precursor cells undergo apoptosis. In ARPKD there is abnormal formation of bile ducts

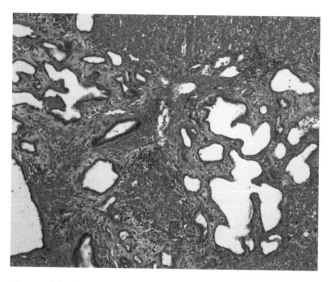

**Figure 26.18** Light microscopy of liver from a patient with ADPKD. There are multiple ectatic, angulated, and branching bile ducts known as bile duct hamartomas (von Meyenburg complex). (H&E, ×40.)

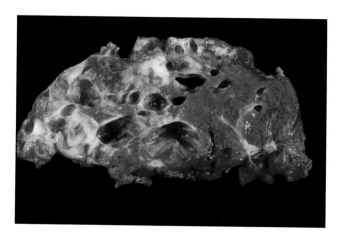

**Figure 26.16** Segmental liver resection from a 47-year-old man with ADPKD reveals cysts associated with fibrosis.

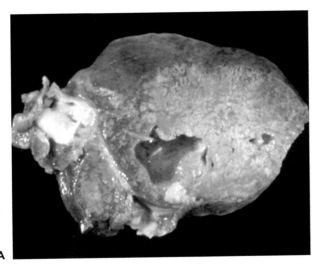
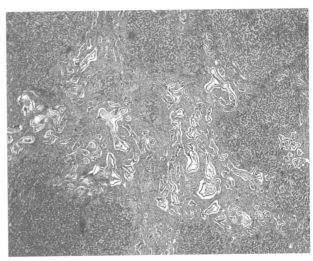

**Figure 26.19** Hepatic fibrosis in neonatal ARPKD from a 15-month-old baby girl who died from acute cholangitis and sepsis owing to *Pseudomonas aeruginosa*. **A:** The liver is enlarged (weight 560 g; normal for age is 331 g), firm, and diffusely nodular. Purulent material filled many cysts. **B:** Microscopically proliferating bile ductules abound and are filled with neutrophils.

and defective apoptosis of excess precursor cells, leading to more bile ducts, abnormal branching, and invariably periportal hepatic fibrosis. Septic cholangitis and death from septicemia is a severe complication in neonates (Fig. 26.19). Malignancy is rare, but a case of cholangiocarcinoma developing in polycystic liver disease in an adult is reported (74).

*Differential Diagnosis.* The differential diagnosis of polycystic liver disease includes Caroli's disease and a newly recognized autosomal dominant polycystic liver disease (ADPLD) not associated with polycystic kidney disease (77). Caroli's disease was described in 1958 as a rare congenital saclike or fusiform dilation of intrahepatic bile ducts not associated with obstruction (78). It usually affects the entire liver, but one lobe or a segment may be involved. It is now recognized that this disease is in the spectrum of ductal plate malformations that represent persistence of embryologic structures at the ductal plate forming focal or diffuse anastomosing channels. Fibrosis and duct ectasia result from local tissue remodeling. Diagnosis of Caroli's disease depends on demonstrating continuity of the cysts with the biliary tree by percutaneous cholangiography. In ARPKD, biliary cysts only rarely communicate with the bile ducts. However, some authors use the term "Caroli's disease" generically to describe nonobstructive intrahepatic biliary dilatation on ultrasound or CT. Cysts in isolated ADLPD arise from biliary microhamartomas. Findings in isolated ADLPD simulate liver involvement in ADPKD, and patients may also have mitral valve abnormalities, but there are no kidney cysts. Pathogenesis of the cysts in ADLPD is not related to PKD1 or PKD2 mutations (76,77).

The diagnosis of entities that combine hepatic fibrosis with hereditary renal cysts can be very complex (78,79). ARPKD is the most likely unifying diagnosis, but renal dysplasia, glomerulocystic kidney disease (GCKD), early-onset ADPKD, and juvenile nephronophthisis must also be considered. ADPKD is typically associated with hepatic cysts rather than hepatic fibrosis. However, a young child with early-onset ADPKD who presented with severe portal hypertension was reported recently. Kidneys were initially normal, but autosomal dominant polycystic kidney disease developed in this child in adolescence (80).

## Pathogenesis

Cysts in ARPKD may have similar pathogenesis with ADPKD cysts. For example fibrocystin has a three-dimensional structure similar to that of polycystin. Fibrocystin normally localizes in collecting ducts and the ureteric bud of the developing kidney and in distal tubules of adult kidney. Immunohistochemistry in normal kidney tissue sections and cultured kidney cells demonstrated that fibrocystin localizes in primary cilia of the branching ureteric bud and collecting ducts and concentrates on the basal bodies in both kidney tissue sections and cultured kidney cells (81). In the liver, fibrocystin staining is found in biliary duct epithelia and also in developing pancreas and testis. Localization of fibrocystin to cilia further strengthens the proposed mechanism of the primary defect in ARPKD being linked to ciliary dysfunction. It is possible that mutant fibrocystin in ARPKD may alter ciliary function, leading to aberrant flow signaling that results in dedifferentiation with dilation of the renal collecting ducts and biliary ducts.

## Clinical Management, Prognosis, and Therapy of ADPKD and ARPKD

Recognition of treatable complications of autosomal dominant polycystic kidney disease (ADPKD) in recent decades facilitated early diagnosis and better management. Fast kidney enlargement detected by ultrasound occurs in some but not all individuals. Those with slower renal growth have fewer associated risk factors such as hypertension and decreased glomerular filtration rate (82). Progressive disease manifests with increased overall kidney and individual cyst size; therefore, potential new therapies target minimizing cyst size and renal growth by selective surgery or with experimental drugs that exploit new molecules as revealed by molecular and animal studies (26,83,84).

## Glomerulocystic Kidney Disease (GCKD)

GCKD is defined as glomerular cysts in more than 5% of glomeruli (85). The term GCKD is used here generically as this is not a single entity and the term "disease" may be suitable only for the familial type that is a dominantly transmitted disease (ADGCKD). Five categories can be devised: (i) familial GCKD; (ii) GCKD associated with heritable diseases such as ADPKD/ARPKD, but also tuberous sclerosis; (iii) syndromic, nonhereditary GCKD; (iv) sporadic GCKD; and (v) acquired GCKD. Kidneys may be enlarged, normal sized, or small. For example, kidneys in familial ADGCKD are either normal or hypoplastic. ADGCKD is clinically heterogeneous and includes families that have mild chronic disease with hypoplastic kidneys in some individuals and normal-sized kidneys in others; separate families are characterized by maturity-onset diabetes of the young (MODY) (<25 years of age) and renal cysts (4). ADGCKD with normal or smaller-than-normal kidneys was described in an Italian family with glomerular cysts, no extrarenal cysts, and an overall benign course with stable renal failure (5,6). A missense mutation (c315R) in the gene for uromodulin (UMOD), also known as Tamm-Horsfall protein, was found in some family members (86). Subsequently, a separate family with ADGCKD and UMOD mutations was reported independently (87). Interestingly, all members of this unique family had severe impairment of urine-concentration ability and hyperuricemia resembling the phenotype of NPH-MCDK complex, and severe reduction of excreted uromodulin. Immunohistochemistry with antibodies to uromodulin revealed dense intracellular accumulation of uromodulin in tubular epithelia of the thick ascending limb of Henle's loop in kidney biopsies. Dense fibrillar material was observed by electron microscopy, the biochemical nature of which remains to be further investigated (86). Older studies describe accumulation of uromodulin within glomerular cysts; however, molecular genetics were not available at the time and such findings were not confirmed in recent GCKD cases that are genetically characterized (88).

The syndrome known as MODY is due to mutations in many factors including those in the hepatocyte nuclear factor (HNF) family. Mutation in one of these factors, HNF 1β, combines renal disease with type II diabetes (4,87–91). Glomerular cysts are found in renal biopsy but with no evidence of diabetic nephropathy. Although glomerular cysts are characteristic in a fraction of patients with HNF-1β mutations, other patients have small kidneys with oligomeganephronia (few but large glomeruli) or renal dysplasia and anomalies of the lower genitourinary tract. The reasons for phenotypic variability in MODY remain unclear. Further molecular genetic testing and exploration of modifying factors is currently being pursued.

### Pathology and Differential Diagnosis

Cysts in GCKD involve the Bowman's space and sometimes the origin of the proximal tubule (85). Cysts may be focal or diffuse. An example of diffuse GCKD is shown in Fig. 26.20. This is a wedge biopsy from a 2-month-old boy who presented with rapid bilateral kidney enlargement. The great majority of glomeruli are cystic, but interestingly, orderly arranged in rows. There are no tubular cysts, and the intervening stroma is not fibrotic (Fig. 26.20). Liver biopsy was also submitted to rule out liver mass suggested by ultrasound. Portal triads were expanded with prominent bile duct proliferation in a pattern of hepatic fibrosis. This case of GCKD associated with hepatic fibrosis simulates the presentation of infantile ARPKD. Other GCKD entities cannot be excluded based solely on pathology. For example, all nine cases of GCKD reported by Guay-Woodford were associated with concurrent hepatic fibrosis, but only a fraction were ARPKD and two were ADPKD by gene analysis (37).

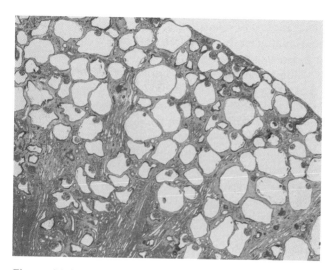

**Figure 26.20** Glomerulocystic kidney disease. Wedge biopsy from a 2-month-old boy who presented with rapidly increasing abdominal girth and a liver mass detected by CT. Glomerular cysts involve most glomeruli. There are no tubular cysts. (×100.)

### TABLE 26.3
## PATHOLOGIC FEATURES OF MOST COMMON HEREDITARY POLYCYSTIC KIDNEY DISEASES

| | Kidney Size | Inheritance | Chromosome | Gene | Protein | Cyst Shape | Cyst Origin | Lining | Liver Disease |
|---|---|---|---|---|---|---|---|---|---|
| ADPKD | ↑ | AD | 16p13.3<br>4q13–q23 | PKD1<br>PKD2 | Polycystin 1<br>Polycystin 2 | Oval | All<br>Nephron | Cuboidal<br>Flat<br>Papillary | Cysts |
| ARPKD | ↑ | AR | 6p21–23 | PKHD1 | Fibrocystin | Cylindrical | CD | Flat | Hepatic Fibrosis |
| GCKD | ↑<br>↓ | AD<br>AR | 16p<br>17q | PKD1<br>HNF-1β | Polycystin 1<br>LFB3 | GL cysts | GL | None | Cysts<br>Hepatic fibrosis |
| NPH-MCKD | Normal | AR<br>AR<br>AR<br>AR<br>AD<br>AD | 2q12–13<br>9q22–31<br>3q21–22<br>1q21<br>16p12<br>? | NPH 1<br>NPH 2<br>NPH 3<br>NPH 4<br>NPH 5<br>MCKD1<br>MCKD 2<br>MCKD3 | Nephrocystin 1<br>Inversin<br>Nephrocystin 3<br>Nephrocystin 4<br>Nephroretinin 5<br>?<br>Uromodulin<br>? | Oval | DT-CD<br>Papilla<br>IMCD | Flat | NPH1<br>NPH3<br>None |

ADPKD, autosomal dominant polycystic kidney disease; ARPKD, autosomal recessive polycystic kidney disease; GCKD, glomerulocystic kidney disease; NPH-MCKD, nephronophthisis–medullary cystic kidney disease; CD, collecting ducts; GL, glomeruli; DT, distal tubules; IMCD, intramedullary collecting ducts.

Glomerular cysts are often seen in kidneys of children with chromosomal anomalies such as trisomy 21 or trisomy 18, or with heritable syndromes such as tuberous sclerosis, oral-facial-digital dysplasia, glutaric aciduria type II, cystic renal dysplasia, or sporadic GCKD (Table 26.3). The oral-facial-digital syndrome (OFD1) has an incidence of 1:250,000, is transmitted by X-linked dominant inheritance, and is caused by mutations of the OFD1 gene localized on chromosome Xp22. The syndrome is characterized by highly variable manifestations that include malformations of the brain, face, mouth, and digits; deafness; and renal anomalies such as bifid kidneys with double ureters and renal agenesis or dysplasia plus embryonic lethality in affected boys (52,89–91).

Glomerular cysts in renal dysplasia, either sporadic type or associated with malformation syndromes, are usually side-by-side associated with other features such as fibromuscular collars and metaplastic cartilage that lead to the diagnosis (Fig. 26.21). Dysplastic kidneys are often associated with urine flow obstruction that may cause both tubular and Bowman's space dilation. Evidence for such a mechanism derives from experimental ureteral ligation in neonatal animals. Urine flow obstruction induces glomerular cysts and disrupts orderly glomerulogenesis (92).

Isolated glomerular cysts in kidneys from children may be difficult to interpret, but a good point of reference is to start by assessing kidney size (Table 26.3). Glomerular cysts in enlarged kidneys likely indicate ADPKD or ARPKD. The differential diagnosis in normal or hypoplastic kidneys in-

cludes autosomal dominant GCKD and sporadic or syndromal renal dysplasia, discussed in detail later. As previously mentioned, an effort to exclude common entities is important. The remaining cases can be designated as "GCKD not otherwise specified." GCKD cases that cannot be easily assessed by gene analysis or that have yet to be linked to a specific gene may present as unilateral or bilateral. Dilated Bowman's space in more than 5% of glomeruli is

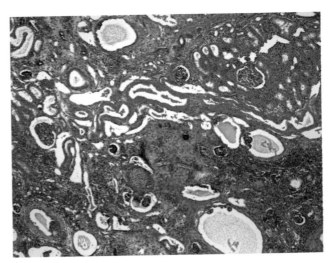

**Figure 26.21** Glomerular cysts in renal dysplasia. The renal parenchyma is disorganized. There are both glomerular and tubular ectasia and significant stromal fibrosis and inflammation. An island of hyaline cartilage is diagnostic of renal dysplasia excluding other causes of GCKD. (×40.)

## TABLE 26.4

### DIFFERENTIAL DIAGNOSIS OF GLOMERULOCYSTIC KIDNEY DISEASE

| | |
|---|---|
| Early-onset ADPKD | AD |
| Autosomal dominant | |
| ARPKD | AR |
| GCKD with renal hypoplasia and HNF-1b mutations | AD |
| Familial GCKD of unknown genetic defect | ? |
| Oral-facial-digital syndrome 1 | X-L |
| Trisomy 21 and trisomy 18 | — |
| Hereditary dysplasia and fibrosis | ? |
| Sporadic renal dysplasia | AD |
| Tuberous sclerosis | AD |
| Short-rib polydactyly syndrome | — |
| Hemolytic uremic syndrome | — |

ADPKD, autosomal dominant polycystic kidney disease; ARPKD, autosomal recessive polycystic kidney disease; GCKD, glomerulocystic kidney; X-L, X-Linked.

sometimes seen in renal biopsies of patients with acquired renal disease, and most often in association with vascular ischemia, for example, in thrombotic microangiopathy associated with hemolytic uremic syndrome (HUS) or concurrent with lupus nephritis, vascular disease, or both (93).

In summary, when one examines kidneys with glomerular cysts, the most common heritable entities in the differential diagnosis include early-onset ADPKD, childhood ARPKD, followed by HNF-1β, OFD1, slowly progressing autosomal dominant GCKD associated with or without UMOD mutations, renal dysplasia (sporadic, heritable, and syndromic), and acquired ischemia (HUS). Genetic counseling and molecular genetic testing are important to exclude ADPKD/ARPKD, HNF-1β, and other genetic abnormalities (Table 26.4).

## Medullary Nephronophthisis

### Medullary Nephronophthisis–Medullary Cystic Kidney Disease Complex (NPH-MCKD)

#### Incidence, Clinical Presentation, and Genetics

Prior to the availability of genetic testing, the NPH-MCKD complex was divided into two diseases known as nephronophthisis, a disease of the young, and medullary cystic kidney disease, which usually presented in adulthood. These diseases share clinical and pathologic features, but they are inherited differently and have distinct extrarenal associations. Juvenile nephronophthisis was first recognized in the mid-1940s as a childhood disorder of decreased urine-concentrating capacity, with polyuria and polydipsia that typically preceded the onset of ESRD (94–99). It is an autosomal recessive disorder and affects an

estimated 6% to 15% of children with ESRD. Renal failure may be the first presenting symptom, but symptoms of polydipsia and polyuria are often uncovered on close questioning. Furthermore, diagnosis can be missed because of nonspecific radiologic findings. Typical findings on renal ultrasound include hyperechogenicity, blurring of the corticomedullary junction, and normal or slightly decreased kidney size with variable numbers of bilateral or unilateral cysts (100–101). Cysts are not a constant finding, however, and the absence of cysts does not rule out juvenile nephronophthisis or medullary cystic kidney disease. In one follow-up study of 10 children over a 7-year period, only 2 children had a single cyst initially, whereas 3 developed cysts 4 to 7 years later (100).

Molecular genetics has now taken the lead in diagnosis of these conditions with at least seven different genes implicated thus far: an infantile, juvenile, and adolescent NPH are recognized (96,97). These are referred to by the corresponding gene name as NPH1, NPH2, NPH3, and so on. The gene products are as follows: NPHP1/nephrocystin-1 for nephronophthisis type 1, NPHP2/inversin for nephronophthisis type 2, NPHP3/nephrocystin-3 for nephronophthisis type 3, NPHP4/nephrocystin-4 for nephronophthisis type 4, and NPHP5/nephrocystin-5 for nephronophthisis type 5 (94–99,102). The genetic defect in most patients with juvenile nephronophthisis is in the NPH1 gene, but a second gene, designated NPH4, was recently identified in families with a mean ESRD onset of 13 years (96). NPH2 is the infantile form characterized by anemia and growth retardation that develop in a short interval after birth with ESRD at 1 to 3 years of age. An adolescent type is known as NPH3, in which ESRD develops at about 19 years. NPH1 is a distinct type that may be associated with exclusive extrarenal symptoms. About 10% to 15% of patients will also have retinitis pigmentosa known as Senior-Loken syndrome, or ocular motor ataxia (Cogan type), hepatic fibrosis, and epiphyseal bone defects (Mainzer-Saldino syndrome), or mental retardation and optic nerve coloboma and cerebellar vermis ataxia (Joubert's syndrome)(103–105). Children with some of these disorders seem to carry the same mutations as those with isolated kidney disease; in fact NPH5 is implicated in Senior-Loken syndrome (99). Notably, hepatic fibrosis is mild in NPH1 unlike in infantile and juvenile ARPKD (Table 26.4).

NPH2 kindreds have a distinct clinical phenotype that combines features of NPH with infantile polycystic kidney disease (106). This phenotype was found in a large Bedouin family. Affected individuals had enlarged echogenic kidneys that lacked corticomedullary differentiation. All patients developed anemia, hyperkalemic metabolic acidosis, and increased serum creatinine and reached end-stage renal failure rapidly. None of the affected had polyuria, polydipsia, or associated ocular or hepatic complications. NPH2 gene is localized on chromosome 9q22-31 and codes for a unique protein called inversin that is involved in left-right axis determination in the body (102,107); hence, NPH2 patients may also have situs inversus by random chance.

The NPH1 gene is localized on chromosome 2q12-q13. Eighty percent of affected children have a large homozygous deletion in this region. Homozygous mutations are considered diagnostic for NPH1. The remaining 20% of children with juvenile onset are heterozygotes and carry point mutations. The NPH1 gene spans 20 exons and from over 100 families reported so far it appears that methodical pedigree analysis coupled with molecular genetics can provide accurate diagnosis in most patients. Prenatal testing is possible if a sibling is affected (95,96). It is expected that there will be more genes discovered that cause nephronophthisis and the existing subcategories will continue to be modified.

MCKD has autosomal dominant inheritance and is relatively rare with an annual incidence of 34 to 56 new cases per year reported at the United States Renal Database. The main clinical symptoms that NPH and MCKD share are decreased urine-concentrating capacity, polydipsia and polyuria, and renal cyst formation in the corticomedullary junction or the medulla. An association with hyperuricemia and gout is recognized. Clinical presentation still

varies greatly across these groups, however; for example, polydipsia/polyuria may be mild or absent and renal cysts may be found only at autopsy and not by ultrasound or CT (108,109). Ultrasound detects cysts in only 40% of patients. Patients with no cysts may not be diagnosed until late in life or at autopsy. Cysts are unilateral or bilateral and they vary in number. In a large 186-member Cypriot family, bilateral cysts were found in only 12.5% of carriers (Fig. 26.22) (108). Less than half of these patients had hyperuricemia, and clinical gout was reported in only five (108). Therefore, although clinical symptoms and presence of cysts are part of the disease phenotype, none are sensitive enough for diagnosis. Heredity may not be apparent at first either. There are two genes (and perhaps a third) designated as MCKD1 and MCKD2 (110,111). ESRD in MCKD1 develops at about 62 years and in MCKD2 at about 32 years. A father-to-son transmission suggests an autosomal dominant mode. Patients often develop hypertension early, but paradoxically, some develop hypotension later owing to salt wasting. There are also associations such as hypogonadism, epilepsy, and spastic quadriparesis among others. A locus on chromosome 1q21 for MCKD 1 was identified in the Cypriot family presenting with very late onset of ESRD (110). A second locus on chromosome

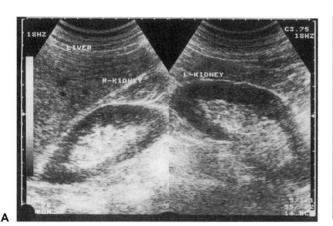

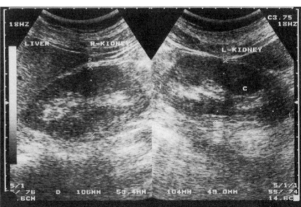

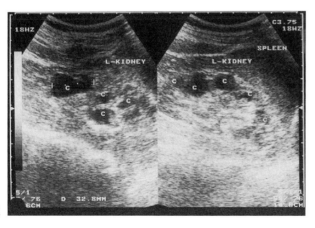

**Figure 26.22** Ultrasound in MCKD patients who were members of Cypriot families positively identified by linkage analysis. **A:** A 42-year-old woman with normal echogenicity and normal kidney size and no cysts. **B:** A 51-year-old man with solitary corticomedullary cyst in left kidney. **C:** A 53-year-old man with multiple corticomedullary cysts in left kidney. (Courtesy Drs. Zouvani, Pieridis, Kyriakou, and Deltas, University of Cyprus.)

16p12 for MCKD2 that encodes for uromodulin was found in an Italian family and confirmed by independent investigators in a Welsh family in the United Kingdom (111,112). A third MCKD gene is thought possible by Kroiss et al (113). To complicate things further, familial hyperuricemic nephropathy presenting during childhood was recently described in two Czech families and one Belgian family (114,115). The gene in these families is located close to 16q12 (16q11 locus, in fact) suggesting that more loci will be identified in families with a combination of MCDK symptoms and variable ESRD onset.

## Pathology and Pathogenesis

The pathology of NPH and MCKD is similar, characterized by the triad of tubular basement membrane disruption, interstitial fibrosis, and cyst formation. Glomerulosclerosis is invariably present but varies between 20% to 50%. In juvenile nephronophthisis, kidneys are grossly normal or slightly small. Typically, a few corticomedullary or medullary cysts are visible (Fig. 26.23). Histologically, there is diffuse interstitial inflammatory infiltrate associated with tubular dilatation (Fig. 26.24A and B). Cystic

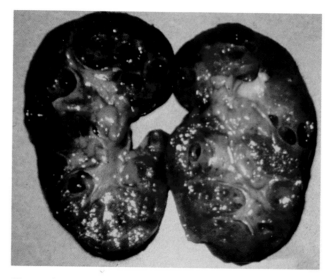

**Figure 26.23** Gross pathology in nephronophthisis. Kidney is slightly small. Cysts are characteristically located at the corticomedullary junction. The patient was an 8-year-old boy who first presented with cerebellar ataxia at the age of 2 years, and at age 6 years he developed polyuria and polydipsia and progressed rapidly to ESRD. His mother had microphthalmia and extremely poor vision of unknown cause.

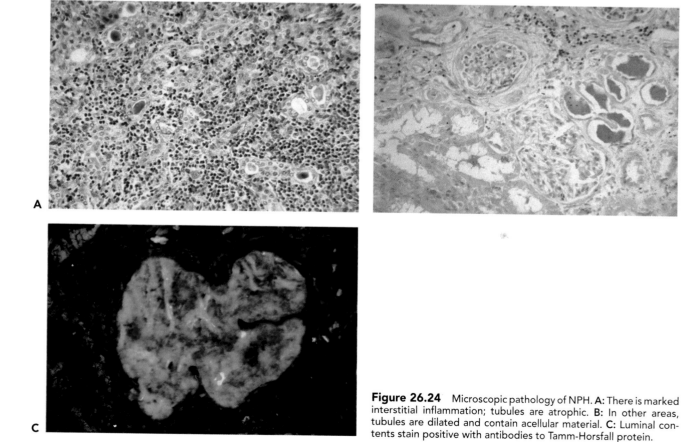

A

B

C

**Figure 26.24** Microscopic pathology of NPH. **A:** There is marked interstitial inflammation; tubules are atrophic. **B:** In other areas, tubules are dilated and contain acellular material. **C:** Luminal contents stain positive with antibodies to Tamm-Horsfall protein.

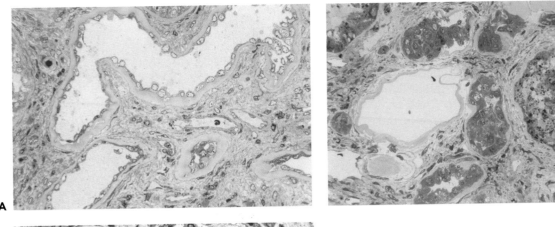

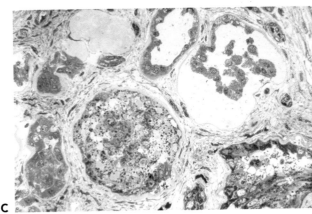

**Figure 26.25** Electron microscopy of NPH. **A:** Dilated tubules are lined by cuboidal epithelium. **B:** Cystic tubules show thickening and thinning of tubular basement membrane and are devoid of epithelium and disintegration. **C:** Tubular epithelial cells are detached and partially collapsed. (Thick sections, ×40.)

dilation involves distal tubules and collecting ducts. Dilated tubules often contain acellular material that stains positive with antibodies to Tamm-Horsfall protein (THP) (Fig. 26.24C). THP (uromodulin) was initially proposed as a hallmark of this disease and the result of an intrinsic tubular defect that allows it to escape into the lumen or the interstitium. However, THP accumulation is often seen in association with increased intratubular pressure in obstructive and reflux nephropathy in which tubular basement membrane disruption is not the primary defect. Nonetheless, an important finding in NPH-MCKD is disintegration of the tubular basement membrane. Electron microscopy reveals dilated tubules with irregular outpouching and tubular basement membrane thickening, splitting, and replication, alternating with thin or absent segments (Figs. 26.25 and 26.26). Thick tubular basement membrane segments are composed of layers of homogenous matrix with intervening lucencies mimicking changes of Alport's syndrome. Unlike with Alport's, however, collagen IV and laminin expression is generally maintained (116). Furthermore, the stigmata of Alport's (hematuria, sensorineural deafness) are absent. Thick and attenuated tubular basement membranes seen concurrently in NPH kidneys are thought to represent reparative changes (117). Studies focusing on cell–matrix adhesion have described loss of organization at the basal aspect of tubular epithe-

lial cells and unique expression of $\alpha 5$ integrin receptor in tubules of NPH-MCKD, suggesting that altered adhesion to substratum contributes to disintegration of tubular basement membrane (118). Pathogenesis of cyst formation and predilection of the corticomedullary junction in NPH-MCKD continues to be an enigma, but several hypotheses are now actively being explored. Because of genetic variability, cyst formation may have a different mechanism in each NPH-MCKD subtype. For example, the products of the five known genes, the nephrocystins, and inversin may play different roles. However, a common link in cyst formation and between nephrocystins and inversin as well as polycystins in ADPKD and fibrocystin in ARPKD is their localization to cilia of tubular epithelial cells (119). These new findings and the molecular biology of uromodulin open up new windows in understanding: perhaps cilia-generated pathways that lead to cyst formation in hereditary cystic kidney disorders (119,120). Uromodulin is thought to inhibit water permeability by epithelial cells in the ascending loop of Henle. Using antiuromodulin antibodies immunoelectron microscopy, accumulation of uromodulin within the endoplasmic reticulum (ER) was demonstrated. It is proposed that such an accumulation within the ER may interfere with appropriate localization of the mutant protein within the physiologic site in the basal aspect of tubular epithelial cells. However, immunolocalization of uromodulin in two

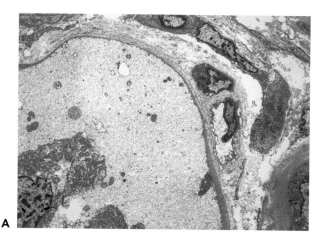

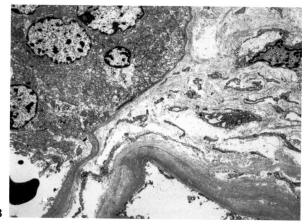

**Figure 26.26** Nephronophthisis. Electron microscopy shows **(A)** thinning and lamellation of the tubular basement membrane and granular disintegration of the cytoplasm of epithelial cells alternating with tubular basement membrane thickening **(B)**. (Thin sections, ×6000.)

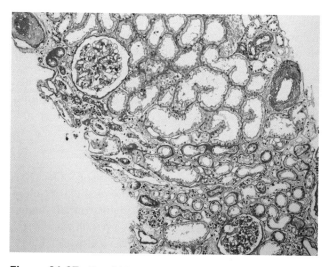

**Figure 26.27** Renal biopsy in MCKD from a 56-year-old man, confirmed by linkage analysis. Focal tubular atrophy in about 15% of surface area is associated with mild chronic inflammation, mild arteriolonephrosclerosis, and increased glomerulosclerosis involving 30% of glomeruli. (Courtesy Drs. Zouvani, Pieridis, Kyriakou, and Deltas, University of Cyprus.)

patients with uromodulin mutations did not confirm this hypothesis (86). Alternatively, cysts in MCKD2 may be mediated by altered water permeability and increased influx of water owing to mutant uromodulin (81).

On renal biopsy of patients with potential NPH-MCKD, one should be aware of the nonspecific findings of tubulointerstitial atrophy and inflammation and focally thick tubular basement membranes (Fig. 26.27). Glomeruli are devoid of immune deposits and are ultrastructurally normal. On electron microscopy, the findings are in the tubules that show lamellated thickening and thinning of the basement membrane (Fig. 26.26).

### Differential Diagnosis

Children who lack active urinary sediment or heavy proteinuria and do not have polydipsia and polyuria may be diagnosed only if they have renal cysts detected by ultrasound. In adults who have no specific symptoms and a nondiagnostic renal ultrasound, diagnosis of NPH-MCKD is very frequently missed. For example, in a recently pub-

lished study of a pedigree of Native Americans living in North Carolina, the diagnosis was not made until family members of a middle-aged man were screened for living related kidney donation (109). Similarly, in the Cypriot series most patients were not diagnosed until late in life (108). Presence of renal cysts and history of familial kidney disease are very helpful, but cysts, as mentioned earlier, are usually few and the size of the kidney is normal or slightly decreased. Notably, NPH-MCKD patients do not develop flank pain, hematuria, or lithiasis as in ADPKD. Furthermore, kidneys in ADPKD are enlarged. On gross examination, cysts are in the corticomedullary or medullary region of the kidney in contrast to diffuse cysts in ADPKD that occupy the entire kidney. Microscopically, there are no papillary proliferations in the cysts of NPH-MCKD. The pathologic findings in NPH-MCKD are of tubulointerstitial nephritis. Luminal Tamm-Horsfall protein in a subset of patients may be a helpful hint. Other entities to be excluded are chronic pyelonephritis, but thyroidization of tubules is usually absent in NPH-MCKD. Hyperuricemia in children or young adults with nephronophthisislike presentation raise the differential diagnosis of inherited deficiencies of purine degradation enzymes such as X-linked hypoxanthine-guanine and autosomal dominant adenine phosphoribosyltransferase (Pribose P synthase) deficiency (121,122). Approximately one third of patients have uromodulin mutations (122). We have seen a renal biopsy from a 29-year-old man with gout and chronic renal failure who additionally had a family history of kidney disease. There were no cysts detected in his kidneys by ultrasound. About 30% of glomeruli were globally sclerosed in the biopsy and there were mild tubular atrophy and interstitial inflammation. On the patient's initiative, genetic studies were performed; and linkage analysis revealed a unique uromodulin mutation in this family (unpublished), testifying to the problematic histologic appearance of progressive kidney diseases associated with hyperuricemia. HNF1β mutations can also mimic hyperuricemic nephropathy (4,89).

## Medullary Sponge Kidney (MSK)

Medullary sponge kidney is a cystic disease of adults. Cysts that may reach 8 to 10 cm arise in the medullary collecting ducts and in at least 50% of patients contain intense calcium deposits or stones. Patients present with hematuria, infection of the urinary tract, or obstruction. On radiologic investigation, bilateral nephrolithiasis is found in most individuals (8,123). A typical example is shown in Fig. 26.28. The excretory ureterogram shows filling defects in the medulla without hydronephrosis. Lithiasis often takes interesting shapes and has been likened to a flower bouquet by radiologists.

Unilateral or segmental disease is rare. MSK in most patients is a nonhereditary disorder, but a small number of patients (approximately 5%) appear to have familial disease. Disease in young children with congenital hemihypertrophy, Wilms' tumors, and neuroendocrine neoplasia syndrome (MEN II) is also reported (124–127). Rarely, focal segmental glomerulonephritis may complicate MSK, but it is unclear whether this is coincidental or secondary to obstruction and hyperinfiltration-induced focal segmental glomerulosclerosis (FSGS) (128). Whether specific metabolic abnormalities are related to nephrolithiasis in

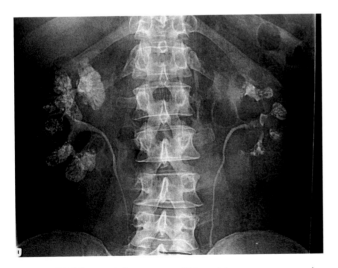

**Figure 26.28** Medullary sponge kidney. Intravenous urography (at 4 minutes) demonstrates markedly dilated collecting ducts greater in the right than the left. The calyceal system is normal. There is no hydronephrosis or hydroureter. From a 34-year-old man who presented with flank pain. (Courtesy Dr. Cary Lynn Siegel, Mallinckrodt Institute of Radiology, Washington University, St. Louis, MO.)

patients with MSK is unknown, but low urinary excretion of citrate and magnesium are typical metabolic abnormalities in MSK patients that distinguish these patients from those with idiopathic calcium stone forming (129).

## Renal Cysts in Hereditary Syndromes

## von Hippel-Lindau Disease

### Incidence, Clinical Presentation, and Genetics

von Hippel-Lindau (VHL) disease is an autosomal dominant hereditary disorder with an incidence of 1:30,000 to 1:50,000 live births (130). VHL is caused by germline mutations of the *VHL* tumor suppressor gene located on 3p25-26 chromosome. Both men and women are affected. The hallmarks of the disease are cysts and benign and malignant tumors in multiple organs. Tumors involve the central nervous system (hemangioblastomas), retina (angiomas), inner ear (endolymphatic sac tumor), kidney, pancreas (islet cell tumors), epididymis in men or broad ligament in women (cystadenomas), and pheochromocytomas (130). A characteristic feature of all tumors associated with VHL is the high degree of vascularization and the presence of a clear cell component. The frequency of lesions varies in different families, and at a minimum, one characteristic tumor (central nervous system [CNS] hemangioblastoma or clear cell tumor in a visceral organ) suffices for diagnosis, if definitive family history exists. In the absence of family history, two characteristic (clear cell) tumors are required for diagnosis. Kidney cysts predominate and are found in approximately 75% of the cases. Pancreatic cysts affect 26% of patients, but cysts in the liver are rare. Characteristically, cysts are bilateral but usually focal. Very rarely, multiple bilateral cysts may simulate ADPKD. Because presence of a few cysts in the kidney is a common occurrence, cysts are not a required criterion for diagnosis of VHL. Renal failure is rare, but when it occurs, it is because of diffuse replacement of the renal parenchyma by multiple cysts. Other organs that may develop cysts include the spleen, lungs, bone, and skin. Kidney tumors are typically renal cell adenocarcinoma (RCC) clear cell type. RCC is the main cause of morbidity and mortality and affects 75% of patients by the age of 60 years; it may also be the first manifestation of the disease. Other symptoms are hematuria and urinary tract infections, but hypertension is rare unless there is a pheochromocytoma. Most studies show that only a few patients have the full set of manifestations. Phenotypic variability is now understood through genetic studies to relate to specific VHL mutations. For example, renal disease is more frequent in patients who have VHL mutations that lead to truncation of the protein (pVHL) or large rearrangements as opposed to patients who have missense mutations (131). Patients with truncating mutations are designated as having VHL type 1 and characteristically develop all manifestations except pheochromocytoma. Patients with missense mutations have a predominant risk to develop pheochromocytoma and are designated as VHL type 2. VHL type 2 is further subdivided into type 2A (low risk for RCC and pancreas tumors), B (susceptible to all tumors from the VHL menu), and C (almost exclusively developing pheochromocytomas) (132). Germ-line mutations are detected in 100% of VHL patients (133). More than 150 germ-line mutations have been identified so far. Fluorescence in situ hybridization (FISH), which may detect the entire deletion or a large gene rearrangement, is a useful adjunct test (134).

### Kidney Pathology

VHL cysts are grossly small and do not transform the kidneys into the giant organs as in ADPKD (Fig. 26.29). Bilateral or unilateral cysts are few in number ranging from microscopic to a few centimeters. Histologically, cysts may be denuded or lined by low epithelium. Intracystic tumor nodules are typically clear cell type RCC (Fig. 26.30). Papillary RCC is sometimes found, but cells lining the papillae are clear cell type. Kidney tumors are usually incidentally found on routine screening for occult disease. Metastatic RCC in the liver, lung, and bones accounts for at least 50% of VHL-associated deaths. A lesion in the CNS or the spinal cord is more likely to be hemangioblastoma than RCC. If abdominal lesions originate outside the kidney, pheochromocytoma should be excluded. Distinguishing VHL from ADPKD and tuberous sclerosis as well as other hereditary cystic diseases may at times be difficult. For example, bilateral cystic kidneys without CNS or eye angiomas and presence of bilateral cystic kidney disease may mimic ADPKD (9,15,135). Differences such as kidney size, frequency of cysts, and extrarenal associations are helpful diagnostic clues. On imaging studies, VHL kidneys are usually either normal or slightly enlarged. Solid nodules within cysts are common in VHL and rare in ADPKD. Cysts in other organs

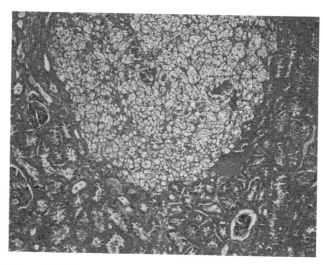

**Figure 26.30**   Renal cell carcinoma clear cell type is present in a von Hippel-Lindau cyst. (×100.)

are primarily in the pancreas (Fig. 26.31). Liver cysts are rare in VHL in contrast to ADPKD. Distinguishing VHL from adult TSC is easier based on the fact that the most common tumor is angiomyolipoma and extrarenal manifestations are distinct from VHL (see below). Diagnosis may be particularly difficult in young children when the first presentation is bilateral renal cell carcinoma. Such tumors may be very low histologic grade with individual tumor cells resembling closely normal tubules or tubular hyperplasia. An example of an extraordinary case from a 7-year-old boy is shown in Fig. 26.32A and B. Kidneys were bilaterally enlarged and occupied by heterogeneous masses with cystic and solid components. CT confirmed multiple renal cysts 1 to 4 cm wide. Renal biopsy revealed benign-appearing

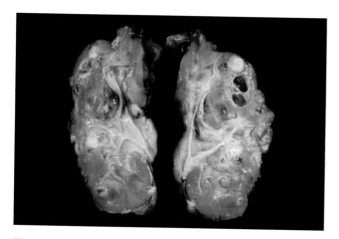

**Figure 26.29**   Von Hippel-Lindau kidneys with bilateral renal cell carcinoma.

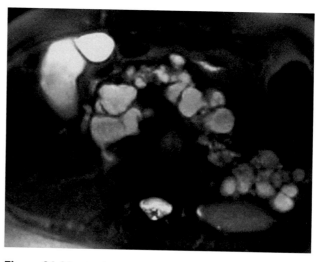

**Figure 26.31**   Axial T2-weighted fat-saturated image demonstrates innumerable cysts in the pancreas of patient with von Hippel-Lindau. (Courtesy Dr. Cary Lynn Siegel, Mallinckrodt Institute of Radiology, Washington University, St. Louis, MO.)

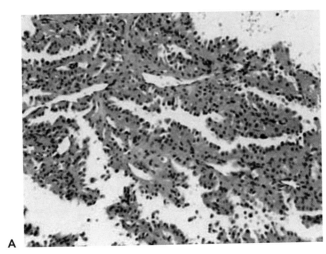
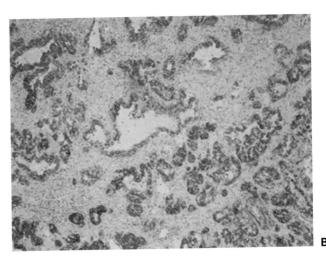

**Figure 26.32** **A:** Papillary RCC in a young child who presented with bilaterally enlarged kidneys. Tumor cell nuclei are low grade and difficult to distinguish from renal tubules on H&E staining. **B:** Cytokeratin and vimentin stains highlight the proliferative process and facilitate the diagnosis. (Vimentin immunohistochemistry, ×100.)

papillary proliferations (Fig. 26.32). Nuclei had very low grade atypia. Immunohistochemistry for vimentin and pancytokeratin were both positive, confirming the diagnosis of RCC (Fig. 26.32). Family history was negative for VHL and TSC in this child, but one should be aware of the possibility of de novo mutations and/or newly described types of hereditary clear cell RCC that are not related to VHL or TSC genes (136–138).

### Pathogenesis

The *VHL* gene targets the hypoxia-inducible factor (HIF)1 that regulates expression of hypoxia-inducible genes including the vascular endothelial growth factors such as VEGF, platelet-derived growth factor B, Flik-1, and Tie-2, and also erythropoietin and transforming growth factor α (TGF α). VHL also regulates genes related to cell cycle, epithelial cell differentiation, and fibronectin assembly in the extracellular matrix (138–144). As a tumor suppressor gene, biallelic *VHL* inactivation leads to uncontrolled cell growth, neoplastic transformation, and overexpression of VEGF in tumor cells and neoangiogenesis. A two-hit mechanism is thought to operate in this disease similarly to ADPKD and TSC. The *VHL* gene has only three exons and codes for three proteins, two of which are owing to an internal translational initiation start site at codon 54. Both proteins are thought to be wild (functional) type. A third protein is derived from exon 1 spliced into exon 3 and is not a tumor suppressor. However, there are at least three HIFa subunits (1a, 2a, and 3a) that are targeted by pVHL; hence, regulation of hypoxia-inducible genes is not straightforward.

### Prognosis and Management

Optimization of surgical treatment has changed the long-term prognosis of VHL patients. Nephron-sparing proce-

dures for lesions greater than 3.5 cm that have solid intracystic nodules are preferred in patients with a few lesions. Bilateral nephrectomy and transplantation is an acceptable alternative in those with multiple lesions.

## Tuberous Sclerosis

### Incidence, Clinical Presentation, and Genetics

Tuberous sclerosis (TSC) is a systemic phacomatosis characterized by hamartomatous proliferative lesions in almost every organ, including the brain, skin, retina, heart, endocrine glands, digestive system, lung, and kidney. Renal lesions include angiomyolipomas, cysts, and renal cell carcinoma. It is estimated to affect 1/10,000 to 1/15,000 live births and is inherited as an autosomal dominant trait. Up to 60% of cases are sporadic with no family history of TSC and are thought to represent new mutations. Both men and women are affected. Development of symptoms varies, but most patients are diagnosed in the first two decades. The heart, kidney, skin, and brain are frequently affected. Angiomyolipomas affect 75% of patients and renal cysts about 50% (145). Angiomyolipomas are composed of variable combinations of fat, vessels, and smooth muscle, and they tend to be numerous and bilateral in TSC in contrast to sporadic tumors. Unusual nuclear pleomorphism or epithelioid variants have been described, and these should be considered potentially malignant. Renal cell carcinomas are less frequent, affecting 1% to 5% of patients; usually these are clear cell type, but rarely papillary or chromophobe forms occur (9). Renal cysts usually coexist with tumors. Cystic-only kidney involvement is less frequent, affecting about 17% of patients, and these cysts are often asymptomatic (145). Renal failure and hypertension may develop because of enlarging lesions and replacement of the renal parenchyma. Pulmonary lymphangiomatosis, a lesion associated with TSC, may on occasion be concurrent with renal cysts (146).

Two tumor suppressor genes, TSC1 and TSC2, located at 9q34 and 16p13.3, respectively, have been identified (147). Development of tumors requires a second (somatic) mutation in addition to the germ-line mutation. Truncating intragenic mutations that affect the corresponding allele were also detected by genetic analysis of hamartomas and malignant tumors of TSC patients. Mutations spanning the entire length of the genes are reported. TSC2 mutations are more frequent in patients who have no family history of TSC (new mutations) and are associated more with mental retardation. Lung disease (lymphangiomatosis) occurs with both TSC1 and TSC2 mutations but is very rare (only 3/150 patients in one study) (146,147). TSC1 encodes for hamartin and TSC2 for tuberin, a putative GTPase that appears to interact with hamartin in vitro, suggesting that they function in the same cellular pathway (148).

Ultrasound is the gold standard for follow-up of patients who carry the diagnosis (149). Cysts are detected more frequently in children. Both cysts and angiomyolipomas increase in size with age. MRI demonstrates coexisting bright and dark signal intensities that correspond to cysts and fat, respectively. TSC tumors are usually treated conservatively unless they are complicated by bleeding. Rapid growth and young age are an exception to watchful waiting. The fact that both VHL and TSC are complicated by renal cell carcinoma may at times cause diagnostic difficulties in patients who lack extra renal stigmata. Analysis of RCC tumors from TSC patients has not so far detected VHL mutations, suggesting potential use of in situ hybridization for diagnostic purposes (150–152). A potential perplexing differential diagnosis in children is the exclusion of the contiguous TSC/ADPKD syndrome (see above under ADPKD). Such children may present with bilaterally enlarged kidneys, negative family ADPKD history, and CNS lesions of tuberous sclerosis (39,153).

## Pathology

Kidney resection is performed for enlarging angiomyolipoma, renal cell carcinoma, or persistent hematuria. Cystic kidneys from TSC patients are not seen in surgical pathology except rarely in children. In such cases diagnosis is often a surprise, because cystic kidneys may be the only and first manifestation of TSC. Cysts may be unilateral or bilateral, diffuse or localized. Kidneys may appear segmentally or diffusely cystic containing cysts of variable size and shape (Fig. 26.33). In childhood TSC, gross pathology is nonspecific and multicystic renal dysplasia is the most likely presumptive clinical diagnosis in the absence of relevant history. However, TSC cysts have unique microscopic features that set them apart from all other cystic diseases, including von Hippel-Lindau disease and renal dysplasia. The lining epithelium is composed of cuboidal

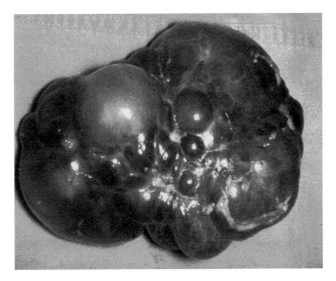

**Figure 26.33** Cystic kidney from a child with tuberous sclerosis.

large cells with deeply eosinophilic cytoplasm in either a single or multiple layers (Fig. 26.34A). Cysts may contain eosinophilic thyroidlike secretions and/or intracystic masses resembling neoplastic proliferations (Fig. 26.34). Nuclear pleomorphism and atypia may be present, suggesting that these are likely precursors of renal cell carcinoma. Both tubular and glomerular cysts have sometimes been the predominant feature in the form of glomerulocystic disease. The unique features may be accompanied by an intraglomerular collection of cuboidal or polygonal proliferating epithelial cells filled with lipid vacuoles known as *glomerular microhamartomas* (154).

Immunohistochemistry with antibodies to tuberin stain cystic epithelia weakly in contrast to normal tubular epithelial cells. Angiomyolipomas and related clear cell RCC do not express tuberin (9).

Cystic disease is usually mild in adults. Cysts are small, focal, and often adjacent to angiomyolipomas (Fig. 26.35A). Cyst lining is usually a monolayer of epithelial cells (Fig. 26.35B). Even though these cysts may resemble cysts in von Hippel-Lindau disease, concurrent angiomyolipomas make the distinction easy, but it should be noted that TSC cysts are not always associated with angiomyolipoma. In summary, histopathologic features that suggest tuberous sclerosis include characteristic cuboidal eosinophilic cyst-lining epithelium, glomerular cysts, glomerular hamartomas, multifocal or bilateral angiomyolipomas, cysts associated with angiomyolipoma or renal cell carcinoma, and or pulmonary lymphangiomatosis (9).

## Differential Diagnosis

In children, multicystic renal dysplasia, early onset ADPKD and or the recently recognized contiguous TSC-ADPKD syndrome are the main entities to consider (39). Von

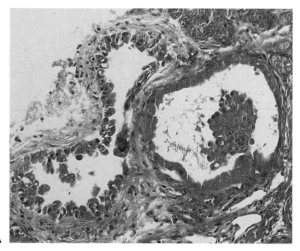 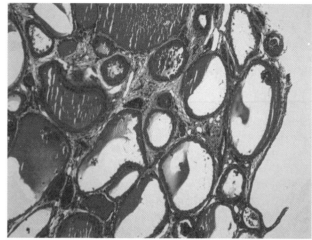

**Figure 26.34** **A:** Tuberous sclerosis cysts are lined by proliferating epithelium composed of large eosinophilic cells with atypical nuclei. (×200.) **B:** Many of the cysts in this case are glomerular and contain collapsed capillary tufts. (×100.)

Hippel-Lindau disease also enters the differential diagnosis, and it may be impossible at times to exclude without molecular genetics (see case discussed under Fig. 26.32).

### Pathogenesis

The mechanisms through which TSC1 and TSC2 mediate cellular growth control are only partially understood. TSC2 was directly linked to cell-size regulation by the discovery that mutation in *dTsc2* leads to the gigas (large cell) phenotype in the fly (155). Recent genetic studies suggest that TSC2 targets the rapamycin (TOR) pathway via phosphotidylinositol-3-kinase (PI3K), whereas the TSC1–TSC2 complex functions downstream of Akt and upstream of TOR to restrict cell growth and cell proliferation (156). Although a role in cell cycle control is found for tuberin, similar cellular specific roles are not proven for hamartin.

The fact that the two interact in vivo suggests similar functions and is consistent with the phenotypic manifestations in patients who carry mutations of either TSC1 or TSC2. Phenotype-genotype correlations and current work into the molecular signaling of these genes suggest that abnormalities in additional pathways, for example, β-catenin signaling, may be responsible for variability in TSC manifestations (157).

### Multilocular Renal Cyst (Multilocular Cystic Nephroma)

### Clinical Presentation

Multilocular cystic nephroma (MCN) is an infrequent lesion seen both in children and adults. Overall, MCN

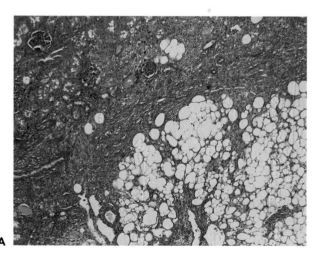 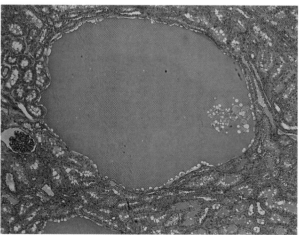

**Figure 26.35** **A:** Tuberous sclerosis cysts in an adult with angiomyolipoma. **B:** Cysts are small, lined by single epithelial layer. (×200.)

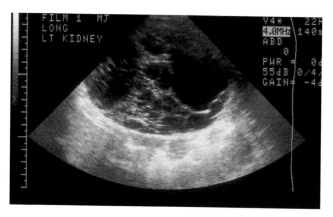

**Figure 26.36** Longitudinal ultrasound image demonstrating large cystic mass involving most of the left kidney with small and large cysts of cystic nephroma.

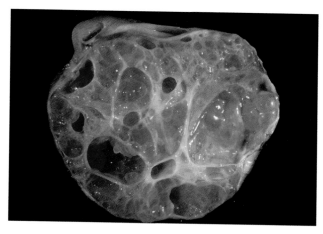

**Figure 26.37** Multilocular cystic nephroma. Multiloculated cysts are filled with gelatinous fluid.

accounts for about 5% of pediatric neoplasms. Children younger than 4 years of age and men and women older than 30 years of age are affected (158). Most cases are sporadic and unilateral, even though at least two familial and a few bilateral cases are reported (11). Congenital presentation in newborns and young infants is usually with an abdominal mass, abdominal pain, and hematuria mimicking Wilms' tumor, a much more frequent entity in infancy. MCN is usually a slow-growing lesion in both children and adults, but occasionally rapid growth is observed. Ultrasound, CT, or MRI is helpful in revealing the cystic nature of the lesion and its multilocular consistency (Fig. 26.36), but cannot distinguish MCN from entities with similar presentation such as unilateral early-onset ADPKD, multicystic dysplasia, malignancy, and a benign, nonfamilial condition known as "localized cystic disease." Pathologic evaluation is the best approach to diagnosis.

## Pathology

MCN usually presents as a large lesion occupying most of the kidney. The tumor is often encapsulated and consists of noncommunicating multiloculated lobules that are filled with gelatinous or clear fluid (Fig. 26.37). The lobules measure a few millimeters to 3 to 4 cm and are separated by thin septae. Septae may fold into the cysts, but nodular proliferations within the cysts are not a feature of MCN. The renal pelvis may be involved. Microscopically, cyst lining is quite characteristic, composed of a single layer of flat or hobnail-appearing cells. The septae contain connective tissue and focally atrophic tubules (Fig. 26.38). Presence of undifferentiated mesenchymal cells (blastema) is not part of benign MCN and is considered to confer malignant potential. The term *partially differentiated nephroblastoma* is coined for these lesions. In spite of the worrisome features, there have been no reported metastases or recurrences following surgical resection in this variant. In 29 pa-

tients with benign MCN, follow-up study of 3½ years post-surgery revealed that surgical removal is adequate therapy (158).

## Localized Cystic Disease

This is an uncommon presentation of renal cystic disease that has been mistaken for unilateral ADPKD, multilocular cystic nephroma, and cystic neoplasms. Some of the described cases have been mistaken diagnoses (159,160). Clinically, localized cystic disease may present with flank pain, hematuria, abdominal mass, or as an incidental finding. Most patients are men. The median age of diagnosis is 50 years (range 24 to 83 years). It may involve a segment or the entire kidney. Depending on the extent of renal involvement, it has been called segmental cystic disease of

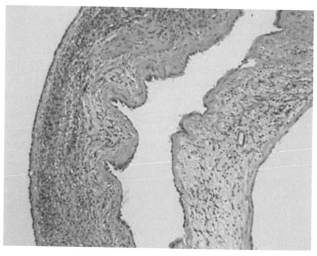

**Figure 26.38** Cysts in multilocular cystic nephroma consist of connective tissue septae lined by a single layer of epithelial cells with a flat or hobnail appearance. (×100.)

the kidney, unilateral cystic disease, or unilateral polycystic disease. Obviously, the latter term is to be avoided, because this entity is not familial, it involves only the kidney, and bears no resemblance to ADPKD, which is a hereditary and systemic disease. We have seen an initially perplexing case from a 73-year-old man who presented with gross hematuria. The right kidney was replaced by a cluster of cysts filled with clear or yellow fluid. The largest cyst measured 5 cm, and the wall of all cysts was smooth. The intervening renal parenchyma grossly appeared normal. Microscopically, the cysts were denuded of epithelium or lined by flat nondescript epithelium. The features resembled multiple simple cortical cysts. The pathogenesis of this entity is poorly understood and has received little attention. Nonetheless, it is important to distinguish it from unilateral ADPKD because this is a nonprogressive and benign condition. More than half of the reported cases were treated conservatively and only 4/18 (approximately 20%) had a nephrectomy (160).

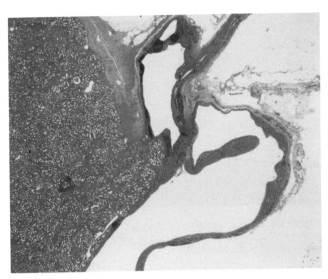

**Figure 26.39**  Simple cortical cyst devoid of epithelial lining located on the cortical surface. (×40.)

## Simple Cortical Cysts

Simple cysts are discrete lesions that may develop within the kidney or on its surface. Their prevalence is reported to be 12% to 25% in the adult population (161). These are common findings in autopsy of older men, but they are a rare phenomenon in children. For example, in a study of 6521 consecutive pediatric autopsies, only seven cases were identified (<1%). A predominant male occurrence is documented in the literature (161).

Simple cysts are usually oval or round with a smooth outline and are filled with clear or yellow fluid. They are acquired and thought to originate from diverticula of the distal convoluted or collecting tubules (162). The proposed pathogenesis is that diverticula increase in number with age, probably as a result of weakening of tubular basement membranes. Enlargement of size and number of cortical cysts was found to increase with age from 5.1% in the fourth to 36.1% in the eighth decade of life (161). The average increase in size and the rate of enlargement were 2.82 mm, and 6.3% yearly, respectively. An interesting observation by Terada et al (161) was that cysts in patients younger than 50 years grew more rapidly than those in patients older than 50 years. However, the results of this study may have been flawed by including patients with multilocular cysts, which reportedly progressed more rapidly than simple cysts. Histopathologic features of a simple cortical cyst are typically of an empty space, often without lining, surrounded by compressed, fibrotic interstitium (Fig. 26.39).

## Acquired Cystic Kidney Disease

Acquired renal cysts by definition occur in the native kidneys of patients with ESRD who are treated for uremia with

hemodialysis or peritoneal dialysis who did not have hereditary cystic kidney disease prior to dialysis. Diagnostic criteria require three or more cysts per kidney in a dialysis patient (163,164). Acquired cysts may manifest even prior to dialysis in about 8 to 13% of patients (163). This complication was first recognized in 1977 in an autopsy study of patients on hemodialysis whose cysts had by that time become widespread. It was later found in peritoneal dialysis patients and in transplanted patients with chronic rejection (164). In contrast, successful transplantation decreases the number of cysts in the native kidneys. The number of cysts increases with time on dialysis, and it is estimated that more than 50% of patients develop cysts within 5 years of dialysis and about 90% by 10 years. Once again, men are more susceptible than women. Children on dialysis are not exempt from this risk: in one study, 25% acquired cysts over a period of 16 years (165).

Two to seven percent of patients with acquired renal cystic disease develop intracystic renal cell carcinoma (9,163). These tumors are often bilateral and may be metastatic at the time of diagnosis. The risk of developing renal cell carcinoma is estimated to be 40 to 100 times higher compared with the general population. Tumors tend to be more aggressive in younger men on dialysis. Periodic radiologic evaluation of all patients on dialysis is recommended to prevent fatal complications (166,167).

## Pathology

Cysts often involve more than 25% of the renal parenchyma but, in contrast to PKD, kidneys with acquired renal cystic disease tend to be either of normal size or slightly small. Occasionally they may be enlarged and difficult to distinguish clinically or radiologically from ADPKD.

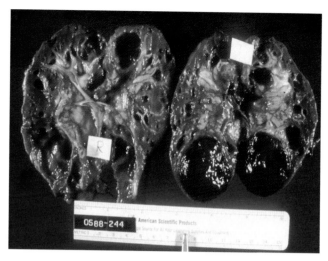

**Figure 26.40** Hemodialysis-induced acquired cystic kidney disease. Cysts occupy more than 25% of the renal parenchyma, but the overall size of the kidneys is not increased.

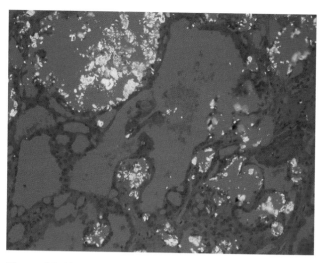

**Figure 26.42** Oxalate deposits are a frequent and distinct feature of acquired cystic disease and in a subset of associated renal cell carcinomas. (×40.) (Courtesy Dr. Luan Truong, Baylor College of Medicine, Houston, TX.)

The cysts often display fresh intracystic bleeding and are lined by cuboidal or hobnail epithelial cells arranged in single or multiple layers (Figs. 26.40 and 26.41). The cytoplasm is granular or deeply eosinophilic and nuclei are enlarged, containing prominent nucleoli appearing bizarre and/or highly atypical. Flat epithelium and micropapillary proliferation forming small adenomas (<5 mm in diameter) are frequent findings in the same specimen, suggesting a malignant predisposition of the lining epithelial cells. In addition, oxalate crystals are common within the cysts and/or in the interstitium and appear to be a distinct finding of these cysts (Fig. 26.42). Furthermore, in a recent

study of RCC associated with acquired cystic renal disease, the authors noted that oxalate crystals are a unique feature in a subset of RCCs associated with bilaterality and multifocality (168). They proposed that that oxalate deposits may promote malignancy or alternatively that the genetic changes that predispose to oxalate crystal formation also promote malignant transformation in acquired cystic epithelia (168). It is generally thought that pathogenesis of acquired renal cystic disease is a consequence of sustained uremia, but recognition of oxalate crystals as a hallmark of this disease brings a new insight that irrespective of its pathogenetic significance may be a helpful radiologic feature to follow-up dialysis patients at risk of developing aggressive tumors. Oxalate deposits may also be a helpful histologic feature in resolving questions on the pathogenesis of RCC in patients with autosomal polycystic kidney disease who develop tumors while on dialysis. The question in this instance may be whether RCC is owing to dialysis or the inherent proliferative activity of the lining epithelia in ADPKD.

## Miscellaneous Renal Cysts

Pyelocalyceal diverticula, perinephric pseudocysts, and hygroma renalis are conditions that may present diagnostic difficulty on radiologic examination and sometimes clinically. They rarely require the pathologist's attention, however, and therefore will be briefly discussed here.

## Pyelocaliceal Diverticula

These appear as circular or ovoid filling defects of the renal pelvis or the calyces on intravenous pyelogram

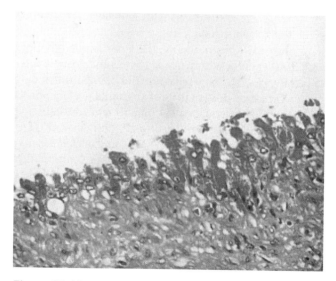

**Figure 26.41** Cysts in acquired cystic disease are lined by hobnail epithelial cells with atypical appearing nuclei. The cytoplasm is eosinophilic and also pigmented because of intracystic hemorrhage (H&E, ×200.)

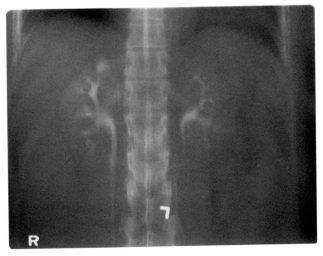

**Figure 26.43** Tomogram from an intravenous urogram demonstrating a collection of contrast material above the upper pole calyces indicating a calyceal diverticulum.

(Fig. 26.43). They are more common in children and are often solitary (169,170). They may be found incidentally during excretory urography or provoke severe acute flank pain and gross hematuria or urinary infection. Stone formation is a late complication and a rare cause of renal colic in adults (170). Isolated pyelocaliceal diverticula are rare in adults, if one excludes postoperative damage of the lining epithelium. Their presence in young children has prompted speculation that they represent ureteric bud branches that failed to induce nephrons and/or to be integrated into the normal tubulocaliceal system (170). Rarely, diverticula may loose their connection to calyx and present as a simple cortical cyst (171). Recently, an association with xanthogranulomatous pyelonephritis was reported (172). Current management of pyelocaliceal diverticula has evolved from open surgery to a minimally invasive retroperitoneal laparoscopic ablation with good results (169).

Histologically, the cavity is lined by flat epithelium surrounded by a thin layer of smooth muscle. Inflammation and squamous metaplasia or calcifications may be present.

### Perinephric Pseudocysts

Perinephric pseudocysts represent urine accumulation within the perinephric fat. They consist of reactive variably inflamed fibrous tissue and fat without a lining epithelium. These lesions are usually localized and rarely cause kidney displacement in the retroperitoneal space. Blunt trauma to the kidney or a surgical procedure that caused damage to the renal capsule is the most frequent cause. Clinically, they may present with flank or abdominal pain or be discovered incidentally long after the event as localized calcified lesions in the perinephric fat.

### Hygroma Renalis

This condition consists of ectasia of the lymphatics in the renal capsule and is also known as *pericaliceal lymphangiomatosis*. It presents as a circumscribed cystic mass that consists of dilated lymphatics containing eosinophilic fluid and encircles the renal pelvis or extends to the renal capsule. The kidney may appear enlarged and diffusely cystic, resembling cysts in polycystic kidneys. However, cysts consist of thin fibrous walls lined by endothelial cells.

Pericaliceal lymphangiomatosis is primarily diagnosed in adults who may be asymptomatic or experience symptoms of urinary obstruction. The condition resembles cystic hygroma of the head and neck. In fact, there is an interesting case report of hygroma renalis affecting one sibling in a single family and hygroma of the face affecting her sister (173). Conservative management with partial nephrectomy to remove the lesion but to preserve residual renal parenchyma serves most patients well.

## DEVELOPMENTAL KIDNEY DEFECTS

### Terminology

The spectrum of congenital anomalies of the kidney and urinary tract (CAKUT) is estimated to affect approximately 10% of births. CAKUT, a term recently proposed by Ichikawa et al (174), is currently favored in the literature instead of the term "renal malformations." CAKUT includes a wide range of kidney anomalies including aplasia, hypoplasia, adysplasia, multicystic dysplasia, and ureteric anomalies such as megaureter, ureteropelvic junction obstruction (UPJ), ureterovesical junction (UVJ) obstruction or incompetence, duplex kidneys/ureters, and anomalies of the bladder and urethra (174). Approximately half of the CAKUT cases associated with end-stage renal failure in children have patent urinary tracts, whereas the rest have obstructive nephropathy; the latter are mainly boys with bladder outflow obstruction (BOO) and posterior urethral valves (175). Some renal functional impairment may be superimposed postnatally from bacterial pyelonephritis and/or persistent urinary flow impairment causing renal atrophy and fibrosis, but the primary "hit" in CAKUT is clearly a developmental one. UPJ, UVJ, and related anomalies are discussed in Chapter 22 under Reflux Nephropathy. This chapter focuses mainly on developmental anomalies of the kidney proper. There is no accepted classification scheme for these anomalies, many of which are now linked to specific gene mutations. Hence, the categories of common kidney anomalies based on gross and microscopic pathology is used (Table 26.5).

### Cell Biology

In the last decade there have been major advances in the understanding of cellular and molecular pathogenesis of

## TABLE 26.5

### DEVELOPMENTAL KIDNEY DEFECTS

Renal agenesis/aplasia
Adysplasia
Renal dysplasia
Renal hypoplasia
   Oligomeganephronia
   Simple hypoplasia
Renal ectopia/malrotation
Renal fusion
Renal duplication
Supernumerary kidney
Tubular dysgenesis

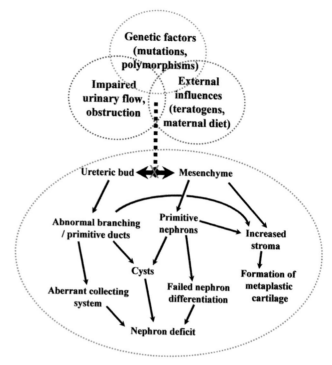

**Figure 26.44** Proposed mechanisms of developmental kidney disease.

CAKUT. To interpret these new developments, one must understand the processes involved in normal nephrogenesis. This is described fully in Chapter 2, but a brief overview is given here. Kidney formation involves a balance between basic cellular and tissue processes such as proliferation, death, differentiation, and morphogenesis, all controlled by regulated gene expression. Cell proliferation predominates as the kidney develops from less than a thousand cells at its inception to many millions in the mature organ, but after the initial stages, this is mainly confined to the periphery of the kidney, particularly the narrow rim of outer cortex containing actively branching ureteric bud tips and adjacent condensing mesenchyme (42). Fine tuning of cell numbers occurs by apoptosis, with as many as 50% of the cells produced in the developing kidney deleted via this process (42,176). Apoptosis occurs in different sites, primarily in early nephron precursors such as comma- and S-shaped bodies and the medulla, locations in which cell death may be important for morphogenesis and collecting duct remodeling. Several levels of differentiation occur during normal nephrogenesis ranging from early mesenchymal-epithelial differentiation to form renal vesicles to terminal differentiation in which different cells in the same nephron segments acquire different functions (for example α and β-intercalated and principal cells in collecting ducts). *Morphogenesis* is the process whereby groups of cells acquire complex three-dimensional shapes. This is clearly important in the kidney where there is such an intimate relationship between different nephron and collecting duct segments and the renal vasculature, but little is known about controlling factors.

Direct perturbation of expression of important nephrogenic genes by either mutations or transgenic technology can result in diverse kidney malformations in both man and experimental animals, but similar disrupted expression is also generated by extrinsic factors, such as teratogens or maternal diet, and physical or functional obstruction of the developing urinary tract. Moreover, these mechanisms can overlap to generate compound effects: genetic factors might generate urinary flow impairment, for example, with secondary effects in the kidney, or there may be altered gene activity in both upper and lower urinary tract. The latter gives rise to a "field effect" and has been postulated for genes such as BMP4 and AT2, which have widespread expression in the developing kidney and urinary tract (177,178). Similarly, in the renal cysts and diabetes (RCAD) syndrome there are genetic defects in hepatocyte nuclear factor (HNF)-1β, which is expressed in nephrogenesis, and there is a predisposition to diabetes, if the mother is a carrier with consequent poorly regulated blood sugars during the pregnancy (179). The proposed pathogenesis of dysplastic kidneys is represented schematically in Figure 26.44, with a central mechanism being disruption of mutual induction between ureteric bud and mesenchymal lineages in many cases. This leads to abnormal collecting duct development/branching and loss of potential functioning nephrons, plus formation of aberrant structures such as cysts and metaplastic cartilage and stromal expansion, with the net effect being a significant nephron deficit. Parts of this pathogenetic schema may also apply to other renal malformations.

## Pathology

### Genetic Causes of Renal Malformations

There are several genetic causes of renal malformations in humans (mainly mirrored in experimental mice), both in isolated renal conditions and as part of multisystem syndromes as listed in Table 26.6. It is beyond the scope of

## TABLE 26.6
## GENETIC CAUSES OF HUMAN RENAL AND URINARY TRACT MALFORMATIONS (CAKUT)

| Disorder | Genetic Mutation | Description |
|---|---|---|
| Apert syndrome | FGFR2 mutation—growth factor receptor | Hydronephrosis and duplicated renal pelvis with premature fusion of cranial sutures and digital anomalies |
| Bardet-Biedl syndrome | Several loci/genes implicated; includes a chaperonin and a centrosomal protein | Renal dysplasia and calyceal malformations with retinopathy, digit anomalies, obesity, diabetes mellitus, and male hypogonadism |
| Beckwith-Wiedemann syndrome | In a few patients, p57KIP2 mutation—cell cycle gene | Widespread somatic overgrowth with large kidneys, cysts, and dysplasia |
| Branchio-otorenal syndrome | EYA1 mutation—transcription factor-like protein | Renal agenesis and dysplasia with deafness and branchial arch defects such as neck fistulae |
| Camptomelic dysplasia | SOX9 mutation—transcription factor | Diverse renal and skeletal malformations |
| Carnitine palmitoyltransferase II deficiency | Gene for enzyme mutated | Renal dysplasia |
| CHARGE association | Unknown | Coloboma, heart malformation, choanal atresia, retardation, genital and ear anomalies; diverse urinary tract malformations can occur |
| Congenital anomalies of the kidney and urinary tract (CAKUT) syndrome | AT2 polymorphism—growth factor receptor | Diverse, nonsyndromic, renal, and lower urinary tract malformations |
| Denys-Drash syndrome | WT1 mutation—transcription/splicing factor | Mesangial cell sclerosis and calyceal defects |
| DiGeorge syndrome | Microdeletion at 22q11; probably several genes involved | Renal agenesis, dysplasia, vesicoureteric reflux, with heart and branchial arch defects |
| Duplex kidney and ureter | Loci and genes unknown | Nonsyndromic familial cases are recognized |
| Glutaric aciduria type II | Glutaryl-CoA dehydrogenase mutation | Cystic and dysplastic disease |
| Hypoparathyroidism, sensorineural deafness, and renal anomalies (HDR) syndrome | GATA3 mutation—transcription factor | Renal agenesis, dysplasia, and vesicoureteric reflux |
| Fanconi's anemia | Six mutant genes reported; involves DNA repair | Renal agenesis, ectopic/horseshoe kidney, anemia, and limb malformations |
| Fraser syndrome | FRAS1 mutation—putative cell adhesion molecule | Renal agenesis and dysplasia, digit and ocular malformations |
| Kallmann's syndrome | X-linked form: KAL1 mutation—cell adhesion molecule. Autosomal form: FGFR1 mutation—growth factor receptor | Renal agenesis and dysplasia in X-linked form |
| Meckel's syndrome | Loci at 11q and 17q; genes unknown | Cystic renal dysplasia, central nervous system and digital malformations |
| Nail-patella syndrome | LMX1B mutation—transcription factor | Malformation of the glomerulus and renal agenesis |
| Oral-facial-digital syndrome type 1 | OFD1 mutation—centrosomal protein | Glomerular cysts with facial and digital anomalies |
| Renal adysplasia | Some cases have de novo heterozygous mutations in uroplakin IIIa | Severe bilateral dysplasia and vesicoureteric reflux, persistent cloaca |
| Renal-coloboma syndrome | PAX2 mutation—transcription factor | Renal hypoplasia and vesicoureteric reflux |
| Renal cysts and diabetes syndrome | HNF1β mutation—transcription factor | Renal dysplasia, cysts, and hypoplasia |
| Simpson-Golabi-Behmel syndrome | GPC3 mutation—proteoglycan | Renal overgrowth, cysts, and dysplasia |
| Situs inversus and nephronophthisis type 2 | Inversin mutations affecting function of primary cilia | Cystic renal malformations with increased risk of situs inversus |
| Smith-Lemli-Opitz syndrome | δ 7-dehydrocholesterol reductase mutation—cholesterol biosynthesis | Renal cysts and dysplasia |
| Townes-Brocks syndrome | SALL1 mutation—transcription factor | Renal dysplasia and lower urinary tract malformations |
| Urofacial (Ochoa) syndrome | Locus on 10q; gene undefined | Congenital obstructive bladder and kidney malformation with abnormal facial expression |
| Urogenital adysplasia syndrome | Some cases have HNF1β mutation | Renal dysplasia and uterine anomalies |
| VACTERL association | Basis unknown apart from one report of mitochondrial gene mutation | Vertebral, cardiac, tracheoesophageal, renal, radial, and other limb anomalies |
| Vesicoureteric reflux | Genetically heterogeneous; one locus on chromosome 1 but gene undefined | Nonsyndromic familial cases with no secondary cause (e.g., urinary flow impairment) are recognized |
| von Hippel-Lindau disease | VHL mutation—tumor suppressor gene | Renal and pancreatic cysts, renal tumors |
| WAGR syndrome | WT1 and PAX6 contiguous gene defect—transcription factors | Wilms' tumor, aniridia, and genital and renal malformations |
| Zellweger syndrome | Peroxisomal protein mutation | Cystic dysplastic kidneys |

this chapter to describe all of these in detail; hence, we will focus on a selected few where more is known about their functional roles in nephrogenesis. These factors can be divided into groups such as transcription factors, growth factors, survival factors, and adhesion molecules, but these categories are not mutually exclusive since certain molecules fall into two categories; for example, both PAX2, a transcription factor, and epidermal growth factor (EGF) also promote cell survival.

Transcription factors are the conductors of the "developmental orchestra," regulating expression of other genes to set up embryonic patterning. Most contain DNA sequence-specific binding domains that modulate target gene mRNA transcription, although precise targets are often unknown. One of the earliest factors linked to renal development and disease was the Wilms' tumor (WT) 1 gene, which was discovered in these tumors but is paradoxically mutated in only a small percentage. WT1 encodes a transcription factor protein containing four zinc-finger DNA binding motifs (180) that is expressed at low levels in mesenchyme and then in comma- and S-shaped bodies, persisting in the mature kidney in podocytes (42). Lack of WT1 causes death in utero in null-mutant mice secondary to defects in mesothelial-derived components such as the heart and lungs (181). In humans, three syndromes arise from WT1 disruption: (i) point mutations, particularly in the zinc-finger DNA-binding domains, can cause the Denys-Drash syndrome of genitourinary abnormalities, including ambiguous genitalia in 46 XY males, nephrotic syndrome with mesangial sclerosis leading to renal failure, and a predisposition to Wilms' tumor (182); (ii) intronic mutations, which affect the balance between different WT1 splice isoforms, can cause Frasier syndrome of focal segmental glomerular sclerosis with progressive renal failure and gonadal dysgenesis (183); and (iii) large deletions with the contiguous PAX-6 gene cause the WAGR syndrome of Wilms' tumor, aniridia, genitourinary abnormalities including gonadoblastoma, and mental retardation.

Expression of another transcription factor, PAX-2, is intimately associated with WT-1 with diverse experiments suggesting both upstream and downstream activation and suppression interactions, and this molecule is also essential for kidney development. PAX2 is expressed in intermediate mesoderm, the nephric duct, then the mesonephric duct, and finally in the tips of the ureteric bud and the condensing mesenchyme in the metanephros (184). Abnormal kidney phenotypes result from perturbed expression: for example, kidneys do not develop in pax-2 null-mutant mice, are hypoplastic in heterozygous mutants, and develop cysts when pax-2 is overexpressed (185,186). Similarly, in humans, too little PAX2 leads to aberrant development. Mutations involving a single nucleotide deletion within the conserved octapeptide sequence in exon five have been linked to the renal-coloboma syndrome, which consists of optic nerve colobomas, renal anomalies, and

vesicoureteral reflux (187,188). Moreover, increased PAX-2 expression is observed in dysplastic kidneys and may contribute to epithelial cell survival and proliferation, which is essential for cyst development (42).

Another transcription factor involved in kidney and eye developments is EYA1, the mammalian homologue of the transcriptional coactivator "eyes absent" gene, which is required for normal eye specification in *Drosophila*. Eya-1 is widely expressed in the ear, branchial arches, and metanephric mesenchyme during mammalian development, and mutations of the human EYA-1 gene occur in 20% to 25% of patients with branchio-otorenal syndrome (189). This is characterized by a combination of hearing loss, preauricular pits, branchial fistulae, and variable renal anomalies including agenesis, hypoplasia, and dysplasia. Intriguingly, there appears to be an evolutionarily conserved regulatory cascade involving Pax family genes (i.e., Pax-6 in the eye, Pax-2 in the kidney), EYA1 and homologues of the *Drosophila* sine oculus (so) gene in the "six" family (190).

Mutations of the transcription factor hepatocyte nuclear factor 1β cause the renal cysts and diabetes (RCAD) syndrome in humans (179). HNF-1β is expressed widely during embryogenesis, including the mesonephric duct, ureteric bud lineage and early nephron epithelia, and adjacent paramesonephric ducts that should differentiate into the uterus and fallopian tubes (179,191). Renal malformations in RCAD are variable, but include cystic dysplastic kidneys, hypoplasia with oligomeganephronia, and unilateral agenesis; females may also have uterine abnormalities.

Growth factors have important functions in nephrogenesis via three potential roles: as paracrine factors secreted by one cell and acting on neighboring cells, as autocrine factors acting on the producing cell, and as juxtacrine factors that become inserted into the plasma membrane of the producing cell to interact with receptors on adjoining cells. The growth factors bind to specific cell-surface receptors, mainly receptor tyrosine kinases, which dimerize and become autophosphorylated and transduce signals into the cell. These signals may stimulate many different processes including cell division, cell survival, apoptosis, differentiation, and morphogenesis. Many of the signaling systems are structurally related; several, for example, belong to the transforming growth factor (TGF) β superfamily such as glial cell line–derived neurotrophic factor (GDNF), bone morphogenetic proteins (BMPs), and TGFβ1 itself. A great number of mouse growth factor mutants have abnormal kidneys, but surprisingly few human conditions have been reported thus far. This may result from genetic background effects since most human populations are relatively heterogeneous whereas mice are often inbred; hence, double mutants are less likely in humans. There may also be polymorphisms/mutations of other genes in the same pathway that alter expression and compensate for loss of the original molecule, particularly as there is frequent promiscuity between growth factor ligands and receptors, with several ligands potentially activating multiple receptors (192). Growth factor/receptor systems in murine development include the GDNF/RET/GFRα pathway where genetic ablation of any one of these factors causes either complete failure of metanephric development or severe dysplasia (193,194). Mutations in bone morphogenetic proteins (BMPs), particularly BMP4 and 7, cause hypoplastic or absent kidney development. The WNT family of secreted signaling molecules, including Wnt2b, Wnt4, Wnt6, Wnt7b, and Wnt11, has been implicated in normal nephrogenesis (195). In humans, increased expression of TGFβ1 has been reported in congenital renal malformations (196), and increased β-catenin/SMAD1 signaling, which is believed to result from BMP activation, is also observed in dysplastic kidneys (197).

Several survival and proliferation-related genes are critical for renal development in mice, but again there is very little evidence linking reduced expression to malformations in humans. BCL2 is the original member of a large family of related genes implicated in control of apoptosis (198). BCL2 and homologues prevent death, whereas BH3-only family members heterodimerize with them and block antiapoptotic activity. BCL2 is up-regulated in the mesenchyme as it condenses around the ureteric bud tips during nephrogenesis, but is then rapidly down-regulated in the comma- and S-shaped bodies and is barely detectable in the adult organ (42,199). Homozygous Bcl2 null-mutant mice have defects in hematopoiesis and hair development and have small hypoplastic kidneys with fewer nephrons and smaller nephrogenic zones antenatally (200), whereas multiple cysts develop postnatally (201). These changes can be abrogated by concurrently knocking out either one or both alleles of the proapoptotic partner BIM (202). The effects of reduced BCL2 are not known in humans, but this antiapoptotic factor is up-regulated in cystic epithelia in dysplastic kidneys (42), which also express PAX2; hence, these epithelia are exposed to concurrent stimuli to survive and proliferate, providing at least one mechanism for cyst expansion.

Cyclin-dependent kinases (CDKs) regulate the cell cycle and proliferation. Cyclin kinase inhibitors (also termed CDKN1C) block proliferation by binding to the CDKs in G1/S phase. One such molecule, p57-KIP2, is expressed in glomeruli and stromal cells between the renal tubules during nephrogenesis; moreover, p57-KIP2 null mutants have fewer renal tubules and small inner medullary pyramids (203). A similar phenotype of poorly formed medullary pyramids is sometimes seen in human Beckwith-Wiedemann syndrome, and the p57-KIP2 gene is close to the region with loss of the imprinted, expressed maternal allele on chromosome 11p15.5 in Beckwith-Wiedemann patients. Hence, defects in p57-KIP2 function have been questioned in this syndrome, but there could

equally be other genes from the imprinted region involved (204).

Adhesion molecules mediate cell–cell and cell–matrix adhesion (205). Examples of the former are the calcium-independent neural cell adhesion molecule (NCAM) (206,207) and calcium-dependent E-cadherin (also known as uvomorulin) (208), whereas molecules involved in cell–matrix adhesion include the collagens, fibronectin (206), and integrin cell-surface receptors (181,209). Many of these molecules also have additional non–adhesion-related functions, particularly proteoglycans that can modulate binding of growth factors to their receptors. GDNF signaling, for example, requires cell-surface heparan sulphate glycosaminoglycans, and mice with a gene trap mutation in the enzyme heparan sulphate 2-sulphotransferase have renal agenesis (210).

KAL-1 is the gene mutated in the X-linked form of Kallmann's syndrome (KS), which comprises hypogonadotrophic hypogonadism and anosmia. It affects 1:8,000 males and 1:40,000 females, with other forms of inheritance also described (211). Renal aplasia, generally unilateral, occurs in 40% of patients (212), but cystic dysplastic kidneys are also reported (213). KAL-1 encodes the extracellular matrix protein, anosmin-1. KAL-1 transcripts occur in the human metanephros and olfactory bulb from 45 days' gestation (214,215), sites consistent with organs affected in KS, whereas the protein anosmin-1 immunolocalizes to basement membrane of human ureteric bud (UB) branches (216). Anosmin-1 is modular, containing several domains including four contiguous fibronectinlike type III (FnIII) repeats, and these are predicted to mediate interactions between anosmin-1 and heparan sulphate, which is essential for kidney development. Loss of function mutations in FGF receptor 1 have been reported in dominantly inherited Kallmann's syndrome, and binding of heparan sulphate to FGF and its receptors is also required for FGF signaling (215,217).

The glypican family consists of heparan sulfate proteoglycans linked to the cell surface through a glycosylphosphatidylinositol anchor. The first member linked to renal development was glypican-3. The gene encoding this protein is mutated in patients with the Simpson-Golabi-Behmel syndrome, which consists of prenatal and postnatal overgrowth and organ abnormalities including renal malformations. Glypican-3–deficient mice replicate many of these features including cystic and dysplastic kidneys (218), with underlying dysregulation of proliferation and apoptosis during ureteric bud branching and medullary differentiation (219).

Another potentially important matrix/adhesion protein is FRAS1. This is mutated in some patients with Fraser syndrome (not to be confused with Frasier syndrome, which involves WT1 mutations), a multisystem disorder comprising cryptophthalmos, syndactyly, and renal defects (220). FRAS1 belongs to a family of novel proteins related to an extracellular matrix (ECM) blastocoelar protein found in sea urchins and contains several domains with potential binding sites for FGF2, BMPs, and TGFβ1. Mutations in a related protein, FREM2, have also recently been described in human Fraser syndrome and FREM2-deficient mice develop cystic kidney disease (221).

## Renal Malformations Associated With Urinary Tract Obstruction

Isolated renal dysplasia is the most important cause of childhood renal failure requiring long-term dialysis and kidney transplantation, but the second largest group is dysplasia associated with urinary tract obstruction, with posterior urethral valves being the most common specific diagnosis (222,223). Other associations include urethral atresia, obstructive lesions at the pelviureteric and ureterovesical junctions, the latter category including obstructive megaureters and ureteroceles (224). In addition, multicystic dysplastic kidneys are classically reported to be connected to atretic (i.e., nonpatent) ureters, and obstruction has been invoked in the early etiopathogenesis of the prune belly syndrome, a condition in boys with urinary tract dilatation and dysplasia, plus cryptorchidism and incomplete development of the abdominal wall muscles.

Renal malformations can also be generated experimentally by obstruction of the developing urinary tract. Over 30 years ago, Beck (225) demonstrated that surgically generated obstruction of fetal sheep perturbed kidney development and replicated many features of dysplasia. More recent studies used similar models to investigate the molecular pathogenesis of this process (226–228). It is intriguing that common patterns of dysregulation of proliferation/apoptosis, plus up-regulation of key nephrogenic molecules such as PAX2 and TGFβ1, occur in these models and both sporadic and obstructed human cases since this implies a common sequence of maldevelopment, irrespective of the underlying cause (228,229). A more recent example reflecting this commonality concerns the secreted matrix metalloproteinase matrilysin, a target gene of Wnt signaling, which is up-regulated in cystic kidneys, toxin-induced nephropathy, and obstruction (64).

Several other obstruction models have also been used. Opossum metanephroi have been experimentally obstructed in neonates in the marsupial pouch to generate broadly similar changes to the ovine studies (93), but these experiments also allowed therapeutic intervention. Administration of insulinlike growth factor (IGF), for example, ameliorates renal fibrosis, tubular cystic changes, and calyceal dilatation that follow obstruction (230). Similarly, Chevalier et al (231) have extensively investigated ureteric obstruction in neonatal rats in which nephrogenesis continues for 2 weeks after birth; once again, obstructive nephropathy is attenuated by EGF or IGF. Animal models have also been used to assess whether decompression of the developing urinary tract can improve renal outcome. In sheep, Glick et al (232) found that in utero decompression prevents renal dysplasia, but this conflicts with reports of Chevalier et all (233) on neonatal rats in which relief of obstruction attenuated but did not reverse renal injury resulting from 5 days' ureteric obstruction. These data are consistent with the generally poor results for in utero intervention to relieve obstruction in humans (234,235) since the kidneys may well be too far advanced along the path of maldevelopment before the abnormalities are detectable.

## Renal Malformations Associated With Teratogens and Altered Maternal Diet

Teratogens have been implicated in the pathogenesis of diverse kidney and lower urinary tract malformations (236) and can be divided into two broad categories: exogenous factors such as drugs and endogenous factors that become teratogenic when present in excess. A classic drug example is angiotensin-converting enzyme inhibitors (ACE-I) which, when used to treat hypertension during pregnancy, can cause skull malformations termed *hypocalvaria* plus neonatal renal failure from a combination of hemodynamic compromise and renal tubular dysgenesis (237). These effects are unsurprising when one considers the widespread expression of components of the renin–angiotensin system in kidney development (238,239). Moreover, Ichikawa et al (174) described ureteric/renal abnormalities in angiotensin type 2 receptor mutant mice and an association between CAKUT and a nucleotide transition within the lariat branchpoint motif of intron 1, which perturbs AGTR2 mRNA splicing efficiency in two human cohorts. This association has been subsequently confirmed in some (240) but not all populations (241). Mutations in the renin–angiotensin pathway have also recently been described in autosomal recessive renal tubular dysgenesis (discussed later).

High glucose levels in diabetic mothers are associated with an increased incidence of kidney and lower urinary tract malformations, plus abnormalities in the nervous, cardiovascular, and skeletal systems (242). Experimental exposure of embryonic kidneys to high glucose alters the expression of laminin β2 in the basement membrane (243) and expression of IGF receptors (244), but at least two other factors may contribute to congenital diabetic nephropathy. First, there is often an association with caudal regression syndrome that causes reduction of distal structures such as the sacrum and hind limbs and might clearly affect the lower urinary tract. Second, it is likely that many of the cases ascribed to maternal diabetes had HNF1β mutations as reported in the RCAD syndrome above. High doses of vitamin A and its derivative retinoids have also been linked to human and rodent renal malformations such as renal agenesis (245), although these are also sometimes associated with caudal regression (246). Too little vitamin A also perturbs renal development, however, via multiple effects including modulation of GDNF/Ret, Wnt11, and WT1 signaling in the metanephros (247,248), and interaction with the GDNF receptor Ret, which patterns distal ureter and bladder trigone development (249). Intriguingly, some of these effects are potentially reversible, at least in vitro (248). Fetal kidney development is abrogated when pregnant mice are exposed to all-*trans*-retinoic acid or the retinoic acid receptor agonist Am580, but nephrogenesis can be rescued by culture in serum-containing media (248).

Maternal diet may have a more subtle effect on nephrogenesis, affecting nephron number rather than inducing gross changes. This hypothesis arose from epidemiologic data suggesting that individuals born to mothers with poor diets are prone to develop hypertension and cardiovascular disease in adulthood (250,251) and proposing a link between congenital nephron deficits and later hypertension (252). Using animal experiments, it is now well established that moderate to severe dietary protein restriction during pregnancy impairs somatic growth and reduces numbers of glomeruli per kidney (253), and this has been linked to early deletion of renal mesenchymal cells by apoptosis, with subsequent reduction in the pool of renal precursor cells (254). Vitamin A may also have a regulatory effect on nephron number (255). Other factors such as dietary iron may be important. Maternal iron restriction, for example, causes hypertension that has been linked in part to a deficit in nephron number (256), which is consistent with proposed roles for iron in development of renal epithelial (229). Expression of many other nephrogenic genes can also be perturbed by altered maternal diet (257).

## Renal Agenesis and Renal Aplasia

*Renal agenesis* is defined as complete unilateral or bilateral absence of the kidney. Studies in animals and human embryos indicate that this anomaly results from failure of initiation of the pronephros–mesonephros sequence and failure of the ureteric bud to develop. In contrast, *renal aplasia* is defined as absent kidneys that were initially induced, but further stages of nephrogenesis were halted and the kidney eventually involuted. These definitions appear distinct in their pathogenesis and cell biology, but in reality, there is crossover when discussed clinically because an absent kidney in any given patient may result from either process.

## Bilateral Renal Agenesis

Absence of both kidneys is rare, with a suggested incidence of 1:7000 to 1:10,000 births and occurring more frequently in boys (258,259). It is almost always incompatible with life, with a sharply increased incidence of premature labor and miscarriage. Neonatal death is due to severe lung hy-

poplasia secondary to oligohydramnios. Kidneys produce most of the amniotic fluid from the second trimester of pregnancy, which is essential for lung and skin development. Oligohydramnios is associated with multiple other anomalies that include limb and face deformities such as wideset eyes, prominent epicanthic folds, receding chin, and flat nose and ears. These abnormalities are known as Potter's sequence (1). The facial/limb features are thought to result from pressure of the uterine wall on the fetus because of decreased amniotic fluid. Typically, the adrenal glands appear enlarged and dislike probably from the lack of compression from the kidney below. Occasionally, the adrenal glands are completely absent. Bilateral renal agenesis is often accompanied by genital anomalies including absent phallus, ectopic testes, hypospadias, small or abnormal uterus and imperforate anus, and urethral and bladder agenesis. These anomalies may form part of a developmental field effect involving the entire caudal end of the embryo including the hindgut and lower extremities to cause sirenomelia (Fig. 26.45). Renal conditions other

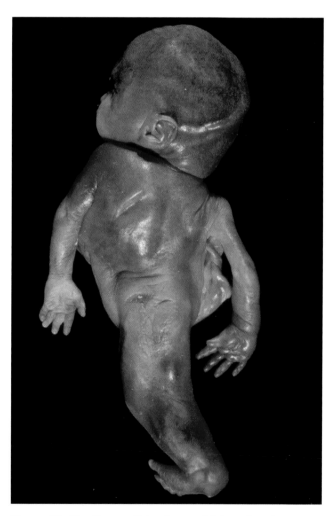

**Figure 26.45**   Sirenomelia in a fetus with bilateral renal agenesis.

than bilateral agenesis such as renal dysplasia, severe infantile polycystic kidney disease, or bilateral renal hypoplasia can also cause Potter's sequence if they are associated with severely decreased urine production (260).

Renal agenesis can be diagnosed by ultrasound as early as the first trimester. Therapeutic abortion is often considered at this stage because of dismal prognosis. It should be noted, however, that there are two reported cases of postnatal survivors demonstrating that lung development and survival of the fetus may proceed without kidneys in some cases (261).

## Unilateral Renal Agenesis

Unilateral absence of the kidney is common, affecting up to 1 in 1000 individuals (262). It occurs equally in both sexes, with the left kidney affected more often. Uncomplicated unilateral agenesis may not be diagnosed until later in life when it is found incidentally or because of a palpable contralateral kidney owing to compensatory hypertrophy. However, a great number of patients (50% to 70%) have an associated urogenital anomaly and are diagnosed early in life either by fetal ultrasound or because of genitourinary complications after birth.

Clinical studies using prenatal and postnatal ultrasound show that in humans, most solitary kidneys represent cases of unilateral renal aplasia that regresses rapidly after birth. For example, fetal ultrasound demonstrated small reniform kidneys that disappeared in a short period after birth (263).

The most frequent association of unilateral renal agenesis is with reflux nephropathy. In one study of 46 consecutive cases of unilateral renal agenesis, approximately half had UVJ or UPJ obstruction in the contralateral kidney (262). Other associated anomalies include contralateral renal dysplasia, absence of vas deferens, absent adrenals, and pelvic renal ectopy. In adults, solitary kidneys are frequently found incidentally; the high incidence in the general population dictates that presence of two kidneys be documented prior to required nephrectomy. The outcome for solitary kidneys has been regarded as benign with only a moderately increased long term risk of proteinuria and hypertension. This may be true if there has been sufficient opportunity for compensatory hypertrophy to develop in utero, but the Brenner hyperfiltration/renal injury model predicts that any reduction in overall renal functional mass may eventually lead to accelerated renal disease (252). In addition, the benign prognosis only applies when there are no abnormalities in the "normal" opposite kidney. Solitary kidneys are not immune to random kidney disease. For example, membranous glomerulonephritis, autosomal dominant polycystic kidney disease, renal cell carcinoma, and renal failure accelerated by obesity and or hypertension have been reported in solitary kidneys (264–266).

Bilateral or unilateral renal agenesis accompanies many syndromes such as the branchio-otorenal syndrome,

RCAD, and the hypoparathyroidism, sensorineural deafness, and renal anomalies (HDR) syndrome, Fanconi's anemia, Fraser and Kallmann's syndrome, DiGeorge syndrome, Smith-Lemli-Opitz syndrome, and Klinefelter's syndrome (47,XXY) (Table 26.6). Perhaps the most intriguing type of renal agenesis is familial disease, occurring either as bilateral or unilateral agenesis/aplasia or in combination with contralateral dysplasia in members of the same family known as hereditary renal adysplasia (267,268).

## Hereditary Renal Adysplasia

*Renal adysplasia* is defined as unilateral renal agenesis in association with dysplasia of the contralateral kidney (Fig. 26.46). The term *adysplasia* is often used more broadly to include dysplasia, absent kidneys, and almost any other structural or positional kidney/lower urinary tract defect (269–272). However, hereditary renal adysplasia should be confined to renal dysplasia, renal adysplasia, or renal agenesis in any combination, in different members of the same family. The genetic link between renal agenesis and some types of renal dysplasia points to a common pathogenetic mechanism for these anomalies and perhaps relates to the degree of failure of the ureteric bud in its inductive function on the metanephric blastema (271). The dysplastic kidneys in renal adysplasia are usually rudimentary (renal aplasia) or multicystic (Fig. 26.47). Most cases of hereditary adysplasia are recognized at autopsy for investigation of perinatal death. Retrospective family studies then reveal unilateral renal agenesis or dysplasia in parents or living siblings. Deaths from bilateral renal agenesis also may have occurred in siblings and sometimes in other generations of the same family (270,273,274). An autosomal dominant mode of

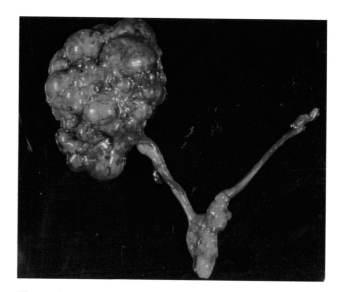

**Figure 26.46** Renal adysplasia. Right kidney is multicystic dysplastic. Left kidney is a knoblike structure (aplastic).

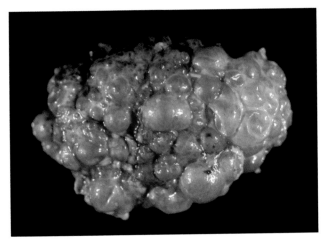

**Figure 26.47** Multicystic dysplastic kidney from a newborn. Notice that the kidney is diffusely cystic but not enlarged.

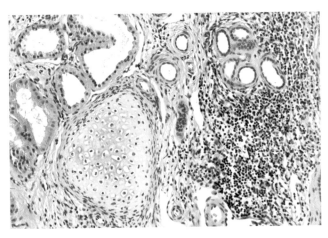

**Figure 26.49** Metaplastic cartilage is a unique feature of renal dysplasia. Significant inflammation is present as well. (×400.)

inheritance with variable expression in familial renal adysplasia is reported, but the occasional cases of agenesis or dysplasia affecting siblings with normal parents suggests that there are other types of inheritance. Moerman et al (271) described a patient with hereditary renal adysplasia exhibiting a de novo autosomal 6p/l9q translocation with breakpoints at 6p21.3 and 19q13.4. The authors suggested 6p as the likely locus for at least one defective gene involved in hereditary renal adysplasia.

## Renal Dysplasia

In the strictest terms, renal dysplasia can be diagnosed only on the basis of histology. The malformed kidney can be either larger or smaller than normal and diffusely or partly cystic (Fig. 26.48). Histologically, though, there are distinct features: disrupted organization and primi-

tive, poorly branched ducts with smooth muscle collars (Figs. 26.47 to 26.51). Cartilage is present in only one third of the cases, but smooth muscle collars enclosing primitive ducts are invariably present. The latter two are the most specific histologic features that are essential for diagnosis of renal dysplasia. Glomeruli may be focally or even diffusely cystic, imitating glomerulocystic kidney disease (GCKD) (Figs. 26.52 to 26.53). The degree of dysplasia within the kidney can vary: for example, it may affect cortex and medulla or predominantly the medulla alone and it may involve a segment or the entire kidney. Segmental dysplasia is most frequently seen in children with duplicate ureters immediately above the duplication (Fig. 26.54) and very rarely in adults (275). Renal cortex is reduced in thickness owing to decreased nephron formation. Nephrogenic rests are sometimes encountered (Fig. 26.55), but Wilms' tumor

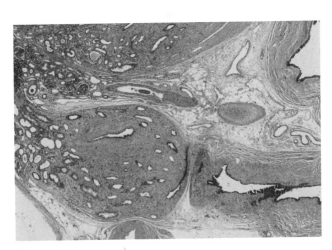

**Figure 26.48** Diagnostic features of renal dysplasia. Kidney parenchyma is disorganized, tubules are primitive, and there is metaplastic cartilage. There is also hydronephrosis with dilated pelvis and calyces. (×100.)

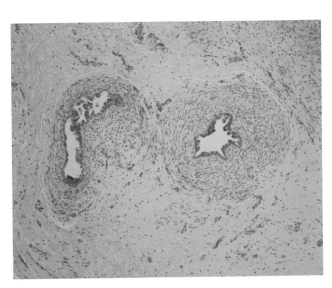

**Figure 26.50** Characteristic smooth muscle collars around primitive ducts. (×200.)

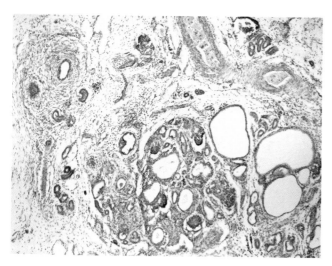

**Figure 26.51**  Complete loss of orderly nephrogenesis in renal dysplasia. Glomerali are immature, tabules are cystic and vessels are thickened. (×40.)

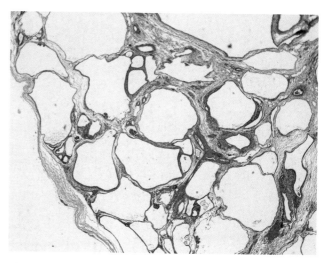

**Figure 26.53**  Glomerulocystic kidney disease associated with obstruction but without histologic features of renal dysplasia.

is a very rare occurrence. In fact, earlier speculations and hypotheses that implied a malignant potential of nephrogenic rests in dysplastic kidneys have not been substantiated by long-term studies (277–282). Renal cell carcinoma developing in an atrophic kidney was the subject of a single case report (283). Atrophic and rudimentary dysplastic kidneys (Fig. 26.56) are sometimes erroneously called hypoplastic from which they should be distinguished (see below). Variations in gross appearance have prompted investigators to distinguish dysplasia in different types such as cystic (multicystic), hypoplastic, hypodysplastic, segmental or obstructive dysplasia when associated with urine flow obstruction (Fig. 26.57). Such distinctions and terminology may have diagnostic value, but with an ever-increasing new literature from cell biology, seem to have lost their luster.

Unilateral dysplasia is more common than bilateral. Both can be associated with Potter's syndrome because of frequent anomalies in the contralateral kidney. Coexisting abnormalities of the urinary tract occur in 50% to 75% of patients with unilateral dysplasia; hence they fall into the CAKUT spectrum (284,285). Renal dysplasia is frequently found in renal ectopias including horseshoe kidney, kidneys with ureteral duplication, hydroureters, UPJ and UVJ obstruction, reflux, and superimposed pyelonephritis also referred to as obstructive nephropathy (Figs. 26.52, 26.54, 26.56, and 26.57). The role of obstruction in the pathogenesis of human renal dysplasia is substantiated by numerous studies that show tubular dilation and cyst formation owing to fluid accumulation in humans and animal models (discussed under Cell Biology above) (286). In obstructed kidneys, the main differential diagnosis is from pure hydronephrosis. In pure hydronephrosis,

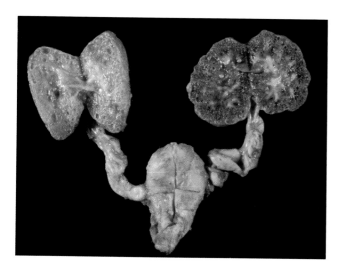

**Figure 26.52**  Fetal kidneys diffusely cystic associated with bilateral hydroureters. Bladder is hypertrophic.

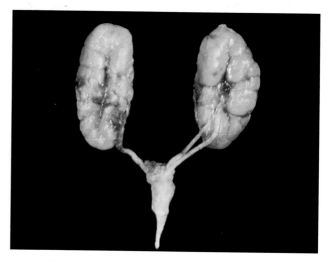

**Figure 26.54**  Ureteral duplication in left kidney.

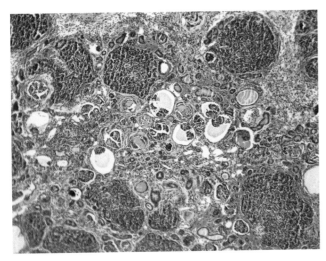

**Figure 26.55** Nephrogenic rests in dysplastic kidney; glomerular cysts are also present. (×200.)

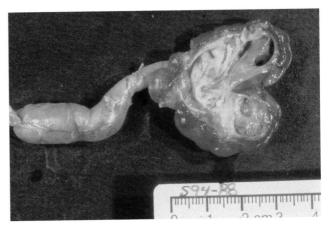

**Figure 26.57** Obstructive renal dysplasia associated with hydroureter and pelvic hydronephrosis.

thinning of the medulla is usually more extreme than that of the cortex, whereas in a hydronephrotic dysplastic kidney, the reverse is more frequent. In addition, primitive comma-shaped ducts and smooth muscle collars are not a feature of pure hydronephrosis (discussed in Chapter 22).

The fact that dysplasia occurs in kidneys without evidence of obstruction has raised alternative hypotheses that include loss of local gene transcriptions (224,287). As discussed under Adysplasia, multicystic dysplasia can be part of related familial kidney anomalies, but unilateral dysplasia without other genitourinary anomalies has been reported with an autosomal dominant mode of inheritance. For example, Srivastava et al (288) reported a woman with unilateral multicystic dysplasia who presented with ab-

dominal mass in infancy; both of her children had unilateral dysplasia detected with prenatal ultrasound. A father-to-son transmission is found in independent families with isolated unilateral cystic dysplasia, further supporting an autosomal dominant mode of inheritance (275,289,290). Search for specific genes revealed mutations in PAX2 as part of the familial renal coloboma syndrome (291) and CDC5L gene rearrangement on chromosome 6p at (6;19) (p21;q13.1) in a Belgian family (292). A de novo uroplakin IIIa heterozygous point mutation was found in 4 of 17 children with varied phenotypes of dysplasia (adysplasia) with no evidence of mutations in all sets of parents (293). These genetic studies reveal complex and variant genetic pathogenesis and are important for genetic counseling of affected individuals, but most often unilateral renal dysplasia appears sporadic rather than familial.

The differential diagnosis of multicystic dysplastic kidneys in childhood includes unilateral or bilateral tumors (38). The overall prognosis of unilateral dysplasia depends on presence of other anomalies that sometimes may be more severe and overshadow the kidney problem. Isolated unilateral disease has good prognosis with appropriate conservative management to prevent infections or treat hypertension. A few patients may experience renin-dependent hypertension owing to increased ectopic renin production in the dysplastic kidney that is curable with surgery (294,295). However, renin is generally decreased in dysplastic kidneys, which is a feature that may contribute to abnormally thick and malformed vessels (Fig. 26.58) (296). Routine surgical removal of the dysplastic kidney is not recommended. At least one third of dysplastic kidneys undergo rapid involution postnatally (297,298).

### Renal Hypoplasia

Hypoplastic kidneys are defined as small kidneys that weigh less than 50% of the normal mean for age and

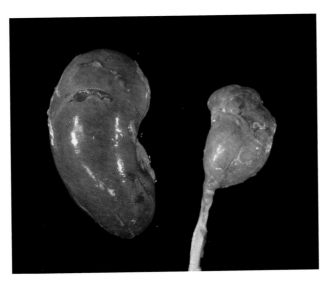

**Figure 26.56** Atrophic (hypoplastic) renal dysplasia in left kidney associated with ipsilateral hydronephrosis (notice dilated pelvis) and hydroureter from a 22-week fetus.

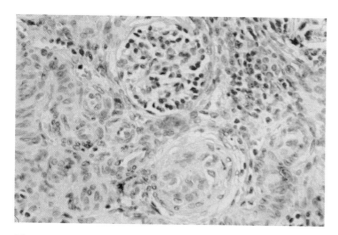

**Figure 26.58** Renin immunohistochemistry in dysplastic kidney reveals sparse renin-positive cells in dysplastic arterioles.

have no histologic abnormality other than secondary FSGS, simple hypoplasia, or hypertrophy of nephrons (oligomeganephronic hypoplasia). Hypoplasia is difficult to distinguish from secondary atrophy as part of acquired or congenital disease in infancy and childhood when reduced renal mass is concurrent with anomalies of the urinary tract such as obstruction and vesicoureteral reflux, hydronephrotic atrophy, renal dysplasia, and segmental pyelonephritic scarring, all of which may interfere with renal growth. Distinguishing features in renal hypoplasia are the reduced number of renal lobes and a narrowed and hypoplastic main renal artery. Routine pathology using a single slice through the long axis of the kidney is seldom sufficient for this assessment. The number of renal lobes is best established by opening the pelvicaliceal system and slicing the kidney to establish the numbers of lobes drained by each papilla. Boissonnat (299) has shown that the normal kidney possesses at least 10 lobes, whereas hypoplastic kidneys usually have 5 or fewer and occasionally only a single lobe. Excluding secondary renal damage in a small kidney requires radiographic examination with contrast media to exclude segmental scarring and calyceal clubbing, a change diagnostic of reflux and congenital renal artery stenosis. A narrow renal artery in acquired renal disease retains a wide, funnel-shaped segment at its origin from the aorta as an indication of its previously wider overall caliber (300,301). Adequate histologic examination of the kidney is required to exclude evidence of dysplasia. Parenchymal maldifferentiation is lacking in the purely hypoplastic kidney. Furthermore, kidneys that are small entirely because of acquired disease should not be described as hypoplastic. An entity that may be relevant at this point is the so-called Ask-Upmark kidney, a type of small kidney associated with hypertension in childhood (discussed in Chapter 22), and small kidneys associated with arteriovenous malformations at the renal hilus (302).

Although the true incidence of renal hypoplasia is difficult to establish, apparently it is much rarer than for-merly thought, and most cases are bilateral. Two main varieties can be distinguished: oligonephronic hypoplasia (oligomeganephronia) and simple hypoplasia.

## Oligomeganephronia

This is a distinct form of nonfamilial bilateral renal hypoplasia in which the combined kidneys weigh 12 to 45 g and always less than 50% of the expected weight. The number of renal lobes is reduced, and sometimes only one or two pyramids can be identified. The parenchyma is typically firm and pale, and the renal surfaces are smooth or finely granular. Microscopically, the striking feature is the reduced number of nephrons, but those present are hypertrophied. The glomeruli are clearly enlarged by up to three times the normal diameter; and the tubules are dilated and lined by enlarged epithelial cells. Children with oligonephronia develop polyuria and polydipsia, a urine-concentrating defect, and often salt wasting in the first 2 years of life. Dehydration, vomiting, unexplained fever, and growth retardation are also common features, and the clinical picture may resemble that of juvenile nephronophthisis. However, significant proteinuria is more frequent with oligonephronia, and the absence of a family history may help to distinguish it from familial juvenile nephronophthisis, which is inherited as an autosomal recessive trait. Although oligonephronia is usually a sporadic isolated anomaly, Park and Chi (303) in 1993 described two infants with this condition and other major congenital abnormalities. One exhibited a chromosome 4p deletion and the other a 4p ring. Salomon et al (304) found PAX2 mutations implicated in three patients with oligomeganephronia. This rare disease characterized by nephron deficit in premature babies and/or infants is gaining increasing interest, particularly in regard to the association of low birth weight with low nephron numbers and subsequent increased risk for hypertension and heart disease in adulthood (305). Premature babies or small–for-age infants have a high incidence of cardiovascular disease, hypertension, hyperlipidemia, diabetes, and renal failure in adulthood. Computer-assisted histomorphometry and radial glomerular counts in one premature infant with low birth weight revealed approximately 50% decrease in glomerular generations compared with normal control and a significant increase in the size of glomeruli. Glomerulomegaly, a hallmark of hyperfiltration, appears to play a role in the renal failure developing later in life of low–birth-weight premature babies and may be due to decreased renal mass (306).

## Simple Hypoplasia

Simple hypoplasia may be bilateral or, much less frequently, unilateral, and it differs from oligonephronic hypoplasia chiefly in that nephronic hypertrophy is not a feature. Histologic examination reveals a reduced volume of normally differentiated renal parenchyma. Secondary glomerular sclerosis with focal tubulointerstitial damage may be apparent, particularly with more extreme reduction in renal size.

Bilateral small kidneys with less than 50% of the expected mean combined renal mass are sometimes encountered in children with multiple congenital malformations, Down's syndrome, or long-standing disease or anomalies of the central nervous system. In this situation, the number of renal lobes is often normal, and the reduced renal size possibly represents a failure of normal postnatal growth rather than an intrinsic deficiency in renal parenchymal mass. Some ectopic or malrotated kidneys may be smaller than expected, even when histologic signs of dysplastic parenchymal differentiation are absent. The blood supply to such kidneys is often anomalous, but it is uncertain whether this is a primary or secondary event (307).

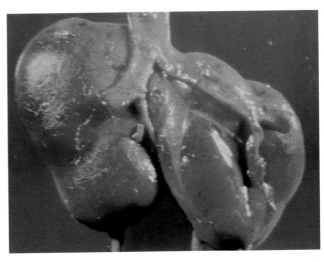

**Figure 26.59**   Fused renal ectopia. Both kidneys were in the left side. Fusion is in the upper poles. (Courtesy Dr. John Kissane, Washington University, St. Louis, MO.)

## Ectopia and Malrotation

Permanent malposition of the kidney outside its normal lumbar site constitutes renal ectopia, a condition that may affect one or both kidneys or a solitary kidney in unilateral agenesis. Ectopia is seen in about 1 in 800 radiologic examinations of the kidney. Ectopic kidneys need to be distinguished from abnormally mobile, ptotic ("droopy") kidneys, which are less firmly anchored than normal to the posterior abdominal wall by their peritoneal covering and may therefore change position excessively during respiration. They are not permanently displaced, however, and they have a normal blood supply.

During development, the kidneys ascend to a progressively higher level; they form at a level equivalent to the pelvis and ultimately end in the lumbar region between the 12th thoracic and 3rd lumbar vertebral bodies. During the ascent, which is largely a result of differential growth of the caudal end of the embryo, the kidney rotates medially through 90°, so the renal hilus and pelvis, which are at first located anteriorly, come to be on the medial aspect. Interference with this process results in renal ectopia below the normal position, usually in the pelvis. Such ectopic kidneys are almost always malrotated with an anteriorly directed pelvis, and their shape is often discoid or lumpy rather than reniform. Rarely, reversed (lateral) rotation of the kidney occurs, with a laterally facing renal pelvis, and exceptionally, the kidney may rotate through 180° so the pelvis is anterior. Ectopic kidneys are very rarely found at a higher level than normal, although they have been described in the thorax in association with a diaphragmatic defect. The blood supply to ectopic kidneys is generally anomalous and is derived from single or multiple branches of the common iliac artery or lower abdominal aorta.

Renal ectopia may be simple or crossed. In simple ectopia, the kidney and ureter are on the correct side of the body. The ureter is short and may be inserted ectopically in the bladder neck, urethra, seminal vesicle, or vagina; sometimes it is subject to vesicoureteral reflux. In crossed ectopia, the kidney is situated on the opposite side of the body of the urethral orifice with the ureter crossing the midline. The two kidneys are thus located on the same side of the body, with the ectopic kidney generally below the orthotopic kidney. The two kidneys may be fused together, a condition known as crossed fused ectopia (Fig. 26.59). Ectopic kidneys are often dysplastic, and distortion or kinking of the renal pelvis or obstruction by blood vessels crossing anterior to the renal pelvis may lead to intermittent obstruction and hydronephrosis. This condition, particularly if accompanied by vesicoureteral reflux, predisposes to renal infection. In about 25%, renal calculi are present. Pelvic renal ectopia can be associated with anorectal anomalies, particularly rectal atresia, or with congenital absence or atresia of the vagina in female patients.

## Renal Fusion

In renal fusion, the two kidneys are joined and the parenchyma is continuous between them. Each kidney has a separate collecting system and ureter that are inserted orthotopically on the two sides. Renal fusion should be distinguished from ureteral duplication, in which two ureters, even if completely separate, are inserted on the same side of the bladder. Most commonly, the kidneys are fused by their lower poles across the midline, the horseshoe kidney, which is seen in approximately 1 in 600 radiologic examinations. Horseshoe kidneys are often situated lower than normal and so can be regarded as ectopic as well as

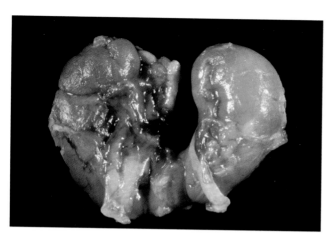

**Figure 26.60**    Horseshoe kidney found in the pelvis of 24-week male embryo.

fused (Fig. 26.60). The renal pelves are usually located anteriorly, and hydronephrosis resulting from a high ureteropelvic junction or compression by aberrant renal arteries is not uncommon. Midline fusion is about twice as common in males as in females. It is not infrequently associated with other congenital malformations and is common in Turner's syndrome. Although usually asymptomatic, the presence of hydronephrosis predisposes to renal infection and calculus formation. Occasionally, the fused renal tissue may be palpable as an apparently pulsatile midline mass that has been mistaken for an aortic aneurysm.

## Renal Duplication

Some degree of duplication of the renal pelvis and ureter (duplex kidney) is common, occurring in about 5% of unselected autopsies. The extent of the duplication varies from mere bifurcation of the extrarenal renal pelvis to complete duplication of the whole system with two completely separate ureters with separate orifices (Fig. 26.54). Complete ureteral duplication is rare (1% of all duplications) and may be associated with segmental renal dysplasia, ectopia of one of the ureters, and ureterocele. The conjoint ureter, in which separate renal pelves and upper ureters join to form a single lower ureter, is relatively common. Rarely, triplication and even quadruplication of the ureter occur.

## Supernumerary Kidney

This rare anomaly is characterized by the presence of a third kidney morphologically separate from the other two, with its own pelvicaliceal system and blood supply. The extra kidney is ectopic, usually situated beneath the lower pole of a normal kidney, and its ureter may join one of the other two or may drain separately. Sometimes it is inserted ectopically. Exceptionally, multiple supernumerary kidneys have

been described. The condition is usually asymptomatic, but renal infection, obstruction, and stone formation may occur.

## Renal Tubular Dysgenesis (RTD)

This syndrome is characterized clinically by oligohydramnios, widely separated cranial sutures and fontanelles, Potter's sequence, and premature stillbirth or neonatal death from respiratory failure. Originally described in two stillborn siblings, RTD was subsequently reported in approximately more than 70 cases (308–310). Voland et al (310) described two affected male siblings and suggested an X-linked recessive inheritance, but other reports include female siblings and consanguineous parents, indicating an autosomal recessive trait. Recent studies by Gribouval et al (309) demonstrated mutations in the genes coding for renin, angiotensin-converting enzyme, or angiotensin II receptor type I. Eleven individuals from nine families, some of whom were consanguineous, had RTD (309). Histologically, all kidneys had typical findings of RTD with absent proximal tubule differentiation and some had intense renin expression detected by immunohistochemistry. The authors proposed that enhanced renin production may be triggered by low blood perfusion in the developing kidney in utero, something that Bernstein and Barajas also noted in 1994 (311). Interestingly, studies in mice show focal renin expressing cells in the fetal kidney suggesting that they may be precursors for a subset of proximal epithelial cells (312). These studies may further explain the acquired RTD lesion in infants of mothers receiving angiotensin-converting enzyme (ACE) inhibitors for hypertension during pregnancy who have widened cranial sutures and RTD in entities causing hypoperfusion of the fetal kidneys (237). The latter include twin–twin transfusion in monochorionic twins in which the donor fetus develops RTD, congenital cardiac anomalies, and severe liver disease (313). Abnormal tubular differentiation has also been described in the infants of mothers receiving nonsteroidal anti-inflammatory drugs (314–316). The lesions in these patients differ from those of hereditary renal tubular dysgenesis by the presence of glomerular cysts and by some limited degree of proximal tubular differentiation. Bale et al (317) reported three infants who died of renal tubular dysgenesis and who also had severe hemosiderotic liver disease.

## Pathology

Grossly, the kidneys are normal sized or enlarged. Histologically, the glomeruli appear crowded together, and the tubules are lined by small, darkly staining cells that cannot be differentiated histologically into proximal and distal convoluted tubules (Fig. 26.61). Lack of differentiation is highlighted by immunohistochemical staining for epithelial membrane antigen that normally stains only

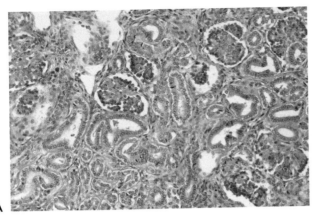
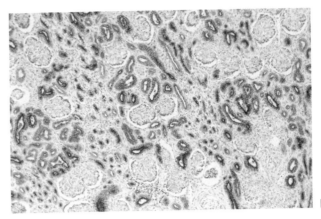

**Figure 26.61**    Renal tubular dysgenesis. **A:** Glomeruli appear crowded together. Proximal tubules lack brush borders and cannot be distinguished from distal. **B:** Epithelial membrane antigen (EMA) stains all tubules (normally only distal tubules stain). (×200.) (Courtesy Dr. David Brink, Department of Pathology, St. Louis University, St. Louis, MO.)

distal tubules. In RTD there is uniform positive staining of all tubules (Fig. 26.61B). Similarly, lectin staining with *Arachis hypogaea* (peanut) lectin shows uniform apical staining of tubular cells, a characteristic of distal tubules and collecting ducts. Electron microscopy may demonstrate occasional tubular segments with brush borders. Earlier studies noted increased renin staining in preglomerular arterioles and suggested that vasoconstriction and decreased glomerular perfusion leading to cortical ischemia could be a factor responsible for defective tubular differentiation (311).

In the infants of mothers given ACE inhibitors, some degree of glomerular and tubular dilatation may be seen, but the condition is not necessarily fatal. The variability of the drug-related lesions, with recovery in some patients, suggests a possible dose-related effect (314).

## REFERENCES

1. Potter E. Normal and Abnormal Development of the Kidney. Chicago: Year Book Medical Publishers, 1972:124.
2. Bernstein J. A classification of renal cysts. In: Gardner KD, Bernstein J, eds. The Cystic Kidney. Dordrecht, The Netherlands: Kluwer Academic, 1990:149.
3. Wilson PD, Falkenstein D. The pathology of human renal cystic disease. Curr Top Pathol 1995;88:1.
4. Bingham C, Bulman MP, Ellard S, et al. Mutations in the hepatocyte nuclear factor-1beta gene are associated with familial hypoplastic glomerulocystic kidney disease. Am J Hum Genet 2001;68:219.
5. Rizzoni G, Loirat C, Levy M, et al. Familial hypoplastic glomerulocystic kidney. A new entity? Clin Nephrol 1982;18:263.
6. Gusmano R, Caridi G, Marini M, et al. Glomerulocystic kidney disease in a family. Nephrol Dial Transplant 2002;17:813.
7. Hildebrandt F, Waldherr R, Kutt R, Brandis M. The nephronophthisis complex: Clinical and genetic aspects. Clin Invest 1992;70:802.
8. Ginalski JM, Schnyder P, Portmann L, Jaeger P. Medullary sponge kidney on axial computed tomography: Comparison with excretory urography. Eur J Radiol 1991;12:104.
9. Truong LD, Choi YJ, Shen SS, et al. Renal cystic neoplasms and renal neoplasms associated with cystic renal diseases: Pathogenetic and molecular links. Adv Anat Pathol 2003;10:135.
10. Davila RM, Kissane JM, Crouch EC. Multilocular renal cyst. Immunohistochemical and lectin-binding study. Am J Surg Pathol 1992;16:508.
11. Sodhi KS, Suri S, Samujh R, et al. Case report: Bilateral multilocular cystic nephromas: A rare occurrence. Br J Radiol 2005;78:450.
12. Gabow PA. Autosomal dominant polycystic kidney disease. N Engl J Med 1993;29;329:332.
13. Johnson AM, Gabow PA. Identification of patients with autosomal dominant polycystic kidney disease at highest risk for end-stage renal disease. J Am Soc Nephrol 1997;8:1560.
14. Ong AC, Harris PC. Molecular pathogenesis of ADPKD: The polycystin complex gets complex. Kidney Int 2005;67:1234.
15. Chatha RK, Johnson AM, Rothberg PG, et al. Von Hippel-Lindau disease masquerading as autosomal dominant polycystic kidney disease. Am J Kidney Dis 2001;37:852.
16. Fain PR, McFann KK, Taylor MR, et al. Modifier genes play a significant role in the phenotypic expression of PKD1. Kidney Int 2005;67:1256.
17. Hateboer N, v Dijk MA, Bogdanova N, et al. Comparison of phenotypes of polycystic kidney disease types 1 and 2. European PKD1-PKD2 Study Group. Lancet 1999;353:103.
18. Koptides M, Constantinides R, Kyriakides G, et al. Loss of heterozygosity in polycystic kidney disease with a missense mutation in the repeated region of PKD1. Hum Genet 1998;103:709.
19. Calvet JP, Grantham JJ. The genetics and physiology of polycystic kidney disease. Semin Nephrol 2001;21:107.
20. Magistroni R, He N, Wang K, et al. Genotype-renal function correlation in type 2 autosomal dominant polycystic kidney disease. J Am Soc Nephrol 2003;14:1164.
21. Tee JB, Acott PD, McLellan DH, Crocker JF. Phenotypic heterogeneity in pediatric autosomal dominant polycystic kidney disease at first presentation: A single-center, 20-year review. Am J Kidney Dis 2004;43:296.
22. Qian F, Watnick TJ, Onuchic LF, Germino GG. The molecular basis of focal cyst formation in human autosomal dominant polycystic kidney disease type I. Cell 1996;13;87:979.
23. Ong AC, Wheatley DN. Polycystic kidney disease–the ciliary connection. Lancet 2003;361:774.
24. Verlinsky Y, Rechitsky S, Verlinsky O, et al. Preimplantation genetic diagnosis for polycystic kidney disease. Fertil Steril 2004;82:926.
25. Nicolau C, Torra R, Badenas C, et al. Autosomal dominant polycystic kidney disease types 1 and 2: Assessment of US sensitivity for diagnosis. Radiology 1999;213:273.

26. Chapman AB, Guay-Woodford LM, Grantham JJ, et al. Renal structure in early autosomal-dominant polycystic kidney disease (ADPKD): The Consortium for Radiologic Imaging Studies of Polycystic Kidney Disease (CRISP) cohort. Kidney Int 2003;64:1035.

27. Gabow PA, Kimberling WJ, Strain JD, et al. Utility of ultrasonography in the diagnosis of autosomal dominant polycystic kidney disease in children. J Am Soc Nephrol 1997;8:105.

28. Avni FE, Guissard G, Hall M, et al. Hereditary polycystic kidney diseases in children: Changing sonographic patterns through childhood. Pediatr Radiol 2002;32:169.

29. Faraggiana T, Bernstein J, Strauss L, Churg J. Use of lectins in the study of histogenesis of renal cysts. Lab Invest 1985;53:575.

30. Peters DJ, Spruit L, Klingel R, et al. Adult, fetal, and polycystic kidney expression of polycystin, the polycystic kidney disease-1 gene product. Lab Invest 1006;75:221.

31. Bernstein J, Evan AP, Gardner KD Jr. Epithelial hyperplasia in human polycystic kidney diseases. Its role in pathogenesis and risk of neoplasia. Am J Pathol 1987;129:92.

32. Cuppage FE, Huseman RA, Chapman A, Grantham JJ. Ultrastructure and function of cysts from human adult polycystic kidneys. Kidney Int 1980;17:372.

33. Nadasdy T, Laszik Z, Lajoie G, et al. Proliferative activity of cyst epithelium in human renal cystic diseases. J Am Soc Nephrol 1995;5:1462.

34. Barisoni L, Trudel M, Chretien N, et al. Analysis of the role of membrane polarity in polycystic kidney disease of transgenic SBM mice. Am J Pathol 1995;147:1728.

35. Grantham JJ, Geiser JL, Evan AP. Cyst formation and growth in autosomal dominant polycystic kidney disease. Kidney Int 1987;31:1145.

36. Grantham JJ. Mechanisms of progression in autosomal dominant polycystic kidney disease. Kidney Int 1997;63(suppl): S93.

37. Guay-Woodford LM, Galliani CA, Musulman-Mroczek E, et al. Diffuse renal cystic disease in children: Morphologic and genetic correlations. Pediatr Nephrol 1998;12:173.

38. Kissane JM, Dehner LP. Renal tumors and tumor-like lesions in pediatric patients. Pediatr Nephrol 1992;6:365.

39. Martignoni G, Bonetti F, Pea M, et al. Renal disease in adults with TSC2/PKD1 contiguous gene syndrome. Am J Surg Pathol 2002;26:198.

40. Rottenberg GT, Gordon I, De Bruyn R. The natural history of the multicystic dysplastic kidney in children. Br J Radiol 1997;70:347.

41. Neufeld TK, Douglass D, Grant M, et al. In vitro formation and expansion of cysts derived from human renal cortex epithelial cells. Kidney Int 1992;41:1222.

42. Winyard PJ, Nauta J, Lirenman DS, et al. Deregulation of cell survival in cystic and dysplastic renal development. Kidney Int 1996;49:135.

43. Wilson PD, Burrow CR. Cystic diseases of the kidney: Role of adhesion molecules in normal and abnormal tubulogenesis. Exp Nephrol 1999;7:114.

44. Wilson PD. Polycystic kidney disease: New understanding in the pathogenesis. Int J Biochem Cell Biol 2004;36:1868.

45. Lubarsky B, Krasnow MA. Tube morphogenesis: Making and shaping biological tubes. Cell 2003;10;112:19.

46. Nadasdy T, Laszik Z, Blick KE, et al. Proliferative activity of intrinsic cell populations in the normal human kidney. J Am Soc Nephrol 1994;4:2032.

47. Harrington EA, Bennett MR, Fanidi A, Evan GI. c-Myc-induced apoptosis in fibroblasts is inhibited by specific cytokines. Embo J 1994;13:3286.

48. Lanoix J, D'Agati V, Szabolcs M, Trudel M. Dysregulation of cellular proliferation and apoptosis mediates human autosomal dominant polycystic kidney disease (ADPKD). Oncogene 1996;13:1153.

49. Woo D. Apoptosis and loss of renal tissue in polycystic kidney diseases. N Engl J Med 1995;6;333:18.

50. Veis DJ, Sorenson CM, Shutter JR, Korsmeyer SJ. Bcl-2-deficient mice demonstrate fulminant lymphoid apoptosis, polycystic kidneys, and hypopigmented hair. Cell 1993;22;75:229.

51. Richards WG, Sweeney WE, Yoder BK, et al. Epidermal growth factor receptor activity mediates renal cyst formation in polycystic kidney disease. J Clin Invest. 1998;101:935.

52. Wilson PD. A plethora of epidermal growth factor-like proteins in polycystic kidneys. Kidney Int 2004;65:2441.

53. MacRae Dell K, Nemo R, Sweeney WE Jr, Avner ED. EGF-related growth factors in the pathogenesis of murine ARPKD. Kidney Int 2004;65:2018.

54. Ma R, Li WP, Rundle D, et al. PKD2 functions as an epidermal growth factor-activated plasma membrane channel. Mol Cell Biol 2005;25:8285.

55. Hillman KA, Woolf AS, Johnson TM, et al. The P2X7 ATP receptor modulates renal cyst development in vitro. Biochem Biophys Res Commun 2004;17;322:434.

56. Romio L, Fry AM, Winyard PJ, et al. OFD1 is a centrosomal/basal body protein expressed during mesenchymal-epithelial transition in human nephrogenesis. J Am Soc Nephrol 2004;15:2556.

57. Snell WJ, Pan J, Wang Q. Cilia and flagella revealed: from flagellar assembly in *Chlamydomonas* to human obesity disorders. Cell 2004;11;117:693.

58. Murcia NS, Richards WG, Yoder BK, et al. The Oak Ridge Polycystic Kidney (orpk) disease gene is required for left-right axis determination. Development 2000;127:2347.

59. Brown NE, Murcia NS. Delayed cystogenesis and increased ciliogenesis associated with the re-expression of polaris in Tg737 mutant mice. Kidney Int 2003;63:1220.

60. Nauli SM, Alenghat FJ, Luo Y, et al. Polycystins 1 and 2 mediate mechanosensation in the primary cilium of kidney cells. Nat Genet 2003;33:129.

61. Ward CJ, Turley H, Ong AC, et al. Polycystin, the polycystic kidney disease 1 protein, is expressed by epithelial cells in fetal, adult, and polycystic kidney. Proc Natl Acad Sci U S A 1996;93:1524.

62. Ong AC, Harris PC, Davies DR, et al. Polycystin-1 expression in PKD1, early-onset PKD1, and TSC2/PKD1 cystic tissue. Kidney Int 1999;56:1324.

63. Obermuller N, Morente N, Kranzlin B, et al. A possible role for metalloproteinases in renal cyst development. Am J Physiol Renal Physiol 2001;280:F540.

64. Surendran K, Simon TC, Liapis H, McGuire JK. Matrilysin (MMP-7) expression in renal tubular damage: Association with Wnt4. Kidney Int 2004;65:2212.

65. Shannon MB, Miner JH. Insertional mutation in laminin α5: A new mouse model for polycystic kidney disease. J Am Soc Nephrol 2004;15:652A

66. Guay-Woodford LM, Desmond RA. Autosomal recessive polycystic kidney disease: The clinical experience in North America. Pediatrics 2003;111(Pt 1):1072.

67. Roy S, Dillon MJ, Trompeter RS, Barratt TM. Autosomal recessive polycystic kidney disease: Long-term outcome of neonatal survivors. Pediatr Nephrol 1997;11:302.

68. Harris PC, Rossetti S. Molecular genetics of autosomal recessive polycystic kidney disease. Mol Genet Metab 2004;81:75.

69. Bergmann C, Senderek J, Schneider F, et al. PKHD1 mutations in families requesting prenatal diagnosis for autosomal recessive polycystic kidney disease (ARPKD). Hum Mutat 2004;23:487.

70. Fonck C, Chauveau D, Gagnadoux MF, et al. Autosomal recessive polycystic kidney disease in adulthood. Nephrol Dial Transplant 2001;16:1648.

71. Parfrey PS. Autosomal-recessive polycystic kidney disease. Kidney Int 2005;67:1638.

72. Blankenberg TA, Ruebner BH, Ellis WG, et al. Pathology of renal and hepatic anomalies in Meckel syndrome. Am J Med Genet 1987;3(suppl):395.

73. Holthofer H, Kumpulainen T, Rapola J. Polycystic disease of the kidney. Evaluation and classification based on nephron segment and cell-type specific markers. Lab Invest 1990;62:363.

74. Everson GT, Taylor MR, Doctor RB. Polycystic disease of the liver. Hepatology.2004;40:774.

75. Levy AD, Rohrmann CA Jr. Biliary cystic disease. Curr Probl Diagn Radiol 2003;32:233.

76. Desmet VJ. Ludwig symposium on biliary disorders–part I. Pathogenesis of ductal plate abnormalities. Mayo Clin Proc 1998;73:80.

77. Qian Q, Li A, King BF, et al. Clinical profile of autosomal dominant polycystic liver disease. Hepatology 2003;37:164.

78. Bernstein J. Hepatic involvement in hereditary renal syndromes. Birth Defects Orig Artic Ser 1987;23:115.

79. Landing BH, Wells TR, Lipsey AI, Oyemade OA. Morphometric studies of cystic and tubulointerstitial kidney diseases with hepatic fibrosis in children. Pediatr Pathol 1990;10:959.

80. Lipschitz B, Berdon WE, Defelice AR, Levy J. Association of congenital hepatic fibrosis with autosomal dominant polycystic kidney disease. Report of a family with review of literature. Pediatr Radiol 1993;23:131.

81. Ward CJ, Yuan D, Masyuk TV, et al. Cellular and subcellular localization of the ARPKD protein; fibrocystin is expressed on primary cilia. Hum Mol Genet 2003;15;12:2703.

82. Fick-Brosnahan GM, Tran ZV, Johnson AM, et al. Progression of autosomal-dominant polycystic kidney disease in children. Kidney Int 2001;59:1654.

83. Torres VE. Therapies to slow polycystic kidney disease. Nephron Exp Nephrol 2004;98:e1.

84. Sweeney WE, Chen Y, Nakanishi K, et al. Treatment of polycystic kidney disease with a novel tyrosine kinase inhibitor. Kidney Int 2000;57:33.

85. Bernstein J. Glomerulocystic kidney disease–nosological considerations. Pediatr Nephrol 1993;7:464.

86. Scolari F, Caridi G, Rampoldi L, et al. Uromodulin storage diseases: Clinical aspects and mechanisms. Am J Kidney Dis 2004;44:987.

87. Rampoldi L, Caridi G, Santon D, et al. Allelism of MCKD, FJHN and GCKD caused by impairment of uromodulin export dynamics. Hum Mol Genet 2003;15;12:3369.

88. Resnick JS, Sisson S, Vernier RL. Tamm-Horsfall protein. Abnormal localization in renal disease. Lab Invest 1978;38:550.

89. Woolf AS, Feather SA, Bingham C. Recent insights into kidney diseases associated with glomerular cysts. Pediatr Nephrol 2002;17:229.

90. Ferrante MI, Giorgio G, Feather SA, et al. Identification of the gene for oral-facial-digital type I syndrome. Am J Hum Genet 2001;68:569.

91. Pierides AM, Athanasiou Y, Demetriou K, et al. A family with the branchio-oto-renal syndrome: clinical and genetic correlations. Nephrol Dial Transplant 2002;17:1014.

92. Liapis H, Yu H, Steinhardt GF. Cell proliferation, apoptosis, Bcl-2 and Bax expression in obstructed opossum early metanephroi. J Urol 2000;164:511.

93. Emma F, Muda AO, Rinaldi S, et al. Acquired glomerulocystic kidney disease following hemolytic uremic syndrome. Pediatr Nephrol 2001;16:557.

94. Hildebrandt F, Omram H. New insights: Nephronophthisis-medullary cystic kidney disease. Pediatr Nephrol 2001;16:168.

95. Saunier S, Salomon R, Antignac C. Nephronophthisis. Curr Opin Genet Dev 2005;15:324.

96. Hildebrandt F, Otto E. Molecular genetics of nephronophthisis and medullary cystic kidney disease. J Am Soc Nephrol 2000;11:1753.

97. Hildebrandt F, Rensing C, Betz R, et al. Establishing an algorithm for molecular genetic diagnostics in 127 families with juvenile nephronophthisis. Kidney Int 2001;59:434.

98. Hoefele J, Sudbrak R, Reinhardt R, et al. Mutational analysis of the NPHP4 gene in 250 patients with nephronophthisis. Hum Mutat 2005;25:411.

99. Otto EA, Loeys B, Khanna H, et al. Nephrocystin-5, a ciliary IQ domain protein, is mutated in Senior-Loken syndrome and interacts with RPGR and calmodulin. Nat Genet 2005;37:282.

100. Blowey DL, Querfeld U, Geary D, et al. Ultrasound findings in juvenile nephronophthisis. Pediatr Nephrol 1996;10:22.

101. Chuang YF, Tsai TC. Sonographic findings in familial juvenile nephronophthisis-medullary cystic disease complex. J Clin Ultrasound 1998;26:203.

102. Phillips CL, Miller KJ, Filson AJ, et al. Renal cysts of inv/inv mice resemble early infantile nephronophthisis. J Am Soc Nephrol 2004;15:1744.

103. Senior B, Friedmann AI, Braudo JL. Juvenile familial nephropathy with tapetoretinal degeneration. A new oculorenal dystrophy. Am J Ophthalmol 1061;52:625.

104. Loken AC, Hanssen O, Halvorsen S, Jolster NJ. Hereditary renal dysplasia and blindness. Acta Paediatr 1961;50:177.

105. Betz R, Rensing C, Otto E, et al. Children with ocular motor apraxia type Cogan carry deletions in the gene (NPHP1) for juvenile nephronophthisis. J Pediatr 2000;136:828.

106. Haider NB, Carmi R, Shalev H, et al. A Bedouin kindred with infantile nephronophthisis demonstrates linkage to chromosome 9 by homozygosity mapping. Am J Hum Genet 1998;63:1404.

107. Otto EA, Schermer B, Obara T, et al. Mutations in INVS encoding inversin cause nephronophthisis type 2, linking renal cystic disease to the function of primary cilia and left-right axis determination. Nat Genet 2003;34:413.

108. Stavrou C, Koptides M, Tombazos C, et al. Autosomal-dominant medullary cystic kidney disease type 1: Clinical and molecular findings in six large Cypriot families. Kidney Int 2002;62:1385.

109. Kiser RL, Wolf MT, Martin JL, et al. Medullary cystic kidney disease type 1 in a large Native-American kindred. Am J Kidney Dis 2004;44:611.

110. Christodoulou K, Tsingis M, Stavrou C, et al. Chromosome 1 localization of a gene for autosomal dominant medullary cystic kidney disease. Hum Mol Genet 1998;7:905.

111. Scolari F, Puzzer D, Amoroso A, et al. Identification of a new locus for medullary cystic disease, on chromosome 16p12. Am J Hum Genet 1999;64:1655.

112. Hateboer N, Gumbs C, Teare MD, et al. Confirmation of a gene locus for medullary cystic kidney disease (MCKD2) on chromosome 16p12. Kidney Int 2001;60:1233.

113. Kroiss S, Huck K, Berthold S, et al. Evidence of further genetic heterogeneity in autosomal dominant medullary cystic kidney disease. Nephrol Dial Transplant 2000;15:818.

114. Dahan K, Fuchshuber A, Adamis S, et al. Familial juvenile hyperuricemic nephropathy and autosomal dominant medullary cystic kidney disease type 2: Two facets of the same disease? J Am Soc Nephrol 2001;12:2348.

115. Dahan K, Devuyst O, Smaers M, et al. A cluster of mutations in the UMOD gene causes familial juvenile hyperuricemic nephropathy with abnormal expression of uromodulin. J Am Soc Nephrol 2003;14:2883.

116. Cohen AH, Hoyer JR. Nephronophthisis. A primary tubular basement membrane defect. Lab Invest 1986;55:564.

117. Zollinger HU, Mihatsch MJ, Edefonti A, et al. Nephronophthisis (medullary cystic disease of the kidney). A study using electron microscopy, immunofluorescence, and a review of the morphological findings. Helv Paediatr Acta 1980;35:509.

118. Rahilly MA, Fleming S. Abnormal integrin receptor expression in two cases of familial nephronophthisis. Histopathology 1995;26:345.

119. Pan J, Wang Q, Snell WJ. Cilium-generated signaling and cilia-related disorders. Lab Invest 2005;85:452.

120. Devuyst O, Dahan K, Pirson Y. Tamm-Horsfall protein or uromodulin: New ideas about an old molecule. Nephrol Dial Transplant 2005;20:1290.

121. Cameron JS, Moro F, Simmonds HA. Gout, uric acid and purine metabolism in paediatric nephrology. Pediatr Nephrol 1993;7:105.

122. Cameron JS, Simmonds HA. Hereditary hyperuricemia and renal disease. Semin Nephrol 2005;25:9.

123. EL-Merhi FM, Bae KT. Cystic renal disease. Magn Reson Imaging Clin N Am 2004;12:449.

124. Rommel D, Pirson Y. Medullary sponge kidney–part of a congenital syndrome. Nephrol Dial Transplant 2001;16:634.

125. Proesmans W, Van Molhem S, Lateur L. A 16-year-old boy with medullary sponge kidneys, osteoporosis, and premature loss of all teeth. Pediatr Nephrol 2000;14:259 discussion, 263.

126. Gambaro G, Fabris A, Citron L, et al. An unusual association of contralateral congenital small kidney, reduced renal function and hyperparathyroidism in sponge kidney patients: On the track of the molecular basis. Nephrol Dial Transplant 2005;20:1042.

127. Diouf B, Ka EH, Calender A, et al. Association of medullary sponge kidney disease and multiple endocrine neoplasia type

IIA due to RET gene mutation: Iis there a causal relationship? Nephrol Dial Transplant 2000;15:2062.

128. Prencipe MA, Biancofiore F, Di Giorgio G, et al. Medullary sponge kidney (MSK) in association with glomerulonephritis (GNP) [in Italian]. G Ital Nefrol 2003;20:414.

129. Yagisawa T, Kobayashi C, Hayashi T, et al. Contributory metabolic factors in the development of nephrolithiasis in patients with medullary sponge kidney. Am J Kidney Dis 2001;37:1140.

130. Chauveau D, Duvic C, Chretien Y, et al. Renal involvement in von Hippel-Lindau disease. Kidney Int 1996;50:944.

131. Gallou C, Chauveau D, Richard S, et al. Genotype-phenotype correlation in von Hippel-Lindau families with renal lesions. Hum Mutat 2004;24:215.

132. Richard S, Lidereau R, Giraud S. The growing family of hereditary renal cell carcinoma. Nephrol Dial Transplant 2004;19:2954.

133. Stolle C, Glenn G, Zbar B, et al. Improved detection of germline mutations in the von Hippel-Lindau disease tumor suppressor gene. Hum Mutat 1998;12:417.

134. Pack SD, Zbar B, Pak E, et al. Constitutional von Hippel-Lindau (VHL) gene deletions detected in VHL families by fluorescence in situ hybridization. Cancer Res 1999;1;59:5560.

135. Browne G, Jefferson JA, Wright GD, et al. Von Hippel-Lindau disease: An important differential diagnosis of polycystic kidney disease. Nephrol Dial Transplant 1997;12:1132.

136. Linehan WM, Vasselli J, Srinivasan R et al. Genetic basis of cancer of the kidney: Disease-specific approaches to therapy. Clin Cancer Res 2004;15;10(Pt 2):6282S.

137. Nagashima Y, Inayama Y, Kato Y, et al. Pathological and molecular biological aspects of the renal epithelial neoplasms, up-to-date. Pathol Int 2004;54:377.

138. Woodward ER. Familial non-syndromic clear cell renal cell carcinoma. Curr Mol Med 2004;4:843.

139. Kaelin WG Jr. Molecular basis of the VHL hereditary cancer syndrome. Nat Rev Cancer 2002;2:673.

140. Maxwell PH, Wiesener MS, Chang GW, et al. The tumour suppressor protein VHL targets hypoxia-inducible factors for oxygen-dependent proteolysis. Nature 1999;20;399:271.

141. Maynard MA, Ohh M. Von Hippel-Lindau tumor suppressor protein and hypoxia-inducible factor in kidney cancer. Am J Nephrol 2004;24:1.

142. Mohr VH, Vortmeyer AO, Zhuang Z, et al. Histopathology and molecular genetics of multiple cysts and microcystic (serous) adenomas of the pancreas in von Hippel-Lindau patients. Am J Pathol 2000;157:1615.

143. Paraf F, Chauveau D, Chretien Y, et al. Renal lesions in von Hippel-Lindau disease: immunohistochemical expression of nephron differentiation molecules, adhesion molecules and apoptosis proteins. Histopathology 2000;36:457.

144. Sano T, Horiguchi H. Von Hippel-Lindau disease. Microsc Res Tech 2003;1;60:159.

145. Ewalt DH, Sheffield E, Sparagana SP, et al. Renal lesion growth in children with tuberous sclerosis complex. J Urol 1998;160:141.

146. Hancock E, Tomkins S, Sampson J, Osborne J. Lymphangioleiomyomatosis and tuberous sclerosis. Respir Med 2002;96:7.

147. Jones AC, Shyamsundar MM, Thomas MW, et al. Comprehensive mutation analysis of TSC1 and TSC2-and phenotypic correlations in 150 families with tuberous sclerosis. Am J Hum Genet 1999;64:1305.

148. van Slegtenhorst M, Nellist M, Nagelkerken B, et al. Interaction between hamartin and tuberin, the TSC1 and TSC2 gene products. Hum Mol Genet 1998;7:1053.

149. Casper KA, Donnelly LF, Chen B, Bissler JJ. Tuberous sclerosis complex: Renal imaging findings. Radiology 2002;225:451.

150. Cook JA, Oliver K, Mueller RF, Sampson J. A cross sectional study of renal involvement in tuberous sclerosis. J Med Genet 1996;33:480.

151. Duffy K, Al-Saleem T, Karbowniczek M, et al. Mutational analysis of the von Hippel Lindau gene in clear cell renal carcinomas from tuberous sclerosis complex patients. Mod Pathol 2002;15:205.

152. Parry L, Maynard JH, Patel A, et al. Analysis of the TSC1 and TSC2 genes in sporadic renal cell carcinomas. Br J Cancer 2001;85:1226.

153. Torra R, Badenas C, Darnell A, et al. Facilitated diagnosis of the contiguous gene syndrome: Tuberous sclerosis and polycystic kidneys by means of haplotype studies. Am J Kidney Dis 1998;31:1038.

154. Nagashima Y, Ohaki Y, Tanaka Y, et al. A case of renal angiomyolipomas associated with multiple and various hamartomatous microlesions. Virchows Arch A Pathol Anat Histopathol 1988;413:177.

155. Ito N, Rubin GM. gigas, a Drosophila homolog of tuberous sclerosis gene product-2, regulates the cell cycle. Cell 1999;96:529.

156. Potter CJ, Huang H, Xu T. Drosophila Tsc1 functions with Tsc2 to antagonize insulin signaling in regulating cell growth, cell proliferation, and organ size. Cell 2001;105:357.

157. Mak BC, Kenerson HL, Aicher LD, et al. Aberrant beta-catenin signaling in tuberous sclerosis. Am J Pathol 2005;167:107.

158. Castillo OA, Boyle ET Jr, Kramer SA. Multilocular cysts of kidney. A study of 29 patients and review of literature. Urology 1991;37:156.

159. Hwang DY, Ahn C, Lee JG, et al. Unilateral renal cystic disease in adults. Nephrol Dial Transplant 1999;14:1999.

160. Slywotzky CM, Bosniak MA. Localized cystic disease of the kidney. AJR Am J Roentgenol 2001;176:843.

161. Terada N, Ichioka K, Matsuta Y, et al. The natural history of simple renal cysts. J Urol 2002;167:21.

162. Baert L, Steg A. Is the diverticulum of the distal and collecting tubules a preliminary stage of the simple cyst in the adult? J Urol 1977;118:707.

163. Choyke PL. Acquired cystic kidney disease. Eur Radiol 2000;10:1716.

164. Neureiter D, Frank H, Kunzendorf U, et al. Dialysis-associated acquired cystic kidney disease imitating autosomal dominant polycystic kidney disease in a patient receiving long-term peritoneal dialysis. Nephrol Dial Transplant 2002;17:500.

165. Mattoo TK, Greifer I, Geva P, Spitzer A. Acquired renal cystic disease in children and young adults on maintenance dialysis. Pediatr Nephrol 2997;11:447.

166. Ishikawa I, Saito Y, Asaka M, et al. Twenty-year follow-up of acquired renal cystic disease. Clin Nephrol 2003;59:153.

167. Ishikawa I. Present status of renal cell carcinoma in dialysis patients in Japan: Questionnaire study in 2002. Nephron Clin Pract 2004;97:c11.

168. Sule N, Yakupoglu U, Shen SS, et al. Calcium oxalate deposition in renal cell carcinoma associated with acquired cystic kidney disease: A comprehensive study. Am J Surg Pathol 2005;29:443.

169. Casale P, Grady RW, Feng WC, et al. The pediatric calyceal diverticulum: Diagnosis and laparoscopic management. J Endourol 2004;18:668.

170. Wulfsohn MA. Pyelocaliceal diverticula. J Urol 1980;123:1.

171. Mosli H, MacDonald P, Schillinger J. Calyceal diverticula developing into simple renal cyst. J Urol 1986;136:658.

172. DeMarco RT, Cain MP, Davis MM. Xanthogranulomatous pyelonephritis associated with a congenital calyceal diverticulum. Urology 2001;57:168.

173. Mullins JR, Shield CF 3rd, Porter MG. Hygroma renalis: Two cases within a family and a literature review. Surgery 1992;111:339.

174. Ichikawa I, Kuwayama F, Pope JC 4th, et al. Paradigm shift from classic anatomic theories to contemporary cell biological views of CAKUT. Kidney Int 2002;61:889.

175. Woolf AS, Winyard PJ. Molecular mechanisms of human embryogenesis: Developmental pathogenesis of renal tract malformations. Pediatr Dev Pathol 2002;5:108.

176. Coles HS, Burne JF, Raff MC. Large-scale normal cell death in the developing rat kidney and its reduction by epidermal growth factor. Development 1993;118:777.

177. Miyazaki Y, Oshima K, Fogo A, Ichikawa I. Evidence that bone morphogenetic protein 4 has multiple biological functions during kidney and urinary tract development. Kidney Int 2003;63:835.

178. Nishimura H, Yerkes E, Hohenfellner K, et al. Role of the angiotensin type 2 receptor gene in congenital anomalies of the

kidney and urinary tract, CAKUT, of mice and men. Mol Cell 1999;3:1.

179. Kolatsi-Joannou M, Bingham C, Ellard S, et al. Hepatocyte nuclear factor-1beta: A new kindred with renal cysts and diabetes and gene expression in normal human development. J Am Soc Nephrol 2001;12:2175.

180. Pritchard-Jones K, Hawkins MM. Biology of Wilms' tumour. Lancet 1997;349:663.

181. Kreidberg JA, Sariola H, Loring JM, et al. WT-1 is required for early kidney development. Cell 1993;74:679.

182. Little M, Wells C. A clinical overview of WT1 gene mutations. Hum Mutat 1997;9:209.

183. Klamt B, Koziell A, Poulat F, et al. Frasier syndrome is caused by defective alternative splicing of WT1 leading to an altered ratio of WT1 +/−KTS splice isoforms. Hum Mol Genet 1998;7:709.

184. Dressler GR, Deutsch U, Chowdhury K, et al. Pax2, a new murine paired-box-containing gene and its expression in the developing excretory system. Development 1990;109:787.

185. Dressler GR, Wilkinson JE, Rothenpieler UW, et al. Deregulation of Pax-2 expression in transgenic mice generates severe kidney abnormalities. Nature 1993;4;362:65.

186. Torres M, Gomez-Pardo E, Dressler GR, Gruss P. Pax-2 controls multiple steps of urogenital development. Development 1995;121:4057.

187. Sanyanusin P, Schimmenti LA, McNoe LA, et al. Mutation of the PAX2 gene in a family with optic nerve colobomas, renal anomalies and vesicoureteral reflux. Nat Genet 1995;9:358.

188. Eccles MR, He S, Legge M, et al. PAX genes in development and disease: The role of PAX2 in urogenital tract development. Int J Dev Biol 2002;46:535.

189. Abdelhak S, Kalatzis V, Heilig R, et al. Clustering of mutations responsible for brachio-oto-renal (BOR) syndrome in the eyes absent homologous region (eyaHR) of EYA1. Hum Mol Genet 1997;6:2247.

190. Xu PX, Adams J, Peters H, et al. Eya1-deficient mice lack ears and kidneys and show abnormal apoptosis of organ primordia. Nat Genet 1999;23:113.

191. Coffinier C, Barra J, Babinet C, Yaniv M. Expression of the vHNF1/HNF1beta homeoprotein gene during mouse organogenesis. Mech Dev 1999;89:211.

192. Jain S, Naughton CK, Yang M, et al. Mice expressing a dominant-negative Ret mutation phenocopy human Hirschsprung disease and delineate a direct role of Ret in spermatogenesis. Development 2004;131:5503.

193. Schuchardt A, D'Agati V, Larsson-Blomberg L, et al. Defects in the kidney and enteric nervous system of mice lacking the tyrosine kinase receptor Ret. Nature 1994;367:380.

194. Pichel JG, Shen L, Sheng HZ, et al. GDNF is required for kidney development and enteric innervation. Cold Spring Harb Symp Quant Biol 1996;61:445.

195. Vainio SJ. Nephrogenesis regulated by Wnt signaling. J Nephrol 2003;16:279.

196. Yang SP, Woolf AS, Yuan HT, et al. Potential biological role of transforming growth factor-beta1 in human congenital kidney malformations. Am J Pathol 2000;157:1633.

197. Hu MC, Piscione TD, Rosenblum ND. Elevated SMAD1/beta-catenin molecular complexes and renal medullary cystic dysplasia in ALK3 transgenic mice. Development 2003;130:2753.

198. Knudson CM, Korsmeyer SJ. Bcl-2 and Bax function independently to regulate cell death. Nat Genet 1997;16:358.

199. LeBrun DP, Warnke RA, Cleary ML. Expression of bcl-2 in fetal tissues suggests a role in morphogenesis. Am J Pathol 1993;142:743.

200. Sorenson CM, Rogers SA, Korsmeyer SJ, Hammerman MR. Fulminant metanephric apoptosis and abnormal kidney development in bcl-2-deficient mice. Am J Physiol 1995;268(Pt 2):F73.

201. Sorenson CM, Padanilam BJ, Hammerman MR. Abnormal postpartum renal development and cystogenesis in the bcl-2 (−/−) mouse. Am J Physiol 1996;271(Pt 2):F184.

202. Bouillet P, Cory S, Zhang LC, et al. Degenerative disorders caused by Bcl-2 deficiency prevented by loss of its BH3-only antagonist Bim. Dev Cell 2001;1:645.

203. Zhang P, Liegeois NJ, Wong C, et al. Altered cell differentiation and proliferation in mice lacking p57KIP2 indicates a role in Beckwith-Wiedemann syndrome. Nature 1997;387:151.

204. Goldman M, Smith A, Shuman C, et al. Renal abnormalities in Beckwith-Wiedemann syndrome are associated with 11p15.5 uniparental disomy. J Am Soc Nephrol 2002;13:2077.

205. Kanwar YS, Wada J, Lin S, et al. Update of extracellular matrix, its receptors, and cell adhesion molecules in mammalian nephrogenesis. Am J Physiol Renal Physiol 2004;286:F202.

206. Bellairs R, Lear P, Yamada KM, et al. Posterior extension of the chick nephric (Wolffian) duct: The role of fibronectin and NCAM polysialic acid. Dev Dyn 1995;202:333.

207. Klein G, Langegger M, Goridis C, Ekblom P. Neural cell adhesion molecules during embryonic induction and development of the kidney. Development 1998;102:749.

208. Vestweber D, Kemler R. Identification of a putative cell adhesion domain of uvomorulin. Embo J 1985;4:3393.

209. Muller U, Wang D, Denda S, et al. Integrin alpha8beta1 is critically important for epithelial-mesenchymal interactions during kidney morphogenesis. Cell 1997;88:603.

210. Bullock SL, Fletcher JM, Beddington RS, Wilson VA. Renal agenesis in mice homozygous for a gene trap mutation in the gene encoding heparan sulfate 2-sulfotransferase. Genes Dev 1998;12:1894.

211. Hu Y, Tanriverdi F, MacColl GS, Bouloux PM. Kallmann's syndrome: Molecular pathogenesis. Int J Biochem Cell Biol 2003;35:1157.

212. Kirk JM, Grant DB, Besser GM, et al. Unilateral renal aplasia in X-linked Kallmann's syndrome. Clin Genet 2004;46:260.

213. Deeb A, Robertson A, MacColl G, et al. Multicystic dysplastic kidney and Kallmann's syndrome: A new association? Nephrol Dial Transplant 2001;16:1170.

214. Duke VM, Winyard PJ, Thorogood P, et al. KAL, a gene mutated in Kallmann's syndrome, is expressed in the first trimester of human development. Mol Cell Endocrinol 1995;110:73.

215. Gonzalez-Martinez D, Kim SH, Hu Y, et al. Anosmin-1 modulates fibroblast growth factor receptor 1 signaling in human gonadotropin-releasing hormone olfactory neuroblasts through a heparan sulfate-dependent mechanism. J Neurosci 2004;24:10384.

216. Hardelin JP, Julliard AK, Moniot B, et al. Anosmin-1 is a regionally restricted component of basement membranes and interstitial matrices during organogenesis: Implications for the developmental anomalies of X chromosome-linked Kallmann syndrome. Dev Dyn 1999;215:26.

217. Dode C, Levilliers J, Dupont JM, et al. Loss-of-function mutations in FGFR1 cause autosomal dominant Kallmann syndrome. Nat Genet 2003;33:463.

218. Cano-Gauci DF, Song HH, Yang H, et al. Glypican-3-deficient mice exhibit developmental overgrowth and some of the abnormalities typical of Simpson-Golabi-Behmel syndrome. J Cell Biol 1999;146:255.

219. Grisaru S, Cano-Gauci D, Tee J, et al. Glypican-3 modulates BMP- and FGF-mediated effects during renal branching morphogenesis. Dev Biol 2001;231:31.

220. McGregor L, Makela V, Darling SM, et al. Fraser syndrome and mouse blebbed phenotype caused by mutations in FRAS1/Fras1 encoding a putative extracellular matrix protein. Nat Genet 2003;34:203.

221. Jadeja S, Smyth I, Pitera JE, et al. Identification of a new gene mutated in Fraser syndrome and mouse myelencephalic blebs. Nat Genet 2005;37:520.

222. Lewis M. Report of the Paediatric Renal Registry 1999. In: UK Renal Registry. The Second Annual Report. Aansell D, et al, eds. city: publisher, year:175.

223. Woolf AS, Thiruchelvam N. Congenital obstructive uropathy: Its origin and contribution to end stage renal disease in children. Adv Ren Replac Ther 2001;8:157.

224. Woolf AS, Price KL, Scambler PJ, Winyard PJ. Evolving concepts in human renal dysplasia. J Am Soc Nephrol 2004;15:998

225. Beck AD. The effect of intra-uterine urinary obstruction upon the development of the fetal kidney. J Urol 1971;105:784.

226. Attar R, Quinn F, Winyard PJ, et al. Short-term urinary flow impairment deregulates PAX2 and PCNA expression and cell survival in fetal sheep kidneys. Am J Pathol 1998;152:1225.

227. Peters CA, Carr MC, Lais A, et al. The response of the fetal kidney to obstruction. J Urol 1992;148(Pt 2):503.

228. Yang SP, Woolf AS, Quinn F, Winyard PJ. Deregulation of renal transforming growth factor-beta1 after experimental short-term ureteric obstruction in fetal sheep. Am J Pathol 2001;159:109.

229. Yang SP, Woolf AS, Yuan HT, et al. Potential biological role of transforming growth factor-beta1 in human congenital kidney malformations. Am J Pathol 2000;157:1633.

230. Steinhardt GF, Liapis H, Phillips B, et al. Insulin-like growth factor improves renal architecture of fetal kidneys with complete ureteral obstruction. J Urol 1995;154(Pt 2):690.

231. Chevalier RL, Goyal S, Wolstenholme JT, Thornhill BA. Obstructive nephropathy in the neonatal rat is attenuated by epidermal growth factor. Kidney Int 1998;54:38.

232. Glick PL, Harrison MR, Adzick NS, et al. Correction of congenital hydronephrosis in utero IV: In utero decompression prevents renal dysplasia. J Pediatr Surg 1984;19:649.

233. Chevalier RL, Thornhill BA, Chang AY, et al. Recovery from release of ureteral obstruction in the rat: relationship to nephrogenesis. Kidney Int. 2002;61:2033.

234. Holmes N, Harrison MR, Baskin LS. Fetal surgery for posterior urethral valves: Long-term postnatal outcomes. Pediatrics 2001;108:E7.

235. Chevalier RL. Perinatal obstructive nephropathy. Semin Perinatol 2004;28:124.

236. Solhaug MJ, Bolger PM, Jose PA. The developing kidney and environmental toxins. Pediatrics 2004;113(suppl):1084.

237. Barr M Jr, Cohen MM Jr. ACE inhibitor fetopathy and hypocalvaria: The kidney-skull connection. Teratology 1991;44:485.

238. Gomez RA, Lynch KR, Chevalier RL, et al. Renin and angiotensinogen gene expression in maturing rat kidney. Am J Physiol 1988;254(Pt 2):F582.

239. Sequeira Lopez ML, Gomez RA. The role of angiotensin II in kidney embryogenesis and kidney abnormalities. Curr Opin Nephrol Hypertens 2004;13:117.

240. Rigoli L, Chimenz R, di Bella C, et al. Angiotensin-converting enzyme and angiotensin type 2 receptor gene genotype distributions in Italian children with congenital uropathies. Pediatr Res 2004;56:988.

241. Hiraoka M, Taniguchi T, Nakai H, et al. No evidence for AT2R gene derangement in human urinary tract anomalies. Kidney Int 2001;59:1244, 2001.

242. Chugh SS, Wallner EI, Kanwar YS. Renal development in high-glucose ambience and diabetic embryopathy. Semin Nephrol 2003;23:583.

243. Abrass CK, Spicer D, Berfield AK, et al. Diabetes induces changes in glomerular development and laminin-beta 2 (s-laminin) expression. Am J Pathol 1997;151:1131.

244. Duong Van Huyen, J P, Amri, K, Belair, MF, et al. Spatiotemporal distribution of insulin like growth factor receptors during nephrogenesis in fetuses from normal and diabetic rats. Cell Tissue Res 2003;314:367.

245. Rothman KJ, Moore LL, Singer MR, et al. Teratogenicity of high vitamin A intake. N Engl J Med 1995;333:1369.

246. Padmanabhan R. Retinoic acid-induced caudal regression syndrome in the mouse fetus. Reprod Toxicol 1998;12:139.

247. Vilar J, Lalou C, Duong VH, et al. Midkine is involved in kidney development and in its regulation by retinoids. J Am Soc Nephrol 2002;13:668.

248. Tse HK, Leung MB, Woolf AS, et al. Implication of Wt1 in the pathogenesis of nephrogenic failure in a mouse model of retinoic acid-induced caudal regression syndrome. Am J Pathol 2005;166:1295.

249. Batourina E, Choi C, Paragas N, et al. Distal ureter morphogenesis depends on epithelial cell remodeling mediated by vitamin A and Ret. Nat Genet 2002;32:109.

250. Barker DJ, Osmond C, Golding J, et al. Growth in utero, blood pressure in childhood and adult life, and mortality from cardiovascular disease. BJM 1989;298:564.

251. Barker DJ. The developmental origins of well-being. Philos Trans R Soc Lond B Biol Sci 2004;359:1359.

252. Brenner BM, Garcia DL, Anderson S. Glomeruli and blood pressure. Less of one, more the other? Am J Hypertens 1988;1(Pt 1):335.

253. Langley-Evans SC, Welham SJ, Jackson AA. Fetal exposure to a maternal low protein diet impairs nephrogenesis and promotes hypertension in the rat. Life Sci 1999;64:965.

254. Welham SJ, Wade A, Woolf AS. Protein restriction in pregnancy is associated with increased apoptosis of mesenchymal cells at the start of rat metanephrogenesis. Kidney Int 2002;61:1231.

255. Gilbert T, Merlet-Benichou C. Retinoids and nephron mass control. Pediatr Nephrol 2000;14:1137.

256. Lisle SJ, Lewis RM, Petry CJ, et al. Effect of maternal iron restriction during pregnancy on renal morphology in the adult rat offspring. Br J Nutr 2003;90:33.

257. Welham SJ, Riley PR, Wade A, et al. Maternal diet programs embryonic kidney gene expression. Physiol Genomics 2005;22:48.

258. Favorito LA, Cardinot TM, Morais AR, Sampaio FJ. Urogenital anomalies in human male fetuses. Early Hum Dev 2004;79:41.

259. Carbillon L, Seince N, Largilliere C, et al. First-trimester diagnosis of sirenomelia. A case report. Fetal Diagn Ther 2001;16:284.

260. Boyd T, Rosen S, Redline RW, Genest DR . Nondysplastic fetal renal hypoplasia associated with severe oligohydramnios: Clinical, pathologic, and morphometric findings. Pediatr Pathol Lab Med 1995;15:485.

261. Murphy JJ, Fraser GC, Blair GK. Sirenomelia: Case of the surviving mermaid. J Pediatr Surg 1992;27:1265.

262. Cascio S, Paran S, Puri P. Associated urological anomalies in children with unilateral renal agenesis. J Urol 1999;162:1081.

263. Hiraoka M, Tsukahara H, Ohshima Y, et al. Renal aplasia is the predominant cause of congenital solitary kidneys. Kidney Int 2002;61:1840.

264. Watanabe T. Membranous glomerulonephritis in a patient with unilateral renal agenesis. Nephron 2002;91:159.

265. Ghavamian R, Cheville JC, Lohse CM et al. Renal cell carcinoma in the solitary kidney: An analysis of complications and outcome after nephron sparing surgery. J Urol 2002;168:454.

266. Jeong GH, Park BS, Jeong TK, et al. Unilateral autosomal polycystic kidney disease with contralateral renal agenesis: A case report. J Korean Med Sci 2003;18:284.

267. Carter CO, Evans K, Pescia G. A family study of renal agenesis. J Med Genet 1979;16:176.

268. Roodhooft AM, Birnholz JC, Holmes LB. Familial nature of congenital absence and severe dysgenesis of both kidneys. N Engl J Med 1984;310:1341.

269. McPherson E, Carey J, Kramer A, et al. Dominantly inherited renal adysplasia, Am J Med Genet 1987;863.

270. Murugasu B, Cole BR, Hawkins EP, et al. Familial renal adysplasia, Am J Kidney Dis 1991;18:495.

271. Moerman P, Fryns JP, Sastrowijoto SH, et al. Hereditary renal adysplasia: New observations and hypotheses. Pediatr Pathol 1994;14:405.

272. Squiers EC, Morden RS, Bernstein J. Renal multicystic dysplasia: An occasional manifestation of the hereditary adysplasia syndrome. Am J Med Genet 1987;3(suppl):279.

273. Buchta RM, Viseskul C, Gilbert EF, et al. Familial bilateral renal agenesis and hereditary renal adysplasia. Z Kinderheilkd 1973;115:111.

274. Battin J, Lacombe D, Leng JJ. Familial occurrence of hereditary renal adysplasia with mullerian anomalies. Clin Genet 1993;43:23.

275. Suzuki K, Kurokawa S, Muraishi O, Tokue A. Segmental multicystic dysplastic kidney in an adult woman. Urol Int 2001;66:51.

276. Hsueh C, Hsueh W, Gonzalez-Crussi F. Bilateral renal dysplasia with features of nephroblastomatosis. Pediatr Pathol 1987;7:437.

277. Dimmick JE, Johnson HW, Coleman GU, Carter M. Wilms tumorlet, nodular renal blastema and multicystic renal dysplasia. J Urol 1989;142(Pt 2):484; discussion, 489..

278. Vlachos J, Tsakraklides V. A case of renal dysplasia and relation to "bilateral nephroblastomatosis. 489" J Pathol Bacteriol 1968;95:560.

279. Marsden HB, Lawler W. Wilm's tumour and renal dysplasia: An hypothesis. J Clin Pathol 1982;35:1069.

280. Belk RA, Thomas DF, Mueller RF, et al. A family study and the natural history of prenatally detected unilateral multicystic dysplastic kidney. J Urol 2002;167(Pt 1):666.

281. Blew B, Carpenter B, Leonard MP. Incidentally detected nephrogenic rests in the setting of congenital obstructive uropathy. Can J Urol 2002;9:1595.

282. Narchi H. Risk of Wilms' tumour with multicystic kidney disease: A systematic review. Arch Dis Child 2005;90:147.

283. Rackley RR, Angermeier KW, Levin H, et al. Renal cell carcinoma arising in a regressed multicystic dysplastic kidney. J Urol 1994;152(Pt 1):1543.

284. Pope JC, Brock JW III, Adams MC, et al. How they begin and how they end: Classic and new theories for the development and deterioration of congenital anomalies of the kidney and urinary tract, CAKUT. J Am Soc Nephrol 1999;10:2018.

285. Damen-Elias HA, Stoutenbeek PH, Visser GH, et al. Concomitant anomalies in 100 children with unilateral multicystic kidney. Ultrasound Obstet Gynecol 2005;25:384.

286. Shibata S, Nagata M. Pathogenesis of human renal dysplasia: An alternative scenario to the major theories. Pediatr Int 2003;45:605.

287. Liapis H. Biology of congenital obstructive nephropathy. Nephron Exp Nephrol 2003;93:e87.

288. Srivastava T, Garola RE, Hellerstein S. Autosomal dominant inheritance of multicystic dysplastic kidney. Pediatr Nephrol 1999;13:481.

289. Sekine T, Namai Y, Yanagisawa A, et al. A familial case of multicystic dysplastic kidney. Pediatr Nephrol 2005;20:1245.

290. Li Volti S, Faiella A, Perrotta S, et al. Non-allelic heterogeneity in familial unilateral renal adysplasia. Ann Genet 2002;45:123.

291. Fletcher J, Hu M, Berman Y, et al. Multicystic dysplastic kidney and variable phenotype in a family with a novel deletion mutation of PAX2. J Am Soc Nephrol 2005;16:2754.

292. Groenen PM, Vanderlinden G, Devriendt K, et al. Rearrangement of the human CDC5L gene a t(6;19)(p21;q13.1) in a patient with multicystic renal dysplasia. Genomics 1998;49:218.

293. Jenkins D, Bitner-Glindzicz M, Malcolm S, et al. De novo uroplakin IIIa heterozygous mutations cause human renal adysplasia leading to severe kidney failure. J Am Soc Nephrol 2005;16:2141.

294. Konda R, Sato H, Ito S, et al. Renin containing cells are present predominantly in scarred areas but not in dysplastic regions in multicystic dysplastic kidney. J Urol 2001;166:1910.

295. Narchi H. Risk of hypertension with multicystic kidney disease: A systematic review. Arch Dis Child 2005;90:921.

296. Liapis H, Doshi RH, Watson MA Reduced renin expression and altered gene transcript profiles in multicystic dysplastic kidneys. J Urol 2002;168:1816.

297. Eckoldt F, Woderich R, Wolke S, et al. Follow-up of unilateral multicystic kidney dysplasia after prenatal diagnosis. J Matern Fetal Neonatal Med 2003;14:177.

298. Ylinen E, Ahonen S, Ala-Houhala M, Wikstrom S. Nephrectomy for multicystic dysplastic kidney: If and when? Urology 2004;63:768.

299. Boissonnat T. What to call hypoplastic kidney? Arch Dis Child 1962;7:142.

300. Portsman W. Renal angiography in children. Prog Pediatr Radiology 1970;3:51.

301. Norton KI. New imaging applications in the evaluation of pediatric renal disease. Curr Opin Pediatr 2003;15:186.

302. Riedlinger WF, Kissane JM, Gibfried M, Liapis H. Congenital bilateral renal arteriovenous malformation: An unrecognized cause of renal failure. Pediatr Dev Pathol 2004;7:285.

303. Park SH, Chi JG. Oligomeganephronia associated with 4p deletion type chromosomal anomaly. Pediatr Pathol 1993;13:731.

304. Salomon R, Tellier AL, Attie-Bitach T, et al. PAX2 mutations in oligomeganephronia. Kidney Int 2001;59:457.

305. Drukker A. Oligonephropathy: From a rare childhood disorder to a possible health problem in the adult. Isr Med Assoc J 2002;4:191.

306. Rodriguez MM, Gomez A, Abitbol C, et al. Comparative renal histomorphometry: A case study of oligonephropathy of prematurity. Pediatr Nephrol 2005;20:945

307. Risdon RA, Young LW, Chrispin AR. Renal hypoplasia and dysplasia: A radiological and pathological correlation. Pediatr Radiol 1975;15;3:213.

308. Allanson JE, Pantzar JT, MacLeod PM. Possible new autosomal recessive syndrome with unusual renal histopathological changes. Am J Med Genet 1983;16:57.

309. Gribouval O, Gonzales M, Neuhaus T, et al. Mutations in genes in the renin-angiotensin system are associated with autosomal recessive renal tubular dysgenesis. Nat Genet 2005;37:964.

310. Voland JR, Hawkins EP, Wells TR, et al. Congenital hypernephronic nephromegaly with tubular dysgenesis: A distinctive inherited renal anomaly. Pediatr Pathol 1985;4:231.

311. Benstein J, Barajas L. Renal tubular dysgenesis: Evidence of abnormality in the renin-angiotensin system. J Am Soc Nephrol 1994;5:224.

312. Sequeira Lopez ML, Pentz ES, et al. Renin cells are precursors for multiple cell types that switch to the renin phenotype when homeostasis is threatened. Dev Cell 2004;6:719.

313. Restaino I, Kaplan BS, Kaplan P, et al. Renal dysgenesis in a monozygotic twin: Association with in utero exposure to indomethacin. Am J Med Genet 1991;39:252.

314. Cunniff C, Jones KL, Phillipson J et al. Oligohydramnios sequence and renal tubular malformation associated with maternal enalapril use. Am J Obstet Gynecol 1990;162:187.

315. Voyer LE, Drut R, Mendez JH. Fetal renal maldevelopment with oligohydramnios following maternal use of piroxicam. Pediatr Nephrol 1994;8:592.

316. Norton ME, Merrill J, Cooper BA, et al. Neonatal complications after the administration of indomethacin for preterm labor. N Engl J Med 1993;329:1602.

317. Bale PM, Kan AE, Dorney SF. Renal proximal tubular dysgenesis associated with severe neonatal hemosiderotic liver disease. Pediatr Pathol 1994;14:479.

# End-Stage Renal Disease  27

*Michael D. Hughson*

End-stage renal disease (ESRD) is the terminal phase of a chronic kidney disease (CKD) that has caused a progressive deterioration of kidney function. The Kidney Disease Outcomes Quality Initiative (K/DOQI) of the National Kidney Foundation recently proposed that CKD be defined as the presence for more than 3 months of kidney damage with or without a decreased glomerular filtration rate (GFR) of less than 60 mL/min/1.73 m$^2$ or of less than 60 mL/min/1.73 m$^2$ without evidence of kidney damage (1). Evidence of kidney damage includes radiologic abnormalities and abnormalities in urine or blood tests with proteinuria and albuminuria being the best studied of these markers. On the basis of this definition, 11% of the United States adult population has been estimated to have CKD (2). Chronically diseased kidneys have some capacity to adapt to the loss of functional tissue, and unless renal perfusion is decreased as a result of a physiologic challenge such as dehydration, most patients with CKD have sufficient renal function to eliminate metabolic wastes and maintain water and solute homeostasis. When GFR is less than 15 mL/min/1.73 m², patients are defined by the K/DOQI as being in chronic kidney failure, and it is estimated that 0.2% of the United States adult population may have this level of renal insufficiency (2). In most cases, patients in chronic kidney failure require renal replacement therapy, either dialysis or kidney transplantation, to sustain life. If the patients require sustained renal replacement therapy, they are administratively defined by the Medicare ESRD program as having ESRD and become eligible for Medicare benefits (1).

Long-term peritoneal and hemodialysis were technically possible by the late 1960s, and in 1972 funding for the treatment of ESRD was enacted as part of the Medicare program (3). This legislation made maintenance dialysis or transplantation financially available to virtually any renal failure patient who was a United States citizen. Early after the ESRD program was established, the prognosis for patients older than age 50 years with end-stage diabetic nephropathy was so poor that they tended to be excluded from maintenance dialysis. Today dialysis is largely a therapy of the elderly. Between 1997 and 2001, the median age of all ESRD patients in the United States was 64.2 years, 48% were older than 65 years of age, and 44% were diabetic (3). Although the elderly constitute the majority of ESRD patients, a substantial number begin dialysis or receive a renal transplant at a young age. The cumulative lifetime risk for developing ESRD in the United States for a 20-year-old has been estimated at 7.8% for black women, 7.3% for black men, 2.5% for white men, and 1.8% for white women (4). For a 20-year-old black man, the cumulative years of lost life because of ESRD is estimated to be greater than what he would lose for carcinoma of the colon or prostate. For a 20-year-old black woman, it approaches the numbers of years of lost life attributed to carcinoma of the breast (4).

There has been a steady increase in the number of patients being funded for the treatment of ESRD. During the year 1978, 14,474 patients began treatment, and the total ESRD population was 42,324. Between 1984 and 1991, the number of ESRD patients in the United States increased by 9% to 13% a year, and in 1991, 201,458 patients were being treated under the Medicare program (3). Although the growth rate has slowed to 4.2% since 2000, between 1991 and 2001, the total population doubled with 406,081 patients being treated during the year 2001 (3).

End-stage dialysis kidney has been used in reference to the kidneys of patients treated by maintenance dialysis. These kidneys are sometimes very small, and single organ weights as low as 5 g have been reported (5). In contrast, some kidneys acquire cystic changes and can be larger than normal. End-stage dialysis kidney implies that the pathology occurring with long-term dialysis is limited to patients undergoing this therapy. This is probably true of kidneys that have stopped all urine production and show severe atrophy. But most, if not all, of the other changes found with long-term dialysis can be seen in CKD patients who have

not required dialysis or who have been dialyzed for short periods of time (6,7).

An end-stage kidney is sometimes diagnosed when patients undergo renal biopsy for unexplained renal failure. The recognition that a final point has been reached in a disease process allows patients to be placed on dialysis and to avoid unneeded diagnostic or therapeutic measures. In addition, the specific disease that has lead to renal failure can often be identified. When patients have been supported by dialysis for several years, the original renal disease may be obscured by the advanced degree of tissue changes. But even among these cases, the cause can often be assigned to at least one of five major categories of disease (hypertension, diabetes, glomerulonephritis, interstitial nephritis, and ischemic nephropathy). It also may be possible to discriminate specific forms of glomerulonephritis and interstitial nephritis.

## ETIOLOGY

Diabetes mellitus and hypertension together account for 70% of patients being treated for ESRD (3). Other common causes are glomerulonephritis, interstitial nephritis, hereditary conditions, and malignancy. Very rarely ESRD is the result of irreversible acute renal injury such as cortical necrosis or chemical nephrotoxicity. Primary glomerulonephritis may be the most common cause of CKD outside of North America, Europe, and Australia, but hypertension and diabetes are becoming commonplace and are increasing rates of ESRD throughout Asia, Latin America, and large parts of sub-Saharan Africa (3).

The percentage of the diseases leading to entry into ESRD programs between 1998 and 2002 and the racial and gender differences as reported in the USRDS 2004 Annual Data Report are shown in Table 27.1. The proportion of males for all ESRD was 53.7%. There is a disproportionate incidence of diabetes as a cause of ESRD in Native Americans at 72% and Hispanics at 59%. Also notable is the nearly 40% greater incidence of ESRD in blacks compared with whites that is attributed to hypertension and large vessel disease. This is almost entirely due to hypertension rather than disease of the large renal arteries. A 1997 survey found that large vessel disease was the assigned cause of renal failure in 2.1% of ESRD patients (8).

The category of glomerulonephritis currently accounts for less than 9% of ESRD in the United States. Focal segmental glomerulosclerosis (FSGS) and focal glomerulonephritis together composed 2.4%, membranous nephropathy 0.5%, membranoproliferative glomerulonephritis 0.4%, IgA nephropathy 0.7%, rapidly progressive glomerulonephritis 0.4%, and Goodpasture's syndrome 0.1% of ESRD cases. Most glomerulonephritis, representing 4.0% of ESRD cases, was not subcategorized as a specific primary glomerular disease. Lupus erythematosus was the major

## TABLE 27.1

**INCIDENCE OF MAJOR CATEGORIES OF DISEASE LEADING TO ENTRY INTO ESRD PROGRAMS BETWEEN 1998 AND 2002**

| Disease | Age (yr) | Male (%) | All Races (%) | White (%) | Black (%) | Native American (%) | Hispanic (%) | Asian (%) |
|---|---|---|---|---|---|---|---|---|
| All | 64 | 53.7 | — | 64.8 | 28.6 | 1.2 | 11.9 | 3.5 |
| Diabetes | 64 | 49.8 | 44.6 | 44.3 | 43.3 | 72.1 | 59.0 | 48.0 |
| Hypertension/large vessel disease | 70 | 56.3 | 26.9 | 24.5 | 33.9 | 9.3 | 17.1 | 24.1 |
| Glomerulonephritis | 53 | 60.7 | 8.9 | 9.1 | 7.8 | 8.1 | 8.0 | 14.4 |
| Secondary glomerulonephritis/vasculitis | 47 | 32.1 | 2.2 | 2.1 | 2.4 | 1.7 | 2.2 | 2.1 |
| Interstitial nephritis/pyelonephritis | 65 | 56.8 | 3.8 | 4.8 | 1.9 | 1.9 | 2.4 | 2.8 |
| Cystic/hereditary/congenital disease | 50 | 57.0 | 3.2 | 4.1 | 1.5 | 1.5 | 2.6 | 2.1 |
| Neoplasms/tumors | 69 | 60.2 | 2.0 | 2.5 | 1.3 | 0.9 | 0.9 | 0.9 |
| Miscellaneous | 59 | 61.8 | 4.2 | 4.1 | 4.9 | 1.7 | 2.2 | 1.6 |
| Cause uncertain | 67 | 58.0 | 4.1 | 4.6 | 3.1 | 2.7 | 3.7 | 4.1 |
| Cause missing | 55 | 54.6 | 1.5 | 1.5 | 1.4 | 0.4 | 1.9 | 1.2 |

The percentages of all diseases by race are greater than 100% because Hispanics were reported as white (85.1%), black (3.0%), Native American (1.2%), and Asian (0.7%).
From the U.S. Renal Data System 2004 Annual Data Report [www.usrds.org]. The data reported here have been supplied by the United States Renal Data System. The reporting of these data is the responsibility of the author and should not be seen as an official policy or interpretation of the U.S. government.

disease in the category that included secondary glomerulonephritis and vasculitis and accounted for 1.1% of patients entering the ESRD program.

Autosomal dominant polycystic kidney disease was responsible for 70.3% of the conditions categorized as cystic, hereditary, or congenital, and in the category of neoplasms and tumors 53.2% were due to multiple myeloma and another 18.5% to amyloidosis or light chain nephropathy. Tubulointerstitial nephritis was responsible for 3.8% of cases of ESRD, and 1.4% of ESRD or 35.6% of the category of tubulointerstitial nephritis was attributed to nephrolithiasis. Analgesic nephropathy remained the cause of 0.2% of cases despite the 20-year absence of phenacetin from the pharmaceutical market, and 0.9% of ESRD or 23.9% of the category was classified as chronic interstitial nephritis without a specified cause.

It is controversial whether or not analgesics that do not contain phenacetin can cause renal failure. In a case-control study, Fored et al (9), found that regular users of acetaminophen and aspirin had a 2.5-fold greater risk of chronic renal failure than sporadic users or nonusers. The design of the study has been criticized, because the increase in regular analgesic use was found among patients who were initially identified as being in chronic renal failure. They were matched against a control group with normal renal function, and it was not clear whether the analgesic use caused renal failure or the conditions leading to chronic renal failure triggered the analgesic use. The Physician's

Health Survey followed participants for 14 years and could find no detrimental effect of regular analgesic use on the kidney function of men who had normal serum creatinine levels at the beginning of the study period (10).

Since 1980, focal segmental glomerulosclerosis has been increasing as an identified cause of nephrotic syndrome and ESRD (11). In 1980, 0.2% of ESRD was estimated to be caused by FSGS; in 2000, the estimate was 2.3%. FSGS is currently the most common primary glomerular disease causing chronic kidney failure and is disproportionately represented among blacks. Between 1995 and 2000, 3% of ESRD among blacks was attributed to FSGS compared with 2% for whites. When extrapolated to the populations at risk, blacks had a fourfold greater risk of developing ESRD owing to FSGS than whites, and the ESRD occurred at a peak age of 40 to 49 years compared with 70 to 79 years for whites (11).

The increased recognition of FSGS as a cause of ESRD may be the result of the greater use of renal biopsies and the routine application of immunofluorescent microscopy since 1980. This may also account for the increased frequency that IgA nephropathy has been identified as a cause of ESRD. IgA nephropathy is rare in blacks, but accounts for 0.9% of ESRD in whites. IgA nephropathy is more common in Asians, Native Americans, and Hispanics than whites, and in this nonwhite, nonblack population, the incidence of ESRD caused by IgA nephropathy from 1995 to 2000 was between 1.3% and 1.7% (11).

# PROGRESSION OF RENAL DISEASE

## Glomerulonephritis

In many primary glomerular diseases including focal segmental glomerulosclerosis, mesangial proliferative glomerulonephritis, IgA nephropathy, membranous nephropathy, and membranoproliferative glomerulonephritis, the pathologic process continues in a progressive fashion over a period of many years (12,13). The late phase of these diseases has been referred to as *chronic glomerulonephritis*, because renal failure develops slowly. The term is also used in reference to chronic pathologic changes that suggest the primary disease was a form of glomerulonephritis but in which a specific diagnosis cannot be made.

In diseases such as primary crescentic glomerulonephritis, Goodpasture's syndrome, and glomerulonephritis associated with systemic vasculitis, glomerular injury tends to be severe and the progression to renal failure more rapid. Some patients can recover completely, but when a large proportion of glomeruli are involved, renal failure usually develops within a few weeks or months (12). Clinically, these diseases have been termed *rapidly progressive glomerulonephritis*, although in some patients, the onset of renal failure is slower and more closely resembles chronic glomerulonephritis.

A third category of glomerular disease has a variable course in different patients. Acute post-streptococcal glomerulonephritis is an example. The great majority of patients recover from the initial episode of nephritis and have no further evidence of renal disease. A few cases develop diffuse crescents and have a clinical course resembling a rapidly progressive glomerulonephritis (14). Some patients with acute glomerulonephritis have persistent hypertension, proteinuria, and hematuria and in rare instances develop chronic renal insufficiency. Rodriguez-Iturbe and Parra (15) reviewed reported series of post-streptococcal glomerulonephritis that included more than 900 patients and estimated that such chronicity is seen in less than 1% of cases.

## Essential Hypertension

The course of hypertensive vascular disease is related, at least in part, to the severity of the elevation in blood pressure. In a 1959 British study of untreated malignant hypertension, it was found that virtually all patients died within 5 years and that 55% developed renal failure within 1 to 3 years (15). The risk of developing renal failure at lower levels of blood pressure is small, but because of the enormous size of the population at risk, many persons with mild or moderate hypertension enter ESRD programs. The NIH Hypertension Detection and Follow-up Program (16) identified 12 deaths caused by renal failure among 7825 patients (0.15%) with mild hypertension (diastolic blood pressure between 90 mm Hg and 104 mm Hg) and 13 renal failure deaths among 3115 patients (0.42%) with diastolic blood pressures greater than 105 mm Hg.

The Multiple Risk Factor Intervention Trial (MRFIT) followed a total of 332,544 men over a mean follow-up period of 16 years and found a graded relationship between blood pressure and the risk of ESRD (18). The age-adjusted relative risk (with 95% confidence intervals [CI]) for ESRD was 3.1 (CI, 2.3 to 4.3) for mild hypertension, 6.0 (CI, 4.3 to 8.4) for moderate hypertension, 11.2 (CI, 7.7 to 16.2) for severe hypertension, and 22.1 (CI, 14.2 to 34.3) for very severe hypertension.

MRFIT additionally identified race and lower socioeconomic status as well as higher blood pressure as risk factors for ESRD (19). In comparison with white men, the 16-year age-adjusted relative risk of black men was 3.20 (CI, 2.62 to 3.91) for all ESRD and 5.16 (CI, 3.64 to 7.31) for hypertensive ESRD. Higher systolic blood pressure and lower income were associated with a higher risk of ESRD in both racial groups, but had a greater impact on blacks. When adjusted for blood pressure, income, previous myocardial infarction, diabetes, cholesterol level, and cigarette smoking, the relative risk of black as compared with white men was reduced but was still 1.87 (CI, 1.47 to 2.39) and 2.42 (CI, 1.52 to 3.84) for all ESRD and hypertensive ESRD, respectively (19).

In a 20-year study of risk factors for CKD in Washington County, Maryland, a graded relationship was found between levels of blood pressure and the development of CKD that was as strong in women as it was in men (20). Current cigarette smoking was also associated with the risk of CKD having a hazard ratio of 2.9 (CI, 1.7 to 5.0) for women and 2.4 (CI, 1.5 to 4.0) for men. The share of the attributed risk of CKD associated with cigarette use was 31%.

The treatment of severe hypertension is clearly beneficial and reduces morbidity and mortality by two thirds or more (16,21,22). The treatment of benign essential hypertension prevents blood pressure from rising to increasingly elevated levels and lowers the risk of cardiovascular disease, but a sizable number of patients progress to ESRD despite what appears to be adequate blood pressure control (23,24,25). A decline in renal function from a baseline normal serum creatinine or normal GFR to CKD has been seen in 15% of patients with treated essential hypertension who were followed from 1 year to more than 10 years (25,26). The Hypertension Detection and Follow-up Program showed that adequate blood pressure control in patients with mild hypertension reduced deaths owing to cardiovascular disease and stroke by 20% (17,27). The number of patients developing terminal renal failure, however, was nearly equal between a group receiving optimized treatment in special clinics and a group receiving community-based care whose blood pressures were not as well controlled (17).

Rostand et al (25) followed up on four patients with essential hypertension and initially normal serum creatinine levels who had good blood pressure control and found that twice as many blacks (23%) as whites (11%) had a deterioration in renal function. The African American Study of Kidney Disease and Hypertension Study Group (AASK) evaluated blood pressure control on the decline of renal function in 1094 blacks with chronic hypertensive kidney disease and an initial GFR between 20 and 65 mL/min/1.73 m$^2$ (28). The effect of lowering blood pressure to an average of 128/78 mm Hg in one group of patients achieved no benefit over an average blood pressure of 141/85 mm Hg in the other group. In both groups, proteinuria, as evidence of kidney damage, was strongly predictive of a loss of GFR. Patients having a urine protein to creatinine ratio of 0.22 or less had an average 12-month decline in GFR of 1.73 mL/min/1.73 m$^2$, whereas, patients having a ratio greater than 0.22 had an average decline of 4.09 mL/min/1.73 m$^2$ per year.

The question is frequently raised as to whether blacks with hypertension have more severe end-organ damage than whites (29,30). Patients with clinically uncomplicated hypertension are rarely biopsied, and it is likely that some patients diagnosed as having essential hypertension who progress to ESRD have a slowly progressive glomerulonephritis (31,32). Nevertheless, a biopsy study by Fogo et al (31) as part of AASK indicated that the great majority of hypertensive blacks who developed renal insufficiency and who were not diabetic did, in fact, have hypertensive nephrosclerosis.

In a separate study, the biopsies from the previously cited study by Fogo et al (31) were compared with biopsies from white patients who had a clinical diagnosis of hypertensive nephrosclerosis (33). The proportion of obsolescent glomeruli was approximately the same in both races. However, solidified global sclerosis, which is thought to be the result of a more severe form of injury than glomerular obsolescence, was significantly more common in blacks. The mean arterial blood pressures of the two groups did not differ, and the authors concluded that blacks suffered a greater degree of kidney damage for any level of hypertension (33).

## Diabetes Mellitus

Diabetic nephropathy develops in 25% to 40% of patients with type 1 diabetes, and the progression to ESRD usually occurs over a period of 20 to 40 years after the onset of disease (34,35). With type 2 diabetes mellitus, diabetic nephropathy has been reported in 5% to 10% of patients at the time diabetes was diagnosed and in 25% to 60% of patients who have been diabetic for more than 20 years (35,36). Most patients with type 2 diabetes die of the complications of atherosclerotic cardiovascular disease, but those who survive 15 years develop diabetic nephropathy

and ESRD at a rate that is similar to patients with type 1 diabetes (35,37). Higher blood pressure, albuminuria, degree of retinopathy, and elevated HgbA1c levels closely predict the progression to ESRD in patients with type 1 and type 2 diabetes (36,38). With both types of diabetes, the treatment of hypertension and better control of hyperglycemia reduces the risk of developing nephropathy and slows the decline in GFR once nephropathy is present (35–42). Approximately one third of the cases of ESRD in diabetics is attributed to nondiabetic renal disease (43). In this subset of patients, hypertension is the most frequently assigned cause of renal failure with other causes being congenital abnormalities, pyelonephritis, and glomerulonephritis.

## Effects of Secondary Hypertension

Blood pressure is elevated in 75% to 90% of renal disease patients as they progress to ESRD and can be difficult to control in half of the cases (44,45). The treatment of blood pressure slows the progression of chronic renal insufficiency in diabetic nephropathy and proteinuric nondiabetic renal disease including glomerulonephritis but does not seem to significantly protect renal function in polycystic kidney disease (18,45–50).

Several studies have found that angiotensin-converting enzyme inhibitors, angiotensin II receptor antagonists, or both together are particularly effective in preserving the renal function of patients with CKD. The effect appears to be independent of the degree of blood pressure control and may not be seen with other classes of antihypertensive agents (28,39,47,48,50,51). The findings suggest that it may be the suppression of the renin-angiotensin system (RAS) rather than just the lowering of blood pressure that benefits the kidney. (28,52–56).

## Hyperperfusion Injury: A Possible Factor in Progressive Renal Injury

As patients with CKD lose GFR, blood pressure tends to become increasingly elevated. Intrarenal arteries show fibrous intimal thickening, and the degree of intimal thickening of arcuate and interlobular arteries has been related to the severity of hypertension and to the degree of glomerulosclerosis (49,57,58). Two patterns of glomerulosclerosis have been associated with hypertension (59). One, termed *ischemic obsolescence*, consists of a collapsed glomerular tuft that becomes surrounded by intracapsular fibrosis filling Bowman's space beneath an intact capsular basement membrane (Fig. 27.1) (60). It is usually, although not always, found distal to arteriolosclerosis in the preglomerular arteries and arterioles and is thought to be caused by a reduction in blood flow to the involved glomerulus. The other pattern of glomerulosclerosis is referred to as *glomerular solidification* (33,59,60). This

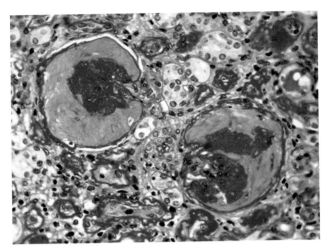

**Figure 27.1** Late stage of ischemic glomerular obsolescence. The tufts of two glomeruli are contracted into small hyaline knots and are surrounded by lightly staining collagen that has formed inside of Bowman's capsule. (PAS-hematoxylin stains, ×200.)

produces global glomerulosclerosis in which the glomerulus is expanded by an increase in mesangial matrix and hyalinosis lesions are frequently present in the sclerotic tufts (Fig. 27.2). Bowman's capsule is fragmented, and the solidified tuft merges with the surrounding interstitial fibrous tissue.

It has been proposed that solidification is caused by loss of the autoregulatory changes in afferent arteriolar tone, which maintains a constant glomerular hydrostatic pressure (59,61). This loss of autoregulatory tone is seen in remnant kidney models of hypertension and in Dahl spontaneously hypertensive rats (61,62). At lower levels of hypertension, autoregulatory afferent arteriolar vasoconstric-

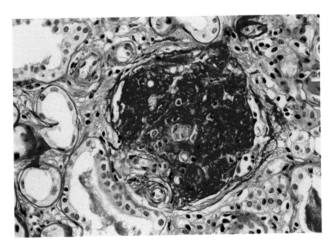

**Figure 27.2** Solidified glomerulus in a patient with focal segmental glomerulosclerosis. The glomerular tuft is expanded by an increase in mesangial matrix that effaces the glomerular capillaries. The basement membrane of Bowman's capsule is fragmented, and the solidified tuft merges with the surrounding connective tissue. (PAS-hematoxylin stains, ×200.)

tion protects glomeruli. But when higher levels of blood pressure are attained, afferent arteriolar tone fails to increase with increasing blood pressure, and glomeruli are subjected to abnormally high filtration pressures with the potential for hyperperfusion injury (62,63).

Several experimental models of glomerular hyperperfusion injury have been described. In these models, when there is a loss of functional renal tissue, a compensatory hypertrophy occurs in the remaining kidney, and the spared or remnant glomeruli are subjected to abnormally elevated plasma flow rates. The resulting increase in glomerular capillary pressure results in hyperperfusion injury that is manifested histologically as focal segmental glomerulosclerosis with hyalinosis (64–67).

The role hyperperfusion glomerular injury plays in the progression of renal disease in man still has not been clarified. Although hyperperfusion produces focal segmental glomerulosclerosis and hyalinosis and causes the decompensation of renal function in experimental models, it is not certain whether the equivalent glomerular lesions occur in humans.

Focal segmental glomerulosclerosis with or without hyalinosis lesions is not commonly seen in essential hypertension. Marcantoni et al (33) found segmental sclerosis in just 7% of glomeruli in renal biopsies of essential hypertension from 19 blacks and in 4% of glomeruli in biopsies from 43 whites. Segmental sclerosis was not found in renal biopsies from 13 patients with essential hypertension by Hughson et al (60). In an autopsy study, Hughson et al (68) evaluated the relationships between aging, obesity, glomerular number, and glomerulosclerosis in 45 adults. Blacks constituted 66% of the patients, many were hypertensive, and a large proportion of blacks and whites were obese. Glomerular obsolescence was the only form of glomerulosclerosis that was identified.

Focal glomerulosclerosis, suggesting hyperperfusion injury, has been reported in patients with unilateral renal agenesis and with solitary kidneys following nephrectomy for an acquired disease (69–74). In some instances, the patients have become proteinuric and have progressed to renal failure (69,71,73). In human renal diseases, hyperperfusion injury seems best established as a complication of overperfusing the remaining kidney in unilateral renal agenesis. Nevertheless, unilateral renal agenesis is relatively common, occurring in approximately 1 in 1100 live births, and clinical renal disease including focal segmental glomerulosclerosis is not unusually prevalent among individuals having this condition (71,75,76). Heptinstall pointed out that patients with solitary kidneys who develop renal failure may be reported selectively because of interest in the pathophysiologic significance of the glomerular lesions (76). Several studies have not shown any long-term deterioration of renal function among patients who have undergone unilateral nephrectomy for acquired disease or to donate transplant kidneys (72,74,76).

## Recovery of Renal Function

Eligibility for Medicare coverage usually begins 60 to 90 days after beginning ESRD therapy (77). After this period, recovery of renal function adequate for survival without dialysis or transplantation rarely occurs. In the year 2000, 3754 patients were reported to recover renal function from the 275,053 patients being treated by dialysis (78). In the Michigan Kidney Registry, renal functional recovery was observed in 211 of 7404 ESRD patients (2.8%) who had been dialyzed for at least 30 days in the 10-year period 1976 to 1985 (79). Recovery lasted 1 year in 75% of patients and for more than 3 years in 50%. Among 14,318 ESRD patients in the Canadian Organ Replacement Register, 342 (2.4%) were observed to recover renal function after being dialyzed for more than 45 days (80). In this study, 67% of patients with recovered function had not returned to dialysis in 6.5 years.

Recovery is seen most frequently in patients with multiple myeloma, systemic lupus erythematosus, vasculitis, crescentic glomerulonephritis, thrombotic microangiopathies, and drug-induced disease. Among those particularly likely to recover are women with systemic lupus erythematosus, scleroderma, or hemolytic uremic syndrome. Recovery is least likely to occur in those with diabetes and polycystic kidney disease. Some reports have suggested that patients treated by continuous ambulatory peritoneal dialysis (CAPD) were more likely to regain function than hemodialysis patients (81). This was not supported by data in either the Michigan or Canadian Registries where recoveries were seen slightly more often in hemodialysis patients (79,80).

# VISCERAL MANIFESTATIONS OF CHRONIC RENAL FAILURE

## Clinical Features

An early sign of chronic renal failure is dependent edema that presents first as ankle or periorbital edema. Uremic patients frequently develop congestive heart failure, in which case dependent edema becomes increasingly severe and may progress to anasarca. The skin of uremic patients has a sallow, yellow appearance because it is pigmented with carotene. When blood urea levels are greater than 80 mg/dL, urea is secreted through the skin where it dries into a white uremic frost, and the patient's breath has a uriniferous odor because of urea being metabolized to ammonia by mouth bacteria. In terminal stages, uremic patients become delirious and lapse into coma before death.

Because of the nearly universal access to renal replacement therapy, cases of fully developed uremia are rare. Nevertheless, ESRD patients have a high prevalence of nonrenal comorbid disease. With prolonged survival on dialysis, pathologic changes occur in virtually all organs of the body.

The ESRD patient is faced with a broad spectrum of cardiovascular, endocrine, osteoarticular, and infectious disease, and longevity is determined in large part by pre-existing cardiovascular disease or the cardiovascular complications of chronic uremia.

## Cardiovascular

Diabetes and hypertension bring a large burden of cardiovascular disease into the population that begins treatment for ESRD, and both all-cause and cardiovascular mortality rates are increased for ESRD patients who have a diagnosis of cardiovascular disease (78). The relationship between cardiovascular and renal disease begins during the early stages of CKD. A population study of over 1,000,000 adults with an average age of 52 years in the Kaiser Permanente Health System found a graded association between a reduction in GFR and the risk of cardiovascular events and death (82). The adjusted hazard ratio for cardiovascular events was 1.4 (CI, 1.4 to 1.5) for a GFR of 45 to 50 mL/min/1.73 m$^2$, 2.0 (CI, 1.9 to 2.1) for 30 to 44 mL/min/1.73 m$^2$, 2.8 (CI, 2.6 to 2.9) for 15 to 29 mL/min/1.73 m$^2$, and 3.4 (CI, 3.1 to 3.8) for a GFR less than 15 mL/min/1.73 m$^2$. The risk of death for persons having a GFR less than 15 mL/min/1.73 m$^2$ was 5.9 times greater than for those without CKD.

McClellan et al (83) observed that patents hospitalized for myocardial infarction or congestive heart failure who also had CKD had a high rate of progression to ESRD in a 12-month period following the cardiovascular event. These authors emphasized the increased risk of ESRD that was associated with cardiovascular disease. Current clinical practice guidelines target the treatment of the risk factors of hypertension, hyperlipidemia, and tobacco use not only for the prevention of cardiovascular disease but also to retard the progression of CKD (1).

## Cardiomyopathies of End-Stage Renal Disease

A large part of the cardiovascular morbidity of ESRD is due to a cardiomyopathy in which there may or may not be coexisting coronary atherosclerosis. The cardiomyopathies of ESRD are classified into two major types (84,85):

1. Dilated cardiomyopathy is characterized by enlargement of the chamber of the left ventricle but without an increase in the thickness of the left ventricular free wall or interventricular septum. Dilated cardiomyopathy is clinically associated with impaired systolic function and a low left ventricular ejection fraction.
2. Hypertrophic cardiomyopathy is characterized by left ventricular hypertrophy. Concentric left ventricular hypertrophy is the most common form of hypertrophic cardiomyopathy in the patient with ESRD and consists of an increased thickness of both the interventricular

septum and left ventricular free wall. Eccentric hypertrophy and asymmetric septal hypertrophy do occur but are less common than concentric hypertrophy. Hypertrophic cardiomyopathy is clinically associated with diastolic dysfunction consisting of impaired left ventricular relaxation and filling in which there is an increased left ventricular end diastolic pressure.

A dilated cardiomyopathy precedes dialysis in 16% of ESRD patients and develops in another 15% during the course of dialytic therapy (84,85). Dilated cardiomyopathy seems to occur most frequently in hypertensive patients who have hyperparathyroidism and high-turnover bone disease (86). It is suggested that an excessive entry of calcium into myocardial cells limits their capacity to hypertrophy in response to elevated blood pressure. To compensate for the increased workload, the heart is forced to dilate to maintain cardiac output.

Hypertrophic cardiomyopathy is found in 27% of ESRD patients at the time dialysis is started and develops in 16% of patients after treatment begins (84,85). Left ventricular hypertrophy is primarily the result of hypertension, but the degree of hypertrophy is not always proportional to the severity and duration of the elevation in blood pressure. The anemia of chronic renal failure, hyperparathyroidism, and the growth factor effect of angiotensin II have been implicated as factors contributing to the myocardial hypertrophy, and hypertrophy has been seen to increase in some patients whose blood pressure appears to be adequately controlled (87,88). Hypertension tends to be better controlled with CAPD than hemodialysis, and Leenan et al (89) suggested that CAPD might reduce the severity of cardiac hypertrophy. Parfrey et al (90) found that progressive cardiac hypertrophy will occur among patients treated by CAPD at a frequency similar to that seen with hemodialysis.

A hypertrophic cardiomyopathy at the onset of renal replacement therapy confers a nearly four times greater risk for all-cause and cardiac mortality in the ESRD patient (91). Patients with cardiac hypertrophy have a high prevalence of known coronary artery disease, but many have clinical symptoms of ischemic heart disease without significant coronary artery stenosis (85,92). Rostand and Rutsky (93) studied 81 ESRD patients with angina pectoris by coronary angiography and found that 73% had over 50% narrowing but 27% had normal or slightly stenotic arteries. Inadequate myocardial perfusion relative to cardiac mass and oxygen demand certainly plays a role in the symptoms of patients without significant coronary atherosclerosis. Hypertrophy of the small intramural cardiac arteries may contribute to the ischemia (92).

## Atherosclerotic Coronary Artery Disease

Atherosclerotic cardiovascular disease is the principal cause of morbidity and mortality in ESRD patients. This largely reflects the prevalence of hypertension and diabetes mellitus in the population and the severity of the atherosclerotic vascular disease that is part of the natural history of these diseases. Nevertheless, severe atherosclerosis can be seen at an unusually young age. In 1974, Lindner et al (94) reported their experience with 39 patients who began maintenance dialysis at an average age of 39 years. The mortality rate was 56.4% by the end of 13 years with 14 of the 23 deaths being caused by arteriosclerotic vascular disease. In eight patients, death was specifically attributed to coronary artery disease. This was a coronary artery disease death rate many times higher than for normal individuals or even hypertensive patients without CKD of a comparable age. The authors used the term "accelerated atherosclerosis" for this early appearance of vascular disease and proposed that chronic dialysis itself contributed to its development (94).

Braun et al (95) measured cardiac and coronary artery calcification by electron beam computed tomography to assess coronary artery disease in 49 chronic hemodialysis patients aged 39 to 74 years. The results were compared with 102 age-matched nondialysis patients with known coronary artery disease who had undergone coronary angiography. A 2.5- to 5-fold higher coronary artery calcification score was found in the dialysis patients, and the scores significantly increased when the patients were re-examined after 1 year.

It has been suggested that when dialysis patients are matched with the general population for age, hypertension, cigarette smoking, hyperlipidemia, and disease diagnosis, differences in the severity of arteriosclerosis may not be so apparent (96,97). Owen et al (97) evaluated the cardiovascular risk factors of 17 patients who began dialysis at an average age of $38.4 \pm 14.5$ years and survived 15 years or more. These patients maintained a low risk profile throughout the period of treatment, and it was thought that the absence of risk factors might have contributed to their longevity.

In contrast, frequent and progressive coronary artery calcification was found by Goodman et al (98) in young adult patients between 20 and 30 years of age who began dialysis at an average age of $13 \pm 4$ years. Coronary calcification was rare in a control group of normal subjects of the same age, and the presence of coronary calcification in the dialysis patients could not be related to blood pressure. This study supported the concept of accelerated atherosclerosis, and the authors proposed that the disturbances in calcium metabolism during chronic dialysis promoted the vascular disease (98).

The elevated serum phosphorus that accompanies ESRD results in metastatic calcification when the product of serum phosphorus and calcium ($Ca \times PO_4$) is elevated. Block et al (99) found a mortality risk of 1.34 ($P < .01$) for ESRD patients having a $Ca \times PO_4$ product higher than 72 $mg^2/dL^2$ when compared with patients having a $Ca \times PO_4$ product of 42 to 52 $mg^2/dL^2$. The increased risk was associated with hyperphosphatemia, although not with serum parathormone levels. Ganesh et al (100) related hyperphosphatemia and an elevated Ca × PO₄ product specifically to an increased risk of cardiac mortality and did find the risk associated with elevated parathormone levels.

The severity of calcification in atherosclerotic plaques can be related to plaque size (101,102). Although calcification can be found in small plaques, it is most pronounced in larger, complicated plaques having a necrotic lipid core and varying amounts of inflammation (103). Calcification also occurs along the media of coronary arteries as Mönckeberg's medial calcific sclerosis in which there is little intimal thickening or luminal narrowing (104). The bone matrix proteins osteopontin, osteocalcin, and osteoblastic differentiation factor Cbfa1 are expressed in areas of medial and plaque calcification. The presence of these locally produced bone matrix stimulating factors indicates that metastatic calcification is an active, cell-mediated process similar to osteogenesis rather than a passive deposition of minerals (105,106). Moe et al (106,107) and Chen et al (105) have suggested that chronic uremia may up-regulate the local deposition of bone matrix proteins and promote atherosclerotic plaque growth.

Most investigators have found cardiac arterial calcification to be related to hyperphosphatemia and elevation of the Ca × PO₄ product. In some of these studies, the calcification was related to elevated parathormone levels whereas in others it was not. The calcification has been inversely associated with bone density, and London et al (108) observed that the highest coronary artery calcification scores were found in ESRD patients having adynamic bone disease and low serum parathormone levels. In their study, bone histomorphometry revealed low numbers of osteoblasts and osteoclasts along the surfaces of bone trabeculae and small or absent double tetracycline labeling. A large percentage of the patients had evidence of aluminum bone disease. The findings were interpreted as indicating that excessive lowering of parathormone activity by calcium salts or aluminum phosphate binders may enhance rather than inhibit cardiac calcification (108).

## Valvular Calcification

The cardiac valves of ESRD patients are frequently calcified. Valvular calcification is closely related to coexisting atherosclerotic coronary artery disease, and the extent of valvular calcification has been found to predict cardiovascular mortality (95,109–111). The mitral valve is calcified in 10% to 59% and the aortic valve in 28% to 55% of dialysis patients. The calcification most severely affects the annulus (Figs. 27.3 and 27.4). Although involvement of the aortic valve cusps and mitral leaflets can produce clinically significant stenosis, this is not common, and the relationship between valvular calcification and cardiac death is

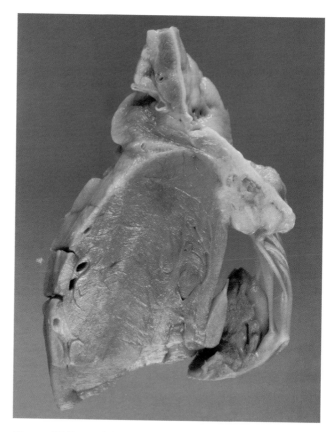

**Figure 27.3** Nodular calcification of the annulus and base of the mitral valve in a 55-year-old hemodialysis patient.

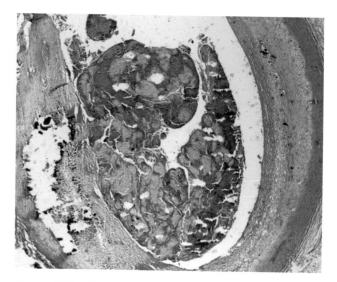

**Figure 27.4** Thrombosis over a calcified plaque of the left anterior descending coronary artery in the hemodialysis patient with the mitral valve calcification shown in Figure 27.3. Note the fissuring of the plaque over the necrotic and calcified core. (H&E, ×4.)

primarily owing to the close association of valvular calcification with coronary artery disease (95,111).

Calcification of the mitral valve can cause heart block or other arrhythmias when the calcification of the annulus extends into the adjacent ventricular wall. Oxalosis is sometimes found in the hearts of ESRD patients as a result of the secondary oxalosis of chronic renal failure. It can extensively involve the coronary arteries or be deposited in the AV node and conducting bundles.

## Calcemic Uremic Arteriopathy

Calcemic uremic arteriopathy (CUA) is a clinical condition that occurs in some patients with long-standing ESRD in which calcification of arterioles in the dermis and subcutaneous tissues produces painful red skin nodules that frequently undergo ischemic necrosis and ulceration (Fig. 27.5) (112,113). CUA is preferred over the previously used term *calciphylaxis*, because in the original description by Selye of an experimentally induced condition, calciphylaxis was characterized by metastatic calcification in the dermis but not in blood vessels (113).

The lesions are most commonly found on the thighs, buttocks, and abdomen. When the hands or feet are affected, there may be gangrene of the fingers or toes. Involvement of the mesenteric artery has also been reported (114). Histologically, the skin shows medial calcification and intimal fibrosis of arterioles and small arteries. The intimal fibrosis may be occlusive or accompanied by thrombosis, and coagulative necrosis is found in the dermis and subcutaneous tissue. Ulceration frequently develops, and a necrotizing panniculitis is sometimes seen that is often complicated by septicemia.

Female gender, white race, obesity, hypoalbuminemia, hyperphosphatemia, and an elevated Ca × PO$_4$ product are predisposing factors for CUA (113). Diabetics and patients receiving Coumadin may also be at higher risk. Elevated parathormone levels are seen in some but by no means all patients, and in a bone biopsy study of seven patients with CUA by Mawad et al (115), five patients had adynamic bone disease and low parathormone levels. This is similar to the bone biopsy findings by London et al (108) that were associated with coronary artery calcification.

When patients have only nonulcerated lesions, the mortality rate is approximately 30%. This increases to more than 80% when ulceration develops. CUA is treated by controlling hyperphosphatemia, debriding necrotic tissues, antibiotic treatment of infection, and by parathyroidectomy if parathormone levels are elevated (112).

## Pericardium

Pericarditis unrelated to infections or autoimmune disease is seen in ESRD patients (116,117). Uremia appears to increase the permeability of small blood vessels and allows a fibrinous exudate to leak across the pericardium. This is referred to as *uremic pericarditis*. The gross examination of the heart shows easily broken bands of fibrin producing the bread and butter appearance described in the standard pathology textbooks (Fig. 27.6). The histopathology of uremic pericarditis reveals a fibrinous exudate accompanied by sparse inflammatory cells covering the visceral and parietal surfaces of the pericardium.

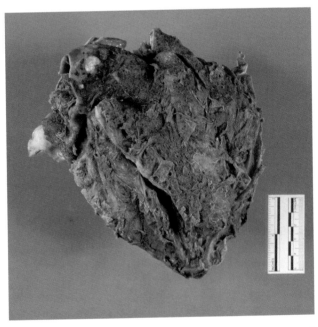

**Figure 27.6** Dialysis-associated pericarditis from an autopsy of a 58-year-old diabetic hemodialysis patient who died of septicemia. The heart is coated with a fibrinous exudate.

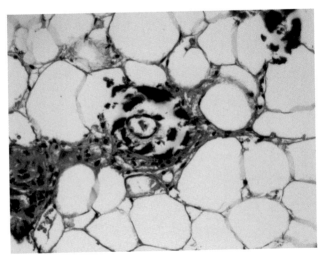

**Figure 27.5** Calcemic uremic arteriopathy. An arteriole in the dermis of a painful skin nodule on the lower leg of a hemodialysis patient is calcified. (H&E, ×400.)

A fibrinous pericarditis can also be seen in acute renal failure and occasionally in patients on dialysis who are thought to be adequately treated. When it occurs 1 month or more after beginning dialysis, it is diagnosed as dialysis-associated pericarditis (116,117). It is a general impression that dialysis-associated pericarditis and uremic pericarditis represent the same pathologic condition. It often is seen when dialysis patients become infected or when they are under increased metabolic stress, such as following surgery. In most cases, dialysis-associated pericarditis clears after treatment schedules are intensified (116,117).

Clinically, uremic or dialysis-associated pericarditis is associated with chest pain and, if a significant amount of fluid accumulates, with cardiac tamponade (116,117). Hemorrhage can occur into the pericardium and is an additional cause of cardiac tamponade in the uremic patient. In hemodialysis patients, this may sometimes be a complication of anticoagulation with heparin. In long-standing pericarditis, the fibrinous exudate is organized into fibrous tissue that produces a constrictive pericarditis (116,117). Constrictive pericarditis is usually a complication of chronic renal failure but has been described with acute renal failure following a single episode of pericarditis (118).

## Lung

As a result of anemia and fluid retention, the cardiomyopathy of ESRD frequently decompensates into congestive heart failure. Patients develop pulmonary edema when the passive accumulation of blood within the pulmonary vasculature causes alveolar intracapillary hydrostatic pressure to exceed oncotic pressure. First, a protein-rich fluid leaks into the interstitium and then into alveoli. Grossly, lungs involved by pulmonary edema are heavy and their sectioned surfaces are covered by frothy, blood-tinged fluid. Microscopically, alveolar capillaries are distended with blood. The perivascular interstitium and interlobular septae are edematous and lymphatics are dilated. Alveoli become filled with amorphous slightly eosinophilic edema fluid that can contain a few red blood cells. If patients have been in congestive heart failure for several days, some hyaline membrane formation may be present (119).

In late-stage uremia, proteinaceous fluid sometimes leaks into the alveoli, producing what has been referred to as uremic pneumonitis. Uremic pneumonitis is not an inflammatory disorder, and the use of the term is discouraged. The condition is regarded as a form of pulmonary edema that is caused by injury to and increased permeability of the alveolar capillaries (119,120). Undefined uremic "toxins" have been implicated in the vascular damage, although the onset and severity of the changes do not always correlate with the degree of uremia (120). The pathology resembles the adult respiratory distress syndrome, and coexisting shock or septicemia may play a role in its pathogenesis. Grossly, the lungs have a stiff, rubbery consistency,

and the sectioned surfaces have a dark, reddish color. Histologically, the earliest stage reveals a hemorrhagic fibrinous fluid filling alveoli with hyaline membranes being formed along alveolar walls and alveolar ducts. If the process does not resolve, fibrin in the alveolar fluid and hyaline membranes is organized into whorls of fibrous tissue referred to as *Masson bodies* (76).

Congestive heart failure is one of the most common causes of death among ESRD patients. Passive pulmonary congestion and acute pulmonary edema are expected autopsy findings. The presence of pathology resembling an adult respiratory distress syndrome suggests a mechanism of death other than heart failure. There will be some overlap in the pathology of these two forms of pulmonary edema, and some cases may not be clearly assigned to one specific condition. ESRD patients often tire of the effort required to continue dialysis regimens. They voluntarily withdraw from dialysis, and in the last days of life, develop uremia and congestive heart failure.

Congestive heart failure is commonly accompanied by pleural effusions that are transudates with low protein concentrations and a specific gravity of less than 1.015. When patients are uremic, they can develop a fibrinous pleuritis that is histologically identical to uremic pericarditis. It is a hemorrhagic exudate with a high protein content and a specific gravity of greater than 1.015 (121). Like uremic pericarditis, it is treated by intensifying dialysis regimens. Occasional patients develop pleural effusions shortly after beginning peritoneal dialysis. These effusions represent an accumulation of the dialysate solution and have a low protein content and very high glucose concentrations (121).

When chronic renal failure is complicated by metastatic calcification, it is usually found in the lung (122). The calcification may be focal or diffuse and tends to affect the upper lobes most severely. Both lungs can be involved. Metastatic pulmonary calcification is usually clinically asymptomatic, and the pattern of deposition may be so delicate that it will not be detected by routine chest radiographs (122). Nevertheless, if the calcification is extensive it can lead to respiratory failure. Grossly, the involved areas of lung have a firm but brittle consistency and a fine netlike appearance that exaggerates the outlines of open alveoli. The areas are gray to pale yellow in color and typically contrast sharply with the adjacent normal or congested lung. Histologically, linear calcifications outline basement membranes within the alveolar septae. Calcifications also are seen along the elastica of arteries, veins, bronchi, and bronchioles and in fibrotic nodules within the lung parenchyma (122).

## Beta-2-Microglobulin Amyloidosis

Beta-2-microglobulin is the light chain of class I HLA antigens. It is an 11,800-dalton protein that enters the bloodstream when HLA antigens are degraded and shed from the surfaces of cell membranes. Beta-2-microglobulin

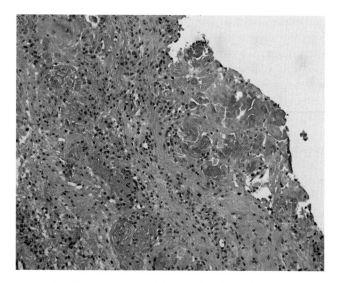

**Figure 27.7** Beta-2-microglobulin–related amyloidosis in the synovium from the right hand of a 54-year-old long-term hemodialysis patient who had a several-week history of interphalangeal joint pain and swelling. Nodular deposits of amorphous hyalin material are seen in the synovial connective tissue. (H&E, ×200.)

accumulates in the plasma of ESRD patients and is deposited as insoluble amyloid fibrils in the articular surfaces of bone, in periarticular connective tissue (Fig. 27.7), and in nerve sheaths in as many as 80% of hemodialysis patients after 10 years of treatment (123). It causes carpal tunnel syndrome and a destructive arthropathy of medium- and large-sized joints, mainly of the shoulders and knees (124). Dialysis-associated amyloid tumors of breast and ovary, nodular skin masses particularly of the buttocks, and nodules of the tongue are additionally described (125–129). Beta-2-microglobulin amyloid was found in the hearts of 7 of 18 hemodialysis patients who had been dialyzed for more than 10 years (130). Amyloid was present in the endocardium and myocardium of the left atrium. In the left ventricle, it was localized to the walls of blood vessels and around areas of calcification of the mitral valve.

Beta-2-microglobulin amyloid is found within bone of 19% of hemodialysis patients after 10 years of treatment (131). These bone deposits are responsible for cysts that develop in the femur and femoral head and possibly for the unusually high prevalence of pathologic femoral neck fractures in hemodialysis patients (Figs. 27.8 and 27.9). Onishi et al (131) observed that 62% of patients had femoral neck fractures when periosteal amyloid deposits were found in posterior iliac crest bone biopsies. Only 4% of a control group of hemodialysis patients having biopsies who did not show periosteal amyloid had femoral neck fractures.

Beta-2-microglobulin amyloid shows Congo red-positive staining and apple-green birefringence under polarized light. By electron microscopy, it is composed of fine fibrils 80 to 100 angstroms in diameter having a curvilinear structure that is thought to be characteristic of beta-

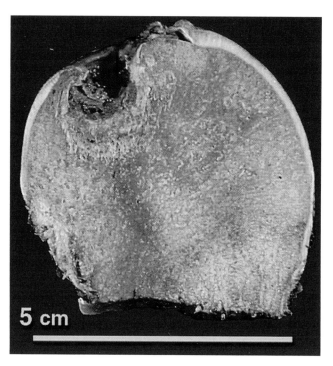

**Figure 27.8** Beta-2-microglobulin–related amyloidosis of the femoral head removed from a 37-year-old long-term hemodialysis patient who had a femoral neck fracture. A necrotic cyst surrounded by a rim of solid white material is present beneath the insertion of the ligamentum teres.

2-microglobulin (Fig. 27.10) (131). Beta-2-microglobulin is cleared to some extent through the peritoneum, and the amyloidosis does not seem to be as prevalent with CAPD as it is with hemodialysis (123). The addition of beta-2-microglobulin absorption columns in series with high-flux dialyzers is being investigated as a therapy for

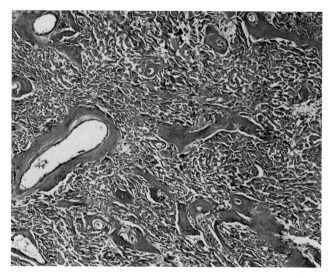

**Figure 27.9** Histologic section from the solid area surrounding the femoral head cyst shown in Figure 27.7. Amyloid is present in the walls of blood vessels and in the interstitium. (Congo red, ×100.)

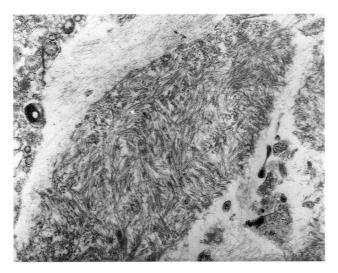

**Figure 27.10** Electron microscopic photomicrograph of the synovial tissue shown in Figure 27.9. Curvilinear fibrils characteristic of beta-2-microglobulin amyloidosis are demonstrated. (×18,000.)

dialysis-associated amyloidosis, but currently little can be done for the condition (132).

## Gastrointestinal Tract and Pancreas

Although it is uncommon now because of the availability of dialysis, terminal uremia is accompanied by edema, inflammation, mucosal erosions, and ulcerations of the entire gastrointestinal tract (76). Gastrointestinal bleeding is a common clinical problem among dialysis patients and most frequently originates in a hemorrhagic gastritis (133). Many dialysis patients have a mild gastritis, duodenitis, or peptic ulcer disease in which *Helicobacter pylori* can sometimes be found; although, these findings may be not be any more common than in the general population (134).

Colonic bleeding can originate from cecal ulcers, stercoral ulcers, angiodysplasia, diverticulosis, or ischemic colitis (133,135). Multiple shallow ulcers attributed to uremia may be found in the cecum and ascending colon. Constipation and fecal impaction, resulting from the use of oral phosphate binders as well as other medications, produce stercoral ulcers in the transverse and rectosigmoid colon. Angiodysplasia consisting of clusters of abnormally dilated mucosal and submucosal blood vessels is found primarily in the cecum and ascending colon. Angiodysplasia is more prevalent in dialysis patients than in the general population, and in some series, it is the most frequent cause of gastrointestinal hemorrhage among ESRD patients (133,135,136). Diverticulosis, diverticulitis, pericolic abscesses, and colonic perforation may be more common in autosomal dominant polycystic kidney disease than with other categories of renal disease (137).

The severe atherosclerosis of diabetes and hypertension places ESRD patients at high risk for ischemic colitis and in-

testinal infarction (135). Hemodialysis patients with beta-2-microglobulin amyloidosis may have amyloid deposited in the connective tissue and small blood vessels of the mucosa and submucosa of the GI tract (138). The gastrointestinal amyloid is usually an incidental finding, but massive involvement of the muscularis propria of the colon has been identified as a cause of bleeding and intestinal infarction (139).

Patients dying of uremia develop an acute pancreatitis in which pancreatic ductules and acini are dilated and contain inspissated eosinophilic material (140,141). The dilated acini become disrupted and surrounded by an acute inflammatory reaction. Pancreatitis is also seen in patients who are well maintained on long-term peritoneal and hemodialysis. Padilla et al (142) reported pancreatitis developing in 4.3% of ESRD patients after the start of dialysis. Alcohol use was the most common predisposing factor, but non–alcohol-related pancreatitis was seen in 2.5% of patients, a figure similar to a 2.3% 10-year incidence reported by Rutsky et al (143). The pancreas may show focal or generalized fibrosis. Sometimes, fibrosis may be the sequela of episodes of acute pancreatitis, but it also has been related to hyperphosphatemia and to ischemic atrophy secondary to the marked arteriolosclerosis that is often found in the small pancreatic arteries (141).

Ascites referred to as nephrogenic or dialysis-associated occurs in a small proportion of hemodialysis patients (144). Some of these patients had been treated by peritoneal dialysis, and histologic studies of the peritoneum have shown fibrosis and chronic inflammation. Congestive heart failure, pancreatitis, and liver cirrhosis are etiologic factors in some cases.

## Hematopoietic System

Chronic renal failure causes a hypoplastic anemia that is caused by a relative deficiency of erythropoietin. In uremic patients, plasma erythropoietin activity is approximately twice that found in normal individuals, but the diseased kidneys do not make enough erythropoietin to stimulate the level of red cell production needed to compensate for the severity of the anemia (145). A shortened red blood cell life span also contributes to the anemia of chronic renal failure. This is reflected in peripheral blood smears that show numerous poikilocytes. These misshapen cells are the result of extrinsic factors that fragment or metabolically alter the erythrocyte. The anemia of chronic renal failure is usually normocytic and normochromic. Since red blood cell production and iron utilization is low, bone marrow examinations of patients with the typical anemia of chronic renal failure show normal to increased amounts of iron. Gastrointestinal bleeding and poor dietary intake, however, can lead to iron deficiency and a microcytic hypochromic anemia. Aluminum toxicity causes a microcytic hypochromic anemia in which adequate iron stores are present (145).

Prior to the availability of human recombinant erythropoietin (EPO), the anemia of chronic renal failure was treated by red blood cell transfusions (146). EPO and intravenous iron therapy is now used to maintain hemoglobin levels in the K/DOQI recommended range of 11 to 12 g/dL (3). Correction of anemia provides relief from many of the debilitating symptoms of chronic renal failure (146,147). These include improvement in sleep, cognitive function, and exercise tolerance. The response to EPO is poor in some ESRD patients, and they require high doses of EPO to raise their hemoglobin levels. There are disease differences in EPO requirements (3,78). Patients with IgA nephropathy and polycystic kidney disease have lower requirements than other patients, and patients with hypertension appear to need higher doses than diabetics (3). The differences may be partly explained by underlying inflammatory conditions or infections. Patients with ESRD owing to SLE, vasculitis, and AIDS require relatively high doses, and EPO resistance is more common in blacks than whites (3). EPO dose requirements and hematocrit levels have both been shown to predict the risk of mortality (148).

Elevated hematocrit levels are accompanied by an elevation of blood pressure in approximately one-third of patients (149,150). Nevertheless, the hypertrophic cardiomyopathy of ESRD has been observed to regress after EPO therapy, and hemodynamic improvement has been seen with dilated cardiomyopathy (151–154). Some centers have experienced an increased frequency of vascular access thrombosis (155). Most centers have not, and coronary and cerebrovascular thrombosis and pulmonary embolization have not been found to complicate the correction of anemia (156).

Hemorrhage into skin, mucous membranes, and gastrointestinal tract is a common problem in the patient with ESRD. The bleeding tendency is attributed to platelet dysfunction. Platelets are normal in number but appear unable to adequately adhere to damaged blood vessels and form hemostatic plugs (157).

## Chronic Hepatitis

The screening of blood products for hepatitis B, the implementation of anti-hepatitis B vaccination programs, and the availability of EPO for the treatment of the anemia has reduced the number of HBsAg carriers in the ESRD population. At the time of a 1995 survey by the Centers for Disease Control, the prevalence of HBsAg carriers among U.S. dialysis patients was 1.1% (158). Hepatitis C virus is the most common cause of chronic liver disease in ESRD, and antibody to hepatitis C virus (anti-HCV) can be detected in 10 to 40% of hemodialysis patients (159,160). The prevalence of seropositivity is related to the number of transfusions that the patients have received.

Liver biopsies have demonstrated chronic liver disease in 50% to 100% of anti-HCV–positive patients (161,162). Martin et al (162) found mild or moderate necroinflammatory changes in all of 28 anti-HCV–positive patients who had liver biopsies while being referred for transplantation. Fibrosis was seen in 79%, and 3 of the 28 (11%) had cirrhosis. Neither hepatitis B or C infection seems to change mortality rates of dialysis patients (160,163,164).

## Central Nervous System

Central nervous system disorders in ESRD have been defined clinically as cerebrovascular disease, uremic encephalopathy, dialysis disequilibrium syndromes, and dialysis dementia (165). Cerebrovascular disease is responsible for the deaths of 5% of ESRD patients. Cerebral infarction accounts for most of these deaths with smaller numbers being the result of cerebral hemorrhage or subdural hematomas. The clinical manifestations of uremic encephalopathy are lethargy, confusion, obtundation, and coma (165). The signs and symptoms can evolve rapidly in patients with acute renal failure and are less often seen in patients who slowly progress to chronic renal failure. If patients have been severely hypertensive, the brain at autopsy may show fibrinoid necrosis of small arteries and provide evidence of a hypertensive encephalopathy. Otherwise, the brain may reveal only nonspecific changes of cerebral edema, or if patients have been dehydrated, the brain may be dry and reduced in size. The dialysis disequilibrium syndrome is characterized by nausea, vomiting, tremor, muscle cramps, dizziness, and blurred vision (165). It is seen in new dialysis patients who develop cerebral edema with intensive hemodialysis. Dialysis dementia is caused by the chronic toxicity of aluminum absorbed from oral phosphate binders or dialysate water. Aluminum exposure is now closely controlled, and dialysis dementia has almost disappeared as a clinical syndrome (165).

## Secondary Parathyroid Hyperplasia

As kidney function is lost, inorganic phosphate normally excreted by the kidneys is retained and serum phosphate levels become elevated. Because calcium and phosphate are present in serum near their solubility product, the rise in phosphate lowers calcium levels, and low ionized calcium stimulates the parathyroid glands to secrete parathyroid hormone. Parathyroid hormone levels, reaching eight to ten times normal, promote osteoclastic activity and the release of mineralized calcium from bone (166).

The kidney is the main tissue that converts 25(OH)-vitamin $D_3$ into 1,25(OH)$_2$-vitamin $D_3$ or calcitriol, the most metabolically active form of vitamin D, which promotes intestinal calcium absorption. The diseased kidney is unable to maintain normal calcitriol levels. This reduces the intestinal absorption of calcium and further contributes to

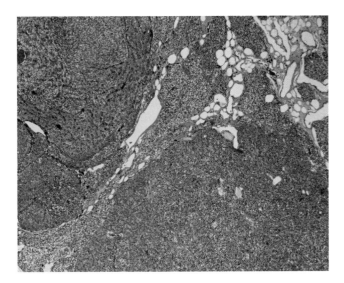

**Figure 27.11** Secondary parathyroid hyperplasia in a 47-year-old chronic hemodialysis patient. Nodules of oxyphil cells are separated by chief cells in a parathyroid gland that weighed 1.12 g. (H&E, ×40.)

secondary parathyroid hyperplasia. In addition, calcitriol normally acts through the vitamin D receptor to inhibit parathyroid hormone transcription and growth of parathyroid cells (167). Low serum levels of calcitriol, by loss of this inhibitory activity, directly contribute to the increased secretion of parathyroid hormone and promote parathyroid hyperplasia. Calcitriol or synthetic vitamin D analogs are administered with calcium salts to many ESRD patients to suppress secondary hyperparathyroidism.

All four parathyroid glands and any accessory glands are enlarged in cases of secondary hyperplasia, although there can be considerable variation in the size of each gland. Single gland weights can range from less than 100 mg to more than 2 g (normal combined gland weight is 50 to 300 mg). The enlargement may be diffuse or nodular. Histologically, the hyperplasia is composed of a mixture of chief cells and oxyphil cells with chief cells usually predominating (Fig. 27.11).

In cases of refractory secondary hyperparathyroidism, clonal chromosomal changes have been detected in the parathyroid glands of 61% of dialysis patients (168). The most common abnormality was a deletion of 1p that was found in 71% of the glands having chromosomal abnormalities. A deletion of 1p is the most common cytogenetic abnormality found in parathyroid adenomas, and the recurring clonality of the deletion in secondary hyperplasia suggests a neoplastic process and the involvement of a tumor suppressor gene (168).

## Renal Osteodystrophy

The term *renal osteodystrophy* encompasses the disorders osteitis fibrosa, osteomalacia, mixed patterns of osteitis fi-

brosa and osteomalacia, and adynamic bone disease (166). Osteitis fibrosa is caused by secondary hyperparathyroidism. It is characterized by a high rate of bone formation and resorption and is referred to as *high-turnover bone disease*. Parathyroid hormone activates bone remodeling by stimulating marrow stromal cells to proliferate and differentiate into osteoblasts and fibroblasts (166). Parathyroid hormone also promotes a proliferation of osteoclasts either directly or through cytokines and growth factors produced by marrow stromal cells and osteoblasts (169). The most important of these locally produced factors appear to be macrophage colony-stimulating factor, interleukin-6, osteoprotegerin, and receptor activator of NF-κB ligand (RANKL).

The bones then undergo a continuing process of resorption and deposition that is not under the normal control of local mechanical strain. The cortex of long bones becomes more porous, and the trabecular bone of the medulla becomes thicker as a result of an increase in unmineralized woven bone or osteoid. Histologically, bone biopsies show an increased number of trabeculae composed of lamellar, mineralized bone of irregular shape and thickness lined by increased amounts of osteoid (166) (Fig. 27.12). Osteoblasts are prominently clustered along the osteoid. Trabeculae are surrounded by fibrous tissue and are scalloped by osteoclasts within Howship's lacunae (Fig. 27.13). Unconnected trabecular islands can be seen within the medullary fibrous tissue emphasizing the lack of organization to the remodeling. The bones are susceptible to spontaneous fractures and, in advanced cases, develop medullary cysts and become markedly deformed.

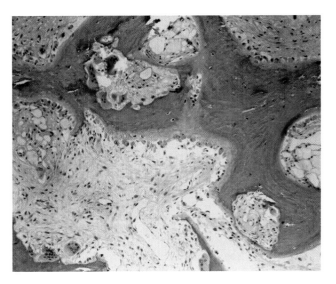

**Figure 27.12** Osteitis fibrosa in a 27-year-old hemodialysis patient with secondary hyperparathyroidism. Fibrous tissue surrounds irregularly shaped trabeculae with numerous multinucleated osteoclasts. Undecalcified section. (H&E, ×100.)

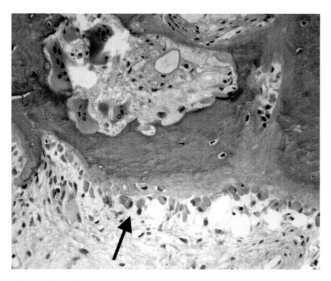

**Figure 27.13**   Higher magnification of Figure 27.12. Irregularly shaped trabeculae with a widened zone of unmineralized osteoid are lined on the lower edge by osteoblasts (*arrow*). Osteoclasts are identified in Howship's lacunae in the center. (Undecalcified section; H&E, ×200.)

Osteomalacia is a low-turnover bone disease and in most cases is the result of aluminum toxicity (166). Osteomalacia softens the bones that can then become deformed and fracture with mild mechanical stress. Bone biopsies show normal numbers of abnormally thickened trabeculae (166). The trabeculae consist of a core of irregularly thickened and thinned lamellar bone surrounded by a markedly widened zone of osteoid (Fig. 27.14). Osteoblasts and osteoclasts are reduced below the number found in normal

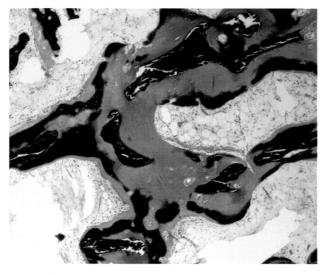

**Figure 27.14**   Osteomalacia in a long-term hemodialysis patient with low-turnover bone disease. There is a marked excess of pink-staining osteoid and no osteoblastic or osteoclastic activity. The mineralized parts of the trabeculae are stained black. (Undecalcified section; von Kossa, ×100.)

bone and are sparsely seen in histologic sections. Mixed bone disease shows a background of osteomalacia with foci of osteitis fibrosa in which there is increased osteoblastic and osteoclastic activity (166).

Adynamic bone disease is also a low-turnover state (166). It can be caused by aluminum overload, but nearly two thirds of the patients have no evidence of bone aluminum deposition (170). Patients with adynamic bone disease have bone pain of uncertain cause. In some patients, pain may be the result of microfractures of trabecular bone. In cases of aluminum overload, bone pain can sometimes be rapidly relieved by treatment with deferoxamine. Bone biopsies of adynamic bone disease show normal to decreased numbers of normal appearing or thinned trabeculae composed of lamellar bone with reduced numbers of osteocytes (166,170,171). The trabeculae show little or no osteoid and few osteoblasts or osteoclasts.

Rates of bone turnover in a renal osteodystrophy can be measured histomorphometrically by double tetracycline labeling in which a bone biopsy is done after two doses of tetracycline, with the doses being administered 2 weeks apart. The tetracycline is deposited in the matrix of newly formed bone, and under ultraviolet light, the autofluorescent tetracycline can be seen along lines at which bone was forming at the time the antibiotic was given. Widely spaced lines of red-green fluorescence along lamellar bone indicate a high rate of bone turnover. Alternatively, narrowly spaced lines of fluorescence indicate low rates of bone formation. Histochemical stains such as alizarin red react stoichiometrically with aluminum. Aluminum bone disease can be diagnosed when a biopsy shows osteomalacia or normal-to-thinned bone, a low rate of bone turnover, and aluminum histochemical staining over 25% or more of the trabecular surfaces (171,172) (Fig. 27.15).

Current practice avoids the use of aluminum phosphate binders. Oral calcium carbonate and calcium acetate are used to bind dietary phosphate. The calcium salts are also used to increase gastrointestinal calcium absorption, and for patients who have more severe secondary hyperparathyroidism, oral calcium is given together with active vitamin D sterols (166,170). Parathyroid hormone secretion is controlled by the increased intestinal calcium absorption and by using dialysate solutions with calcium concentrations that allow a net calcium ion movement toward the patient (170).

These strategies usually suppress parathyroid hormone secretion and have greatly reduced the prevalence of osteitis fibrosa and aluminum bone disease as well as the need for parathyroidectomy. Some patients are unusually susceptible to developing hypercalcemia-associated muscle weakness, hypertension, or metastatic tissue calcification. They are unable to take oral calcium preparations and must still use aluminum gels. Osteitis fibrosa can still be seen in these patients, and parathyroidectomy may be needed to treat the bone disease (170). Vitamin D administration

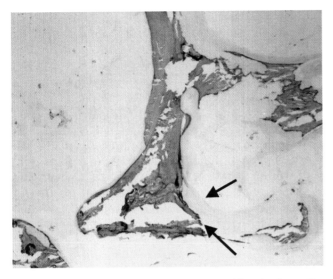

**Figure 27.15** Iliac crest bone biopsy stained for aluminum. Osteomalacia is diagnosed by the wide osteoid seams, represented by the pale-staining areas outside the mineralized bone (*arrows*). The aluminum histochemical reaction product is the red line at the interface between mineralized bone and osteoid. (Undecalcified section; alizarin red, ×200.)

has been associated with excessive soft tissue and vascular calcifications and is not recommended if serum calcium, corrected for albumin, is greater than 9.5 mg/dL or serum phosphorus is more than 4.5 mg/gL (173).

## Hypertension in End-Stage Renal Disease

Three types of hypertension have been recognized in ESRD (174,175). The least common is malignant hypertension in which patients have very high plasma renin levels. The patients often have an exaggerated rise in blood pressure when they are dialyzed. This is presumably caused by an increase in renin excretion that follows the reduction in intravascular volume. Bilateral nephrectomy usually is required for blood pressure control. Because of pharmacologic improvements in the treatment of high blood pressure, this type of hypertension is rarely seen today (175).

The most common type of hypertension is volume dependent (175). In hemodialysis patients, volume-dependent high blood pressure develops between dialysis sessions as a result of dietary salt and fluid intake. When patients are dialyzed to a dry weight and dry weight is maintained in the interdialytic period, blood pressure can be normalized. This is not easily attained, and 53% of hemodialysis patients have been reported to have predialysis systolic blood pressures of 150 mm Hg or greater (174). There is another common form of hypertension that does not respond well to dialysis, but it is not associated with elevated plasma renin levels. This type of hypertension has been related to secondary hyperparathyroidism and high serum and intracellular calcium concentrations (174,175).

Treatment of the hyperparathyroidism with vitamin D or parathyroidectomy has reduced blood pressure in some, but not all, series of such patients (174,176).

Weight gain and the expansion of intravascular volume between dialysis treatments often makes blood pressure control difficult during long-term hemodialysis. CAPD uses the diffusion and osmotic gradients created by glucose solutions continuously in place in the peritoneal cavity to steadily reduce total body sodium and water without the rapid volume shifts that accompany hemodialysis. Although CAPD patients have a greater elevation of plasma renin activity than hemodialysis patients, their hypertension tends to be more easily controlled (87,177).

## PATHOLOGY OF THE END-STAGE KIDNEY

### Background

In the late 1960s and during the 1970s, bilateral nephrectomies frequently were performed on ESRD patients to treat severe hypertension intractable to medical therapy or to prepare the patients for transplantation. A pathologic diagnosis of end-stage kidney would be rendered on many of these nephrectomy specimens or on end-stage autopsy kidneys, and little attempt would be made to clarify the underlying disease. In 1976, Schwartz and Cotran (178) examined 95 pretransplant nephrectomies by light and immunofluorescent microscopy and were able to diagnose the primary disease in 90 cases. By studying glomeruli that were not in an advanced state of sclerosis, they were able to classify 34 of 47 cases of chronic glomerulonephritis as a specific glomerular disease. The study showed that the original disease could be determined in many end-stage kidneys.

In 1977, Dunnill et al (179) reported the striking cystic change of kidneys from 14 hemodialysis patients who were known not to have had renal cystic disease prior to the onset of renal failure. These authors coined the term *acquired renal cystic disease* (ARCD) and identified renal cell carcinomas or adenomas in six cases.

The early descriptions of the end-stage kidney emphasized the severe arteriosclerosis of the intrarenal arteries (76). Heptinstall referred to the arterial thickening as a "disuse endarteritis" and related its development to the reduced perfusion of the kidneys (76). Despite the reduced blood flow, the arteries and arterioles of kidneys removed to control hypertension showed the effects of the prior elevated blood pressure (180). The histologic examination of some cases demonstrated hyperplasia of renin-containing cells in the juxtaglomerular apparatus and afferent arterioles and helped clarify the pathogenesis of the hypertension.

Gross and microscopic criteria will be provided below for placing an end-stage kidney into one of six major categories of disease: hypertension, diabetes, glomerulonephritis, ischemic nephropathy, and obstructive and nonobstructive interstitial nephritis. Much of the material in the following sections will describe more general features of the end-stage kidney. It will point out the rather remarkable degree of cellular proliferation that occurs in this background of chronic disease and will emphasize the development of ARCD- and ESRD-associated renal cell carcinomas.

## Gross Pathology

End-stage kidneys are usually reduced in size unless they are involved by ARCD. Most end-stage kidneys that have not undergone any degree of cystic change weigh in the range of 40 to 120 g, but some are very small (5). The kidneys frequently contain cysts filled with clear yellow to cloudy green fluid. Some of the subcapsular cysts project through the renal capsule, and many will rupture if the capsules are stripped from the kidneys.

## Hypertension, Diabetes, and Glomerulonephritis

The subcapsular surface of kidneys from patients with hypertension, diabetes, and glomerulonephritis has a granular appearance (Fig. 27.16). End-stage diabetic kidneys are frequently larger than expected and may show no apparent reduction in size. In contrast, the kidneys of patients with end-stage glomerulonephritis are often severely contacted and can weigh as little as 5 g (5). In all three conditions, the kidneys have conically shaped renal pyramids and a pelvicaliceal system that is not dilated and that is lined by a normal transitional mucosa. Kidneys removed for malignant hypertension may show some hemorrhages in the

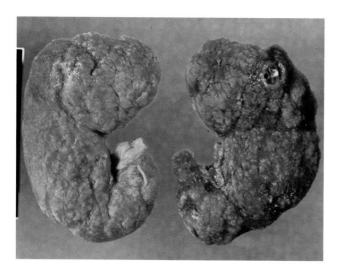

**Figure 27.16**  Kidney from a patient with end-stage chronic glomerulonephritis. Both kidneys were markedly reduced in size (40 g each). The subcapsular surface is coarsely granular.

subcapsular cortex and pelvic mucosa, but more often such hemorrhages are inconspicuous or are not present in the end-stage kidney (32,76). Small arteries stand out prominently at the corticomedullary junction and as radially oriented cordlike structures in the lower cortex. The interlobar arteries are concentrically thickened and lumens may be reduced to pinpoint size. The main renal artery of kidneys from younger patients may not be appreciably thickened, but atherosclerotic plaques will frequently be found in the proximal parts of the main renal artery in kidneys from patients with diabetes and hypertension. In diabetics and other patients with hypercholesterolemia, yellow atheromatous plaques may be seen in segmental and interlobar arteries.

## Ischemic Nephropathy

Ischemic nephropathy is caused by renal vascular disease. Most cases occur after 50 years of age and are the result of aortic or renal artery atherosclerosis. It is also seen with large vessel vasculitis (Takayasu disease and giant cell arteritis), polyarteritis nodosa, fibromuscular dysplasia, and Kawasaki disease in children (181,182). Aortic atherosclerosis, with or without an abdominal aneurysm, can produce stenosis of the renal artery ostia, and atherosclerotic narrowing of the proximal renal artery can reduce and, in some cases, completely obstruct the flow of blood to the kidneys.

Atherosclerotic renal artery stenosis is often bilateral, but one kidney typically is affected more severely than the other (182,183). Ischemic nephropathy produces irregular scarring of the renal cortex (Fig. 27.17). Kidneys with accessory renal arteries show marked contraction of the part of the kidney supplied by a narrowed or occluded artery and preservation or relative preservation of the part supplied by a nonstenotic accessory artery.

Atheromatous material mechanically disrupted by operative or invasive intravascular procedures or spontaneously dislodged from the surface of ulcerated atheromatous plaques can embolize into the kidney (184). These emboli can be associated with deep, broad-based cortical scars that in some instances represent old infarcts and in other instances areas of ischemic atrophy.

## Interstitial Nephritis

Interstitial nephritis or tubulointerstitial nephritis comprises those renal diseases in which the pathologic changes are directed primarily toward the interstitial compartment of the kidney and its tubules. The classification of tubulointerstitial nephritis consists of a long list of disorders that are discussed in Chapter 23. This section will consider the pathology of those diseases that cause a substantial number of cases of ESRD. These are chronic obstructive and nonobstructive pyelonephritis and chronic drug-induced

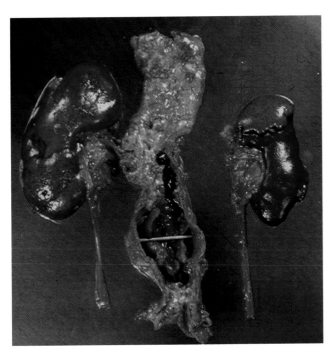

**Figure 27.17** Ischemic nephropathy. The patient died of a myocardial infarct after being treated for renal failure by hemodialysis for 3 months. Parts of both kidneys are contracted or scarred owing to bilateral atherosclerotic renal artery stenosis above a large abdominal aneurysm.

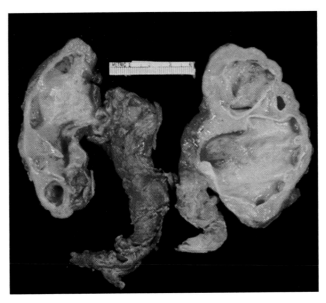

**Figure 27.18** End-stage chronic obstructive pyelonephritis. Ureters and the pelvicaliceal system are thickened and dilated. The renal papillae are blunted, and the renal cortex is markedly thinned.

interstitial nephritis (77). The myeloma kidney and other renal diseases found in plasma cell dyscrasias are covered in detail in Chapter 19.

Chronic pyelonephritis is the late result of bacterial infections that have reached the kidney from the lower urinary tract (185). As a cause of ESRD, chronic obstructive pyelonephritis is most common in older males with benign hyperplasia or carcinoma of the prostate. It is seen with bladder stones, and in women, it is a frequent complication of uterine malignancy.

The kidneys of chronic obstructive pyelonephritis show dilatation of the ureter, renal pelvis, and caliceal system (Fig. 27.18). The collecting system is lined by a transitional mucosa thickened by chronic inflammation and fibrosis (185). Renal pyramids entering the dilated calices are blunted, and the overlying renal cortex is contracted into broad-based scars owing to chronic tubulointerstitial inflammation.

Struvite renal stones are commonly present in the chronically infected kidney, and large staghorn calculi are formed in some cases (186). In many patients, it is the nephrolithiasis rather than the extent of inflammatory damage that seems to lead to ESRD. Nephrolithiasis was considered to be responsible for the ESRD of 3.2% of patients entering dialysis programs at the Necker Hospital, Paris, France, from 1989 through 1990, and 42% of the nephrolithiasis was owing to underlying kidney infections (186).

Patients with chronic nonobstructive pyelonephritis have vesicoureteral reflux, but they do not have obstruction to urine flow in the lower urinary tract (185). The kidney shows dilatation of one or more calices and large, flattened scars deforming the overlying cortex. This most commonly occurs at the poles of the kidney where compound papillae drain fused renal lobes (185).

Analgesic nephropathy is seen in patients who over time consume hundreds of grams or thousands of pills of an analgesic (187,188). The condition was originally described in phenacetin abusers, but after phenacetin was removed from a large part of the world market in the 1970s, analgesic nephropathy continued to be seen with mixtures containing acetaminophen and aspirin (188,189). It is seen with acetaminophen alone and in patients who take large amounts of nonsteroidal anti-inflammatory drugs (188, 189,190). Cigarette smoking, excessive caffeine consumption, and chronic alcoholism have been suggested as contributing factors (188).

The gross appearance of analgesic nephropathy can be similar to that of chronic nonobstructive pyelonephritis. Both are characterized by scarring and inflammation of the renal cortex and by alterations of the underlying papillae. In analgesic nephropathy, papillary necrosis is invariably present, and most of the pyramids are involved (see Chapter 23). Some are partially necrotic and show a central pale discoloration. Others are completely necrotic and may have sloughed from the kidney, leaving a cavitary defect beneath the cortex. Necrotic remnants of papillae may be found lying free within the pelvis. Necrotic papillae that remain attached to the kidney often contain gross calcifications.

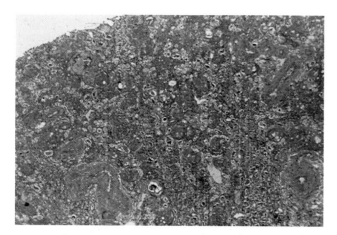

**Figure 27.19** Low-power view of kidney with great reduction in size. There is diffuse glomerular solidification and generalized tubular atrophy. From a 22-year-old woman with end-stage glomerulonephritis who had been on dialysis for 15 months. She had been anuric for a year and had developed accelerated hypertension. (H&E, ×40.)

## Microscopic Pathology

The end-stage kidney is characterized by advanced glomerulosclerosis, tubular loss and atrophy, and some degree of cystic change. The renal blood vessels are thickened, and many end-stage kidneys contain extensive oxalate crystal deposits. The granular appearance of kidneys from patients with hypertension, chronic glomerulonephritis, and diabetes is produced by depressed areas of atrophy that alternate with cortex having normal or hypertrophied nephrons. In some cases of chronic glomerulonephritis, there is a diffuse pattern of glomerular solidification with generalized tubular atrophy and loss in which the cortex is smooth rather than granular (Fig. 27.19).

## Glomeruli

Chronically diseased kidneys show patterns of glomerulosclerosis that lead to the effacement of normal glomerular capillary structure. This is referred to as glomerular obsolescence, and the final structure is termed a *hyalinized* or *obsolete glomerulus*. Different patterns of glomerular obsolescence as well as pathologic changes in less severely involved glomeruli can be used to classify the renal disease that has led to ESRD.

### Hypertension and Ischemic Glomerular Obsolescence

Hypertension and ischemic nephropathy produce a type of glomerular loss termed *ischemic glomerular obsolescence* (32,60). In its early stages, glomerular capillary basement membranes are thickened because of wrinkling. The glomerular tuft then contracts toward the hilar pole and becomes simplified into fewer capillary loops. At the same

time, fibrous connective tissue builds up on the inside of the basement membrane of Bowman's capsule. This process, termed *intracapsular fibrosis*, eventually fills Bowman's space with acellular fibrous tissue having the staining characteristics of collagen. The structure of the ischemic glomerulus is best studied with the PAS stain. The intracapsular fibrosis is pale pink and is encircled by the bright magenta staining basement membrane of Bowman's capsule. The glomerular tuft also stains a deep magenta and is contracted into a small hyalinized knot at the vascular pole where it is surrounded by the intracapsular fibrosis. The basement membrane of Bowman's capsule remains relatively intact until late stages of glomerular obsolescence when it becomes disrupted into small fragments and the glomerulus gradually disappears.

In patients with hypertension, perfusion of the renal cortex is reduced by arteriosclerotic intimal thickening of the interlobular and arcuate arteries (57,58). This leads to the development of scars in the subcapsular cortex that contain clusters of glomeruli showing ischemic obsolescence (32). These areas of scarring may be small and identified only by the presence of a few obsolete glomeruli, or they can be larger and show increased amounts of interstitial fibrous tissue where tubules have been lost. Atrophic, colloid-containing tubules are found in the fibrous scars, and adjacent tubules are frequently hypertrophic and dilated. Some chronic inflammation is usually present. It may be quite intense and notably conspicuous beside hyalinized glomeruli.

### Ischemic Nephropathy

Ischemic nephropathy is caused by the reduction of renal blood flow through the large renal arteries. Histologically, the grossly angular or broad-based cortical scars of an ischemic nephropathy show wide areas of atrophy that contain many ischemic glomeruli reflecting the larger size of the involved vessels. Evidence of cholesterol embolization may be seen (Fig. 27.20), and cortical infarcts sometimes are found (184). Patients with ischemic nephropathy frequently have secondary renovascular hypertension or they may have coexisting essential hypertension (182). The high blood pressure produces intimal thickening in the interlobular and arcuate arteries, and areas of subcapsular fibrosis, attributable to the small artery arteriosclerosis, develop in the kidney or parts of kidneys exposed to the elevated blood pressure (182).

### Diabetes

End-stage diabetes reveals diabetic glomerulosclerosis involving most of the glomeruli in the kidney. Glomeruli not in an advanced state of obsolescence show diffuse thickening of glomerular capillary basement membranes, increased mesangial matrix, and an expansion of mesangial matrix into intercapillary (Kimmelstiel-Wilson) nodules (Fig. 27.21). As these diabetic changes progress, they

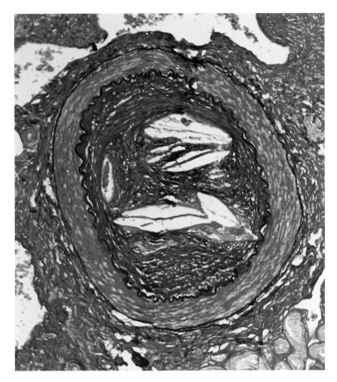

**Figure 27.20** Kidney from a patient with renal failure owing to ischemic nephropathy showing an arcuate artery occluded by cholesterol emboli and intimal fibrous tissue. (Aldehyde fuchsin–Van Gieson, ×100.)

solidify glomeruli into large hyalinized structures about the size of a normal glomerulus (60). With a PAS stain or with the Jones methenamine silver method, Kimmelstiel-Wilson nodules and hyalinosis lesions can be observed in glomeruli in late stages of obsolescence. In addition

to large solidified glomeruli, a variable number of hyalinized glomeruli will be found that are contracted and show ischemic changes. Arterio-arteriolosclerosis is severe in the late-stage diabetic kidney. Afferent arterioles are thickened and hyalinized, and when the hilum of the glomerulus is cut in cross section, both afferent and efferent arteriolar hyalinization can be seen. In diabetes, the renal tubules show basement membrane thickening, and there is a degree of tubular loss and atrophy that corresponds to the severity of glomerulosclerosis.

## Glomerulonephritis

Glomerulonephritis results in a pattern of obsolescence that solidifies glomerular tufts in a manner that, unlike ischemia, results in little reduction in their size (60,76). Glomerular capsular adhesions are created in most forms of glomerulonephritis. During the development of the solidified tuft, the basement membrane of Bowman's capsule is fragmented and partially lost, and the sclerotic glomerulus becomes surrounded by small tubular structures termed *pseudo-tubules* or *adenomatoid lesions* (Fig. 27.22). Cases of membranous glomerulopathy sometimes retain glomeruli showing diffuse basement membrane thickening within an open Bowman's space while the tubulointerstitial compartment is severely atrophic (76). Silver stains may reveal spikes or holes in the glomerular basement membranes. Membranoproliferative glomerulonephritis often shows a prominent lobular pattern into late stages of obsolescence (76).

Immunofluorescence and electron microscopy are helpful in making a diagnosis of a specific type of glomerulonephritis. Immunofluorescence microscopy is required to distinguish IgA nephropathy from other types of sclerosing glomerular diseases, although a predominantly

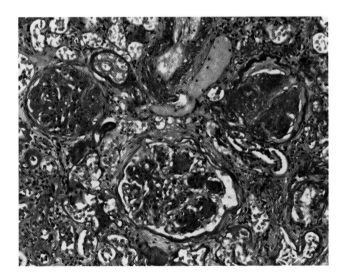

**Figure 27.21** Glomerular obsolescence in an end-stage diabetic nephropathy. Solidified glomeruli lie beside a less severely involved glomerulus showing basement membrane thickening, expansion of the mesangium, and intercapillary (Kimmelstiel-Wilson) nodules. (PAS, ×150.)

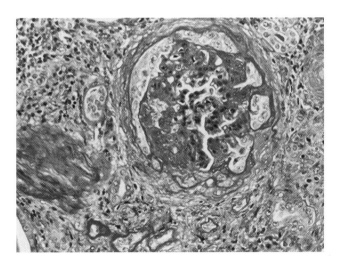

**Figure 27.22** Sclerotic, partially solidified glomerulus from a case of end-stage glomerulonephritis. Tubulelike structures lined by epithelial cells are present over the sclerotic tuft and separated by adhesions to Bowman's capsule. (Alcian blue–PAS, ×200.)

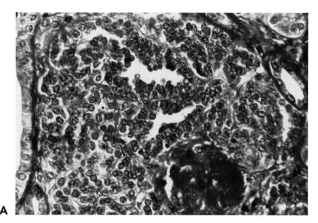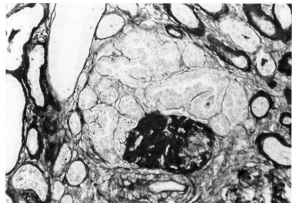

**Figure 27.23**    **A:** Embryonal hyperplasia of Bowman's capsular epithelium forms delicate tubulopapillary structures beside a hyalinized glomerulus. (Luxol fast blue–hematoxylin, ×200.) **B:** The hyalinized remnant of the glomerulus is emphasized in this micrograph, which shows the embryonal hyperplasia of Bowman's capsular epithelium surrounding an obsolete glomerular tuft. (PAS, ×200.)

mesangioproliferative pattern may be seen in less severely affected glomeruli. IgA nephropathy shows prominent mesangial electron-dense deposits when examined by electron microscopy and predominant or codominant staining for IgA by immunofluorescent microscopy.

Many hyalinosis lesions and an absence of electron microscopic and immunofluorescent findings characteristic of another type of glomerulonephritis is consistent with idiopathic focal segmental glomerulosclerosis. Hyalinosis lesions in all forms of glomerular disease show immunofluorescence staining with IgM and C3. The diagnostic immunofluorescence and electron microscopic features of a specific type of glomerular disease are found in the parts of glomeruli still retaining patent capillary loops away from the hyalinosis lesions (178).

### Pyelonephritis

Four types of glomerular injury can be found in chronic pyelonephritis. For a detailed discussion of their significance and histologic appearance, the reader is referred to Chapter 22. The most characteristic is periglomerular fibrosis. Bowman's space is open and the glomerular tuft and parietal epithelium are not notably changed, but the basement membrane of Bowman's capsule is thickened and surrounded by loose layers of connective tissue in a lamellar arrangement. Arteriosclerosis of large and small renal arteries is invariably present in long-standing chronic pyelonephritis, and a considerable amount of glomerular loss is the result of ischemic glomerular obsolescence. Focal and segmental glomerulosclerosis with hyalinosis can be seen, particularly if the patient has significant proteinuria (191). Cases of end-stage chronic pyelonephritis as well as other diseases complicated by malignant hypertension can show fibrinoid necrosis of glomeruli, and some of the affected glomeruli develop cellular crescents.

### Embryonal Hyperplasia of Bowman's Capsular Epithelium

As many as one third of end-stage kidneys reveals a proliferation of small dark embryonal-appearing cells that surround obsolete glomeruli (192) (Fig. 27.23). These cellular proliferations have been termed *embryonal hyperplasia of Bowman's capsular epithelium* (EHBCE). In early stages, the cells line pseudotubular structures, but larger lesions form cell clusters that can be more than twice the size of a normal glomerulus (192). Serial histologic sections may be needed to demonstrate the association of EHBCE with a remnant of a glomerulus.

Kishani et al (193) reported EHBCE in the bilateral nephrectomies of a 9 year-old male with end-stage FSGS. A 1 cm tumor was present in one kidney that resembled a metanephric adenoma. The authors observed that EHBCE morphologically, immunohistochemically, and ultrastructurally resembled the metanephric adenoma and proposed that both originated from the same cell type. Interstitial epithelial proliferations composed of small dark cells indistinguishable from those of EHBCE are found in tubules that seem to have no association with obsolete glomeruli. Ogata (194) identified these interstitial lesions in one third of pediatric end-stage kidneys.

### Unusual Epithelial Growth or Endothelial Metaplasia

McManus et al (195,196) studied serial sections of end-stage kidneys and found unusual patterns of cell growth that were limited to single specimens but reinforced the idea that a remarkable degree of regeneration was occurring in these chronically and severely injured kidneys. Under the title "Dialysis Enhances Epithelial Proliferation," a complex structure was described that resembled EHBCE by originating near a glomerulus (195). The lesion grew

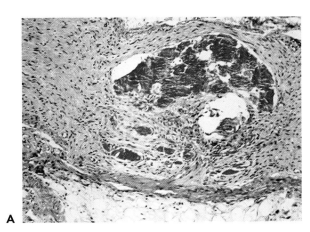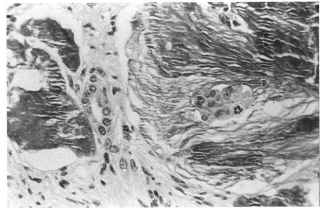

**Figure 27.24** **A:** Nerve containing epithelial inclusions within an extracellular PAS-positive material. The section was taken from the hilum of an end-stage kidney of a patient on hemodialysis for more than 2 years. (PAS–hematoxylin, ×100.) **B:** High magnification of the nerve showing a glandlike inclusion with a mitotic figure within the PAS-positive mucinous material. (PAS-hematoxylin, ×400.)

within a tubule lumen creating branching nests of cells with multiple outpouchings and blind ends. The same kidney contained a tubule that grew along and then into a large myelinated renal nerve at the renal hilum and formed nests of loosely cohesive and mitotically active cells (Fig. 27.24). Another kidney demonstrated metaplastic squamous epithelium in tubules adjacent to an infarct (196). By itself, this would not be an unexpected response in the urinary tract since it commonly occurs in the prostate gland. But more remarkable was the presence of cells resembling cuboidal tubular epithelium that lined the lumen of an artery (Fig. 27.25). From the artery, the epithelial-like cells extended into the more peripheral arterioles and then into the lumens of the glomerular capillaries. In some glomeruli, the intracapillary cells assumed features of squamous epithelium with distinct intercellular bridges.

## Juxtaglomerular Apparatus

End-stage kidneys removed from patients with malignant hypertension and high plasma renin levels show hyperplasia of granular cells in the juxtaglomerular apparatus of obsolete glomeruli (180) (Fig. 27.26). Granules also can be seen in hypertrophied smooth muscle cells along most of the length of afferent arterioles where the modification of cells is termed *granular cell metaplasia.*

Faraggiana et al (197) studied the immunohistochemical staining and distribution of renin in the end-stage kidneys of five patients with nondiabetic renal disease who had severe hypertension that could not be readily lowered by dialysis. Also studied were three cases of end-stage diabetic glomerulosclerosis in which patients were mildly hypertensive. Intense renin immunoreactivity was found in the glomeruli and afferent arterioles of the patients with severe dialysis-resistant hypertension. In two of the cases, the degree of renal atrophy was so advanced that most of

the glomeruli had disappeared. In these cases, many arterioles showed the strong renin staining. In contrast, the kidneys of diabetic patients demonstrated only minimal renin immunoreactivity that was even less than the staining in normal control kidneys (197). This anatomic finding correlates with the clinical observation that diabetics rarely develop high plasma renin activity and malignant hypertension (37).

## Blood Vessels

The intrarenal arteries of end-stage kidneys are markedly thickened and the lumens severely narrowed. This is referred to as *obliterative intimal fibrosis* because of the concentric thickening of the arterial intima by collagenous connective tissue containing moderate numbers of spindle cells (76). The spindle cells are identified as myointimal cells by their positive immunohistochemical staining for smooth muscle actin. Electron microscopy of the intimal cells demonstrates thin cytoplasmic filaments and cytoplasmic membrane-dense bodies characteristic of smooth muscle (76). Obliterative intimal fibrosis is considered to be an adaptive change to increased vascular resistance resulting from the loss of the peripheral microvascular bed (76).

The intrarenal arteries of kidneys removed for severe hypertension show a pronounced intimal thickening composed of mucoid ground substance and many myointimal cells (180,198) (Fig. 27.27). If there has not been a history of chronic hypertension, the internal elastic lamina may show minimal, if any, duplication. Mucoid ground substance focally involves the media, and in such areas, medial smooth muscle cells can be found crossing the internal elastic lamina where they appear to be migrating into the intima. Intimal smooth muscle frequently is oriented tightly around the narrowed arterial lumen in the fashion of a new internalized media (199) (Fig. 27.28).

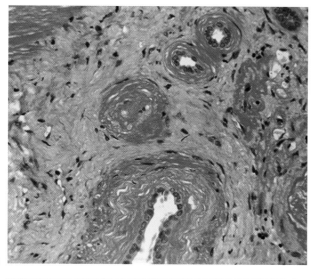

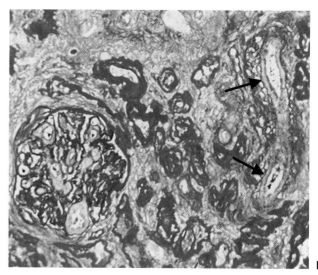

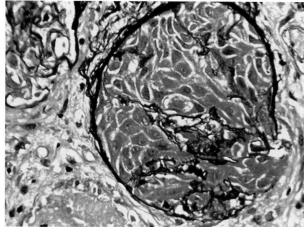

**Figure 27.25**   A 64-g kidney of a 27-year-old hemodialysis patient with end-stage hypertensive renal disease. **A:** Cuboidal epithelial-like cells line the lumen of a small artery and a segment of arteriole. (PAS–hematoxylin, ×200.) **B:** An arteriole (*arrows*) is lined by cuboidal tubularlike cells that are also present within a nearby glomerulus. (Alcian blue–PAS, ×200.) **C:** Squamous epithelial metaplasia lies within the capillaries of a glomerulus. (Periodic acid–methenamine silver–hematoxylin, ×400.)

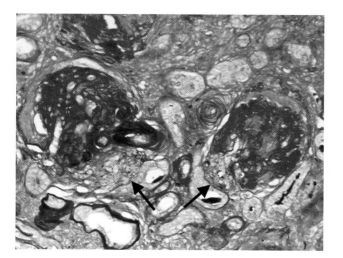

**Figure 27.26**   Prominent granular cells (*arrows*) are seen in the hyperplastic juxtaglomerular apparatus of two obsolete glomeruli. The specimen was from a bilateral nephrectomy performed to treat pharmacologically intractable malignant hypertension. The patient had been treated by hemodialysis for 6 weeks and had very high plasma renin levels. (Luxol fast blue–PAS, ×200.)

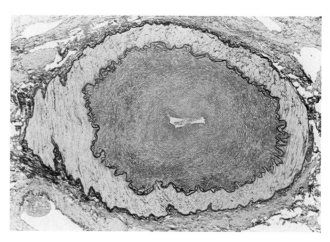

**Figure 27.27**   Musculomucoid intimal hyperplasia of an interlobar artery. The intima is markedly thickened by dark-staining mucoid ground substance. There is minimal reduplication of the internal elastic lamina. (Aldehyde fuchsin–Weigert's hematoxylin–Van Gieson, ×100.)

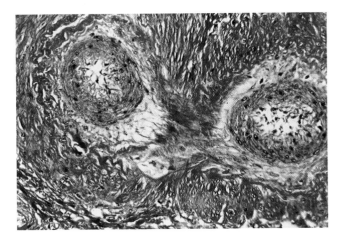

**Figure 27.28** Remodeling or remedialization of an interlobular artery in a hemodialysis patient. Smooth muscle is rearranged within the intima to form a collar of cells resembling a second media around the lumen. (H&E, ×400.)

This type of vascular change was termed *musculomucoid intimal hyperplasia* by Pitcock et al (198), who described its occurrence in blacks with malignant hypertension. The histopathology resembles or is identical to the arterial pathology of malignant hypertension and acute scleroderma. The arteries most severely affected in scleroderma and malignant hypertension, however, measure less than 200 μm in diameter (distal arcuate and interlobular arteries), whereas musculomucoid intimal hyperplasia in dialysis kidneys involves intrarenal arteries of all sizes (76).

Obliterative intimal fibrosis and musculomucoid intimal hyperplasia probably represent a continuum of arterial pathology rather than different types of vascular disease. Musculomucoid intimal hyperplasia is likely to change into the picture of obliterative intimal fibrosis when myointimal cells begin to synthesize increased amounts of collagen and the intimal mucopolysaccharide content is reduced.

In the series of Pitcock et al (198), the patients rapidly developed malignant hypertension, but musculomucoid intimal hyperplasia was not accompanied by arterial necrosis. Many of the patients had no prior history of benign hypertension, and it was suggested that musculomucoid intimal hyperplasia may have been the cause of hypertension. McManus et al (180) reported on 12 dialysis patients with high plasma renin levels who underwent bilateral nephrectomy for malignant hypertension. The kidneys showed hyperplasia of the juxtaglomerular apparatus of obsolete glomeruli, musculomucoid intimal hyperplasia of intrarenal arteries, and fibrinoid necrosis of arteries and arterioles. Five of the patients had end-stage glomerulonephritis and one had chronic pyelonephritis. In these cases, malignant hypertension was considered to be secondary to parenchymal renal disease.

In musculomucoid intimal hyperplasia with arterial necrosis, the interlobular arteries show an insudate of fi-

brin and red cells that dissects along the mucoid intima and focally extends into the media (180,199). Fibrinoid necrosis is found in afferent arterioles, and in some arterioles, the cells of the vessel wall proliferate to form arteriolar nodules (Figs. 27.29). Many are solid smooth muscle nodules and resemble small leiomyomas. Others are vascular and resemble the plexiform lesions of the lung that are found in the small pulmonary arteries of patients with high grades of pulmonary hypertension. Arteriolar nodules are also seen in organs other than the kidney (pancreas, adrenal capsule, heart, paravertebral ganglia) of patients with treated malignant hypertension (200) (Fig. 27.30).

The veins of end-stage kidneys are thickened by bundles of smooth muscle and fibrous tissue (199). The bundles of smooth muscle are frequently oriented parallel to the long axis of the vein in a configuration that has been termed *nodular phlebosclerosis*. The walls of the thickened veins sometimes enclose tubules lined by cuboidal clear cells (Fig. 27.31). The tubules seem to be entrapped atrophic tubules, although the epithelium sometimes demonstrates mitoses (199).

## Tubules and Interstitium

Injury to the tubules and interstitium can be primary when the disease is directed toward tubules and interstitium or secondary when the initiating pathology principally involves glomeruli and blood vessels. In either case, the kidneys of ESRD patients show marked interstitial fibrosis, tubular atrophy, and some amount of chronic interstitial inflammation.

### Interstitial Nephritis, Differential Diagnosis

Chronic pyelonephritis shows inflammation of the renal parenchyma that consists mainly of lymphocytes, macrophages, and plasma cells (185). The lymphoid infiltrate is frequently arranged in follicles with prominent germinal centers. Some eosinophils are present, and in some cases, neutrophils may be numerous. The inflammation is primarily interstitial, but neutrophil infiltrates and casts may be found in tubules. Areas of chronic inflammation are seen that contain atrophic tubules having a thyroidlike appearance. Tamm-Horsfall protein extravasates from tubules into the interstitium and elicits an inflammatory reaction consisting of mononuclear cells and eosinophils. The protein can be identified as amorphous to fibrillar eosinophilic material that stains brightly with the PAS stain.

It needs to be emphasized that these inflammatory changes are not specific for chronic pyelonephritis. Chronic inflammation usually is not striking in hypertension or diabetes unless there is coexisting pyelonephritis, but collections of small lymphocytes can be prominent in ischemic nephropathy. Chronic inflammation with many plasma cells is frequently pronounced in the renal cortex of glomerulonephritis. In both glomerulonephritis and

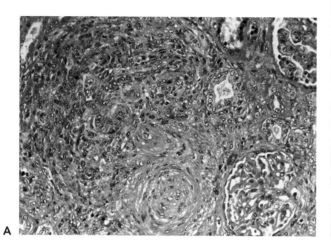

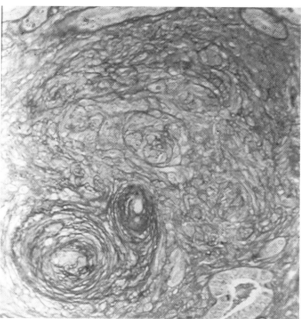

A                                                                                      B

**Figure 27.29**   The kidney of a hemodialysis patient with malignant hypertension. **A:** A cellular arteriolar nodule originates in an arteriole at the bottom of the micrograph. (H&E, ×200.) **B:** The origin of another nodule is demonstrated in an arteriole showing fibrinoid necrosis. (Alcian blue–PAS, ×200.)

ischemic nephropathy, the intensity of the inflammation can lead to a mistaken diagnosis of chronic pyelonephritis. The characteristic feature of chronic pyelonephritis is a "pyelitis" consisting of lymphoplasmacytic inflammation in the mucosa of the pelvis and calices and blunting of the associated renal papillae (185). Reactive lymphoid follicles are frequently seen in the pelvicaliceal inflammation.

In the absence of these pelvicaliceal changes, other forms of interstitial nephritis should be considered, includ-

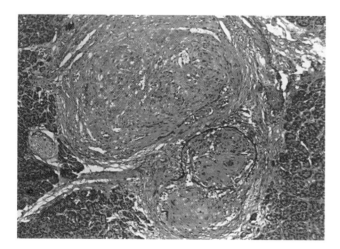

**Figure 27.30**   Arteriolar nodule in the pancreas of a hemodialysis with poorly controlled malignant hypertension. (Aldehyde fuchsin–hematoxylin, ×100.)

ing antibody and cell-mediated immune diseases. If a large number of eosinophils or granulomas are present, the differential diagnosis should include a drug-induced hypersensitivity disease. Sarcoidosis and tuberculosis need to be ruled out when the inflammation is granulomatous.

Papillary necrosis is present in cases of analgesic nephropathy (189). Histologically, the necrotic papillae show ghostlike remnants of collecting tubules and a deeply eosinophilic staining interstitium. In long-standing cases, the necrotic papillae are frequently calcified and heterotopic bone formation may be present. In analgesic nephropathy, there is little or no inflammation adjacent to the necrotic papillae, and, in most cases, there is a pronounced thickening of the capillary walls in the submucosa of the renal pelvis and ureter. The thickened capillary wall consists of concentric lamellae of basement membrane material that stain brightly with the PAS method (see Chapter 23).

Renal papillary necrosis is also found in acute pyelonephritis and is particularly common in diabetics. In these kidneys, there is a band of intense acute inflammation in the upper papillae between the viable and necrotic tissue. These kidneys also show interstitial and intratubular collections of neutrophils as additional evidence of acute pyelonephritis. Acute interstitial nephritis is not a feature of analgesic nephropathy unless there is superimposed infection.

Malacoplakia and xanthogranulomatous pyelonephritis are forms of chronic pyelonephritis that present

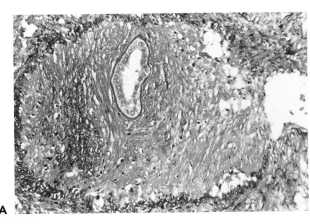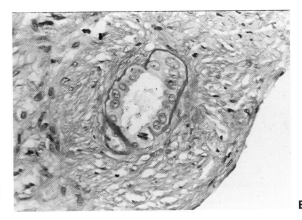

**A**    **B**

**Figure 27.31**    **A:** Thickened vein wall in an end-stage kidney of a chronic hemodialysis patient. A tubule is enclosed within the thickened vein whose original wall is outlined by elastic tissue. (Aldehyde fuchsin hematoxylin, ×200.) **B:** A mitotic figure is seen in the tubule in further sections of the vein shown in **(A):** (H&E, ×200.)

special histologic features (201,202). In xanthogranulomatous pyelonephritis, sheets of large foamy histiocytes efface the renal parenchyma. This often has a tumorous appearance that can be confused with clear cell carcinoma of the kidney. In malacoplakia, histiocytes with somewhat granular basophilic cytoplasm are found in the renal interstitium. The histiocytes contain PAS-positive Michaelis-Gutmann bodies that are calcospherites and stain with the Von Kossa technique for calcium.

## Tubular Atrophy

Tubular atrophy in the end-stage kidney has been classified into three types: classic atrophy, endocrine tubules, and tubular thyroidization (203). Classic atrophy is the most common and consists of tubules with small lumens containing eosinophilic and PAS-positive hyaline casts. The tubular basement membrane is thick and often duplicated. The epithelium of classic atrophic tubules is cuboidal, and the cytoplasm often contains lipofuscin pigment. Lectin histochemistry has shown that the cells of most of these tubules stain with markers that in the normal kidney bind preferentially with proximal renal tubules (203). A few of the tubules of classic atrophy demonstrate staining with distal tubular markers.

Endocrine tubules consist of cells having pale to slightly granular cytoplasm that are surrounded by thin basement membranes. Lumens are inconspicuous, and epithelial cell nuclei have a round to slightly oval appearance with finely granular chromatin and small nucleoli. Endocrine tubular cells stain primarily with distal tubular markers, but proximal tubular staining also is seen occasionally (203).

The endocrine tubule is named after similar appearing tubules that develop in the two-kidney, one-clip model of hypertension in the rat (32,203). The clipped kidney is reduced in size and becomes the endocrine kidney. Tubules lose their proximal and distal tubular histologic features

and acquire a uniform appearance consisting of cords of pale cells that do not form perceptible lumens. The tubules of this experimental model were initially thought to be the source of a pressor substance that caused the hypertension. The pressor substance was subsequently shown to be renin derived from the juxtaglomerular apparatus of glomeruli in the ischemic kidney (32). The name "endocrine tubule" has been retained, but the tubules do not have neurosecretory granules and are not known to have any endocrine function.

Thyroid tubules are small, round cystic structures filled with eosinophilic colloid, resembling follicles of the thyroid gland (203). Thyroid tubules are lined by a flattened simple epithelium and are surrounded by a basement membrane that is normal to slightly increased in thickness. Thyroidization is often a conspicuous feature of chronic pyelonephritis, but it is not diagnostic of this condition. It is found in the late stages of all chronic renal diseases.

In addition to atrophic tubules, the end-stage kidney contains tubules that are hypertrophied and dilated (203). These are mainly proximal tubules, and they display proximal tubular staining with lectin stains and by immunohistochemistry (203). These tubules are lined by columnar eosinophilic cells sometimes containing hyaline protein resorption droplets (32,203). The droplets frequently collect at the apex of cells and are shed into tubular lumens in a manner similar to apocrine secretory activity. The nuclei contain prominent nucleoli, and the chromatin is marginated along the nuclear membranes.

## Oxalosis

Oxalate crystals can be seen in most end-stage kidneys, and in some kidneys the crystal deposits can be quite extensive. Oxalate deposits are found within tubule lumens, embedded within interstitial connective tissue, or intermixed with the epithelium of cysts and tubules. The crystals are birefringent with polarized light in routinely processed histologic sections and can be stained histochemically with Alcian blue. Oxalate is normally excreted by the kidneys, and plasma oxalate levels become elevated with uremia. The severity of the oxalate deposition has been related to the duration of chronic renal failure (76). Oxalate may be seen in disorders such as primary hyperoxaluria and ethylene glycol toxicity, and ESRD can be a complication of these conditions.

## Miscellaneous Interstitial Changes

In some cases with well-advanced atrophy, aldehyde fuchsin, orcein, and Verhoeff-Van Gieson stains show areas of interstitial fibrosis having the staining properties of elastic tissue. By means of aldehyde fuchsin and Giemsa stains, large numbers of mast cells are frequently seen within interstitial inflammatory infiltrates (180). Occasional end-stage kidneys contain focal collections of interstitial myxoid connective tissue. Metaplastic cartilage and woven bone can be seen in such foci (Fig 27.32) (199).

The renal medullae of chronically diseased kidneys are often fibrotic. Interstitial fibrosis in which collagen fibril formation appeared to be derived from medullary interstitial cells was described in benign nephrosclerosis by Haggitt et al (204). In this study, medullary fibrosis increased with age, blood pressure, and the degree of arterio-arteriolosclerosis. The loss of the normal loose ground substance that composes the medullary interstitium in younger persons may be pathophysiologically significant, because it may interfere with the function of prostaglandin $E_2$ and other vasodepressor lipids that are produced by medullary interstitial cells (205). There may also be a loss of medullary interstitial cells with advanced fibrosis. Medullary fibrosis is seen in many end-stage kidneys, but in some kidneys, the renal medulla is occupied by spindle cells having features

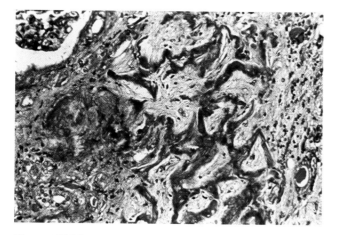

**Figure 27.32**   Osteoid forming within a focus of myxoid tissue in the interstitium of an end-stage dialysis kidney. (Masson's trichrome, ×200.)

of smooth muscle that tend to be oriented circumferentially around collecting ducts (206).

In addition to hyperplasia of granular cells of the juxtaglomerular apparatus of obsolete glomeruli, end-stage kidneys removed for high-renin hypertension show a prominence of medullary interstitial cells that contain large amounts of glycogen (206). This pattern of glycogen deposition is different from that seen in the Armanni-Ebstein phenomenon of diabetes or with glycogen storage diseases. The physiologic significance is not known, but it may be caused by a disruption of metabolic pathways in the medulla that convert glycogen to interstitial glycans (206).

## Acquired Renal Cystic Disease

Radiologic studies of hemodialysis patients have shown that during the 3 years after beginning dialysis, diseased kidneys continue to atrophy, but that at approximately 4 years, the size of the kidneys increases as ARCD begins to develop (207–209). ARCD has been reported to occur in 10% to 67% of dialysis patients (210). Some studies have indicated that men develop ARCD at a 3:1 to 6:1 ratio over women and that cystic change is more frequent in hypertension and glomerulonephritis than diabetes (211,212). Using radiologic criteria, ARCD has been diagnosed in 60% to 90% of patients who had been dialyzed for 5 to 10 years (209,213). In these studies, the prevalence of cystic disease is related to the duration of dialysis and not to sex or diagnosis.

ARCD develops in both hemodialysis and CAPD patients. Park et al (214) investigated the prevalence of ARCD by ultrasonography in 49 hemodialysis and 49 CAPD patients. ARCD was defined as three or more cysts in each kidney. ARCD developed in 31% of patients at an average duration of 74 months, and no difference in prevalence was seen between the methods of dialysis. This had been the experience of Matson and Cohen (213) and Ishikawa et al (215), who could also find no differences between hemodialysis and CAPD in the severity of ARCD.

The presence of several renal cysts and even many small cysts has been recognized in chronically diseased kidneys since the last century and certainly is not limited to the situation seen after renal dialysis (216). The marked cystic transformation of end-stage kidneys, described by Dunnill et al (179) is quite different from the development of a few cysts or small cysts and deserves recognition as a unique pathologic condition. Radiologically, ARCD has been defined as the presence of five or more cysts in each kidney in some studies and three or more cysts in others (213,214). For the pathologist, Feiner et al (217) suggested that ARCD should be defined as the cystic change of at least 40% of the volume of the kidney. This creates some discrepancy between radiologic and pathologic diagnoses, which might account for differences in the frequency with which ARCD is reported by different observers. Ishikawa et al (218) graded the degree of cystic change and measured kidney volumes by computerized tomography in 19 men and 17 women hemodialysis patients over a period of 20 years. Grade 1 cystic change consisted of 1 to 3 cysts and grade 4 more than 20 cysts per kidney, with grades 2 and 3 being in between. At 10 years, the degree of cystic change and the increase in kidney volumes between sexes were approximately equal, but at 15 years, males had significantly more grade 4 changes. At 20 years, the kidney volumes of males were twice that of females.

Intrarenal hemorrhage has been observed in 17% of cystic end-stage kidneys (209). Hemorrhage has been associated with heparinization during hemodialysis, but it is actually seen more frequently between dialysis periods when patients are not heparinized. In these cases, platelet dysfunction secondary to uremia is suggested as the etiologic factor. In some patients, intrarenal hemorrhage ruptures into the retroperitoneum and can be life threatening (207,209).

The cause of acquired cystic disease is not known. It has been proposed that following a loss of renal tissue a renotropic growth factor is produced that promotes renal hypertrophy (210). In the end-stage kidney, the factor or factors may act on remaining tubular segments and stimulate cyst growth.

Epidermal growth factor and transforming growth factor alpha promote in vitro cyst development of human renal cortical epithelial cells dispersed in a collagenous matrix (219). Transforming growth factor alpha is a ligand for epidermal growth factor receptor. The ligand and receptor are proto-oncogenes that form a feedback loop in the regulation of renal epithelial cell growth (220). The aberrant up-regulation of transforming growth factor alpha and epidermal growth factor receptor has been found in renal cell carcinoma (221). This growth factor and receptor overexpression is probably involved in the development of ARCD and may be involved in the tumorigenesis that accompanies the condition (211,219).

Hepatocyte growth factor and its receptor c-met are additional proto-oncogenes involved in the regulation of epithelial cell growth (222). Konda et al (223) have shown that both hepatocyte growth factor and c-met are overexpressed in the cystic epithelium of ARCD with the increased expression being predominantly in hyperplastic, multilayered cysts. In this study, the inhibition of apoptosis by the increased expression of bcl-2 was also thought to play a role in cyst growth.

## Gross Pathology

In a review of published case series, single organ weights of kidneys involved by ARCD have been found to average 134 grams with a range of up to 800 grams (5). In some cases, the cysts are small and evenly distributed, giv-

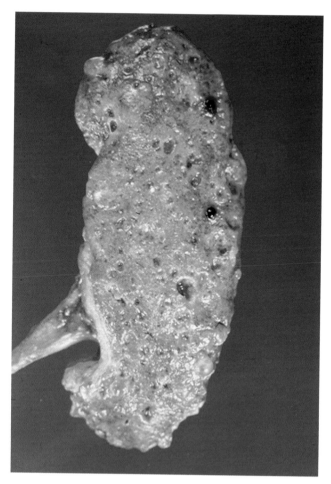

**Figure 27.33** Acquired cystic disease in a 42-year-old man supported by hemodialysis for 4 years. This 120-g kidney contained many small cysts.

ing the kidney a spongy texture (Fig. 27.33). Cysts can be localized to part of the kidney, or large cysts, many more than 2 cm in diameter, can involve the entire kidney. Extensive cystic transformation is not uncommonly accompanied by the development of renal cell carcinoma (Fig. 27.34). Cysts are located mainly in the cortex but can be found in the renal medulla. Most cysts are filled with clear to slightly cloudy straw-colored serous fluid, but the contents may have a gelatinous consistency. When there has been intrarenal hemorrhage, cysts are filled with liquid or clotted blood.

The gross appearance of the very large examples of ARCD can resemble autosomal dominant polycystic kidney disease (ADPKD) (224). Usually, however, the size of the kidneys in the two conditions is quite different. Although examples of ADPKD with single kidney weights of 300 to 400 g or less have been observed when patients were not in renal failure, the single kidney weights of symptomatic ADPKD range from 2000 to 4000 g (225). The largest kidneys reported for ARCD are just at 800 g, and the

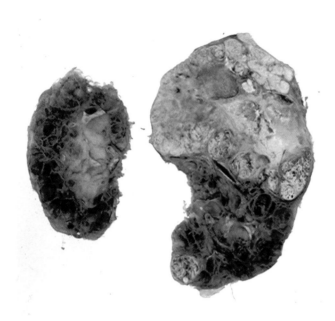

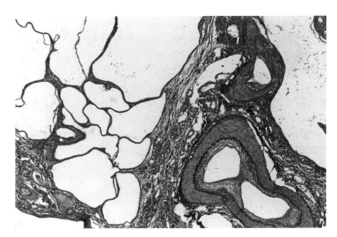

**Figure 27.35**    Micrograph from a case of acquired cystic disease. The cysts are lined by a flattened simple epithelium. (H&E, ×100.)

**Figure 27.34**    Acquired cystic disease in a man supported by hemodialysis for 9 years. The kidneys are enlarged by extensive cystic change and had a combined weight of 680 g. The kidney on the right has two renal cell carcinomas. A small tumor is in the lower pole. (Courtesy of Dr. M.S. Dunnill, Oxford University.)

great majority are less than 300 g (5). To help discriminate between the two diseases, the anatomic findings should be correlated with the clinical history. Cases of ARCD are found in patients with chronic renal failure who have not reached the point of requiring dialysis, but most patients have been on dialysis for many months and more often years (6,7). A prior history of noncystic renal disease will establish a diagnosis of ARCD, and a family history of autosomal dominant disease inheritance will allow ADPKD to be diagnosed. The presence of cysts in the liver and pancreas can be helpful, but liver cysts have been described with ARCD (224).

Although the two genes involved in the development of 90 to 95% of ADPKD are known, they are very large and mutations are widely distributed throughout their many exons (226–228). This makes molecular genetic testing impractical for the diagnosis of any individual case of presumed ARCD that may resemble ADPKD.

## Microscopic Pathology

Most cysts of ARCD are lined by a flat, nondescript epithelium (Fig. 27.35). Some are lined by tall proximal tubular cells containing prominent hyaline droplets that are identical to those seen in hypertrophied tubules (Fig. 27.36). Other cysts are lined by small cuboidal cells resembling distal tubular epithelium, and the small cuboidal cells stain with lectins or immunohistochemical markers (*Arachis hypogaea* and epithelial membrane antigen) that bind pref-

erentially with distal tubule in the normal kidney (229). In some cases, cystic dilatation of glomeruli is widespread and contributes to the cystic appearance of the kidneys.

Cysts lined by both tall columnar and small cuboidal cells often develop a papillary and multilayered hyperplasia (Fig. 27.37). These hyperplastic, multilayered cysts, or atypical cysts, are seen in approximately 30% of end-stage kidneys (230). The epithelium of atypical cysts frequently shows dysplastic cytologic features and loss of nuclear polarity. Atypical cysts are seen with increased frequency in kidneys with renal cortical tumors and appear to be preneoplastic lesions (230).

Lectin histochemistry and immunohistochemistry using markers for proximal and distal tubular epithelium have shown that the cysts of ARCD are derived from both

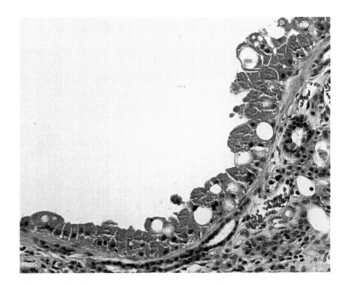

**Figure 27.36**    Acquired cystic disease. This cyst is lined by proximal tubular cells that contain hyalin colloid droplets. The cells focally pile on one another along the cyst's wall. (H&E, ×200.)

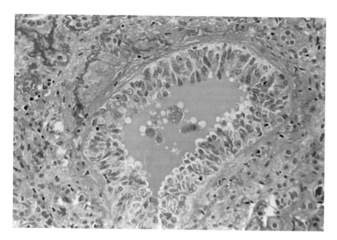

**Figure 27.37** An atypical cyst in a dialysis kidney. The cyst is lined by hyperplastic cells showing loss of stratification. (PAS–hematoxylin, ×200.)

proximal and distal tubules (229,231). This confirms earlier nephron dissection studies in which cysts were found to develop from all levels of the nephron (217). These nephron dissection techniques demonstrated that many cysts begin as outpouchings or sacculations of intact tubular segments. Histologically, nodules of collagen, elastic tissue fibers, and duplicated tubular basement membranes are formed at points of cyst outpouching (230). As a result of old intracystic hemorrhage, some cysts contain a large amount of hemosiderin in the epithelium and connective tissue of the cyst wall.

The kidneys of ARCD invariably show the background of obsolete glomeruli, tubular atrophy, and obliterative intimal fibrosis of arteries that characterize end-stage kidneys. The renal parenchyma between the cysts of ADPKD, in contrast, remains remarkably normal, even when patients are becoming uremic. After dialysis, however, secondary atrophic changes will often be found in ADPKD, and the microscopic differences between ADPKD and ARCD can become obscure (232). The cysts of ADPKD, like those of ARCD, are derived from all levels of the nephron, and immunohistochemical studies do not distinguish between the two types of cystic diseases (231).

## Renal Cell Tumors of Acquired Renal Cystic Disease

Renal cortical tumors of varying size are found in approximately 17% of end-stage kidneys and are multiple in approximately 9% of cases (5). Renal cell carcinoma (RCC) has been reported in 3.8% of prospectively screened candidates for renal transplantation and in 3.9% of patients after transplantation (233,234). Denton et al (235) examined 260 consecutive pretransplant nephrectomies of native end-stage kidneys. Adenomas were found in 14% and carcinomas in 4.2% of the specimens. The approximately

4% detection rate for RCC in these studies compares with a 0.04% detection rate among nonrenal patients undergoing ultrasonography and a 17.3 per 100,000 male age standardized population rate (0.017%) for RCC in the general United States population (236,237).

In an analysis of data from the United States, Europe, Australia, and New Zealand registries, Stewart et al (238) calculated the risk for kidney cancer among dialysis patients as standardized incidence ratios (SIR) of the background risk in those countries. The SIR of all dialysis patients was 3.6 (CI, 3.5 to 3.8) and increased from 3.2 (CI, 3.0 to 3.5) during the first year of dialysis to 6.8 (CI, 5.1 to 8.9) after 10 years. The increased risk was seen in all renal diseases but was greatest for congenital diseases, toxic and analgesic nephropathies, and Balkan nephropathy, with the SIR of analgesic nephropathy being 16.7 (CI, 14.1 to 19.6) and Balkan nephropathy 26.2 (CI, 13.1 to 46.9). The type of kidney cancer was not specified, and the very high SIR for analgesic and Balkan nephropathy was probably owing to the increased prevalence of transitional cell carcinoma of the renal pelvis that is seen in these conditions. This was reflected in bladder cancer SIR rates for analgesic nephropathy of 13.3 (CI, 11.3 to 15.7) and Balkan nephropathy of 18.2 (CI, 9.4 to 31.8) (238).

RCC occurs in both cystic and noncystic kidneys, but patients with ARCD appear to develop RCC approximately six times more frequently and at an average age that is 10 to 12 years younger than persons not in ESRD (5,209,230,239,240). MacDougall et al (241) found that the degree of cystic change, as determined by kidney weight, correlated with the development of RCC.

Many of the tumors of end-stage kidneys are small, well-circumscribed, yellow-to-white lesions of the subcapsular cortex lying just under the renal capsule. Most of these tumors are papillary neoplasms that can be considered adenomas. Less frequently, the tumors are clear cell neoplasms. Although any size tumor of this histopathologic type is considered a clear cell carcinoma, the risk of metastasis is low when the tumor is less than 2 to 3 cm in diameter and well-confined within the kidney (see Chapter 29).

All clinical stages of renal cell carcinomas have been identified in end-stage kidneys. Those discovered at advanced stages involve a large proportion of the kidney, invade the renal vein and perinephric tissues, and metastasize to lymph nodes and distant sites.

The tumors of the end-stage kidney are histologically identical to sporadically occurring neoplasms (179,242) (Figs. 27.38 and 27.39). Papillary RCCs are overrepresented in the end-stage kidney compared with clear cell carcinomas (242,243). Ishikawa and Kovacs (242) classified 18 of 44 (41%) and Hughson et al (243) classified 15 of 21 (71%) RCC in end-stage kidneys as papillary neoplasms. However, papillary carcinoma represents only 10% to 15% of sporadically occurring RCC. Cases of ESRD-associated oncocytoma, oncocytomatosis, and at least one case of

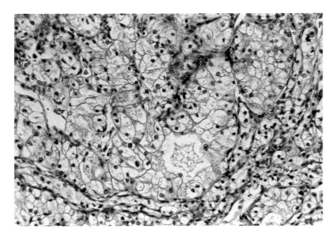

**Figure 27.38** This clear cell carcinoma developed in a dialysis kidney that was also involved by acquired cystic disease. (H&E, ×100.)

chromophobe carcinoma have been reported (235,244–246). Denton et al (235) found oncocytoma in 0.6% of their series of pretransplant nephrectomies.

The different types of RCC have distinctively characteristic cytogenetic changes (247). Sporadic papillary RCC is characterized by numerical chromosomal abnormalities with trisomy or tetrasomy of chromosome 7 being found in 45% to 88% and trisomy of 17 in 64% to 88% of tumors (247). In contrast to papillary tumors, sporadic clear cell RCCs demonstrate a deletion of the short arm of the chromosome 3 (3p) in more than 90% and mutations of the von-Hippel Lindau tumor suppressor gene (*VHL*) at 3p25-26 in 50% to 60% of tumors (248). *VHL* mutations do not occur in papillary RCC (247).

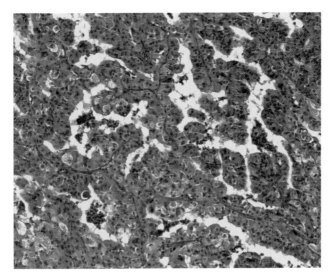

**Figure 27.39** A papillary renal cell carcinoma that had developed in acquired cystic disease. This tumor is composed of columnar, eosinophilic cells. (H&E, ×100.)

Genetic analyses have been performed on several papillary RCC of ESRD (211,249–251). Numerical chromosomal changes were found in all studies. Chudek et al (249) found trisomies of chromosomes 3, 5, 7, 8, or 16 in four of five tumors but trisomy of 17 in only one. Ishikawa et al (251) found trisomies of 3, 8, 16, and 20 without involvement of 7 or 17. Hughson et al (211) identified duplications of 7 and/or 17 in 6 of 14 tumors with 8 of the 14 papillary RCC showing involvement of neither chromosome 7 nor 17. Although these findings show that some of the papillary RCC of ESRD have the genetic changes commonly found in sporadic papillary RCC, a disproportionate number apparently do not.

Deletions of 3p have been detected in eight of 16 ESRD clear cell RCC. This represents the number analyzed in three separate studies of ESRD tumors (243,249,252). Yoshida et al (252) detected *VHL* mutations in three of the seven tumors included in these reports. Although a role for *VHL* is shown for some of the clear cell RCC, the relative infrequency with which clear cell RCC have been reported in ESRD indicates that the increased overall prevalence of RCC does not depend on an unusually high *VHL* mutation rate.

The high prevalence of papillary RCC in ESRD suggests that an increased frequency of nondisjunction may be the abnormal event leading to tumor development (243). The presence of extra gene copies, or increased gene dosage owing to the increased number of chromosomes, may provide a selective growth advantage and result in a transformed cell type (243). The *MET* protooncogene at 7q31 is mutated and duplicated in hereditary papillary RCC and in 7% to 13% of sporadic papillary RCC (222). The hereditary and sporadic tumors with *MET* mutations are composed of small basophilic cells, the type I papillary RCC in the classification of Delahunt and Eble (222). The large majority of the tumors in ESRD are composed of eosinophilic granular cells, the type II papillary RCC (243). *MET* mutations have not been found in type II papillary RCC and probably do not play a developmental role in the renal tumors of ESRD (222).

In some centers, it has been observed that a functional renal transplant can reverse or retard the development of ARCD in the native kidneys and may prevent the growth of tumors (253,254). This has not been everyone's experience, and the clinical studies on which these assertions were based preceded the use of cyclosporin in the management of rejection. More recently, a 2% incidence of death from RCC has been described in kidney transplant patients, and it is thought that cyclosporin may play a role in promoting tumor formation (255,256). Kasiske et al (257) calculated the rates of malignancy among 35,765 first time renal transplant recipients and found that kidney cancer was 15-fold more common than in the general population. This compared with the common cancers of breast, prostate, lung, and colon that were twice as common and the immunosuppression-associated non-Hodgkin lymphomas and Kaposi's sarcoma that are 20-fold more common than in the general population. Cystic change and RCC also have been described in the transplant kidney itself (258–262).

The major factors affecting longevity on dialysis are age and cardiovascular disease (3,78). Nevertheless, cancer is a common cause of death among ESRD patients (239). This is mainly because of an increased prevalence of invasive carcinomas of the kidney and uterus, but because of the preponderant influence of cardiovascular disease, the increased risk of cancer does not have a notable statistical effect on the survival of ESRD patients (209,239,263). The biologic behavior of end-stage kidney tumors seems to be more indolent than that of sporadic renal cancers. Metastases have been observed in 17% of chronic hemodialysis patients with renal carcinomas (239). This contrasts with sporadic RCC in which 30% are metastatic at the time of diagnosis.

## PERITONEUM IN PERITONEAL DIALYSIS

Peritonitis occurs in approximately 15% of CAPD patients every 12 months (87). Staphylococci are the most common etiologic agents, and the most frequent source of the infection is contamination by skin contact through the dialysis catheter. Peritonitis presents as a cloudy dialysate being returned from the abdomen, loss of dialytic clearance, and a steady rise in serum creatinine. A low-grade fever may be present but is surprisingly infrequent. Mesothelial cells lose contact with each other and slough from the peritoneal membranes that then become covered with fibrin (264,265). Within 2 to 4 weeks after successful antibiotic therapy, the mesothelial layer recovers and the dialyzing capacity of the peritoneum is usually restored.

The relationship between the integrity of the mesothelium and the dialyzing capacity of the peritoneum is not quite clear, because the mesothelium is probably not an osmotic barrier. It is more likely that the capillaries of the peritoneum provide the barrier to the transport of solutes and the ultrafiltration capacity of the peritoneum (266,267). Peritonitis probably causes the loss of the ultrafiltration capacity of the peritoneum by damaging the vasculature and making it hyperpermeable to small solutes.

Peritoneal clearances become inadequate in 20% to 30% of CAPD patients after 5 years (267). The reason for this declining function is not clear. Repeated infections may play a role in some patients, but in most, the poor biocompatibility of the dialysis solutions and the reaction it provokes in the peritoneum seems to be more important. The most widely used dialysates are acidic, lactate buffered solutions having high glucose concentrations. These solutions are heat sterilized creating glucose degradation products that consist primarily of low–molecular-weight aldehydes (268).

The high-glucose solutions up-regulate vascular endothelial growth factor (VEGF) in the peritoneal vasculature and produce diabeticlike vascular changes in which there is colocalization of VEGF and advanced glycosylation end products (269–272). Zweers et al (272) found evidence for the local production of both TGF-β1 and VEGF by the peritoneum of CAPD patients, and in viral transfection experiments, Margetts et al (273) demonstrated that TGF-β1 induced peritoneal VEGF production. This is analogous to diabetic microangiopathy. VEGF is thought to be a principal factor mediating the structural and functional changes of the microvascular and the hyperpermeabiltity of the peritoneum (272,273).

Peritoneal biopsies from CAPD patients and experimental studies of the peritoneum have shown similar findings that consist of fibrous thickening, increased myofibroblast cellularity, and increased vascular density (269–274). The peritoneal biopsies and autopsies on nondiabetic CAPD patients have additionally shown thickening and hyalinization of the walls of small arteries and thickening of capillary basement membranes that are identical to diabetic microangiopathy (271,275). Honda et al (271) demonstrated advanced glycosylation end products (AGEs) in the altered vessels and found that the AGE accumulation, vascular sclerosis, and interstitial fibrosis corresponded to the degree of ultrafiltration failure.

Some patients develop a diffusely thickened peritoneum with widespread adhesions that cause intermittent, recurrent, or persistent bowel obstruction (276). This condition of encapsulating peritoneal sclerosis (EPS) has a reported incidence of 0.7% to 7.3% among peritoneal dialysis patients and a mortality rate as high as 69%. Kawanishi et al (276), in a multicenter study, followed 1959 peritoneal dialysis patients for four years. EPS occurred in 48 patients (2.5%). The incidence was 0.0% at 3 years but increased to 17.2% among patients who had been on dialysis for more than 15 years. The EPS was attributed to peritonitis in 25% of the patients. This was similar to the findings of Rigby and Hawley (277) who found that 38% of EPS in Australian peritoneal dialysis patients was related to peritonitis. Kawanishi et al (276) found an overall mortality rate owing to perforating peritonitis or sepsis of 37.5%, but there was also a 45.8% recovery rate following treatment with total parenteral nutrition, corticosteroids, and surgery.

## TREATMENT OUTCOME

In 2001, 65% of U.S. ESRD patients were being treated by in-center hemodialysis, 28% with a functional renal transplant, and 7% by peritoneal dialysis (3). The 2-year survival rate adjusted for age, sex, race, and primary renal disease is 25% higher for patients with functional transplants

**TABLE 27.2**

**DISTRIBUTION OF CAUSES OF DEATH FOR ESRD PATIENTS BY AGE GROUP BETWEEN 2000 AND 2002**

| Causes of Death | Average (%) | Age (%) | | |
|---|---|---|---|---|
| | | 20–44 yr | 45–64 yr | ≥65 yr |
| Acute myocardial infarct | 8.3 | 5.4 | 8.9 | 8.3 |
| Cardiac arrest, arrhythmia | 26 | 24.9 | 25.9 | 26.2 |
| Cardiomyopathy | 3.5 | 2.0 | 2.7 | 4.1 |
| Other Cardiac | 3.6 | 2.0 | 2.7 | 4.2 |
| Pericarditis | 0.1 | 0.4 | 0.2 | 0.1 |
| Pulmonary edema | 0.8 | 0.9 | 0.8 | 0.9 |
| Cerebrovascular | 5.0 | 5.2 | 5.4 | 4.8 |
| GI hemorrhage | 0.7 | 0.5 | 0.7 | 0.8 |
| Other hemorrhage | 0.9 | 1.4 | 1.0 | 0.8 |
| Septicemia | 11.2 | 11.6 | 12.4 | 10.6 |
| Pulmonary infection | 2.2 | 1.4 | 1.7 | 2.5 |
| Other infection | 0.7 | 1.0 | 0.8 | 0.6 |
| Hyperkalemia | 1.4 | 1.8 | 1.1 | 1.5 |
| Malignancy | 3.6 | 2.0 | 3.6 | 4.0 |
| Cachexia | 1.0 | 0.4 | 0.6 | 1.2 |
| Other | 24.1 | 27.9 | 24.4 | 22.9 |
| Cause unknown | 6.7 | 11.4 | 6.9 | 6.5 |

Adapted from the U.S. Renal Data System 2004 Annual Data Report [www.usrds.org]. The data reported here have been supplied by the United States Renal Data System. The reporting of these data is the responsibility of the author and should not be seen as an official policy or interpretation of the U.S. government.

than for patients treated by dialysis (263). The distribution of causes of death among treated ESRD patients between 2000 and 2002 are given by age group in Table 27.2. Myocardial infarction is responsible for 8% to 9% of cardiac deaths. Most cardiac deaths are caused by cardiac arrhythmias or classified as cardiac arrest. This accounts for 25% to 26% of deaths and remains nearly the same for the different age groups from 20 to older than 65 years.

Infections are the next most frequent causes of death. Fatal infections are most commonly the result of septicemia from infected access sites. Hemodialysis patients with arteriovenous grafts have higher infection rates than patients with arteriovenous fistulas (7). CAPD patients develop peritoneal catheter-related infections that can be categorized as peritonitis or as infections of the skin and soft tissue tunnel at the catheter exit site. Peritonitis is responsible for 1.3% to 1.6% of deaths of CAPD patients (7,177). The organisms responsible for fatal peritonitis are commonly fungi. Most access site infections including hemodialysis fistula or graft infections are caused by *Staphylococcus aureus* or by *Staphylococcus epidermidis*, and an increased susceptibility to infection can be predicted by positive *S. aureus* nasal cultures (7). Except for peritonitis, infection rates are similar for CAPD and hemodialysis patients and the morbidity and mortality is predicted by low socioeconomic status and malnutrition (7). Serum albumin is often used as a measure of nutritional status. Patients with a serum albumin of less than 3.0 g/dL have a 2.5 times greater risk of developing an infection during a 12-month period than patients whose serum albumin is greater than 3.0 g/dL.

Mortality rates vary according to the diagnosis of the primary renal disease (263). Adjusted for age, race, and sex, 5-year survival estimates are 17.4% for diabetes, 29.9% for hypertension, and 36.6% for chronic glomerulonephritis. The mortality rate of diabetics owing to cardiac disease and stroke even in younger age groups is three times that of nondiabetics, and septicemia is twice as frequent (278).

## REFERENCES

1. National Kidney Foundation. Kidney Disease Outcome Quality Initiative (K/DOQI). Part 4. Definition and classification of stages of chronic kidney disease. Am J Kidney Dis 2002;39 (suppl 1):S46.
2. Coresh J, Astor BC, Greene T, et al. Prevalence of chronic kidney disease and decreased kidney function in the adult U.S. population: Third National Health and Nutrition Examination Survey. Am J Kidney Dis 2003;41:1.

3. United States Renal Data System 2003 Annual Report. Am J Kidney Dis 2003;42(suppl 5):S1.
4. Kiberd BA, Clase CM. Cumulative risk for developing end-stage renal disease in the U.S. population. J Am Soc Nephrol 2002;13:1635.
5. Hughson MD, Buchwald D, Fox M. Renal neoplasia and acquired cystic disease in patients receiving long-term dialysis. Arch Pathol Lab Med 1986;110:592.
6. Chung-Park M, Ricanati E, Lankerani M, Kedia K. Acquired renal cysts and multiple renal cell and urothelial tumors. Am J Clin Pathol 1983;141:238.
7. Hogg RJ. Acquired renal cystic disease in children prior to the start of dialysis. Pediatr Nephrol 1992;6:176.
8. Faticia RA, Port FK, Young EW. Incidence trends and mortality in end-stage renal disease attributed to renovascular disease in the United States. Am J Kidney Dis 2001;37:1184.
9. Fored CM, Ejerblad E, Linblad P, et al. Acetaminophen, aspirin, and chronic renal disease. N Engl J Med 2001;345:1801.
10. Kurth T, Glynn RJ, Walker AM, et al. Analgesic use and change in kidney function in apparently healthy men. Am J Kidney Dis 2003;42:234.
11. Kitiyakara C, Eggers P, Kopp JB. Twenty-one year trend in ESRD due to focal segmental glomerulosclerosis in the United States. Am J Kidney Dis 2004;44:815.
12. Cameron JS. The natural history of glomerulonephritis. In: Black D, Jones NF, eds. Renal Disease, 4th ed. Oxford, UK: Blackwell, 1979:329.
13. D'Amico G, Imbrasciati E, Barbiano di Belgioioso G, et al. Idiopathic IgA mesangial nephropathy: Clinical and histological study of 374 patients. Medicine (Baltimore) 1985;64:49.
14. Silva FG. Acute postinfectious glomerulonephritis and glomerulonephritis complicating persistent bacterial infection. In: Jennette CJ, Olson JL, Schwartz MM, Silva FG, eds. Heptinstall's Pathology of the Kidney, 5th ed. New York, Philadelphia: Lippincott-Raven Publishers, 1998:389.
15. Rodriquez-Iturbe B, Parra, G. Post-streptococcal glomerulonephritis. In: Massry SG, Glassock RJ, eds. Textbook of Nephrology, 4th ed. Philadelphia: Lippincott Williams & Wilkins, 2001:667.
16. Leishman AW. Hypertension: Treated and untreated; a study of 400 cases. Br Med J 1959;15:1361.
17. Hypertension Detection and Follow-up Program Cooperative Group: Five year findings of the hypertension and detection and follow-up program. I. Reduction in mortality of persons with high blood pressure, including mild hypertension. JAMA 1979;242:2562.
18. Klagg MJ, Whelton PK, Randall BL, et al. Blood pressure and end-stage renal disease in men. N Engl J Med 1996;334:13.
19. Klagg MJ, Whelton PK, Randall BL, et al. End-stage renal disease in African American and white men. 16-year MRFIT findings. JAMA 1997;277:1293.
20. Haroun MK, Jaar BG, Hoffman SC, et al. Risk factors for chronic kidney disease: A prospective study of 23,534 men and women in Washington County, Maryland. J Am Soc Nephrol 2003;14:2934.
21. Veterans Administration Cooperative Study Group on antihypertensive agents. Effects of treatment on morbidity in hypertension. Results in patients with diastolic blood pressures averaging 115 through 129 mm Hg. JAMA 1967;202:1028.
22. Hamilton M, Thompson EM, Wisniewski TK. The role of blood-pressure control in preventing complications of hypertension. Lancet 1964;41:235.
23. Blyth WB, Maddux FW. Hypertension as a causative diagnosis of patients entering end-stage renal disease programs in the United States from 1980 to 1986. Am J Kidney Dis 1981;18:33.
24. McClellan W, Tuttle E, Issa A. Racial differences in the incidence of hypertensive end-stage renal disease (ESRD) are not entirely explained by differences in the prevalence of hypertension. Am J Kidney Dis 1988;12:285.
25. Rostand SG, Brown G, Kirk KA, et al. Renal insufficiency in treated essential hypertension. N Engl J Med 1989;320:684.
26. Segura J, Campoc C, Gil P, et al. Development of chronic kidney disease and cardiovascular prognosis in essential hypertensive patients. J Am Soc Nephrol 2004;15:1616.
27. Hypertension Detection and Follow-up Cooperative Group. The effect of treatment on mortality in "mild" hypertension. Results of the Hypertension Detection and Follow-up Program. N Engl J Med 1982;307:976.
28. Wright JT, Bakris G, Greene T, et al. Effect of blood pressure lowering and antihypertensive drug class on progression of hypertensive kidney disease. Results from the AASK trial. JAMA 2002;288:2421.
29. Perneger TV, Whelton PK, Klagg MJ, Rossiter KA. Diagnosis of hypertensive end-stage renal disease: effect of patient's race. Am J Epidemiol 1995;141:10.
30. Schlessinger SD, Tankersley MR, Curtis JJ. Clinical documentation of end-stage renal disease due to hypertension. Am J Kidney Dis 1994;23:655.
31. Fogo A, Breyer JA, Smith MC, et al, AASK Pilot Study Investigators. Accuracy of the diagnosis of hypertensive nephrosclerosis in African Americans: A report from the African American Study of Kidney Disease Trial. Kidney Int 1977;51:244.
32. Heptinstall RH. Hypertension I. Essential hypertension. In: Heptinstall RH, ed. Pathology of the Kidney, 4th ed. Boston: Little, Brown and Company, 1992:951.
33. Marcatoni C, Ma L-T, Federspeil C, Fogo AB. Hypertensive nephrosclerosis in African Americans versus caucasians. Kidney Int 2002;62:172.
34. Christensen JS, Gammelgard J, Tronier B, et al. Kidney function and size before and after initial insulin treatment. Kidney Int 1982;21:683.
35. Selby JV, Fitzsimmons SC, Newman JM, et al. The natural history and epidemiology of diabetic nephropathy: Implications for prevention and control. JAMA 1990;263:1954.
36. Cusick M, Chew EY, Hoogwerf B, et al, and the Early Treatment Diabetic Retinopathy Study Research Group. Risk factors for renal replacement therapy in the Early Treatment Diabetic Retinopathy Study Report No. 26. Kidney Int 2004;66:1173.
37. Ritz E, Hasslacher C, Tschope W, et al. Hypertension in diabetes mellitus. Contrib Nephrol 1987;54:77.
38. Rossing K, Christensen PK, Hovind P, et al. Progression of nephropathy in type 2 diabetic patients. Kidney Int 2004;66:1596.
39. Bakris GL, Copley JB, Vicknair N, et al. Calcium channel blockers versus other antihypertensive therapies on progression of NIDDM associated nephropathy. Kidney Int 1996;50:1641.
40. Breyer JA. Diabetic nephropathy in insulin-dependent patients: In depth review. Am J Kidney Dis 1992;20:533.
41. Christlieb AR, Warram JH, Krolewski AS, et al. Hypertension: The major risk factor in juvenile-onset insulin-dependent diabetics. Diabetes 1981;30(suppl 2):90.
42. Parving, H-H, Jacobsen P, Smidt UM, et al. Benefits of long-term antihypertensive treatment on prognosis in diabetic nephropathy. Kidney Int 1996;49:1778.
43. Brancati FL, Whelton PK, Randall BL, et al. Risk of end-stage renal disease in diabetes mellitus. A prospective cohort study of men screened for MRFIT. JAMA 1997;278:2069.
44. Acosta JH. Hypertension in chronic renal disease. Kidney Int 1982;22:702.
45. Oldrizzi L, Rugiu C, DeBiase V, Maschio, G. The place of hypertension among the risk factors for renal function in chronic renal failure. Am J Kidney Dis 1993;21:119.
46. Brazy PC, Stead WW, Fitzwilliam JF. Progression of renal insufficiency: Role of blood pressure. Kidney Int 1989;35:670.
47. Hannedouche T, Landais P, Goldfarb B, et al. Randomized controlled trial of enalapril and beta-blockers in non-diabetic chronic renal failure. BMJ 1994;309:833.
48. Maschio G, Alberti D, Janin G, et al. Effect of the angiotensin-converting-enzyme inhibitor on the progression of chronic renal insufficiency. N Engl J Med 1996;334:939.
49. Walser M. Progression of chronic renal failure in man. Kidney Int 1990;37:1195.
50. Zucchelli P, Zuccala A, Borghi M, et al. Long-term comparison between captopril and nifedipine in the progression of renal insufficiency. Kidney Int 1992;42:452.

51. Kasiske BL, Kalil RS, Ma JZ, et al. Effect of antihypertensive therapy on the kidney in patients with diabetes: A meta-regression analysis. Ann Intern Med 1993;118:129.

52. Brenner BM, Cooper ME, deZeeuw D, et al. Effects of losartan on renal and cardiovascular outcomes in patients with type 2 diabetes and nephropathy. N Engl J Med 2001;345:861.

53. Ferrari P, Marti H, Pfister M, et al. Additive proteinuric effect of combined ACE inhibition and angiotensin II receptor blockade. J Hypertens 2002;20:125.

54. Lewis EJ, Hunsicker LG, Clarke WR, et al. Renoprotective effect of the angiotensin-receptor antagonist irbesartan in patients with nephropathy due to type 2 diabetes. N Engl J Med 2001;345:851.

55. Mann JF, Gerstein H, Pogue J, et al. Renal insufficiency as a predictor of cardiovascular outcomes and the impact of ramipril: The HOPE randomized trial. Ann Intern Med 2001;134:629.

56. Noris M, Remuzzi G. ACE inhibitors and AT1 receptor antagonist: Is two better than one? Kidney Int 2002;61:1545.

57. Kasiske BL. Relationship between vascular disease and age associated changes in the human kidney. Kidney Int 1987;31:1153.

58. Tracy RE. Blood pressure related separately to parenchymal fibrosis and vasculopathy of the kidney. Am J Kidney Dis 1992;20:2.

59. Luke RG, Reif MC. Hypertension. In: Massry SG, Glassock RG, eds. Textbook of Nephrology, 4th ed. Philadelphia: Lippincott Williams & Wilkins, 2001:1305.

60. Hughson MD, Johnson K, Young RJ, et al. Glomerular size and glomerular sclerosis: Relationship to disease categories, glomerular solidification, and ischemic obsolescence. Am J Kidney Dis 2002;39:649.

61. Bidani AK, Griffin KA. Pathophysiology of hypertensive damage: Implication for therapy. Hypertension 2004;44:595.

62. Bidani AK, Griffin KA, Picken M, Lansky DM. Continuous telemetric BP monitoring and glomerular injury in the rat remnant kidney model. Am J Physiol 1993;265:F391.

63. Karlsen FM, Andersen CB, Leyssac PP, Holstein-RathlouN-H. Dynamic autoregulation and renal injury in Dahl rats. Hypertension 1997;30:975.

64. Hostetler TH, Olson JL, Rennke HG, et al. Hyperfiltration in remnant nephrons: A potentially adverse response to renal ablation. Am J Physiol 1981;241:F85.

65. Olson, JL, Heptinstall RH. Biology of disease: Nonimmunological mechanisms of glomerular injury. Lab Invest 1988;59:564.

66. Olson JL, Wilson SK, Heptinstall RH. Relationship of glomerular injury to preglomerular resistance in experimental hypertension. Kidney Int 1986;29:849.

67. Rennke HG, Klein PS. Pathogenesis and significance of nonprimary focal and segmental glomerulosclerosis: In depth review. Am J Kidney Dis 1989;13:443.

68. Hughson MD, Farris AB, Douglas-Denton R, et al. Glomerular number and size in autopsy kidneys: The relationship to birth weight. Kidney Int 2003;63:2113.

69. Bhathena DB, Julian BA, McMorrow RG, Baehler RW. Focal sclerosis of hypertrophied glomeruli in solitary functioning kidneys of humans. Am J Kidney Dis 1985;5:226.

70. Guttierrez-Millett V, Nieto J, Praga M, et al. Focal glomerulosclerosis and proteinuria in patients with solitary kidneys. Arch Intern Med 1986;146:705.

71. Kiprov DD, Colvin RB, McClusky RT. Focal and segmental glomerulosclerosis and proteinuria associated with unilateral renal agenesis. Lab Invest 1982;46:275.

72. Robittaille P, Mongeau J-G, Lortie L, Sinnassamy P. Long-term follow-up of patients who underwent unilateral nephrectomy in childhood. Lancet 1985;1:1297.

73. Thorner PS, Arbus GS, Celemajer DS, Baumal R. Focal segmental glomerulosclerosis and progressive renal failure associated with a unilateral kidney. Pediatrics 1984;73:806.

74. Zucchelli P, Cagnoli L, Casanova S, et al. Focal glomerulosclerosis in patients with unilateral nephrectomy. Kidney Int 1983;24:649.

75. Atala A. Congenital urologic abnormalities. In: Schrier RW, ed. Diseases of the Kidney and Urinary Tract, 7th ed. Philadelphia: Lippincott Williams & Wilkins, 2001:649.

76. Heptinstall RH. End-stage renal disease. In: Heptinstall RH, ed. Pathology of the Kidney, 4th ed. Boston: Little, Brown and Company 1993:713.

77. United States Renal Data System 1996 Annual Data Report. Am J Kidney Dis 1996;28(suppl 3):S1.

78. United States Renal Data System 2002 Annual Data Report. Am J Kidney Dis 2003;41(suppl 2):S1.

79. Sekkerie MA, Port FK, Wolfe RA, et al. Recovery from end-stage renal disease. Am J Kidney Dis 1990;15:61.

80. Pichette V, Querin S, Desmeules M, et al. Renal functional recovery in end-stage renal disease. Amer J Kidney Dis 1993;22:398.

81. Rottembourg J. Residual renal function and recovery of renal function in patients treated by CAPD. Kidney Int 1993;43(suppl 40):S106.

82. Go AS, Chertow GM, Fan D, et al. Chronic kidney disease and the risk of death, cardiovascular events, and hospitalization. N Engl J Med 2004;351:1296.

83. McClellan WM, Langston RD, Presley R. Medicare patients with cardiovascular disease have a high prevalence of chronic kidney disease and a high rate of progression to end-stage renal disease. J Am Soc Nephrol 2004;15:1912.

84. Foley RN, Parfrey PS, Hartnett JD, et al. Clinical and echocardiographic disease in patients starting end-stage renal disease therapy. Kidney Int 1995;47:186.

85. Parfrey PS, Hartnett JD, Barre PE. The natural history of myocardial disease in dialysis patients. J Am Soc Nephrol 1991;2:2.

86. London GM, Fabiani F, Marchais SJ, et al. Uremic cardiomyopathy, an inadequate left ventricular hypertrophy. Kidney Int 1987;31:973.

87. Churchill DN. Comparative morbidity and mortality among hemodialysis and continuous ambulatory dialysis patients. Kidney Int 1993;43(suppl 40):S16.

88. Vlahakos DV, Hahalis G, Vassilakos P, et al. Relationship between left ventricular hypertrophy and plasma renin activity in chronic dialysis patients. J Am Soc Nephrol 1997;8:1764.

89. Leenen FH, Smith DL, Khanna R, Oreopoulos DG. Changes in left ventricular hypertrophy and function in hypertensive patients started on continuous ambulatory peritoneal dialysis. Am Heart J 1985;110:102.

90. Parfrey PS, Hartnett JD, Griffiths SM, et al. The clinical course of left ventricular hypertrophy in dialysis patients. Nephron 1990;55:114.

91. Silberberg JS, Barre PE, Prichard SS, Sniderman AD. Impact of left ventricular hypertrophy on survival in end-stage renal disease. Kidney Int 1989;36:286.

92. Rostand SG, Branzell JD, Cannon RO, Victor RG. Cardiovascular complications in renal failure. J Am Soc Nephrol 1991;2:1053.

93. Rostand SG, Rutsky EA. Ischemic heart disease in chronic renal failure: Management considerations. Semin Dial 1989;2:98.

94. Linder A, Charra B, Sherrard DJ, Scribner BH. Accelerated atherosclerosis in prolonged maintenance hemodialysis. N Engl J Med 1974;290:697.

95. Braun J, Oldendorf, Moshage W, et al. Electron beam computed tomography in the evaluation of cardiac calcifications in chronic dialysis patients. Am J Kidney Dis 1996;27:394.

96. Lemeire N, Bernaert P, Lambert, M-C, Vijt D. Cardiovascular risk factors and their management in patients on continuous ambulatory peritoneal dialysis. Kidney Int 1994;46(suppl 48):S31.

97. Owen WF, Madore F, Brenner BM. An observational study of cardiovascular characteristics of long-term end-stage renal disease survivors. Am J Kidney Dis 1996;28:931.

98. Goodman WG, Goldin J, Kuizon BD, et al. Coronary artery calcification in young adults with end-stage renal disease who are undergoing dialysis. N Engl J Med 2000;342:1478.

99. Block GA, Hulbert-Shearon TE, Levin NW, Port FK. Association of serum phosphorus and calcium x phosphate product with mortality risk in chronic hemodialysis patients: A national study. Am J Kidney Dis 1998;31:607.

100. Ganesh SK, Stack AG, Levin NW, et al. Association of elevated serum $PO_4$, $Ca \times PO_4$ product and parathormone levels with cardiac mortality in chronic hemodialysis patients. J Am Soc Nephrol 2001;12:2131.

101. Rumberger JA, Simons DB, Fitzpatrick LA, et al. Coronary artery calcium area by electron-beam computed tomography and

coronary atherosclerosis plaque area: A histopathologic correlative study. Circulation 1995;93:2157.

102. Sangiorgi G, Rumberger JA, Severson A, et al. Arterial calcification and not lumenal stenosis is highly correlated with atherosclerotic plaque burden: A histopathologic study of 723 coronary artery segments using non-decalcifying methodology. J Am Coll Cardiol 1998;31:126.

103. Gotleib AI, Silver MD. Atherosclerosis: Pathology and pathogenesis. In: Silver MD, Gotleib AI, Schoen FJ, eds. Cardiovascular Pathology, 3rd ed. New York: Churchill Livingstone, 2001:68.

104. McCullough PA, Soman, S. Cardiovascular calcification in patients with chronic renal failure. Are we on target with this risk factor? Kidney Int 2004;66(suppl 90):S18.

105. Chen NX, O'Neill KD, Duan D, Moe SM. Phophorus and uremic serum up-regulate osteopontin expression in vascular smooth muscle cells. Kidney Int 2002;62:1724.

106. Moe SM, O'Neill KD, Duan D, et al. Medial artery calcification in ESRD patients is associated with deposition of bone matrix proteins. Kidney Int 2002;61:638.

107. Moe SM, Duan D, Doehle BP, et al. Uremia induces the osteoblastic differentiation factor Cbfa 1 in human blood vessels. Kidney Int 2003;63:1003.

108. London GM, Marty C, Marchaio SJ, et al. Arterial calcification and bone histomorphometry in end-stage renal disease. J Am Soc Nephrol 2004;15:1943.

109. Adler Y, Vaturi M, Herz I, et al. Nonobstructive aortic valve calcification: A window to significant coronary artery disease. Atherosclerosis 2002;161:193.

110. Raggi P, Boulay A, Chasan-Taber S, et al. Cardiac calcification in adult hemodialysis patients: A link between end-stage renal disease and cardiovascular disease? J Am Coll. Cardiol. 2002;39:695.

111. Wang AY, Wang M, Woo J, et al. Cardiac valve calcifications as an important predictor for mortality and cardiovascular mortality in long-term peritoneal dialysis patients: A prospective study. J Am Soc Nephrol 2003;13:159.

112. Duh, Q-Y, Lim RC, Clark OH. Calciphylaxis in secondary hyperparathyroidism: Diagnosis and parathyroidectomy. Arch Surg. 1991;126:1213.

113. Moe SM. Calcemic uremic arteriopathy: A new look at an old disorder. NephSAP (Nephrology Self-Assessment Program) 2004;3:77.

114. Brown DF, Denny CF, Burns DK. Systemic calciphylaxis associated with massive gastrointestinal hemorrhage. Arch Pathol Lab Med 1998;122:656.

115. Mawad HW, Sawaya BP, Sarin R, Mallucki HH. Calcific uremic arteriopathy in association with low turnover bone disease. Clin Nephrol 1999;52:160.

116. Rostand SG, Rutsky EA. Pericarditis in end-stage renal disease. Cardiol Clin 1990;8:701.

117. Rutsky EA, Rostand SG. Pericarditis in end-stage renal disease: Clinical characteristics and management. Semin Dialysis 1989;2:25.

118. Weiss SW, Taw RL, Hutchins GM. Constrictive uremic pericarditis following hemodialysis for acute renal failure. Johns Hopkins Med J 1973;132:301.

119. Wagenvort CA, Mooi WJ. Vascular diseases. In: Dail DH, Hammer SP, eds. Pulmonary Pathology, 2nd ed. New York: Springer-Verlag, 1993:985.

120. Kuhn C, West WW, Craighead JE, Gibbs AR. Lungs. In: Damjanov I, Linder J, eds Anderson's Pathology, 10th ed. St. Louis, MO: Mosby–Yearbook, 1996:1470.

121. Hammar SP. Pleural diseases. In: Dail DH, Hammer SP, eds. Pulmonary Pathology, 2nd ed. New York: Springer-Verlag, 1993:1463.

122. Dail DH. Metabolic and other diseases. In: Dail DH, Hammer SP, eds. Pulmonary Pathology, 2nd ed. New York: Springer–Verlag, 1993:707.

123. McCarthy JT, Williams AW, Johnson WJ. Serum beta-2-microglobulin concentration in dialysis patients: Importance of intrinsic renal function. J Lab Clin Med 1994;123:495.

124. Manske CL. Dialysis-related amyloidosis. J Lab Clin Med 1994;123:458.

125. Baudini S, Bergesio F, Conti P, et al. Nodular macroglossia with combined light chain and β-2 microglobulin deposition in a long-term dialysis patient. J Nephrol 2001;14:128.

126. Fleury AM, Buetens OW, Campassi C, Argani P. Pathologic quiz case: A 77-year-old woman with bilateral breast masses. Amyloidosis involving the breast. Arch Pathol Lab Med 2004;128:e67.

127. Mount SL, Eltabbakh GH, Hardin NJ. β-2-microglobulin amyloidosis presenting as bilateral ovarian masses: A case report and review of the literature. Am J Surg Pathol 2002;26:130.

128. Shimizu S, Yasui C, Yasukawa K, et al. Subcutaneous nodules on the buttocks as a manifestation of dialysis related amyloidosis: A clinicopathologic entity? Br J Dermatopathol 2003;149:400.

129. Yusa H, Yoshida H, Kikuchi H, Onizawa K. Dialysis-related amyloidosis of the tongue. J Oral Maxillofacial Surg. 2001;59:947.

130. Takayama F, Miyazaki S, Morita T, et al. Dialysis related amyloidosis of the heart in long-term dialysis patients. Kidney Int 2001;78(suppl):8172.

131. Onishi S, Andress DL, Maloney NA, et al. Beta-2-microglobulin deposition in bone in chronic renal failure. Kidney Int 1991;39:990.

132. Abe T, Uchita K, Orita H, et al. Effects of β-2 microglobulin absorption on dialysis related amyloidosis. Kidney Int 2003;64:1522.

133. Milito G, Taccone-Galluci M, Brancaleone C, et al. The gastrointestinal tract in uremic patients on long-term hemodialysis. Kidney Int 1985;28:S157.

134. Rowe PA, El Nujumi AM, Williams C, et al. The diagnosis of Helicobacter pylori in uremic patients. Am J Kidney Dis 1992;20:574.

135. Vaziri ND, Dure Smith B, Miller R, Mirhmadi MK. Pathology of the gastrointestinal tract in chronic hemodialysis patients: An autopsy study of 78 cases. Am J Gastroenterol 1985;80:608.

136. Navab F, Masters P, Siubrami R, et al. Angiodysplasia in patients with renal insufficiency. Am J Gastroenterol 1989;84:1297.

137. Scheff RT, Zuckerman G, Hartner H, et al. Diverticular disease in patients with chronic renal failure due to polycystic kidney disease. Ann Intern Med 1980;92:202.

138. Takahashi S, Morita T, Koda Y, et al. Gastrointestinal involvement of dialysis-related amyloidosis. Clin Nephrol 1988;30:168.

139. Choi H-S, Heller D, Picken MM, et al. Infarction of the intestine with massive amyloid deposition in two patients on long-term hemodialysis. Gastroenterology 1989;96:230.

140. Abu-Alfa A, Ivanovitch P, Mujais SK. Uremic exocrine pancreopathy. Nephron 1988;48:94.

141. Avram RM, Iancu M. Pancreatic disease in uremia and parathyroid hormone excess. Nephron 1982;32:60.

142. Padilla B, Pollak VE, Pesce A, et al. Pancreatitis in patients with end-stage renal disease. Medicine 1994;73:8.

143. Rutsky EA, Robards M, Van Dyke JA, Rostand SG. Acute pancreatitis in patients with end-stage renal disease without transplantation. Arch Intern. Med 1986;146:1741.

144. Gluck Z, Nolph KD. Ascites associated with end-stage renal disease. Am J Kidney Dis 1987;10:8.

145. Eschbach JW, Adamson JW. Anemia of end-stage renal disease (ESRD). Kidney Int 1985;28:1.

146. Eschbach JW, Egrie JC, Downing MR, et al. Correction of the anemia of end-stage renal disease with recombinant erythropoietin: Results of a combined phase I and phase II trial. N Engl J Med 1987;316:73.

147. Eschbach JW, Haley NR, Egrie JC, Adamson JW. A comparison of the responses to recombinant human erythropoietin in normal and uremic subjects. Kidney Int 1992;42:407.

148. Zhang Y, Thamer M, Stefanik K, et al. Epoetin requirements predict mortality in hemodialysis patients. Am J Kidney Dis 2004;44:866.

149. Abraham PA, Macres MG. Blood pressure in hemodialysis patients during amelioration of anemia with erythropoietin. J Am Soc Nephrol 1991;2:927.

150. Buckner FS, Eschbach JW, Haley NR, et al. Hypertension following erythropoietin therapy in anemic hemodialysis patients. Am J Hypertens 1990;3:947.

151. Cannella G, La Canna G, Sandrini M, et al. Renormalization of high cardiac output and of left ventricular size following long-term recombinant erythropoietin treatment of anemic, dialyzed uremic patients. Clin Nephrol 1990;34:272.

152. Fernandez A, Vega N, Jimenez F, et al. Effect of recombinant human erythropoietin treatment on hemodynamic parameters in continuous ambulatory peritoneal patients and hemodialysis patients. Am J Nephrol 1992;12:207.

153. Hayashi T, Suzuki A, Shoji T, et al. Cardiovascular effect of normalizing the hematocrit during erythropoietin therapy in predialysis patients with chronic renal failure. Am J Kidney Dis 2000;35:250.

154. Portoles J, Torralbo A, Martin P, et al. Cardiovascular effects of recombinant human erythropoietin in predialysis patients. Am J Kidney Dis 1997;29:541.

155. Muirhead N. Erythropoietin is a cause of access thrombosis. Semin Dialysis 1993;6:188.

156. Eschbach JW. Erythropoietin is not a cause of access thrombosis. Semin Dialysis 1993;6:180.

157. Remuzzi G, Pusineri F. Coagulation defects in uremia. Kidney Int 1988;33(suppl 24):S13.

158. Tokars JI, Miller ER, Alter MJ, Arduino MJ. National surveillance of hemodialysis associated diseases in the United States, 1995. ASAIO J 1998;44:98.

159. Fabrizi F, Martin P, Lunghi G, Locatelli F. Liver disease in dialysis patients. Int J Artif Organs 2000;23:736.

160. Roth D. Hepatitis C virus: The nephrologist's view. Am J Kidney Dis 1995;25:3.

161. Caramelo C, Ortiz A, Aguilera B, et al. Liver disease patterns in hemodialysis patients with antibodies to hepatitis C virus. Am J Kidney Dis 1993;22:822.

162. Martin P, Carter D, Fabrizi F, et al. Histopathologic features of hepatitis C in renal transplant candidates. Transplantation 2000;69:1479.

163. Parfrey P, Farge D, Forbes R, et al. Chronic hepatitis in end-stage renal disease: Comparison of HBsAg-negative and HBsAg-positive patients. Kidney Int 1985;28:959.

164. Rao KV, Anderson WR. Liver disease after renal transplantation. Am J Kidney Dis 1992;19:496.

165. Fraser CL, Arieff AL. Nervous system manifestations of renal failure. In: Schrier RW, ed. Diseases of the Kidney, 7th ed. Philadelphia: Lippincott Williams & Wilkins, 2001:2769.

166. Hruska KA, Teitelbaum SL. Renal osteodystrophy. N Engl J Med 1995;333:166.

167. Dusso AS. Vitamin D receptor: Mechanisms for vitamin D resistance in renal failure. Kidney Int 2003;63(suppl 85):S6.

168. Alphonso S, Santamaria I, Guinsburg ME, et al. Chromosomal abberrations, the consequence refractory hyperparathyroidism: Its relationship with biochemical parameters. Kidney Int 2003;63(suppl 85):S32.

169. Boyce BF, Xing L, Shakespeare W, et al. Regulation of bone remodeling and emerging breakthrough drugs for osteoporosis and osteolytic bone metastasis. Kidney Int 2003;63(suppl 85):S2.

170. Coburn JW. Mineral metabolism and renal bone disease: Effects of CAPD versus hemodialysis. Kidney Int 1993;43(suppl 40):S92.

171. Pei Y, Herez G, Greenwood C, et al. Non-invasive prediction of aluminum bone disease in hemo- and peritoneal dialysis patients. Kidney Int 1992;41:1374.

172. O'Connor MO, Garrett P, Dockery M, et al. Aluminum-related bone disease. Am J Clin Pathol 1986;86:168.

173. Coburn JW, Maung HM. Use of active vitamin D sterols in patients with chronic kidney disease, stages 3 and 4. Kidney Int 2003;63(suppl 85):S49.

174. Mailloux LU, Haley WE. Hypertension in the ESRD patient: Pathophysiology, therapy, outcomes, and future directions. Am J Kidney Dis 1998;32:705.

175. Zucchelli P, Zuccala A, Degli Esposti E, et al. Pathophysiology and management of hypertension in hemodialysis patients. Contrib Nephrol 1987;54:209.

176. Ifudu O, Matthew JJ, Macey LJ, et al. Parathyroidectomy does not correct hypertension in patients on maintenance dialysis. Am J Nephrol 1998;18:28.

177. Maiorca R, Caucarini GC, Brunori G, et al. Morbidity and mortality of CAPD and hemodialysis. Kidney Int 1993;43(suppl 40):S4.

178. Schwartz, M. M, Cotran RS. Primary renal disease in transplant recipients. Hum Pathol 1976;7:445.

179. Dunnill MS, Millard PR, Oliver D. Acquired cystic disease of the kidneys: A hazard of long-term intermittent maintenance haemodialysis. J Clin Pathol 1977;30:868.

180. McManus JF, Hughson MD, Fitts CT, Williams AV. Studies on end-stage kidneys. I. Nodule formation in intrarenal arteries and arterioles. Lab Invest 1977;37:339.

181. Mailloux LV, Napolitano B, Bellucci AG, et al. Renal vascular disease causing end-stage renal disease, incidence, clinical correlates, and outcomes: A 20 year experience. Am J Kidney Dis 1994;24:662.

182. Rimmer JM, Gennari FJ. Atherosclerotic renovascular disease and progressive renal failure. Ann Intern Med 1993;118:712.

183. Textor SC. Ischemic nephropathy: Where are we now? J Am Soc Nephrol 2004;15:1974.

184. Lajoie G, Laszik Z, Nadasdy T, Silva FG. The renal-cardiac connection: Renal parenchymal alterations in patients with heart disease. Semin Nephrol 1994;14:441.

185. Heptinstall RH. Urinary tract infection, pyelonephritis, reflux nephropathy. In: Jennette JC, Olson JL, Schwartz MM, Silva FG, eds. Heptinstall's Pathology of the Kidney, 5th ed. Philadelphia: Lippincott-Raven Publishers, 1998:725.

186. Jungers P, Joly D, Barbey F, et al. ESRD caused by nephrolithiasis: Prevalence, mechanisms, and prevention. Am J Kidney Dis 2004;44:799.

187. Perneger TV, Whelton PK, Klag MJ. Risk of kidney failure associated with the use of acetaminophen, aspirin, and nonsteroidal antiinflammatory drugs. N Engl J Med 1994;331:1675.

188. Nanra RS. Renal effects of antipyretic analgesics. Am J Med 1983;75(Suppl):70.

189. Buckalew VM Jr, Shey HM. Renal disease from habitual antipyretic analgesic consumption: An assessment of the epidemiological evidence. Medicine 1986;11:291.

190. Henrich WL, Agoda LE, Barrett B, et al. National Kidney Foundation position paper: Analgesics and the kidney: Summary and recommendations to the Scientific Advisory Board of the National Kidney Foundation. Am J Kidney Dis 1996;27:162.

191. Cotran RS. Glomerulosclerosis in reflux nephropathy. Kidney Int 1982;21:528.

192. Hughson MD, McManus JF, Hennigar GR. Studies on end-stage kidneys. II. Embryonal hyperplasia of Bowman's capsular epithelium. Am J Pathol 1978;91:71.

193. deSilva K, Tobias V, Kainer G, Beckwith B. Metanephric adenoma with embryonal hyperplasia of Bowman's capsular epithelium: Previously unreported association. Pediatr Dev Pathol 2000;3:472.

194. Ogata K. Clinicopathologic study of kidneys from patients on chronic dialysis. Kidney Int 1990;37:1333.

195. McManus JFA, Hughson MD, Hennigar GR, et al. Dialysis enhances renal epithelial proliferations. Arch Pathol Lab Med 1980;104:192.

196. McManus JFA, Hughson MD. Studies on end-stage kidneys. V. Unusual epithelial activity or remarkable endothelial metaplasia: Findings in a dialyzed kidney. Am J Surg. Pathol 1979;3:229.

197. Faraggiana T, Venkataseshan VS, Inagami T, Churg J Immunohistochemical localization of renin in end-stage kidneys. Am J Kidney Dis 1988;12:194.

198. Pitcock JA, Johnson JG, Share L, Hatch FE, et al. Malignant hypertension due to musculo-mucoid intimal hyperplasia of intrarenal arteries. Circ Res 1975;36(suppl 1):S33.

199. Hughson MD, Fox M, Garvin AJ. Pathology of the end-stage kidney after dialysis. Progress Reprod Urinary Tract Pathol 1990;2:157.

200. Hughson MD, Harley RA, Hennigar GR. Cellular arteriolar nodules: Their presence in heart, pancreas, and kidney of patients with treated malignant hypertension. Arch Pathol Lab Med 1982;106:71.

201. Dobyan DC, Truong LD, Eknoyan G. Renal malakoplakia reappraised. Am J Kidney Dis 1993;33:243.
202. Parsons MA, Harris SC, Longstaff AJ, Granger RG. Xanthogranulomatous pyelonephritis: A pathological, clinical and aetiological analysis of 87 cases. Diag Histopathol 1985;6:203.
203. Nadasdy T, Laszik Z, Blick KE, et al. Tubular atrophy in the end-stage kidney: A lectin and immunohistochemical study. Hum Pathol 1994;25:22.
204. Haggitt RC, Pitcock JA, Muirhead EE. Renal medullary fibrosis in hypertension. Hum. Pathol 2:587.
205. Muirhead EE, Germain GS, Leach BE, et al. Renomedullary interstitial cells, prostaglandins and the antihypertensive function of the kidney. Prostaglandins 1973;3:581.
206. Hughson MD, McManus JFA, Fitts CT, Williams AV. Studies on end-stage kidneys. III. Glycogen deposition in interstitial cells of the renal medulla. Am J Clin Pathol 1979;72:400.
207. Ishikawa I. Uremic acquired cystic disease of the kidney. Urology 1985;26:101.
208. Ishikawa I, Saito Y, Onouchi Z, et al. Development of acquired cystic kidney disease and adenocarcinoma of the kidney in glomerulonephritic hemodialysis patients. Clin Nephrol 1980;14:1.
209. Levine E, Slusher SL, Grantham JJ, Wetzel LH. Natural history of acquired renal cystic disease in dialysis patients: A prospective longitudinal CT study. Am J Radiol 1991;156:501.
210. Grantham JJ. Acquired cystic kidney disease. Kidney Int 1991;40:143.
211. Hughson MD, Bigler S, Dickman K, Kovacs G. Renal cell carcinoma of end-stage renal disease: An analysis of chromosomes 3, 7, and 17 abnormalities by microsatellite amplification. Mod Pathol 1999;12:301.
212. Ishikawa I, Onouchi Z, Saito Y, et al. Sex differences in acquired cystic disease of the kidney on long-term dialysis. Nephron 1985;39:336.
213. Matson MA, Cohen EP. Acquired cystic disease: Occurrence, prevalence, and renal cancers. Medicine 1990;69:217.
214. Park JH, Kim YO, Park JH, et al. Comparison of acquired cystic disease between hemodialysis and continuous ambulatory peritoneal dialysis. Korean J Med 2000;15:51.
215. Ishikawa I, Shikura N, Nagahara M, et al. Comparison of the severity of acquired renal cysts between CAPD and hemodialysis. Adv Perit Dialysis 1991;7:91.
216. Bommer J, Waldherr R, Van Kaick G, et al. Acquired renal cysts in uremic patient—in vivo demonstration by computed tomography. Clin Nephrol 1980;14:299.
217. Feiner HD, Katz LA, Gallo GR. Acquired cystic disease of the kidney in chronic dialysis patients. Urology 1981;12:260.
218. Ishikawa I, Saito Y, Askara M, et al. Twenty-year follow-up of acquired cystic disease. Clin Nephrol 2003;59:153.
219. Neufeld TK, Douglass D, Grant M, et al. In vitro formation and expansion of cysts derived from human renal cortex epithelial cells. Kidney Int 1992;41:1222.
220. Humes HD, Beals TF, Cielinski DA, et al. Effects of transforming growth factor-β, transforming growth factor-α, and other growth factors on proximal tubule cells. Lab Invest 1991;64:538.
221. Atlas I, Mendelsohn J, Baselga J, et al. Growth factor regulation of human renal carcinoma cells: The role of transforming growth factor-α. Cancer Res 1992;52:3335.
222. Lubensky IA, Schmidt L, Zhuang Z, et al. Hereditary and sporadic papillary renal cell carcinomas with c-met mutations share a distinct morphologic phenotype. Am J Pathol 1999;155:517.
223. Konda R, Sato H, Hatafuku F, et al. Expression of hepatocyte growth factor and its receptor c-met in acquired renal cystic disease associated with renal cell carcinoma. J Urol 2004;171:2166.
224. Bakir AA, Hasnain M, Young S, Dunea G. Dialysis associated renal cystic disease resembling autosomal dominant polycystic kidney disease: A report of two cases. Am J Nephrol 1999;19:519.
225. Risdon RA, Woolf AS. Developmental defects and cystic diseases of the kidney. In: Jennette JC, Olson JL, Schwartz MM, Silva FG, eds. Heptinstall's Pathology of the kidney, 5th ed. Philadelphia: Lippincott-Raven Publishers, 1998:1149.
226. The European Polycystic Kidney Disease Consortium. The polycystic kidney disease 1 gene encodes a 14 kb transcript and lies within a duplicated region on chromosome 16. Cell 1994;77:881.
227. Qian F, Watnik TJ, Onuchic LF, Germino GG. The molecular basis of focal cyst formation in human autosomal dominant polycystic disease type 1. Cell 1996;87:979.
228. Torra R, Viribay M, Telleria D, et al. Seven novel mutations of the PKD2 gene in families with autosomal dominant polycystic kidney disease. Kidney Int 1999;56:28.
229. Deck MA, Verani R, Silva FG, et al. Histogenesis of renal cysts in end-stage renal disease (acquired cystic kidney disease): An immunohistochemical and lectin study. Surg Pathol 1988;1:391.
230. Hughson MD, Hennigar GR, McManus JF. A. Atypical cysts, acquired cystic disease and renal cell tumors in end-stage dialysis kidneys. Lab Invest 1980;42:475.
231. Farragiana T, Bernstein J, Strauss L, Churg J. Use of lectins in the study of histogenesis of renal cysts. Lab Invest 1985;53:575.
232. Zeir M, Fehrenbach P, Geberth S, et al. Renal histology in polycystic disease with incipient and advanced renal failure. Kidney Int 1992;42:1259.
233. Doublet JD, Peraldi MN, Gattengo B, et al. Renal cell carcinomas of native kidneys: Prospective study of 129 renal transplant patients. J Urol 1997;158:42.
234. Gulanikar AC, Dailey PP, Hamrich-Turner JE, Butkis DE. Prospective pretransplant ultrasound screening in 206 patients for acquired renal cysts and renal cell carcinoma. Transplant 1998;66:1669.
235. Denton MD, Magee CC, Ovuworie C, et al. Prevalence of renal cell carcinoma in patients with ESRD pre-transplantation: A pathologic analysis. Kidney Int 2002;61:2201.
236. Tosaka A, Ohya D, Yamada K, et al. Incidence and properties of renal masses and symptomatic renal cell carcinoma detected by abdominal ultrasound. J Urol 1990;144:1097.
237. United States Cancer Statistics. 1999–2001 Incidence and Mortality Data. Web-based Incidents and Mortality Reports. National Program of Cancer Registries. Atlanta: Department of Health and Human Services. Centers for Disease Control and Prevention.
238. Stewart JH, Buccianti G, Agoda L, et al. Cancers of the kidney and urinary tract in patients on dialysis for end-stage renal disease: An analysis of data from the United States, Europe, and Australia and New Zealand. J Am Soc Nephrol 2003;14:197.
239. Ishikawa I. Renal carcinoma in chronic hemodialysis patients: A 1990 questionnaire study in Japan. Kidney Int 1993;43(suppl 41):S167.
240. Port FK, Ragheb NE, Schwartz AG, Hawthorne VM. Neoplasms in dialysis patients: A population based study. Am J Kidney Dis 1989;14:119.
241. MacDougall ML, Welling LW, Weighman TB. Prediction of carcinoma in acquired cystic disease as a function of kidney weight. J Am Soc Nephrol 1990;1:828.
242. Ishikawa I, Kovacs G. High incidence of papillary renal cell tumors in patients on chronic hemodialysis. Histopathology 1993;22:135.
243. Hughson MD, Schmidt L, Zbar B, et al. Renal carcinoma of end-stage renal disease: A histopathologic and molecular genetic study. J Am Soc Nephrol 1996;7:2461.
244. Basile JJ, McCullough DL, Harrison LH, Dyer RB. End-stage renal disease associated with acquired cystic disease and neoplasia. J Urol 1988;140:938.
245. Fujimoto K, Anai S, Okajima E, et al. Chromophobe cell renal carcinoma with acquired cystic disease of the kidney in a long-term hemodialysis patient. Int J Urol. 2003;10:99.
246. Shiga Y, Suzuki K, Tsutsumi M, et al. Renal oncocytomatosis in a long-term hemodialysis patient treated by laparoscopic surgery. Int J Urol 2002;9:646.
247. Kovacs G, Akhtar M, Beckwith B, et al. The Heidelberg classification of renal cell tumors. J Pathol 1997;183:131.
248. Gnarra JR, Tory K, Weng Y, et al. Mutations of the VHL tumor suppressor gene in renal carcinoma. Nature Genet 1994;7:85.
249. Chudek J, Herbers J, Wilhelm M, et al. The genetics of renal tumors of end-stage renal dialysis differs from those occurring in the general population. J Am Soc Nephrol 1998;9:1045.

250. Hughson MD, Meloni AM, Silva FG, Sandberg AA. Renal cell carcinoma in an end-stage kidney of a patient with a functional transplant: Cytogenetic and molecular genetic findings. Cancer Genet Cytogenet 1996;89:65.

251. Ishikawa I, Shikura N, Ozaki, M. Papillary renal cell carcinoma with numeric changes of chromosomes in a long-term hemodialysis patient: A karyotype analysis. Am J Kidney Dis 1993;21:553.

252. Yoshida M, Yao M, Ishikawa I, et al. Somatic von Hippel-Lindau disease gene mutations in clear-cell carcinomas associated with end-stage renal disease/acquired cystic disease of the kidney. Genes Chromosomes Cancer 2002;35:359.

253. Ishikawa I, Yuri T, Kitada H, Shinoda, A. Regression of acquired cystic disease of the kidney after successful renal transplantation. Am J Nephrol 1983;3:310.

254. Vaziri ND, Darwish R, Martin DC, Hostetler MJ. Acquired renal cystic disease in renal transplant recipients. Nephron 1984;37:203.

255. Dlugosz BA, Bretan PN, Novick AC, et al. Causes of death in kidney transplant recipients: 1970 to present. Transplant Proc 1989;21:2168.

256. Penn I, Brunson ME. Cancers after cyclosporin therapy. Transplant Proc 1988;20:885.

257. Kasiske BL, Snyder JJ, Gilbertson DT, Wang C. Cancer after kidney transplantation in the United States. Am J Transplant 2004;4:905.

258. Birkeland SA. Cancer in transplant patients: The Scandiatransplant material. Transplant Proc 1983;15:1071.

259. Chung WY, Nast CC, Ettenger RB, et al. Acquired cystic disease in chronically rejected renal transplants. J Am Soc Nephrol 1992;2:1298.

260. Ishikawa I, Shikura N, Kitada H, et al. Severity of acquired renal cysts in native kidneys and renal allograft with long-standing poor function. Am J Kidney Dis 1989;14:18.

261. Lien, Y-H, Kam I, Shanley PF, Schroter GPJ. Metastatic renal cell carcinoma associated with acquired cystic disease 15 years after successful renal transplantation. Am J Kidney Dis 1991;18:711.

262. Shingleton WB, Sewell PE. Percutaneous cryoablation of renal cell carcinoma in a transplant kidney. BJU Int 2002;90:137.

263. United States Renal Data System 1994 Annual Data Report. Am J Kidney Dis 1994;18(Suppl 2):S48.

264. Dobbie JW. Monitoring peritoneal histopathology in peritoneal dialysis: The role of a biopsy registry. Dial Transplant 1989;18:319.

265. Dobbie JW. Pathogenesis of peritoneal fibrosing syndromes (sclerosing peritonitis) in peritoneal dialysis. Perit Dial Int 1992;12:14.

266. Flessner MF. Osmotic barrier of the parietal peritoneum. Am J Physiol 1994;267:F861.

267. Krediet RT. The peritoneal membrane in chronic peritoneal dialysis. Kidney Int 1999;55:341.

268. Witowsky J, Wisniewska J, Korybalska K, et al. Prolonged exposure to glucose degradation products impairs viability and function of human peritoneal mesothelial cells. J Am Soc Nephrol 2001;12:2434.

269. Combet S, Miyata T, Moulin P, et al. Vascular proliferation and enhanced expression of nitric oxide synthetase in human peritoneum exposed to long-term peritoneal dialysis. J Am Soc Nephrol 2000;11:717.

270. DeVriese AS, Tilton RG, Stephan CC, Lameire NH. Vascular endothelial growth factor is essential for hyperglycemia-induced structural and functional alterations of the peritoneal membrane. J Am Soc Nephrol 2001;12:1734.

271. Honda K, Nitta K, Horita S, et al. Accumulation of advanced glycation end-products in the peritoneal vasculature of continuous ambulatory peritoneal dialysis patients with low ultra-filtration. Nephrol Dial Transplant 1999;14:1541.

272. Zweers MM, deWaart DR, Smit W, et al. Growth factors VEGF and TGFβ-1 in peritoneal dialysis. J Lab Clin Med 1999;134:124.

273. Margetts PJ, Kolb M, Galt T, et al. Gene transfer of transforming growth factor-β1 to the rat peritoneum: Effect on membrane function. J Am Soc Nephrol 2001;12:2029.

274. Williams JD, Craig KG, von Ruhland C, et al, for the Biopsy Registry Study Group. The natural course of peritoneal membrane biology during peritoneal dialysis. Kidney Int 2003;64(suppl 88):S43.

275. Mateijsen MAM, van der Wal AC, Hendriks PMEM, et al. Vascular and interstitial changes in the peritoneum of CAPD patients with peritoneal sclerosis. Perit Dial Int 1999;19:517.

276. Kawanishi H, Kawaguchi Y, Fukui H, et al, for the Long-Term Peritoneal Dialysis Study Group. Encapsulating peritoneal sclerosis in Japan: A prospective controlled, multicultural study. Am J Kidney Dis 2004;44:729.

277. Rigby RJ, Hawley CM. Sclerosing peritonitis: The experience in Australia. Nephrol Dial Transplant 1998;13:154.

278. United States Renal Data System 1989 Annual Data Report. V. Survival probabilities and causes of death. Am J Kidney Dis 1991;18(suppl 2):S49.

# Renal Transplant Pathology

28

*Robert B. Colvin    Volker Nickeleit*

## BACKGROUND

Renal transplantation provides a cost-effective therapy that improves survival and quality of life for patients with end-stage renal disease (1). In 2002, 14,232 renal transplants were performed in the United States (2) and probably over 30,000 worldwide. Expansion of the number of recipients is constrained primarily by the number of donors. The most common indications for renal transplantation are diabetes, nephrosclerosis associated with hypertension (probably a heterogeneous group), polycystic kidney disease, and various types of glomerular diseases, most commonly IgA nephropathy (2).

Therapy for graft dysfunction is based primarily on renal biopsy findings. These biopsies provide urgent and perplexing challenges for the pathologist, because there is little time for consultation, several diseases can impinge on the graft simultaneously, and a wide range of potent therapy is possible, whose appropriate selection rests firmly on the accuracy of the diagnosis. We hope that this chapter will provide a practical resource to pathologists and clinicians trying to solve clinical dilemmas and to investigators seeking innovative solutions to prevent graft loss. The extensive, exciting, and ever-expanding literature has been cited as much as space permits.

### Brief History of Transplantation (3)

The first public demonstration of a successful renal transplant was by Emerich Ullmann, on March 7, 1902, in the lecture hall of the Society of Physicians in Vienna. He showed a dog with an autotransplant in the neck that produced visible urine from the ureter in the skin, which lasted for 5 days; 12 days later he reported his findings in the medical literature (4). In 1902 Dr. Ullmann also attempted the first kidney transplant (from a pig) to a patient, but this was technically unsuccessful (5). Alexis Carrel, working in Lyon, France, developed the end-to-end vascular suture techniques in 1902 that are widely used in transplantation, and for this and his subsequent work on organ preservation at the Rockefeller Institute in New York, received the Nobel prize in 1912 (6). In 1906, Mathieu Jaboulay, also from Lyon, used Carrel's technique to transplant a xenograft kidney (pig or goat) to the limbs of two patients with chronic renal failure; both grafts failed within an hour (7). Three years later, Ernest Unger in Berlin transplanted a monkey kidney to a girl dying of renal failure; no urine was produced, and Unger concluded that the biochemical barrier was insoluble (8). Working in some obscurity, Dr. Yu Yu Voronoy, in 1936 in Kherson, Ukraine, transplanted the first human kidney. The donor died from a head injury, and the recipient had acute renal failure from mercuric chloride poisoning. The kidney was ABO-incompatible (B to O) and the kidney never worked, but the vessels were patent at autopsy 2 days later (9).

In 1945 Drs. Charles Hufnagel (research fellow), Ernest Landsteiner (chief resident in urology), and David Hume (assistant professor of surgery) at the Peter Bent Brigham Hospital and Harvard Medical School in Boston transplanted a human cadaver kidney to the axilla of a young woman comatose from acute renal failure owing to septicemia (10). The kidney worked for several days and was then removed after the woman regained consciousness; her own kidneys then made a full recovery. Seven other cases of temporary implants were reported from Paris in 1951 (11). One received the first living related kidney (mother to son, who lost a single kidney in a traffic accident); the kidney functioned without any immunosuppression for 22 days before rejecting. In 1951 to 1953, Dr. Hume continued this approach, transplanting kidneys into the thighs of nine patients without immunosuppression; one graft functioned for 6 months (12).

Mastery of the surgical aspects encouraged surgeons to begin transplanting kidneys from identical twins, who do not require immunosuppression. The first such operation was performed on December 23, 1954, by Drs. Hume, Joseph Murray, and Hartwell Harrison (13). The recipient survived 8 years, succumbing to recurrent disease, the major risk in twin recipients.

Broad clinical application awaited the definition of the underlying immunologic events and the means to thwart immunologic rejection. The need for skin graft treatment of war burn wounds motivated the scientific efforts of the young Peter Medawar to ponder "why it was not possible to graft skin from one human being to another, and what could be done about it." Medawar did indeed do something about it, showing in 1953 that injection of lymphoid cells in neonatal mice established a lifelong, specific tolerance to subsequent transplanted skin from the same donor, for which he received the Nobel Prize in 1960 (14). The discovery of the immunosuppressive ability of 6-mercaptopurine by Robert Schwartz and William Dameshek in Boston in 1959 (15) was soon applied in humans in 1960. Gertrude Elion and George Hitchings (Nobel Prize, 1988) at Burroughs Wellcome discovered azathioprine (Imuran), which Roy Calne in Cambridge proved beneficial and less toxic in dog kidney grafts (16). Joseph Murray (Nobel Prize, 1992) first tried azathioprine in humans and added corticosteroids to the regimen (13). The improved results obtained by combination of azathioprine with corticosteroids ushered in the era of clinical renal transplantation in the early 1960s, through the successful studies of Thomas Starzl (17), Murray (13), and colleagues. Innovative therapies, such as antithymocyte globulin (ATG or ALG) (1970s); cyclosporin A (cyclosporine, CsA), anti-CD3 monoclonal antibody (OKT3) (1980s); mycophenolate, tacrolimus (1990s); and others have markedly increased success. Recent clinical trials with protocols to induce transient mixed chimerism have shown promise of achieving Medawar's goal of specific tolerance without immunosuppression (18).

The pathologic literature on renal grafts began with the photomicrographs of canine allograft rejection, published by Carl Williamson of the Mayo Clinic in 1926. He illustrated a "marked lymphocytic infiltration" and "intense glomerulitis" in the dog and attributed graft loss to "atypical glomerular nephritis" (19). He noted that recipients responded differently to autografts and allografts and hoped that "in the future it may be possible to work out a satisfactory way of determining the reaction of the recipient's blood serum or tissues" (19). Subsequent work reported in 1953 by William Dempster in London (20) and Morten Simonsen in Denmark (21) showed that canine grafts are infiltrated by pyroninophilic mononuclear cells, which they concluded were donor-derived plasma cells and their precursors, a "response of the renal mesenchyma to the recipients' individual-specific antibodies and antigens" (22). The infiltrating cells were later shown to be of recipient origin using radiolabeled cells (23). Simonsen illustrated an example of endarteritis in a small artery in a dog, but did not appreciate its distinctiveness, interpreting the lesions, which also had fibrinoid necrosis, as "periarteritis nodosa" (21).

The pathology of human renal transplants was initially described in the 1960s, particularly by Gustav Dammin at Harvard and Kendrick Porter at St. Mary's Hospital in London. Among the early discoveries were the descriptions of endarteritis in acute rejection by Dammin, which he attributed correctly to recipient mononuclear cells (24), chronic transplant arteriopathy (25) and chronic transplant glomerulopathy were reported by Porter (26,27), the relationship of the arteriopathy to anti-HLA antibodies by Paul Russell et al (28), and the pathology of hyperacute rejection and its relationship to humoral antibodies by Kissmeyer-Nielsen et al (29). The recurrence of glomerulonephritis in transplants was first described in isografts by Richard Glassock et al (30). Perhaps most important to pathologists, Priscilla Kincaid-Smith demonstrated the value of the renal biopsy in clinical management, concluding that "the renal biopsy provides a clear-cut diagnosis of rejection and indicates which patients should receive prompt treatment for rejection" (31). Our goal is to make this always true!

## Surgical Procedure

Renal transplant surgical techniques have been standardized (32). The donor kidney is usually placed in the right iliac fossa, which has the advantages of simplicity and accessibility for observation and biopsy. The main renal artery is anastomosed end-to-end to the right hypogastric artery (or end-to-side to the iliac artery with a cuff of donor aorta). When the renal arteries are multiple, various procedures have been devised, making sure the lower pole artery is not sacrificed because it usually also supplies the ureter. Endarterectomy may be necessary in atherosclerotic vessels. The renal vein is anastomosed end-to-side to the iliac vein. Two alternative techniques are commonly used for the ureter, either implantation of the donor ureter into the recipient bladder or anastomosis of the donor pelvis to the recipient ureter. The advantages of the former are that the recipient kidney does not have to be removed and a normal recipient ureter is not required. The main disadvantage is that the blood supply to the ureter can be compromised and later stenosis can result; reflux may also develop. The pyeloureteral anastomosis minimizes the risk of ureteral ischemia and stenosis (33), but urine leaks are more common, if not done properly. Pyeloureteral anastomosis requires a recipient nephrectomy, which provides the potential benefit to determine the primary disease and exclude malignancy in the end-stage kidney. Double kidney transplants from marginal donors have also been performed with success (34,35). Kidneys taken by laparoscopic nephrectomy have more subcapsular cortical injury, including fibrin, necrosis, and hemorrhage, than those harvested by conventional nephrectomy (36). Initial function is slightly worse, but 1-year graft survival is the same as kidneys taken by open procedures (37).

## Standard Immunosuppression

Calcineurin inhibitors (CNI; cyclosporine or tacrolimus) are the mainstay of most standard protocols, usually with corticosteroids (prednisolone or prednisone) and mycophenolate mofetil (MMF) or azathioprine (*triple therapy*). The drugs are tapered in the initial 3 to 6 months to baseline maintenance levels, which in adults are typically approximately 100 ng/mL of cyclosporine and 5 to 15 ng/mL of tacrolimus at the trough level, depending on the other drugs in the regimen and the immunologic risk (38). OKT3 or ATG can substitute for calcineurin inhibitors in patients with delayed graft function (DGF). For treatment of acute rejection episodes, the usual first defense is a short course (2 to 3 days) of high-dose steroids orally (prednisolone) or intravenously (methylprednisolone), followed if necessary by rescue with OKT3 or ATG. Newer FDA-approved drugs include rapamycin (sirolimus; a blocker of IL-2 signaling and cell proliferation) and monoclonal antibodies to the IL-2 receptor (basiliximab; Simulect), CD52 (daclizumab; CAMPATH1), and CD20 (Rituxan, rituximab) and inhibitors of costimulatory signals (e.g., CTLA4Ig mutated protein LWA29Y, belatacept). All of these drugs have the potential for complications related to immunosuppression, and some cause nephrotoxicity.

## Clinical Outcome

Graft and patient survival curves have improved dramatically over the last three decades (Fig. 28.1) (39). The biggest improvement is in the first year, with a lower frequency of rejection, improved response to antirejection therapy, and fewer infectious complications. The long-term loss of grafts has shown only modest improvement, with almost parallel curves of attrition in the last decade. The improvement has been primarily in patients who did not have an episode of acute rejection (40) and those with a retransplant (41). There has been no recent improvement in long-term survival of first transplants from the 1988 to 1995 era (41).

The outcome of the graft depends on the source of the graft (deceased, living related, living nonrelated) and the histocompatibility between the donor and recipient (Figs. 28.1 and 28.2). In the United States from 1992 to 2002, the number of cadaveric kidneys transplanted increased only 8% to 8087, entirely due to an increased number of expanded criteria donors; the number of living donor kidneys increased 146% to 6236 (2).

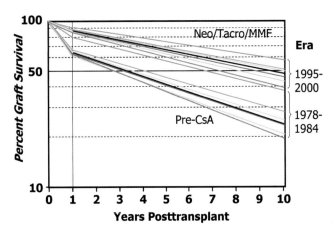

**Figure 28.1** Graft survival by HLA mismatch and era of transplantation from 1978 to 2000 (47). Number of mismatches (HLA-A, B, DR): red, 6; light blue, 5; pink, 4; purple, 3; yellow, 2; blue, 1; green, 0. Most of the improvement over the last two decades has occurred in the 1-year graft survival. The best match (0 mismatches) in the early cohort has a lower survival than the worst match (6 mismatches) in the later group. Beyond 1 year the curves are almost but not quite parallel, indicating that the factors that affect late graft loss have not been affected by improvements in management. (From Danovitch GM, and Cecka JM. Allocation of deceased donor kidneys: past, present and future. Am J Kidney Dis 2003;42:882.)

## Living Donors

*Isografts* (between monozygotic twins) are not immunologically rejected, and no immunosuppression is required. However, isografts are lost from recurrence of the original disease. In the largest compilation, 5-year graft survival was

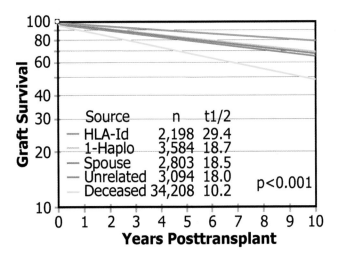

**Figure 28.2** Graft survival by donor source and HLA match (2). The strong effect of the MHC (HLA locus) can be seen by the increased half-life ($t_{1/2}$) of the HLA-identical (HLA-Id) versus the one-haplotype match (1-haplo) related donors (29.4 versus 18.7 years). Unrelated donor kidneys have a similar outcome as one-haplotype family member but a much better survival than deceased donor kidneys (half-life of 18.0 versus 10.2 years). (From Cecka JM. The OPTN/VNOS Renal Transplant Registry 2003. Clin Trans 2003;17:1, with permission.)

70% (42). After 5 years, graft survival was quite stable, with 55% surviving 27 years. Eight of the graft failures (27%) were due to recurrent glomerulonephritis or vasculitis 3 months to 20 years after transplantation, and 18% were lost in the first year.

*HLA-identical grafts* from siblings have identical HLA genes in the major histocompatibility complex (MHC) on chromosome 6, but differ randomly in non-MHC (minor) histocompatibility antigens encoded by genes that segregate independently. These grafts do well, with a 96% 1-year graft survival and a slow chronic loss yielding a graft half-life ($t_{1/2}$) of 29.4 years (Fig. 28.2) (2). However, grafts do develop acute rejection (46% in one series of 108 recipients) (43), but this is usually responsive to steroids; chronic rejection occurs in about 2% over 10 years, about half the rate of haplo-identical grafts (44–46). These results demonstrate that non-MHC antigens can elicit a strong recipient immune response for acute rejection, but have relatively little role in chronic rejection.

*HLA-haplo-identical grafts* (from parent, child, or sibling) have a common chromosome 6 region of one MHC locus, but differ in the other MHC and non-MHC antigens. These grafts have a half-life of 18.7 years, significantly worse than the HLA-identical grafts (Fig. 28.2) (2). The 10-year survival difference compared with MHC identical grafts demonstrates the importance of the MHC as a target in the immune response in chronic rejection.

*Living unrelated grafts*, typically from a spouse or friend, have been tried more commonly recently because of the shortage of deceased donor kidneys. Despite the fact that the MHC is usually mismatched, the results are excellent and almost as good as haplo-identical grafts, with a half-life of 18.0 to 18.5 years (Fig. 28.2) (2). Thus, the condition of the donor (living versus. deceased) is more important than the MHC match.

## Deceased Donors

Deceased donors represent most grafts used worldwide. One-year graft survival has increased from 77% (1987 to 1988) to 89% (1998 to 2001), close to the 95% 1-year graft survival for living donor grafts (2). During this time, the graft half-life ($t_{1/2}$) has risen from 7.9 years to 10.2 years, yielding a projected 10-year survival of 51% (versus 68% with living donors) (2). Graft survival is a function of the number of mismatched antigens (Fig. 28.1) (2,47). With zero HLA-A, -B, or -DR mismatches, the long-term survival approaches that of living donors, with a graft half-life of 14.0 years, compared with six mismatches with a half-life of 8.0 years (2). The estimated overall 19% improvement of survival at 10 years justifies the cost of HLA matching by the United Network of Organ Sharing (UNOS) (48).

Because of the shortage of donors, the standards for accepting a graft are becoming less stringent. Expanded criteria donors (ECD) are defined by UNOS as those older than age 60 years or aged 51 to 59 years with any two additional risk factors (cerebrovascular death, hypertension, serum creatinine level greater than 1.5 mg/dL). Grafts from these donors have a poorer outcome, but still have a 70% 1-year graft survival (2). Selection of older donor kidneys based on histologic criteria leads to graft survival equivalent to grafts from young donors (49). Kidneys from donors whose heart stopped before the kidney was harvested (asystolic donors) have a striking increase in the requirement of dialysis posttransplant (delayed graft function, DGF) (93% versus 17%), but a satisfactory long-term outcome (50). Protocol biopsies at 6 to 12 months show these kidneys have no increase in fibrosis compared with those from heart-beating deceased donors (51).

## Factors That Affect Graft Survival

In addition to the type of immunosuppression, kidney source, and MHC match, the key factors that affect outcome are acute rejection episodes, presensitization, DGF, donor and recipient race and age, and transplant center. DGF is an adverse complication primarily because of the associated increased risk of acute rejection (2,52,53). Black race of recipient is an adverse risk factor, whether the donor is white or black. The survival of HLA-identical sibling kidneys is the same in blacks, but survival of grafts with a one-haplotype match is no different than deceased donor grafts. Outcome varies by transplant group (the center effect) with a 10 to 15% difference in 1-year graft survival (54). Nephron mass has a significant effect (e.g., when a young child's kidney is transplanted to an adult recipient) (55). The nature of the primary disease influences graft survival (e.g., diabetes, hypertension, oxalosis, hemolytic uremic syndrome). Other factors no longer considered important are donor sex, recipient O blood group, blood transfusion, and time on dialysis.

# THE RENAL ALLOGRAFT BIOPSY

## Diagnostic Value

Renal biopsies remain the gold standard to determine the cause of graft dysfunction episodes, which occur in 30% to 60% of patients after transplantation. Biopsies are particularly useful to guide treatment in ambiguous clinical situations and can distinguish acute rejection from acute tubular necrosis, polyomavirus infections, recurrence of original disease, calcineurin inhibitor toxicity, and chronic rejection (56,57). Biopsy findings change the clinical diagnosis in an average of 36% of patients (27% to 46%) and therapy in 59%, with no obvious diminishing value in the last 20 years (56–63) (Table 28.1). Biopsy results change therapy in both the early and late (more than

| TABLE 28.1 | | | | |
|---|---|---|---|---|
| **CLINICAL IMPACT OF THE RENAL ALLOGRAFT BIOPSY** | | | | |
| No. Biopsies | Changed Clinical Diagnosis (%) | Changed Therapy (%) | Avoided Immuno-suppression (%) | Reference |
| 89 | 46 | | | 58 |
| 35 | 46 | 46 | | 57 |
| 64 | 42 | 42 | 30 | 56 |
| 240 | | 83 | | 59 |
| 95 | 30 | 38 | 18 | 60 |
| 263 | | 55 | | 61 |
| 100 | 27 | | | 63 |
| 82 | | 42 | 19 | 62 |
| **Total 968** | **36** | **59** | **22** | |

1 year) posttransplant periods with approximately equal frequency (61,62). Most important, biopsy findings lead to reduced immunosuppression in 22% (19% to 30%) of patients.

## Sensitivity and Specificity

The sensitivity of the biopsy depends on the size, number, and content of the cores. In a study of 130 biopsies with multiple cores, acute rejection was found in only one core in 10% of the cases (64). Thus, the sensitivity of a single core is approximately 90%. In another study, 10% of 79 paired biopsy cores had one core that was insufficient for the diagnosis of rejection (65). The sensitivity of "$n$" biopsy cores can be calculated as $1-(1-\text{sensitivity of a single core})^n$. Accordingly, if one core has a sensitivity of 90%, two cores have a predicted sensitivity of 99%. Thus, the conventional wisdom that recommends two cores is substantiated.

The specificity of the biopsy is impossible to measure because no higher standard for comparison is available. One study showed a specificity of 87% compared with a blinded retrospective clinical review (66). The results that show the biopsy results correlate with the clinical course in 80% to 89% of cases is also reassuring (59,64). However, the short-term clinical course is not the final arbiter, because rejection may be occult or delayed. The issue of clinically silent rejection is discussed in the section on protocol biopsies.

## Safety

Most renal biopsies are done with ultrasound guided Biopty "guns" with 16- or 18-gauge needles (67,68). Gun biopsies have an excellent record of safety in experienced hands; none of the large series reported any deaths caused by biopsy (0 of 5026) (59,67–71). The gun technique has fewer graft losses (1 of 3996, 0.03%) than the hand operated Tru-cut (4 of 1229, 0.3%). A multicenter audited series of 2127 protocol biopsies reported no patient deaths and one potentially avoidable graft loss (71). Ultrasound guidance increases the probability of obtaining cortex from 75% to 91%; guidance by on-site examination by a dissecting microscope increases adequacy to 100% (72).

A 16-gauge needle appears to be the best compromise between tissue yield and complications. Among 1171 protocol biopsies in adults with an automated 16- or 18-gauge needle, no graft losses occurred (73). The 16-gauge needle had no worse major complication rate (73,74) and a better yield of tissue than the 18-gauge needle (76% versus 53% yielded more than seven glomeruli and one or more arteries) (73). The 16-gauge needle had a higher hematoma rate than the 18-gauge needle in children (75). Pediatric transplant biopsies have a similar low complication rate: of 212 biopsies from 19 centers, there were no deaths or graft losses, and only one required surgical exploration for bleeding (76). The types of complication are the same as from biopsies of native kidneys, namely hematuria, ureteral obstruction from clots, hemorrhage, shock, and arteriovenous fistula. Follow-up showed 75% of the fistulas spontaneously closed and none had an impact on renal function requiring intervention (77). Some centers use 15-gauge needles with success.

## Diagnostic Approach to Biopsies

Two cores are divided for light and immunofluorescence microscopy, with most of both cores going for light microscopy. Electron microscopy is processed if glomerular disease is suspected, but usually not otherwise. We prepare about 15 sections stained with hematoxylin and eosin (H&E) (three levels) and 5 for trichrome and 5 cut at 2 microns and stained with periodic acid–Schiff reagent

---

**TABLE 28.2**

**PATHOLOGIC CLASSIFICATION OF RENAL ALLOGRAFT DISEASES**

**I. Immunologic rejection**
  A. Hyperacute rejection (pre-existing alloreactivity to donor)
    1. Antibody mediated (usual)
    2. T-cell mediated (rare)
  B. Acute rejection
    1. Acute T-cell–mediated rejection (acute cellular rejection)
      a. Tubulointerstitial (Banff type I)
      b. Endarteritis/endothelialitis (Banff type II)
      c. Arterial fibrinoid necrosis/transmural inflammation (Banff type III)
      d. Glomerular (transplant glomerulitis (no Banff type)
    2. Acute antibody-mediated rejection (acute humoral rejection, C4d+)
      a. Tubular injury (Banff type I)
      b. Capillaritis/thrombotic microangiopathy (Banff type II)
      c. Arterial fibrinoid necrosis (Banff type III)
  C. Chronic rejection
    1. Chronic T-cell–mediated rejection (with signs of T-cell activity)
      a. Tubulointerstitial (Banff I + fibrosis)
      b. Transplant arteriopathy (Banff II + intimal fibrosis/foam cells)
      c. Transplant glomerulopathy (GBM duplication with glomerulitis)
    2. Chronic antibody-mediated rejection (with signs of antibody mediation, C4d+)
      a. Transplant glomerulopathy (GBM duplication associated with C4d+)
      b. Peritubular transplant capillaropathy (BM duplication and C4d+)
      c. Transplant arteriopathy (intimal fibrosis, C4d+)

**II. Alloantibody/autoantibody-mediated diseases of allografts**
      a. Anti-GBM disease in Alport's syndrome
      b. Nephrotic syndrome in nephrin-deficient recipients
      c. Anti-TBM disease in TBM antigen–deficient recipients
      d. De novo membranous glomerulonephritis
      e. Anti-angiotensin II receptor autoantibody syndrome

**III. Nonrejection injury**
  A. Acute ischemic injury (ATN)
  B. Drug toxicity
      a. Calcineurin inhibitor (cyclosporine, tacrolimus)
      b. OKT3
      c. Sirolimus/rapamycin
  C. Acute tubulointerstitial nephritis (drug allergy)
  D. Infection (viral, bacterial, fungal)
  E. Major artery/vein thrombosis
  F. Mechanical
    1. Obstruction
    2. Urine leak
  G. Renal artery stenosis
  H. Arteriosclerosis
  I. De novo glomerular disease
  J. Posttransplant lymphoproliferative disease
  K. Chronic allograft nephropathy, not otherwise classified: interstitial fibrosis and tubular atrophy

**IV. Recurrent primary disease**
  A. Immunologic: IgA nephropathy, lupus nephritis, anti-GBM disease, and others
  B. Metabolic: amyloidosis, diabetes, oxalosis, and others
  C. Idiopathic: dense-deposit disease, focal segmental glomerulosclerosis, and others

---

(total of 5 slides). Elastin stains are recommended for evaluation of intimal fibrosis. Each section is carefully examined for (a) the nature and degree of the interstitial cellular infiltrate (e.g., activated mononuclear cells, edema, intracapillary cells; (b) arterial and arteriolar lesions (e.g., endarteritis, myocyte necrosis, thrombi, nodular hyaline); (c) tubular injury, inflammation (tubulitis), and nuclear atypia; and (d) glomerular lesions. Further levels are obtained if no diagnosis is evident. We recommend that all biopsies be stained for C4d, as well as IgG, IgA, IgM, C3, lambda, kappa, albumin, and fibrin (by immunofluorescence or immunohistochemistry).

Frozen sections for light microscopy are of limited value, but can be prepared in urgent situations; the diagnostic accuracy was reported to be 89% compared with permanent sections (78). The errors in frozen sections were missing acute cellular rejection owing to sampling and not detecting microthrombi, vascular inflammation, or glomerular lesions. Rapid (2 to 4 hour) permanent sections are used at our centers and provide quite satisfactory preparations.

The recommended requirements are at least seven nonsclerotic glomeruli and two arteries (with two or more medial layers) (64,79). However, the adequacy of the biopsy sample depends entirely on the lesions seen. One artery with endarteritis is sufficient for the diagnosis of acute rejection, even if no glomerulus is present; similarly, immunofluorescence or electron microscopy of one glomerulus is adequate to diagnose membranous glomerulonephritis. In contrast, a large portion of cortex with ten glomeruli and a minimal infiltrate does not exclude rejection. A normal medulla does not rule out rejection (80), because medulla has a lower sensitivity for rejection than cortex (77%) (81). However, when a prominent mononuclear infiltrate and tubulitis are present in the medulla, rejection is highly likely, if not certain (100% specificity) (81), provided infection, obstruction, and drug allergy are excluded. Furthermore, medulla is satisfactory for C4d stains. Subcapsular biopsies often show inflammation and fibrosis within 1 to 2 mm of the capsule; these are caused by the transplantation procedure and are not representative.

## Diagnostic Classification

Jean Hamburger emphasized that graft rejection could not be attributed merely to different intensities of a single type of immune response (82). This has proved to be true, with many different immunologic mechanisms of injury to each of the cellular targets in the graft. The principal alloreactive initiators of graft rejection are T-cells and antibodies (cellular or humoral rejection), which trigger various secondary mediators (e.g., activation of macrophages, complement). The ideal diagnostic classification should be based on pathogenesis, have therapeutic relevance, and be reproducible. The classification in Table 28.2 is our current attempt to meet these criteria.

## DONOR BIOPSY

### Intrinsic Disease

The pathologist may be asked to advise whether a particular kidney from a deceased donor is suitable for transplantation, sometimes in the middle of the night. The most common questions are (a) the degree of scarring owing to vascular disease in the marginal donor, (b) the presence of active renal disease, and (c) the clinical significance of incidentally discovered neoplasms. Another type of donor biopsy, implantation or zero-hour, is used in clinical trials to document underlying disease that might be confused with chronic rejection or drug toxicity.

The extent to which pathologic findings in donor kidneys are predictive of the fate of a graft has not been extensively studied in controlled trials. No study has established an absolute, validated threshold of glomerular sclerosis, fibrosis, or vascular disease beyond which a donor kidney must not be used. In two series, the outcome of the transplants at 1 to 5 years was not measurably different in those with or without pathologic lesions (83,84). It is clear that some abnormalities do not measurably affect outcome, in part because of the other causes of graft loss (rejection, cardiovascular disease, infection). A great concern of setting arbitrary criteria is that kidneys will be discarded needlessly. The number of discarded kidneys per year is half of the number of deaths on the kidney wait-lists (1442 discarded versus 2929 deaths on the waiting list in the year 2000) (85). Each kidney used saves approximately $21,000 over 2 years versus dialysis. Prospective trials that include donor biopsies but do not use that information to discard kidneys would be useful.

Most examinations of donor kidneys are limited to frozen sections, which have numerous pitfalls in the interpretation. Frozen sections have prominent interstitial space (lack of the usual shrinkage artifact owing to fixation), which can be mistaken for fibrosis or edema. Glomerular cellularity cannot be reliably assessed, although thrombi and crescents can be identified. Although the reproducibility of counting sclerotic glomeruli should be excellent, even in frozen sections, the sample size is typically small. The minimum number of glomeruli needed to correlate with outcome was found to be 25; the minimum number to obtain consistent results from paired biopsies was 15 (86). In our opinion, at least 25 glomeruli should be studied, from as deep in the cortex as is feasible. If a scar is sampled, as indicated by clusters of globally sclerotic glomeruli, this area should be noted but treated separately in the analysis to avoid overstating the percentage of sclerosis. Most important, a wedge biopsy is not representative, since it includes mostly outer cortex, the zone where glomerulosclerosis and fibrosis owing to vascular disease is most severe. Intimal fibrosis, in contrast, affects the arcuate and larger arteries more than the interlobular arteries and therefore is underrepresented in a wedge biopsy (87). Reproducibility of visual scoring of interstitial fibrosis, intimal fibrosis, and hyalinosis is notoriously poor (88). Acute tubular injury is not readily assessed in frozen sections, and even in permanent sections, the prediction of recovery is hazardous. With regard to tumors, among the pitfalls in the frozen section interpretation of a possible clear cell carcinoma are epithelioid angiolipoma, intrarenal adrenals (89), and cystic renal cell carcinoma with scant epithelial lining.

## Donor Vascular, Glomerular, and Interstitial Disease (Table 28.3)

The question of donor vascular disease (hypertensive and age-related nephrosclerosis) arises more often now because of increasing use of older donors (90). The use of "harvest" biopsies increases with donor age: 5% at age 20, to 20% at age 45, 40% at age 55, and 60% at age 65 (2). Most studies show a correlation of glomerulosclerosis (91), interstitial fibrosis (92), and intimal fibrosis (93,94) with donor age. Before 40 years of age, 54% of deceased donor biopsies are normal, whereas only 7% of donor kidneys after age 40 are normal (84). However, even septuagenarians have kidneys with glomerulosclerosis that varies from 1.5% to 23% (95); among a group of marginal donors aged 60 to

75 years, 57% had less than 10% glomerulosclerosis (94). The use of histologic evaluation of kidneys from donors older than 60 years of age is recommended because it can result in a graft survival rate similar to that of grafts from younger patients (49).

*Glomerulosclerosis* has been evaluated in many studies with contradictory results. A seminal study showed that allografts with good function at 6 months had less global glomerulosclerosis in the donor biopsy than those with poor function (2% versus 20%) (91). A threshold of less than 20% glomerulosclerosis distinguished a group with a lower rate of DGF (33% versus 87%) and graft loss (7% versus 38%). The proposed 20% cutoff has had subsequent support. Randhawa found among 78 donor biopsies, kidneys with more than 20% glomerulosclerosis had a worse outcome at 6 months (94). The odds ratio remained significant after adjustment for donor age, rejection episodes, or panel reactive antibody. Similarly, others reported that graft survival was strikingly diminished in recipients of grafts with more than 20% glomerulosclerosis, compared

### TABLE 28.3
### DONOR BIOPSY: PREDICTORS OF OUTCOME

| N | Feature | Predictive Value of Feature | References |
|---|---------|------------------------------|------------|
| **Arteriosclerosis** | | | |
| 130 | Any | Graft loss at 2 years, 34% vs. 28%, $P < .05$ | 93 |
| 113 | Any | Elevated creatinine (Cr) at last follow-up 1.9 versus 1.4, $P < .01$ | 99 |
| 50 | Any | 4.6 increased risk of fibrosis at 18 months | 100 |
| 114 | Severe | 100% incidence of DGF; 40% higher Cr at 1 year $P < .05$ | 101 |
| **Globally sclerotic glomeruli** | | | |
| 65 | >20% versus ≤20% | ↑ DGF 87% versus 33%<br>↑ Graft loss 38% versus 7% | 91 |
| 387 | >20% versus ≤20% | ↑ Cr 3–24 months; no change in graft survival. Not independent of donor age | 97 |
| 210 | >20% versus 0% | ↓ 5-year graft survival 35% versus 80%) $P < .04$ | 96 |
| 78 | 4 grades: 0–30% | ↑ Risk of adverse outcome at 6 months. Independent of donor age, rejection episodes | 94 |
| 3444 | >20% versus <20% | Small decrease in 1-year graft survival, 82.7% to 79.4%, but only if creatinine clearance is ≤80 mL/min<br>Age >50 years also risk factor | 85 |
| **Glomerular hypertrophy** | | | |
| 96 | Maximum planar area by point counting | ↓ Creatinine clearance at >2 years | 104 |
| | Maximum planar area | ↓ Creatinine clearance at 0.5–4 years | 105 |
| **Interstitial fibrosis** | | | |
| 78 | Banff ci > 0 | ↑ Risk of adverse outcome at 6 months, 1.9 times beyond prediction by age alone | 94 |
| 43 | Morphometric interstitial volume | Graft function at 1 year | 92 |
| 199 | Banff ci | No predictive value; not reproducible | 86 |

DGF, delayed graft function (dialysis required.)

with those with 0% sclerosis (35% versus 80% 5-year graft survival) (96). However, a large study of 387 donor biopsies found that donor glomerulosclerosis was not an independent predictor of function, if age were included in a multivariate analysis (97). Recipients of grafts with more than 20% glomerulosclerosis had a decreased glomerular filtration rate (GFR) at 2 years, but no difference in graft survival. In a large, well-analyzed UNOS study of 3444 deceased donor kidney biopsies, glomerulosclerosis of more than 20% predicted decreased graft survival only when associated with decreased creatinine clearance in the donor, and then only to a minor degree (3.4% more graft loss) (85). According to this result, glomerulosclerosis should not be the sole criterion for discarding donor kidneys. A preliminary report of UNOS donor biopsies (approximately 25% of more than 23,000 donors) found that donors with more than 10% glomerulosclerosis had a significantly increased rate of DGF, primary nonfunction, and graft loss, even when adjusted for donor age or race (98). The adverse effect was ameliorated by a better HLA match, a nonsensitized recipient, and a first transplant, suggesting that the effect is due to increased susceptibility of a previously damaged kidney to the effects of rejection.

## Other Features

Arteriosclerosis in the donor biopsy correlates with a 6% increase in graft loss at 2 years (93), a 30% increase in creatinine on follow-up (99), and a 4.6-fold increased risk of interstitial fibrosis at 18 months (100). In another series, recipients of grafts with severe arteriosclerosis had a 100% incidence of DGF and a 40% increase in creatinine at 1 year (101). Interstitial fibrosis correlated with outcome in some but not all studies (86,92,94); but its predictive value is not independent of donor age (94). If more than 40% of the cortex has chronic injury (glomerulosclerosis, tubular atrophy, interstitial fibrosis, or occluded vessels), these grafts have an increased risk of graft loss, but this was found in only 3.7% of donor kidneys (102). Increased interstitial alpha–smooth muscle actin (103) and glomerular hypertrophy (104,105) correlate with decreased renal function over 3 to 4 years, but cannot be readily evaluated in frozen sections.

Glomerular thrombi are found in 3% to 7% of donor biopsies, particularly those dying of head trauma (97,106,107). The published data are mixed on the suitability of these kidneys. Thrombi in less than 50% of glomeruli after reperfusion had no effect on graft outcome in one series (108), but in another series of nine donor kidneys with glomerular thrombi (of unspecified extent), three had primary nonfunction (97). Among eight cases of thrombotic microangiopathy in 230 consecutive donor biopsies, DGF was twice as frequent (63%) but graft function and survival at 2 years were not affected (107). The small number of cases prevents meaningful correlation with the extent (five

had less than 25%, one 25% to 50% and two had more than 50% glomerular thrombi; all survived). Thrombi disappeared in all five recipients with subsequent biopsies, even 8 days later in a kidney that previously contained more than 50% glomerular thrombi (107). It is not established whether an occasional atheromatous embolus is a contraindication. Eclamptic kidneys have also recovered fully (106) (and personal experience with one case).

## Primary Renal Disease

The implantation (zero-hour) or 1-hour reperfusion donor biopsy provides a unique view of subclinical renal lesions in healthy individuals. These lesions require a full renal biopsy workup for diagnosis (not just a rapid frozen section), and thus are detected in retrospect after transplantation is completed.

The most common specific glomerular finding is IgA deposition, present in 11% of 108 living donors (two had mesangial sclerosis; the others were normal by light microscopy) (109) and 9% of deceased donors (110). In a large series from Nanking, 24% of 342 donor kidneys had IgA deposits (111). Even considering that IgA nephropathy has a high incidence in Asia, this suggests either that subclinical IgA nephropathy is quite common or that mesangial IgA without proliferation is not a disease. Donor-derived IgA disappears on follow-up biopsy (106,112–114), and graft survival is no different from those without IgA (111). In the Chinese series, recipients of kidneys with mesangioproliferative IgA nephropathy developed transient edema, nephrotic-range proteinuria, microhematuria, hypertension, and DGF and also had a higher rate of acute rejection (31.3% versus 19.3% $P < .001$) (111).

Rarely, kidneys with membranous glomerulonephritis have been transplanted; one survived to at least 3 years (115) and in another, almost complete resolution of the deposits with residual basement membrane spikes was documented at 20 months posttransplant (116). In a personal case, renal vein thrombosis developed acutely and may have been related to the donor disease (Colvin, unpublished). Other diseases that resolved without obvious ill effects include lupus nephritis (117), acute postinfectious glomerulonephritis (98), membranoproliferative glomerulonephritis (type I) (118), and hepatorenal syndrome (119).

## Prediction of Rejection or Ischemic Injury

Several studies have attempted to correlate the presence of neutrophils in the 1-hour postperfusion biopsies in permanent sections with outcome. Neutrophils in both glomerular and peritubular capillaries predicted hyperacute rejection. Neutrophils may reflect an increased ability of the endothelium to promote an active immune response by increased expression of adhesion molecules, MHC antigens, or cytokines or possibly the presence of subclinical donor reactive antibodies. Neutrophils in peritubular capillaries predicted acute rejection, and neutrophils in glomeruli correlated with cold ischemia time and subsequent graft loss (108). Macrophages or platelets in capillaries also are associated with a twofold to threefold increased risk of acute rejection (120). Widespread loss of glomerular endothelial cells is also associated with transiently impaired function (121). C4d in peritubular capillaries predicts later acute antibody-mediated rejection (122). The presence of casts or tubular degeneration correlates with increased ischemic time but not DGF (93). Deceased donor kidneys that later develop DGF have increased tubular cell apoptosis (TUNEL staining) (123,124) and ICAM-1 expression by immunohistochemistry (IHC) (125), compared with those without DGF. Morphology is not very accurate in identifying the severity of ischemic injury, and gene expression signatures may provide a more sensitive method (126).

## Malignancy

Renal cell carcinoma of one of the kidneys has been reported in about 0.9% of donors (127). Occasionally these kidneys are used after wide excision of the tumor. The published data that address this issue come largely from the transplant tumor registry started by the late Israel Penn at Cincinnati. Renal carcinoma was found in 16 kidneys at the time of harvest (128). When the neoplasm was removed completely early posttransplantation, there were no recurrences (14 of 14 recipients). The tumor was not completely removed in two other recipients, and both died of metastases. Sixteen patients received kidneys from donors in whom the opposite kidney had a renal carcinoma. Fifteen remained tumor free, and one had allograft nephrectomy for rejection 3 months posttransplantation and an incidental carcinoma was discovered (127,128). In 17 other recipients, the renal cell carcinoma was not recognized during transplantation, but was first detected at graft nephrectomy an average of 3 months posttransplant (9 cases) or as a metastasis an average of 1 year posttransplant (7 cases) (128). The other was detected by routine ultrasonography, as a hypoechogenic lesion that progressively increased in size. The data support using a kidney with a small primary renal cell carcinoma that can be excised, but the clinical experience is very limited. No kidney with metastatic tumor should be accepted nor any kidney from a donor with known malignancy, except for low-grade tumors of the skin (not melanoma) and possibly the brain (129).

## ACUTE T-CELL–MEDIATED REJECTION

Acute rejection is defined as the rapid (days) loss of graft function due to recipient T-cell or antibody reactiv-

ity to donor alloantigens. These two immunologic pathways, which have distinctive pathologic, immunopathologic, and clinical features, can be active separately, although they not uncommonly occur together. The literature prior to 1999 did not distinguish T-cell and antibody-mediated rejection reliably and is therefore difficult to interpret.

Acute T-cell–mediated rejection (also known as acute cellular rejection, ACR) is the form of rejection that develops most commonly in the first few weeks after transplantation. The frequency of acute rejection episodes declines sharply after the first 6 months, but may arise at any time in stable grafts (130,131). The classical clinical features are an abrupt rise in serum creatinine that progresses over several days, a declining urine output, weight gain, fever, malaise, graft tenderness, and swelling (the last three are muted or absent in patients on calcineurin inhibitors). Rarely, acute rejection can present with the nephrotic syndrome (132). The primary risk factors for acute rejection are the degree of histocompatibility between the donor and the recipient and the presence of prior antigen exposure (previous graft, pregnancy, blood transfusions) (2). Other factors of importance are immunosuppressive drugs used; recipient age, race, sex; patient compliance; and ischemic damage to the graft. Current immunosuppression regimens with calcineurin inhibitors, steroids, and mycophenolate mofetil have considerably reduced the frequency of acute rejection episodes (133). Clinically evident acute rejection currently affects 12% to 18% of recipients of living donor kidneys and 14% to 30% of deceased donor kidneys in the first 6 months (134). Acute rejection now accounts for 11% to 16% of graft failures in the first year and 7% to 11% of failures after the first year (134).

## Pathologic Findings

T-cells react to donor histocompatibility antigens in the kidney, affecting the interstitium, tubules, vessels, and glomeruli, separately or in combination. The approximate relative frequencies of the different patterns of acute cellular rejection are 45% to 70% tubulointerstitial, 30% to 55% vascular, and 2% to 4% glomerular, with considerable variation by center.

## Gross Pathology

Kidneys with severe rejection are swollen and pale, indicative of edema and ischemia, with up to threefold increase in weight (135). In cross section, the cortex is pale and the medulla is congested; the main renal vessels are patent. Also present are marked congestion, petechiae, and focal cortical infarction; acute rupture can occur (Fig. 28.3). The donor ureter shows similar changes, with edema, pallor, and in severe cases, hemorrhagic necrosis.

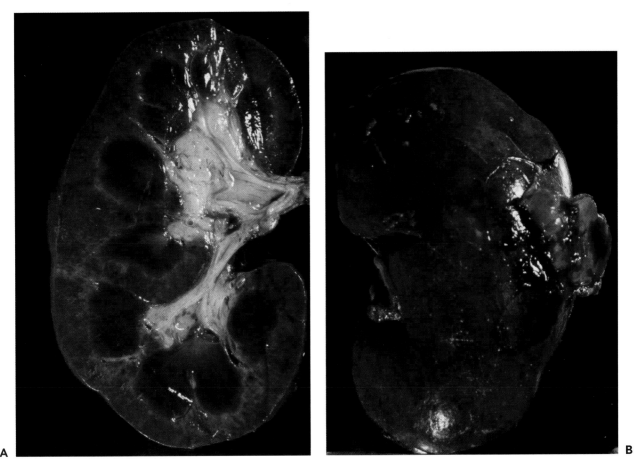

A

B

**Figure 28.3**   Gross photographs of a kidney removed 6 weeks posttransplant for graft failure owing to acute rejection (type III) and rupture (**A** and **B**). The cut surface of the cortex is congested and hemorrhagic (**A**). The hemorrhagic area on the capsule is the site of rupture (**B**). This was the second transplant.

## Light Microscopy

The usual major findings in acute cellular rejection are an infiltrate of activated T lymphocytes and monocytes in the edematous interstitium and tubules and in more severe cases, a similar infiltrate of the arterial intima and glomeruli. This is accompanied by signs of injury of the target cells, such as endothelial swelling and loss, tubular cell apoptosis, and interstitial edema. Hemorrhage and necrosis are found in more severe cases.

## Glomeruli

Mononuclear cells are present in glomeruli to some degree in about 10% of biopsies of acute cellular rejection (136), accompanied by mild, focal endothelial injury or reactive changes (swelling) (Fig. 28.4) (137–140). This mild glomerulitis consists primarily of T-cells and occasional a few neutrophils. This change, although it may represent a T-cell–mediated response in the glomerulus, is not considered a defining or important feature of acute rejection.

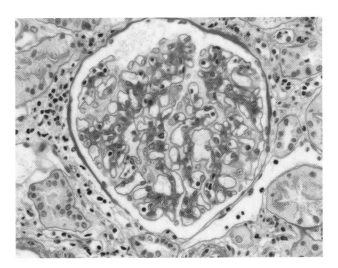

**Figure 28.4**   Several mononuclear cells are present in glomerular capillaries. This is below the threshold of transplant glomerulitis (acute allograft glomerulopathy). (PAS, ×400.)

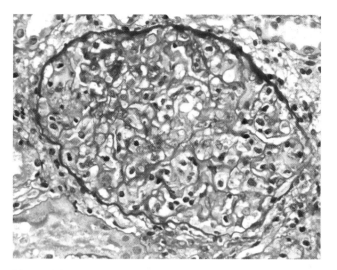

**Figure 28.5** Acute cellular rejection with transplant glomerulitis (acute allograft glomerulopathy) 73 days posttransplant. The C4d stain was negative and type II rejection was present. In contrast to Figure 28.4, the endothelial cells are markedly swollen, occluding the capillaries. (PAS, ×400.)

In contrast, in about 2% to 4% of biopsies, a severe form of glomerular injury dominates the histologic pattern, typically arising in the first 1 to 4 months posttransplant (139,141–144), although it may arise several years after transplant (140,145). In this condition, termed *transplant glomerulitis* or *acute allograft glomerulopathy*, most or all glomeruli show hypercellularity, injury and enlargement of endothelial cells, infiltration of glomeruli by mononuclear cells, and webs of periodic acid-Schiff (PAS)–positive material (Fig. 28.5) (144). Focal and segmental lesions can also be found with the same features, including dilation of capillaries filled with inflammatory cells and swollen endothelial cells. This lesion is best appreciated in 2-μm

PAS-stained sections, which reveals the webbing pattern in capillaries and mesangiolysis. Occasional endothelial necrosis can be found, and the endothelial cells appear activated (increased basophilic cytoplasm and enlarged open nuclei with nucleoli). The mononuclear cells also have an activated appearance. Crescents are not found and thrombi are rare. The glomerular lesions are commonly accompanied by infiltration of arterial endothelium by mononuclear cells and intimal proliferation (56,139–142,146,147). In one series of 12 patients, 92% had associated endarteritis (146). However, glomeruli can be affected in the absence of tubulointerstitial cellular infiltrates or other evidence of rejection (139,140,144). In one large series, 40% lacked other evidence of rejection (140).

### Tubules

In acute cellular rejection, T-cells and macrophages invade tubules and insinuate between tubular epithelial cells, a process termed *tubulitis* (Figs. 28.6 to 28.8). This is best demonstrated in PAS-stained slides to define the tubular basement membrane (TBM). Tubulitis is normally recognized by increased numbers of small dark nuclei in tubules or an irregular distribution of the nuclei. Normal tubular epithelial cells have larger and less dense nuclei than lymphocytes. However, it is sometimes difficult to distinguish infiltrating mononuclear cells from apoptotic or degenerating tubular epithelial cells. Sometimes a clear area surrounds the mononuclear cell. A CD3 stain can be combined with PAS to help demonstrate tubulitis (148). Both proximal and distal tubules are affected, although some have reported that the distal tubules are most frequently infiltrated (149–151). The degree of tubulitis of the proximal but not the distal tubules correlates with the extent of the interstitial infiltrate (150). The medulla may also show

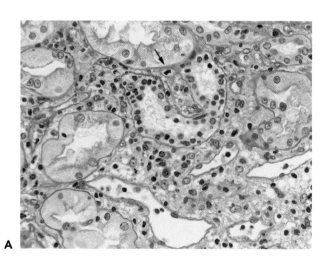
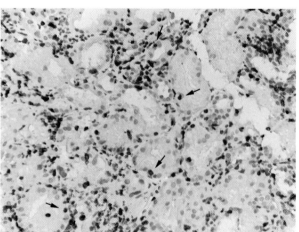

**Figure 28.6** Acute cellular rejection, type I, with tubulitis. **A:** Activated mononuclear cells and edema are present in the interstitium. A mitotic figure is present in the infiltrate (*arrow*). (PAS, ×40.) **B:** A CD3 stain in another case shows that T-cells are the predominant interstitial and intratubular mononuclear cells (*arrows*). (Immunoperoxidase, × 200.)

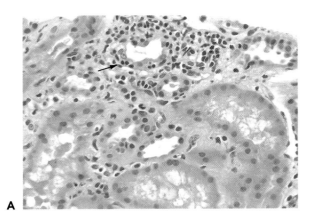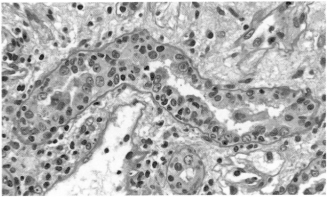

A    B

**Figure 28.7**    Tubulitis in acute cellular rejection (Type I). **A:** More than 10 mononuclear cells are on one tubular cross section (*arrow*). Surrounding tubules have 0 to 2 infiltrating cells. (H&E, ×400.) **B:** Extreme tubulitis in a longitudinal section. (PAS, ×400.)

tubulitis. Rarely a few neutrophils can be found in tubular lumens in acute rejection, but these are more typical of acute bacterial infection or humoral rejection (152,153). Eosinophils are rarely found in tubules in acute rejection. Disruption of the TBM (Fig. 28.8) and leakage of Tamm-Horsfall protein into the interstitium may be evident on PAS stains (154). Occasionally, granulomas are present, associated with ruptured tubules (Fig. 28.8).

### Interstitium

Acute cellular rejection has a pleomorphic interstitial infiltrate of mononuclear cells, accompanied by interstitial edema and sometimes hemorrhage (Fig. 28.6). The earliest lesion in our experience is a rather inconspicuous intertubular infiltrate (probably within peritubular capillaries) without edema. The interstitial infiltrate is probably actually focused on the peritubular capillaries, whose en-

dothelium represents an important target of the immune response.

The infiltrating mononuclear cells are almost exclusively T-cells and macrophages (Fig. 28.6). The T-cells are typically activated (lymphoblasts), with increased basophilic cytoplasm, occasional nucleoli, and occasional mitotic figures, indicative of increased synthetic and proliferative activity (Fig. 28.6). Small lymphocytes with dense nuclear chromatin and little cytoplasm are also present. Macrophages/monocytes may account for up to half of the cells (137,155), and may be the major cell type if T-cell depleting agents are used, such as CAMPATH1 (156). B-cells were traditionally described as uncommon in the acute phase of graft rejection (137,139,157–160). However, more recent studies indicate that a subset of acute rejection has CD20+ B-cells, a finding that is correlated with poor prognosis (161). Plasma cells may be prominent, especially in acute rejection episodes that occur after several months

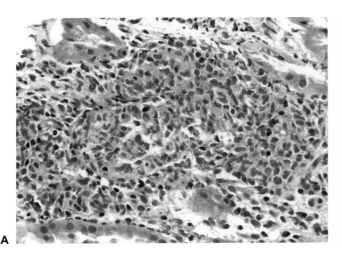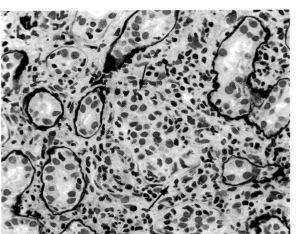

A    B

**Figure 28.8**    Severe tubulitis. **A:** Acute cellular rejection with tubular rupture and granuloma formation. (H&E, ×400.) **B:** Partial dissolution and rupture of the tubular basement membrane can be appreciated in periodic acid–silver stains (*arrows*). (×400.)

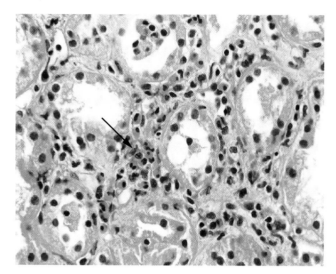

**Figure 28.9** Acute cellular rejection with abundant eosinophils. Eosinophils (*arrow*) are about 20% of the infiltrate in this field. (H&E, ×400.)

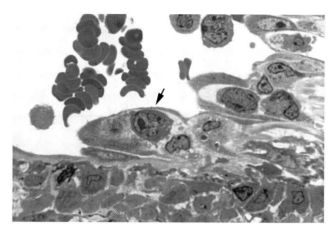

**Figure 28.11** Acute cellular rejection with endarteritis (type II). One-micron Epon-embedded sections show the subendothelial activated mononuclear cells (*arrow*). (Giemsa, ×1000.)

(162–166). Mast cells are present in increased numbers in acute rejection, as judged by tryptase content, and correlate with edema (167).

Granulocytes are not uncommonly present, but are rarely more than a few percent of the infiltrate. If granulocytes are noted, perhaps the most useful conclusion is that the process is currently active, since their lifespan is 2 to 4 days. When neutrophils are abundant, the possibility of a humoral rejection or pyelonephritis should be considered. Eosinophils are present in about 30% of biopsies with acute rejection, but are rarely more than 2% to 3% of the infiltrate (Fig. 28.9) (168–172). Abundant eosinophils (more than 10% of the infiltrate) are commonly found in rejected kidneys that have endarteritis (Banff type II) (173). Degranulated eosinophils can be detected by free major ba-

sic protein in the tissues (174). Basophils constitute a minor component of the infiltrate; these cells can also invade tubules and be up to 5% of the infiltrate (175).

### Vessels

Infiltration of mononuclear cells under arterial and arteriolar endothelium is the pathognomic lesion of acute cellular rejection (Figs. 28.10 to 28.15). Many terms have been used for this process, including "endothelialitis," "endotheliitis," "endovasculitis," "intimal arteritis," and "endarteritis." We prefer "endarteritis" because it emphasizes the type of vessel involved and the site of inflammation; also, more than the intima can be involved. The biologic and diagnostic significance of endarteritis was probably first noted and illustrated by Dammin in 1960 (24). The importance of this lesion has been emphasized for many years (176), and it is now widely accepted as a key pathogenetic feature of

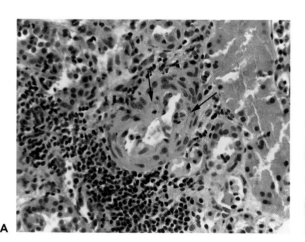

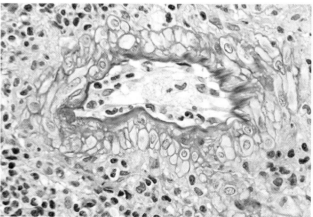

**Figure 28.10** Acute cellular rejection with endarteritis (type II). **A:** Small artery with subendothelial mononuclear cells (*arrows*). A prominent perivascular infiltrate is also present. (H&E, ×400.) **B:** Small artery with many subendothelial mononuclear cells. The endothelial layer is not clearly defined and is probably partially denuded. (PAS, ×400.)

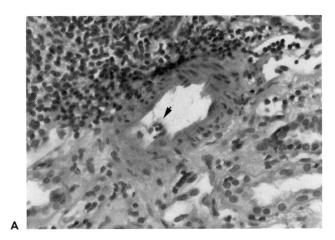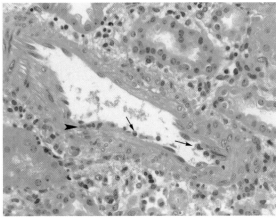

A

B

**Figure 28.12** Acute cellular rejection with endarteritis (type II). **A:** Minimum endarteritis. A single subendothelial cell is evident. (PAS, ×400.) **B:** Mononuclear cells stick to endothelium (*arrows*) and focally are underneath endothelium (*arrowhead*). Only subendothelial lymphocytes are counted for type II rejection.

acute T-cell–mediated rejection (64,170,177). Endarteritis can occur in cases with minimal or no interstitial infiltrate and no tubulitis, arguing that it has a distinct pathogenetic mechanism.

Endarteritis has been reported in 18% to 56% of renal biopsies with acute cellular rejection (64,170,178–181). Frequencies may be affected by sampling, timing of the biopsy with respect to antirejection therapy, HLA matching, and level of immunosuppression. Endarteritis tends to affect larger arteries preferentially, although arteries of all sizes including the arterioles can be involved. Cases have been noted in which the lesion is restricted to the arcuate-sized arteries, making sampling particularly difficult. The prevalence of endarteritis is about twice as high in arteries (27% of cross sections) as in arterioles (13% of cross sections) (170). Mural inflammation in arterioles (arteri-

olitis) has the same significance as endarteritis (Fig. 28.13) (182).

Arterial endothelial cells show increased disruption and lifting from supporting stroma by infiltrating inflammatory cells, consisting of T-cells and macrophages (Figs. 28.10 to 28.13) (183). One mononuclear cell under the arterial endothelium is considered by the Banff and the National Institutes of Health (NIH) Cooperative Clinical Trials in Transplantation (CCTT) systems to be sufficient for the diagnosis of endarteritis (Fig. 28.12) (64,177). Endothelial cells that are lifted off the basement membrane without undermining mononuclear cells cannot be distinguished from artifact. Mononuclear cells that are attached to the surface are probably the early phase of this lesion, but are not sufficient for diagnosis of endarteritis (Fig. 28.12). The endothelial cells appear activated with enlarged and

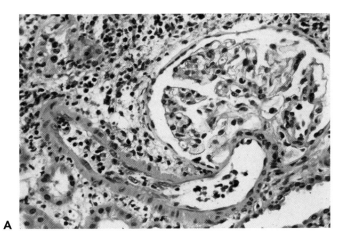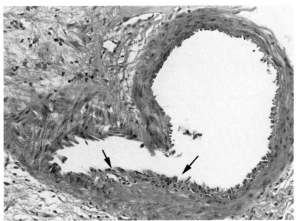

A

B

**Figure 28.13** Acute cellular rejection with endarteritis (type II). **A:** An afferent arteriole has a prominent mononuclear infiltration. This is of similar significance as endarteritis affecting larger arteries. (H&E, ×400.) **B:** Arcuate-sized artery with endarteritis (*arrows*). (PAS, ×200.)

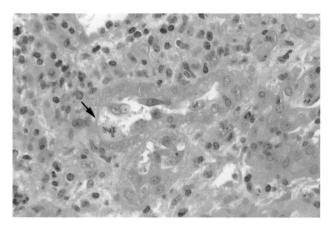

**Figure 28.14** Acute cellular rejection with endarteritis (type II). Small artery with reactive, enlarged, basophilic endothelial cytoplasm. An endothelial mitosis is present (*arrow*). Eosinophils are in the surrounding mixed mononuclear interstitial infiltrate. (H&E, ×600.)

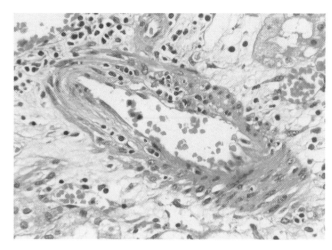

**Figure 28.16** Acute cellular rejection with endarteritis (type III). A small artery has transmural infiltration of mononuclear cells (through the media), one of the criteria for type III rejection. The C4d stain was negative, indicating the process is independent of antibody and probably mediated by T-cells and macrophages. (H&E, ×400.)

basophilic cytoplasm. Rarely endothelial cells are apoptotic, absent, or show mitotic figures (Fig. 28.14). Despite the obvious endothelial injury, thrombosis is rare. Acute intimal lesions can occur in arteries with pre-existing arteriosclerosis (Fig. 28.15), sometimes confused with the chronic lesion of transplant arteriopathy. The media usually shows little change. In severe cases, a transmural mononuclear infiltrate can be found affecting the media, with focal necrosis of the myocytes (Figs. 28.16 and 28.17), features that constitute type III rejection (transmural inflammation or fibrinoid necrosis). Fibrinoid necrosis is usually associated with acute humoral rejection.

Peritubular capillaries in acute cellular rejection usually contain increased numbers of mononuclear cells and sometimes a few neutrophils (184,185). The endothelium is difficult to visualize in standard preparations, but with

1-micron Epon sections, peritubular capillary endothelial activation and injury can be appreciated. Small veins and lymphatics also sometimes contain loose thrombi and Tamm-Horsfall protein. Infiltration of mononuclear cells into the media of veins is found in about 10% of biopsies with acute cellular rejection, but has no prognostic significance (186). These lesions can be found in inflammatory processes other than rejection.

### Ureter and Pelvis

The donor ureter and pelvis are targets of acute cellular rejection. Lymphocytes infiltrate the urothelium, which is often exfoliated and sometimes ulcerated (Fig. 28.18) (135,187,188). Mononuclear cells and plasma cells

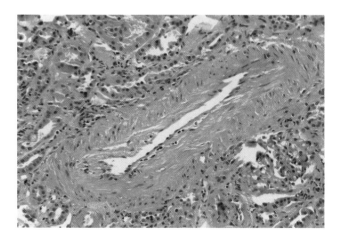

**Figure 28.15** Acute cellular rejection with endarteritis (type II). Subendothelial mononuclear cells are present in an artery superimposed on pre-existing arteriosclerosis (donor disease). This can be confused with chronic rejection, but is actually an acute process. (H&E, ×200.)

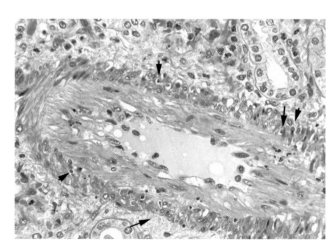

**Figure 28.17** Acute cellular rejection with endarteritis (type III). Transmural inflammation of a small artery with apoptosis of many medial smooth muscle cells (*arrows*), probably the beginning of fibrinoid necrosis. (H&E, ×400.)

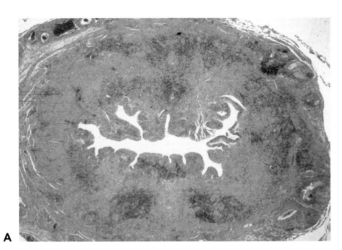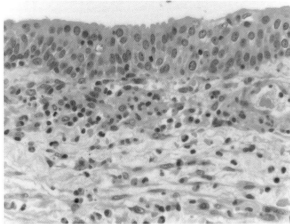

A                                                                                                    B

**Figure 28.18** **A:** Ureter with acute cellular rejection. At low power, dense lymphocytic submucosal infiltrates can be seen. (H&E, ×25.) **B:** Urothelial invasion of mononuclear cells in acute rejection involving the caliceal mucosa. Lymphocytes and eosinophils are in the submucosa. (H&E, ×400.)

infiltrate the edematous submucosa. The ureters develop marked luminal narrowing because of edema and hemorrhage. Complete necrosis of the ureter can occur from vascular compromise (189). Small arteries in the ureter can also be affected by endarteritis and fibrinoid necrosis (135,190). Of 26 ureters from irreversibly rejected kidneys, 80% had acute rejection of the ureter (187). The inflammatory reaction corresponded to that in the kidney, although occasionally there was a difference in degree.

## Immunofluorescence Microscopy

Little, if any, immunoglobulin deposition is found by immunofluorescence in acute cellular rejection. Extravascular fibrin is typically present in the interstitium, and not uncommonly, C3 is prominent along the TBM. By definition, peritubular capillaries lack C4d deposition in "pure" cellular rejection; the presence of C4d indicates a component of humoral rejection.

### Glomeruli

In transplant glomerulitis (acute allograft glomerulopathy), fibrin, scant immunoglobulin (especially IgM), and C3 deposits are found in glomeruli along the GBM (144). Some of the glomerular C3 derives from donor cells, as shown by the C3 allotypes expressed (191).

### Tubules

A characteristic feature of acute cellular rejection (which persists in later biopsies) is abundant C3 deposition along the TBM in a segmental linear pattern, which exceeds the "normal" pattern found in native kidneys. C3 is often pronounced in atrophic tubules. Peritubular C3 is largely derived from tubular cells, as judged by C3 allotype antibodies; donor-specific C3 mRNA can be detected in rejecting renal allografts by polymerase chain reaction (PCR) (191).

Proximal tubular cells in culture synthesize C3 in vitro in response to IL-2 (192). C5b-9 is also deposited along the TBM in about 30% of acute cellular rejection cases (193).

### Interstitium

Fibrin is typically present in the interstitium (194–196). The fibrin-rich interstitial edema probably causes the allograft swelling, analogous to the fibrin gel that causes induration in delayed hypersensitivity reactions (197). The fibrin deposition derives from peritubular capillary disruption and activation of the clotting system, probably by cytokine induction of macrophage procoagulants (198).

### Vessels

Most investigators, including these authors, find no significant immunoglobulin or C3 deposits in the arterial vessels in acute cellular rejection (beyond the usual IgM and C3 in arterioles seen in native kidneys) (183); focal fibrin deposition is sometimes seen. Diffuse peritubular capillary C4d deposits or arterial accumulation of IgG, IgM, and C3 are evidence for a concurrent humoral rejection (199,200).

## Electron Microscopy

Electron microscopy is generally not performed for diagnostic purposes in acute rejection. However, it may be indicated if the glomeruli are notably involved.

### Glomeruli

In transplant glomerulitis, many endothelial cells are enlarged and reactive, with a marked increase in cytoplasmic organelles (ribosomes, mitochondria, endoplasmic reticulum) and enlarged nuclei with open chromatin and prominent nucleoli (Fig. 28.19). The enlargement may fill and obstruct the lumen. The endothelial cells typically

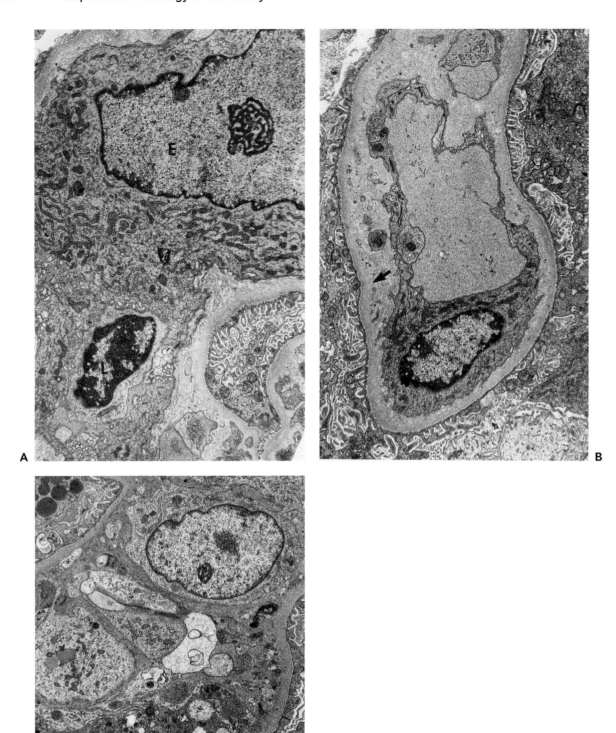

**Figure 28.19** Transplant glomerulitis/acute allograft glomerulopathy. **A:** A lymphocyte (L) is in contact with an activated glomerular endothelial cell (E). **B:** An activated endothelial cell has lost fenestrations and is separated from the original basement membrane (*arrow*) by an expanded subendothelial space that contains loose matrix, cell processes, and debris. **C:** Platelets are numerous in a capillary loop that has denuded endothelium. (Electron micrographs, **A:** ×6360; **B:** ×5225; **C:** ×6000.)

lose their fenestrations and are often separated from the GBM by loose, amorphous material. The capillaries contain monocytes and activated lymphocytes, with occasional neutrophils, platelets, and fibrin. Some GBM may be bare of endothelium or wrinkled and collapsed. The mesangium has loose matrix and sometimes monocytes. Amorphous electron-dense deposits are sparse and limited to subendothelial spaces and the mesangium (144). Podocytes may show segmental or rarely global foot process effacement.

### Tubules

Lymphocytes in the tubules accumulate between the epithelium and the TBM, frequently surrounded by a clear zone (201). The tubular epithelial cells remain in contact with the basement membrane, but the lymphocytes are separated from it by a thin layer of epithelial cytoplasm; breaks in the basement membrane are rarely found by electron microscopy (Fig. 28.20) (149). Occasional leakage of Tamm-Horsfall protein into the interstitium through fractured TBM has been described; the deposits contain 4-nm-thick filaments, tending to be arranged in parallel clusters and sometimes herniating into vessels (154). The tubular epithelial cells in the vicinity of mononuclear cells often show signs of injury, including vacuolization (201), necrosis, or apoptosis (149). In contrast, the tubular epithelium in drug-induced interstitial nephritis is reported not to be injured in the vicinity of the lymphocytes (202).

### Interstitium

The interstitium is expanded by edema and a mixed infiltrate of activated lymphocytes and macrophages. Granulocytes are occasionally encountered. The fibroblasts may appear active with fibrils, typical of myofibroblasts. The mononuclear cells are often apposed to the TBM.

### Vessels

Mononuclear cells accumulate in the peritubular capillary lumen, sometimes to the point of apparent obstruction. The intracapillary cells consist mostly of lymphocytes, which are sometimes in contact with the endothelium or emigrating through the wall (Fig. 28.21) (203). The endothelium shows signs of activation, as judged by cytoplasmic and nuclear enlargement, increased ribosomes, endoplasmic reticulum, mitochondria, and Golgi profiles (203). The fenestrations almost completely disappear (203). By morphometric analysis, the endothelial thickness doubles (from about 400 to 750 nm) and the endothelial cross-sectional area increases (from 18 to 28 $\mu m^2$), without a change in the diameter of the vessels (mean 27 $\mu m$) (203). Loss of endothelium and balloon degeneration occurs focally in association with the mononuclear leukocytes (201,203). The basement membrane can be disrupted, associated with lymphocytes and edema (204). Deposition of fibrin is sometimes found in these defects (195,203). Sim-

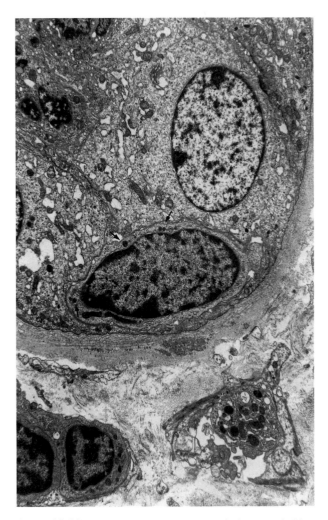

**Figure 28.20**   Acute cellular rejection. A tubule is invaded by a lymphocyte with a few dense cytotoxic granules (*arrows*) that are oriented toward the epithelial cells. The tubular basement membrane has fine laminations, but does not appear disrupted. (Electron micrograph, ×5200.)

ilar microvascular endothelial activation and injury have been described in human skin grafts (205). The endothelial hypertrophy has been compared with normal postcapillary venules, which are otherwise not anatomically recognized in the kidney (203). Which of these features are specifically related to T-cell versus antibody-mediated rejection has not been determined. The endarteritis lesions have been little studied ultrastructurally because of the difficulty in sampling.

## Etiology and Pathogenesis

### Antigens

#### Major Histocompatibility Complex (MHC) Antigens
Major histocompatibility complex (MHC) antigens, present in all vertebrates, were first identified in mice in

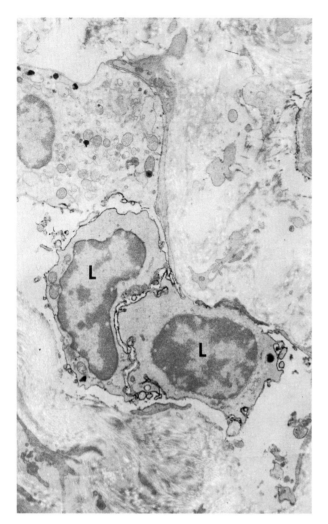

**Figure 28.21** Acute cellular rejection. Two lymphocytes (L) in a peritubular capillary stained with anti-CD4 using immunoelectron microscopy; the capillary endothelium is focally absent. (×6800.) (Courtesy of Eveline Schneeberger.)

experiments that showed that one genetic locus (the MHC) was the major determinant of graft survival. Two chemically and functionally different classes (I and II) of histocompatibility molecules are encoded in the MHC. Disparity of either alone is sufficient to cause graft rejection in mice (206). The exquisite sensitivity of the immune system to these antigens has been elegantly demonstrated using $K^{bm}$ mutant mice. Skin grafts from donors that differ from the recipient in only one to three amino acids in a single MHC molecule are promptly rejected (206,207). The human MHC (termed HLA for Human Leukocyte Antigen) spans 4000 kilobases on the short arm of chromosome 6 and contains multiple genes (208). The dominance of HLA antigen mismatch in determining outcome is supported by the observation that grafts from an HLA-identical sibling survive longer than those from a non–HLA-identical sibling (Fig. 28.2).

Class I MHC antigens consist of highly polymorphic transmembrane 45-kDa glycoprotein α chains associated with monomorphic 12-kDa β2-microglobulin. About 100 alleles of the A, B, or C class I loci have been defined with alloantibodies and more than 1000 with genetic probes (207). Class I antigens are widely distributed on all nucleated cells, but their concentration on the cell surface varies widely, even to the point of undetectability by standard immunohistochemical techniques (e.g., placental and Langerhans cells). In normal human tissues, the vascular endothelium (arteries, veins, capillaries) stains most intensely for class I antigens; the parenchymal cells are moderately positive (209).

Class II MHC antigens contain noncovalently associated transmembrane α and β chains of 25 to 28 and 29 to 34 kd, respectively, with most of the polymorphism on the smaller β chain. Three gene families (DP, DQ, DR), each with multiple α and β genes, have been identified. Class II antigens are more restricted in distribution than class I and vary by species and class II family. In humans, class II antigens are normally found on B-cells, dendritic cells, capillary endothelium, monocytes, Langerhans cells, and activated T-cells (209). DR but not DQ is demonstrable on capillary endothelium; both are on dendritic cells. Parenchymal cells normally have less intense staining for HLA-DR, and no DQ or DP (139,210,211). Normal arterial endothelium has little or no detectable class II antigens.

The expression of MHC molecules is regulated on the cell surface, under the control of inflammatory mediators, such as the interferons and tumor necrosis factor (212,213). IFNγ, produced by antigen-activated T-cells and natual killer (NK) cells, induces both class I and class II MHC antigens on epithelial and endothelial cells (214). Increased surface density of MHC molecules enhances the susceptibility to T-cell–mediated lysis and the ability to present antigen (215). However, induction of graft MHC molecules is not necessary to promote rejection. IFNγ-deficient mice reject kidney allografts as quickly as normal mice without induction of MHC molecules (216). Paradoxically, class I and II deficient grafts are also rejected efficiently, with MHC expression undetectable by immunoperoxidase techniques (217,218).

The normal function of MHC class I and II molecules is to present antigen to T-cells. MHC molecules bind certain peptide antigens more avidly and thereby present these antigens more effectively. T-cells are positively selected in the thymus for recognition of self-MHC molecules, so that they are normally restricted to antigen presented by self-MHC antigens. Cells with a high reactivity to self-MHC or no affinity for MHC are deleted. The T-cells recognize an altered conformation of self-MHC molecules plus the associated antigen. Antigen not associated with MHC molecules is invisible to T-cells. Graft rejection thus occurs in part because the T-cells recognize the foreign MHC antigens as if they were self-MHC molecules altered by association with some X antigen (the altered self-hypothesis) (219) or because of their intrinsic affinity for the MHC. These theories explain the high clonal frequency of T-cells directly reactive to any nonrelated individual cells (1 to 2 per 1000) and why the MHC is the major determinant of allograft survival (220).

Direct recognition of HLA antigens on graft cells can result in cell-mediated cytotoxicity and release of cytokines. T-cells can also react with MHC alloantigens from the graft that are processed and presented by autologous dendritic cells or infiltrating macrophages, as with other protein antigens (221). This response is termed the *indirect pathway* to distinguish it from the direct recognition of antigens on the donor cell surface. Indirect responses cause rejection by the action of lymphokines or through activation of B-cells or macrophages associated with dendritic cells. In addition, if grafts share an HLA antigen with the recipient, graft alloantigens can be presented as peptides associated with MHC by graft cells, as in a normal immune response to micro-organisms or perhaps in a tolerogenic manner (without costimulatory activation) (221).

### Non-MHC antigens

Non-MHC histocompatibility antigens (*minor antigens*) are defined simply by their ability to elicit graft rejection and a genetic locus outside the MHC. These antigens are responsible for graft rejection between MHC-identical congenic mice and HLA-identical siblings. Their chemical nature and distribution are largely unknown. In the mouse, 30 to 50 minor loci are calculated to trigger skin graft rejection (222). Some minor antigens are tissue specific. Graft-infiltrating T-cells can be isolated that recognize minor antigens on donor tubular epithelium but do not react with donor lymphocytes (223). The vascular endothelium expresses polymorphic non-MHC histocompatibility antigens, which have not yet been characterized at a molecular level (224).

### Antigen Response by T-Cells

Engagement of MHC-associated antigen by the specific T-cell receptor leads to expression of IL-2 receptor on the cell surface. Second (costimulatory) signals from the antigen presenting cell are required to move the T-cell to produce T-cell growth factors, such as IL-2, IL-4, or IL-15. Costimulatory signals, including CD86, CD40, and OX40L, are provided by "professional" antigen-presenting cells, such as dendritic cells and monocytes. These bind to CD28, CD40L (CD154), and OX40 on T-cells, respectively. T-cells that see antigen without the second signal are rendered anergic, i.e., refractory to specific antigen stimulus in the future. The conditions that promote such an outcome are of considerable clinical interest as a strategy to produce tolerance.

On recognition of antigen on a cell surface with sufficient costimulatory signals, the T-cells make two types of responses: secretion of cytokines and chemokines, which affect the behavior of nearby cells, and the development of cytotoxic effector functions that kill cells that express the relevant MHC. Delayed-type hypersensitivity to exogenous protein antigens is mediated by the former mechanism, whereas resistance to viral infection is dependent on the latter. These are the two nonexclusive mechanisms proposed for acute cellular graft rejection.

T-cells are heterogeneous in function. CD4 cells, which recognize peptide antigens (typically antigens exogenous to the cell) presented by self class II molecules, are critically important for graft rejection. Deficiency of CD4 cells prevents heart or skin graft rejection in mice (225). CD4 cells can be divided according to their cytokine production into Th1 and Th2 cells, as proposed by Mosman (226), although some cells have overlapping cytokine profiles. Th1 cells produce interferon gamma (IFNγ), interleukin-2 (IL-2), and tumor necrosis factor alpha (TNFα) and express CXCR3 and CCR5 chemokine receptors. Th1 cells activate macrophages, mediate delayed hypersensitivity reactions, mediate cytotoxicity via Fas ligand/Fas, and are typically present in the infiltrate of acutely rejecting grafts. IFNγ and TNFα activate macrophages to produce nitric oxide, which causes vasodilation and edema, reactive oxygen species, and more TNFα. TNFα in turn induces apoptosis via activation of caspases. IL-12 produced by other cells (e.g., dendritic cells and macrophages) promote Th1 cell activity and inhibit Th2 cytokines. IL-10 and IL-13 produced by macrophages and other cells promote Th2 activity and inhibit production of Th1 cytokines.

Th2 cells synthesize IL4, IL-5, IL-10, and TNFα and have the chemokine receptors CCR3, CCR4, and CCR8. These cells provide help for B-cells and production of IgE and IgG4 antibodies (227). Th2 cytokines promote eosinophil production and infiltration. IL-4 and IL-13 stimulate the production of eotaxins (CCL11,24,26) by parenchymal cells, including endothelial cells (228). Th2 cells are sufficient to mediate cardiac allograft rejection in mice and promote a heavy infiltrate of eosinophils (229). It is likely that some of the variation in morphology of acute graft rejection is owing to differences in the proportionate contribution of Th1 and Th2 cells in the infiltrate.

CD8 cells, which recognize peptide antigens presented by class I MHC molecules, produce IFNγ and mediate direct cytotoxicity via granzyme A and B and perforin, and by Fas ligand (230,231). Perforin forms a membrane channel that allows the granzymes into the target cell cytoplasm, where they activate Bid and caspases that trigger apoptosis (232). Expression of granzyme B, but not perforin, depends on IL-12 and correlates strongly with cytolytic activity. Across an isolated class I mismatch, perforin deficiency prolongs survival of heart or skin grafts (233). However, fully mismatched recipients that lack either perforin or granzymes

A and B reject kidneys with equal efficiency and develop tubulitis and endarteritis, arguing against a necessary role for either mediator (234).

A subpopulation of T-cells, termed *regulatory T-cells* (Treg), inhibit activation of effector T-cells. Treg are antigen specific and can suppress memory CD8 cells, apparently via a CD30-dependent pathway (235). Activation of Treg function requires engagement of the TCR (i.e., is antigen specific), but can affect other cells through soluble mediators (antigen nonspecific). Most Treg are CD4+CD25+CD152+ and produce IL-10 and TGFβ, but not IL-2 or IL-4 (236,237). Differentiation into Treg is promoted by TGFβ and is mediated by the master transcription factor, Foxp3, which continues to be expressed in Treg cells and serves as a distinctive marker of these cells in tissues.

## Chemokines

A burgeoning, complex, and confusing literature is emerging on the role of chemokines in transplantation (238). In acutely rejecting human kidney grafts, various chemokines are produced (IP-10, RANTES, macrophage inflammatory protein-1α [MIP-1α], MIP-1β, lymphotactin, MCP-1) and the infiltrating cells express several chemokine receptors (CXCR4, CXCR3, CCR5, CCR2) (239–244). CCR5 is mostly in the diffuse infiltrate (240), whereas CXCR4 is in nodular aggregates of mononuclear cells (245). The pattern of expression suggests a predominance of Th1 over Th2 cells (i.e., CCR5 and not CCR3 or CCR8) (240). Tubules synthesize RANTES (246), IL-8 (247), CXC₃L1 (245), and IL-6 (248) in acute rejection; none of these is detected in normal kidneys. These may be a response to local T-cell production of IL-17 (249). MCP-1, MIP-1α MIP-1β, and RANTES are increased in the basolateral surface of tubules (242,246,250). Heparan sulfate in the TBM may provide sites for chemokines, such as CCL4, to bind and create gradients (251). MCP-1 and MIP-1β levels are higher in type II than in type I rejection (250).

## Pathogenetic Mechanisms

The various components of the kidney are affected to differing degrees in individual episodes of acute rejection. Although each of these targets is believed to be affected by T-cells, macrophages, and their cytokines, the pathogenesis may vary somewhat. Immunohistochemistry, in situ hybridization, and laser capture microdissection are yielding new insights into the cells and molecules that participate in rejection.

### Infiltrating Cells

Both CD8+ and CD4+ T-cell subsets are present in varying proportions, as well as a minor population of CD4+CD8+ cells (252,253). Typically, the CD8+ cells are enriched in the graft and are found permeating diffusely in the renal

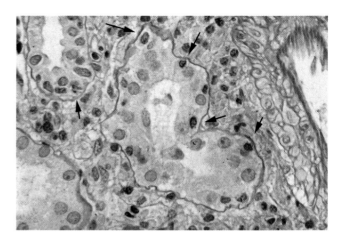

**Figure 28.22**   Acute cellular rejection, type I. Lymphocytes in tubules express the cytotoxic granule associated protein TIA-1 (GMP17). (PAS combined with anti-TIA-1 antibody/immunoperoxidase technique, ×400.)

cortex (139,160,254). CD4+ cells are usually selectively concentrated in perivascular aggregates (139,157,254). T-cells in the infiltrate express the CD45RO isoform of activated memory cells (255). Most infiltrating CD3+ T-cells express the usual α/β TCR (256,257); occasionally more than 10% of T-cells are γ/δ+ (257). A skewed distribution of TCR gene rearrangements has been reported, suggesting local selection of specificities (258–262).

Many infiltrating T-cells express cytotoxic molecules, namely perforin (263,264), FasL (264,265), granzyme A and B (264,266–268), and TIA-1/GMP-17 (159,268) (Fig. 28.22). About 30% of the infiltrating cells are TIA-1/GMP-17+ (159); most of these express CD8, but 12% are CD4 (159). Thus some cytotoxicity may be mediated by CD4+ T-cells, consistent with the observation that donor-specific cytotoxic CD4+ T-cells can be cultured from grafts (269). The infiltrating cells also express TNFβ (lymphotoxin) and. TNF receptors (270). Foxp3+ cells, presumably Tregs, are present in variable numbers in the infiltrate (271) (Fig. 28.23). Foxp3+ Treg cells are known to suppress cell-mediated reactions and may serve to dampen T-cell–mediated graft rejection. Supporting this role in vivo, Foxp3+ cells infiltrate grafts in certain experimental conditions that promote tolerance (272).

Activation of the infiltrating T-cells has been demonstrated by the presence of IL-2 (270) and its receptor CD25 (155,273,274). In situ hybridization studies show cytokines are typically synthesized by a minority of the cells (presumably the specific alloreactive cells) (275). IFNγ is synthesized in the graft (163,276,277) and is detected in lymphocytes scattered throughout the infiltrate (273). Other markers of activation expressed by the infiltrate are the transferrin receptor (278), CD38 (137), and CD69 (279). Some CD8 cells express CD152, and a few CD4 cells express CD40L.

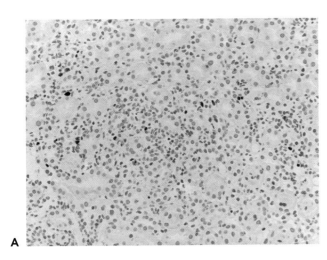
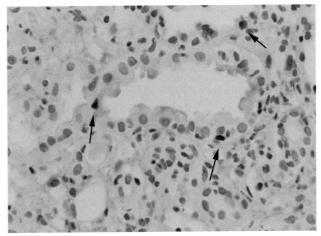

**Figure 28.23** Acute cellular rejection, type I. **A:** Cells in the infiltrate stain for Foxp3, a transcription factor for T regulatory cells. **B:** Foxp3 cells are present in the tubules (*arrows*). (Anti-Foxp3 immunoperoxidase, **A:** ×200; **B:** ×600.)

Apoptosis of the infiltrating T-cells can be demonstrated with the TdT-uridine-nick end label (TUNEL) technique (159,280–282) and may occur at a frequency comparable to that in the normal thymus (1.8% of cells in a section) (159). Apoptosis probably occurs in infiltrating T-cells as a result of activation-induced cell death and would thereby serve to limit the immune reaction (159).

Macrophages expressing CD14 or CD68 sometimes rival T-cells in abundance and may be the predominant leukocyte (160,283,284). Macrophages are characteristically present in a peritubular location applied in a linear fashion along tubular borders (285). Macrophages display markers of activation, including the tissue factor procoagulant-related antigen (155,286), receptors for VCAM-1 and fibronectin (CD49d, VLA-4) and Fas ligand (287). Macrophages expressing the tissue procoagulant-related antigen are associated with interstitial fibrin deposits (155). Endothelin, IL-6, and vascular endothelial growth factor (VEGF) can also be detected in macrophages in rejection, but not in normal kidneys (248,288,289). TNFα mRNA and protein is expressed by mononuclear cells, especially at the corticomedullary junction and peritubular, perivascular, and periglomerular sites (248,273,290). Macrophages express costimulatory molecules CD80 and CD86, but not CD40 (274). Plasminogen activator inhibitor-1 (PAI-1) synthesis is detected in infiltrating cells, especially in hemorrhagic areas, perhaps serving a protective role (291). Urokinase plasminogen activator and its receptor are also produced by the infiltrating cells (292). In animal models, intravascular monocytes are increased 10-fold in allografts and have been shown to actively produce TNFα, iNOS, and tissue factor (293).

B-cells can be present, even in early biopsies. The local synthesis of CXCL13 and expression of its receptor CXCR5 in B-cell clusters has been noted in patients who developed rejection in the first 9 days (294). NK cells are difficult to measure in tissues, since no common specific marker has been identified. About 2% to 30% of the infiltrating mononuclear cells have been reported to express CD57 (HNK-1) (139,155,160,210). Numerous CD56+ cells (also considered to be NK cells) have been reported (266), but using a panel of three "NK" antibodies (PEN 5, CD57, and CD56), positive mononuclear cells were rare (<1%) (159); similar results were noted by others (158).

### Tubules

Tubulitis is an important mechanism of graft rejection that involves both CD8+ and CD4+ cells (139). Intratubular T-cells with cytotoxic granules accumulate selectively in the tubules, compared with the interstitial infiltrate (159) (Fig. 28.22). These cells account for 65% of the mononuclear cells in tubules compared with about 30% of the interstitial cells. Lymphocytes expressing perforin mRNA and perforin protein are closely associated with tubular epithelial cells (295). Intratubular T-cells express CD103 (αEβ7), the integrin that binds to E-cadherin, which is normally on the surface of tubular cells (296–298). CD103+ cells are found exclusively in the tubules (298). CD103 probably contributes to their concentration within tubules (159): mouse T-cells deficient in CD103 do not effectively mediate tubulitis or tubular injury (299). Surprisingly, cyclosporine increases the expression of CD103 in the infiltrate (299). T-cells proliferate once inside the tubule, as judged by the marker Ki67 (MIB-1), which labels 15% of the intratubular lymphocytes (300).

Increased numbers of TUNEL+ tubular cells are present in acute rejection, compared with normal kidneys (159,280–282), calcineurin inhibitor toxicity, or ATN (159). Tubular cells have increased Bax and p53 and less

Bcl-2 (301). The degree of apoptosis correlates with the number of cytotoxic cells and macrophages in the infiltrate, consistent with a pathogenetic relationship (159,281). Apoptosis of murine tubular cells can be induced in vitro by IL-2 or IFNγ, both present in acute rejection (302). Tubular epithelial cell proliferation can also be detected with Ki67, which labels 1.5% ± 2.3% of the epithelial cells (300).

Tubular cells can process and present antigen to activated T-cells in vivo and in vitro (303) and express the co-stimulatory molecules CD80 and CD86 in acute rejection (304). Increased tubular epithelial cell expression of HLA-DR is characteristic, but not diagnostic, of acute cellular rejection (137,210,278,305–308). Increased tubular HLA-DR antigen expression correlates strongly with the presence of a T-cell infiltrate and presumably is a local response to IFNγ produced by these cells (137,210,277,309). Proximal and distal tubules express the IFNγ receptor, detectable with immunoperoxidase in acute rejection (270,310). Tubular synthesis of C3 (191) correlates with local IFNγ production (277) and exposure to Il-17 (249). Tubules also synthesize TNFα (290), TGFβ1, IL-15, osteopontin, and VEGF (289,297,310). Expression of osteopontin correlates with CD68+ cell infiltration and tubular cell regeneration (Ki67+).

Several adhesion molecules are increased on tubular cells during acute rejection. ICAM-1 (CD54) is increased (311–313) and closely correlated with HLA-DR. VCAM-1 is increased, mostly on the basal surface of tubular cells, and correlates with the degree of T-cell infiltration (283) and CD25+ cells (312). Decreased staining for urokinase and antithrombin III occurs in proximal tubular cells (314). Tubules also produce urokinase plasminogen activator and its receptor (292). Increased expression of the calcium binding protein S100 4A may signal the process of epithelial to mesenchymal transition (315).

Some molecules and cells in tubules have the potential to inhibit acute rejection. Protease inhibitor-9 (PI-9), the only known inhibitor of granzyme B, is synthesized by tubules in acute rejection, suggesting this may suppress tubular injury by cytoxic T-cells (267). IL-15 produced by tubular cells inhibits expression of perforin (297). Tubules also produce the complement inhibitor clusterin (316), which is colocalized in the TBM with the C5b-9 complex and vitronectin (317). Foxp3+ (T regulatory cells) (271) are concentrated in tubules, which may be a result of local TGFβ1 (318). This raises the heretical possibility that the tubulitis may have beneficial consequences.

### Vessels

Endarteritis is a common and significant manifestation of cellular rejection, observed in all allograft organs. In kidney transplants endarteritis can affect intra- as well as extraparenchymal vessels (i.e., hilar or periureteral arteries) (563). The evidence is quite convincing that acute cellular endarteritis is mediated by T-cells rather than an-

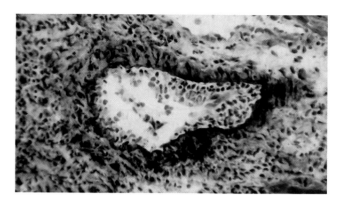

**Figure 28.24**    Endarteritis in a cardiac allograft in a mouse deficient in B-cells. This shows that endarteritis lesions can occur without the participation of antibody (319). (Elastic tissue stain of a cryostat section, ×400.)

tibodies. Cellular arteritis occurs in the absence of humoral antibody (B-cell knock-out mice) (Fig. 28.24) (319) and has not been produced by passive transfer of antibodies in animals. As further evidence, in humans, rejection with intimal infiltrates can usually be reversed with OKT3 (179,320,321). The cells infiltrating the endothelium and intima are T-cells and monocytes, but not B-cells (139,183,563). Macrophages (CD68+) can be abundant and cell proliferation (KI-67+) conspicuous (563). Scattered myofibroblasts can already be seen during the early "insudative" phase of transplant endarteritis; they become much more prominent in "transplant arteriolopathy" (see below) (563). Both CD8+ and CD4+ cells invade the intima in early grafts, but later, CD8+ cells predominate (139), suggesting that class I antigens are the primary target. Some of the T-cells express a cytotoxic phenotype (159). TNF receptors are detectable in the endothelium of arteries (270). Apoptosis of vascular endothelial cells can be detected in sites of endarteritis (159,280), and increased numbers of endothelial cells appear in the circulation (322).

Normal arterial endothelial cells express class I antigens, weak ICAM-1, and few or no class II antigens, or VCAM-1. During acute rejection, the endothelium of arteries expresses increased HLA-DR (139,210) and ICAM-1 and VCAM-1 (311,313), and endothelial synthesis of ICAM-1 and VCAM-1 can be demonstrated by in situ hybridization (323). The up-regulation of the adhesion molecules occurs in association with CD3+ (283) and CD25+ (312) infiltrating mononuclear cells. Endothelium also up-regulates ligands for L-selectin (sialyl-Lewis x and lactosamine) (324). The endothelium of arteries with acute cellular rejection shows a striking increase in platelet-derived growth factor (PDGF) A chain mRNA and protein (325). PDGF B chain, in contrast, is largely limited to the CD68+ inflammatory cells, probably macrophages, under the endothelium and probably promotes myofibroblast proliferation. IL-6 is also increased in the media and endothelium of vessels in acute rejection (248). In type II rejection, the endothelium expresses PAI-1 mRNA (291) and the urokinase plasminogen activator receptor (292); the arterial media shows increased urokinase plasminogen activator (292).

Normal peritubular capillary endothelial cells express prominent HLA-DR, HLA-class I antigens, LFA-3 (CD58), PECAM-1 (CD31), factor VIII antigen, and low levels of ICAM-1 and ICAM-2 (158,312,326). During acute cellular rejection, the capillary pattern for HLA-DR and ICAM-1 antigens is lost, probably because of disruption and necrosis of the endothelium (158,326). This was confirmed using a monoclonal antibody that reacted selectively with donor class I (HLA-A2) in six cases (326). Endothelial cells also have decreased endothelin expression in rejection with endarteritis but not in tubulointerstitial rejection (327). Peritubular capillaries express a decoy receptor for chemokines, Duffy antigen receptor for chemokines (DARC), during acute rejection, which may serve to inhibit CCR5-dependent T-cell accumulation (328,329).

## Glomeruli

In transplant glomerulitis, intraglomerular mononuclear cells are primarily CD8+ (139,330) accompanied by fewer macrophages (Fig. 28.5B,C). The lymphocytes have an activated phenotype, as judged by expression of CD25 and HLA-DR. The glomeruli have increased staining for HLA class I antigens (139). Mesangial cells may have increased (331) or decreased (314) staining for $\alpha$-smooth muscle actin. TNF$\alpha$ protein is detectable in glomerular endothelial cells (290), which normally have TNF receptors (270). Thromboxane synthetase and IL-6 increases in glomeruli in rejection, probably because of intraglomerular macrophages (248,332).

It is not known why rejection occasionally becomes focused on glomerular components, sometimes exclusively. Florid glomerulopathy may occur with little interstitial inflammation, although cellular endarteritis is common (139,140,144,333). This argues that the common element is a process directed at the endothelium. Perhaps interferons or other cytokines activate the endothelium and render the glomerulus more susceptible to rejection (139,334). Some cases have been attributed to cytomegalovirus (CMV) (144,146,335,336) or hepatitis C virus (HCV) infections (337,338), although most cases do not have a viral association (141–143).

## Differential Diagnosis

## Tubulointerstitial Inflammation

Interstitial mononuclear inflammation and tubulitis occur in various diseases other than acute rejection, such as infection, posttransplant lymphoproliferative disease (PTLD), drug-induced allergic tubulointerstitial nephritis, and is-

chemic injury, and are not sufficient per se to prove the existence of rejection.

### Infection See pages 1441–1449 and Table 28.16)
Viral infection is suggested initially by nuclear inclusions and confirmed by specific viral stains (e.g., polyoma, CMV, adenovirus). Features that favor polyoma are prominent tubular cell lysis, and plasma cell–rich infiltrates (sometimes even invading tubules). Tubular HLA-DR expression is typically not increased (308) and C4d is not detected along peritubular capillaries (348). Neutrophils outnumbering lymphocytes in tubules favor pyelonephritis (152). Frank abscesses (collections of abundant neutrophils with destruction of tissue) do not occur in rejection alone. However, neutrophils in peritubular capillaries and tubules do occur in antibody-mediated rejection and occasionally also in calcineurin inhibitor toxicity. Granulomas are extremely rare in allograft biopsies owing to rejection alone, although they may occur in response to ruptured tubules. Granulomas have been associated with miliary tuberculosis, adenovirus, *E. coli* urinary tract infection, and *Candida albicans*, generally with the organism demonstrable in the lesions (339). Drug allergy may also produce granulomatous interstitial nephritis.

### Posttransplant Lymphoproliferative Disease (PTLD)
PTLD is fully discussed later (page 1458). In contrast to acute cellular rejection, PTLD typically has a monotonous mononuclear infiltrate of enlarged lymphocytes (with few macrophages and granulocytes) and little edema. Tubulitis, even transmural vascular inflammation and necrosis of the infiltrate, may be found in PTLD (340). However, the infiltrate is primarily B-cells, expressing CD20 or PAX5. Epstein-Barr virus (EBV) infection can usually be demonstrated by in situ hybridization for EBV-encoded RNA 1 (EBER). However, rare PTLD cases have a rich infiltrate of EBER-negative polyclonal plasma cells or T-cells difficult to distinguish from rejection (166).

### Drug Allergy (See page 1440)
Definitive distinction between drug allergy and cellular rejection is not generally possible. If eosinophils are prominent (more than 5%), and especially if they invade tubules, the possibility of drug allergy should be strongly considered. In fact, drug allergy should always be included in differential diagnosis, if there is no definitive evidence of rejection (endarteritis or C4d deposition).

### Calcineurin Inhibitor Toxicity and Ischemic Injury
If tubular injury extends widely outside areas of infiltrate, other causes should be considered (drug toxicity, vascular compromise, obstruction, urine leak). The threshold of 25% for interstitial infiltrate in the Banff system is adequate to exclude cases with acute tubular injury (ATI) caused by ischemia (150). Even a 10% infiltrate is probably unusual

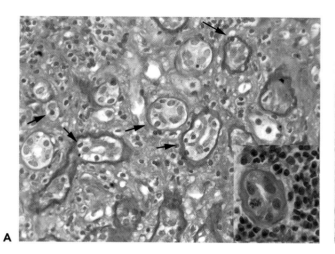
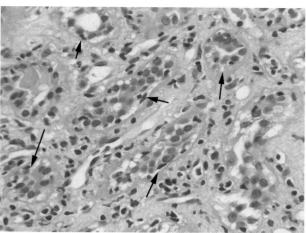

**Figure 28.25** Tubulitis in atrophic tubules is not considered for the diagnosis of acute rejection. **A:** Mononuclear cells (*arrows*) are in small tubules with a clear cytoplasm and thickened basement membrane. (PAS, ×400.) The presence of occasional mitotic figures in "atrophic" tubules belies their designation of atrophy. (*Insert*, ×600). **B:** Tubulitis is present in these smaller tubules with simplified, clear cytoplasm, but the TBM is not particularly thickened. This is probably active rejection. The rejection process itself leads to tubular atrophy, and the line of distinction between active and inactive is not definitive. (H&E, ×400.)

in ATI. Compared with ATI, tubulitis is more prominent in rejection, particularly in proximal tubules (150). Intratubular lymphocytes express cytotoxic granule proteins and are associated with tubular cell apoptosis more often in acute rejection than in ATI or calcineurin inhibitor toxicity (159). Less prominent tubular HLA-DR is found in ATI (278) and calcineurin inhibitor toxicity than in rejection (341). Unfortunately, it is not uncommon for acute rejection and signs of calcineurin inhibitor toxicity to be present simultaneously (17% in one series) (63). If isometric vacuolization is found in biopsies that also meet the criteria for acute rejection, these cases generally have improved function after treatment for rejection, suggesting that rejection may be the main cause of graft dysfunction (342). Calcineurin inhibitor toxicity is discussed in detail below (page 1427).

### Plasma Cell–Rich Infiltrates
When plasma cells are prominent, the differential diagnosis includes antibody-mediated rejection (especially in late grafts) (343), polyomavirus nephropathy, and PTLD. Certain systemic infections, for example, CMV, EBV (164), and HCV, may also be associated with plasma cell and B-cell–rich infiltrates.

### Other Conditions
Other causes of tubulitis have been documented in renal transplants with dysfunction, including lymphocele (obstruction) and systemic infection (pneumonia) (344). Among patients with suspicious/borderline scores for rejection, 12% had evidence of obstruction (345). Tubulitis in atrophic tubules should not be considered evidence of

acute rejection (Fig. 28.25). Interstitial inflammation in the subcapsular cortex is common in renal transplant biopsies and is also not evidence for active rejection.

### Vascular Lesions

Detection of endarteritis permits a definitive diagnosis of active rejection (178,252). The issue is exactly what constitutes endarteritis. When lymphocytes are present only on the surface of the endothelium, their significance is uncertain. Reactive endothelial cells (enlarged nuclei) and interstitial hemorrhage are associated with endarteritis and may be a clue that endarteritis is present (170). Mononuclear cells attached to the endothelium are highly suggestive of active cellular rejection and should prompt an even more diligent search for endarteritis. Lymphocytes also commonly surround vessels, a nonspecific feature, unless the lymphocytes also invade the media. At least three levels with multiple sections must be examined (346). The diagnostic accuracy improves with increasing numbers of arteries (170). Using the probability of 27% per artery sampled, a negative biopsy does not rule out endarteritis with a $P < .05$, unless 10 or more arteries are included ($P_{\text{no. arteries involved}} = [1 - 0.27]^n$, where $n$ = number of arteries sampled) (64). Of course, the usual biopsy samples far fewer arteries.

Endarteritis must not be confused with necrotizing arteritis, which is more characteristic of C4d+ antibody-mediated rejection. Transmural cellular inflammation is regarded as a form of cellular rejection, provided the C4d stain is negative in peritubular capillaries. However, fibrinoid arterial necrosis may be found in the absence

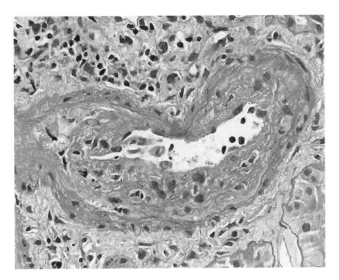

**Figure 28.26** The differential diagnosis of endarteritis includes thrombotic microangiopathy (TMA) as illustrated in this case. The loose, thickened intima of TMA may contain a few mononuclear cells. Clues that favor TMA are trapped red cells, mucoid change, lack of C4d in peritubular capillaries, and involvement of the glomerular vascular pole. (PAS, ×400.)

of any evidence for antibody-mediated rejection (20% to 50% of cases with fibrinoid necrosis in our experience), presumably because of severe cell-mediated inflammation. Thrombotic microangiopathy can also resemble endarteritis, because some mononuclear cells may be present in the edematous, thickened intima (Fig. 28.26). Detection of other features of thrombotic microangiopathy, such as red cell entrapment and fragmentation and thrombi are helpful in this differential, as is a C4d stain to exclude humoral rejection.

## Glomerular Lesions

Transplant glomerulitis is more common in humoral than cellular rejection (136,153,347–349), and a diagnosis of humoral rejection can be made by the C4d stain. Predominance of intraglomerular T-cells over macrophages favors cell-mediated rejection. In C4d negative glomerulitis, T-cells outnumber macrophages at least 2:1 (350) (Fig. 28.5). Neutrophils are found in a few pure cellular rejection biopsies (less than 10%) and are more typical of acute humoral rejection (153). Thrombotic microangiopathy is the other major cause of an acute glomerulopathy in transplants. The presence of vascular thrombi, red cells trapped in the loose expanded intima of arteries, and the absence of C4d deposition in peritubular capillaries favor thrombotic microangiopathy (TMA). A rare cause of TMA with glomerular lesions is complement factor H deficiency, which leads to the uncontrolled activation of the alterative pathway (351). Crescents or prominent immune complexes in glomeruli are rarely, if ever, found in cell-

mediated acute allograft glomerulopathy. Either strongly suggests de novo glomerulonephritis, for example, related to endocarditis (352), or recurrent disease.

## Banff/CCTT Criteria and Scoring System

Several grading systems have been proposed over the years to codify renal allograft rejection (64,79,215,353). At the present time the most widely used system is called the *Banff working schema* ("Banff" for short). Banff started as a collaborative effort of investigators meeting in Banff, Canada, with the leadership of Kim Solez, Philip Halloran, and Lorraine Racusen, to achieve a consensus that would be acceptable to the FDA for drug trials and useful for routine diagnostic use (79). This system has gone through a number of significant revisions and modifications over the years since it was published in 1993. The most important of these were the incorporation of the NIH Cooperative Clinical Trials in Transplantation (CCTT) criteria (64) in 1999, which separated the category of endarteritis (177), and the addition of antibody-mediated rejection in 2003 (185). Banff scores the individual elements of the biopsy by light microscopy and uses these to classify rejection (Table 28.4). The four elements scored to assess acute rejection are tubulitis (t), the extent of cortical mononuclear infiltrate (i), vascular inflammation (intimal arteritis or transmural inflammation) (v), and mononuclear cell glomerulitis (g).

Banff recognizes three major categories of acute T-cell–mediated rejection, derived from the NIH-CCTT categories (Table 28.5). The Banff threshold of infiltrate sufficient for the diagnosis of type I (tubulointerstitial) acute cellular rejection is more than 25%, provided tubulitis of at least t2 (5 to 10 cells per tubule) is present (177). Cases with 10 to 25% infiltrate are classified as suspicious for rejection or borderline in the Banff system, as long as tubulitis is present. Cases with no tubulitis, regardless of the extent of infiltrate, are not considered acute cellular rejection. The threshold for acute cellular rejection in the CCTT system is lower, more than 5% infiltrate and three or more lymphocytes in tubules in 10 high-power fields, combined with two of three other features: tubular injury, lymphocyte activation, and/or edema. The CCTT system has no suspicious/borderline category (64). Biopsies with C4d+ peritubular capillaries are considered to have an additional component of antibody-mediated rejection, which occurs in 20% to 30% of cases (354). Glomerular inflammation is not currently used for the diagnosis or classification of rejection, so that transplant glomerulitis (acute allograft glomerulopathy) per se is not considered rejection by the Banff system.

One area of debate is the clinical implication of suspicious/borderline lesions. Many, but not all, of these cases are indeed rejection. Two large studies have shown that 75% to 88% of patients with suspicious/borderline category and graft dysfunction improve renal function with

## TABLE 28.4
### BANFF ACUTE REJECTION SCORES (79,177)

| Interstitial inflammation | i0 | i1 | i2 | i3 |
|---|---|---|---|---|
| % of cortex[a] | <10% | 10–25% | 26–50% | >50% |
| **Tubulitis** | t0 | t1 | t2 | t3 |
| Cells/tubular cross section[b] | 0 | 1–4 | 5–10 | >10 |
| **Glomerular inflammation** | g0 | g1 | g2 | g3 |
| % of glomeruli[c] | 0 | <25% | 25–75% | >75% |
| **Arterial inflammation** | v0 | v1 | v2 | v3 |
| Intimal or transmural[d] | 0 | Intima <25% lumen | Intima ≥25% lumen | Transmural inflammation or fibrinoid necrosis |

[a]Scoring of unscarred cortex only. Cells in areas of fibrosis are not counted nor cells in subcapsular or around large veins or lymphatics. If more than 5% of the cells are neutrophils, eosinophils, or plasma cells, an asterisk is added.
[b]The number of cells in two or more tubular cross sections (or group of 10 tubular cells). Cells in atrophic tubules (less than half the normal diameter) are not counted. If t2 lesions are associated with at least two foci of TBM breaks ("vanishing tubules") and inflammation, the score is increased to t3 as per the Third Banff Conference.
[c]Mononuclear cells only. The glomerular score is not used for diagnosis of rejection.
[d]One subendothelial mononuclear cell is sufficient for v1. Hemorrhage or infarction is no longer sufficient for v3.

## TABLE 28.5
### BANFF/CCTT TYPES OF ACUTE T-CELL–MEDIATED REJECTION (185)[a]

| Type | Description |
|---|---|
| Suspicious/ borderline[b] | Any tubulitis + infiltrate of 10%–25%, or Any infiltrate of ≥10% + tubulitis of 1–4 cells per tubule |
| Type I[c] | Tubulitis >4 cells per tubule + infiltrate >25% A: with 5–10 cells per tubule (t2), or B: with >10 cells per tubule (t3) |
| Type II | Mononuclear cells under arterial endothelium A: <25% luminal area, or B: ≥ 25% luminal area |
| Type III | Transmural arterial inflammation, or fibrinoid arterial necrosis with accompanying lymphocytic inflammation[d] |

[a]All cases should be analyzed for C4d deposition. If C4d is present, an additional diagnosis of concurrent antibody-mediated rejection is made.
[b]The CCTT categories do not include suspicious, which is incorporated into type I rejection.
[c]The threshold for acute cellular rejection in the CCTT system is lower, >5% infiltrate and three or more lymphocytes in tubules in 10 high-power fields, combined with two of three other features: tubular injury, lymphocyte activation, and/or edema.
[d]Cases with these features are often due to alloantibody. To use as a category of T-cell–mediated rejection requires C4d in peritubular capillaries to be negative.

increased immunosuppression (355,356), comparable to the response rate in type I rejection (86%) (355). In follow-up biopsies 1 month later, the histology often progressed to florid rejection (33% type I; 46% type II or III) (356). Others find that a minority (28%) untreated suspicious/borderline cases progress to frank acute rejection in 40 days (345). Thus the biopsy that shows suspicious/borderline features should be interpreted in the context of the clinical situation (356). If there is any other evidence that favors rejection (e.g., a rise in creatinine), the diagnosis of rejection with a suspicious biopsy is highly likely. Almost all with suspicious/borderline findings do well, provided there is no element of concurrent antibody-mediated rejection (which may occur in biopsies with a suspicious/borderline pattern). The suspicious category is not counted as acute rejection in most clinical trials, a major omission in our opinion.

The interobserver reproducibility of the present Banff classification improved after the incorporation of the CCTT system (64,357). In a Canadian series of 184 protocol biopsies, the agreement rate for rejection was 74%, but there was only 43% agreement on the suspicious/borderline cases (358). A recent European series reached similar conclusions (359). CCTT has a 91% agreement rate on acute rejection (64). Even experienced pathologists do not reproducibly score certain Banff features. Among a group of 21 European pathologists, the agreement rate was poor for all of the acute Banff scores (t, i, v, g) in transplant biopsy slides (all kappa scores <0.4) (88). Agreement for t and v scores improved significantly when participants were asked to grade a lesion in a photograph (kappa scores of 0.61 and

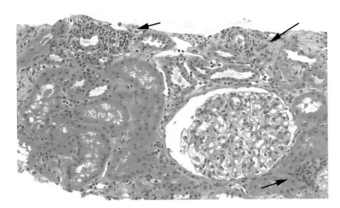

**Figure 28.27** The extent of the interstitial infiltrate is difficult to quantitate because the threshold of what is considered an infiltrate varies. In this field some might consider the infiltrate just to be in areas marked with the *arrows*, whereas others score the mononuclear cells between the tubules in most of the rest of the cortex. (H&E, ×20.)

0.69, respectively), arguing that the challenge is primarily finding the lesion in the glass slide. The fact that glomerulitis (g) and interstitial inflammation (i) scores were not improved in a photograph (kappa 0.22 and 0.31, respectively), indicates that the problem probably rests in their definitions (Fig. 28.27). Even if grading were reproducible, the sampling problem in core biopsies, particularly for vessels, will make fine distinctions hazardous. Perhaps these limitations will lead to new validated mathematical combinations of elements that will improve the accuracy of diagnosis, as suggested by initial experience with a computer Bayesian belief network (360).

Finally, we need to be aware that the criteria for diagnosis of rejection are not absolute, but based on the patterns observed in clinicopathologic correlations in patients on specific maintenance therapy in the past. Drugs have the ability to modify rejection, for example, a decrease in the intensity of infiltrate and edema with cyclosporine or a decrease in eosinophils with steroids. Some of the newer drugs may have other effects. For example, CAMPATH1, which profoundly depletes T- and B-cells, can lead to episodes that clinically behave like rejection, yet do not meet the criteria of Banff, owing to sparse mononuclear infiltrates (361). To the extent that our criteria correspond to mechanisms of the rejection process itself (tubulitis, endarteritis), the criteria will be robust. Nonetheless, we have to be prepared to identify novel features and mechanisms of rejection that might occur with new drugs.

Although many details are still being refined, Banff has had a beneficial effect in the standardization of definitions for publications and provides a stimulus for consensus development and translational research. Among the remaining issues for the future are to define markers that distinguish rejection from potential beneficial infiltrates in the

suspicious category and fully recognize glomerular lesions as acute rejection.

In practice, at our institutions we normally do not provide detailed Banff scores, except for clinical trials. We do indicate the percent infiltrate, percent fibrosis, vascular and glomerular lesions, and the presence and extent of tubulitis. When the biopsy is in the borderline/suspicious Banff range, but meets the CCTT criteria for acute rejection (edema, activated lymphocytes, and/or tubular injury), we favor the diagnosis of acute rejection. In these cases, we indicate that other causes should be excluded (e.g., vascular compromise, obstruction, urine leak).

## Clinical Course, Prognosis, Therapy, and Clinicopathologic Correlations

The first-line treatment for acute cellular rejection is bolus steroids for up to 3 days. In patients who do not respond, the standard rescue therapy is OKT3, a murine monoclonal antibody to CD3, or polyclonal antithymocyte antibody (horse ATGAM or rabbit Thymoglobulin). Antibody treatment is continued typically for 10 to 14 days. As noted above, cellular rejection involving the arteries is less responsive to steroids (170), but does respond to OKT3 (179); transplant glomerulitis also sometimes responds to OKT3 (362).

Following treatment of acute cellular rejection with pulse steroids, ATG, or OKT3, a marked decrease in the interstitial infiltrate occurs, although the intratubular cells may remain, along with considerable edema. Functional inactivation has most clearly been demonstrated during OKT3 therapy, in which modulation of CD3 from the cell surface occurs in the graft as well as the blood (321,363). The staining of infiltrating cells in sections for CD3 during OKT3 therapy may be attributable to intracytoplasmic CD3 (364). Sometimes the interstitial infiltrate persists, despite functional improvement. It is difficult to judge whether the rejection is still active by histologic criteria, and here molecular studies are likely to be useful.

Certain pathologic features of acute rejection have prognostic significance either individually or in combination (Table 28.6). The most important predictors of outcome are the arterial lesions. Endarteritis (intimal arteritis), which defines type II rejection, has an adverse effect on prognosis, compared with tubulointerstitial rejection without arterial involvement. Several studies have demonstrated decreased survival or reversibility of type II rejection. Bates and colleagues studied the outcome in 293 patients with biopsies (181). Those with type II rejection had a 75% 1-year graft survival versus more than 90% among those with type I, suspicious, or no rejection (Fig. 28.28). Endarteritis was the only determinate in the Banff classification to predict graft failure (hazard ratio of 1.85) (365), similar to that in another series, in which endarteritis doubled the rate of graft loss (31% versus 15%) (366). A large multicenter trial

## TABLE 28.6

### BIOPSY FEATURES IN ACUTE REJECTION THAT CORRELATE WITH SUBSEQUENT GRAFT LOSS[a]

| Feature | Selected References |
|---|---|
| **Glomeruli** | |
| Thrombosis | 372 |
| Necrosis | 58,353,371 |
| Endothelial swelling | 58,375 |
| Tranplant glomerulitis | 143,144,146,755 |
| CD3+ or CD8+ lymphocytes | 137,139 |
| Monocytes | 138,1323 |
| **Vessels** | |
| Arterial/arteriolar thrombosis | 372,375 |
| Medial (fibrinoid) necrosis | 181,353,371,375,376,508 |
| Infarction | 372,373 |
| Endarteritis | 170,179,181,182,320, 365,366 |
| C4d in peritubular capillaries | 153,347,348,354,391, 400,1324 |
| **Interstitium** | |
| Hemorrhage | 58,353,371,375 |
| CD8+ cells | 114,137,139 |
| Cytotoxic cells granzyme B | 238 |
| Eosinophils | 168,169,174,378 |
| Monocytes/macrophages | 279,379 |
| Plasma cell rich | 162–164 |
| **Tubules** | |
| Severe disruption | 58 |
| Severe tubulitis t3 | 380 |
| HLA-DR expression | 210 |
| TBM breaks | 381 |

[a]Not all studies have confirmed these findings (see text).

found that endarteritis increased the risk of a clinically severe rejection sixfold (64). Graft survival at 1 year (71% to 75% versus 51% to 58%) (179) is higher for type I than type II rejection, and steroid resistance is more often found in the latter (170,367,368). Those with 25% or more of the luminal area involved (Banff IIB) have a worse response to antirejection therapy and a twofold increased risk of graft loss, compared with those with endarteritis involving less than 25% of the luminal area (369). Endarteritis is associated with subsequent arterial intimal fibrosis at 3 months (370). Arteriolitis is associated with endarteritis and has a similar adverse effect on prognosis (182). Type III rejection (necrotizing arteritis) has much worse prognosis than endarteritis (20% to 32% 1-year survival) (170,181,215,368,371), although these results, no doubt, include cases of humoral rejection (pre–C4d studies).

Infarction is an ominous finding in graft biopsies, if surgical trauma can be excluded (372,373). In a series of 59 cases with infarction, the graft survival was 47% if the infarct was in a biopsy in the first 2 months and only 22% if the infarct was present in a biopsy after 2 months (graft survival was 71% in patients with severe rejection without infarction) (373). Infarction was associated with infection, especially disseminated CMV. In these studies, humoral rejection was not assessed. Old infarcts are occasionally found in well-functioning grafts, dating from the time of transplantation; these are of no significance (374). Interstitial hemorrhage correlates with development of chronic rejection (375) and is a morphologic predictor of return to dialysis in 1 year (58).

The intensity of the interstitial infiltrate has no correlation with the outcome of the rejection episode (58,64,170,215,320,353,367,371,372,376). Similarly, the numbers of CD3+ or CD2+ cells in the interstitial infiltrate correlate with the presence, but not the prognosis, of rejection (137,278,377). In some studies, those with greater infiltrates had an even better outcome than those with focal infiltrates (215). Thus grading the rejection on the basis of the extent of the infiltrate is of dubious value. The

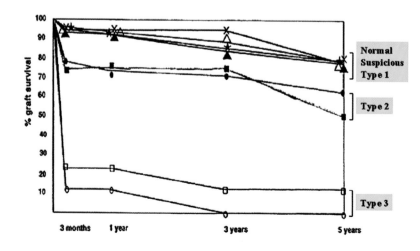

**Figure 28.28** The Banff/CCTT type of rejection correlates well with graft survival (181). Type I does not significantly affect prognosis, but both type II and especially type III do diminish graft survival. This study was done before C4d stains were widely used (compare with Fig. 28.47). (Modified from Bates WD, Davies DR, Welsh K, et al. An evaluation of the Banff classification of early renal allograft biopsies and correlation with outcome. Nephrol Dial Transplant 1999;14:2364, with permission from Oxford University Press.)

proportion of CD8+ cells correlates with a poorer response to immunosuppressive therapy in some (137,139,254) but not all studies (320). By multivariate analysis, type I rejection with diffuse cortical CD8+ infiltrate was associated with a 46-fold increase in risk of graft loss within 10 weeks (254). Expression of granzyme B by more than 2% or CD40 by more than 25% of the infiltrating cells has been associated with shorter allograft survival (268). The reason for this is not clear; the CD8+ cells may be relatively resistant to immunosuppressive drugs or may mediate more severe injury. Eosinophil-rich infiltrates (more than 2%) have been associated with graft loss (86% versus 37%) (168). One explanation may be the association of eosinophils (more than 10/mm$^2$) with type II rejection (378). An increased number of interstitial macrophages have also been associated with an adverse outcome (279,379). Plasma cell–rich acute rejection has been reported to have a poorer prognosis in most (162–165) but not all series (166). When three studies (162,165,343) are combined in a meta-analysis, plasma cell infiltrates in acute rejection affect prognosis only in the first 6 months (increasing graft loss from 23% to 53%); after 6 months, the outcomes of acute rejection with or without plasma cells are equally poor (graft loss in 67% to 68%) (343).

The predictive value of tubulitis is debatable. Severe tubulitis (Banff t3) was associated with a significant increase in graft loss compared with those with lesser degree of tubulitis (t1, t2) (380). The adverse effect of t3 was the same as endarteritis (v1, v2). Severe TBM disruption was an adverse feature (58), and more extensive TBM breaks (more than 10/mm$^2$) correlated with later graft dysfunction and increased tubular atrophy on follow-up biopsy (381). However, in other studies neither the extent nor the Banff grade of tubulitis was predictive of outcome (64,170,366–368), nor was TBM disruption (154).

The prognostic significance of transplant glomerulitis (acute allograft glomerulopathy) in pure T-cell–mediated rejection has not been settled, because past studies have not discriminated between mild and severe forms or glomerulitis-caused by antibodies. Most studies report a poor prognosis, e.g., 67% graft loss (139,141, 142,144,146,382), although two large series failed to demonstrate an adverse impact (140,366). Rarely, severe transplant glomerulitis persists on repeated biopsies with little apparent consequence on graft function (145).

## ACUTE ANTIBODY-MEDIATED REJECTION

Acute antibody-mediated rejection (or acute humoral rejection, AHR) has only recently become a well-defined diagnostic category. In the past, cases with fibrinoid necrosis were believed to be related to antibody and termed "accelerated acute," "delayed humoral rejection," "delayed hy-

peracute," or "vascular" rejection (a very confusing term that should be avoided) (21). However, evidence of antibody reaction in the tissues was sparse, and, except for fibrinoid necrosis and hyperacute rejection, the concept of antibody-mediated rejection was not widely accepted. AHR occurs in patients who develop a threshold level of antidonor antibodies after transplantation, as opposed to hyperacute rejection in which pre-existing antibodies damage the graft immediately after reperfusion. The histologic features of AHR are quite variable and not sufficient for definitive diagnosis (199,383). Detection of C4d in vessel walls as a marker, pioneered by Feucht et al (384), and the new solid phase methods for detecting antidonor antibody (385) have led to better diagnosis of this condition. AHR may occur in the absence of features of T-cell–mediated rejection, although it commonly is accompanied by a cellular component (i.e., mixed cellular and antibody mediated rejection).

In 1970, Jeannet et al (28) reported that de novo anti-HLA antibodies to donor cells correlated strongly with acute and chronic rejection of renal allografts (28). Halloran et al (386,387) observed a short-term worse outcome in patients who developed acute rejection in the presence of circulating antibodies to donor HLA class I antigens. Certain morphologic features (neutrophils in peritubular capillaries, thrombi, fibrinoid necrosis) were more common in patients with anti-HLA antibodies, but none was a specific or sensitive indicator of circulating antibodies (136). Deposition of immunoglobulin or C3 was not conspicuous in these cases, and a diagnostically useful immunologic marker of humoral rejection was not identified (388).

Feucht at al (384,389) reported in the early 1990s that deposition of complement split fragments C4d and C3d in peritubular capillaries could be detected in most transplanted kidneys with "cell-mediated rejection." C4d deposition was associated with "high immunological risk" (i.e., previous transplants or circulating anti-HLA-antibodies) and with a poor prognosis. These authors suggested that humoral rejection should be considered, despite negative cross-match before transplantation and paucity of immunoglobulin deposition. We later documented the strong association of C4d deposition in peritubular capillaries with circulating antidonor-specific antibodies and with certain pathologic features (neutrophils in capillaries and fibrinoid necrosis of arteries) that are not common in pure cellular rejection (153,390,391). These observations have been confirmed in many centers, and criteria are now widely accepted for the definition of AHR (185,388).

The clinical presentation of AHR (with or without a cellular component) is generally that of severe rejection, with more frequent oliguria (35% versus 10% without antibodies) and need of dialysis (40% versus 10%), compared with rejection in the absence of HLA class I antibodies (386). However, there are no reliable clinical features that permit distinction from pure T-cell–mediated acute rejection.

| TABLE 28.7 | | |
|---|---|---|
| **PREVALENCE OF ACUTE HUMORAL REJECTION (388)[a]** | | |
| Patients | N | % |
| Crespo et al, Boston (391) | 232 | 8.2% |
| Rocha et al, Durham (476) | 286 | 5.6% |
| Abe et al, Tokyo (497) | 640 | 6.5% |
| **TOTAL** | **1158** | **6.6%** |
| Biopsies for acute rejection | | |
| Mauiyyedi et al, Boston (153) | 67 | 29% |
| Nickeleit et al, Basel (348) | 265 | 35% |
| Herzenberg et al, Vancouver (354) | 93 | 37% |
| Mengel et al, Hanover (456) | 377 | 21% |
| Lorenz et al, Vienna (393) | 388 | 17% |
| **TOTAL** | **1190** | **24%** |

[a]These data include all cases that were C4d+, whether or not a concurrent component of acute cellular rejection was present. From Rotman S, Collins AB, Colvin RB. C4d deposition in allografts: Current concepts and interpretation. Transplant Rev 2005;19:65.

AHR is most common 1 to 3 weeks after transplantation, but can develop suddenly at any time. In one series, the mean day of onset was 15 ± 11 days (earliest 3 days), not different from that of acute cellular rejection (14 ± 10; earliest 6 days) (153). Late onset is often associated with decreased immunosuppression or noncompliance (392).

Overall, about 5% to 7% of patients develop an episode of AHR, and evidence for an AHR component is detected in about 24% of biopsies for acute rejection (Table 28.7). AHR occurs with all current drug regimens (e.g., cyclosporine, tacrolimus, mycophenolate mofetil, sirolimus, or CAM-PATH1), without obvious differences (393), even in protocols that cause profound T-cell depletion (394,395). The primary risk factor for AHR is presensitization (blood transfusion, pregnancy, prior transplant) as judged by a historical positive cross-match or high levels of panel-reactive antibody (PRA) (393). However, most patients who develop AHR have a negative cross-match at the time of transplantation, since ordinarily that is a requirement for transplantation. AHR does not correlate with HLA match, ischemic time, or donor age (393). AHR may be associated with alpha interferon therapy in HCV (396). ABO incompatible grafts recipients treated with special protocols to reduce isoagglutinin titers have a higher risk of AHR, with about 30% of recipients developing clinical AHR (397,398). Certain pathologic features are found in association with circulating antibody and C4d deposition, whether or not a component of T-cell–mediated rejection is present. These features are considered to be due to AHR and are described below.

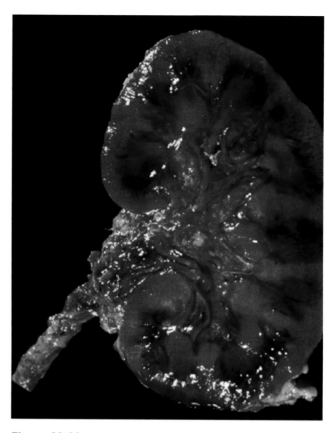

**Figure 28.29** Gross appearance of an allograft with severe acute humoral rejection 16 days after transplantation that failed after initially functioning for several days; ABO-incompatible graft (A2 into O) (1325).

## Pathologic Findings

### Gross Pathology

The kidneys are swollen and congested. In severe cases, widespread hemorrhage and patchy infarction are present (Fig. 28.29).

### Light Microscopy

#### Glomeruli

Glomerular capillaries have neutrophils in 10% to 55% of cases (136,153,347,386) and mononuclear glomerulitis in 19% to 90% (136,153,347,348) (Fig. 28.30). Intraglomerular mononuclear cells are mostly monocytes/macrophages (CD68+) (349,399), in contrast to T-cell predominance in acute cellular rejection (350) (Fig. 28.30). Fibrin thrombi or necrosis are present in about 20% of cases (136,153,386).

#### Tubules

Evidence of acute tubular injury is common (loss of brush borders, thinning of cytoplasm, paucity of nuclei); in one

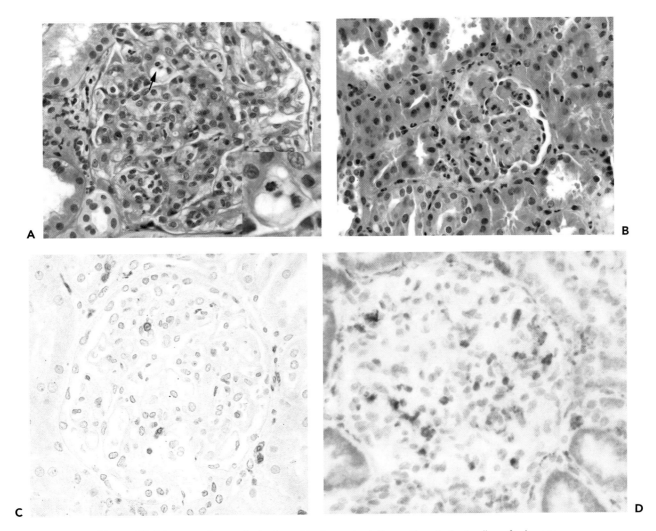

**Figure 28.30** Acute humoral rejection with glomerular inflammation. **A:** Acute allograft glomerulopathy with mononuclear cells, neutrophils, and reactive endothelial cells. An endothelial mitosis is shown (*arrow*, and *insert*) C4d stain was positive. (PAS, ×400.) **B:** Acute glomerulitis with neutrophils and thrombi. (H&E, ×20.) **C:** Transplant glomerulitis in acute humoral rejection with a few CD3+ cells (T cells). **D:** Same graft showing many CD68 cells (macrophages). The graft had prominent C4d deposition. Compare with Figure 28.5. (**C** and **D** immunoperoxidase stains courtesy of Alex Magil, Vancouver.)

series, these were found in 75% of cases (153). Acute tubular injury may be the only manifestation of AHR (Fig. 28.31) (153). Focal coagulative necrosis of tubules is found in a few cases (Fig. 28.32) (153). Neutrophilic tubulitis is a distinctive feature, found more often in antibody than T-cell–mediated rejection (55% versus 9%) (Fig. 28.33) (153). Mononuclear tubulitis is found in 30 to 80% of cases and is considered evidence of a concurrent T-cell–mediated component (136,153,347), as is increased expression of HLA-DR (383).

## Interstitium

Edema with a scant mononuclear infiltrate may be present in the interstitium, insufficient for the diagnosis of acute

cellular rejection. In one series, most fell within the suspicious/borderline range (347). Whether this represents a subthreshold component of T-cell–mediated rejection or is caused by the antibody/complement interaction with the tissue is not known. Macrophages infiltrate more in C4d+ than in C4d– rejection (349). Interstitial hemorrhage can be prominent (Fig. 28.33), but is not necessarily indicative of an antibody component (153,343). Frank cortical infarction is present in a few cases (5%) (153). Some have reported that plasma cells are more abundant in acute antibody-mediated rejection, either early (164) or late (163,343) after transplantation (Fig. 28.34). Plasma cell infiltrates with antidonor antibodies have also been associated with massive edema and increased IFNγ

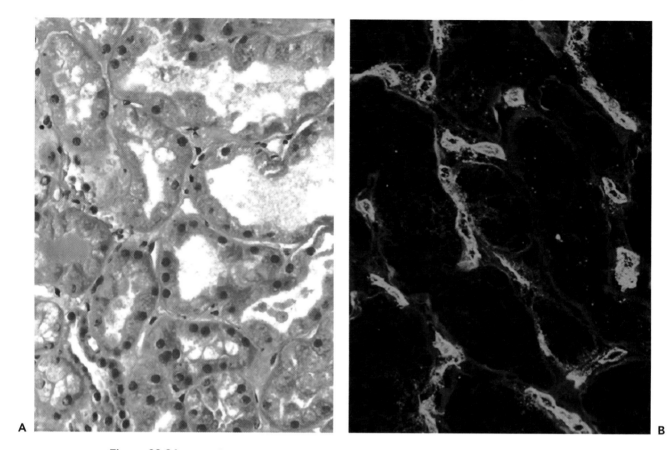

**Figure 28.31** Acute humoral rejection present on day 9 of DGF. **A:** Pattern of acute tubular injury without evidence of inflammation. (H&E, ×400.) **B:** Immunofluorescence C4d stain on cryostat section shows widespread staining of peritubular capillaries. (×400.)

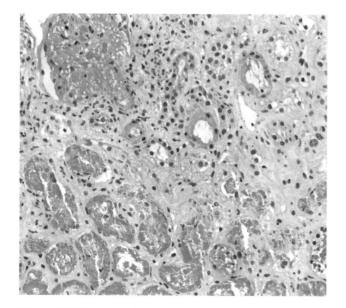

**Figure 28.32** Acute humoral rejection with glomerular and tubular necrosis. (H&E, ×200.)

production in the graft (163). B-cells also can be present in aggregates (Fig. 28.35), although an association with antibody-mediated rejection has not been shown.

### Vessels

Trpkov et al (136) pointed out the association of neutrophils in peritubular capillaries and AHR, a feature long recognized in hyperacute rejection (Fig. 28.36). In three series totalling 78 cases, 54% had neutrophils in peritubular capillaries (136,153,400). However, neutrophils were rarely (less than 3%) found in a series from Vienna (347). Mononuclear cells, especially monocytes/macrophages, are also present (Fig. 28.36). The peritubular capillaries are often markedly dilated (136).

In a few cases (10% to 25%), the arterial media shows myocyte necrosis, fragmentation of elastica, and accumulation of brightly eosinophilic material called "fibrinoid" with little mononuclear infiltrate in the intima or adventitia (Fig. 28.37). This lesion is not dissimilar to necrotizing arteritis in native kidneys, for example, caused by microscopic polyangiitis. Among the patients with anti–class I antibody, 25% had fibrinoid necrosis (versus 5% of those without such antibodies) (136). Another study noted 53%

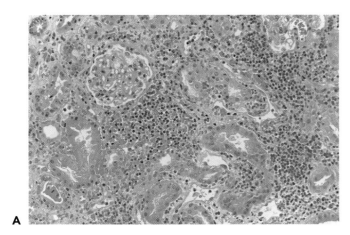
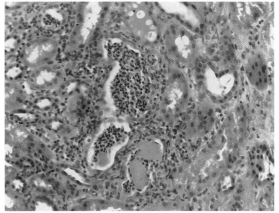

**A**

**B**

**Figure 28.33**  Acute humoral rejection. **A:** Widespread interstitial hemorrhage is present. **B:** Neutrophils are in tubules, resembling acute pyelonephritis. (H&E, **A:** ×400; **B:** ×200.)

of 17 patients had either fibrinoid necrosis (24%), transmural arterial inflammation (18%), or both (12%) (401). Arterial thrombosis occurs in a few (10% in one series) (401). A pattern resembling thrombotic microangiopathy has also been seen, with mucoid intima thickening and trapped red cells (Fig. 28.37). An infiltrate of neutrophils and eosinophils may be present. Eosinophil cationic protein deposits have been demonstrated in the necrotic vascular walls (402).

## Immunofluorescence Microscopy and Immunohistochemistry

### Glomeruli

No distinctive patterns are found by immunofluorescence for immunoglobulins in glomeruli (153). Mesangial IgM and IgG may be more prominent than in non–antibody-

mediated rejection, but the difference (43% versus 17%) is not diagnostically useful (136). Glomerular staining for C4d in glomeruli occurs in about one third of cases of AHR (347) and is best evaluated by immunohistochemistry of formalin-fixed tissue, because no C4d is found in normal glomeruli in formalin-fixed, paraffin-embedded sections, whereas the normal mesangium stains for C4d in frozen sections (Figs. 28.38 and 28.39). C3 components (C3c, C3d), C-reactive protein (CRP), and vitronectin have also been reported (403,404).

### Tubules

C3 and C5b-9 (membrane attack complex, MAC) deposits have been reported primarily in tubular basement membranes (TBM), rather than peritular capillaries (PTC) (193). The reason for this is not clear, but may relate to the relative expression of the inhibitor of MAC formation,

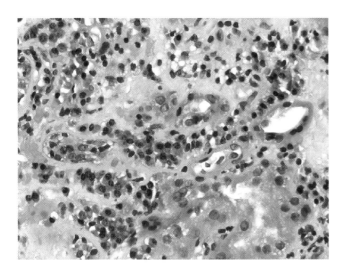

**Figure 28.34**  Plasma cell–rich late acute rejection with positive C4d. The combination of plasma cell infiltrates and acute humoral rejection has been reported to have a poor prognosis, although it is uncommon (163,343). (H&E, ×400.)

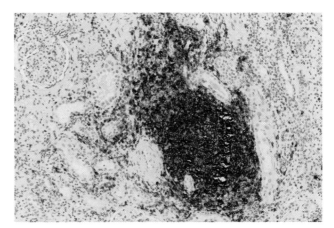

**Figure 28.35**  Acute humoral rejection with a nodule of B-cells, a finding that has been reported to carry an adverse prognostic significance (161). At present there is no direct linkage between the B-cells in the infiltrate and the presence of anti-donor antibodies. (Immunohistochemical stain for CD20, ×100.)

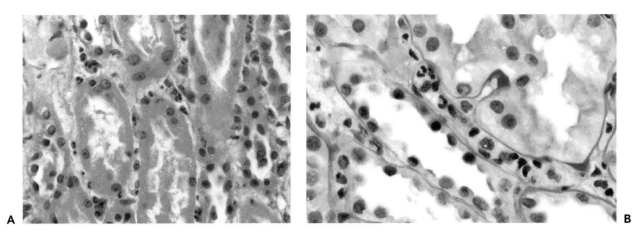

**Figure 28.36**  Acute humoral rejection with characteristic intraluminal peritubular capillary leukocytes. **A:** Primarily neutrophils. **B:** primarily mononuclear cells. (**A:** H&E, ×400; **B:** PAS, ×600.)

CD59. C5b-9 and C3 also are deposited in ACR along the TBM (193). CRP has been detected in tubular cytoplasm (404). C4d is occasionally present segmentally along the TBM, in both AHR and ACR.

### Peritubular Capillaries

Immunoglobulin is usually not demonstrable in peritubular capillaries (348); however, in a few anti-class I antibody cases, IgM and IgG are present (136,153). IgM was reported in 20% and IgG in 0% of patients with anti-HLA class I or II antibodies (390). In contrast, IgM is usually present in ABO-incompatible grafts with AHR (405) (see below).

Intense immunofluorescence staining for C4d is usually detected in a widespread uniform distribution in the peritubular capillaries (384,390) (Fig. 28.40). Focal deposition may also be found, but is of uncertain significance. In classic cases, at low power the smaller oval and elongated ringlike fluorescent profiles of dilated peritubular

capillaries are readily evident between the larger negative tubular cross sections. The capillary staining is crisp, linear, and continuous, but also may have a finely granular pattern at high power, which extends into the lumen from the more linear deposits (Fig. 28.40). Medullary vessels are also generally positive. In paraffin sections with immunohistochemistry, C4d has a similar pattern, diffuse, linear, and circumferential in the peritubular capillary wall, although the intensity varies (Fig. 28.39). Intraluminal and interstitial C4d staining may also be seen and is an artifact of fixation.

C4d is present in most peritubular capillaries, even those that lack endothelial cell markers, and colocalizes with anti-type IV collagen and endothelial cells in frozen tissue, suggesting that some C4d is bound to the basement membrane (390). This location fits with the known ability of C4 to cross-link to nearby proteins at the site of complement activation. The covalent linkage of C4d to structural proteins

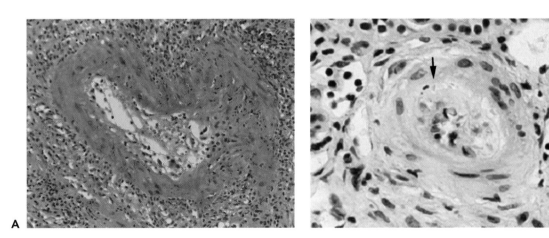

**Figure 28.37**  Acute humoral rejection. **A:** Fibrinoid arterial necrosis (Banff type III). Neutrophils and fibrin are seen in the wall of the arcuate-sized artery. Nephrectomy specimen. C4d-positive. (H&E, ×200.) **B:** Mucoid intimal thickening resembling TMA. Patient had anti-class I antibodies (136) and red cell fragment in intima (*arrow*) (H&E.) (Case courtesy of Kim Solez.)

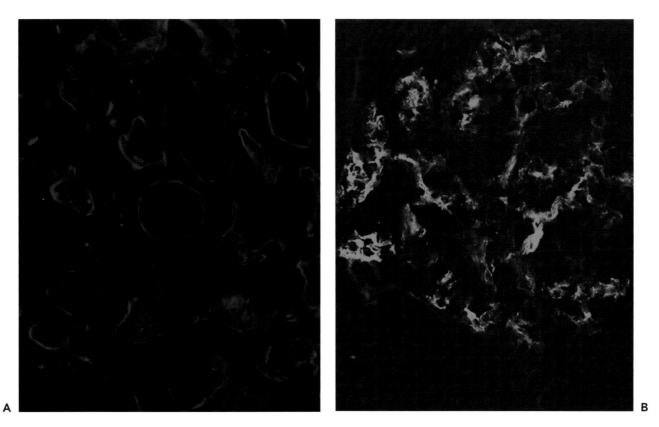

**Figure 28.38** Normal kidneys stained for C4d using a monoclonal antibody in cryostat sections. **A:** Negative peritubular capillaries and faint staining along the TBM. **B:** Prominent mesangial deposits are present in normal glomeruli, making it difficult to discern glomerular deposits due to humoral rejection. (×400.)

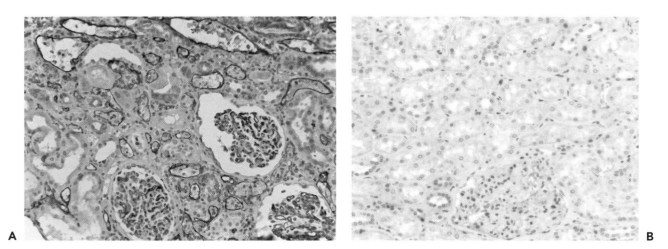

**Figure 28.39** Paraffin sections stained using a polyclonal anti-C4d (347). **A:** Acute humoral rejection showing widespread, circumferential deposits in characteristically dilated peritubular capillaries containing leukocytes. The glomerular capillary walls also stain prominently. **B:** Normal kidney, stained with the same technique, demonstrates the absence of C4d in the glomeruli in paraffin sections (compare with Figure 28.38B). (×200.)

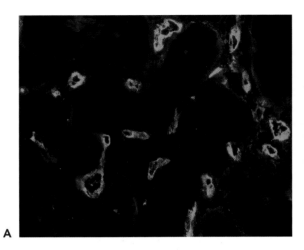 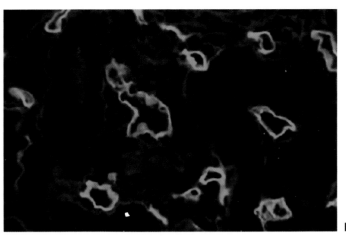

**A**                                                                    **B**

**Figure 28.40**  Acute humoral rejection, C4d stain using monoclonal antibody to C4d in cryostat sections (390). Bright widespread circumferential staining is present in **(A)** and **(B)**. **A** has a slightly granular appearance and **(B)** is purely linear. Both patients had antibodies to donor HLA antigens. (×400.)

may explain why C4d remains for several days after alloantibody disappears, since antibody binds to cell-surface antigens that can be lost by modulation, shedding, or cell death. Reduced CD34 expression has been described, as well as platelet fragments that stain for CD61 (also found in ACR) (406). C3d deposits in PTC with or without C4d. Of 26 C3d+ cases, 81% were also C4d+; of the 35 C4d+ cases, 60% were C3d+ (200); in another series, 44% of the C4d cases had C3 (390). C4d deposition does not persist long after the antibody disappears, as judged by a few repeat biopsies. Loss of C4d has been observed in repeat biopsies 7 to 8 days after a positive biopsy (348)(and unpublished data).

## Arteries

The fibrinoid deposits in arteries usually stain for IgG and/or IgM, C3, C4d, and fibrin (195,196,390). Follow-up biopsies have been reported in a few instances in which immunoglobulin, complement, and fibrin staining became negative (196). Nondiagnostic C4d deposition occurs along endothelial surfaces of arteries and arterioles and in thickened intima of arteries and arteriolar hyaline, whether or not AHR is present (seen also in native kidneys).

## Electron Microscopy

### Glomeruli

The appearance may resemble thrombotic microangiopathy, with platelets, fibrin, and neutrophils in glomerular capillaries (Fig. 28.41). The glomerular endothelium is reactive and separated from the GBM by a widened lucent space. Swelling of endothelial cells (136) and loss of endothelial fenestrations may be present, indicative of injury.

Other cases have mononuclear inflammatory cells (transplant glomerulitis/acute allograft glomerulopathy) or even little ultrastructural change. Later biopsies (1 month) may begin to show a new layer of GBM, the early change of transplant glomerulopathy (407).

## Peritubular Capillaries

Neutrophils and monocytes can be found in peritubular capillaries with platelets, fibrin, and mononuclear cells (Fig. 28.41) (407,408). Interstitial edema and red cell extravasation can be found. Intact platelets are few, but microvesicles presumably derived from platelets are common (406). Endothelial cells show swelling, detachment, and expansion of the subendothelial space with electron-lucent fluffy material and sometimes trapped red cells (408). Lysis, apoptosis, and fragmentation of endothelial cells are evident (407). These changes are more severe and extensive than the endothelial swelling and apoptosis that occur in ischemic renal injury (407). C4d can be detected on the surface of the endothelial cells and in intracytoplasmic vesicles by immunoelectron microscopy (409). Apparent new capillary sprouts have been illustrated (407). After 2 to 4 weeks, the endothelial cells show cytoplasmic processes extending into the lumen and some multilayering of the basement membrane (407,408). In severe cases, after 2 to 3 months, some capillaries are completely destroyed, with disappearance of the endothelial lining and remnants of the basement membrane; those that remain have a thickened, multilayered basement membrane (408).

## Arteries

The small arteries with fibrinoid necrosis show marked endothelial injury and loss, smooth muscle necrosis, and deposition of fibrin tactoids.

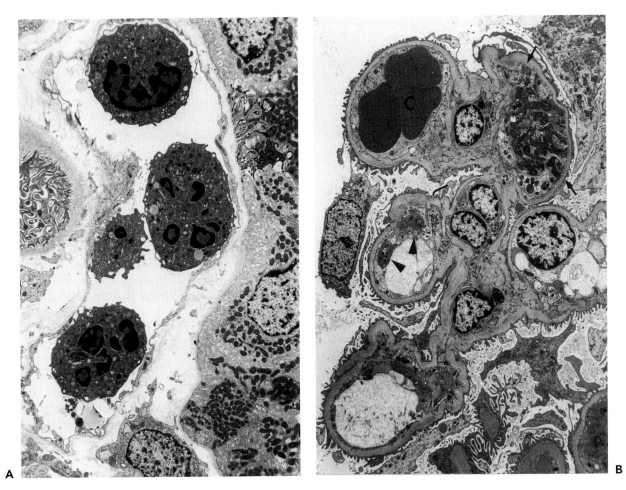

**Figure 28.41**  Acute humoral rejection. **A:** Neutrophils are in peritubular capillaries whose endothelium shows the subtle changes of injury (loss of fenestrations). **B:** A glomerulus has one capillary plugged with fibrin (*arrows*) and another filled with compacted red cells surrounded by a reactive endothelial cell (labeled C); a third loop has a few platelets (*arrowheads*). (Electron micrographs, **A:** ×3700; **B:** ×3300.)

## Etiology and Pathogenesis

### Antigens (410)

The usual antigenic targets of antibody-mediated rejection are MHC antigens (class I and II) (386,391,411) and, less often, the ABO blood group antigens (412). Production of HLA alloantibodies depends on exposure to HLA antigens from pregnancy, blood transfusion, or transplantation; these antibodies are predominately IgG. In contrast, ABO antibodies arise naturally in response to exogenous cross-reactive carbohydrate antigens. In addition, nonclassic MHC antigens, such as MICA (MHC class I-related chain A) are potential polymorphic endothelial surface alloantigens. Antibodies to MICA can be detected in renal allograft recipients and are associated with later rejection and graft loss (413,414).

Non-MHC antigens other than ABO are potentially important, as evidenced by the occasional HLA-identical graft that develops AHR (415–417). We have observed two cases

of putative antibody-mediated rejection (C4d+) in HLA-identical grafts (Chicano et al, unpublished), and non-MHC alloantibodies have been eluted from rejected HLA-identical kidneys (418). Pretransplant serum antibodies to peritubular capillary endothelium can be detected by immunoperoxidase techniques in some patients and are associated with decreased graft survival (419). Endothelial antibody was detected by granular staining of cultured umbilical vein endothelial cells with serum from three cross-match–negative patients with acute humoral rejection; however, no evidence was provided that they reacted to surface alloantigens (420). Non-MHC antigens, such as the endothelial-monocyte alloantigen (415), remain undefined at the molecular level.

Autoantigens may occasionally be a target of AHR. In 16 cases reported from Berlin, IgG autoantibodies to angiotensin II type 1 receptor (AT1) were detected in patients who presented with malignant hypertension and graft dysfunction; three had seizures (421). None had antidonor

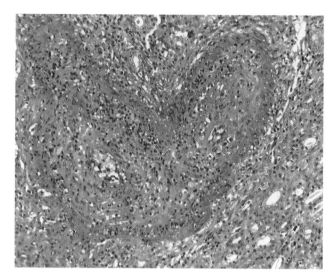

**Figure 28.42** Artery with fibrinoid necrosis and cellular infiltration of intima associated with antibodies to angiotensin II type 1 receptor (421). (Provided by Duska Dragun, Berlin.)

HLA antibodies. IgG1 and IgG3 autoantibodies recognized two different nonpolymorphic epitopes on the second extracellular loop of AT1, which activated the receptor in cultured vascular smooth muscle cells. Grafts showed fibrinoid necrosis of arteries and acute rejection with increased expression of tissue factor (Fig. 28.42). Peritubular capillaries had C4d in 33% of cases. Curiously, the AT1 antibodies did not affect vessels in native organs, suggesting a component of rejection is necessary to manifest this effect. This was confirmed in passive transfer of the AT1 antibody to rats, which caused lesions only in allografts. It would appear that the AT1 receptor antibody is "piling on" vascular lesions caused by alloreactive processes. The explanation for this cluster of patients is not obvious. The syndrome of malignant hypertension and fibrinoid necrosis is quite unusual and awaits confirmation at other centers. Treatment with losartan or plasmapheresis may be beneficial (421).

Although not reported in humans, in some experimental models endothelial damage in ischemic organs is mediated by natural IgM autoantibodies and complement fixation (422). This might provide another potential mechanism of AHR.

## B-Cells and Plasma Cells (410,423)

An IgG alloantibody response requires CD4⁺ T-cell reactivity through the indirect pathway (424,425). By contrast, IgM alloantibodies specific for MHC antigens (424) and carbohydrate antigens (ABO) (424) may not require T-cell help. Activated T-cells provide help for B-cell memory, isotype switching, and affinity maturation through various T-cell–derived cytokines and costimulatory factors that recognize receptors on B-cells (such as CD80/CD86, CD40L, and ICOS). The B-cell response leads to the production of

long-lived plasma cells, which migrate to the bone marrow and continue to produce antibodies indefinitely, without requiring T-cell help (426). It is not known whether antibodies specific for graft antigens are maintained due to the longevity of plasma cells or to the continuous generation of new-memory B-cells.

## Effector Mechanisms (410,427)

Complement fixation by antibody seems to be essential for antibody to provoke acute rejection (428). Complement-fixing antibody isotypes are required for passive transfer of AHR in mouse cardiac allografts (429,430). Furthermore, complement antagonists inhibit acute and hyperacute antibody-mediated rejection (431,432). One study has noted a specific increase in antidonor HLA antibodies of the IgG3 subclass (strong complement activator) in three patients with acute rejection (433).

The pathways that lead to complement activation and C4d deposition are diagrammed in Figure 28.43 (388). Complement mediates acute graft injury by attracting inflammatory cells mainly through the chemoattractants C3a and C5a and by lysis of endothelial cells (410). C3a also promotes vasospasm through the release of PGE2 from macrophages, and C5a causes edema through the release of histamine from mast cells. Both cause endothelial cell release of IL-6, IL-8, IL-1α and CCL5 and increased expression of adhesion molecules E-selectin, VCAM-1, and ICAM-1 (434,435). MAC causes lysis and apoptosis of endothelial cells, a process dependent on C6 (436,437). In sublytic concentrations, soluble MAC increases expression of adhesion molecules, such as E-selectin, ICAM-1, and VCAM-1 on cultured endothelial cells and synthesis and secretion of IL-8, MCP-1, CCL2, and CCL5 (438,439). Finally, C5a and MAC trigger endothelial synthesis of tissue factor (a part of the extrinsic clotting system) (440,441) and can have growth-promotin effects.

Several molecules control the activation of the cascade. Plasma factor I inactivates C4b to C4d, which remains bound covalently to the tissue and is thereby a durable in situ marker of complement activation, in contrast to C1q or antibody. So far, no reports indicate functional activity for C4d, whose structure has been ascertained by x-ray crystallography (442). Theoretically, graft injury might be prevented if activation stops at C4 without C3 activation (manifested by C4d but no C3d deposition in the graft) (443,444), although this has not yet been shown to be true in clinical samples. Four major cell-surface inhibitors of complement activation are known: decay-accelerating factor (DAF, CD55), which dissociates C4b/C3b; membrane cofactor protein (MCP, CD46) and CR1 (C4b/C3b receptor, CD35), which catalyze the cleavage of C4b/C3b by factor I; and protectin (CD59), which inhibits the formation of MAC (C5b-9) (445–447). All complement-regulatory proteins are expressed in the glomerulus, probably providing

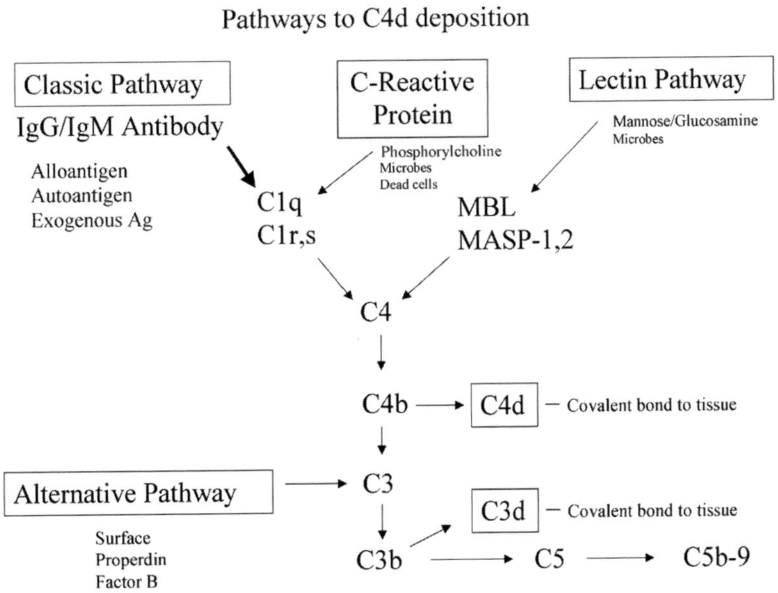

Pathways to C4d deposition

**Figure 28.43**  Pathways of C4 activation (388). Activation of C1 (composed of C1q, C1r, and C1s) is initiated by interaction of C1q with IgG or IgM bound to epitopes on the graft endothelium. C4 is cleaved by C1s into C4a and C4b, exposing a sulfhydryl group. The reactive sulfhydryl group of C4b rapidly forms an ester or amide bond with nearby molecules containing hydroxyl or amino groups. C4b combines with the enzymatically active fragment C2a to form C4bC2a, which is known as the classic pathway C3 convertase. C4bC2a cleaves C3 into C3a and C3b (which also has a reactive sulfhydryl group) and with the C3b molecule covalently deposited in the immediate vicinity, forms the C5 convertase C4bC2aC3b. Cleavage of C5 releases a bioactive peptide C5a, and C5b. C5b initiates formation of the membrane-attack complex (MAC; membrane-bound C5b-9), which causes cell lysis (437). The lectin pathway is stimulated when mannan-binding lectin (MBL), L-ficolin, or H-ficolin binds to the appropriate carbohydrate (typically on pathogens or apoptotic cells) (468). MBL binds to mannose (or glucosamine), and the ficolins bind to N-acetylglucosamine. L-ficolin also binds to elastin and lipoteichoic acid, and H-ficolin also binds N-acetyl galactosamine. MBL, L-ficolin, and H-ficolin (all homologous to C1q and fibrinogen) activate C4 via their associated serine proteases, MASP-1 and -2 (homologous to C1r and C1s). C4 is also activated via the binding of C-reactive protein (CRP) to the carbohydrate phosphorylcholine with participation of C1q (1326). Few or no terminal components (C5b-9) are generated, because CRP simultaneously recruits factor H, and may thus provide an anti-inflammatory effect. (From Rotman S, Collins AB, Colvin RB. C4d deposition in allografts: Current concepts and interpretation. Transplant Rev 2005;19:65.)

protection from the spontaneous "ticking over" of C4 and C3 that exposes their reactive thiol group (448) and from other potential harmful immunologic events. The normal accumulation of C4d in the glomerulus can be taken as evidence for this process. Only CD59 is prominent in normal cortical peritubular capillaries in frozen sections (445,449,450). Thus at the peritubular capillary surface, the classic pathway activation and generation of C4d is relatively unopposed; the inhibition of complement occurs at only the level of C5b-9.

Antibodies can also lyse endothelial cells by complement-independent pathways through the $Fc\gamma IIA$ receptor (CD16) on NK cells and macrophages (antibody-dependent cellular cytotoxicity, ADCC) (451). The contribution of this mechanism to graft rejection remains uncertain due to a lack of in vivo experimental studies.

It is intriguing, however, that $Fc\gamma IIA$ polymorphisms in recipients of renal allografts correlate with risk of acute rejection (452). Antibodies also have direct effects on endothelial cells, independent of complement and cells, and can stimulate production of tissue factor by cultured endothelial cells (453).

## Differential Diagnosis

### Criteria and Classification

The criteria for acute humoral rejection proposed by Mauiyyedi (153) were incorporated with minor modification by Banff (185) (Table 28.8). These include (a) histologic evidence of acute injury (neutrophils in capillaries,

## TABLE 28.8

### CRITERIA FOR ACUTE ANTIBODY-MEDIATED REJECTION (AHR)ᵃ

1. Morphologic evidence of acute tissue injury, such as
   a. Acute tubular injury, or
   b. Neutrophils and/or mononuclear cells in peritubular capillaries and/or glomeruli, and/or capillary thrombosis, or
   c. Fibrinoid necrosis/intramural or transmural inflammation in arteries
2. Immunopathologic evidence for antibody action, such as
   a. C4d and/or (rarely) immunoglobulin in peritubular capillaries, or
   b. Immunoglobulin and complement in arterial fibrinoid necrosis
3. Serologic evidence of circulating antibodies to donor HLA or other antidonor endothelial antigens.

ᵃCases that meet only two of the three numbered criteria are considered suspicious for acute humoral rejection. Acute cellular rejection may also be present as judged by the criteria in Table 28.5. From Racusen LC, Colvin RB, Solez K, et al. Antibody-mediated rejection criteria—an addition to the Banff 97 classification of renal allograft rejection. Am J Transplant 2003;3:708.

acute tubular injury, fibrinoid necrosis), (b) evidence of antibody interaction with tissue (typically C4d in peritubular capillaries), and (c) serologic evidence of circulating antibodies to antigens expressed by donor endothelium (typically HLA, ABO). If only two of the three major criteria are established (for example, when no HLA cross-match is available or when C4d staining is not done), the diagnosis should be considered suspicious for AHR. A negative C4d stain or a negative serology does not rule out AHR. Histology by itself is insufficient to rule AHR in or out (185).

AHR has been divided into three types based on light microscopy (153,185): type I, acute tubular injury; type II, neutrophils in capillaries; and type III, fibrinoid necrosis of arteries (185) (Table 28.2). Biopsies that meet the criteria for both AHR and ACR type I or II are considered to have both forms of rejection (i.e., mixed cellular and humoral rejection). C4d+ biopsies without acute inflammation but with chronic injury (GBM duplication, arteriopathy, interstitial fibrosis, and tubular atrophy) are considered to be chronic antibody-mediated rejection. Biopsies with C4d and no pathology may be a manifestation of accommodation.

No single histologic feature consistently distinguishes biopsies with AHR (136,199). Lesions that favor humoral rejection compared with pure cellular rejection are neutrophils in peritubular capillaries (46% to 65% versus 5% to 9%), fibrinoid necrosis of arteries (25% versus 0 to 5%), glomerulitis (35% to 55% versus 4% to 10%), thrombi (20% to 46% versus 0% to 15%) and infarction (5% to 38% versus 0% to 2%) (136,199,348). Of these criteria, we find peritubular neutrophils to be the most useful; however, neutrophils can be observed in peritubular capillaries in ACR and calcineurin inhibitor toxicity, even to a quite prominent degree, with no circulating HLA antibodies.

A positive C4d stain with the immunofluorescence technique is defined as "widespread, strong linear circumferential peritubular capillary staining in cortex or medulla, excluding scar or necrotic areas," according to a consensus at the 2003 Banff Conference (454). For positivity with immunohistochemistry of paraffin-embedded tissues, "strong staining is not required as tissue pretreatment influences staining intensity (454)." "Widespread" was intentionally left undefined because of the lack of any systematic study of thresholds. In practice, more than 50% is often used in publications for widespread or diffuse.

Interpretation of focal capillary staining (i.e., less than 50%) is problematic (Fig. 28.44). There is no consensus for the minimum amount of staining to qualify as focal positive: some suggestions have been 10 positive peritubular capillaries (348,455), more than 5% or more

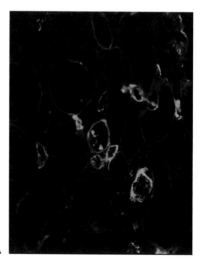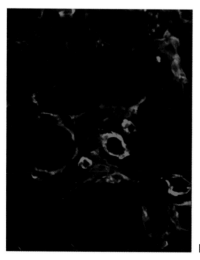

**A**  **B**

**Figure 28.44** Focal C4d in two samples (**A** and **B**) stained as in Figure 28.39. Less than 50% of the capillaries are stained. The significance of this is uncertain; some find no adverse effect (343), but occasionally these cases will be otherwise typical acute humoral rejection (personal observations). (×400.)

than 25% of capillaries (343,456). Focal patterns were considered an early phase of the more extensive deposition by Feucht (389). Indeed, early biopsies may show focal or no C4d deposition, but then become positive after 1 to 3 days (unpublished data). Two studies have failed to show any significant clinical or pathologic difference in cases of focal and diffuse C4d staining (348,455). In contrast, late rejection episodes (after 6 months) with focal C4d staining (about 5 to 50% of capillaries) behaved clinically better than those with diffuse C4d (over 50% of capillaries) and had the same outcome as those with negative C4d (343). C4d (mostly focal) can be found in histologically normal appearing graft biopsies taken for dysfunction. These C4d positive cases seem to benefit from anti-rejection therapy despite the lack of apparent morphologic signs of rejection (457). Although the reported findings have to be confirmed in larger series, they support the notion that C4d positivity in dysfunctioning grafts—regardless of morphology—indicates an active rejection process (348,383,457). Little is known of the correlation of focal C4d with donor-specific antibodies. Antibodies to donor class II antigens were found in two of three patients tested with focal C4d, arguing that this pattern is owing to circulating antibodies (455).

Protocol biopsies have shown that C4d deposition can precede histologic evidence of AHR. Haas et al (122) found focal or diffuse C4d staining in two of 82 1-hour biopsies taken at the time of transplantation after reperfusion. Both patients later developed an acute humoral rejection (day 5 and 34). The recipients had been treated with plasmapheresis before transplantation because of a positive cross-match and had a weakly positive flow cross-match at the time of transplantation (122). In 1-week protocol kidney biopsies, Sund showed PTC endothelial C4d deposition in 30% of cases, of which 82% later experienced clinical acute rejection (67% of these also met histologic criteria of acute rejection) (399). Koo (458) reported C4d in 13% of 48 1-week protocol biopsies. C4d was present in 33% of samples with rejection and 3% of samples without rejection; all five with C4d and rejection had donor-reactive antibodies (458). Outcome at 1 year was not affected by C4d status at 7 days, despite the lack of specific treatment.

## Diseases That Mimic Acute Humoral Rejection

Fibrinoid necrosis may occur in the absence of C4d deposition. Compiling the results of four small series, 27% (7/26) of biopsies with fibrinoid necrosis were C4d-negative (136,153,348,400). Presumably the fibrinoid necrosis in these cases is due to T-cell–mediated mechanisms, severe hypertension, or other factors. Argument for a T-cell component is also provided by the rare case of fibrinoid necrosis that responds to OKT3 therapy (320). As described above, antibodies to the angiotensin II type 1 receptor have appar-

ently caused fibrinoid necrosis in arteries in acute rejection in the absence of C4d deposition in capillaries (421).

One of the common diagnostic dilemmas in transplant biopsies is the distinction between thrombotic microangiopathy (TMA, hemolytic uremic syndrome [HUS]) due to calcineurin inhibitor toxicity or recurrent disease and AHR. Fortunately, C4d is negative in peritubular capillaries in thrombotic microangiopathy in native kidneys. We have tested 26 cases of thrombotic microangiopathy/HUS in native kidneys and found none with positive C4d, including cases with lupus anticoagulant and antiphospholipid antibodies (388). In five reported cases of recurrent HUS in a transplant, C4d was also negative (459). Thus, although the arterial and glomerular lesions overlap, peritubular capillary C4d provides a useful discriminator between AHR and TMA/HUS (Fig. 28.45) (347). C4d was also not found in glomerular capillaries in paraffin sections in TMA in six cases (347). Unpublished studies from our laboratory (two native kidneys and three transplants; Colvin, unpublished) and from others (12 cases, including native and transplant cases; Regele, personal communication) also showed no C4d in glomeruli in paraffin in TMA. Increased staining for CD61, a marker of platelets, in peritubular capillaries favors acute rejection over TMA, but does not distinguish AHR and ACR (406).

Many studies have sought evidence for C4d peritubular capillary deposition in other diseases in native kidneys. Ischemia does not usually have C4d deposition. A study of seven cases of acute tubular necrosis in native kidneys revealed no C4d deposition in peritubular capillaries (460). We have studied 30 zero-hour biopsies (after 20 minutes of reperfusion) and four non–heart-beating donor kidneys with histologic changes of ischemia injury and found no C4d deposition (388). In five ANCA-related glomerulonephritis in native kidneys, we also found no examples of peritubular capillary C4d deposition (388). Bright peritubular capillary C4d staining can be seen in lupus nephritis cases in either a granular or linear pattern (388,461) and in endocarditis (461). In frozen sections, C4d deposition is common in the mesangium and not specific for AHR. Additional staining along the GBM occurs in AHR, but is difficult to score. Granular glomerular C4d is typical in immune complex diseases (e.g., membranous glomerulonephritis).

## C4d Interpretation and Pitfalls (388)

### Sensitivity and Specificity

C4d+ cases have circulating antidonor antibodies detectable at the time of the biopsy in about 80% of recipients (63% to 90%) (153,462,463). In contrast, biopsies without C4d have circulating antidonor antibody in an average of 35% of the recipients (2%–53%). The widely varying rates of detection probably relate to the sensitivity of the

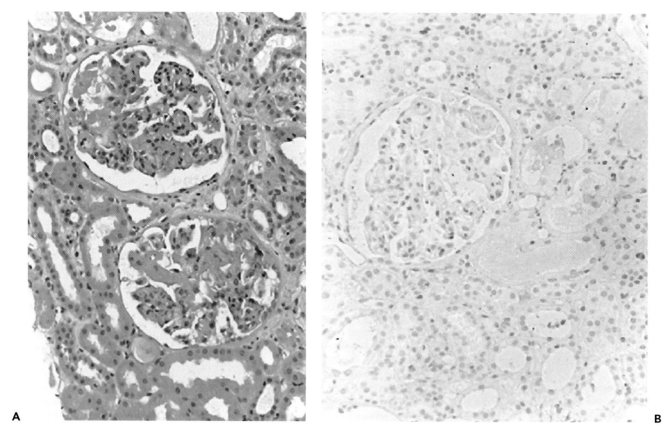

**Figure 28.45**  Allograft with thrombotic microangiopathy. **A:** Fibrin thrombi in glomeruli. (H&E.) **B:** C4d stain by immunohistochemistry (paraffin section). No C4d is detected in peritubular capillaries or glomeruli. (**A** and **B:** ×200.)

antibody assays, with some, such as AHG, highly specific and others, such as flow cytometry, less specific (more false-positives). In the first study to compare the two tests, C4d was a highly specific (96%) and sensitive (95%) marker of AHR, using circulating antidonor HLA-specific antibodies by the anti-human globulin cytotoxicity test (AHG) as the gold standard (153). By flow cytometry cross-match, 88% of recipients with C4d+ had circulating donor-specific antibodies detectable, similar to the 90% with AHG tests (463). However, approximately 50% of those without C4d deposition also had evidence of donor-specific antibodies by flow cytometry; whether this is related to false-positives, increased sensitivity, or non–complement-fixing antibodies is not clear. Using antibodies to donor type HLA-DR as the standard, Lederer et al (462) found that C4d staining had a sensitivity of 78% and specificity of 63% (37% of the HLA-DR antibody-negative patients had C4d deposition, due, presumably to HLA class I antibodies). C4d deposition does not correlate well with panel-reactive antibodies (PRA), which do not measure specific antidonor reactivity.

Direct comparison of the sensitivity of immunofluorescence (IF) using monoclonal antibody to C4d in frozen sections (IF) with immunoperoxidase stains using polyclonal antibody in paraffin-embedded tissue (IHC) has been reported, although the data are limited (347,388,464,465). Assuming a true positive is one with either IHC or IF positive staining, the false-negative rate of IHC is roughly about 10% to 20% and that of IF is 5% to 10%, probably in part related to sampling a different core. The triple-layer immunofluorescence technique proved the most sensitive in a systematic study (465). Different laboratories may find one or the other to be optimal, based on their proficiency with the techniques.

### Adequacy of Sample

The minimal adequacy is for viable cortical or medullary tissue. No glomeruli are required. This means that if tissue is sparse, the portion with medulla can be used for C4d staining. However, distinction between tubular basement membrane and vascular C4d deposits is more difficult in the medulla. Necrotic and scarred areas are not sufficient, since they are commonly negative, even in samples positive elsewhere. No formal studies of adequacy of sample size or number of cores have been given, but considering that cellular rejection has a false-negative rate of about 10% for one core, and that stains of individual portions or cores with IHC and IF have a false-negative rate of 10% to 20%, it is recommended that two cores be studied in cases suspicious on other grounds for humoral rejection.

## Artifacts

Immunofluorescence has fewer artifacts than IHC. Not uncommonly, the plasma in the capillaries is fixed by the formalin processing and also stains for C4d, which interferes with interpretation. Extravasation of C4d into the connective tissue is also common and should not be mistaken for capillary wall deposition. If extensive, these samples are not interpretable. In one series, 8% of the samples showed this pattern, which can be alleviated by decreasing the microwave treatment time (343). Granular staining of PTC by IHC is of uncertain significance.

## C4d Deposition in Other Sites

In unfixed cryostat sections, normal kidneys always show C4d in the glomerular mesangium and with variable commonly weak intensity along the glomerular basement membrane. The cause is not known, but occurs in other species (466) and may be due either to spontaneous activation of C4 in the circulation or deposition of "normal" immune complexes from infections and other stimuli. In fixed paraffin-embedded tissues, normal glomeruli are entirely negative (463). This difference may be because of fixation blocking access to C4d embedded in the mesangial matrix or GBM (as opposed to cell surfaces). Support for this theory comes from anti-GBM nephritis, in which the antibody (and presumably complement fixation) occurs in the GBM matrix. In this disease, C4d cannot be demonstrated along the GBM in paraffin sections but can in frozen sections, although it is often much weaker than IgG (unpublished). In contrast, the deposits in membranous glomerulonephritis stain intensely for C4d in frozen or paraffin sections and are a useful positive staining control. Arterial endothelial surfaces and thickened intima in arteriosclerosis and hyaline arteriolar deposits in native kidneys are often C4d-positive in frozen sections. The mechanism is not known, but it is tempting to speculate that this involves either CRP, which binds to altered lipoproteins and activates C4 (467), or L-ficolin, which binds to elastin (468).

## C4d Deposition Without Circulating Antibodies

About 10% to 40% of recipients with C4d+ acute rejection have no detectable circulating donor-reactive HLA antibodies. These may be caused by non-HLA specificities (e.g., MICA or autoantigens) or adsorption of antibody by the graft. Antidonor HLA antibodies can be eluted from about 70% of rejected grafts, even though only 30% of the patients have detectable serum antibodies (469); adsorption is the most likely explanation for most antibody-negative cases, in our opinion. Alternatively, C4 may be activated by antibody-independent pathways (Fig. 28.43). The lectin pathway has been shown to be relevant to renal ischemia in the mouse (470), in which extensive mannan-binding lectin (MBL) deposition occurs in peritubular capillaries and tubular epithelial cells. However, at present there is little or no evidence for MBL/MASP (MBL-associated serine protease) deposition in human renal allografts (471).

## Clinical Course, Prognosis, Therapy, and Clinicopathologic Correlations

### Outcome (199)

In most series, the overall graft loss at 1 year after AHR (with or without ACR) is considerably worse than after ACR. In one series, 4% of ACR were lost versus 30% of AHR (153). Acute rejection associated with cytotoxic IgG anti-HLA class I antibodies (401) or antibodies to endothelial antigens (180) had a 1-year graft survival of 16% and 25%, respectively. These data are quite comparable to those of other recent series who have reported 3% to 7% graft loss after a C4d-negative acute rejection episode and 16% to 50% graft loss after C4d-positive acute rejection (354,463,472). Most recent series emphasize that the majority of graft losses in the first year have been attributable to humoral rejection. Notably, 75% of the overall 1-year graft losses from acute rejection were in the C4d+AHR group (153). A uniformly poor prognosis of the cases with fibrinoid necrosis (type III) in the older literature has been reported, with about 25% graft survival at 1 year (215,353,371,376). In a large, well-analyzed study, the presence of C4d strikingly and adversely impacted the outcome of either type I or II acute rejection (354) (Fig. 28.46). C3d deposition in peritubular capillaries is also a risk factor for graft loss, but its contribution as distinct from C4d is not clear (200). C3d in peritubular capillaries was not associated with circulating antidonor antibodies or neutrophils in peritubular capillaries (400). Curiously, glomerulitis with C4d deposition can persist on repeated biopsies with continuing normal function (473). Those patients who survive an AHR episode do not seem to have an adverse long-term outcome, emphasizing the importance of vigorous initial treatment (136,153,348,383,391).

### Treatment (199,410)

Treatment of acute antibody-mediated rejection is still evolving, and randomized, controlled trials of therapies are yet to be reported. The most common strategies are based on the quick reduction of antibody titers with plasmapheresis plus immunosuppression with drugs such as tacrolimus and mycophenolate mofetil (385,474–476). Treatment of any T-cell–mediated component may also be needed. Pascual et al (477) reported successful reversal of acute humoral rejection with plasmapheresis, tacrolimus, and MMF. A follow-up study reported additional patients who were treated similarly with successful reversal of humoral

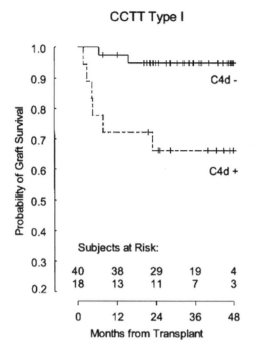

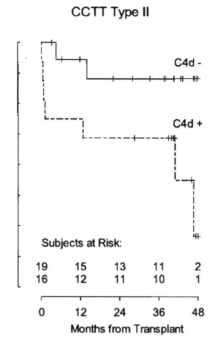

**Figure 28.46** Graft survival as a function of the type of cellular rejection (type I or II) and the presence or absence of C4d deposition in peritubular capillaries. In both types of rejection, C4d is a poor prognostic feature. (From Herzenberg AM, Gill JS, Djurdjev O, Magil AB. C4d deposition in acute rejection: An independent long-term prognostic factor. J Am Soc Nephrol 2002;13:234.)

rejection and return to normal graft function (391). Intravenous human gamma globulin (IVIG) is often used because of its immunomodulatory effects, especially on B-cells, antibody, and complement (476,478–480). Selective interference with the complement system using infusion of soluble (481) or membrane-targeted complement regulators (482) or antibodies to C5 (483) may be useful in the acute management of AHR. Immunoadsorption therapy with protein A, which binds mainly to IgG, successfully reversed acute humoral rejection in nine of ten cases with 80% graft survival over a 14-month follow-up period (484) and rendered nine sensitized patients cross-match–negative before transplantation (485).

No therapeutic small molecules are available that interfere selectively with B-cell or plasma cell function. The most specific drug, rituximab, reacts with CD20 on premature and mature B-cells and leads to transient B-cell depletion with B-cell recovery after 6 to 9 months. Preliminary studies indicate that rituximab decreases the level of pre-existing and posttransplant antibodies (486–489). Conclusions and extrapolations are limited, however, because rituximab was usually combined with other therapies in these small and uncontrolled trials. Normal plasma cells express little or no CD20 and therefore are resistant to rituximab-mediated depletion.

## ABO-Incompatible Grafts (388)

ABO-incompatible (ABOi) grafts have special features that warrant separate consideration. Blood group antigens, most importantly the A and B antigens, are carbohydrate epitopes on glycolipids and glycoproteins, which are present on most tissues, including erythrocytes and the endothelium. In the kidney, the ABO antigens are on the endothelium and distal convoluted tubules (and on the collecting ducts of secretors) (490). Antibodies to A or B antigens arise naturally in normal individuals without A or B blood groups in response to antigens in the environment (isoagglutinins) and are usually of the IgM isotype. Antibodies to blood group A2, which accounts for about 20% of type A, are present at lower levels, and tissues express less of the blood group glycolipid, making allografts less vulnerable to rejection than allografts in patients with other ABO incompatibilities.

Removal of circulating ABO antibodies by extracorporeal immunoabsorption or plasmapheresis has permitted successful transplantation of ABO-incompatible kidneys from HLA-identical siblings (491,492). Some of these protocols also use splenectomy or rituximab (493). Even with these treatments, AHR has developed in 30% to 50% of recipients. A recent innovative approach is to perform paired exchanges of living donor organs so that ABO matching can be achieved (494).

One-hour postperfusion biopsies have shown C4d in 57% of 14 ABOi grafts, usually also with IgM (88%) and occasionally with IgG (40%); however, only 37% of patients with C4d deposition developed acute rejection in the first month (405). Among 19 recipients of ABO-incompatible grafts, 52% were C4d+ in the first 90 days, compared with 16% of recipients with acute rejection in ABO-compatible grafts (397). AHRs due to ABO antibodies more commonly has IgM and C3 in peritubular capillaries than those due to HLA antibodies (Fig. 28.47). One of the larger and most systematic studies of ABO-incompatible grafts included

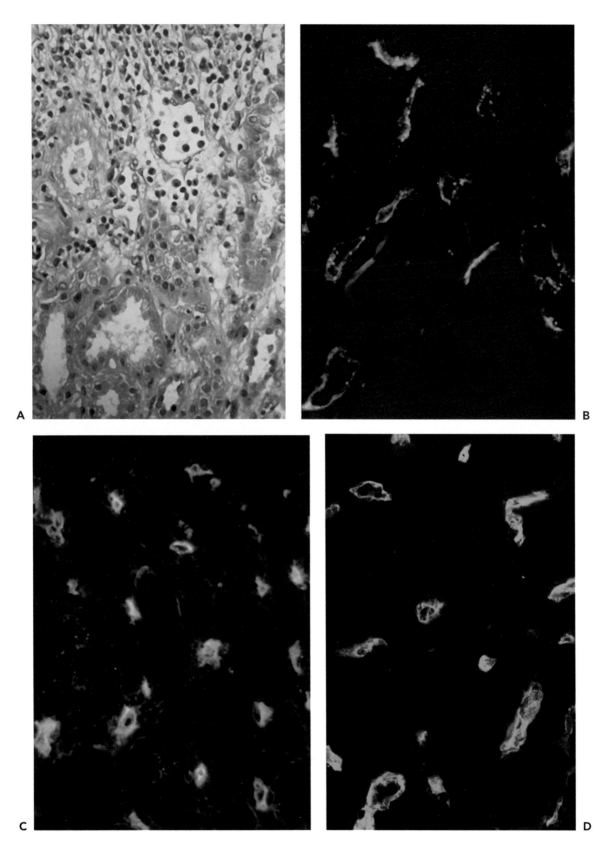

**Figure 28.47**  ABO-incompatible graft with acute humoral rejection (same patient as in Fig. 28.29).
A: Neutrophils are prominent in dilated peritubular capillaries. IgM (B), C3 (C), and C4d (D) are
deposited in peritubular capillaries, as shown by immunofluorescence stains of cryostat sections.

protocol biopsies in 32 patients (398). Overall, 28% developed acute rejection: C4d was present in 56%, often with neutrophil infiltration (67%), glomerular (78%) or arterial (33%) thrombi, mesangiolysis (78%), interstitial hemorrhage and necrosis (56%), and arteriolar thrombi (33%). IgM usually accompanied C4d deposition (405). Subclinical AHR was diagnosed by protocol biopsies in 12% of patients that showed C4d and glomerular thrombi (398).

ABOi grafts have had a significantly higher rate of early graft loss (21% in the first year), than ABO-compatible grafts, but then have a similar outcome, with 5-year graft survival of 75% (495). Other series that include A2 donors have reported lower graft loss (496). Curiously, survival has been achieved even though high titers of IgG and IgM antibodies returned in the circulation after 1 year, a phenomenon termed *graft accommodation*. Protocol biopsies performed 214 to 420 days posttransplant in stable recipients showed mild mesangiolysis in 12% and C4d immunostaining in 25%. Recovery from AHR in ABO-incompatible grafts correlates with a decrease in ABO titer but not with a disappearance of C4d, in contrast to AHR caused by HLA antibodies in which recovery is associated with loss of both antibody titer and C4d (497). This and the observation of C4d without graft pathology suggest that accommodation may be more easily achieved with ABO antibodies and antigens.

## HYPERACUTE REJECTION

### Clinical Presentation

*Hyperacute rejection* refers to immediate rejection of the kidney on perfusion with recipient blood (typically within 10 to 60 minutes), a process that requires the recipient to be presensitized to alloantigens on the surface of the graft endothelium. Hyperacute rejection is a variant of acute humoral rejection in which antibody titers are sufficient at the time of transplantation to cause immediate rejection. Some cases first become evident postoperatively, from 8 hours to 2 days (498), presumably because the circulating antibodies are of insufficient titer at the time of grafting. The graft rapidly becomes cyanotic and flaccid despite good pulses at the hilum and swells poorly on venous compression (499). In the first 10 minutes, the graft sequesters platelets, neutrophils, complement, fibrinogen, and coagulation factors II, V, and VIII, and the level of circulating antidonor antibodies decreases (500). The usual postoperative clinical signs are anuria, high fever, and no perfusion on renal scan; sometimes thrombocytopenia and increased circulating fibrin split products occur (501). Microangiopathic hemolytic anemia can develop, which reverses on removal of the graft (501). The clinical presentation can also resemble acute tubular necrosis and be mistaken for DGF (387). Hyperacute rejection is now rare, encountered

in about 0.5% of transplants due to effective cross-match screening (502). A higher prevalence may be concealed in the category of primary nonfunction, which is about 5% higher in second grafts (502).

## Pathologic Changes

### Gross Pathology

The kidney becomes livid, mottled, and cyanotic soon after reperfusion in the operating room (29,498,503,504). The kidney is initially flabby and soft, but subsequently swells and develops widespread hemorrhagic cortical necrosis with medullary congestion (Fig. 28.48). The large vessels are sometimes thrombosed. Dystrophic calcification can occur (499).

### Light Microscopy

The pathologic features are similar to those in severe acute antibody-mediated rejection (Fig. 28.49). In fact, the

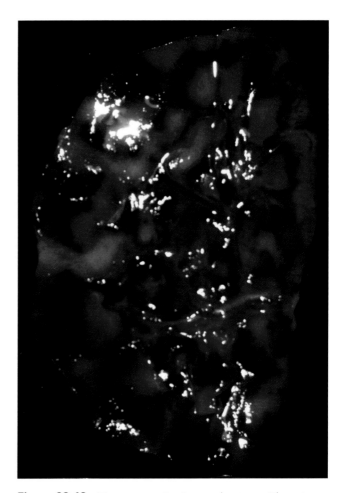

**Figure 28.48**  Hyperacute rejection, nephrectomy. The cut surface of the markedly swollen kidney is grossly hemorrhagic and glistening with edema fluid (hence the reflections).

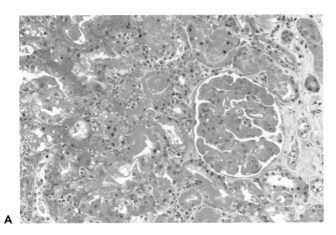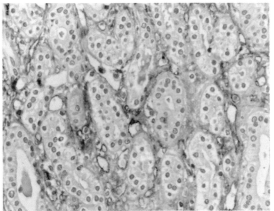

A                                                    B

**Figure 28.49** Hyperacute rejection due to pre-existing anti-donor class II HLA antibodies (509). **A:** Interstitial edema and hemorrhage is conspicuous as are neutrophils in peritubular capillaries. Glomeruli are congested and have lost endothelial nuclei. (H&E, ×200.) **B:** C4d on paraffin section shows widespread circumferential deposition along the peritubular capillaries (stain done on an unstained paraffin section stored for 25 years). (C4d immunohistochemistry, ×400.)

earliest stages of antibody-mediated rejection were first observed in hyperacute rejection. Neutrophil and platelet margination occurs in the first hour along damaged endothelium of glomerular and peritubular capillaries, and the capillaries fill with sludged, compacted red cells and fibrin (499). Neutrophils do not infiltrate initially, but form chainlike figures in the peritubular capillaries without obvious thrombi (499). The endothelium is stripped off the underlying basal lamina, and the interstitium becomes edematous and hemorrhagic. Intravascular coagulation occurs, and cortical necrosis ensues over 12 to 24 hours. The medulla is relatively spared, but is ultimately affected as the whole kidney becomes necrotic (29). Widespread microthrombi are usually found in the arterioles and glomeruli and can be detected even in totally necrotic samples. The larger arteries may be spared, but small arteries often also show neutrophilic infiltration or fibrinoid necrosis. Mononuclear cell infiltrates are typically sparse. One case showed CD3+ cells in the adventitia of small arteries and in the surrounding interstitium (498).

## Immunofluorescence Microscopy and Immunohistochemistry

In hyperacute rejection, antibodies often cannot be detected in the vessels (503–505), even though antibodies can be eluted from the kidney (506,507). Fibrin, IgM, and C3 are occasionally quite prominent in the vascular and glomerular lesions (195,499,503,508). Mesangial deposition of IgG and properdin are found in some cases (498,499). The nature of the antigen influences the distribution of the staining and the isotype of the antibody. ABO antibodies are primarily IgM and deposit in all vascular endothelium. Anti-HLA class I antibodies cause C3 deposition, neutrophils, and fibrin in the microvascula-

ture (387). Cases with anti-class II antibodies have IgG/IgM primarily in glomerular and peritubular capillaries, where class II is normally conspicuous, but not in arteries (509). IgG deposition associated with anti–endothelial-monocyte antibodies is reported to be primarily in peritubular capillaries (510).

C4d is deposited in the peritubular capillaries and glomeruli, as in acute humoral rejection (Fig. 28.49), and is more useful diagnostically than immunoglobulin deposition. Occasional cases biopsied at the time of operation may be initially negative for C4d (A. H. Cohen, Cedar Sinai Hospital, Los Angeles, personal communication), perhaps related to focally decreased perfusion or insufficient time to generate substantial amounts of C4d.

## Electron Microscopy

Neutrophils are abundant in the glomerular capillaries, where they seem to attach to injured endothelial cells (499) (Fig. 28.50). Electron-dense deposits are rare or absent (499). The endothelium is swollen, separated from the GBM by a lucent space. Capillary loops and peritubular capillaries are often bare of endothelium. Platelet, fibrin thrombi, and trapped erythrocytes occlude capillaries.

### Etiology and Pathogenesis

### Antigens

ABO blood group antigens were the first identified target of hyperacute rejection (499,504). Eluates from the rejected kidney contain anti-ABO IgM or IgG antibodies (511). Other blood group antigens such as MN are on endothelium, but no cases of hyperacute rejection have been reported to that determinant; Lewis blood group antigens are absent from vascular endothelium.

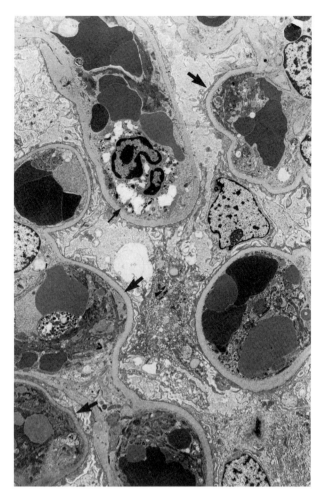

**Figure 28.50**  Hyperacute rejection owing to anti-HLA DR antibodies, biopsied at 24 hours after transplantation. Electron micrograph of glomerular capillaries shows fibrin platelet thrombi (*thick arrows*), a degranulated neutrophil (*arrow*), and compacted red cells; the endothelium is absent from most of the GBM. (×5000.)

HLA class I (29,499,503,504,512) and class II (411,509) antigens can also be targets of hyperacute rejection, and antibodies reactive to donor MHC have been eluted from a few hyperacutely rejected kidneys (507). The rapid graft destruction in humans by anti-MHC antibodies contrasts with that in rodents and may be explained by the fact that normal murine endothelium has less class I and class II antigen expression (214) and a less efficient complement system. Some B-cell antibodies are IgM autoantibodies and react in the cold; these are usually harmless. Warm-reactive IgG anti–B-cell antibodies can portend hyperacute rejection (509).

Non-MHC or non-ABO antigens on endothelium have been implicated in cross-match negative cases of hyperacute rejection (180). These patients are typically multiparous females or recipients of prior transplants (498), and some have received HLA-identical kidneys (513). Antibodies have been eluted from hyperacutely rejected kidneys

that stain the endothelium of peritubular capillaries and arterioles (514–516). Some of these are cross-reactive with monocytes (510,516) and others are not (514). Testing of the pretransplant serum on the donor kidney can show binding of immunoglobulin to the peritubular capillaries in patients with antiendothelial antibodies (180,510), but it is sometimes quite weak (514). Testing of donor skin with recipient serum can also reveal pre-existing complement-fixing antibodies (509). Pre-existing donor kidney–reactive antibodies were detected by immunoperoxidase techniques in 19% of 70 patients who had a negative T-cell cytotoxic cross-match, and 50% reacted with endothelium (some also with epithelium) (419).

Rarely, cold-reactive IgM agglutinins (reactive with recipient red cells) have been implicated in immediate injury in kidneys that are not rewarmed before blood flow is re-established (517,518). The lesions have relatively few neutrophils, resembling ex vivo perfusion injury (see below). These cause immediate graft dysfunction because of intravascular aggregation of recipient erythrocytes and thrombosis, as described in five cases (519).

## Effector Mechanisms

Hyperacute rejection is caused by binding of circulating antibodies to the surface of endothelial cells, complement fixation, platelet activation, lysis of the endothelium, and activation of the clotting system with thrombosis. The sequence of events is similar, if not identical, to that in acute antibody-mediated rejection, only developing more rapidly and vigorously, in a setting with no opportunity for the endothelium to develop resistance (accommodation).

Renal allografts in monkeys presensitized to donor antigens develop a marked reduction in renal blood flow because of vasoconstriction, as the earliest and most abnormal finding (520). At 5 minutes endothelial immunoglobulin and faint C3 deposits were detectable, but never became prominent; fibrin formation was sparse at all times. Glomeruli were the most sensitive, and arterial injury became more prominent at higher antibody titers. Early red cell sequestration and stasis were marked, followed by progressive aggregation of platelets and infiltration of neutrophils. Renal venous studies revealed marked consumption of C3 but no evidence of intrarenal activation of the coagulation, fibrinolytic, or kinin-forming systems. Platelet aggregates in glomeruli and IgM deposition on the surface of glomerular endothelial cells were beautifully demonstrated by electron microscopy in hyperacute rejection in rabbits (521). Platelets were closely adherent to the endothelium of arteries and glomeruli. The damaged endothelium released platelet-activating factor and probably other mediators (521). Increased expression by endothelial cells of leukocyte adhesion molecules CD31 (PECAM-1) and CD62E (E-selectin), increased production of tissue factor, plasminogen activator inhibitor, and decreased thrombomodulin also occur (522). A similar sequence occurs in discordant xenografts (i.e., those in which the recipient has preformed natural IgM antibodies) (523–525).

In general, only the complement-fixing antibodies mediate hyperacute rejection. IgG3 (4% of circulating IgG) and IgM are better complement-fixing antibodies than IgG1 (65% of circulating IgG) or IgG2 (25% of IgG); IgG4 (5% of IgG) does not fix complement. Sera that are positive in microcytotoxicity assays (complement fixation required) contain predominantly IgG3 with or without other IgG isotypes; sera negative by microcytotoxicity but positive by flow cytometry (only antigen binding required) contain predominately IgG2 and IgG4. About 80% of patients with high titers of antidonor cytotoxic antibodies in pretransplant cross-match tests reject their kidney hyperacutely (526). IgM antibodies, the most potent complement-fixing subclass in vitro, curiously do not always trigger hyperacute rejection; only about half of those with IgM anti-class I antibodies have hyperacute rejection. One reason may be the low affinity, which is characteristic of IgM antibodies; affinity maturation by somatic mutation and selection occurs after subclass switch to IgG. As a measure of low affinity, some of these antibodies react only in the cold or dissociate after multiple washes. IgA antibodies have not been associated with hyperacute rejection.

Hyperacute rejection rarely occurs in the absence of demonstrable antidonor antibody, presumably caused by primed cytotoxic T-cells present in the circulation at the time of transplantation. We documented such a phenomenon in presensitized pigs, which reject renal allografts hyperacutely but have no detectable humoral antibody (527). The first visible lesion within 30 minutes consists of lymphocytes attached to the arterial endothelium; after a few hours, the graft develops florid mononuclear infiltrate and necrosis. T-cell–mediated hyperacute rejection of mouse heart allografts has also been described in the absence of pre-existing donor-reactive antibodies (528). Hyperacute rejection is occasionally reversed in humans by anti–T-cell antibody (OKT3) (498), arguing in favor of a T-cell–mediated process in a few cases.

### Differential Diagnosis

The differential diagnosis of hyperacute rejection includes perfusion injury and major vascular thrombosis. Hyperacute rejection typically has more hemorrhage, necrosis, and neutrophil accumulation than perfusion injury. Perfusion injury has prominent loss of endothelium and thrombi. Increased neutrophils in glomeruli and peritubular capillaries were always associated with hyperacute rejection in one series; glomerular neutrophils alone were associated with ischemic injury (108). Grafts lost because of thrombosis of extrarenal arteries owing to technical complications or hypercoagulable states typically show necrosis with little hemorrhage, microthrombi, or widespread

accumulation of neutrophils in peritubular capillaries and glomeruli. Renal vein thrombosis shows marked congestion and relatively little neutrophil response. Antiphospholipid antibodies can predispose to the thrombotic events (529).

The major diagnostic feature of hyperacute rejection is the deposition of C4d in peritubular capillaries and the prominence of neutrophils in capillaries in hyperacute rejection. Although the finding of antibody and C4d deposition in small vessels, including capillaries, is diagnostic when present, negative immunofluorescence stains for IgG, IgM, and C4d do not exclude hyperacute rejection. The pretransplant serum should be retested with the most sensitive techniques against donor antigens (T-cells, B-cells, monocytes, erythrocytes, and antigen-coated beads). Antiendothelial antibodies can be sought by antibody-dependent cytotoxicity or indirect immunofluorescence. If no evidence of antibodies is found, the possibility that T-cells are the cause of the hyperacute rejection should be considered.

Rabbit antithymocyte globulin has been implicated in a rare case of hyperacute rejection: the batch reacted with activated endothelial cells; no C4d was detected in peritubular capillaries (530). In two other cases given equine antithymocyte globulin (ATGAM), acute humoral rejection occurred, with C4d deposition in peritubular capillaries (530). Perfusion of the donor kidney with third party human plasma containing donor-reactive cytotoxic antibodies is a rare cause of hyperacute rejection (531,532), which provides proof that antibody alone is sufficient to initiate this injury, even a single exposure.

### Clinical Course, Prognosis, Therapy, and Clinicopathologic Correlations

Recovery from hyperacute rejection is extraordinarily rare, but has been reported (498). In one case a follow-up biopsy at 30 days showed resolution of the glomerular thrombi and inflammation, but several glomeruli showed ischemic collapse (498). The interstitium had patchy inflammation predominately of neutrophils, which also permeated the tubules. Arteritis, vascular necrosis, and mononuclear cell tubulitis were not observed. At present there are no satisfactory treatment regimens for hyperacute rejection with any degree of success. Total graft necrosis is almost inevitable. Removal of the necrotic graft is often necessary to prevent the development of systemic toxicity.

Preventive desensitization protocols are now being tried that involve various combinations of plasmapheresis, IVIG, rituximab, and immunosuppressive drugs (533,534). Splenectomy is also added in some protocols and immunoabsorption with antigen (ABO) or protein A columns (535,536). If the titer of antibodies diminishes to low or undetectable titers, transplantation has been safely undertaken, even though antibodies were previously present

(533,537). In some patients, the antibodies return with either an episode of acute rejection or no immediate effect on graft function (accommodation). The long-term outcome of these recipients is unknown but of great interest.

## CHRONIC REJECTION AND OTHER LATE GRAFT PATHOLOGIES

### Clinical Presentation

Late graft failure develops at a rate of about 2% to 5% per year, which has changed little over the last decade despite dramatic improvements in short-term graft survival (Fig. 28.1) (134). Patients with progressive loss of renal function commonly have hypertension and proteinuria, often in the nephrotic range (538). Both alloimmune-mediated and non–immune-mediated mechanisms contribute to late graft loss (Table 28.9). Although these may be coexistent and even synergistic, the active mechanisms in a graft need to be distinguished whenever possible to choose appropriate therapy (539–541). By 10 years after transplantation, about 20% of the grafts have been lost to chronic rejection, 8% to recurrent glomerulonephritis, 4% to acute rejection, and 15% to death with a functioning graft (542). Although some have argued that the renal biopsy is not useful in analyzing graft dysfunction after 1 year, published studies show that the biopsy leads to a change in management that improved renal function in 8% to 38% of patients (61,62).

Considerable confusion reigns in the nomenclature of the pathology of late graft loss, largely related to the difficulty in diagnosis and the common occurrence of multiple diseases. Most late allograft loss is attributed to "chronic rejection" or "chronic allograft nephropathy" (CAN), which accounts for 28.32% of graft failures after the first year

(134). We recommend that "chronic rejection" be defined specifically as graft injury due to immunologic reaction to donor antigens. "Chronic" (chronos, time) does not mean inactive, as some have used the term, but rather, that the process progresses slowly (months to years) because of persistent or recurrent activity. This definition requires evidence in the biopsy for *ongoing* immunologic activity due to T-cells and/or alloantibodies, as well as evidence of tissue injury (e.g., tubular atrophy, loss of capillaries) or abnormal production of new tissue components (e.g., fibrosis, new basement membrane). Some use the term "sclerosing chronic rejection" to refer to the active and progressive nature of the lesions (543). In either case, chronic rejection should be distinguished from immunologically inactive sclerosis that is the residua of past activity. The late pathologic features generally attributed to repeated or persistent attack on graft target cells are arterial intimal fibrosis (with or without T-cells in the intima) and glomerular and/or peritubular capillary basement membrane duplication (with or without corresponding C4d deposition) (539,544). Isolated interstitial fibrosis and tubular atrophy that also has signs of immunologic activity, such as a mononuclear infiltrate or C4d deposition in peritubular capillaries, might also be considered sufficient. In the literature before 2001, these distinctions were not made. Therefore, the pathology and clinical features need to be re-evaluated with these more stringent criteria.

Few pathologic terms are misused more than CAN, which entered the medical literature in 1993 as a category in the Banff classification. CAN was intended to include "at least four entities that at present cannot always be distinguished by biopsy (chronic rejection, chronic [calcineurin inhibitor] toxicity, hypertensive vascular disease and chronic infection and/or reflux)" (79). The rationale was that "because it is often impossible to define the precise cause or causes of chronic allograft damage, the term 'chronic/sclerosing allograft nephropathy' is preferable to 'chronic rejection,' which implies allogeneic mechanisms of injury, *unless* there are specific features to incriminate such a rejection process," such as intimal fibrosis with inflammatory cells or duplication of the glomerular basement membrane (GBM) (177). CAN was not intended to replace specific diagnostic categories if these entities could be identified.

Unfortunately, CAN is often misused as a generic term for chronic renal allograft dysfunction and fibrosis or as a synonym for chronic rejection. In fact, the definition of CAN even includes pre-existing donor disease. We have said that applying CAN indiscriminately to all cases with fibrosis inhibits accurate diagnosis and understanding of pathogenetic events and obscures appropriate therapy (540). In our view, and according to the original Banff conception, CAN should be restricted to the few biopsies that are truly nonspecific in their pathology (i.e., CAN, not otherwise specified, or CAN, NOS). The 2005 Banff conference agreed

---

**TABLE 28.9**

## CAUSES OF SLOWLY DETERIORATING GRAFT FUNCTION[a]

Chronic rejection
  T-cell mediated
  Antibody mediated
Structural calcineurin inhibitor toxicity
Infection (e.g., polyomavirus)
Recurrent disease
De novo disease (e.g., diabetic nephropathy)
De novo arteriosclerosis (hypertensive vascular disease)
Renal artery stenosis
Unclassified (chronic allograft nephropathy, not otherwise specified)
Progression of donor disease (arteriosclerosis, fibrosis)

[a]Death with a functioning graft is responsible for about 22% to 25% of graft failures.

by consensus to abolish the term CAN and replace it with a term more clearly descriptive, such as "interstitial fibrosis and tubular atrophy." Here we will use "CAN" in quotes to refer to the results from studies that used this term in the absence of a more specific diagnosis.

## Pathologic Changes

### Gross Pathology

The chronically rejected kidney is pale and fibrotic with a dense, thickened, adherent capsule. The weight may be normal or increased because of previous compensatory hypertrophy. However, if the patient returns to dialysis (or receives another graft), the remaining original graft will become progressively smaller. The cortical surface is typically smooth, indicating uniform atrophy, and the cortex and medulla are proportionately affected. The thickened, obliterated arcuate and interlobar arteries can often be appreciated at the corticomedullary junction (545). The extrarenal arteries, including ureteric vessels, are also commonly affected by the rejection process and show fibrous intimal thickening up to the point of anastomosis with the recipient artery (25).

### Light Microscopy

#### Glomeruli

The morphologic definition of transplant glomerulopathy (also known as chronic allograft glomerulopathy) is widespread duplication or multilayering of the GBM with or without mesangial expansion, in the absence of specific de novo or recurrent glomerular disease (Figs. 28.51 and 28.52). Glomerular abnormalities were first recognized in long-term grafts and related to rejection by Kendrick Porter (26). The GBM is classically duplicated on PAS or silver stains, either segmentally or globally, and may have occasional mesangial cell interposition (Fig. 28.53). The GBM may also appear slightly thickened. There is often mesangial hypercellularity and increased matrix, but this is typically mild and nonspecific (546). Compensatory glomerular hypertrophy can also be sometimes appreciated. Occasionally the glomeruli will have prominent mesangial hypercellularity with a lobular pattern, which can evolve and remodel to a less cellular pattern with the duplication remaining. Signs of activity include prominent mononuclear cells in capillary loops with endothelial swelling (transplant glomerulitis; Fig. 28.52) (547). An infiltrate is sometimes found in Bowman's capsule at the origin of the tubule, which sometimes vaguely resembles a crescent (548). The juxtaglomerular apparatus is commonly prominent, even in patients not on calcineurin inhibitors (549,550).

The glomeruli can develop global or segmental sclerosis and adhesions, either as a secondary phenomenon or as a direct result of the glomerular damage. Focal adhesion of the tip of the glomerular tuft to the origin of the tubule, the so-called glomerular tip lesion, has been described (548). Atubular glomeruli (without a proximal tubular orifice) are increased in grafts with chronic rejection and may constitute most of the glomeruli present (551,552). Atubular glomeruli are about 30% reduced in volume and are hard to distinguish from glomeruli with tubules on single sections except when they form glomerular cysts with dilated Bowman's space (552).

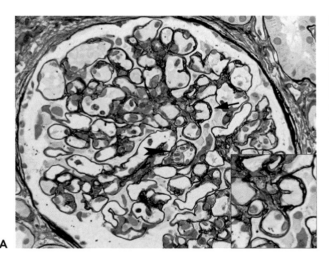
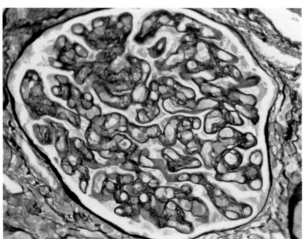

**Figure 28.51** Transplant glomerulopathy. **A:** Segmental duplication of the GBM (*arrow*, shown at higher power in the *insert*) accompanied by mild mesangial hypercellularity and intracapillary mononuclear cells and reactive endothelial cells (*arrowhead*). **B:** Widespread duplication of the GBM affecting more than 90% of the capillaries associated with positive C4d deposition (chronic humoral rejection). Capillaries are compromised by reactive endothelial cells. The mesangium is mildly increased. (**A** and **B:** periodic acid–silver, ×400.)

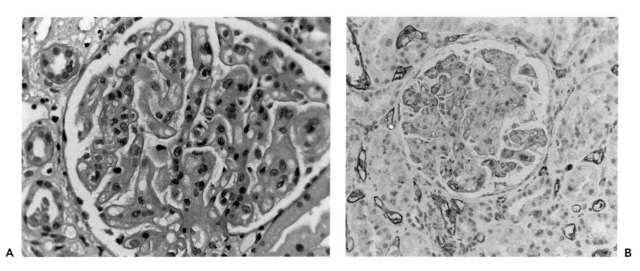

**Figure 28.52** Transplant glomerulopathy with **(A)** prominent mononuclear cells in capillary loops and duplication of the GBM and **(B)** C4d deposition in glomerular and peritubular capillaries. (**A:** PAS, ×400; **B:** C4d immunohistochemical stain on paraffin section, ×200.)

### Tubules

Tubular atrophy is found focally or diffusely and is likely to be caused by ischemia or tubulitis. Atrophic tubules typically have a few intratubular mononuclear cells and mast cells (553), which should not be confused with the tubulitis of acute rejection, because intratubular mononuclear cells are found in atrophic tubules in native kidneys. If tubulitis is found in nonatrophic tubules, this is interpreted as a manifestation of active T-cell–mediated rejection. One may occasionally find numerous lymphocytes in

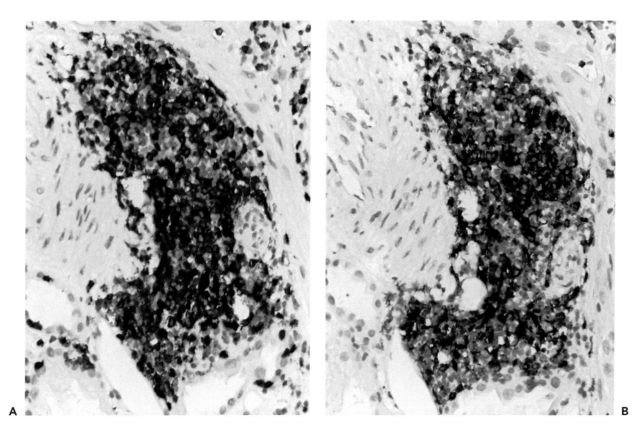

**Figure 28.53** Nodular aggregate of T- **(A)** and B- **(B)** cells in a graft with chronic humoral rejection (C4d+). Some of the small vessels may be lymphatics, as determined in other cases by Kerjaschki and thus represent a site of lymphoid neogenesis (555). Adjacent sections stained immunohistochemically for CD3 **(A)** and CD20 **(B)**.

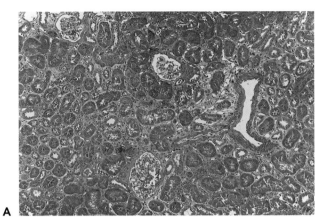

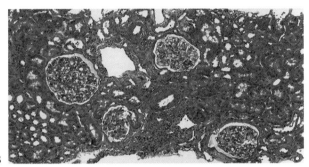

**Figure 28.54** Interstitial fibrosis patterns in late graft biopsies. **A:** Diffuse, fine interstitial fibrosis affecting all of the cortex (100%), but less than half of the cortical area that includes tubules. Some edema is also present. **B:** Focal, broad fibrosis affecting about 40% of the cortex in the field and about 40% of the cortical area. Quantitation of the two patterns differs depending on the criteria. (Trichrome, ×100.)

small damaged tubules, presumably because the lymphocytes are causing the injury. The tubular basement membranes are thickened and duplicated, a finding sometimes even in nonatrophic tubules. Sometimes tubules show pronounced shrinkage and thinning of the TBM.

## Interstitium

The interstitium typically has fibrosis in association with tubular atrophy and a variable mononuclear infiltrate,

with small lymphocytes, plasma cells, and mast cells (175,553,554). The fibrosis can have many different patterns: dense and focal, diffuse and fine, striped, or subcapsular (Fig. 28.54). The lymphocytes generally do not appear activated, and edema is not conspicuous (unless there is a component acute rejection). Lymphocytes may be present in areas with or without fibrosis. Nodular aggregates of lymphoid cells, sometimes with germinal centers, can occur around small arteries, especially at the corticomedullary junction and associated with increased lymphatic vessel density (Fig. 28.53) (555). Abundant plasma cells may also be present (Fig. 28.55) (343). Mast cells, readily detected with tryptase or c-kit antibodies, are associated with fibrosis and are often degranulated (554,556). Evidence of ongoing activity includes edema, tubulitis in nonatrophic tubules, and a mononuclear infiltrate that is extensive enough to meet criteria for T-cell–mediated rejection.

### Peritubular Capillaries

The peritubular capillaries are depleted in chronic rejection, leaving only occasional traces of the original basement membrane behind (326,557). Decreased density of peritubular capillaries correlates with the extent of interstitial fibrosis and graft dysfunction. In favorable silver- or PAS-stained sections, lamination of the basement membrane may be appreciated by light microscopy (Fig. 28.56). Peritubular capillaries may also show accumulation of mononuclear cells and apoptosis, features that probably indicate immunologic activity (557).

### Arteries

As early as 1 month after transplantation, graft arteries may develop severe intimal proliferation and luminal narrowing, sometimes accompanied by a sparse infiltrate of T-cells and macrophages (558) (Fig. 28.57 to 28.60). The intimal change is most prominent in the larger arteries, but extends from the main renal artery to the interlobular arteries, the same distribution as endarteritis in acute rejection. These arterial lesions have been termed "sclerosing

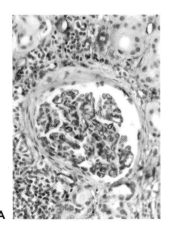

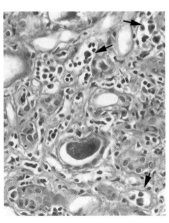

**Figure 28.55** Chronic humoral rejection with **(A)** C4d deposition and **(B)** prominent plasma cells in the infiltrate, some of which are in capillaries (*arrows*). This is a particularly florid case, and is uncommon. (**A:** C4d immunohistochemistry, ×200; **B:** H&E, ×400.)

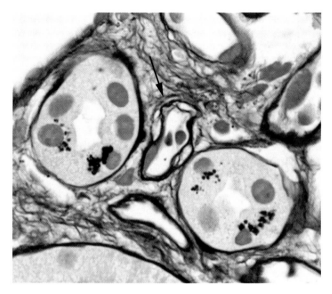

**Figure 28.56** Chronic humoral rejection with duplicated basement membrane of peritubular capillaries evident by light microscopy (*arrow*). Silver-positive protein reabsorption droplets are in the tubules. (Periodic acid–silver, ×600.)

transplant vasculopathy," "graft atherosclerosis," "accelerated atherosclerosis," "chronic allograft arteriosclerosis," "allograft vascular sclerosis," "chronic allograft arteriopathy," and "transplant arteriopathy." We prefer the last term, since the disease affects transplanted arteries (allo- or xeno-incompatible) and is noncommittal on pathogenesis.

The intima shows pronounced, concentric or less commonly eccentric, fibrous thickening without prominent elastic fiber accumulation, in contrast to the multilayering of elastica typical of hypertensive and involutive arteriosclerosis (fibroelastosis) (Fig. 28.57). The elastica interna generally remains intact. The matrix is generally loose, somewhat pale in hematoxylin and eosin–stained sections, and contains acid mucopolysaccarides, collagen, and increased hyaluronic acid (559,563). Fibrin is sometimes deposited in a bandlike subendothelial location. The cells in the intima include spindle-shaped, alpha–smooth actin-positive cells (myofibroblasts or smooth muscle cells) (Fig. 28.60). The media generally shows no obvious abnormality aside from focal loss of smooth muscle. Sometimes a double media is formed, with a concentric rudimentary

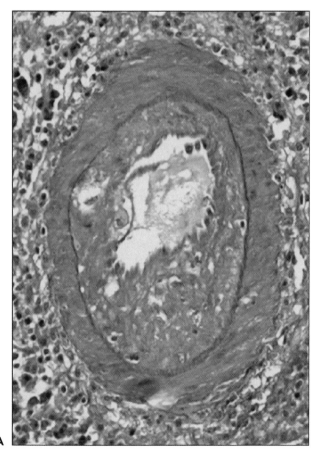

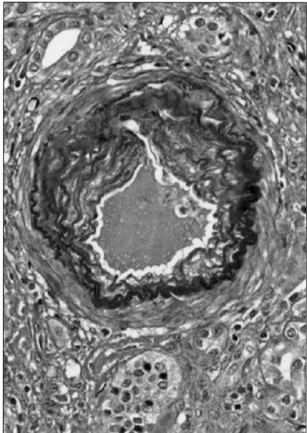

**Figure 28.57** Comparison of chronic arterial sclerosis caussed by aging/hypertension (arteriosclerosis) and chronic rejection. (transplant arteriopathy) **A:** Artery from a graft shows a neointima formation without increased elastic fibers and with a few scattered mononuclear cells. **B:** Artery from a native kidney shows neointima with marked duplication of the internal elastica (elastosis) and few or no inflammatory cells. (Elastic tissue, ×400.)

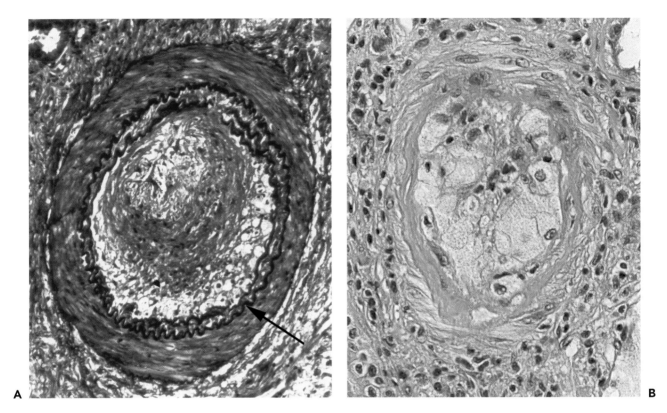

**Figure 28.58** Transplant arteriopathy with foam cells (macrophages) in the intima. **A:** Graft at 2 years shows foam cells lined up along the internal elastica (*arrow*). (Elastic, ×200.) **B:** Occlusive foam cells in intima with mononuclear cells at 2 months after transplantation. (H&E, ×400.)

neomedia containing elastic laminae and smooth muscle cells under the endothelium, inside and separated from the old artery by internal elastic lamina and poorly cellular tissue (544,560,561).

Intimal thickening in the setting of transplant arteriopathy may be inactive or show signs of ongoing activity with inflammatory cells in the intima consisting of T-cells and macrophages (Fig. 28.59) (563). The CD3+ T-cells are generally sparsely distributed in the intima (Fig. 28.59B) and sometimes focally intense immediately subjacent to the endothelium, a feature indicative of endarteritis (562). The presence of T-cells in the intima can be taken as presumptive

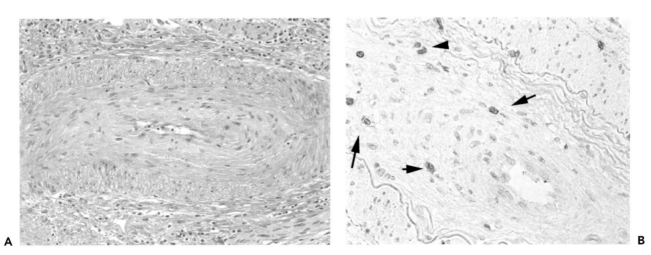

**Figure 28.59** Transplant arteriopathy. **A:** The neointima shows loose fibrous thickening with spindle cells. **B:** Same artery, showing scattered T-cells in the intima. (A: H&E, ×200; B: anti-CD3 immunohistochemistry, ×400.)

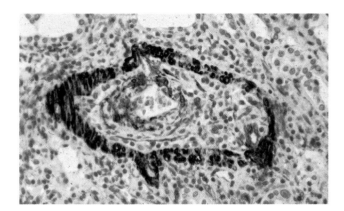

**Figure 28.60** Chronic cellular rejection of a small artery, showing prominent mononuclear cells in the intima with spindle-shaped, alpha-smooth muscle actin positive cells. Graft at 60 days posttransplant. This illustrates the continuity of acute to chronic lesions. (Alpha-smooth muscle actin immunohistochemistry, ×400.)

evidence of active T-cell–mediated rejection, analogous to endarteritis. Macrophages filled with lipid (foam cells) can be found as early as 4 weeks after transplantation and are typically deeper in the intima, applied to the inner surface of the internal elastica (Fig. 28.58). Intermediate stages between acute and chronic lesions are sometimes found, with lymphocytes admixed with fibrin and fibromuscular proliferation (Fig. 28.60). This sequence has been well documented in a nonhuman primate model of chronic rejection (563). At a later stage, the intima may show fibrosis without T-cells, a stage that is presumably inactive and irreversible.

Arterioles generally do not show intimal changes, but may have hyaline deposits. Such lesions are regarded as owing to donor disease, diabetes, hypertension, aging, or chronic calcineurin inhibitor toxicity rather than rejection. In nonhuman primates with severe chronic rejection not on immunosuppressive drugs, hyalinosis is never seen (564).

### Ureter

The donor ureter is also a target of chronic rejection (187,188). Chronic vascular lesions can affect the arteries in the ureter (187,190). Severe submucosal fibrosis and thickening and a moderate mononuclear infiltrate, even lymphoid follicles, can be present. Ureteral stenosis can result from ischemia and fibrosis (187,563,565).

## Immunofluorescence Microscopy and Immunohistochemistry

### Glomeruli

IgM is often present in the mesangium and/or along the GBM, sometimes with C3, but without features typical of any specific diagnosis in native kidneys (27,143,194, 546,566). Immunofluorescence shows few or no granular deposits of immunoglobulin IgG or IgA. With IHC tech-

niques in paraffin sections, C4d is present along the capillary walls in about 10% to 30% of cases (Figs. 28.61 and 28.62) (409,567). Extensive crescents, diffuse granular or linear deposits of IgG, or subepithelial deposits are unusual and suggest recurrent or de novo glomerulonephritis (27,30,568).

### Tubules

The tubular basement membrane in atrophic and nonatrophic tubules not uncommonly has deposition of C3 in a broad segmental pattern. This is an exaggeration of similar changes found in normal kidneys and probably represents a residue from prior episodes of tubular injury and remodeling or possibly persistent chronic injury. Linear IgG TBM deposits and associated circulating anti-TBM antibodies have been reported in the past in a few cases (3% to 10%) (569,570). Granular TBM deposits of IgG and/or C3 were demonstrated in 25% of renal transplants (570) and had a poor long-term prognosis (570). Focal granular IgG and C4d TBM deposits can occasionally be a manifestation of polyomavirus infection (571).

### Peritubular Capillaries

Peritubular capillaries have deposition of C4d in about 50% of the grafts with either transplant arteriopathy or glomerulopathy (Fig. 28.62) (348,409,567,572–574) (Table 28.10). The association is greatest for transplant glomerulopathy. The pattern is linear and circumferential, similar to that in acute humoral rejection; however, fewer positive capillaries are found; and the diffuse and widespread pattern is not so common. The reasons for the difference are not known, but may relate to decreased antigen expression, accommodation, or loss or peritubular capillaries. C4d can even be found on capillary structures with no remaining endothelial cell markers (572).

### Arteries

Immunofluorescence, often but not invariably, shows IgG, IgM, C3, and fibrin in the intima and media, as a diffuse blush or as focal granular deposits (28,194,575). It is not clear whether this is caused by specific antibody deposition, although the granular pattern favors that possibility over nonspecific trapping. C4d is also present in the intima, but does not indicate an antibody-mediated rejection, since native kidneys also have C4d in intimal fibrosis.

## Electron Microscopy

### Glomeruli

The characteristic feature of transplant glomerulopathy (chronic allograft glomerulopathy) is widespread replication of the GBM (26,194,538,576,577) (Fig. 28.63), sometimes with multiple lamina extending around the circumference of the capillary, even between the endothelium and

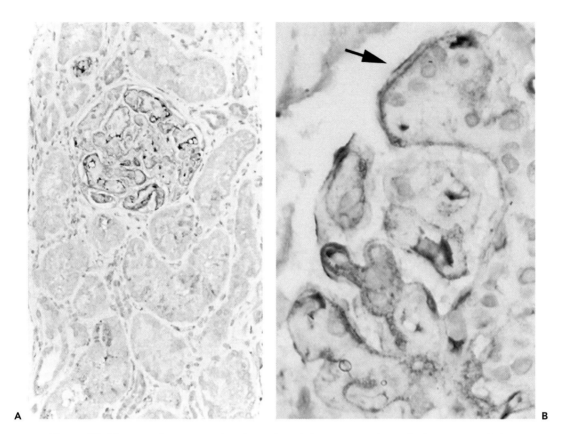

**Figure 28.61** Transplant glomerulopathy, with C4d deposition in glomerular but not peritubular capillaries (**A**) as described (567). A double contour of C4d deposition is evident in some of the glomerular capillaries (*arrow*) **B:** When only glomerular staining is present, the differential includes chronic humoral rejection and other antibody-mediated glomerular diseases (C4d immunohistochemistry, **A:** ×200; **B:** ×600.)

the mesangium, where basement membrane is normally absent (Figs. 28.64 and 28.65) (578). Electron microscopy detects 40% more cases of transplant glomerulopathy than light microscopy (579). Circumferential multilamination of GBM, when present, may be particularly characteristic

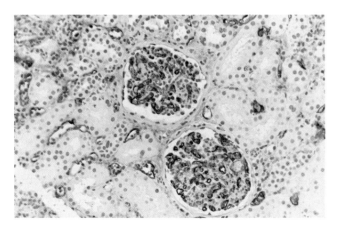

**Figure 28.62** Chronic humoral rejection with both peritubular and glomerular C4d deposition. (C4d immunohistochemistry, ×200.)

of allografts with transplant glomerulopathy, since it is not commonly found in native kidneys with other diseases that cause GBM duplication, such as TMA (578). Endothelial cell dedifferentiation is characteristically present, as manifested by a loss of the normal fenestrations (26,576,580) (Figs. 28.66 to 28.68). The other sign of endothelial damage is the ectopic location of the endothelial nuclei on the free side of the capillary loops; they are normally mainly on the mesangial side of the capillaries. The mesangial matrix is often increased, and sometimes mesangiolysis is present, manifested by dissolution of the mesangial matrix, leaving a loose reticular web (576). Mesangial cells may be interposed between the GBM layers, although this is seldom a prominent feature (Fig. 28.65). Focal effacement of foot processes is common and may be extensive (576). Moderate thickening of the GBM is seen in late allografts and is owinge to normal compensatory hypertrophy. Two reported cases were characterized by the presence of global, diffuse, subepithelial, electron-lucent deposits in addition to the usual features of transplant glomerulopathy and were associated with the nephrotic syndrome, deterioration of renal function, and eventual graft loss (581). This pattern may be a residue of old membranous glomerulonephritis;

**TABLE 28.10**

## PREVALENCE OF C4D IN CHRONIC REJECTION

| Study | N | % of Cases |
|---|---|---|
| Chronic rejection (transplant glomerulopathy and/or transplant arteriopathy)[a] | | |
| Mauiyyedi et al, Boston (572) | 38 | 61 |
| Regele et al, Vienna (409) | 58 | 67 |
| Mróz et al, Warsaw (573) | 6 | 83 |
| Vongwiwatana et al, Edmonton (574) | 24 | 25 |
| Sijpkens et al, Leiden (567) | 10 | 40 |
| Horita et al, Tokyo (615) | 9 | 100 |
| Aly et al, St. Louis (616) | 20 | 0 |
| Total | 165 | 49[b] |
| Control transplant sample (no glomerulopathy or arteripathy) | | |
| Mauiyyedi et al, Boston (572) | 30 | 3 |
| Regele et al, Vienna (409) | 155 | 22 |
| Mróz et al, Warsaw (573) | 14 | 7 |
| Vongwiwatana et al , Edmundton (574) | 19 | 0 |
| Sijpkens et al, Leiden (567) | 14 | 7 |
| Total | 232 | 16 |

[a]All cases with C4d in the biopsy with transplant glomerulopathy (CAG) and/or arteriopathy are included.
[b]P <.01 versus control group, including the study that failed to demonstrate any cases with C4d.
From Rotman S, Colins AB, Colvin RB. C4d deposition in allografts: Current concepts and interpretation. Transplant Rev 2005;19:65.

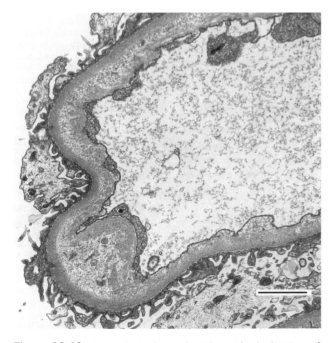

**Figure 28.63** Transplant glomerulopathy with duplication of the GBM separated by loose matrix and some cell debris. The podocytes are normal and the endothelium shows focal loss of fenestrations. (Electron micrograph; bar = 2000 nm.)

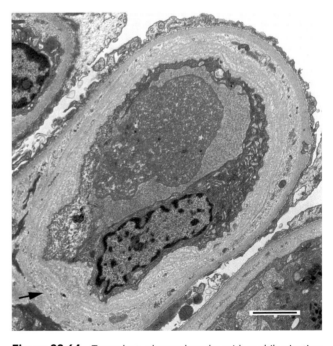

**Figure 28.64** Transplant glomerulopathy with multilamination of the GBM that extends circumferentially around the capillary lumen, including the region that normally has no basement membrane, between the endothelium and the mesangium (*arrow*) (578). The endothelium is reactive (expanded endoplasmic reticulum) and shows loss of fenestrations. Podocytes show focal loss of foot processes. Biopsy showed focal C4d positivity. Same case as Fig. 28.66. (Electron micrograph; bar = 2000 nm.)

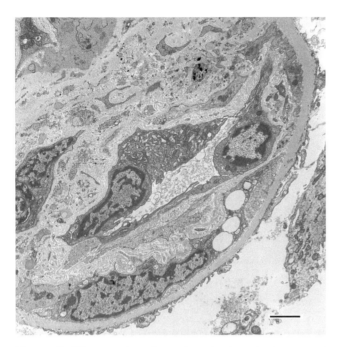

**Figure 28.65** Transplant glomerulopathy. GBM duplication and mesangial cell interposition are present, with marked endothelial cell hypertrophy and loss of fenestrations. No electron-dense deposits are evident. C4d was present focally along the GBM (not shown). (Electron micrograph; bar = 2000 nm.)

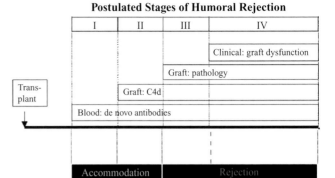

**Postulated Stages of Humoral Rejection**

| | I | II | III | IV |
|---|---|---|---|---|
| Trans-plant | | | | Clinical: graft dysfunction |
| | | | Graft: pathology | |
| | | Graft: C4d | | |
| | Blood: de novo antibodies | | | |
| | Accommodation | | Rejection | |
| | No C4d | With C4d | Subclinical | Clinical |

**Figure 28.67** Postulated stages (or states) of antibody-mediated rejection (410). The process begins with antibody production, followed by C4d fixation in the tissue (if sufficient amounts of complement-fixing antibodies are formed). These two stages have no graft pathology or dysfunction and are therefore states of accommodation to antibody rather than rejection. The third stage has pathologic lesions followed by the fourth stage when graft dysfunction becomes clinically evident. The inevitability of progression has not been proved in humans, although these stages occur in nonhuman primates without immunosuppression (564).

it also resembles the diffuse subepithelial lamination found in pediatric kidneys transplanted to adults (582).

The subendothelial space is widened and contains various rarefactions, fibrils, and deposits categorized by Olsen et al into five ultrastructural types (568). The electron-lucent subendothelial flocculent material (type 1) is

present in 74% of the routine biopsies taken at about 2 years (26). This glomerular change may be seen in the absence of other features of chronic rejection and in acute rejection (26). Similar findings may be seen in TMA, which must be considered in the differential diagnosis. Scattered granular electron-dense deposits (type 2), similar to immune complexes in other diseases, are typically subendothelial or mesangial (333,568,583). In contrast to recurrent or de novo glomerular immune complex diseases, these deposits are typically sparse. Small (type 3) and large

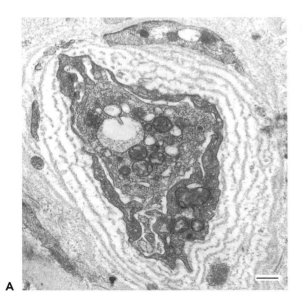

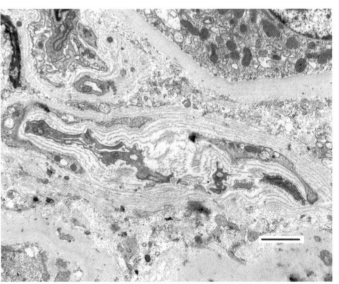

A

B

**Figure 28.66** Chronic humoral rejection. Peritubular capillaries with marked multilayering of the basement membrane. More than six layers are seen in (**A**) and (**B**): (Electron micrographs; bar = 500 nm (**A**) or 2000 nm (**B**).

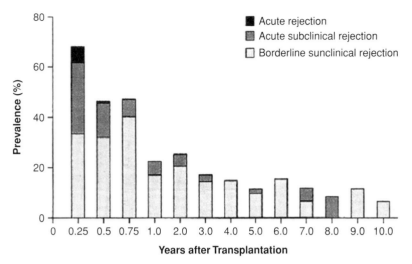

(type 4) vesicles, once thought to be viruses, are probably cell debris, as are the membranous ribbons (type 5).

Elegant scanning electron microscopy studies have shown that many glomeruli in chronic rejection lose their tubular outlet and have transformation of the parietal epithelial cells into podocytes with foot processes (551,552). Transformation to atubular glomeruli with parietal podocytes occurs in other forms of chronic renal disease, including renal artery stenosis, and is thus probably mediated by ischemic changes.

### Tubules and Interstitium

The tubular basement membrane shows pronounced thickening and lamination of the basement membrane (149,584). These changes do not correlate with the deposition of immune reactants (584).

### Peritubular Capillaries

A chronic lesion in the peritubular capillaries was noted by Monga et al (585) and Mazzucco et al (586), consisting of multilayering of the basement membrane (Fig. 28.66). Each ring probably represents the residue of one previous episode of endothelial injury going from oldest (outer) to most recent (inner). Careful quantitation of a median of 14 capillaries per case has revealed that only in chronic rejection were three or more peritubular capillaries found with five to six circumferential layers or one peritubular capillary with seven or more circumferential layers ("marked multilamination") (579). In that series, 59% of biopsies (27/46) with chronic rejection had such features and 85% were accompanied by GBM duplication. The ultrastructural changes in the glomeruli and capillaries were similar, suggesting common pathogenetic mechanisms. Peritubular capillary lamination correlates with transplant glomerulopathy (579,586), C4d deposition (409), and loss of peritubular capillaries (557). In some cases with repeat biopsies, the peritubular capillary lesions have been shown to precede the glomerular lesion. Marked multilamination was found in 50% of cases with interstitial fibrosis that lacked arterial or glomerular changes and may point to past episodes of rejection as the cause of the fibrosis (586).

### Vessels

Scanning electron microscopy shows endothelial cell injury, and disorganization with gaps between endothelial cells, often with leukocytes and platelets (587). The thickened arterial intima consists of smooth muscle cells, collagen fibrils, basement membrane material, and a loose amorphous electron-lucent ground substance (580). Scattered lymphocytes and macrophages are present, the latter sometimes filled with fine lipid droplets, corresponding to the foam cells by light microscopy. Smooth muscle cells also may contain fat droplets in lysosomes (588). The smooth muscle cells have abundant ribosomes and rough endoplasmic reticulum, displaying a secretory phenotype (589,590). With time, the cellularity diminishes and the amount of collagen increases (195,549).

### Etiology and Pathogenesis

Considerable evidence favors a central role for MHC disparity in the subset of cases of late graft injury we term chronic rejection. Glomerular and arterial lesions develop less commonly in HLA-identical sibling grafts (591–593), e.g., in none of 25 HLA-identical sibling grafts in one series (583). Similarly, in 48 HLA-identical renal transplants, 10-year graft survival was 84%; only one failed from chronic rejection (46). In more recent series, living related HLA-identical grafts were found to have no "CAN" in the first 2 to 5 years and half the frequency of "CAN" after 5 years, compared with haplo-identical living related grafts (44,45). Among 10 HLA-identical recipients, none had histologic evidence of chronic rejection in protocol biopsies at 2 years, compared with 50% of those who received cadaveric kidneys

(45). An HLA matching effect is also seen in survival of cadaver donor kidneys (Fig. 28.1). Finally, kidney allografts from mice deficient in the expression of MHC class I and II molecules have greatly reduced infiltrates and chronic damage (594).

Acute rejection episodes, particularly when multiple origins after 60 days, are implicated in the development of chronic rejection (595,596). Chronic rejection developed in 0.8% of recipients of living donor kidneys who did not have an acute rejection episode, in 20% of those with acute rejection within 60 days of transplant, and in 43% of those who had an acute rejection episode after 60 days (595). A similar progression of risk of chronic rejection after acute rejection episodes was noted in recipients of cadaveric grafts (0%, 36%, and 63%, respectively). A history of DGF and a rejection episode correlated with graft loss after 1 year; DGF in the absence of rejection had no impact (53).

Other risk factors are CsA dosage less than 5 mg/kg per day at 1 year and infection (CMV and other microbes), suggesting a contribution by inadequate immunosuppression and systemic immunologic activity (596). Other factors less consistently associated with chronic rejection are ischemia time, cadaveric source, hyperlipidemia, extreme age of donor (young or old), and history of smoking (596–598). These may contribute to the graft injury even in cases with clear evidence of chronic rejection, and separation of the different pathogenetic mechanisms may be difficult or impossible in late biopsies.

## Alloantibody and T-cells

Considerable evidence supports a role for anti-MHC antibodies in chronic graft injury (410). Circulating HLA antibodies are common in patients with functioning organ allografts. In a prospective multicenter trial of 4763 patients, HLA antibodies were detected in 21% of patients with renal allografts (385). Circulating antibodies to donor HLA antigens are highly associated with later graft loss (599–601). Donor-specific antibodies were detected in 51% of renal allograft recipients who developed graft failure, but only 2% of stable controls; these antibodies preceded graft failure in 60% (600). Circulating HLA antibodies are usually evident months to years before graft dysfunction, suggesting that antibody-mediated graft injury is muted within the graft. Even HLA antibodies not reactive to the donor correlate with late graft loss (601–603) and dysfunction (604), provided these arose de novo (the donor-specific antibodies were hypothesized to be selectively adsorbed to the graft). Among 2278 renal allograft recipients followed prospectively, graft failure per year was greater in patients who developed alloantibodies than in those who did not (8.6% versus 3.0%; $P$ <.0001) (385). The difference in graft survival 1 to 2 years later was restricted to those with intermediate graft dysfunction at the time of the antibody measurement (Creatinine [Cr] 2.0 to 3.9 mg/dL) (603). Among 1229 recipients, donor-specific antibodies were found in 5.5% and de novo non–donor-specific antibodies in 11.3% of patients monitored annually over 5 years. These had similar risk factors and clinical associations: both were associated with HLA-DR mismatch, presensitization, acute rejection episodes, increased graft loss, and proteinuria (601). Antibodies to MICA (a polymorphic class I–related antigen) are also associated with late graft failure, even in the absence of measurable HLA antibodies (414). Panel-reactive antibodies in recipients of HLA-identical grafts are also risk factor for late graft loss (605). Elution of late graft nephrectomies with "CAN" recovered antibodies to donor HLA class I or II antigens in 71%, even though only 32% had antibody detectable in the circulation (469). Elution of needle core biopsy specimens has almost as great a recovery rate of antidonor antibody (55% to 65%) (606).

The best evidence for T-cell mechanisms of chronic allograft injury in humans is that subclinical or late clinical cellular rejection is associated with progressive graft fibrosis and dysfunction (539,607,608). For example, 12% to 28% of protocol biopsies 1 year or more after transplantation have acute cellular rejection, a finding that predicted the later progression of interstitial fibrosis and tubular atrophy and graft failure (45,609,610). In studies of late protocol biopsies, concomitant acute cellular rejection with fibrosis predicts the later occurrence of chronic injury (609,611,612). Late acute cellular rejection (after 4 months) was a stronger predictor of "CAN" than rejection in the first 3 months (609). Tubulitis probably indicates ongoing activity, since about 41% of patients respond to increased immunosuppression (613). Patients who develop late graft dysfunction have an increased frequency of indirect T-cell reactivity to donor HLA peptide (604,614). Donor-specific responsiveness by direct recognition for both CD4 and CD8 cells is reduced even in those with "CAN" (614).

## Transplant Glomerulopathy

Transplant glomerulopathy is probably the result of a persistent or repeated immune response directed at the endothelium. In a few cases, repeat biopsies have shown transplant glomerulopathy to be the sequela of an episode of transplant glomerulitis (143,144,409), and this has been observed in nonhuman primates (563,564). Risk factors for transplant glomerulopathy include donor-reactive antibodies (409,572), C4d deposition (400,409,567,574,615), and a previous episode of transplant glomerulitis/acute allograft glomerulopathy (143,144,335,348,538). Overall, about 50% of the cases with transplant glomerulopathy have prominent C4d deposition in peritubular capillaries. Most patients with C4d deposition have circulating antibodies to donor HLA antigens; those without C4d did not have antidonor antibodies (88% versus 0% of controls, P <.001)(572). Others have confirmed and extended these observations. Regele (409) showed that 34% of graft biopsies taken a year or more after transplantation had C4d in peritubular capillaries. C4d was correlated with transplant glomerulopathy, duplication of the peritubular capillary basement membrane, and mononuclear cells in capillaries (transplant glomerulitis). Overall, 66% of the cases with transplant glomerulopathy had C4d deposition. Most important, C4d was found to precede and predict development of the glomerulopathy, arguing that complement fixation in the graft vasculature is related to the pathogenesis and not just an epiphenomenon. Sijpkens et al at Leiden University (567) showed that glomerulopathy could occur with glomerular C4d+ in the absence of peritubular C4d deposition (Fig. 28.61A). Among six reports comprising 388 patients, 49% of those with transplant glomerulopathy or arteriopathy had C4d deposition versus 16% of grafts without these lesions (409,567,572–574,615,616) (Table 28.10). One study failed to demonstrate C4d in any of 20 cases of glomerulopathy, although 2 of 34 cases of "CAN" without glomerulopathy were C4d+ (616). Presumably this difference reflects the frequencies of other causes of glomerulopathy (such as calcineurin inhibitor induced glomerulopathy, TMA or T-cell–mediated injury; see Table 28.15). T-cells and macrophages may also contribute to the pathogenesis, because mononuclear glomerulitis is commonly present. T-cell and macrophage numbers decrease as the sclerosis advances (547,617). Intraglomerular leukocytes stain for ICOS and CXCR3, expressed on activated effector T-cells, and CXCR3 ligands Mig and IP-10 (618).

Cells in glomeruli produce matrix-promoting growth factors, such as acidic fibroblast growth factor (FGF-1) and transforming growth factor (TGFβ). FGF receptors are detected in mesangial and epithelial cells in chronic rejection but not in normal glomeruli. The receptors diminish in more advanced lesions. Antibodies to MHC class I molecules increase expression of FGF-1 receptors on cultured endothelial cells (619). Glomeruli accumulate FGF-1 protein in the nuclei of visceral and parietal epithelial cells and mesangial cells, although FGF-1 mRNA is restricted to leukocytes in glomeruli (617). No mRNA for FGF-1 was detectable in normal human kidneys or in glomerular scarring diseases other than transplants. The mesangium can show increased α-smooth muscle actin, a finding that may predict a worse prognosis (331) and is associated with cell proliferation (PCNA+) (620) and vascular endothelial growth factor (VEGF) production (289). Enhanced PDGF B-type receptor expression is also associated with mesangial proliferation (621). TGFβ1 synthesis is increased in glomeruli isolated from protocol biopsies with fibrosis (622). Nonclassic and non-HLA antigens may also be targets of antibodies. Circulating autoantibodies to agrin, the principal heparan sulfate proteoglycan of the GBM, have

been found in 44% of patients with transplant glomerulopathy (623).

In transplant glomerulopathy, tenascin and the EDA isoform of fibronectin increase in the mesangium (624). The GBM contains granular deposits of tenascin and fibronectin (625), which are associated with GBM duplication, proteinuria, and progressive azotemia (626). Transglutaminase, which cross-links proteins via gamma glutamyl-lysine bonds, is increased in the mesangium (627). Increased cortical synthesis of the α3 chain of type IV collagen, presumably from the glomerulus, has been detected (628).

Loss of endothelial cell fenestrations may relate to insufficient production of VEGF by the podocyte or resistance to its action (629,630). Podocytes, which normally express VEGF, show increased amounts in 41% of patients with "CAN" (289), possibly a reaction to ischemia. Increased glomerular ecto-AMPase activity and a decrease in ecto-ATPase activity have been demonstrated in glomeruli, a response typical of ischemia (631). Loss of endothelial fenestrations should markedly restrict bulk water flow through capillary wall and decrease filtration.

A major secondary pathogenetic mechanism in chronic glomerular damage that has been postulated is hyperfiltration injury (55). Kidneys from young children transplanted to adults do less well that those from other adults. Proteinuria of more than 0.8 g per day is more common at 2 years in adult recipients of kidneys from children younger than 6 years of age than in those who received adult kidneys (50% versus 12%, respectively) (632). Florid focal sclerosis has developed in some of these (633). Studies in rats support the role of hyperfiltration injury, which can be reduced by transplanting two kidneys (634). However, these lesions do not typically show the GBM duplication and can be distinguished from transplant glomerulopathy.

## Transplant Arteriopathy

The pathogenesis of chronic arterial lesions in allografts has been investigated in animal studies quite actively in recent years, and there is now convincing evidence that the process is primarily immunologically mediated (563,564,635). The vast experimental data can be summarized as follows: (a) the lesions do not routinely arise in isografts; (b) the lesions develop in the absence of hypertension or hyperlipidemia, (c) the target antigens can be either major or minor histocompatibility antigens; (d) three separate, but not mutually exclusive, pathways have been identified: T-cells, antibody, and NK cells; (e) the target cell is probably the endothelium; and (f) IFNγ is a key mediator of neointimal proliferation (636). Ultimately the process becomes independent of specific antidonor immunologic activity (637). In mice, antibodies are sufficient to cause arteriopathy without participation of T-cells. Immunodeficient *scid* or RAG1⁻/⁻ mice given repeated doses of anti-class I alloantibodies develop fibrous intimal thickening of coronary arteries in cardiac allografts over 1 to 2 months (638) and C4d deposition in the capillaries (Uehara et al, unpublished data). Pure T-cell–immune reactivity is also sufficient to mediate transplant arteriopathy, e.g., in male to female grafts (639), or in B–cell–deficient recipients. In nonhuman primates, a transition from endarteritis to fibroproliferative intimal thickening has been described, in the absence of C4d deposition during early vascular remodeling, supporting the hypothesis that T-cell reactivity is sufficient to evoke these lesions (563).

Specific risk factors for transplant arteriopathy in humans are episodes of endarteritis (370) and donor-reactive alloantibodies (28,640). Other risk factors for de novo intimal fibrosis are histoincompatibility and hypercholesterolemia (641). Association of HLA antibodies with transplant arteriopathy is more variable than with transplant glomerulopathy, perhaps because of the difficulty in distinguishing rejection from arteriosclerosis and to alternative cellular mechanisms of chronic arterial injury. The mechanisms probably involve stimulation of growth factors by antibody and/or complement and infiltrating macrophages. Complement components and antibody alone can stimulate growth of endothelial cells in culture. C5b-9 (MAC) elicits signals for endothelial cell proliferation, as shown by the release of growth factors, including PDGF and bFGF (642). Antibodies to MHC class I molecules promote endothelial proliferation (643) and expression of FGF-1 receptors and also promote phosphorylation Src (644). Anti-HLA class I antibodies cause up-regulation of the GTP-binding protein RhoA, associated with translocation to the cell membrane, F-actin stress fiber formation, and reorganization of the cytoskeleton (645). Proliferation induced by anti-HLA antibodies is inhibited by simvastatin or C3 exoenzyme, which inhibit RhoA (645). T-cells can also promote proliferation of vascular cells; for example, T-cell supernatants from patients with chronic rejection enhance the proliferative effects of PDGF on cultured smooth muscle cells (646).

A mononuclear infiltrate of T-cells (CD4+, CD8+, CD45RO+) and macrophages (CD68+) is generally present in the intima (562,563,647). B-cells (CD20) are not generally detected (563,647). Attraction of the mononuclear cells to the endothelium is expected to be promoted by the increased adhesion molecules, ICAM-1 and VCAM-1 (648). The T-cells express cytotoxic markers, including perforin (649), and GMP-17 (159), and the chemokine receptor CXCR4 (650). Apoptosis of endothelial cells has been described in allografts and is believed to be an important mechanism of chronic vascular injury (651–653). Deficiency of either perforin or granzyme B inhibits development of chronic arterial lesions in mice (654,655). Blocking Fas ligand pathway of apoptosis with soluble Fas inhibits graft neointimal formation in aortic grafts in rats (287). T-cells and macrophages are accompanied by myofibroblasts that increase in number over time (563). The macrophage, with its broad repertoire of cytokines, degradative enzymes, and cell interaction, is a likely central participant (284). Macrophages are prominent in animal models (656–658). Chronic rejection of kidney allografts in rats is regarded as predominantly a macrophage-dependent event with intense intra-graft up-regulation of macrophage products such as MCP-1, IL-6, and iNOS; RANTES synthesis precedes the macrophage infiltration (659). Proliferation of mononuclear cells, spindle cells, and endothelium is evident with PCNA or MIB-1 stains (563,647).

In humans and nonhuman primates, the intima of affected arteries shows accumulation of myofibroblasts. The myofibroblast cells stain prominently for α-smooth muscle actin, which is a marker of the normal contractile phenotype of adult smooth muscle cells (590,656,660–662). These cells are most numerous close to the elastica interna (563). Many spindle-shaped cells that contribute to the intimal thickening are of recipient origin (663,664), more than 40% in one study using X/Y FISH (fluorescence in situ hybridization) (665). The intimal cells also express β-actin, which is a marker of the synthetic phenotype not expressed in normal adult medial myocytes (589). In support of the synthetic phenotype, electron microscopy reveals that the intimal cells have abundant ribosomes and rough endoplasmic reticulum (589,590). The α-smooth muscle actin positive cells in the neointima are relatively resistant to apoptosis, perhaps because of up-regulation of Bcl-xL; blocking Bcl-xL inhibits neointimal formation in murine allografts (666,667). Endothelin-1 peptide (668) and iNOS (668) is increased in the neointima, localized to smooth muscle cells.

Myofibroblasts are the primary source of the extracellular matrix in the intima, which consists of collagen, fibronectin, tenascin, proteoglycans, and acid mucopolysaccarides (563,624,669). Early on fibronectin and collagen IV predominate; as the lesions advance, fibrillar collagen I and III accumulate in the intimal zones rich in myofibroblasts (563). Collagen deposition progresses from the outer zone to the inner (luminal) zone (563) The fibronectin has the extra domain of cellular fibronectin (EDA), typical of embryonic or wound-healing fibronectin (624). Proteoglycan protein synthesis (biglycan and decorin mRNA) has also been detected in the arterial intima (669). A proteolytic fragment of perlecan, a proteoglycan synthesized by endothelial cells, inhibits apoptosis in smooth muscle cells (670). Plasminogen activator inhibitor 1 (PAI-1) protein and mRNA are expressed by endothelial cells of arterioles and arteries in chronic rejection but not in normal kidneys (291,671). Protease-activated receptor-1, which binds thrombin, is present in endothelium in association with fibrin deposits (671).

Several cytokines believed to be important in the pathogenesis of the fibrosis are synthesized in the intima, including FGF-1, PDGF-A, and PDGF-B (325,617). PDGF A chain protein is synthesized by endothelial cells, whereas the B chain is in macrophages and smooth muscle cells (325). Intimal cells and smooth muscle cells express PDGF B-type and FGF-1 receptors (617,621). Increased synthesis and expression of SPARC (secreted protein acidic and rich in cysteine) was evident in the neointima (672). SPARC is an endogenous inhibitor of proliferation that binds to PDGF and stimulates TGFβ production. TNFα and TGFβ1 are also increased in the arteries (273,673). One of the cytokines that can promote transplant arteriopathy is IFNγ (636). Antibodies to IFNγ inhibit the lesions in coronary arteries in mice (674). Antagonists to endothelial adhesion molecules, up-regulated during rejection, such as ICAM-1 and LFA-1, and antagonists of VLA-4 (α4β1 integrin) also inhibit development of the lesions in mice (675,676).

Nonimmunologic factors likely contribute to vascular injury, as they do in native kidneys. Intimal lipid accumulation in foam cells (macrophages) is a prominent, although not ubiquitous, component of transplant arteriopathy. Apolipoproteins A1, A2, and B1 accumulate, mostly extracellularly (677). Recurrent deposition of mural fibrin-platelet thrombi on the subendothelium exposed by endothelial loss with subsequent organization should promote progression of allograft arteriopathy, analogous to atherosclerosis (678). Ischemia may also promote intimal fibrosis: prolonged ischemia increased the severity of the chronic vascular lesions in rats (679), and DGF is one of the predictors of intimal fibrosis at 3 months (370).

## Chronic Tubulointerstitial Rejection

Chronic tubulointerstitial rejection is characterized by patchy fibrosis, tubular atrophy, and a scanty mononuclear infiltrate. These nonspecific findings may follow almost any significant injury to the kidney. However, in the setting of an allograft and in the absence of any indicators of specific cause, grafts with fibrosis and tubular atrophy behave as chronic rejection. The risk factors for interstitial fibrosis and tubular atrophy (excluding calcineurin inhibitor toxicity or recurrent disease) are immunologic (HLA match, acute rejection episodes de novo after 3 months, and pretransplant panel-reactive antibodies), whether or not arteriopathy is present (680,681). Polyomavirus nephritis can lead to similar pathology. Late acute rejection episodes (after 3 months posttransplantation) were found to be the strongest risk factor for interstitial fibrosis with or without arteriopathy. Prior biopsies with breaks in the TBM were associated with an increased risk of tubular atrophy (381). A history of rejection, calcineurin inhibitory toxicity, or CMV infection were the leading predictors of fibrosis and tubular atrophy in protocol biopsies at 2 years (683).

T-cells in the infiltrate in late-rejecting grafts express the CXCR4 cytokine receptor (650). Other receptors (CCR1,

CCR2, CCR5) and chemokines (CCL2 and CCL5) are expressed in lower amounts than in acute rejection (241). Macrophages contain VEGF and TNFα (289,684).

The interstitium shows increased α-smooth muscle actin+ cells (presumably myofibroblasts), which correlate with type III collagen accumulation (331) and interstitial fibrosis (685). PDGF B-type receptors are on myofibroblasts in the proximity of clusters of infiltrating macrophages and T lymphocytes (621). Increased TGFβ expression in grafts has been associated with interstitial fibrosis (686–688). Extracellular, but not intracellular, TGFβ1 reactivity in 100-day protocol biopsies correlated with increased fibrosis at 3 years and loss of graft function (689). Types I and III collagen both increase (690,691). TGFβ and collagen I and III synthesis in 6- and 12-month protocol biopsies were indistinguishable in cyclosporine- and tacrolimus-treated recipients (692). Tissue transglutaminase is also increased and correlates with fibrosis (627). Angiotensin II receptor protein and mRNA are increased in "CAN" (693), and antagonists such as losartan inhibit expression of TGFβ and the progress of fibrosis (694). One must also consider that some forms of TGFβ are inactive or are precursors and can be rendered inactive by antagonists that bind it, such as decorin (695).

Apoptosis increases in proximal and distal tubules in kidney allografts with chronic rejection, compared with native kidneys in liver transplant recipients (a control for drug effects); no increased apoptosis was detected in the glomeruli or interstitium (682). Loss of specialized tubular cell functions, molecular atrophy, can be detected as a loss of the normal aquaporin-2 expression in collecting ducts (696). Proximal tubules express the protease-activated receptor-1 for thrombin, which causes increased tubular cell TGFβ production in vitro (671).

Experimental models have provided evidence that the tubular epithelium can emigrate from the tubule and become fibroblasts in the interstitium, a process termed *epithelial to mesenchyme transition* (EMT) (697). In rodent kidney allografts with chronic rejection, there is increased synthesis of α-smooth muscle actin and decreased E-cadherin accompanying production of types I and III collagen along with superoxide anion (698). CsA promotes EMT of human renal tubular cells in culture, which involves increased production of TGFβ and protein kinase C pathways (699). Evidence for EMT in allografts includes de novo expression of S1004A in tubular cells; S1004A is a molecule related to cell migration, which can be induced by TGFβ (315). However, the interstitial fibroblasts are predominately of recipient origin, as judged by X/Y FISH (665), arguing against substantial derivation from tubular epithelium.

Senescence in the donor kidney may contribute to an ineffective reparative response and enhance the consequences of ischemia, rejection, or drug toxicity. Conversely, repair of injury may accelerate the aging process by requiring cell replication (700). Cellular senescence, as judged by FISH telomere length or senescence-associated beta-galactosidase, correlates with the severity of chronic allograft damage and donor age but not with prior acute rejection, ATN, or recipient age (701,702). Other markers than can be applied in biopsies to identify senescence are the cyclin-dependent kinase inhibitors p21 (WAF1/CIP1) (701), p16$^{INK4A}$, (703) and p27 (704). p16$^{INK4A}$ was present in tubular nuclei and cytoplasm in amounts greater than predicted by age in grafts with interstitial fibrosis and tubular atrophy and dysfunction; both normal and atrophic tubules were positive (703,704). Grafts with normal function had no increase in p16$^{INK4A}$. Grafts with "CAN" had a calculated biologic age about 15 years older than their chronologic age (704). These data support the hypothesis that graft injury leads to accelerated senescence (700) and that senescence markers may have some prognostic significance.

The lymphatic vessel content of the cortex shows a 50-fold increase in some grafts with chronic rejection (555). The molecules LYVE-1 and podoplanin are expressed by lymphatic but not blood vessel endothelial cells. Neolymphatics were distributed around the periphery of nodular aggregates of T-cells, B-cells, dendritic cells, and macrophages. The lymphoid cells showed evidence of proliferation (Ki67) and macrophages produced VEGF-C (a growth factor for lymphatic endothelium). Lymphatic neoangiogenesis may be involved in the maintenance of a potentially detrimental alloreactive immune response in the graft. Of note the new lymphatic endothelium derives in part from circulating recipient progenitor cells, as judged by XY FISH (705).

Peritubular capillary endothelium is a target of chonic rejection (326,557,586), often mediated by antibodies (409). The endothelium responds by repeated synthesis of basement membrane, analogous to the response of other basement membrane–producing cells. Loss of PTC is found with or without evidence of currently active T-cell or antibody-mediated injury and may be a sequela of prior episodes of acute or subacute rejection (557). Loss of peritubular capillaries correlates with fibrosis, graft dysfunction, and proteinuria (presumably because the glomerular capillaries are also affected) (557). Loss of peritubular capillaries has the potential to create ischemic damage to the tubules, and indeed, tubular atrophy is associated with C4d in peritubular capillaries (409).

## Classification of Chronic Rejection

By definition, as used in this chapter, *chronic rejection* refers to graft injury mediated by immunologic reaction to donor antigens, either by T-cells or antibodies. Either or both of these may be active in the graft, and certain aspects suggest one or the other of the pathogenetic mechanisms. Since these processes occur over a long period of time, probably

as episodic, subclinical events, the chance of catching the active process in any given biopsy (especially those late in the course) may be small.

### Chronic Antibody-Mediated Rejection

A consensus meeting at the NIH proposed draft criteria for chronic antibody-mediated rejection (chronic humoral rejection [CHR]) (392), and the 2005 Banff conference. As in acute antibody-mediated rejection, three elements should be present (Table 28.11): histologic evidence of chronic injury, immunopathologic evidence of antibody action (e.g., C4d), and evidence of antibody reactive to the donor in the circulation. C4d is a marker of current antibody activity, since it is present only transiently, lasting for 1 to 3 weeks after deposition (153,348). CHR is distinct from AHR in that no acute inflammation (neutrophils, edema, necrosis, thrombosis) is present. The reason why some cases with donor-specific antibodies elicit AHR and some lead to CHR is not clear. We have postulated that partial accommodation accounts for the difference, as well as other factors such as titer, avidity, and effector functions (706).

We proposed that chronic humoral rejection arises through a series of stages or states as diagrammed in Figure 28.67. The serologic and pathologic evidence is most consistent with the hypothesis that the first common event typically (but not always) is alloantibody production, then antibody interaction with alloantigens resulting in the deposition of C4d in peritubular capillaries and possibly glomeruli, followed by pathologic changes and graft dysfunction only later. In our series, 21% (3 of 14) of the late alloantibody-positive patients lack C4d in the biopsy (707). Others have shown that C4d deposition occurs before transplant glomerulopathy (409). We have observed this sequence in nonhuman primates with

---

**TABLE 28.11**

**DIAGNOSTIC CRITERIA FOR CHRONIC ACTIVE ANTIBODY MEDIATED REJECTION (CHR)$^a$**

1. Histologic evidence of chronic injury: need two of four
     Arterial intimal fibrosis without elastosis
     Duplication of glomerular basement membrane
     Multilaminated PTC basement membrane$^b$
     Interstitial fibrosis with tubular atrophy
2. Evidence for Ab action/deposition in tissue (e.g., C4d in PTC)
3. Serologic evidence of anti-HLA or other antidonor antibody

$^a$All three major criteria required (392). These parallel those used in the Banff schema for acute antibody-mediated rejection and have been incorporated into the Banff classification (Solez et al, submitted). The presence or absence of graft dysfunction determines whether rejection is clinical or subclinical, as in other forms of rejection.
$^b$Criteria of Ivanyí are recommended (three or more capillaries with five to six layers or one capillary with seven or more layers (see text).

renal allografts that develop donor-reactive antibodies (564). Further studies should identify the significance and appropriate therapy for each of these stages.

## Chronic T-Cell–Mediated Rejection (539)

The criteria used for acute T-cell–mediated rejection (tubulitis, interstitial infiltrate, intimal inflammation) can be used to define an active T-cell component in rejection that also has the histologic features of persistent injury and sclerosis (563). As in CHR, one would require chronic structural change (the same ones as for CHR) and the presence of T-cells in sites of chronic damage, i.e., the arterial intima, glomeruli, tubules, and interstitium. A third criterion, demonstrable T-cell reactivity to donor, cannot be required at present, because tests for antidonor T-cell reactivity are not readily available (in contrast to antidonor antibody assays). Molecular markers are expected to aid in the detection of T-cell activity in the graft.

## Scoring Systems for Chronic Lesions

Chronic lesions are scored subjectively for diagnostic purposes. The Banff system uses four grades of cortical fibrosis, vascular intimal fibrosis, tubular atrophy, and GBM duplication (Table 28.12). The reproducibility of Banff chronic scores is not high (kappa scores of 0.195 to 0.375). Reproducibility improved substantially for intimal fibrosis and hyalinosis when photomicrographs were used, indicating

that the problem for these parameters was identifying the lesion in the glass slides. The reproducibility of interstitial fibrosis did not improve with practice or by supplying photomicrographs (88), indicating that there is a problem with the definition. A small group of pathologists who had worked together had better kappas (0.53 to 0.65) evaluating protocol biopsies for interstitial fibrosis, but transplant glomerulopathy scoring was still not reproducible (358). Sampling problems must also be considered. It has been estimated that 25% of biopsies are overscored or underscored for fibrosis by sampling, based on the observation that 12% of protocol biopsies show a decrease in fibrosis on subsequent sampling, even when seven or more glomeruli are in the sample (708).

### Morphometry

For clinical research and trials, various techniques have been used to obtain more precise quantitation. Most morphometry studies have focused on interstitial fibrosis, which is amenable to morphometry and may be less subject to sampling error than vascular lesions. The markers used for fibrosis include antibodies to collagen (I or III [709]) and special stains (Masson/Mallory trichrome [710] and Sirius/picosirius red [711,712]). Digital images and computerized data analysis are used to calculate cortical interstitial volume fraction ($V_{IF}$). Errors owing to interpretation (but not sampling) can be minimized by using morphometric analysis, although selection of the threshold for positive

## TABLE 28.12

### BANFF SCORING CATEGORIES FOR CHRONIC CHANGES

| | | | | |
|---|---|---|---|---|
| **Interstitial fibrosis** | ci0 | ci1 | ci2 | ci3 |
| % of cortex | ≤5% | 6%–25% | 26%–50% | >50% |
| **Tubular atrophy** | ct0 | ct1 | ct2 | ct3 |
| % of cortex | 0 | ≤25% | 26%–50% | >50% |
| **Allograft glomerulopathy** | cg0 | cg1 | cg2 | cg3 |
| % of peripheral capillaries with double contours[a] | <10% | 10%–25% | 26%–50% | >50% |
| **Mesangial matrix increase[b]** | mm0 | mm1 | mm2 | mm3 |
| % of glomeruli | 0 | <25% | 26%–50% | >50% |
| **Arterial fibrointimal thickening[c]** | cv0 | cv1 | cv2 | cv3 |
| % narrowing of luminal area most severely affected artery | 0 | ≤25% | 26%–50% | >50% |
| **Arteriolar hyalinosis[d]** | ah0 | ah1 | ah2 | ah3 |
| Number of arterioles with hyaline | 0 | 1 | >1 | ≥1 |
| | | Noncircumferential | Noncircumferential | Circumferential |

[a]In most severely affected glomerulus.
[b]Defined as mesangial increase that exceeds two mesangial cells in width between two adjacent capillaries in at least two glomerular lobules.
[c]Note if lesions characteristic of chronic rejection are present (inflammatory cells in intima, formation of neointima without elastosis, foam cells, or breaks in the internal elastica).
[d]Based on the system of Mihatsch, which was found to be more reproducible than the original Banff (mild, moderate, severe) (see Table 28.14). Peripheral nodules should be noted by an asterisk.

staining (segmentation) is itself subjective (713). Since interobserver segmentation thresholds vary, a computer program has been developed that sets the segments automatically for Sirius red staining of interstitial and mesangial areas (713).

Some examples show the power of morphometry. $V_{IF}$ in 6-month protocol biopsies, quantitated with Sirius red-stained protocol biopsies, was highly correlated with time to graft failure (711); similar data were found for $V_{IF}$ measured by IHC for collagen III (709). Measurement of $V_{IF}$ in 12-month biopsies using picrosirius red demonstrated increased fibrosis in patients on cyclosporin (versus tacrolimus) (714). In children, a picrosirius red $V_{IF}$ greater than 10% predicted a decline in GFR at 2 years (712). Sirius red can be used with or without polarization: in one study, nonpolarized measurements correlated better with GFR (715).

The definition of percent fibrosis might be either the percentage of the cortex that has increased fibrosis of any degree (the usual interpretation of pathologists), or an estimate of the percentage of the cortical area that is the fibrotic tissue itself (as with point counting in morphometry), with or without excluding glomeruli and large vessels or subtracting the normal amount of fibrous tissue (Fig. 28.54). For example, the amount of fibrous tissue in normal kidneys by point counting is 26% of cortical volume, which the pathologist would score as "0% fibrosis" (716). Alternatively, the area of fibrosis could be related to the number of glomeruli in the sample, which would serve to mark the area of the original cortex (like surgical clips). Curiously, in a study of 1-year protocol biopsies, the subjective scores of fibrosis were superior to Sirius red morphometry in predicting serum creatinine at 8 to 10 years or late graft loss (717). Perhaps the pathologists took into account features missed by the computer algorithm.

### Combined Scores

Some propose combining the scores for multiple pathologic features to assess the degree of chronic renal damage. For example, the Chronic Allograft Damage Index (CADI) is the arithmetic sum of the six scores for interstitial fibrosis, tubular atrophy, glomerular mesangial expansion, intimal fibrosis, interstitial infiltrates, and glomerulosclerosis (all 0 to 3). CADI scores correlate with graft loss at 3 years (718); the extent of interstitial fibrosis at 6 months was the most predictive of graft loss by multivariate analysis (718). Previous acute cellular rejection predicted elevated CADI at 3 years, and the latter predicted inferior graft function at 5 years. Other combined scores have been used. A chronic graft damage score at 6 months, calculated from the degree of vascular intimal hyperplasia, glomerular mesangial changes, focal lymphocytic infiltration, focal and diffuse interstitial fibrosis, and tubular atrophy, also was strongly associated with graft loss 2 to 3 years after transplantation (719). The Banff Chronic Sum (calculated

as the sum of cg, ci, ct, and cv) was not correlated with morphometric analysis of Sirius red staining, but did correlate with graft failure (711). When predictive variables are combined arithmetically to give a single score, as in the CADI or the Banff "CAN" grade, the individual predictors should ideally be independent and strongly correlated to outcome, while providing some unique contribution to the assessment of the score (720). These markers need to be validated in long-term follow-up to see if changes in the scores correlate with changes in the late outcome.

### Differential Diagnosis

The diagnosis of late graft damage first requires evaluation of whether an active alloimmune process is responsible. Among the established measures of immunologic activity are those related to injury mediated by T-cells (tubulitis, interstitial inflammation, infiltration of arterial intima, and glomeruitis) and antibody (C4d deposition in PTC). Molecular markers should enhance detection of ongoing activity and determine which signaling pathways are most appropriate for therapeutic intervention.

### Glomerulopathy

GBM duplication per se is not specific for chronic graft rejection. Other diseases with similar light and electron microscopic glomerular features also are characterized by endothelial injury (e.g., thrombotic microangiopathy, calcineurin inhibitor toxicity, scleroderma, eclampsia). Whether these conditions can be reliably distinguished has not been proved. One feature found primarily in transplant glomerulopathy is multilamination of the GBM that extends around the entire circumference of the capillary, even between the endothelium and the mesangium, where basement membrane is normally absent (578). This circumferential, multilayered pattern resembles that in the peritubular capillary and was not a feature in native kidneys with other causes of GBM duplication (e.g., TMA, systemic lupus erythematosus [SLE], membranoproliferative glomerulonephritis [MPGN] type I). Most of the cases also have transplant arteriopathy. About half have C4d deposition in peritubular capillaries, which is a strong argument in favor of an alloimmune mechanism versus TMA or calcineurin inhibitor toxicity. Mononuclear glomerulitis is also a common finding in allograft glomerulopathy and is associated with C4d in peritubular capillaries or glomeruli and circulating donor-specific antibodies (348,547). Cases with no C4d represent a diagnostic dilemma. Some may be caused by chronic TMA. Other cases may be the sequelae of antibody-mediated glomerular damage that is currently inactive or T-cell–mediated glomerulitis.

If immune complex deposits are more than occasional, or if in a subepithelial location, recurrent or de novo glomerulonephritis should be suspected. Recurrent MPGN type I typically has prominent mesangial hypercellularity, subendothelial electron-dense deposits, and C3 staining greater than that of IgM, in contrast to transplant glomerulopathy (721). Mesangial hypercellularity associated with IgM and C3 in the absence of GBM duplication has been observed, but is not necessarily related to rejection and may be associated with viral infections (546,566).

Recurrent glomerular disease causes late allograft failure in 8.4% of patients by 10 years (542) and is fully discussed below. The frequency and clinical significance of recurrence varies with the disease. Recurrent glomerular disease is usually recognizable by the same features that permitted the original diagnosis. Membranous glomerulonephritis and focal segmental glomerulosclerosis not uncommonly arise de novo in allografts, but typically appear later than the recurrent forms of these diseases (more than 1 year). De novo focal segmental sclerosis may arise in grafts, probably a manifestion of chronic calcineurin inhibitor toxity (722). The collapsing variant is commonly in association with severe microvascular disease, such as arteriolar hyalinosis (723–725).

Complicating the interpretation may be superimposed hyperfiltration injury, which can be suspected if segmental glomerulosclerosis and/or hypertrophied glomeruli are prominent. Grafts from young pediatric donors to adults can develop diffuse GBM lamellation, probably owing to hyperfiltration injury. However, in this instance, the lamination is subepithelial rather than subendothelial and has a scalloped pattern (582).

## Arteriopathy

Arterial lesions are a cardinal feature of chronic rejection (726), but are often confused with donor or de novo arteriosclerosis. In the first 6 months after transplantation, 44% of the cases originally considered to be chronic rejection were changed on review of all available clinical data, most often to donor arteriosclerosis (558). Findings that we regard as specific for rejection (versus hypertensive, aging, and diabetic changes) are a mononuclear infiltrate in the intima or media, intimal thickening with a lack of accumulation of elastic lamellae, and intimal foam cells against the internal elastica. Radiation therapy can produce a similar foam cell distribution in small arteries. Marked elastic fiber accumulation (fibroelastosis) and a thickened media are features of hypertension (580). In some cases transplant arteriopathy is superimposed on arteriosclerosis; special stains (elastin) can help identify this process. TMA may have a few mononuclear cells in the active phase, and in the healing phase may leave intimal fibrosis that resembles chronic rejection. TMA, however, predominately affects smaller arteries and arterioles, in contrast to rejection. Chronic calcineurin inhibitor toxicity also primarily affects the arterioles.

## Interstitial Fibrosis and Tubular Atrophy

The differential diagnosis of tubular atrophy and interstitial fibrosis is wide and includes chronic rejection, calcineurin inhibitor toxicity, polyoma virus infection, prior ischemia, donor disease, chronic obstruction, and renal artery stenosis. Donor disease is most definitively recognized by implantation biopsies or other biopsies early in the course.

The most useful marker of chronic tubulointerstitial rejection is the multilamination of peritubular capillary basement membranes. Unfortunately, this must be assessed by electron microscopy, and quantitation is necessary to distinguish rejection from other causes. The use of electron microscopy to detect peritubular capillary lamination can reduce the fraction of nonspecific CAN, NOS cases to about 15% (545).

The best evidence for chronic calcineurin inhibitor toxicity in allograft biopsies is the characteristic peripheral nodular hyaline deposition in the periphery of arterioles. Chronic rejection is favored by numerous plasma cells (727). Other features, such as intratubular calcification and striped fibrosis, are of dubious differential diagnostic significance. For example, striped fibrosis was found in 60% of biopsies from patients not on calcineurin inhibitors and 80% of cases of advanced diabetic nephropathy (728). Molecular discriminators that have been proposed to discriminate calcineurin inhibitor toxicity from rejection are laminin β2, TGFβ1 (628), and types I and III collagen (690,691).

Polyomavirus nephropathy (PVN) leads to late interstitial fibrosis and tubular atrophy (disease stage C; Table 28.17). The diagnosis of PVN can be confirmed by detecting intranuclear inclusion bodies and a typical immunohistochemical staining profile (see below) (729).

The features of chronic obstruction include dilated collecting ducts, ruptured tubules with leakage of PAS+ Tamm-Horsfall protein into the interstitium with associated mild inflammation, and dilated lymphatics. Interstitial fibrosis and tubular atrophy with a modest mononuclear infiltrate is common. GBM duplication and neointima formation are not features of chronic obstruction. In most cases, the diagnosis of obstruction cannot be made by biopsy, but requires imaging techniques. Renal artery stenosis can produce severe tubular atrophy, but usually this is not accompanied by marked interstitial fibrosis, small unscarred glomeruli, and no interstitial infiltrate.

## Chronic Allograft Nephropathy, Not Otherwise Specified (CAN, NOS)

Unfortunately, a significant minority of biopsies taken for late graft dysfunction cannot be assigned to a specific diagnosis. In one study, 37% had nonspecific tubulointerstitial fibrosis and tubular atrophy (572); higher frequencies of nonspecific findings have been reported (544,545). This residual group is rightfully defined as "CAN, NOS" until further specific pathologic or pathogenetic features are identified.

## Clinical Course, Prognosis, Therapy, and Clinicopathologic Correlations

Over the last two decades, late graft loss has modestly improved. Of those who survive 1 year, the 4-year graft survival has risen from 80% to 90% (133). In patients with late graft dysfunction, the decline in GFR is gradual, estimated to be 0.5 mL/min/month, similar to other chronic renal diseases (543,733), leading to graft failure in 3 to 4 years (375). Approximately 90% have diastolic hypertension, which is associated with a more rapid loss of renal function (733).

Transplant glomerulopathy develops in 2% to 7% of grafts in adults and children (567,580,734,735). Transplant glomerulopathy is uncommon in the first 6 months (none in 48 biopsies with chronic rejection) (558), but is found in 5% to 13% of protocol biopsies at 1 year (538,736) and 40% of protocol biopsies at 5 years (737). The median time of diagnosis is about 8 years (567). Transplant glomerulopathy is almost always associated with transplant arteriopathy (538), but cases do occur without vascular disease; these may be due to causes other than rejection, such as calcineurin inhibitor toxicity (680).

Transplant glomerulopathy has a poor prognosis. Duplication of the GBM of at least 10% of the capillary loops of the most affected glomerulus (Banff g1 to 3) correlates with a decline in GFR more than the percentage of sclerosed glomeruli (737). Among those in whom subclinical transplant glomerulopathy was detected in a 1-year protocol biopsy, the 3-year graft survival was 85%, worse than in those with normal biopsies or only interstitial fibrosis (612,736). In a third study, glomerulopathy increased the risk of graft loss twofold (546). Patients with transplant glomerulopathy commonly have proteinuria, often in nephrotic range (738). However, glomerulopathy also can be found in biopsies in the absence of proteinuria (25% of cases) (538). Proteinuria itself is associated with decreased graft survival in proportion to its severity (739,740). In patients treated with CsA, the rate of graft loss in the presence of 1 g per day of proteinuria is 25% in the first year and 62% by 5 years (735). Proteinuria owing to recurrent or de novo glomerulonephritis has a better prognosis (17% graft loss in 5 years).

Transplant arteriopathy is uncommon in the first 6 months after transplantation, documented in biopsies in only 2.4% of 1117 grafts (558), but increases to 36% to 41% in protocol biopsies at 1 to 2 years (612,741). Occasionally chronic arteriopathy can be seen as early as 1 month posttransplant (558). The prognostic significance of arteriopathy is variable. In one series, the actuarial survival of grafts with transplant arteriopathy was only 35% (558).

When found in protocol biopsies at 3 months, arterial intimal fibrosis affected long-term survival more than interstitial fibrosis (742). However, a recent large series showed no prognostic effect of arteriopathy in 1-year biopsies separate from interstitial fibrosis, inflammation, or glomerulopathy, a finding the authors attributed to reduced severity of arteriopathy in current drug regimens (612).

Interstitial fibrosis develops over the first year and can remain stable (607). Two recent studies have shown an adverse outcome associated with fibrosis when inflammation is present. Patients with fibrosis at 1 year (ci of 1 or more) had a 5-year survival of 90%, compared with 100% for those with no fibrosis. Those who also had interstitial inflammation had a 60% 5-year graft survival (736). In another study, 10-year graft survival went from 90% to 62% if the patients with "CAN" in protocol biopsies at 1 year also had evidence of acute rejection (609).

Treatment of chronic graft damage depends first on accurate diagnosis. Cases with a component of inflammation (T-cell–mediated rejection) or C4d may respond to increased immunosuppression. The question is whether new therapies can be identified that selectively target processes critical for the pathogenesis of the vascular or glomerular lesions. Prevention of chronic rejection will require sufficient immunosuppression to prevent acute rejection (even subclinical), but with low enough levels to avoid toxicity. Among the promising results are the substitution of mycophenolate mofetil for azathioprine, which reduced the number of patients with CAN at 1 year from 71% to 46% (743). Elimination of calcineurin inhibitors after 3 months was associated with a reduction of "CAN" at 1 year from 70 to 41%, with no increase in subclinical rejection (744). Conversion from cyclosporine to azathioprine at 3 months also led to a fourfold reduced risk of "CAN" at 1 year (745). Ultimately, if reliable methods for tolerance induction are discovered, the chronic vascular and glomerular lesions should be preventable to the extent that they are mediated by responses to alloantigen.

## PROTOCOL BIOPSIES, SURROGATE END POINTS, ACCOMMODATION, AND TOLERANCE

### Protocol Biopsies

Protocol (surveillance) biopsies are taken at predetermined times, in contrast to the usual biopsies taken to diagnose graft dysfunction (indication biopsies). Protocol biopsies can be done safely and have become a common component of multicenter clinical trials. Many centers now routinely perform protocol biopsies, although their ultimate role is debated (746–748). Protocol biopsy studies have shown repeatedly that considerable graft pathology can be present before graft dysfunction is clinically evident and that inflammation in the graft generally portends a worse prognosis. Protocol biopsies thus have the potential to improve clinical care by prompting early interventional therapy (including either an increase or a decrease of immunosuppression). They also are valuable to elucidate pathogenetic mechanisms before the pathologic features become nonspecific or inactive.

## Subclinical Rejection

Protocol biopsies have demonstrated that a mononuclear interstitial infiltrate and tubulitis can be present in stable patients (252,749). When the biopsy findings meet the pathologic criteria for acute rejection in a patient with normal graft function, the term *subclinical rejection* is used. In the first 1 to 6 months, an average of 12% to 17% of patients have subclinical rejection and 21% to 22% have borderline/suspicious inflammation (607,608,736,750–756), which declines thereafter (Table 28.13; Fig. 28.68). However, there is wide variation among studies, probably related to differences in immunosuppression, HLA match, sensitization, and donor organ type. Among 190 patients, acute rejection was detected as often in protocol biopsies (17%) as in biopsies taken for graft dysfunction (13%) (753). Subclinical or clinical acute rejection was a predictor of "CAN" at 12 months. In another study of 120 recipients on CsA and azathioprine, subclinical rejection by Banff criteria was common, detected in about 25% at 1 to 2 years and in 5% to 10% thereafter (607). Among a group of patients treated with either tacrolimus or cyclosporine, the prevalence of acute rejection in 2-year protocol biopsies was 8.9% and 9.2%, respectively (683).

Subclinical acute cellular rejection is a risk factor for progression, arguing that immunologic rejection is a major pathogenetic factor. Among 128 grafts at 2 years, 30% had diffuse inflammation, which correlated with later development of reduced function (741). Similarly, patients who had the least infiltrate in sequential protocol biopsies from 1 to 12 months posttransplant had the best graft function at 12 months (749). In patients with "CAN" in protocol biopsies at 1 year, 50% had subclinical acute rejection; these patients had a worse graft survival at 5 years than those with "CAN" without subclinical acute rejection. These findings were confirmed by a study of 292 recipients with 12-month surveillance biopsies: subsequent graft survival was predicted by fibrosis with inflammation. These data argue that more than a minimal infiltrate in a long-term graft is pathologic.

Protocol biopsies in the first 1 to 2 weeks have revealed acute rejection in 5 to 25% and borderline/suspicious inflammation in 9 to 38% (Table 28.13). Focal interstitial infiltrates, TBM rupture, peritubular macrophages, and C4d each increased the risk of a clinical rejection episode by at least twofold (458,757). Those with subclinical acute rejection at 2 weeks had lower graft survival at 1 to 10 years (736). Suspicious findings did not affect graft survival. Acute rejection was more common in patients with delayed graft function than in those with initial function (18% vs 4%), a strong argument for biopsies in this setting (751).

Protocol biopsies help identify early events mediated by antibodies, including those that lead to accommodation. In a large European multicenter study with 551 protocol biopsies, 4.4% had peritubular capillary deposits of C4d (456). C4d was associated with retransplants and inflammation in peritubular and glomerular capillaries, similar to the C4d associations in indication biopsies. However, C4d deposition had no significant impact on allograft

---

**TABLE 28.13**

**FREQUENCY OF SUBCLINICAL ACUTE REJECTION AND BORDERLINE/SUSPICIOUS INFLAMMATION IN PROTOCOL BIOPSIES IN STABLE PATIENTS BY TIME AFTER TRANSPLANTATION**

| Center | Ref | 1–2 Weeks | | | 4–6 Weeks | | | 3 Months | | | 6 Months | | |
|---|---|---|---|---|---|---|---|---|---|---|---|---|---|
| | | N | AR | B/S | N | AR | B/S | N | AR | B/S | N | AR | B/S |
| Seoul, Korea | 736 | 304 | 13% | 38% | | | | | | | | | |
| Pittsburgh, PA | 750 | 28 | 25% | 21% | | | | | | | | | |
| Oxford, UK | 752 | 76 | 13% | 12% | | | | | | | | | |
| Leicester, UK | 754 | 92 | 5% | 9% | 79 | 8% | 16% | 78 | 1% | 10% | 61 | 0% | 5% |
| Hanover, Germany | 753 | | | | 190 | 13% | 24% | 190 | 11% | 22% | 190 | 10% | 21% |
| Winnipeg, Canada | 608 | | | | 35 | 43% | 11% | 33 | 27% | 21% | 34 | 15% | 29% |
| Westmead, Australia | 607 | | | | | | | 138 | 42% | 33% | 87 | 15% | 31% |
| Barcelona, Spain | 756 | | | | | | | 98 | 4% | 23% | | | |
| **Total/Average** | | **500** | **12%** | **28%** | **304** | **15%** | **21%** | **537** | **17%** | **23%** | **311** | **12%**[a] | **25%** |

N, number of biopsies (patients); AR, acute cellular rejection (Banff criteria; C4d not usually reported); B/S, borderline or suspicious findings (Banff criteria).

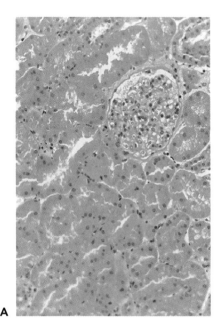

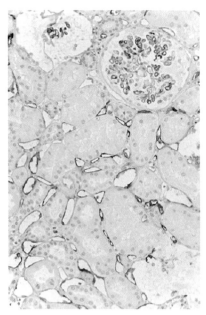

**Figure 28.69** Protocol biopsy with normal graft histology (**A**), but with prominent accumulation of C4d in peritubular and glomerular capillaries (corresponding to stage II in Fig. 28.69). (**A:** H&E; **B:** C4d immunohistochemistry, ×200.)

survival during the time of observation (about 1 year). Histologically, normal protocol biopsies may show C4d deposition (Fig. 28.69). Further follow-up and correlations with circulating antibody will be needed to interpret the clinical significance of incidental C4d deposition. At least we can conclude that incidental C4d deposition does not portend acute humoral rejection and probably represents accommodation. Whether that accommodation is stable or not, and how to ascertain the stability, remains to be determined.

In stable grafts, endarteritis is found rarely (0.3% in one series) (456) and fibrinoid necrosis never (252,758). In one instance, endarteritis was present in a protocol biopsy and the patient developed rejection 3 days later (758). We have seen only two cases in which endarteritis was present on a biopsy with no clinical evidence of rejection at the time of biopsy or later.

## Other Subclinical Diseases

Protocol biopsies at 3 and 12 months have revealed subclinical polyomavirus infection in about 1.2% of recipients (759). These patients had an outcome better than those with polyomavirus first diagnosed with graft dysfunction. Subclinical calcineurin inhibitor toxicity, as manifested by arteriolar hyalinosis, is typically found at 3 years and beyond, reaching 100% of recipients at 7 to 10 years; other features that may be related to calcineurin inhibitor toxicity, striped fibrosis and tubular microcalcification, were found in 88% and 79%, respectively (607,760). Acute, reversible calcineurin inhibitor toxicity (tubulopathy) was found usually in the first 6 months (760). In protocol biopsies at 2 years, chronic (structural) calcineurin in-

hibitor toxicity was found in 24% of patients on tacrolimus and 17% of patients on cyclosporine (683). In a group of 60 tacrolimus-treated recipients, 7% of the protocol biopsies at 1 to 12 months showed unsuspected acute calcineurin inhibitor toxicity and 12% showed acute or borderline rejection, leading to change in therapy in 10% (761).

Nephrocalcinosis is a predictor of later "CAN" (73,762). Intratubular calcium oxalate crystals were found in 52% of biopsies in the first 3 months and were associated with prior acute tubular injury, graft dysfunction, and decreased 10-year graft survival (50% versus 74%) (763). Tubular calcification was progressively more common in protocol biopsies taken from 6 weeks (6%) to 6 months (18%) and was correlated with higher serum parathormone and calcium levels, rather than rejection, acute tubular injury, or calcineurin inhibitor toxicity. Tubular calcification with high parathormone levels predicted inferior graft function 1 year after transplantation (762).

Finally, protocol biopsies can also reveal the normal physiologic response of a transplanted organ, independent of rejection. For example, increased glomerular size can be appreciated with light microscopic morphometry. At 4 months posttransplant, glomerular volume increased 39% from the donor biopsy ($4.1 + 1.4 \times 10^6 \mu m^3$) in histologically normal grafts; those with "CAN" at 4 months had glomeruli that had decreased in mean volume by 7% (764).

## Surrogate End Points

Protocol biopsies have also been used to predict outcome, with the potential benefit of shortening the follow-up time needed to evaluate efficacy in drug trials (720,765). For clinical trials, quantitative pathology generally provides useful data for correlations. Candidates for an early surrogate marker of long-term graft survival rely on protocol biopsies at a time relatively close to transplant (i.e., 3 to 6 months). Among the documented predictors of graft loss at 2 to 10 years are arterial intimal fibrosis and interstitial fibrosis, detected on biopsy at 3 to 6 months posttransplant (718,742,755,766) and CADI scores at 1 year (718). One example of this approach is the finding that patients who had early withdrawal of steroids had increased interstitial fibrosis at 12 months (761).

Molecular studies are also starting to be applied to protocol biopsies. Recipients at 2 to 3 years with high CD3γ chain mRNA by real time reverse transcriptase PCR (RT-PCR) in the biopsy had more proteinuria and a higher serum creatinine 2 years later (767). Increased bFGF, decreased TGFβ1, and increased cytokeratin 15 mRNA at 6 months correlated with later development of interstitial fibrosis (CAN) at 12 months (768).

It should be emphasized that the outcome of a graft is not predetermined by early events alone, but is also influenced by subsequent events that are not always predictable, such as noncompliance, drug toxicity, infections, and recurrent or de novo diseases (720). Routine biopsies at late intervals (6 months, 12 months, and 2 years) are recommended in investigative therapeutic trials, since the pathologic lesions may be silent and the risk of protocol biopsies is minimal (70,73).

## Accommodation, Acceptance, and Tolerance

Acute rejection episodes become less frequent with time, for largely unknown reasons. Graft acceptance probably involves events in the graft and changes in the immune response.

### Events in the Graft

It has been hypothesized that events in the graft are critical to the development of tolerance. Not all infiltrates in the graft lead to graft injury, and some may actually promote acceptance. Individual patients can have biopsies that meet the histologic criteria for rejection, yet remain stable for 6 months even without increased immunosuppression (769). Grafts in animals that are developing tolerance typically have graft infiltrates, which we have termed the *acceptance reaction.* (770). In certain class I disparate murine and pig renal allografts, the intense infiltrate spontaneously disappears and is followed by indefinite graft survival (771,772). Graft biopsies reveal a T-cell and macrophage infiltrate with tubulitis. However, the acceptance infiltrate differed from that in rejecting grafts in certain features, including less infiltration by CD3+ T-cells and macrophages, less T-cell activation (CD25, PCNA), absent endarteritis, and less apoptosis of graft cells. Long-lasting apoptosis of graft-infiltrating T-cells occurred, which may have contributed to the limitation of the immune response. The grafts also expressed less IFNγ and more IL-10 than rejecting grafts (772). Acceptance reactions associated with donor-specific transfusions in rats had mRNA levels for cytotoxic proteins similar to that in rejection reactions (773), suggesting that cytotoxic cells were present but blocked in their effects. Treg cells (identified by the transcription factor Foxp3) were more numerous in mice undergoing certain forms of tolerance induction (costimulatory blockage with anti-CD40L) (272). Foxp3+ cells have also been observed in human grafts with acute cellular rejection in the tubules and in aggregates (271). Although the significance of foxp3+ cells has yet to be determined, it is likely that high numbers of such Treg cells are beneficial, in view of the known suppressor functions of these cells.

Under some conditions, tubular cells can induce specific anergy. Cultured human tubular cells stimulated with IFNγ and TNFα increase the expression of MHC class I and II antigens, LFA-3 and ICAM-1, and have enhanced binding of mononuclear cells. The tubular cells fail to stimulate mitogenesis in normal lymphocytes, and subsequently their proliferative response to donor antigens (but not third party) is inhibited (774). Tubular cells also produce an inhibitor of the cytotoxic protein granzyme B in clinical and especially subclinical rejection (267).

### Accommodation

*Accommodation* is defined as an acquired state in which an organ resists the assault of humoral or cellular rejection (775). For example, grafts from recipients with donor-reactive alloantibodies are considered to show complete accommodation if they show no pathologic changes, such as interstitial fibrosis, glomerulopathy, or arteriopathy. At a cellular level, accommodation may occur via multiple mechanisms, including internalization, down-regulation, inactivation or inhibition of the target antigen. Binding of human natural antibodies to porcine endothelial cells triggers the induction of inducible nitric oxide synthase (iNOS), Bcl-2, and Bcl-xl, which in turn confer resistance to apoptosis (776). Accommodation may also be induced by immunosuppressive regimens, notably after intravenous gamma-globulin (IVIG) in pig to primate xenografts (777). In a small study of pig to baboon renal xenografts, lack of histologic injury was associated with C4d deposition in the absence of C5b or MAC, both of which were present in rejecting grafts (778), suggesting truncation of complement activation was a feature of accommodation. Expression of complement regulatory proteins, CD59 and CD55, is increased in some cases of chronic rejection (706). Microarray gene expression analysis of stable ABO-incompatible renal allografts showed differences in signaling pathways and cytokines but no detectable increase in mRNA for the antiapoptotic molecules (779).

Peritubular capillary C4d deposition has been detected in ABO-incompatible, pathology-free grafts (456) and in several HLA-incompatible grafts (456) (Fig. 28.69). The questions in these cases are whether C4d deposition is a harbinger of chronic rejection or a manifestation of accommodation and how to tell the difference. We advocate no specific treatment in this setting but heightened vigilance, since C4d deposition is an indicator of an active immune response and, in our experience, is a precursor to chronic rejection (564). Stable accommodation has not been documented for HLA antigens, only noncarbohydrate antigens (ABO in humans and the xenoantigen, alpha-[1-3]-galactose in animals). Multicenter studies combining protocol biopsies with serologic monitoring should yield critical information on the significance of either circulating antibody or C4d deposition in stable recipients and lead to clinical trials of early intervention.

## Endothelial Repopulation

One of the proposed mechanisms for accommodation is the replacement of donor endothelium by recipient cells. This has been documented in human organ allografts, but recipient endothelial repopulation is neither common nor predictable. In human renal allografts, 8% had detectable, focal recipient endothelium, as judged by the development of Barr bodies in male to female kidney transplants (780). The Barr body technique is limited, because not all sections are in the right plane and the interpretation is difficult. As judged by the expression of ABO blood group antigens, 23% had partial endothelial replacement (781). The ABO antigen is also not an ideal marker, since the carbohydrate epitopes might be converted on the cell by enzymes supplied by the recipient.

Studies of long-standing renal grafts (26 to 29 years) showed only donor endothelium of vessels, as judged by immunohistochemistry for donor HLA class I antigens in four cases and Y-chromosome in situ hybridization in two cases (782). Only one case had evidence of recipient class I+cells, apparently lining glomerular capillaries and in the mesangium. Studies using XY FISH techniques in 26 sex-mismatched renal allografts showed a strong correlation between the percentage of recipient endothelial cells in the peritubular capillaries and type II rejection; grafts without a history of rejection had only sporadic recipient endothelial cells (783). These data suggest that endothelium damaged by vascular rejection is repaired by circulating cells from the recipient. Low levels of tubular epithelial chimerism (2% to 7%) have been detected by XY FISH or laser capture/short tandem repeat analysis in 88% of patients (784). Lymphatic endothlelial chimerism also can be detected by FISH in long-standing grafts (705). Chimerism in tubules had no correlation to outcome or graft morphology. The main pitfall of the FISH technique is that infiltrating leuko-cytes need to be excluded (by combining FISH with a cell lineage marker).

## Immunologic Alterations

Patients with well-functioning kidneys have decreased precursor cytotoxic T-lymphocyte frequencies in the blood at 3 months posttransplant compared with pretransplant values. This decrease is donor specific and is permanent in a few patients (785). Reversible acute rejection was associated with a marked increase in antidonor precursor cytotoxic T lymphocytes, returning to pretransplant levels. Chronic rejection was also associated with a transient increase in donor-reactive cytotoxic cells. Others have found the loss of donor-specific cytotoxic T-cell precursors in the first 3 months, but this did not correlate with the presence or absence of rejection; neither did antidonor proliferative responses (MLR) (786). The data argue that the establishment of a state of functional clonal inactivation facilitates allograft acceptance, but that reliable detection of such a state is difficult by current techniques. Antidonor antibody may also have paradoxically beneficial effects. In mice, non-complement fixing antibodies to the donor are associated with acceptance of the graft (787). Humans with accepted grafts show late increases of antidonor antibody of the IgG4 subclass (non-complement fixing) (433).

Starzl (788) drew attention to the presence of rare donor-derived cells in the circulation and recipient tissue and proposed that this might be a mechanism of graft acceptance. Peripheral blood microchimerism was found in 7 of 33 kidney allograft recipients 12 to 18 months posttransplant; the frequency of donor cells averaged about 1 in 75,000, but did not correlate with lack of rejection (789). Whether microchimerism (typically detected by PCR) is a cause or an effect of graft acceptance has been debated (790,791). The argument against a causal effect is that the microchimerism disappears shortly after the graft is removed. This is different from mixed chimerism induced by bone marrow transplantation, in which the tolerance is lifelong (792). In any case, the presence of microchimerism may be a useful diagnostic marker of graft acceptance.

## Clinical Tolerance Induction

Specific immunologic tolerance can be defined as acceptance of a histo-incompatible graft without immunosuppressive agents, while retaining full immunologic competence for other antigens. Although this can be done predictably in rodents, it has been achieved only sporadically in patients (793,794). In patients the term *operational tolerance* is preferred, because proof of tolerance by rechallenge with donor and third party grafts cannot be done. A great need is an assay that will predict a state of operational tolerance, to guide immunosuppressive reduction.

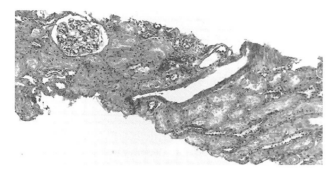

**Figure 28.70** Protocol biopsy from an operationally tolerant patient induced by the mixed chimerism protocol (18). Biopsy taken 18 months after transplantation, with more than 1 year off all immunosuppression. Blood vessels, glomeruli, interstitium, and tubules are normal. There was no interstitial infiltrate. (H&E, ×100.)

A few protocols are currently undergoing clinical development and testing. The most promising at the time of writing is induction of mixed chimerism, using bone marrow cells from the kidney donor and nonmyeloablative treatment that spares the recipient marrow (394,795–797). Stable, fully chimeric recipients of bone marrow transplants have successfully been transplanted years later with kidneys from the same donor without immunosuppression (798) or the converse (794). In most mixed-chimerism protocols, short-term immunosuppression is given at the time of transplantation (cyclosporine, anti–T-cell antibody, cyclophosphamide). In HLA-identical recipients who had end-stage renal failure owing to myeloma cast nephropathy, the approach has shown promise, with six patients off immunosuppression with functioning grafts at up to 7 years (795). In HLA haplo-identical living donor recipients, long-term graft survival has been achieved off immunosuppression in three of four patients (Fig. 28.70) (Kawai et al, unpublished). This approach is being refined in nonhuman primates (799), with the expectation that a combination of costimulatory blockade and other measures might make this approach work, even after an organ has been transplanted under conventional immunosuppression.

## QUANTITATIVE GENE EXPRESSION AND MICROARRAYS

Gene expression analyses of whole graft biopsies, blood, and urine have provided insights into pathogenesis and have potential for diagnosis. These assays offer certain advantages over morphology, including better efficacy for early warning of rejection and response to therapy, objective quantitation, identification of drug targets, and less invasiveness. However, morphology has the edge in sensitivity and specificity of diagnosis, detection of irreversible injury, site of tissue injury, cost, and speed. Each has some advantage in detecting activity of rejection and will have a

significant role in the management of the transplant patient and clinical investigation. Their combination may be the most powerful strategy using specific molecular probes and anatomic localization. Unfortunately, a common missing element from most molecular studies is a systematic pathologic analysis to correlate with the elegant molecular results.

### Graft

Among the more specific and sensitive measures of rejection by PCR are the transcripts for proteins of cytotoxic T lymphocytes (CTLs): granzyme B, perforin, and Fas ligand (800–806). T-bet, a master transcription factor for CTLs, is also elevated in acute rejection (804). Fas ligand, but not perforin or granzyme B, has been associated with therapy-resistant rejection in a small series (806,807). In mice, elevated graft CTL-associated transcripts (CATs) precede tubulitis and remain elevated as the graft develops irreversible necrosis (808). In humans, treatment of rejection is followed by a measurable decrease of CATs in grafts (803).

IFNγ mRNA is detectable in fine-needle aspirate samples taken 1 week before the clinical onset of rejection, consistent with the view that IFNγ is synthesized early in rejection (809) and often distinguishes acute rejection from controls (277,800,809,810). IL-2 mRNA has not proved as useful for diagnosis (800,810,811). Of 72 immune-related genes, the cytokines and chemokines associated with acute rejection were IFNγ, TNFβ, TNFα, RANTES, and MIP-1α (804). No elevation of TGFβ or IL-10 was detected. Complement components are also locally produced, such as C3 and C1q (277,804,812). To date no transcripts yet distinguish type I and type II rejection and none have been found for antibody-mediated rejection (161).

Comprehensive microarrays have great potential to discover novel mechanisms and targets. Sarwal et al (161) at Stanford provided a systematic screening of genes expressed in rejecting grafts. In addition to confirming much of the prior PCR studies for CATs, they also found a signature associated with subsequent graft failure. Interestingly, this turned out to be B-cell transcripts. The investigators translated the molecular test into a simple measurement of B-cells by immunohistochemistry. Microarray studies have also revealed that several members of the family of genes induced by IFNγ are regularly and highly expressed in acute rejection (812,813) and various matrix proteins in chronic rejection (161). Different results have been reported in small microarray series (e.g., no CATs), probably related to the problem of the very small ratio of samples to parameters (812). It will take many samples, sophisticated data analysis, and considerable collaborative effort to define robust transcription patterns from the myriad of idiosyncratic results, influenced by timing, patient population, comparison control groups, and therapy.

Subclinical rejection has gene expression profiles similar to clinically evident acute rejection, which argues that the process is indeed rejection (814). Many of the same potentially injurious molecules are elevated perforin, granzyme B, IFNγ, TNFβ, and TNFα as well as the chemokines, RANTES, and MIP-1α and the costimulatory molecules CD154 (CD40L) and inducible costimulator molecule (ICOS) (804,814,815). The only up-regulated genes that distinguished clinical from subclinical rejection in one study were T-bet, Fas ligand, and CD152 (CTLA4) (804).

In late biopsies, increased TGFβ but not IL-2, IFNγ, IL-4, IL-10, granzyme B, or perforin, correlates with concurrent fibrosis (687,805). TGFβ and laminin β2 mRNA are higher in chronic cyclosporine toxicity than in chronic rejection. In patients with late acute rejection, RT-PCR detected up-regulation of IFNγ, IL-2, IL-4, IL-10, and TNFα transcripts, rather than granzyme B (816). The synthesis of the heat shock protein HDJ-2, as well as Hsp60, is elevated in chronic rejection; neither is detected in normal kidneys (817). The mRNA species that predict later graft loss include CD3γ (767); increased FGF-1, type 1 angiotensin II receptor (818); and cytokeratin 15; and decreased TGFβ1 (768). The last finding fits with the observation that high TGFβ1 in acute rejection predicts later lack of chronic rejection (perhaps related to induction of Treg cells) (628). Evidence for a viral component of late graft dysfunction (e.g., CMV, EBV, human herpesvirus [HHV-6, HHV-7], polyomavirus) can also be revealed by PCR analysis (819).

## Urine

Urine provides a potentially unique, noninvasive window on the graft, especially for those molecules involved in tubular injury. Remarkably, urine mRNA can be retrieved in sufficient quantities for analysis, as pioneered by Suthanthiran (805). Among the mRNA species detected in the urine and correlated with acute rejection are the inhibitor of granzyme B, serine protease inhibitor-9 (PI-9) (820), IP-10 and CXCR3 (821), CD103 (822), granzyme B (823), and granulysin (824). To date, these have good sensitivity and can rise before clinical evidence of rejection. With sufficient specificity (greater than 95%), these will have potential as screening tests. Certain transcripts, such as Foxp3, are predictive of a response to therapy (825).

## Blood

Increased expression of CATs (granzyme B, perforin, fas ligand) (826–828), IL-18 (829), IL-5 and IL-13 (830), HLA-DR (827), CD40L on CD4 cells (831), and decreased IL-10 (830) can be detected in the blood and correlate with those in the graft (828). Elevated CD40L on CD4 cells (831) and Fas ligand (832) are also reported in chronic graft dysfunction. In some cases, elevation in the blood precedes clinically evident rejection by 1 to 2 weeks and is reduced by therapy (826,830) (829). Increased IL-18 (a molecule that up-regulates perforin) also can be detected (829). The sensitivity and specificity varies from around 80% to 90% to 90% to100% depending on whether a single test is used or several are combined, and these tests are still at the research stage.

### Genetic Polymorphisms

Many of the cytokines, chemokines, and their receptors have DNA sequence polymorphisms. These are beginning to be examined to see if they have significant clinical or pathologic effects on the rejection process or response to therapy. For the most part, these studies have been done in single center cohorts and the validity of the associations is unproved. With that caveat, some of the representative observations include the following: the donor T allele of the IFNγ gene is associated with chronic allograft fibrosis (833), high-producer genotypes for IFNγ and TNFα in the recipient increased the risk of early rejection, and high-producer TNFα was associated with type II rejection. High TGFβ1 genotype in the recipient was protective against acute rejection (834). Others have found no correlation with TGFβ, TNFα or IL-10 SNPs (single nucleotide polymorphisms) and chronic graft injury (835).

## ACUTE ISCHEMIC INJURY

Allografts routinely undergo a period of ischemia that can result in graft injury. If transient dialysis is required during the first week posttransplantation, the term *delayed graft function* (DGF) is used, whereas *primary nonfunction* (PNF) indicates that a graft never produced urine. DGF is not uncommon in deceased donor kidneys, which are preserved in the cold for 24 to 48 hours (836). Among 457 adult recipients of primary deceased donor allografts at Minnesota, the incidence of DGF was 23% (53). DGF is more common in renal allografts from asystolic donors (42% to 84%), and PNF occurs in 7% to 18% (837–840). In comparison, PNF is seen in 2% to 3% of conventional deceased donor grafts (838,840). In our series (University of North Carolina), DGF occured in 19% of kidneys from deceased donors and 2% in those from living donors. The average duration of DGF is 10 to 15 days, with a declining incidence over time (14% at 2 weeks, 9.5% at 3 weeks, and 1.7% at 4 weeks posttransplantation) (reviewed in 841).

DGF is purely a clinical term (836). The initial cause is usually acute ischemic injury (acute tubular necrosis, ATN), related to the cold and warm ischemia times. However, DGF can be due to other causes that may occur alone or in conjunction with ischemia, including drug toxicity (calcineurin inhibitors or sirolimus), acute antibody- or T-cell–mediated rejection, glomerular endothelial injury, and surgical complications at the anastomotic sites. If renal function remains poor posttransplantation, a diagnostic biopsy is indicated to render a specific diagnosis. In one series, 18% of patients with DGF had acute rejection on biopsy at 7 days (751). The pathology and pathophysiology of acute ischemic injury are detailed in Chapter 24. Here we will emphasize the features most relevant to transplanted kidneys.

## Pathologic Findings of Acute Ischemic Injury and Differential Diagnosis

As in native kidneys, ATN in renal allografts is characterized by dilatation of proximal tubules accompanied by flattening of the epithelial cell layer, loss of the brush border, and activation of epithelial cell nuclei containing prominent nucleoli. Mitotic figures are sometimes conspicuous (842). Ischemic tubular injury can be associated with non-isometric tubular cell vacuolization. The interstitium can show edema and minimal inflammation, and, especially in the medulla, dilatation of peritubular capillaries filled with mononuclear cells, sludged erythrocytes, and neutrophils. Changes can be most prominent in the vasa recta of the outer medulla and increase over the first days postgrafting. Arteries, arterioles, and glomeruli typically show only minor nonspecific abnormalities (842). Ischemia-reperfusion injury may result in the activation of the alternative or lectin pathways of complement activation. However, ischemic injury and ATN are typically not associated with the accumulation of the complement degradation product C4d along peritubular capillaries (122,348,470). If C4d is found in the setting of ischemia-reperfusion injury, a "pure" antibody-mediated rejection episode has to be considered as the primary cause for graft dysfunction (see above).

Several differences between ATN in normal and transplant kidneys have been described. Nuclear staining for proliferating cell nuclear antigens (PCNA) in proximal tubular epithelium is higher in transplanted kidneys (8.0%) than in native kidneys (4.4%) (844). ATN in 13 transplanted kidneys had tubular injury affecting short tubular segments with necrotic tubular cells, a finding seldom seen in 57 cases of ATN in native kidneys (845). Intratubular cellular debris and neutrophils may be found that resemble acute pyelonephritis. In cases of pyelonephritis, however, the neutrophil casts are typically densely packed and neutrophils are additionally found between tubular epithelial cells and in the adjacent interstitium. In 30 transplanted kidneys with ATN, the number of Tamm-Horsfall–positive casts was substantially lower than in native kidneys with ATN (844).

DGF may also be the result of glomerular injury. The changes associated with ice storage include endothelial swelling and vacuolization with obliteration and collapse of glomerular capillary lumens (846). Increased numbers of glomerular neutrophils are correlated with cold ischemia time and subsequent graft loss (108). Focal intraglomerular fibrin thrombi may contribute to delayed function; however, they did not predict poor outcome (108), presumably owing to rapid lysis by the normal host fibrinolytic system.

Only very severe and prolonged ischemic injury results in interstitial fibrosis, tubular atrophy, and nephron loss, potentially caused in part by the destruction of peritubular capillaries (lesions that should not be misinterpreted as chronic allograft rejection) (847,848). Such changes likely contribute to the high early graft failure rate seen in organs of non–heart-beating donors (15% within 3 months of transplantation reported in one study [849]).

## Pathogenesis

There is mounting evidence that T-cells, in particular CD4+ lymphocytes, natural killer cells, and IFNγ, play a crucial role in the development of ischemia-reperfusion injury likely owing to direct "cross-talk" of activated T lymphocytes with the endothelium of the microvasculature and up-regulation of adhesion molecules (See Chapter 24). T-cell activation and the up-regulation of adhesion molecules may explain the association between ATN, tubular MHC expression, and the increased risk of acute rejection after DGF (53). Also, complement activation by the alternative or lectin pathways appear to play a role in ischemia-reperfusion injury (470,482).

## Clinical Presentation, Prognosis, and Therapy

Patients are maintained on dialysis as needed and calcineurin inhibitors are generally used sparingly in the setting of DGF. Patients with DGF require less dialysis when calcineurin inhibitors are withheld (850). New treatment strategies for ischemia-reperfusion injury include antioxidants, as well as anti-inflammatory drugs (836). Unexpectedly slow functional improvement of DGF warrants a renal biopsy to rule out confounding causes.

By multivariate analysis, DGF by itself is not a significant risk factor for decreased graft survival in patients without rejection (53). Rather, it appears that the adverse prognosis associated with DGF is substantially related to an increased incidence of rejection (53,851). Approximately 95% to 98% of grafts with DGF recover; 50% within 10 days and 83% within 20 days postsurgery (836). In organs from asystolic donors, 10% of the episodes of DGF last for more than 4 weeks (837). In most instances, ATN and ischemia-reperfusion injury heal with resitutio ad integrum. Although DGF is most frequently found in organs from asystolic donors, the 6-year death-censored graft survival of these transplants does not differ significantly from conventional deceased donor organs (838). Renal function was significantly better in patients with only short-term dialysis dependency at 1 year (837).

## CALCINEURIN INHIBITOR TOXICITY

Drugs that inhibit calcineurin have tremendously improved allograft survival of all transplanted organs. Cyclosporine (cyclosporine A, CsA), increased 1-year deceased donor kidney graft survival from less than 60% to more than 80% during the decade of its clinical introduction in the 1980s (852). CsA, the first calcineurin inhibitor, is a cyclic, lipophilic undecapeptide isolated from a soil fungus (*Tolypocladium inflatum Gams*) (853). The peptide ("24–556") was relegated to obscurity as a mediocre antifungal agent until the screening system of Jacques Borel documented its potent immunosuppressive activity in 1976 (854). Clinical trials were soon reported by Calne et al (855) and Powles et al (856) in kidney and bone marrow transplant recipients. The results confirmed the promising animal studies; however, high doses of CsA (20 mg/kg per day) caused profound oliguric renal failure (856). Over the years, CsA drug preparations, as well as dosing and monitoring protocols, have undergone significant adaptations (857). The second currently widely used calcineurin inhibitor is tacrolimus (FK506), a macrolide isolated from the fungus *Streptomyces tsukubaensis* in Japan. It was introduced into clinical transplantation in the early 1990s as an alternative to CsA. Tacrolimus does not share any structural similarities with CsA, but has very similar therapeutic mechanisms and toxicity.

Calcineurin inhibitors still play a major role in the immunosuppression of allograft recipients, although their clinical significance may diminish in the future (858,859). Currently in the United States, tacrolimus is administered more often than CsA (67% of renal transplant recipients in 2003) (860). Tacrolimus is favored by many because it appears to reduce the incidence of acute rejection episodes and because it has a lower incidence of hirsutism and gingival hyperplasia (861–863). Recent studies under current modern dosing regimens do not, however, seem to unequivocally demonstrate a better efficacy of tacrolimus in suppressing acute rejection and improving long-term graft outcome (864,865).

Both CsA and tacrolimus have the same nephrotoxic side effects with indistinguishable histologic lesions primarily involving tubules, arterioles, and glomeruli (760,863,866). A histologic diagnosis of CsA toxicity was made in 61% of renal allograft biopsies in an early series (178) and in 38% almost a decade later (59). There are two major forms of toxicity: functional (owing to vasospasm and lacking morphologic changes) and structural (with various early or late histologic alterations, typically associated with functional toxicity; Fig. 28.71). Nephrotoxicity also occurs in native kidneys of patients treated with CsA or tacrolimus, such as recipients of heart or bone marrow transplants or patients with autoimmune diseases (867). TMA (thrombotic microangiopathy/hemolytic-uremic syndrome) due to CsA was first reported in bone marrow recipients (868)

and subsequently in renal allografts and native kidneys of patients under CsA or tacrolimus therapy (867,869–873). Severe chronic renal failure caused by CsA toxicity was initially observed in heart transplant patients who received CsA for more than 1 year at the time of its introduction when therapeutic trough levels were high (874). The pioneering studies of Michael Mihatsch in Basel have defined most of the key histopathologic features of calcineurin inhibitor–induced toxicity, most notably, the structural changes in arterioles and glomeruli, which Mihatsch terms "cyclosporine-type-arteriolopathy" and "cyclosporine-type-glomerulopathy" (875–878). We will modify his terms to "calcineurin inhibitor–induced" arteriolopathy and glomerulopathy, since they also apply to tacrolimus.

Functional toxicity is typically not associated with any characteristic morphologic changes and is fully reversible on dose reduction (879). Often allograft biopsies display a normal architecture and the diagnosis of "functional toxicity" is made by exclusion only. Other diseases may be superimposed, such as ATN.

Most structural nephrotoxic effects of calcineurin inhibitors in arterioles and glomeruli may be best regarded as manifestations of thrombotic microangiopathies, with different patterns and grades of severity (877). They range from insidious and limited forms (hyaline arteriolopathy) to the florid hemolytic uremic syndrome (Fig. 28.72). Mild forms are without great clinical significance; they are completely or partially reversible on dose reduction. Severe variants with fully developed, systemic thrombotic microangiopathies can result in graft failure. Both calcineurin inhibitor arteriolopathy and glomerulopathy can develop within days to a few weeks, rendering terms such as "acute" and "chronic" toxicity inaccurate. The interstitial compartment shows lesions of uncertain pathogenesis. The following pathology description applies to structural toxic changes.

### Pathologic Findings

#### Tubules

The most common morphologic change in the tubular compartment linked to calcineurin inhibitor toxicity is *isometric vacuolization*, defined as cells filled with uniformly sized small vacuoles (Fig. 28.72). The vacuoles are found in the cytoplasm of tubular epithelial cells, sometimes associated with loss of the brush border. Among over 1000 diagnostic renal transplant biopsies, isometric tubular vacuolization was found in 40% of cases in the first 2 weeks, in 30% at 6 months, in 18% at 1 year, and in about 8% at 3 years (880). Under current therapeutic dose regimens, isometric cytoplasmic vacuolization most often involves only scattered proximal tubules. It predominates in the straight portion of the proximal tubules (881), although it

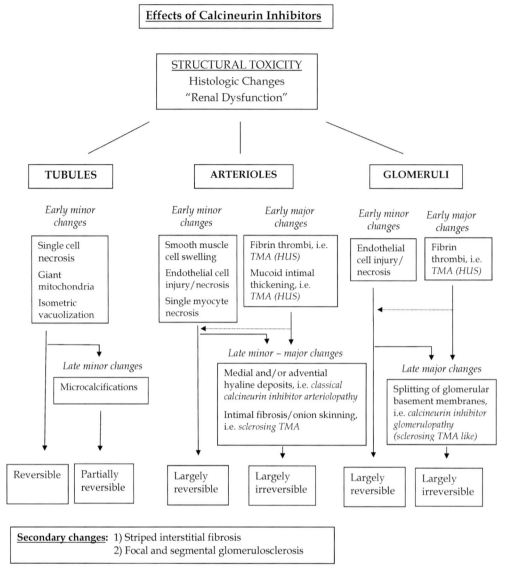

**Figure 28.71**  Schematic of calcineurin inhibitor-induced structural toxicity. (TMA, thrombotic microangiopathy; HUS, hemolytic uremic syndrome.)

also occurs in the convoluted portion and can occasionally be seen in parietal epithelial cells lining Bowman's space. The vacuoles, much smaller than the nucleus, contain clear aqueous fluid (unstained by H&E or PAS). Electron microscopy reveals an empty appearing, markedly dilated smooth endoplasmic reticulum (881). Although typically the entire cytoplasm of an affected tubular cell is densely packed with equal-size vacuoles, they can be less abundant in the early phase of injury. Tubular epithelial cells with isometric vacuolization suggestive of toxic tubulopathy can occasionally also be found in urine cytology specimens (882–885). The degree of vacuolization does not correlate well with calcineurin inhibitor blood levels; the lesions are readily reversible with a reduction of dosage (Fig. 28-71).

Two other pathologic features in tubules have been linked to calcineurin inhibitor toxicity but have little diagnostic value. Giant mitochondria, rarely found even in cases with marked toxicity, are irregularly distributed in proximal tubules. Typically one giant mitochondria per cell is seen that can reach about half the size of a nucleus (Fig. 28.73) (878). By electron microscopy, the giant mitochondria are irregularly outlined, have only few cristae, and can occasionally contain crystalline material. Dystrophic microcalcifications (often not bigger than a tubular cell) can occasionally be found scattered throughout the nephron. They typically have a round or layered egg shell appearance and are believed to arise as dystrophic calcifications from intratubular Tamm-Horsfall protein or secondary from toxic single epithelial cell necrosis (878,886).

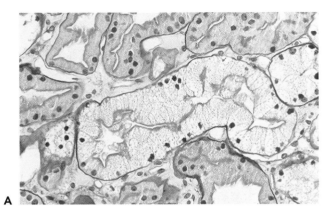
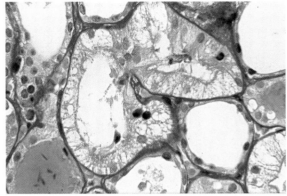

**Figure 28.72** Calcineurin inhibitor–induced toxic tubulopathy **(A)** with isometric vacuolization of the proximal tubular epithelial cell cytoplasm. In comparison, ischemia-induced tubular injury **(B)** with nonisometric vacuolization of the tubular cytoplasm; this change should not be mistaken for toxic tubulopathy. (**A:** PAS, ×150; **B:** trichrome, ×250.)

Microcalcifications are not diagnostic of toxicity, but are seen in many cases of "ATN"; they are rather uncommon under modern calcineurin inhibitor doses (887).

## Arterioles and Arteries

Calcineurin inhibitor–induced vascular lesions are found most characteristically in afferent arterioles. The arteriolar lesions can extend in severe cases into the glomerulus (i.e., toxic glomerulopathy) and into small arteries with up to two layers of smooth muscle cells. Branches of arcuate arteries are characteristically spared. Proliferative arterial intimal fibrosis, fibroelastosis, and transplant endarteritis are not features of toxicity.

Early calcineurin inhibitor–induced arteriolar changes are characterized by marked swelling, so-called balloon-

ing, of medial smooth muscle cells that can obscure the normal vascular architecture (Fig. 28.74). The cytoplasm of the medial cells contains very large, clear vacuoles, caused by marked dilatation of the endoplasmic reticulum. These early changes are fully reversible on dose reduction. They can, however, progress to calcineurin inhibitor arteriolopathy with intramural hyaline deposits (see below; Fig. 28.71). Arteriolar medial ballooning as a sign of early calcineurin inhibitor–induced toxicity should be evaluated only in normal-appearing parenchymal zones, since identical changes are seen in severe ischemic renal injury (ATN) or in some cases of the nephrotic syndrome presenting with nonselective proteinuria.

The classic morphology of late calcineurin inhibitor arteriolopathy has been described as "nodular protein deposits (hyaline deposits) replacing single necrotic smooth

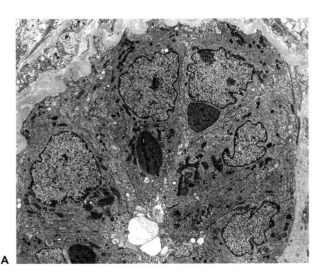
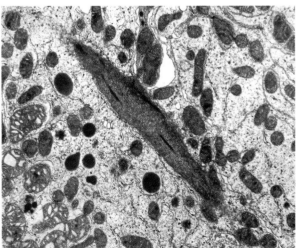

**Figure 28.73** Calcineurin inhibitor–induced toxic tubulopathy with mega-mitochondria (typically one per cell). The mitochondria reach approximately one half the size of the nucleus **(A)** and display distorted cristae **(B)**. (Electron photomicrographs, **A:** ×3000; **B:** ×14,000.) (Courtesy of Michael Mihatsch, Basel, Switzerland.)

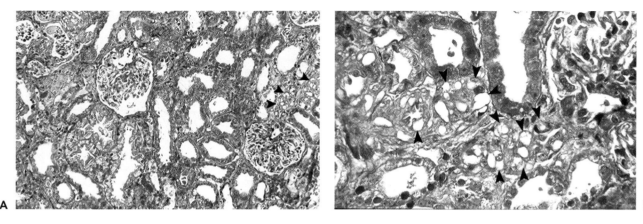

**Figure 28.74**  Calcineurin inhibitor–induced early toxic arteriolopathy with swelling (so-called ballooning) of medial smooth muscle cells, obscuring the vascular architecture (*arrowheads* in **A** and **B**). In this case, early toxic arteriolar changes are associated with isometric vacuolization of the tubular cytoplasm (**A**). (**A**: trichrome, ×100; **B**: trichrome, ×400.)

muscle cells of the media" (877), "occasionally in a pearl-like pattern" (888). Hyaline nodules can be most pronounced along the adventitial layer; they stain intensely with PAS (Fig. 28.75). Hyalinosis is most pronounced in renin-producing smooth muscle cell layers along afferent arterioles and in very small arteries with up to two layers of smooth muscle cells (888–890). The severity of calcineurin inhibitor–induced arteriolopathy varies con-

siderably, even in the same biopsy. Some vessels may show only mild changes with few intramural/advential hyaline nodules whereas others demonstrate advanced arteriolopathies with segmental or circumferential hyalinosis, complete loss of medial smooth muscle cells, and stenosis (Fig. 28.75B). The endothelial cell layers remain typically intact, even in severe cases, and fibrin thrombi are absent. Extensive fibrinoid arteriolar wall necrosis and

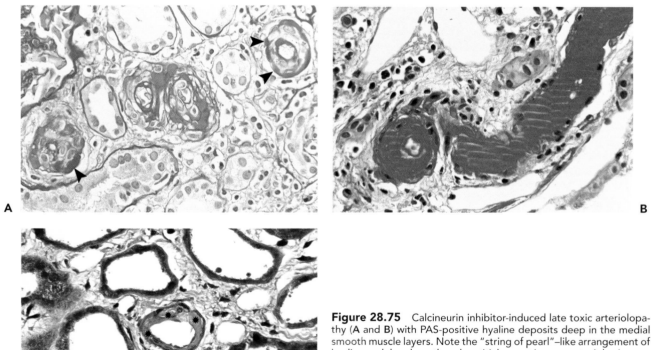

**Figure 28.75**  Calcineurin inhibitor-induced late toxic arteriolopathy (**A** and **B**) with PAS-positive hyaline deposits deep in the medial smooth muscle layers. Note the "string of pearl"–like arrangement of hyaline nodules along the adventitial aspect in some arterioles (*arrowheads* in **A**). **A**: The arteriolopathy is scored as ha 2. **B**: An example of ha 3 with very severe transmural and circumferential hyaline accumulations. **C**: In contrast, hypertension-induced arteriolosclerosis typically demonstrates subendothelial hyaline deposits (*asterisks*) surrounded by (sometimes atrophic) intact medial smooth muscle cells. (**A** and **B**: PAS, ×400; **C**: trichrome, ×400.)

inflammation are typically not found, and if present, a florid thrombotic microangiopathy (i.e., HUS) or severe acute rejection (i.e., Banff type 3) have to be considered in the differential diagnosis. Calcineurin inhibitor arteriolopathy also develops in native kidneys of patients who receive CsA or tacrolimus (710,867,892).

Immunofluorescence microscopy is nonspecific with the accumulation of IgM and the complement factors C1q, C3, C5b-9, and C4d in hyaline deposits (C4d is, however, not detected along peritubular capillaries). Electron microscopy reveals a distinctive replacement of individual smooth muscle cells with amorphous dense, granular material that protrudes into the advential layer (888,889,893). Intercellular junctions are decreased, and extracellular matrix proteins including collagens are increased. Myocytes with two nuclei and mitotic figures can be observed (889). The endothelium sometimes appears vacuolated (889,894).

Calcineurin inhibitor arteriolopathy with medial hyaline nodules can develop fast over days to a few weeks; in one carefully analyzed series of renal transplants in Basel,

the percentage of arterioles affected with the specific lesion, defined as "protein deposits replacing necrotic smooth muscle cells in the afferent arteriole," increased from 5% at 6 months (in all examined arterioles), to 9% at 1 year and 12% at 2 years (891). Similarly, in 38 renal transplant patients on CsA, 15% of protocol biopsies at 6 months showed calcineurin inhibitor type arteriolopathies, which increased to 45% in protocol biopsies 18 months postgrafting (895). The cumulative prevalence of calcineurin inhibitor-induced arteriolopathy reaches 100% at 10 years, i.e. all transplants show structural toxicity (760). Under lower doses of calcineurin inhibitors, the overall prevalence of arteriolopathy has decreased. In 1981 70% of all biopsies demonstrated arteriolopathy, whereas in 1990 the prevalence had decreased to 40%; the average percentage of affected arterioles decreased from 17% to 7% (891).

In most severe cases, calcineurin inhibitors induce a florid thrombotic microangiopathy (TMA/HUS; Fig. 28.76). In TMA arterioles are typically affected in a focal fashion, most pronounced at the glomerular vascular poles with fibrin and platelet thrombi that can extend distally

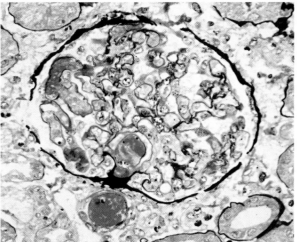

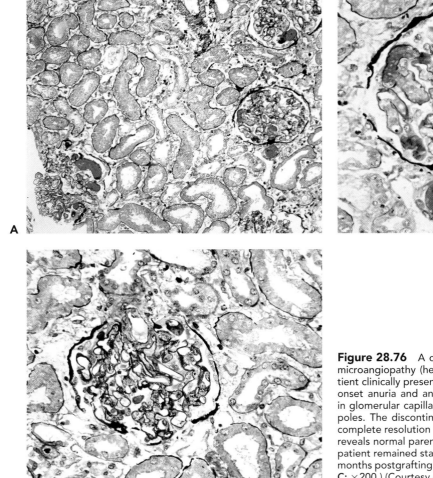

**Figure 28.76** A calcineurin inhibitor-induced florid thrombotic microangiopathy (hemolytic uremic syndrome, **A** and **B**). The patient clinically presented on day 11 after transplantation with new-onset anuria and anemia. The graft biopsy shows fibrin thrombi in glomerular capillaries and arterioles at the glomerular vascular poles. The discontinuation of CsA therapy resulted in rapid and complete resolution of the TMA within 5 days. A repeat biopsy (**C**) reveals normal parenchyma without thrombi. Renal function in the patient remained stable with a serum creatinine level of 1 mg/dL 7 months postgrafting. (**A–C:** methenamine silver, **A:** ×100; **B:** ×250; **C:** ×200.) (Courtesy of Alenka Vizjak and Dusan Ferluga, Ljubljana, Slovenia.)

into glomerular capillaries (often in a segmental pattern) and proximally into prearterioles. Medial smooth muscle layers frequently show single cell necrosis. Arteriolar mucoid intimal thickening and edematous swelling can occur but are uncommon. Similar to other forms of TMA, vascular lesions often undergo remodeling with intimal sclerosis, sometimes concentric with an onion skin appearance. TMA/HUS with fibrin thrombi can undergo resolution with restitutio ad integrum (896) (Fig. 28.76c).

There is no generally accepted scheme for scoring the severity of calcineurin inhibitor–induced arteriolopathy, and the Banff 1997 classification system is ill suited (177). We use and recommend a grading scheme developed by Michael Mihatsch (personal communication, 896a) (Table 28.14).

### Glomeruli

Glomeruli can be affected as part of endothelial injury/thrombosis, or as a later consequence of severe calcineuring inhibitor arteriolopathy resulting in glomerulosclerosis. Intraglomerular fibrin thrombi, typically in a focal and segmental distribution, are found in cases of calcineurin inhibitor-induced florid thrombotic microangiopathies, often associated with mesangiolysis (Fig. 28.76). Sometimes, intraglomerular thrombi may also occur as isolated events without arteriolar thrombi (897). Glomerular endothelial cell injury and activation, without fibrin thrombi,

| Score | Description |
|---|---|
| ha 0 | No hyaline deposits in arterioles |
| ha 1 | Focal hyaline deposits replacing necrotic or degenerated medial smooth muscle cells in one arteriole (without circumferential and transmural involvement) |
| ha 2 | Focal hyaline deposits replacing necrotic or degenerated medial smooth muscle cells in more than one arteriole (without circumferential and transmural involvement) |
| ha 3 | Transmural and circumferential hyaline deposits replacing the entire arteriolar wall, independent of the number of involved vessels |

**TABLE 28.14**

**SCORING OF CALCINEURIN INHIBITOR INDUCED HYALINE ARTERIOLOPATHY**

Adapted from M. Mihatsch personal communication (896, 896a.)

are frequently seen by electron microscopy, they are commonly not associated with morphologic changes by standard light microscopic examination.

Protracted or recurrent glomerular endothelial cell injury caused by calcineurin inhibitors can result in widening of the lamina rara interna and subendothelial new basement membrane formation with duplication of the GBM (Figs. 28.77 and 28.78). GBM duplication typically

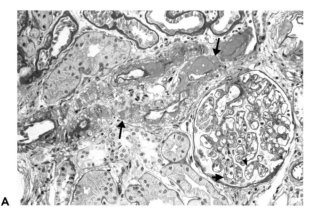

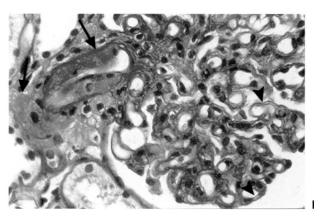

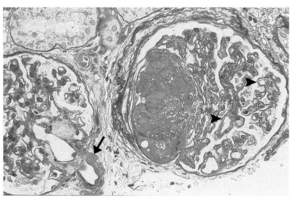

**Figure 28.77** Calcineurin inhibitor-induced late toxic glomerulopathy (A–C). Peripheral glomerular capillary walls show segmental duplication (*arrowheads* in **A**, **B**, and **C**) without conspicuous cell interposition that is only occasionally seen (*short arrow* in **A**). Afferent arterioles feeding the affected glomeruli characteristically demonstrate calcineurin inhibitor–induced toxic arteriolopathy (*long arrows* in **A**, **B**, and **C**). Superimposed on the toxic glomerulopathy is segmental tuft sclerosis (**C**) interpreted to be a secondary phenomenon. (**A**: PAS, ×100; **B**: PAS ×400; **C**: PAS, ×200.)

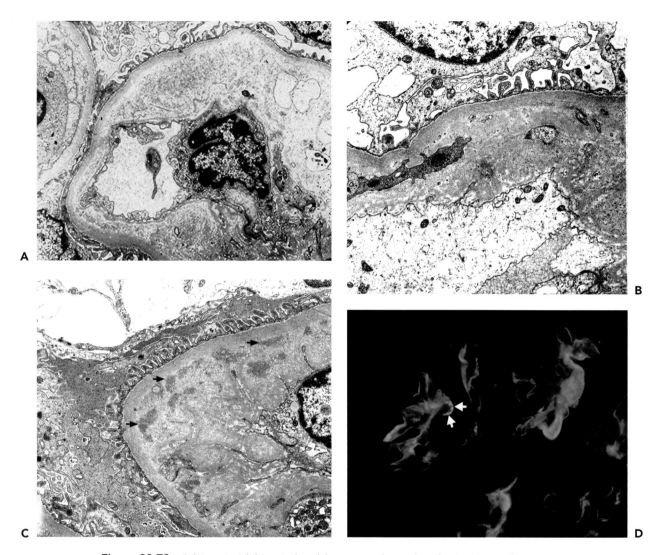

**Figure 28.78**  Calcineurin inhibitor–induced late toxic glomerulopathy (**A–D**). By electron microscopy, widening of the subendothelial compartment, the accumulation of flocculent material, and new basement membrane formation (sometimes wavy appearing, **B**) is noted. Occasionally small focal and segmental electron-dense deposits are seen (*arrows* in **C**) associated with segmental minimal staining by immunofluorescence microscopy (*arrows* in **D**). The deposits are characteristically inconspicuous and should not be misinterpreted as evidence of an immune complex–mediated glomerulonephritis. The overall changes of toxic glomerulopathies are reminiscent of the remodeling phenomena seen in cases of thrombotic microangiopathies (i.e., the hemolytic uremic syndrome). (Electron photomicrographs, **A:** ×6500; **B:** ×10,000; **C:** ×7500; **D:** Immunofluorescence microscopy with an antibody directed against IgG, ×400.) (Parts **B**, **C**, and **D** and Figure 28.77A are from the same case.)

is focal and segmental. Mesangial regions are often slightly expanded owing to matrix deposition. We term this "calcineurin inhibitor glomerulopathy." The glomerular capillary lumens can contain scattered mononuclear cells. However, capillary dilatation and conspicuous intracapillary inflammatory cell aggregates, as well as prominent cell interposition along duplicated capillary walls, are not characteristic of calcineurin inhibitor glomerulopathy (in contrast to transplant glomerulitis or recurrent glomerulonephritis) (Table 28.15). Identical glomerular changes occur in native kidneys in heart and bone marrow transplant recipients on calcineurin inhibitors (878). Calcineurin in-

hibitor glomerulopathy is characteristically associated with calcineurin inhibitor arteriolopathy, typically most severe in the arterioles feeding the affected glomeruli (Fig. 28.77). Calcineurin inhibitor glomerulopathy occurred in 65% of biopsies with severe arteriolopathy, in 25% to 45% with mild to moderate, and in none with no evidence of arteriolopathy (878,897).

Other glomerular lesions related to calcineurin inhibitors include FSGS, which is most often seen in cases with hyaline arteriolopathy or glomerulopathy and probably represents a secondary phenomena caused bt overload (Fig. 28.77C). Distal to afferent arterioles with

**TABLE 28.15**

**DIFFERENTIAL DIAGNOSIS OF CALCINEURIN INHIBITOR–INDUCED TOXICITY**

| Toxic Lesions | Differential Diagnosis | Helpful Features for Excluding Toxicity |
|---|---|---|
| Tubulopathy with isometric vacuolization | Osmotic nephrosis | – Clinical history of previous medications (e.g. mannitol, IVIG solutions)<br>– Electron microscopy showing phagolysosomes |
| Thrombotic microangiopathy (TMA) | Other causes of a TMA | – Clinical history of native kidney disease, other risk factors for TMA (e.g. radiation) |
|  | Antibody-mediated rejection | – C4d positivity along peritubular capillaries<br>– Detection of circulating donor-specific antibodies |
| Calcineurin inhibitor-induced arteriolopathy | Diabetes mellitus | – Clinical history<br>– Other diabetic changes (e.g. glomerular capsular drops or fibrin caps) |
|  | Hypertension | – Clinical history<br>– Concurrent arterial intimal fibroelastosis<br>– Dominant subendothelial arteriolar hyaline deposits (in contrast to medial deposits seen with toxicity) |
|  | Pre-existing donor disease | – Findings in zero-hour implantation biopsies |
|  | Chronic vascular rejection | – Chronic rejection typically affects arteries, not afferent arterioles |
|  | Fabry's disease | – History and glomerular changes |
| Calcineurin inhibitor-induced glomerulopathy | Other causes of a TMA | – Clinical history of native kidney disease, other risk factors for a TMA (e.g. radiation) |
|  | Chronic rejection (transplant glomerulopathy) | – Concurrent chronic allograft arteriopathy<br>– Concurrent transplant glomerulitis<br>– Absence of marked calcineurin inhibitor arteriolopathy<br>– C4d positivity along peritubular capillaries |
|  | Membranoproliferative glomerulonephritis | – Pronounced glomerular hypercellularity, proliferative changes, and cell interposition in a global and diffuse pattern<br>– Marked immune complex type deposits by immunohistochemistry/immunofluorescence microscopy and electron microscopy<br>– Sometimes crescent formation<br>– Often active urine sediment<br>– Decreased serum complement levels |

severe (stenosing) arteriolopathy (i.e., ah-3) glomeruli might reveal atrophy or global sclerosis. In several cases, we have observed the collapsing variant of FSGS in the setting of severe calcineurin arteriolopathy in transplanted (723) or native kidneys (898) (Fig. 28.79).

By immunofluorescence microscopy, glomeruli with calcineurin inhibitor glomerulopathy show non-diagnostic IgM and complement factor C1q, C3, C4d, and C5b-9 deposits. On rare occasions, focal and segmental minimal to mild (non-diagnostic) granular, IgG, IgA, and light chains accumulate along peripheral basement membranes (Fig. 28.78C). C4d is not detected along peritubular capillaries. If peritubular C4d is found (and/or other histologic evidence of acute rejection such as typical transplant endarteritis), a diagnosis of rejection has to be made.

Electron microscopy in calcineurin inhibitor glomerulopathy shows findings typical of thrombotic microangiopathies (Fig. 28.78; see Chapter 16). The endothelium is reactive with increased cytoplasm and loss of fenestrations. The lamina rara interna is widened, and subendothelial new basement membrane is formed, sometimes with a layered appearance owing to repetitive endothelial cell injury and basement membrane production (the ultrastructural correlate of GBM duplication seen by light microscopy). The newly formed subendothelial compartment can contain cell processes and occasional small (non-diagnostic) electron-dense deposits (Fig. 28.78C). Glomerular injury in severe cases shows intracapillary fibrin thrombi typical for florid cases of thrombotic microangiopathies and segmental mesangiolysis.

## Interstitium

In acute toxicity, the interstitium is often normal or demonstrates focal minimal edema. Only cases with toxic tubulopathies associated with acute ischemic injury show marked edema and acute tubular injury. Frank tubular necrosis, however, is typically inconspicuous in the setting of toxicity, unless ATN of other causes is also present (887). Interstitial inflammatory cell infiltrates are

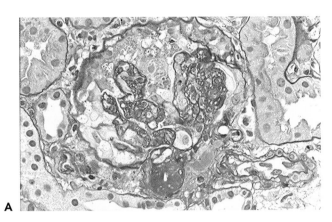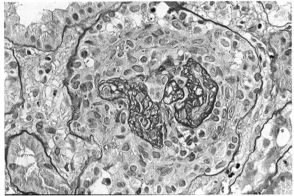

**Figure 28.79**  De novo collapsing focal and segmental glomerulosclerosis (**A** and **B**) in a patient with marked calcineurin inhibitor–induced toxic arteriolopathy, i.e., ha3, 35 months after grafting. Glomerular capillary tufts appear condensed and collapsed with marked activation of the overlying podocytes (illustrated in **B** is a so-called pseudo-crescent caused by podocyte crowding and proliferation). (**A** and **B**: PAS, ×200.)

characteristically very sparse and tubulitis is absent or at best minimal (899,900). If marked mononuclear inflammatory cells and tubulitis are found, a concurrent acute cellular rejection episode has to be considered.

Striped interstitial fibrosis, tubular and global glomerular atrophy, and sclerosis have been described in the setting of calcineurin inhibitor–induced toxicity, mainly in biopsies with conspicuous calcineurin inhibitor arteriolopathies and glomerulopathies (863,867,878). In renal biopsies from 20 patients suffering from psoriasis or uveitis under CsA therapy, significant interstitial fibrosis and tubular atrophy were found, compared with 40 age- and sex-matched controls (901). Tubulointerstitial sclerosis, likely primarily induced by CsA therapy, also reported in native kidneys from various nonrenal transplant recipients (867). Thus, calcineurin inhibitor therapy contributes to interstitial scarring. However, even though the patchy/striped fibrotic interstitial changes observed in renal biopsies are clinically significant and contribute to graft dysfunction, they lack diagnostic specificity (902).

## Etiology and Pathogenesis

CsA and tacrolimus bind to intracytoplasmic receptor proteins, the immunophilins, a family of peptidylprolyl *cis-trans* isomerases that include the cyclophilins (for binding of CsA) and FK binding proteins (for tacrolimus), both with rotamase activity (903–908). The immunophilin/CsA or tacrolimus complexes have a high affinity to bind to and to thereby inhibit calcineurin, a phosphatase. Calcineurin physiologically dephosphorylates intracytoplasmic nuclear regulatory proteins in lymphocytes (i.e., NFAT [nuclear factors of activated T-cells]) and hence facilitates their translocation into the nucleus and activation as intranuclear transcription factors for various mediators (such as IL-2, IL-4, interferon

gamma, and tumor necrosis factor alpha). Calcineurin typically promotes T-cell activation. In therapeutic doses, CsA and tacrolimus block approximately 50% of the calcineurin activity. They do not affect neutrophils, phagocytosis, or the bone marrow, thus still allowing for an effective overall immune response.

A key question is whether the immunosuppressive and nephrotoxic effects of calcineurin inhibitors are related to inhibition of the isomerase enzymatic activity of calcineurin. Elegant studies with dozens of CsA analogs showed that immunosuppression potency and acute nephrotoxicity were inseparable (909). These data suggest that the transduction pathways important for immunosuppressive activity are similar to the ones that cause nephrotoxicity and that there is little hope for finding a variant that separates these effects (909). The likely common mechanism of action for both immunosuppression and toxic side effects is the inhibition of calcineurin.

Nephrotoxicity correlates best with peak blood calcineurin levels (760) and less with trough levels (879). Among patients with renal allograft dysfunction, CsA trough levels averaged 358 ± 167 ng/mL in those 38 with biopsy-confirmed CsA nephrotoxicity, whereas patients with rejection had levels of 220 ± 120 ng/mL using a monoclonal antibody radioimmunoassay (910). CsA trough levels greater than 400 ng/mL predicted CsA toxicity with a specificity of 89% but a sensitivity of only 32%. Dysfunction associated with CsA levels of up to 150 ng/mL was owing to rejection in 91%. 63% of episodes of CsA nephrotoxicity and 59% of the acute rejection episodes occurred at "therapeutic" levels of 150 to 400 ng/mL. Al-Awwa et al (63) reported that more than 75% of all histologic diagnoses of either CsA- or tacrolimus-induced structural toxicity were made in the clinical setting of low or therapeutic blood drug levels. The imperfect correlation between trough levels and histologically diagnosed toxicity may be because the biopsy diagnosis of "late" structural toxicity is established long after peak toxic drug levels caused arteriolar and glomerular injury. In addition, individuals differ in drug metabolism, absorption, and sensitivity to the toxic side-effects. Factors known to contribute to toxicity include polymorphism of P-glycoprotein (911) and variation in the level of cytochrome P450 (900,912,913).

Calcineurin inhibitors significantly affect smooth muscle cells of the media. A major functional consequence is vasoconstriction, which can already be seen after the first oral dose (914). The effects of CsA on vascular smooth muscle cells are complex (915). CsA can cause a slow contraction of isolated aortic smooth muscle cells (916), which can be inhibited by calcium channel blockers (verapamil). CsA causes hypersensitivity to angiotensin II as judged by an increased cytosolic free $Ca^{2+}$ response due to an increased permeability of the plasma membrane for $Ca^{2+}$. Resting levels of $Ca^{2+}$ are not affected, but rather the uptake is increased. The elevation of cytosolic free calcium is associated with an increase in the production of endothelin, *a vasoconstricting polypeptide* (917). In the human, but not the rat, the released endothelin also has proliferative effects on vascular smooth muscle cells. CsA causes a dose dependent release of endothelin from cultured human and rat arterial smooth muscle and endothelial cells (918–923). Plasma levels of endothelin-1 are significantly elevated in bone marrow transplant patients on CsA. CsA at therapeutic levels (0.1 μM) also induces an increased expression of endothelin receptor subtype A mRNA in cultured rat vascular smooth muscle cells.

In addition, calcineurin inhibitors can also cause necrosis of individual smooth muscle cells, as shown in animal studies (924). In one model of calcineurin inhibitor-induced toxicity, injury to muscle cells was first detected at day 10 as an accumulation of eosinophilic granular material in afferent arterioles (925). The disease process progressed over the next 25 days with focal smooth muscle cell vacuolization and the accumulation of discrete hyaline deposits in vessel walls (925,926). Electron microscopy demonstrated an increased accumulation of renin granules in the smooth muscle cell cytoplasm, corresponding to the eosinophilic granular transformation seen histologically. Increased renin was also demonstrated by immunocytochemistry. The inhibition of type I angiotensin II receptors with losartan (but not other antihypertensives, hydralazine and furosemide), inhibited the development of calcineurin inhibitor-induced arteriolopathy in rats (927).

Regeneration is limited in the media of arterioles. Thus, calcineurin inhibitor-induced necrosis of single medial smooth muscle cells is typically "repaired" by insudation of plasma proteins into the necrotic foci. This gives rise to intramural hyaline deposits and the classic morphology of calcineurin inhibitor arteriolopathy. In native kidneys, structural calcineurin inhibitor-induced toxic vascular changes may potentially be enhanced because of the intact sympathetic innervation (867).

Calcineurin inhibitors also affect the endothelium since they shift the balance of arachidonate pathways toward vasoconstriction and thrombosis (increased thromboxane A2 levels) and decreased vasodilation and antithrombosis (decreased prostaglandin and prostacyclin levels) (928,929). Experimentally, CsA toxicity is inhibited by thromboxane A2 antagonists (900). The rise in circulating levels of von Willebrand factor, tissue plasminogen activator, and plasminogen activator inhibitor-1 was correlated with the severity of thrombotic microangiopathy in bone marrow recipients on CsA therapy (932). CsA enhances the thromboplastic response of the endothelium (and monocytes) in vitro to IL1 or tumor necrosis factor alpha (933). Further evidence that CsA causes endothelial injury was the finding of elevation of plasma concentrations of factor VIII-related antigen in renal allograft recipients during calcineurin inhibitor nephrotoxicity, which fell toward normal as the CsA dose of CsA was reduced (934). CsA also promotes epithelial to mesenchyme transition (EMT) of human renal tubular cells in culture, which involves increased production of TGFβ and protein kinase C pathways (699).

## Differential Diagnosis

The major differential diagnoses of calcineurin inhibitor-induced structural toxicities are listed in Table 28.15. To establish the cause of arteriolar hyalinosis, implantation/zero hour and early posttransplant biopsies should be reviewed for pre-existing donor disease. Biopsies taken years after grafting may show combined hypertension-induced and calcineurin inhibitor arteriolopathies (i.e. subendothelial and medial/advential hyaline deposits). Toxic changes can coincide with other disease processes, such as rejection episodes, infections (polyomavirus nephropathy), or glomerulonephritides. The complement degradation product C4d is characteristically not detected along peritubular capillaries in any form of calcineurin inhibitor-induced toxicity including thrombotic microangiopathies; its presence indicates humoral rejection.

## Tubular Lesions

Isometric tubular epithelial vacuolization is characteristic, but not pathognomonic of calcineurin inhibitor-induced tubulopathies, because identical light microscopic changes can be seen in a variety of diseases, including fatty changes in the setting of the nephrotic syndrome or cases of so-called osmotic nephrosis following therapy with plasma expanders (such as mannitol, dextran), radiolabeled contrast media, or sucrose-rich hyperimmune globulin and IVIG solutions (935–937). In contrast to calcineurin inhibitor-induced tubulopathy, however, these cases typically demonstrate dilated phagolysosomes rather than a dilated smooth endoplasmatic reticulum by electron microscopy. Nonisometric and irregular intracytoplasmic tubular vacuoles of different sizes should not be interpreted as evidence of toxic tubulopathy (Fig. 28.72B). They are commonly seen in various forms of tubular injury, mainly ischemia. Late after grafting, tubular vacuolization may be seen in scattered atrophic-appearing tubules located in zones of fibrosis; these changes are of undetermined significance.

Several other morphologic changes can be seen in patients treated with calcineurin inhibitors that are considered to be nondiagnostic of structural toxicity. ATN and congested peritubular capillaries containing mononuclear cell elements are often found in acute renal failure of different causes (899). Giant mitochondria in tubular epithelial cells are present in cases of ischemia; they are typically lysed and empty appearing. Dystrophic calcifications can be seen after pronounced ischemic ATN (donor disease and/or posttransplantation following ischemia/reperfusion injury), in the setting of hypercalcemia, or bowel-cleansing procedures with phosphate-rich solutions (762,938,939). In these latter conditions, the calcifications are often large and irregular and sometimes even involve basement membranes.

## Arteriolopathy

Arteriolar hyalinosis is not only induced by calcineurin inhibitors. It is common in patients suffering from long-standing hypertension or diabetes mellitus. Arteriolosclerosis in the setting of hypertension differs from calcineurin inhibitor-induced arteriolopathy, because it has predominately subendothelial hyaline deposits that are covered by an intact, although sometimes atrophic, medial smooth muscle layer (Fig. 28.75C). Transmural hyaline deposits are less common. Arteriolosclerosis can develop post-grafting as a de novo lesion in the setting of hypertension; it is also seen in zero-hour implantation biopsies representing donor disease. Arteriolar hyalinosis in cases of diabetic nephropathy is very similar to calcineurin inhibitor-induced arteriolopathy and cannot be reliably distinguished (see Table 28.15).

In our experience and that of others intramural and adventitial hyaline nodules are most specific for calcineurin inhibitor induced toxicity (880), however, they are not pathognomonic. These nodules are relatively rare, and detection may require meticulous study of multiple sections. Although some overlap between calcineurin inhibitor-induced and hypertensive arteriolopathies undoubtedly exists, when the hyalinosis has multiple discrete nodules the size and location of the medial smooth muscle cells, classic calcineurin inhibitor type toxicity should be diagnosed. Peripheral nodules are rarely found in non-transplant cases; the only common other setting is un-

treated Fabry's disease (personal observations). Since kidney transplant recipients treated with calcineurin inhibitors often also suffer from arterial hypertension, injury can be synergistic and lead to combination lesions. Mihatsch refers to these late changes as "arteriolopathies of the mixed conventional hypertensive and toxic types (personal communication)."

Arterial intimal sclerosis and/or inflammation (in interlobular, arcuate, or interlobar arteries) are not features of calcineurin inhibitor-induced structural toxicity (differential diagnosis: chronic rejection or hypertension-induced arterionephrosclerosis). Potentially, in the future the detection of elevated m-RNA levels of laminin beta-2 and transforming growth factor (TGF) beta may help to diagnose calcineurin inhibitor-induced toxicity more accurately (940).

## Glomerulopathy

The detection of duplicated peripheral glomerular basement membranes in renal transplants raises three major differential diagnoses (Table 28.15): (a) a late phase of a thrombotic microangiopathy not induced by calcineurin inhibitors (e.g. recurrent disease or caused by other drugs), (b) membranoproliferative glomerulonephritides, and (c) transplant glomerulopathy in the setting of chronic rejection. Thrombotic microangiopathies of other causes can be diagnosed only on clinical grounds including detailed knowledge of the underlying native kidney disease that had resulted in renal failure. Membranoproliferative glomerulonephritides (MPGN) are characterized by glomerular hypercellularity, an accentuation of the tuft lobulation including conspicuous cell interpositions, and the accumulation of immune complex type deposits (Fig. 28.80). Transplant glomerulopathy in the setting of chronic rejection is very similar, but not identical, to calcineurin inhibitor glomerulopathy. Transplant glomerulopathy often shows evidence of concurrent rejection, such as transplant endarteritis, chronic allograft arteriopathy (i.e. chronic vascular rejection) transplant glomerulitis (57% to 90% of cases), or C4d deposits along peritubular capillaries (36 to 53% of cases) (143,348,567). Calcineurin inhibitor glomerulopathy typically does not show evidence of rejection, but rather, demonstrates marked hyalinosis in the afferent arterioles. Combination of chronic rejection and calcineurin inhibitor toxicity also occurs and can be diagnosed by the presence of the distinctive lesions of each type.

### Clinical Presentation, Prognosis, and Therapy

Patients treated with calcineurin inhibitors commonly present (among other signs) with a decreased glomerular filtration rate (because of arteriolar vasospasms) and hypertension. Toxicity in the kidney clinically presents with renal dysfunction and in the setting of calcineurin

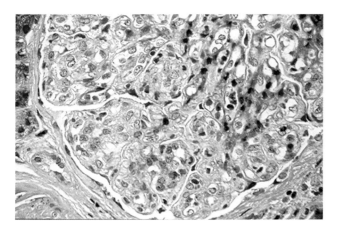

**Figure 28.80** Membranoproliferative glomerulonephritis type I (MPGN-I). The differential diagnosis of a calcineurin inhibitor–induced late toxic glomerulopathy includes a MPGN that usually presents with global hypercellularity of glomerular capillary tufts, accentuation of the tuft lobulation, and conspicuous cell interpositions along duplicated GBM segments. The MPGN pattern is commonly quite different from a toxic glomerulopathy. (Trichrome, ×400.)

inhibitor type glomerulopathy with proteinuria. Functional and early structural toxicity often reverse on reduction or discontinuation of therapy, and even toxicity with protracted oliguria (for 21 to 83 days posttransplantation) usually vanishes (8/9 patients) (941). Isometric vacuolization is readily reversible (942).

Chronic renal failure can occur after long-term use of calcineurin inhibitors (888). Ojo et al (943) found chronic renal failure (defined as a glomerular filtration rate of up to 29 mL/min/1.73 m$^2$ of body surface area) in 16.5% of 69,321 recipients of nonrenal organ transplants during the

period 1990 to 2000; 29% of these patients (3297) went on to end-stage renal disease (dialysis or transplantation). The cumulative rate of chronic renal failure was 20% and 25% at 10 years for heart and liver recipients, respectively. However, no pathology was provided, and the cause was not proved to be calcineurin inhibitors. Other studies indicate that hypertension and hyperlipidemia are probably contributing factors promoting chronic renal failure in patients treated with calcineurin inhibitors (867,943). In pediatric heart transplant patients, 3.2% of 125 recipients developed renal failure years post surgery (944).

Regression of calcineurin inhibitor hyaline arteriolopathy has been reported (760,945,946). In mild to moderate forms, discontinuation of CsA is followed by arteriolar remodeling and morphologic resolution of the intramural hyaline deposits in a substantial number of patients (55% of 20 renal allografts), as judged by repeat biopsies after 6 to 18 months (Fig. 28.81) (946). This arteriolar remodeling is characterized by structural irregularities of the medial layers and an increased deposition of basement membrane–like material ("unorganized appearance," Fig. 28.81B). Even circumferential arteriolar hyaline deposits may sometimes undergo resolution (945). Healing of calcineurin inhibitor–induced arteriolopathy was also found in a rat model following the discontinuation of CsA for 2 months (926).

In general, the detection of calcineurin inhibitor arteriolopathy does not necessarily indicate poor long-term prognosis. Serum creatinine levels improve in most patients on dose reduction (likely in part owing to functional toxicity and vasoconstriction), and drastic changes to the immunosuppressive drug regimens are not always required.

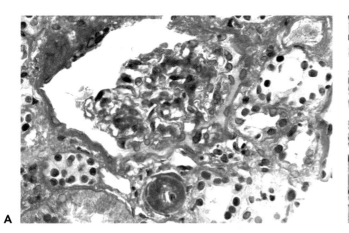
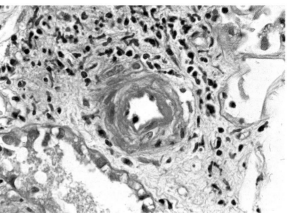

A                                                        B

**Figure 28.81** Regression of a calcineurin inhibitor–induced late toxic arteriolopathy (**A** and **B**). Forty weeks after transplantation, typical signs of a toxic arteriolopathy are seen (red staining hyaline deposits in (**A**) in a patient treated with CsA. Discontinuation of CsA therapy resulted in almost complete resolution of the hyaline deposits (**B**). The repeat biopsy was taken 92 weeks after transplantation; it shows arteriolar wall remodeling with structural changes including irregularly arranged medial smooth muscle cells. (**A:** trichrome, ×200; **B:** PAS, ×400.) (Courtesy of Michael Mihatsch, Basel, Switzerland.)

Calcineurin inhibitor-induced TMA is generally an early event occurring within the first few weeks postgrafting (range 2 to 56 days) (896,947,948) with only sporadic cases seen after months (949,950). Although the precise mechanisms are not known, a causal role of CsA is clear in that rechallenge with CsA can precipitate a recurrence (951). In bone marrow recipients, TMA usually presents as a sudden drop in hematocrit and rising creatinine 3 to 12 months after transplantation (952). In kidney transplant recipients, the TMA may be limited to the renal allograft without systemic symptoms, such as hemolysis, schistocytes, or low platelet counts, and present clinically with rapid onset of graft dysfunction (953). Such limited form was observed in 38% of cases (8/21) in one series and associated with 100% graft survival (872). Among reported cases, thrombocytopenia was present in 33% to 64% and hemolytic anemia in 86%; LDH elevation occurred in 95% (948,954). Sometimes TMA-like symptoms can clinically be missed before biopsy if not specifically searched for (948).

The incidence of TMA has been diminishing since CsA was initially introduced (954). CsA-associated thrombotic microangiopathy caused graft loss in 8% of 200 consecutive renal allografts in the early 1980s (accounting for 40% of those that failed) (871). Series of patients from the last 20 years reported an incidence of 0.9% to 14.1% (872,896,948,953,955–957), representing 26% of all cases of thrombotic microangiopathy after renal transplantation (acute rejection, probably humoral, accounted for 53% and recurrent thrombotic microangiopathy for 16%) (955). TMA-like changes have been reported with a prevalence of 1% to 4.7% in patients under tacrolimus therapy (863,866,949).

The treatment of calcineurin inhibitor-induced thrombotic microangiopathies includes the discontinuance or reduction of CsA/tacrolimus (sometimes with switch to sirolimus), and occasionally plasmapheresis, intravenous immunoglobulin, or thrombolytic agents (947,948,957, 958), with an overall graft salvage rate of 80 to 90% (896,947,958). If outcome is stratified into renal limited forms of a TMA and systemic generalized variants, graft survival rates were 100% in the former group (with reduction, temporary discontinuation, or conversion of calcineurin inhibitor therapy) and 62% to 90% in the latter cohort (including plasmapheresis as a treatment option) (872,957). Calcineurin inhibitor induced TMA is (sometimes) fully reversible with the resolution of fibrin thrombi and restitutio ad integrum, as demonstrated in 27% of grafts in one study (Fig. 28.76) (896). Onion skin lesions disappeared in three of three patients in repeat biopsies, and three of five patients showed loss of subendothelial fibrinoid deposits (942). Other studies, however, reported less favorable outcome of a TMA (even in renal limited forms) with an overall graft survival rate of only 69% (953); 30% of patients presenting with a TMA after liver transplantation died (959).

Interestingly, most renal transplant recipients (60 to 90%) tolerate the reintroduction of calcineurin inhibitors following the diagnosis and therapy of a TMA (896,947,957,960–963); 25% were successfully converted to tacrolimus, with an overall salvage rate of 92% (961). It is curious that switching from CsA to tacrolimus is sometimes successful even through both drugs act via very similar pathways (953,956,964). One recipient responded to intraarterial allograft infusion of streptokinase and subsequent systemic heparinization, and recovered normal renal function. Patients with liver transplants have been successfully treated with plasma exchange.

## OTHER DRUG-INDUCED DISEASE IN ALLOGRAFTS

All drugs known to have nephrotoxic side effects in the native kidneys can induce identical changes in the renal allograft (see Chapter 23). Drugs, such as IVIG or hyperimmune globulin solutions (likely because of the high sucrose content), as well as mannitol or dextran can induce isometric vacuolization of tubular epithelial cells (i.e. osmotic nephrosis) very similar to changes seen with calcineurin inhibitor-induced toxic tubulopathies. Here we will provide limited information relevant for the interpretation of kidney transplant specimens.

### Drug-Induced Acute Tubulointerstitial Nephritis

In general, allergic types of interstitial nephrites induced by various drugs (such as trimethaprim-sulfamethoxazole) can cause great problems for the pathologist since the morphologic changes are identical to those seen in cases of tubulointerstitial cellular rejection. This is one reason why acute allergic interstitial nephritis is rarely recognized after kidney transplantation (965). The other reason is that steroids used for immunosuppression inhibit allergic reactions. The temporal relationship between drug administration, the onset of allograft dysfunction and the development of rash, fever, or eosinophilia may provide some clinical clues for differentiating allergic nephritis from rejection.

Both allergic interstitial nephritis and tubulointerstitial rejection demonstrate patchy mononuclear cell infiltrates (often with small clusters of plasma cells) eosinophils in variable numbers, edema, tubulitis, and tubular injury. Acute rejection occasionally has a prominent eosinophilic infiltrate (168,169,171,172,174,402); conversely, drug-induced interstitial nephritis, especially that due to nonsteroidal anti-inflammatory drugs, may have no eosinophils. If the inflammatory cells predominate at the corticomedullary junction/outer medulla (and spare the cortex), allergic interstitial nephritis is most likely (965). The additional detection of ill-formed, small, nonnecrotizing granulomas may serve as a further diagnostic clue in some cases (see Chapter 23). If tubulointerstitial inflammation is accompanied by additional typical signs of rejection, i.e. transplant endarteritis, glomerulitis, C4d accumulation along peritubular capillaries, a diagnosis of rejection must be made. Often, however, it is impossible to make a clear distinction based on morphologic criteria. In those cases, it seems best to error on the side of rejection and initiate antirejection therapy with bolus steroids that will help to decrease all tubulointerstitial inflammatory cell infiltrates and will prevent the long-term detrimental effects of untreated rejection.

## TMA Owing to Anti-CD3 Monoclonal Antibody (OKT 3)

TMA with glomerular thrombosis caused graft loss in 5% of 93 patients who received 10 mg/day prophylactic OKT3 for 2 weeks in one early series (966). An additional four patients had thrombosis of major renal vessels (one arterial, three venous) (967–969). OKT3 stimulates the release of cytokines from T-cells, especially after the first dose. Among the clinically observed effects of this cytokine-release syndrome are fever, chills, dyspnea, diarrhea, rash, and rarely pulmonary edema, hypotension, or aseptic meningitis with seizures. Serum levels of TNFα, IFNγ, IL-2, IL-8, and IL-10 rise (some peak at 1 to 4 hours after the first dose). Monocytes in the presence of T-cells are activated by OKT3 to produce procoagulants (970); increased tissue factor activity appears as early as 2 hours after the first dose (971). Pretreatment with high-dose corticosteroids and anti-inflammatory drugs inhibit the cytokine release and the development of clinical symptoms (972). Cytokine release is also attenuated by the administration of antibodies to TNF α (973). Currently thrombotic microangiopathy induced by OKT3 occurs very infrequently and is distinguishable from other causes only by its close association with the timing of drug therapy.

## Tubular and Other Toxicities of Rapamycin/Sirolimus

Rapamycin (sirolimus, Rapamune) is a newer immunosuppressive agent increasingly used since the late 1990s to permit decreasing steroid and/or calcineurin inhibitor exposure. It potentially limits the development of "chronic allograft nephropathy" by inhibiting the proliferation of mesenchymal cells (974–976). Rapamycin is a macrolide antibiotic that was isolated from *Streptomyces hygroscopicus*. It binds, in conjunction with the FK binding protein, to a protein named mTOR (mammalian target of Rapamycin), a kinase that controls the phosphorylation of proteins and thereby regulates mRNA translation of cell-cycle regulators. Various cytokine and growth factor-stimulated signals for cell proliferation (mainly regulating the progression from Gl to S phase) and for cell differentiation are inhibited (977). Rapamycin blocks via mTOR the production of vascular endothelial growth factor (VEGF), and it can induce endothelial cell death and thrombosis in tumor vessels (978–980). Potentially, alterations of the VEGF expression in podocytes promote the development of proteinuria seen in some patients (981). By immunohistochemistry, mTOR was found ubiquitously in epithelial, mesenchymal, and epithelial renal cells with the highest staining intensity detected in tubular cells of the distal nephron (841). Clinical and pathologic experience with rapamycin is limited at this time.

In 2003 Smith et al (841) reported a new type of tubular injury that they had observed in 55% (12/22) of patients under rapamycin therapy (Fig. 28.82). All of the patients had experienced prolonged episodes of DGF of more than 3 weeks duration without signs of acute rejection. The tubules demonstrated histologic signs of acute injury, intratubular amorphous eosiniophilic cast material with fracture lines, influx of histiocytes, and the formation of multinucleated giant cells, closely resembling myeloma cast nephropathy. However, incontrast to myeloma, the casts contained keratin (remnants of epithelial cells) rather than light chains. Some intratubular casts appeared less developed with eosinophilic bodies, representing necrotic tubular cells and cellular debris. On withdrawal of rapamycin and tacrolimus, resolution of the casts and functional recovery were noted after 2 weeks in three of three patients.

Proteinuria is another side effect attributed to Rapamycin. Reversible proteinuria, which can be in the

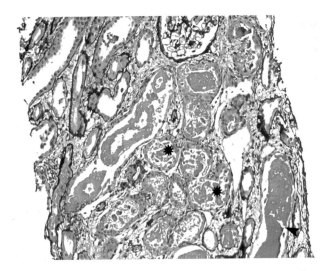

**Figure 28.82** Toxic changes associated with rapamycin therapy. The tubules show signs of acute injury and contain abundant amorphous, proteinaceous cast material, partially coarsely granular (*asterisks*), partially cylindrical with a fracture line (*arrowhead*). (Methenamine silver, ×100.) (Courtesy of Kelly Smith, Seattle, WA.)

nephrotic range, occurs in about 30% of patients (981, 982). One case showed no foot process effacement, arguing of a tubular mechanism (983). This fits with the tubular toxicity noted above and studies of protein overload in the rat, in which Rapamycin increases cast formation (984).

Rapamycin is also associated with thrombotic microangiopathy (873). Four renal allografts from patients on rapamycin (calcineurin inhibitor free) developed TMA. In three patients, the histologic diagnosis of TMA and concurrent cellular rejection was made within 3 months of transplantation; the other patient had TMA in association with chronic rejection (986). On the other hand, rapamycin has been successful in preventing recurrent TMA/HUS (987). Rapamycin can show various other side effects, including leukopenia, anemia and thrombocytopenia, hyperlipidemia, diarrhea, mouth ulcers, cardiac arrythmias, and impaired wound healing (974, 988, 989).

## INFECTIONS

### Polyomavirus Nephropathy (PVN)

Polyomaviruses are double-stranded, non-encapsulated DNA viruses of approximately 5300 base pairs with substantial gene homology. They are ubiquitous and have specifically adapted to their hosts during evolution. Polyomaviruses are of no clinical significance in immune-competent individuals. Disease is only seen in patients with pronounced and long-lasting immunosuppression. The polyomaviruses that are pathogenetic in humans are the BK- and JC strains (the SV40 strain seems to play only a minor role). The BK virus was initially identified by Gardner et al in the urine of "BK," a renal transplant patient from the Sudan with ureteral stenosis (990). Polyomavirus nephropathy (PVN) affecting a kidney transplant was first described as a single case report by Mackenzie et al in 1978 (991). In the 1980s PVN was rarely seen. The clinical scenario changed dramatically in the mid-1990s when high-dose tacrolimus and mycophenolate mofetil were introduced into the routine management of kidney transplant recipients (729,992–996). PVN is currently by far the most important infection involving kidney transplants. The definitive diagnosis of PVN requires a kidney biopsy.

### Pathologic Findings

#### Gross Pathology

Kidneys lost to polyomvirus infections are generally slightly decreased in size, firm with an ill-defined corticomedullary junction and a granular surface. The gross abnormalities are non-specific and similar to changes found in other disease entities associated with fibrosis and atrophy. Infarction and hemorrhage are only seen in cases with concurrent rejection.

### Light Microscopy

Most important for the diagnosis of PVN are virally induced changes in the tubules (Figs. 28.83 and 28.85). Viral replication results in the lysis of inclusion-bearing tubular cells and the denudation of basement membranes (308,729,993,996,997). Despite marked epithelial damage, however, the tubular basement membranes usually remain intact. In exceptional cases, PVN is associated with tubular rupture and the formation of large, non-necrotizing granulomas (personal observation). In addition, parietal epithelial cells lining Bowman's capsule can, on occasion, show signs of viral replication, sometimes in association with the formation of pseudocrescents (729,998). Early cases of PVN may be restricted to the collecting ducts of the medulla. The focal pattern of involvement is an issue for diagnostic accuracy. In one study, 36% of biopsies with multiple cores had cores discordant for virus expression (999).

Four distinct variants of virally induced nuclear changes can be seen (Fig. 28.83) (308,729,997).

> Type 1, the most frequent form, is an amorphous basophilic ground glass inclusion body.
> Type 2, a rare CMV-like type, is a central, eosinophilic, granular inclusion body surrounded by a mostly incomplete halo.
> Type 3 is a finely granular variant without a halo.
> Type 4 is a vesicular variant with clumped, irregular chromatin and occasional nucleoli.

These nuclear changes are, at least in part, caused by different patterns of viral aggregation (i.e. evenly dispersed virions cause type 1 inclusions, and crystalloid aggregates cause types 2 and 4 changes; Fig. 28.84). Most easily discernible are types 1 and 2 inclusion bodies. Types 3 and 4 changes are least specific; similar light microscopic nuclear alterations can also be seen in some cases of tubular injury and regeneration.

Nuclear changes induced by viral replication are found in nearly all the cases of PVN, although they can be limited to collecting ducts in the medulla. PVN typically shows a focal distribution pattern. Often infected tubules containing many inclusion-bearing epithelial cells are located adjacent to normal ducts (Fig. 28.85A and B). Rarely light microscopically discernible inclusions are absent (in our experience less than 3% of cases), presumably representing very early stages of PVN prior to the development of typical nuclear changes. The replication of polyomaviruses does not induce any cytoplasmic inclusion bodies.

*Interstitium.* PVN is associated with varying degrees of interstitial inflammation and fibrosis that are incorporated into the staging of the disease (999–1003) (Table 28.16 and Fig. 28.85). During the early phases of PVN (stage A), the interstitium is normal or only shows minimal inflammation.

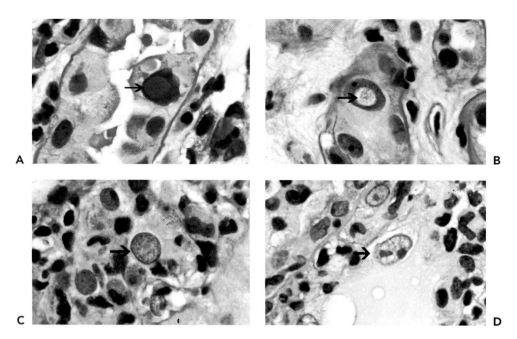

**Figure 28.83** Polyomavirus nephropathy (A–D). Viral replication in epithelial cells can induce different nuclear changes: (A) an amorphous ground glass inclusion body (type 1); (B) a central irregular inclusion body surrounded by a halo (type 2); (C) finely granular nuclear alterations (type 3); (D) vesicular changes (type 4). (A–C: PAS; D: H&E, ×600.)

Florid PVN (stage B) is characterized by marked tubular injury, denudation of the tubular basement membranes, and interstitial edema with a mixed mild to marked inflammatory cell infiltrate (B and T lymphocytes and plasma cells). Neutrophils can be prominent adjacent to severely injured tubules. Inflammation is associated with tubulitis (occa-

sionally plasma cell tubulitis). The sclerosing late phase of PVN (stage C) is characterized by marked fibrosis and tubular atrophy.

No lesions are seen in glomeruli or vessels, except for occasional viral inclusions in the parietal epithelium and small crescents. Signs of a productive polyomavirus

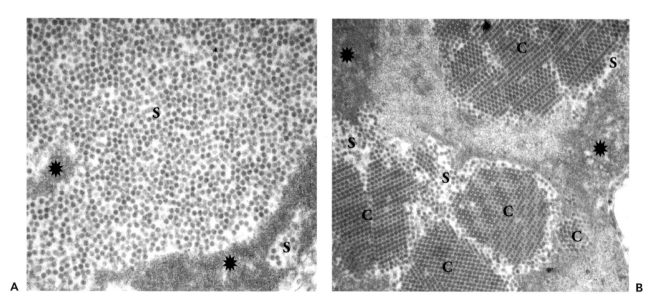

**Figure 28.84** Ultrastructurally polyomaviruses (30 to 50 nm in diameter) are found in nuclei as single viral particles (S) or in crystalloid arrays (C) surrounded by chromatin (*asterisks*). Changes illustrated in (A) are the ultrastructural correlate for amorphous ground glass type of inclusions (compare with Fig. 28.83A); crystalloid viral aggregrates (B) can be associated with types 2 and 4 nuclear changes (compare with Fig. 28.83B and D).

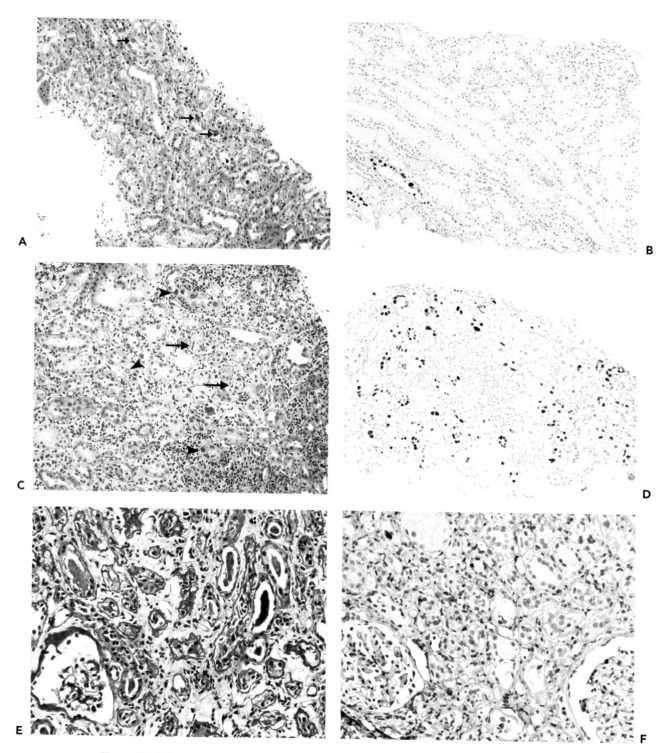

**Figure 28.85** Histologic stages of polyomavirus nephropathy (**A–F**). Stage A (early phase, **A** and **B**) with only few intranuclear inclusion bodies (*arrows* in **A**) and minimal tubular injury (**A** and **B**); the interstitium is without significant changes. Stage B (florid phase, **C** and **D**) with marked viral replication (*arrowheads* in **C**) involving many tubules (**D**), severe tubular injury, and focal denudation of tubular basement membranes (*arrows* in **C**). There is a diffuse inflammatory cell infiltrate in the interstitium and associated tubulitis. Stage C (sclerosing phase, **E** and **F**) with marked interstitial fibrosis and tubular atrophy. Immunohistochemistry (**F**) demonstrates only very focal evidence of viral replication with scattered positive (brown) staining signals in tubular nuclei. (**A, C,** and **E:** H&E and PAS, ×100, ×200, ×250; **B, D,** and **F:** immunohistochemistry to detect the SV-40T antigen shows intranuclear staining in epithelial cells, ×100 and ×250.) (Images **A, B, E,** and **F** are from repeat biopsies of the same patient taken 10 weeks apart.)

**TABLE 28.16**

### HISTOLOGIC STAGES OF POLYOMAVIRUS NEPHROPATHY[a] (999–1003)

**Stage A (Early)**
- Viral activation in cortex and/or medulla with intranuclear inclusion *and/or* positive immunohistochemistry or in situ hybridization
- Minimal tubular epithelial cell lysis
- No denudation of tubular basement membrane (TBM)
- Minimal interstitial inflammation
- Minimal tubular atrophy and interstitial fibrosis (≤10%)

**Stage B (Florid)**
- Marked viral activation in cortex and/or medulla
- Marked virus induced tubular epithelial cell necrosis/lysis and associated denudation of TBM
- Interstitial inflammation (mild to marked)[b]
- Interstitial fibrosis and tubular atrophy (minimal to moderate, ≤50%)
  - *Stage B1 ≤25% of biopsy cores involved*
  - *Stage B2 >25% and <50% of biopsy cores involved*
  - *Stage B3 ≥50% of biopsy cores involved (if interstitial fibrosis and tubular atrophy >50%: stage C)*

**Stage C (Late)**
- Viral activation in cortex and medulla
- Interstitial fibrosis and tubular atrophy >50% of cortex[c]
- Tubular epithelial cell necrosis/lysis and TBM denudation
- Interstitial inflammation (minimal to marked)

[a]Additional signs of BK virus activation are always present such as decoy cells in the urine, BK virus DNA, RNA in the serum and urine, or free virions in the urine by negative-staining electron microscopy.
[b]Interstitial inflammation and tubulitis can in some cases mark concurrent tubulointerstitial cellular rejection; rejection-induced changes are not part of the scoring of polyomavirus nephropathy.
[c]Interpreted to be mostly secondary to protracted virus-induced tubular injury.

infection are also found in the transitional cell layer lining the renal pelvis, the ureters, and/or the urinary bladder (729), where marked inflammation and even ulceration may occur.

### Immunofluorescence and Immunohistochemistry

Polyomavirus is readily detected with commercially available antibodies to the SV-40 T antigen (large T antigen) that cross-react with all polyomaviruses pathogenic in humans (i.e. BK-, JC-, and SV-40) and work in paraffin sections (Fig. 28.85). Because the polyoma T antigen is expressed in abundance only during the early stages of intranuclear viral replication, some types 1 or 4 inclusion-bearing cells representing late phases of virus assembly can be negative by immuno-histochemistry. Furthermore, the expression of the polyoma T antigen precedes the formation of intranuclear viral inclusion bodies, and consequently, a positive staining reaction may be detected in normal-appearing nuclei (308,729,997,1002). Crisp nuclear polyoma T-antigen staining always indicates clinically significant viral replica-

tion and may be the first sign of PVN. Viral replication can also be detected by in situ hybridization or with antibodies directed against outer capsid proteins.

In some patients, PVN is associated with focal granular deposits along tubular basement membranes (staining by immunofluorescence microscopy with various antibodies directed against immunoglobulins and complement factors; Fig. 28.86) (571). In our experience tubular deposits seem to be rare, and they are of undetermined clinical significance. In PVN the complement degradation product C4d is not detected along peritubular capillaries (its presence indicates PVN and a concurrent acute rejection episode) (348). Viral replication in tubular cells is not associated with marked tubular expression of MHC class II (HLA-DR) (308).

### Electron Microscopy

Polyomaviruses present as viral particles 30 to 50 nm in diameter, occasionally forming crystalloid structures (Fig. 28.84). Virions are primarily found in the nucleus, rarely in the cytoplasm. Rare cases of PVN show focal immune complex type deposits along tubular basement membranes with currently undetermined clinical significance (571).

### Etiology and Pathogenesis

PVN is typically caused by activation and replication of the polyoma-BK-virus strain. Only a minotiry of cases (approximately one-third) show activation of BK- and JC-viruses simultaneously with undetermined clinical significance. Nephropathies only induced by JC- or SV-40 viruses are exceptionally rare (1004a,1004b,1004c,1004d).

Polyoma-BK-virus is ubiquitous and rarely causes disease, except in immunodeficient hosts. A renal transplant per se predisposes to PVN, as inferred from the rarity of PVN in similarly immunosuppressed recipients of non-kidney organs (1006). This might be related either to increased renal injury (ischemia, rejection, obstruction) or the lack of self-MHC on the tubular cells (viral sanctuary) in renal allografts.

After a primary infection with polyomaviruses, which occurs in most individuals early in life, the viruses establish lifelong latency in renal tubular and urothelial cells (1007–1010). Latent viruses can only be detected with molecular techniques (e.g. PCR or southern blot analysis). PVN in kidney transplants is probably caused by the reactivation of dormant BK viruses in the urothelium and/or renal parenchyma of the donor organ (308,729,1010–1012). However, risk factors for PVN are incompletely understood (1001). Intense and long lasting immunosuppression, often with tacrolimus and/or mycophenolate-mofetil, plays an important role for the promotion of disease (i.e. the reactivation of latent BK viruses), but it constitutes only one aspect in a multifactorial scenario

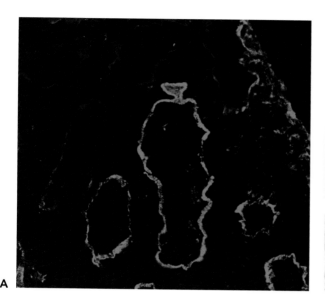
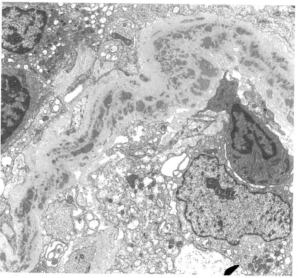

**Figure 28.86** Polyomavirus nephropathy with focal immune complex–type deposits along tubular basement membranes; this finding is of undetermined clinical significance at the present time. **A:** Immunofluorescence microscopy with an antibody directed against IgG demonstrates granular deposits along some tubular basement membranes. (×400.) **B:** Electron microscopy from the same case shows immune complex–type deposits in the TBM. (×10,000.)

(308,992,1014,1015). Good animal models of PVN are currently not available. A closely related polyomavirus that was incidentally detected in non human primates can cause lesions similar to human PVN, with interstitial nephritis of either the native or the transplanted kidney, ureteral stenosis, and graft loss (1016).

Polyomaviruses adhere to their host cells via binding of viral capsid proteins to cell-surface receptors (involving an N-linked glycoprotein containing α (2,3)-linked sialic acid) (1017). After cell entry via caveola-mediated endocytosis (1018), viral particles diffuse through the cytoplasm/microtubules (1019) and the nuclear pores into the host cell nucleus. The host cell is subsequently reprogrammed to produce viral particles; daughter virions are assembled in the nucleus (1005). Ultimately host cells are lysed and mature daughter virions are released.

## Differential Diagnosis

Although the histologic changes are characteristic for PVN, other viral infections caused by herpes simplex virus, adenovirus, or cytomegalovirus must be considered in the differential diagnosis (Table 28.17). Diagnostic confirmation of PVN is achieved by immunohistochemistry with antibodies directed against the T antigen or against VP capsid proteins. In situ hybridization and/or electron microscopy may also provide diagnostic evidence. Additionally, PCR techniques may be used to demonstrate viral DNA or RNA in tissue samples and to confirm the diagnosis of PVN (730,1020,1021). However, PCR results must be interpreted with great caution. Only high levels of viral

DNA (greater than 10 to 50 BK virus copies per cell equivalent), in the setting of histologically or immunohistochemiecallly demonstrable virally induced nuclear changes, can be used to distinguish clinically significant productive from clinically insignificant latent polyomavirus infections (730,1007,1008,1010,1020,1022). PVN is practically never seen in association with a concurrent second viral infection of the kidney. We are only aware of two anecdotal cases, both of which showed dominant activation of either adenovirus (1023) or CMV (1024) and only focal evidence of PVN.

The diagnosis of acute rejection in the setting of PVN is challenging. PVN is associated with varying degrees of interstitial inflammation that can in some instances represent concurrent acute rejection (308,997,1001,1025–1027). Rejection should be diagnosed if transplant endarteritis, transplant glomerulitis, or C4d along peritubular capillaries are found (1027). IHC phenotyping of the inflammatory cells in PVN has shown plasma cell (CD138), B- (CD20), or T-cell (CD3)–dominant infiltrates, so that IHC is not diagnostically helpful (1028–1030).

## Clinical Presentation, Prognosis, and Therapy

PVN is generally limited to the kidney graft and can present with renal dysfunction 6 days to 6 years post transplantation (mean: 380 days) (997,1031,1032). Signs of a generalized infection (e.g. fever) are lacking; only one reported exception had multiorgan involvement (1033). Hematuria and proteinuria are typically absent. In renal allograft recipients PVN has a prevalence of 1% to

**TABLE 28.17**

## DIFFERENTIAL DIAGNOSIS OF SELECTED VIRAL LESIONS IN ALLOGRAFTS

| | BK-Virus | Cytomegalovirus | Adenovirus | EBV-PTLD |
|---|---|---|---|---|
| Viral inclusion type | | | | |
| Smudgy | ++ | + | ++ | − |
| Homogeneous with halo | + | +++ | + | − |
| Sites of viral replication | | | | |
| Tubular epithelial cells | +++ | +++ · | +++ | − |
| Endothelial cells | − | ++ | − | − |
| Mononuclear cells | − | + | ± | +++ |
| Acute tubular injury | +/+++ | +/++ | +++ | ± |
| Focal necrosis | − | ± | ++/+++ | ±/+ |
| Interstitial hemorrhage | − | − | + | − |
| Granuloma formation | −[a] | ± | +/++ | − |
| Interstitial inflammation | −/++ | +/++ | +++ | +++ |

[a]Productive polyomavirus infections of the kidney only very rarely show nonnecrotizing epithelioid granulomas.
From Singh HK, Nickeleit V. Kidney disease caused by viral infections. Curr Diag Pathol 2004;10:11.

9% largely dependent on the administered immunosuppressive drug regimens (6.5% at The University of North Carolina in Chapel Hill and less than 2% at the Massachusetts General Hospital). In disease stage A, kidney function can be normal and the diagnosis may be first made in a protocol biopsy (759). PVN stage A is diagnosed early (8.7 months post transplantation versus 15.9 months for stages B and C) (1033) and responds to therapy with favorable long-term graft function and survival (759,997,999,1025,1026,1034). In one series 11/14 patients (78%), in whom viral nephropathy had been diagnosed early, cleared the virus after 23 months of follow-up (1034).

Antiviral treatment strategies include reduction of the immunosuppression, potentially combined with leflunomide or low dose cidofovir therapy (999,1001,1038–1041). PVN and concurrent acute rejection episodes can respond to transient anti-rejection and subsequent antiviral therapy (i.e. two-step approach) as illustrated in anecdotal cases (308,997,1001,1003,1025–1027). Graft failure rates, especially if PVN is diagnosed late (disease stages B or C) or treatment strategies fail, can reach 50% to 80% within 24 months (1001,1014,1032,1042,1043). In one series, progression from stage B to stage C was observed in 60% of diagnostic follow-up biopsies (1044). If kidney grafts are lost because of progressive viral nephropathy, retransplantation is an option. Small case series have provided encouraging results: recurrent PVN was seen in only approximately 12% of all repeat allografts (1035–1037).

Overall improved graft survival has been reported with vigorous patient screening programs that facilitate

an early diagnosis and intervention (308,997,1001,1003, 1025,1026,1045,1046). Renal allograft recipients at risk for PVN can be identified by detecting signs of polyomavirus activation in the urine and/or plasma. All patients with PVN show high numbers of polyomavirus inclusion-bearing cells in the urine, so-called decoy cells (Fig. 28.87) (308,729,992,993,1000,1025,1047–1049). Decoy cells, presumably mostly of urothelial origin, indicate the

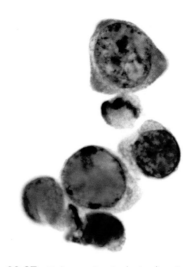

**Figure 28.87** Polyomavirus inclusion bearing cells (so-called decoy cells) in the urine. Decoy cells show glassy appearing intranuclear viral inclusion bodies, sometimes interspersed with dense, granular material. They are a morphologic sign of the activation of polyomaviruses and likely mostly originate from the urothelium. (Liquid-based urine cytology preparation, Papanicolaou, ×600.)

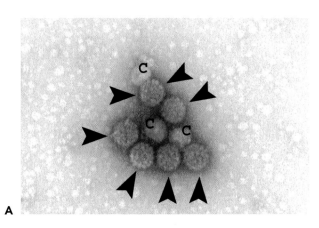

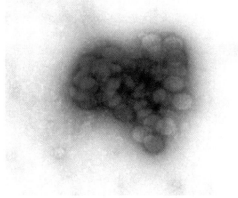

**A**                                                    **B**

**Figure 28.88** Negative-staining electron microscopy on urine samples to detect polyomaviruses. In patients with significant activation of polyomaviruses, free viral particles (*arrowheads* in **A**) are easily detected in urine samples (note the characteristic regular capsid proteins on the surface of the viruses); virions are sometimes adherent to cell fragments (labeled C). Patients with PVN characteristically shed large three-dimensional viral aggregates, so-called "Haufen" (**B**), sometimes resembling casts. (**A**: ×100,000; **B**: ×80,000.)

activation of polyomaviruses in the urogenital tract, but not necessarily PVN. The detection of more than ten decoy cells per ThinPrep slide has an excellent negative predictive value of more than 99% but a positive predictive value of only 27% (308,1049). Also quantitative urine PCR analyses and negative staining electron microscopy on urine samples can show evidence of polyomavirus activation (Fig. 28.88) (994,1001,1050–1052). Quantitative plasma PCR tests have the highest positive predictive value for PVN; plasma viral load levels exceeding 10,000 copies/ml predict disease with more than 80% probability (999,1001,1025,1052,1053). However, thus far quantitative PCR tests have not been standardized and the proposed viral load cutoff levels have not been validated in large multicenter studies. We have occasionally diagnosed PVN in patients with low plasma viral load levels (<3000 copies/ml). Potentially, in the future, the detection of three dimensional polyomavirus aggregates (so-called "Haufen") in the urine by electron microscopy (Fig. 28.88B) can help to diagnose PVN more accurately. In our preliminary experience "Haufen" have a positive predictive value for PVN of greater than 95% and a negative predictive value of greater than 99% (personal observation).

## Cytomegalovirus (CMV)

Cytomegalovirus (CMV), a herpesvirus, is one of the most common pathogens in renal transplant recipients, typically causing a symptomatic infection in the first 2 to 3 months after transplantation, manifested by fever, leukopenia, viremia, and hepatitis or pneumonitis (334) and direct kidney injury in approximately 25% to 30% of symptomatic patients (1054,1055). Effective patient screening and clinical management strategies have made productive CMV infections of the transplanted kidney

exceedingly rare, and we have seen only exceptionally few cases over the last years (in comparison, a polyomavirus nephropathy is currently approximately 50 times more common in western countries). In contrast, CMV nephropathy seems to be more often seen in other parts of the world. A recent series from India reported a prevalence of 1.9% (6 of 321 allograft recipients monitored between 1997 and 2002) (1031).

Lesions induced by the replication of CMV in the kidneys have been described in renal transplants and native kidneys (1054,1055). Cytopathic changes are typically very focal and most often seen in the nuclei and cytoplasm of tubular epithelial cells, sometimes in endothelial cells, and only occasionally in mononuclear inflammatory cells (1054,1055). CMV-infected cells are typically enlarged with nuclei containing a central round inclusion body surrounded by a circumferential halo, i.e. the typical owl's eye appearance. Also homogenous smudgy-appearing intranuclear inclusions are occasionally observed (Table 28.17) Small basophilic lumpy cytoplasmic viral inclusions are frequently (but not always) detected in cells with virally induced intranuclear changes (1054). The replication of CMV in the tubular compartment can be associated with a nodular, sometimes granulomatous-appearing, mononuclear inflammatory cell infiltrate. Interstitial inflammation was absent in two of six cases of CMV nephropathy in one series (1055). Foci of necrosis and microabscesses can occur but are uncommon (1055). Rarely, CMV infects glomerular cells and causes an acute glomerulonephritis with crescents (1056–1059); in one exceptional case, CMV replication was limited to glomerular endothelial cells and not accompanied by inflammation (1058).

Diagnostic confirmation of a productive CMV infection can easily be achieved by immunohistochemistry (e.g. with an antibody directed against the immediate early antigen), in situ hybridization, or by electron microscopy. Ultrastructurally, virions of approximately 150 nm in diameter are found in nuclei and the cytoplasm, often with a central electron-dense core surrounded by an envelope. Immunofluorescence microscopy with a standard panel of antibodies detecting immunoglobulins and complement factors is unrevealing (only sometimes minute glomerular IgG deposits are seen) (1054).

CMV genome was detected by in situ hybridization in the tubular epithelium in about 40% of renal allografts, independent of whether the patient had an active CMV infection at the time (1060). CMV genome is found in the absence of cytopathic changes, and PCR or in situ hybridization studies cannot clearly distinguish between productive and latent infections (1061). Thus, it seems doubtful whether the use of highly sensitive techniques (such as tissue CMV-PCR) really demonstrates a higher prevalence of CMV disease as suggested by some (1062). The minimal criteria to establish the diagnosis of CMV nephropathy should include the demonstration of cytopathic changes, or CMV proteins or mRNA; not just the CMV genome. Once typical cytomegalic changes are histologically noted, the diagnosis is established; it can easily be confirmed in ancillary tests. The differential diagnosis of CMV nephropathy includes other types of viral infections, mainly caused by polyomaviruses or adenovirus (see above; Table 28.17). Since CMV (in contrast to polyomavirus and adenovirus) replicates in endothelial and inflammatory cells, a distinction between rejection-induced changes and infection-driven inflammation is difficult.

CMV infections can stimulate indirect effects on the kidney graft by modulating the immune response and possibly promoting rejection episodes (334). Older reports had described acute allograft glomerulopathy caused by severe CMV infections (144); these glomerular changes are now classified as rejection-induced transplant glomerulopathy. The most convincing evidence that CMV indirectly causes graft injury is reported by Reinke et al (1063), who showed that 85% of patients with late acute rejection responded to ganciclovir therapy. The outcome with conventional immunosuppression was considerably worse, with 80% graft failure at 1 year. The patients had no symptoms of a CMV infection/disease, although virus was detectable in the blood in 80% by PCR and in 42% by the antigenemia test.

## Adenovirus

Productive adenovirus infections of renal allografts are exceptionally rare, however, the incidence may be increasing (1064). Adenovirus infections show a focal necrotizing tubulointerstitial nephritis, as shown originally in native kidneys (1023,1065–1069). The characteristic changes are viral inclusions in tubular epithelial cell nuclei (mostly of the ground glass type); severe tubular destruction with rupture of TBM and foci of necrosis; a marked interstitial mononuclear and plasma cell infiltrate, often nodular and sometimes granulomatous; and focal interstitial hemorrhage and intratubular red blood cell casts (1070,1071) (Fig. 28.89 and Table 28.17). Neutrophils are abundant in areas of necrosis, and even large, wedge-shaped cortical infarcts can occur. Viral replication induces cytopathic changes in tubular epithelial cell nuclei that commonly appear enlarged with smudgy ground glass inclusions. Intranuclear viral inclusion bodies are occasionally surrounded by a clear halo (1023,1065). Glomeruli and blood vessels are generally not affected, except for rare cases with viral cytopathic changes in the parietal epithelium lining Bowman's capsule (1023). Immunohistochemistry with antibodies to adenovirus antigens easily identifies viral particles in tubular cell nuclei, as well as the cytoplasm (Fig. 28.89D). Ultrastructurally virions of approximately 75–80 nanometers are found in nuclei and the cytoplasm. In addition free viral particles can typically be detected in the urine by negative staining electron microscopy. Immunofluorescence microscopy with antibodies to immunoglobulins and complement factors is unremarkable. The complement degradation product C4d is in our experience not found along peritubular capillaries.

Adenovirus replication (versus PVN or CMV) can usually be suspected by light microscopy based on (a) frank tubular destruction with foci of necrosis, (b) granulomatous inflammation with palisading of macrophages around severely injured tubules, and (c) interstitial hemorrhage (Table 28.16). Very rarely, both PVN and productive adenovirus infections occur together (1 in 14 patients in one report) (1023). Most patients with adenovirus nephritis have a surprisingly rapid improvement of renal function and a good long-term prognosis (1066–1069,1072). In one patient, clearance of adenovirus was documented in a repeat graft biopsy taken 26 days after onset of the disease (1073).

## Acute Pyelonephritis

Pyelonephritis is an uncommon but potentially devastating complication of transplantation. Of 1100 consecutive transplants, 1.6% of patients developed acute pyelonephritis; females account for 93% of cases (1074). The presence of vesicoureteral reflux is a significant risk factor (1075) in native kidneys. Patients who develope end-stage renal disease from pyelonephritis are also at a higher risk for disease recurrence post transplantation (1074).

Pyelonephritis can present as acute renal failure (1076,1077) and cause graft loss (1078,1080). It arises most often 1 year or more after transplantation (80% of episodes) (1074). *E. coli* is the most common organism (80%). Rare cases of fatal emphysematous pyelonephritis, owing to gas-producing organisms, have developed even in non-diabetic recipients (1079). Other notable infections that have been described include perinephric abscesses

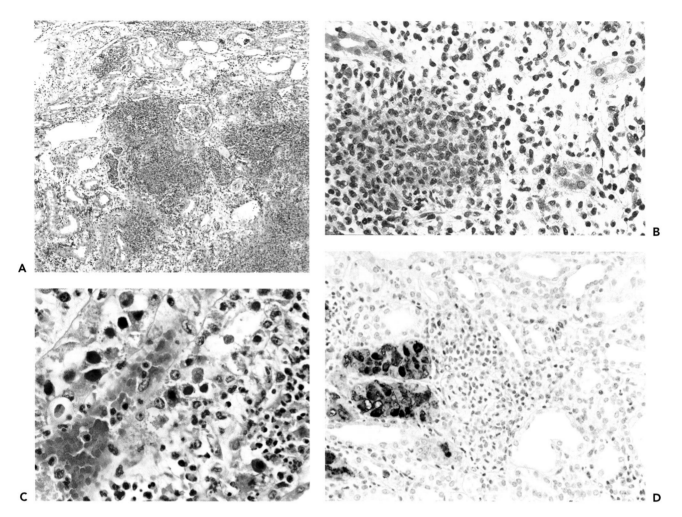

**Figure 28.89** Adenovirus infection. Characteristic for an adenovirus infection is a focal necrotizing tubulointerstitial nephritis (**A**) that may show occasional small granulomas (**B**). On high power examination (**C**) adenovirus infections demonstrate ground glass type intranuclear viral inclusion bodies in tubular epithelial cells, tubular destruction and necrosis, and interstitial hemorrhage. Immunohistochemistry to detect adenovirus antigens (**D**) reveals intranuclear and cytoplasmic staining in tubular epithelial cells (**A, B,** and **C**; H&E, ×40, ×200, and ×400; **D**: Immunohistochemistry to detect adenovirus antigens ×200.)

owing to anaerobic bacteria (1080), pyelitis with obstructive uropathy owing to *Corynebacterium urealyticum* (with negative routine cultures) (1081), "acute lobar nephronia" (acute focal bacterial pyelonephritis presenting as a renal mass radiologically) (1082), fungal and cryptococcal pyelonephritis (1083).

Acute pyelonephritis can be demonstrated on renal biopsy, despite the expectation that the process is patchy in distribution (1076). The diagnosis should be raised by the pathologist when intratubular neutrophils are present, often forming casts. Neutrophils are typically also found between tubular epithelial cells and in the adjacent edematous interstitium. The complement degradation product C4d is characteristically not detected along peritubular capillaries (differential diagnosis: humoral rejection; see above).

## SURGICAL AND MISCELLANEOUS COMPLICATIONS

### Ureteral Obstruction/Leak/Reflux

The proximal ureter derives its blood supply from the renal pelvic vessels and is therefore at risk for ischemic injury after transplantation because of devascularization at time of harvest. Furthermore, the ureterovesical surgical anastomosis must be functional to prevent leakage or reflux. Urine leak can also arise from the ureteropelvic anastomosis. Urologic complications occurred in 6.8% of 1183 consecutive renal transplants performed with bladder anastomoses using various surgical techniques, usually in the first 4 months (84%) (1085). The most common problems were ureterovesical obstruction (4.1%), anastomotic leak (1.0%), and ureteropelvic obstruction (0.4%). Ureteral necrosis was seen in 3.2% of cases (52 of 1629) in another series (1086). These complications are generally treated with temporary percutaneous nephrostomy, dilatation stent placement, or surgical reanastomosis; they rarely cause graft loss (0.1%) (1085) and do not impact 10-year patient or graft survival (1086). Postoperative hematuria from bleeding at the site of the ureteral reimplantation site, symptomatic lymphocele formation, and urinary fistula resulting from necrosis of the distal ureter are other well-known problems occurring postgrafting (1087). Only very limited data are available on histologic changes of injured ureters. In 25 surgically removed necrotic ureteral segments, vascular thrombosis of periureteral vessels was by far the most common observation (80%) followed by signs of productive CMV (16%) and BK virus infections (8%) (1086). Whether CMV or BK viruses played a causative role in the development of ureteral necrosis was undetermined. Although ureteral stenosis is mostly a surgical complication, ureteral ischemia and fibrosis can also be caused by severe rejection episodes with transplant endarteritis involving not only intrarenal but also ureteral graft vessels (563).

## Lymphocele

Lymphoceles are collections of lymphatic fluid (i.e., nonsanguinous and nonpurulent) in the perinephric space. Most lymphoceles are small, clinically insignificant, and detected only by ultrasound. Large lymphoceles can cause obstruction or complications owing to infection (1088). The fluid usually derives from the renal lymphatics at the hilum that are not reanatomosed with the recipient lymphatics during surgery. Intrarenal lymph flow increases during rejection episodes because of increased vascular permeability and intraparencymal edema formation, thereby promoting the formation of lymphoceles. Among 386 consecutive renal transplants, 35 lymphoceles greater than 50 mL were detected by ultrasonography 2 to 11 years posttransplantation, one third of which were associated with rejection episodes (1088). In a more recent analysis involving more than 500 patients, 34% demonstrated lymphoceles greater than 2.5 cm in diameter, and 16% required therapeutic intervention. The highest prevalence was noted in patients treated wih drug regimens containing rapamycin (nearly half of them [45%] had perinephric fluid collections). Other risk factors were obesity and rejection episodes (1089). Lymphoceles often recur; however, long-term graft survival is unaffected.

## Arterial or Venous Thrombosis

Arterial and/or venous thromboses of hilar vessels are caused by technical problems with the anastomoses or a hypercoagulable state. They typically develop early posttransplantation and are limited to the large vessels; smaller intraparencymal arteries and glomeruli are characteristically spared. Thrombus formation in large hilar vessels can cause delayed graft function (DGF), anuria, and potentially infarction. Acute renal vein thrombosis usually presents as sudden pain in the transplant, graft swelling, hematuria, and proteinuria (1090,1091).

The incidence of large vessel thrombosis varies considerably by transplant center. Among 558 consecutive deceased donor kidney recipients, the prevalence of primary renal graft thrombosis was 6% (1.9% arterial, 3.4% venous, and 0.7% both) (1092). In another series, renal artery thrombosis was seen in 0.4% and renal vein thrombosis in 0.1% of patients (1093). The risk factors include surgical technical problems, a history of venous thrombosis and the antiphospholipid syndrome, diabetic nephropathy, the recipient's hemodynamic status perioperatively, right vs left donor kidney (1092), and placement of the graft on the left side (1094,1095).

Thromboses owing to surgical complications have to be distinguished from acute rejection (Banff II and III). The former are limited to the renal artery and/or vein, even in cases of graft infarction. Vascular rejection episodes, on the other hand, do not affect veins, but rather, large and small intraparenchymal arteries and glomerular capillaries with thrombus formation, fibrinoid necrosis, and inflammation. Thrombi in rejection are unevenly distributed in the graft (because of the unimpaired fibrinolytic capacity of the recipient). Cases of acute rejection with thrombosis are nearly always antibody mediated and associated with the deposition of the complement degradation product C4d along peritubular capillaries of the cortex and/or medulla; C4d is not seen in cases of surgical complications. However, C4d is negative in areas of necrosis, even when owing to antibody-mediated rejection.

## Arterial Stenosis

Renal artery stenosis in the transplant recipient, which presents with hypertension and renal dysfunction, can masquerade as rejection or it can be clinically overlooked (1096,1097). Renal artery stenosis is relatively common, and seen in 1% to 23% of patients. Variable incidence rates reflect differences in diagnostic criteria and surgical expertise (1097). Most of the cases are diagnosed between 3 months and 24 months post surgery. Patients are usually treated with percutaneous angioplasty, resulting in a significant although sometimes only transient improvement of blood flow (1097). In one series, the frequency of rejection episodes was twice as high in patients with renal artery stenosis, raising the possibility that transplant endarteritis involving major hilar arteries may have contributed to arterial remodeling and stenosis (1098). The pathology in the kidney is expected to show ischemic atrophy (small, simplified tubules with little interstitial fibrosis). However, we have seen two recent cases

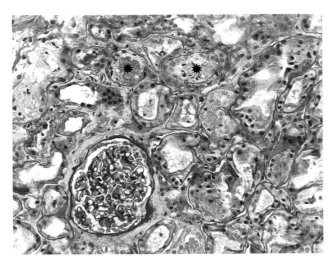

**Figure 28.90** A patient with central renal artery stenosis and persistent allograft dysfunction shows focal acute tubular injury and intratubular proteinaceous cast material (*asterisk*). (PAS, ×150.)

that demonstrated protracted acute tubular injury over several months (Fig. 28.90). Acute changes, i.e. ATN (versus the expected atrophy) may relate to intermittent, variable stenosis.

## Graft Rupture

The classic symptoms of allograft rupture are the sudden onset of severe pain, swelling over the allograft, oliguria, and hypotension. Almost all cases (96%) occur within 3 weeks of transplantation (1099). Graft rupture has occasionally been misinterpreted clinically as renal artery thrombosis (1099). The frequency in published reports ranges from 4.1% (1099,1100) to 0.35% in a recent series of 1682 living donor organs (1101). The usual cause of graft rupture is rejection (accounting for approximately two thirds of the cases), followed by ATN (seen in one quarter), renal vein thrombosis (in approximately 10%), and trauma (diagnosed in only a few instances) (1099–1103). Rupture is an indication for immediate surgical intervention, which can result in graft salvage in about 50% of patients; untreated cases are associated with a high fatality rate (1101,1102).

## DE NOVO AND RECURRENT RENAL DISEASES

Virtually all acquired glomerular diseases known to occur in native kidneys have been detected in renal allografts as de novo or recurrent diseases. Renal transplantation illuminates the early morphologic events during the development of renal diseases, and it can on occasion document the reversibility of pre-existing donor diseases such as early diabetic changes or glomerular IgA deposits. The histologic

criteria to establish the diagnoses are identical to those described in native kidneys, although the clinical course of the patients may differ because of the baseline immunosuppressive drug regimens administered to prevent allograft rejection. Glomerular diseases occurring after transplantation can be superimposed on other changes such as rejection or calcineurin inhibitor–induced toxicity. Indeed, proteinuria in a renal allograft recipient, particularly years after transplantation, is most often a manifestion of chronic allograft nephropathy (60%) rather than recurrent (15%) or de novo (10%) glomerulonephritis (1104).

### De Novo Glomerular Diseases

Three de novo glomerular diseases have special significance to the allograft: membranous glomerulopathy, anti-GBM disease, and recurrent nephrotic syndrome in congenital nephrosis, because the lesions are probably caused by alloantibodies to donor antigens. The fourth, FSGS, is quite common in allografts and has diverse causes.

### Membranous Glomerulopathy (MGN)

De novo MGN in allografts has frequently been reported in patients with stable transplant function (1105–1113). The patients typically present about 2 years after transplantation (range 1 month to more than 10 years) with proteinuria in the nephrotic range, although proteinuria may sometimes be minimal (1107,1109). Light microscopy often shows rather mild GBM changes accompanied by nonspecific mesangial hypercellularity in about 33% of biopsies. The diagnosis can usually be established only by typical immunofluorescence, immunohistochemical, and/or electron microscopic findings. By electron microscopy, the deposits tend to be smaller and more irregular in distribution than in primary MGN; spike formation is often inconspicuous (1112), likely because of an early stage of the disease development. GBM changes of concurrent transplant glomerulopathy with duplication of the basement membranes are present in up to 50% of cases (1112,1114). Repeat biopsies have shown persistence or progression of the deposits in most patients (1109,1114); the resolution of deposits is rare. Most cases of MGN in renal allografts occurr de novo (83% to 90%), often years after surgery (1108,1111,1115,1116). The overall prevalence (de novo and recurrent MGN) is about 0.3% to 2.1% among adult transplant patients in large series (16 of 4913, 19 of 1500, and 21 of 1029 allograft recipients) (1105,1108,1117). The risk for MGN seems to be increased in pediatric kidney transplant recipients (9% in one series of 530 grafts, [1109,1118]).

No specific therapy is effective in cases of posttransplant MGN. CsA does not increase or decrease the frequency of de novo MGN, and steroids seem to have little effect on the disease development. The long-term graft outcome is not different for patients with and without de novo MGN (1105,1106,1108).

Of particular note: de novo MGN can also be associated with a hepatitis C infection (1119). In one series, 18% of allograft biopsies from infected patients had signs of MGN and decreased overall graft survival (1120).

## Anti-GBM Glomerulonephritis in Alport's Syndrome

The common X-linked form of Alport's syndrome is characterized by a genetic defect in the $\alpha5$ chain of type IV collagen encoded on the X chromosome (COL4A5). The $\alpha5$ chain is necessary for the phenotypic expression of the $\alpha3$ (IV) chain in the GBM, whose 26 kd NC1 terminal domain is the usual autoantigen of anti-GBM nephritis. Alport's kidneys fail to express the autoantigen of Goodpasture's syndrome (1124), and thus Alport's patients may lack self-tolerance to certain $\alpha$ chains of type IV collagen. Those can be recognized as a foreign antigen after transplantation and trigger an immune response (1125–1127). Indeed, in one series, after transplantation all 21 patients with Alport's disease developed varying titers of antibodies directed against the $\alpha3$, $\alpha4$, and $\alpha5$ chains of collagen type IV that were associated with linear IgG deposits along glomerular capillary walls in 13 of 21 graft recipients (evaluated by immunofluorescence microscopy). Evidence of a post transplant anti-GBM nephritis was found in 10 of 21 patients, all with signs of linear IgG deposits (1127). Other series showed linear glomerular IgG deposits without glomerulonephritis in approximately 10% of kidney transplant recipients suffering from Alport's syndrome (1128–1130). The 5-year graft survival in these latter patients was equal to that of controls (1128,1131). The reason why anti-GBM disease develops only in a minority of Alport's patient post transplantation is not known.

Overall de novo crescentic and necrotizing glomerulonephritis owing to anti-GBM antibodies after transplantation is uncommon, seen in only 5% of male adult renal allograft recipients with typical Alport's syndrome (1131,1132). The time of onset of the anti-GBM glomerulonephritis varies from a few days to several months postgrafting; three quarters of the grafts with anti-GBM nephritis fail (1131,1132). Retransplantation may be successful in some patients (reported in three cases [1133]); however, anti-GBM nephritis can recur in successive allografts (1134–1136). The second recurrence can be accelerated and develop in the immediate postoperative period (1136).

The morphology of anti-GBM disease occurring posttransplantation is very similar to that observed in native kidneys. It is characterized by the formation of extracellular crescents, segmental fibrinoid glomerular tuft necrosis, and a lack of significant endocapillary proliferations in uninvolved capillary tufts. Tubules show signs of acute injury and intratubular red blood cell casts. By immuno-fluorescence microscopy, typically bright diffuse and global, linear staining for IgG and less pronounced C3 is detected along peripheral glomerular basement membranes. Fibrin is found in areas of tuft necrosis and extracapillary proliferations. Linear, usually minimal to mild, IgG deposits can also be seen along the GBM in cases of transplant glomerulitis and glomerulopathy or diabetes mellitus, the latter associated with bright staining for albumin. This latter staining pattern should not be mistaken for anti-GBM-glomerulonephritis.

## Congenital Nephrotic Syndrome

*Congenital nephrotic syndrome* of the Finnish type, an autosomal recessive disease owing to mutations in the nephrin gene NPHS1, can paradoxically lead to posttransplant nephrotic syndrome (1130,1137). In a large recent series, 13 of 51 transplants developed recurrent nephrotic syndrome; some of the patients had repeated recurrences (1138). All patients with posttransplant nephrotic syndrome had the Fin-major/Fin-major genotype and complete absence of nephrin (1138). Electron microscopy revealed endothelial swelling of the glomerular capillaries and in some cases podocyte foot process effacement resembling minimal change disease (1139,1140), The nature of the recurrent nephrosis is thought to be the development of antibodies to nephrin in the graft to which the patient is not immunologically tolerant (analogous to anti-GBM antibodies in Alport's syndrome).

## De Novo Focal and Segmental Glomerulosclerosis

De novo focal and segmental glomerulosclerosis (FSGS) in allografts has been described in several settings: (a) in longstanding grafts, in which nephron loss and fibrosis has resulted in glomerular hyperfiltration injury; (b) in adult recipients of pediatric kidneys, in whom the presumed pathogenesis is hyperfiltration injury; (c) in grafts with severe vascular disease resulting in presumed glomerular hypoperfusion and (secondary) collapsing FSGS (Fig. 28.79); (d) in grafts with other glomerular lesions (e.g. transplant or calcineurin inhibitor induced glomerulopathies) (Fig. 28.77C); and (e) as new-onset primary FSGS (rare).

Secondary FSGS is frequently seen in late allograft biopsies obtained many months to years after transplantation, associated with nephron loss and glomerular hyperfiltration or in some cases potentially even glomerular hypoperfusion (725). Secondary FSGS is often found in cases of late structural calcineurin inhibitor–induced toxic changes, nephron loss, and fibrosis. Although certain histologic subtypes of FSGS (i.e., perihilar and not otherwise specified) are more common in secondary FSGS variants, a distinction between primary and secondary can typically not be rendered based on morphologic grounds, and even the collapsing variant of FSGS may occur as a secondary phenomenon (724). Similar to observations made in native kidneys, glomerular size also correlates with the presence of FSGS in allografts (although this phenomenon cannot easily be appreciated by standard light microscopic examination) (1141). In biopsies taken 2 or more years from the time of transplant, the mean glomerular diameter increased by 37% from 148 $\mu$m pretransplant to $203 \pm 10$ $\mu$m in kidneys with FSGS versus $158 \pm 8$ $\mu$m in kidneys without FSGS taken at the same time interval $\pm 8$ (p <.05). These results further support the hypothesis that FSGS develops in conjunction with glomerular hypertrophy.

The collapsing variant of FSGS can arise de novo posttransplantation (Fig. 28.79) (723–725,898). These patients have no risk factors (HIV) and may present with modest proteinuria or the nephrotic syndrome. Affected grafts often show severe small-vessel disease including arteriolar hyalinosis related to calcineurin inhibitors, and less commonly, other lesions such as thrombotic microangiopathy, transplant endarteritis or arteriopathy, or transplant glomerulitis. It is likely that one of the pathogenetic factors is vascular stenosis that leads to glomerular hypoperfusion and tuft collapse. The outcome seems to be poor (724), with rapid progression to end-stage renal failure seen in four of five patients within 2 to 12 months in one series (723).

A rare form of rapidly progressive de novo FSGS occurs in adult recipients of kidneys from children younger than 3 years of age. All in a series of four patients developed severe hypertension, heavy proteinuria, and ultimate renal failure after 1 to 9 months (1142). Biopsies disclosed focal and segmental glomerulosclerosis with crescents in three patients; the fourth had only mesangial hypercellularity (1142). The authors concluded that severe hypertension and glomerular hyperperfusion promoted glomerular sclerosis and crescent formation in maturing infant kidneys (1142).

### Recurrent Glomerular Diseases

Kidney transplantation provides unique opportunities for insights into the basic mechanisms of renal disease. Two idiopathic glomerular diseases were first shown to be caused by blood-borne factors because of their recurrence in the graft (FSGS and dense-deposit disease). Conversely, the failure to recur proves that the disease is intrinsic to the kidney (e.g., Alport's disease, autosomal dominant polycystic kidney disease) or that the pathogenetic mechanisms are "burnt-out" (nephritis owing to anti-GBM antibodies).

Recurrent disease is a small but significant problem in renal allografts, estimated to affect 1% to 8% of transplants (1143–1145). The published data, however, are often difficult to interpret because of small case numbers, short follow-up periods postgrafting, unknown and unclassified native kidney diseases, and lack of definitive pathologic studies (1145). Information provided on graft survival does not always demonstrate whether recurrent disease or other causes (such as rejection) resulted in ultimate transplant failure. Thus, the overall impact of recurrent glomerulonephritides on graft survival is not precisely known (1145).

The diagnosis of recurrence requires ideally the accurate classification of the original kidney disease (either in a biopsy or nephrectomy specimen) and proper diagnostic workup of a subsequent graft biopsy including special stains and immunofluoresecence as well as electron microscopic studies. Many different kidney diseases may potentially recur during the lifetime of the graft, e.g. glomerulonephritides, diabetic glomerulosclerosis, or hypertension-induced arterionephrosclerosis, all of which present similarly in native and transplanted kidneys. Here we will focus on a few significant and informative disease entities.

### Focal Segmental Glomerulosclerosis of the Primary Type (FSGS)

Focal segmental glomerulosclerosis of the primary type (FSGS) recurs in about 30% of grafts and is associated with an increased graft failure rate (1108,1146–1152). After a graft is lost to recurrence, the probability of recurrence in a second transplant may increase to up to 80% (1147,1151,1153). The time of diagnosis averages 7.5 months postsurgery in adults (1151) and 2 weeks in children (1150). Occasionally the recurrence is immediate and dramatic, with proteinuria noted in the first drop of urine emerging from the ureter at surgery. The risk factors for recurrence are rapid progression of the original disease (1146,1147,1151,1152,1154,1155), the collapsing variant of FSGS, diffuse mesangial hypercellularity (1147,1152,1156–1158), and preadolescent age (1152,1157).Children have a recurrence rate 5 times that of adolescents and adults (50% versus 11%) (1157). The rate of recurrence seems to be increased in organs of living donation (1159,1160). FSGS recurred in 56% of 16 children who developed renal failure within 3 years of the initial diagnosis and in 9% of 11 children with a longer disease course (1146). Similarly, the mean time to develop end-stage renal disease from FSGS was 33 months in those who had recurrence and 52 months in those who did not (1150). Collapsing FSGS also frequently recurs (1158,1161–1163). Secondary FSGS, arising as a late complication of other native renal diseases, does not recur, as expected from its presumed hyperfiltration mechanism (1164–1166). Hariharan et al (1117) reported from the renal allograft disease registry that FSGS (recurrent and de novo) accounted for 34% of all listed glomerular diseases and resulted in inferior graft survival (34% versus 67% in a control group at 5 years).

The study of renal transplants has allowed insights into the early phase of podocyte injury in FSGS. The pathologic changes in biopsies begin as widespread foot process effacement and villous transformation of the cytoplasm (1 to 2 weeks), followed by podocyte detachment (so-called dropout), segmental tuft sclerosis, and the accumulation of intracapillary foam cells (1 to 2 months) (1169). Displaced slit diaphragms, similar to those in aminonucleoside-treated rats, have been observed (1170). Podocytes show profound changes in adhesion molecules and signs of transdifferentiation into macrophagelike cells (1171,1172). Podocyte foot processes are restored after remission is induced by plasmapheresis (1151).

The evidence from transplantation that FSGS is owing to a circulating factor led to the use of plasmapheresis to treat recurrence. Initial studies demonstrated that plasmapheresis could diminish the proteinuria but had little long-term effect. However, aggressive plasmapheresis for about 2 weeks early in the recurrence led to long-lasting remission (more than 1 year) in 11 of 15 (73%) patients (1173–1176). CsA has little or no effect overall, although occasional cases have apparently responded.

## Membranoproliferative Glomerulonephritis Type I

Membranoproliferative glomerulonephritis type I (MPGN-I) occurs as an idiopathic disease and in association with certain infections (e.g., hepatitis C virus). The rate of recurrence after transplantation is expected to differ depending on the cause. Idiopathic MPGN-I is estimated to recur in the transplant with clinical signs of proteinuria in 20% to 50% of patients usually within the first 4 years (1104,1145,1177) (recurrence was reported in one patient as early as 2 weeks postsurgery [1178]). Graft failure is commonly seen years after diagnosis in 10% to 50% of cases (1104,1145,1177,1178). The recurrence rate is higher in repeat allografts and if the native kidney disease had crescents (1179). No specific treatment strategies for recurrent MPGN-I have been established; most often therapeutic attempts with cyclophosphamide or plasmapheresis are made (1145). Regression of the immune deposits after long-term graft survival has been documented in two anecdotal cases (734).

Chronic hepatitis C virus (HCV) infections and mixed cryoglobulinemia can cause MPGN in native kidneys; HCV is common in patients with end-stage renal disease. Therefore an underlying HCV infection should be considered whenever MPGN-I is found in the allograft (338, 1119,1180). In one recent series, MPGN-I was diagnosed in 36% of renal graft biopsies from HCV-positive patients versus 4% in the HCV-negative control group; graft survival in patients with MPGN-I and HCV was decreased (1120).

Recurrent MPGN-I usually presents morphologically as a global and diffuse glomerular disease process with signs of endocapillary proliferation, mesangial hypercellularity, GBM duplication, cell interposition, and accentuation of the tuft lobulation. Some cases have prominent crescents. Immunofluorescence microscopy demonstrates significant typically global and diffuse complement factor C3, occasional IgG, and light chain accumulations along glomerular capillary walls and in mesangial zones. Ultrastructurally abundant dense deposits with relatively sharp edges are found most often along the lamina rara interna (associated with the interposition of cell processes and new subendothelial basement membrane formation) and in mesangial regions (1178).

Careful morphologic analyses can usually help to render a specific diagnosis and to distinguish MPGN-I from its histologic look-alikes. The pathologic differential diagnosis includes transplant glomerulopathy, calcineurin inhibitor–induced glomerulopathy, or other causes of a thrombotic microangiopathy (Table 28.15). In contrast to MPGN-I, all of the latter lesions show less pronounced endocapillary and mesangial proliferations, GBM duplication with cell interposition, and crescent formation. Transplant and calcineurin inhibitor–induced glomerulopathies, as well as thrombotic microangiopathies, usually only show minimal immune deposits (143,333,1181), and sometimes multilayering of newly formed subendothelial basement membrane material (Fig. 28-78B) (143,333); these changes differ from those seen in MPGN-I.

## Dense-Deposit Disease/Membranoproliferative Glomerulonephritis Type II

Dense-deposit disease/membranoproliferative glomerulonephritis type II (MPGN-II) recurs in nearly all patients after renal transplantation, although recurrence is not inevitable; one recipient had a negative biopsy 8 years after transplantation (1182–1184). The diagnosis is usually (10 of 11 patients) established in the first graft biopsy, taken as early as 12 days after surgery (1183). Serum C3 levels are normal in approximately 35% of patients with morphologic evidence of recurrent disease (1183,1185). The dense deposits, typically intensely and exclusively staining for complement factor C3, can be found either in the mesangial regions and/or in glomerular capillary walls (1183). Additional deposits may be seen in tubular basement membranes and Bowman's capsule (1186). Whether C3 deposits can first be noted by immunofluorescence microscopy followed by the subsequent formation of ultrastructurally identifiable dense deposits (1187) or vice versa is currently undetermined (1188). Over time MPGN-II–associated glomerular changes may persist or sporadically even regress (1188). Follow-up biopsies analyzed in one series failed to demonstrate a significant increase in global glomerulosclerosis compared with control kidney grafts without recurrent disease (1185). Outcome in pediatric renal allograft patients with recurrent MPGN-II did not differ from controls (1189). Crescent formation, however, shows a negative correlation with graft survival (1183,1185). The presence of crescents in native kidney diseaes is also a risk factor for the recurrence rate of MPGN–II (1179).

## Hemolytic-Uremic Syndrome (HUS)/Thrombotic Microangiopathy (TMA)

Hemolytic-uremic syndrome (HUS)/thrombotic microangiopathy (TMA) recurred in 41% of 17 patients at the University of Minnesota, based on strict clinical and histologic features (1190). Other series have reported frequencies of 15% to 29% (873,1191,1192). The cause of the HUS/TMA influences recurrence, with the highest rate seen in familial forms (approximately 100%) (1193) and scleroderma (1194), and the lowest (approximately 0%) in HUS associated with E. coli infections (1195). Recurrent disease typically becomes manifest during the first year post grafting with symptoms noted as early as the first post operative day. TMA can occur in the kidney in the absence of overt clinical symptoms, as described in 18% of patients (1190). The diagnosis of recurrent HUS/TMA is difficult because de novo variants in the transplant have an identical pathology (e.g., calcineurin inhibitor, sirolimus or OKT3 induced; Table 28.15). A focal distribution pattern may favor a diagnosis of calcineurin inhibitor-induced toxic injury, and the lack of C4d deposition excludes acute humoral rejection.

Whether therapy with calcineurin inhibitors and/or sirolimus, which can cause HUS/TMA, is a risk factor for disease recurrence has been debated; clearly recurrence is seen in the absence of these drugs (1196,1197). In classical HUS (with diarrhea), patients seem to benefit from CsA therapy, which resulted in increased graft survival in one study (1195). The recommended treatment for recurrent HUS/TMA is intensive plasmapheresis combined with administration of fresh frozen plasma, as in the primary disease (1198). Recurrent HUS/TMA causes graft loss in most patients (70%) (one patient lost three successive grafts, and another lost two) (1190,1191,1197), and patient survival at 3 years is only 50% (873).

## IgA Nephropathy

IgA nephropathy recurrence is reported with a frequency of 37% to 60% (1108,1178,1199–1203); the frequency increases over time (IgA– biopsies averaged 15 months, whereas IgA+ biopsies averaged 46 months posttransplant) (1201). This suggests that with increasing graft survival time, recurrence of glomerular IgA deposits will become more common. Approximately 13% of patients with recurrent IgA glomerulopathy will exhibit recurrence-related renal graft dysfunction after a mean follow-up of 5 years (1203). Fortunately, only a few patients (approximately 10% to 20%) present with more than microscopic hematuria (proteinuria, hypertension, active urinary sedi-

ment, elevated serum creatinine levels); these cases are histologically characterized by IgA deposits along glomerular capillary walls, endocapillary proliferations, or segments of tuft sclerosis. In the majority of patients recurrent glomerular IgA deposits present with only minor histologic abnormalities including no or mild mesangial hypercellularity, IgA deposits detected by immunofluoresence microscopy or immunohistochemistry, and mesangial electron-dense deposits observed by electron microscopy. Crescents are rare and with diffuse glomerular involvement are associated with graft failure. Overall graft outcome is not appreciably affected by the recurrence of IgA glomerulopathy, at least up to 8 years posttransplant; renal failure is uncommon (2% to 21% of patients) (1202–1205), although with better treatment for other causes of graft loss, recurrent disease may have more significance.

## Membranous Glomerulonephritis (MGN)

The overall frequency of recurrence of MGN is about 10% to 30% (1106,1149,1160,1206,1207). Recurrent MGN can appear within 1 to 2 weeks after transplantation with symptoms of severe proteinuria (1106,1206,1208–1210); 28% of cases develop within 4 months. Later cases of "recurrent" MGN cannot be as reliably distinguished from de novo disease. All forms of MGN have an identical histology. Since renal allograft recipients are monitored closely posttransplantation, proteinuria is typically detected early. In these cases light microscopic studies (including PAS or silver stains) will not demonstrate diagnostic abnormalities, which are detected only by immunofluorescent or immunohistochemical assays and electron microscopy showing "naked" subepithelial immune deposits without GBM spike formation. Only a few (less than 10%) of all cases of MGN in allografts arise as recurrence in patients with a previous history of MGN (1108,1206). No conclusive risk factors have been identified (1211), except for the possible role of HLA matching (1207). Of those that recurred within 4 months, 75% were in kidneys from living related donors (1106,1206).

The overall outcome is not greatly affected by the presence of recurrent MGN. However, graft loss has been reported in about 10% to 50% of patients with recurrence within 10 years (1106,1149,1160,1206,1207,1211); in one series 2 of 3 patients with recurrent MGN lost graft function whereas one patient experienced spontaneous recovery (1116).

## Anti-GBM Disease

Anti-GBM disease recurs if circulating antibodies are present after transplantation. Since the anti-GBM autoantibody response is usually transient, recurrence can be minimized by postponing transplantation for 6 to 12 months after the serum has turned negative for anti-GBM antibodies (1208,1212,1213). In the early experience, 41% of patients (25/68) developed recurrent IgG deposits along the GBM, but only 10% of the grafts failed (580). Thus, IgG deposition along the GBM is by itself insufficient to cause severe glomerular injury if cofactors are lacking (1127). Recent series report recurrence rates of 0 to 5% (1160,1208,1214) and no recurrence-related graft loss (1215). Recurrent glomerulonephritis and graft failure were observed in an unusual patient presenting with IgA autoantibodies directed against the α1/α2 (IV) collagen chains (collagenous domain) (1216). Another case of "recurrence" was diagnosed in a patient 12 years after grafting (1217), potentially representing a second de novo event. Nephrectomy of the native kidneys has no beneficial effect on graft survival (1208,1218).

## Antineutrophil Cytoplasmic Antibody (ANCA)-Mediated Diseases

ANCA-associated renal disease recurred in 17% to 19% of patients regardless of the underlying disease entity (Wegener's granulomatosis, microscopic polyangiitis, or renal limited disease forms), the original ANCA type (elevated MPO versus PR3 antibodies), the presence or absence of circulating ANCAs at the time of transplantation (in clinically asymptomatic patients), the type of graft (living versus deceased donor organs), or cyclosporine therapy (1219–1223). Recurrence can arise at any time (5 days to 89 months postgrafting), but rarely causes graft failure (1215,1219,1224,1225). At the time of recurrence, ANCA titers are generally elevated (1226,1227) although sometimes only marginally (1225). Recurrence has also been reported in extrarenal sites, sparing the allograft (1225). Recurrent ANCA disease responds favorably to therapy including cyclophosphamide or plasmapheresis (1223,1225,1228). Recurrent forms of ANCA-associated small-vessel vasculitis and pauci-immune glomerulonephritis are histologically identical to those seen in native kidneys. The complement degradation product C4d is not deposited along peritubular capillaries (personal observation).

## Systemic Lupus Erythematosus

Systemic lupus erythematosus recurs but not as frequently as might be predicted, given its systemic autoimmune pathogenesis (1208,1229). Recurrence of lupus nephritis is seen in 1% to 8.6% of patients, on average between 1 and 6 years posttransplantation (range: 6 days to 15 years) (1230–1233). In three series, no recurrence was found among 56 patients, 4 of whom presented with positive serologies (1234–1236). Histologically recurrent lupus often shows mesangial hypercellularity (class II) (1232,1237). The true recurrence rate of lupus nephritis may be underestimated, at least of the milder forms, due

to biopsy practice and the lack of special studies including immunofluorescence and electron microscopy (1232). Goral et al (1232) found in 50 transplanted lupus patients an overall recurrence rate of 30% (52% of patients who underwent biopsy). Most common was a mesangioproliferative pattern (class II seen in 8 patients), followed by a focal proliferative pattern (class III, 4 patients) and a membranous glomerulopathy (class V, 3 patients). Class II would be missed in graft biopsies if special studies were not performed.

Recurrence is clinically often associated with an increase in antinuclear antibody (ANA) and dsDNA antibody titers, a decrease of serum complement levels, hematuria, proteinuria, rash, or Raynaud's phenomenon. However, clinical signs in patients with recurrence can be quite bland. Recurrence of lupus nephritis as the cause for graft failure is uncommon (0% to 1.6% of patients) (1233,1238), and transplant outcome in lupus is not appreciably affected (1229,1232,1233,1236–1238).

## Amyloidosis

Amyloidosis recurs in about 10 to 30% of patients 1 to 10 years posttransplantatioin (1239–1242). Recurrence depends on the amyloid type and the progression of the underlying disease; systemic amyloidosis with marked cardiomyopathy is generally considered to be a contraindication for kidney transplantation. Patients with amyloidosis commonly tolerate complications postgrafting poorly. Isoniemi et al (1243) in 1994 reported a 5-year patient survival rate of 49% among 96 patients with amyloidosis who had undergone renal transplantation between 1973 and 1992. Patient death was attributed to amyloidosis in 20% of cases. Experience is largest in patients with AA-type renal amyloid deposits, which infrequently recur in the graft, in particular in patients in whom the acute phase response in the serum is controlled (1239,1242,1244,1245). Five patients with familial Mediterranean fever (FMF), who developed renal failure from amyloidosis, have had recurrences in the graft at 1 to 2 years that did not affect function (1246,1247). A recent series of cases with amyloidosis secondary to FMF reported a recurrence rate of only 5% (1248). Data on outcome post-kidney transplantation in cases of primary AL- or AH-type amyloidoses is sparse; however, it appears that outcome is surprisingly good with overall patient and graft survival rates of approximately 65% (1240,1242).

## Monoclonal Immunoglobulin Deposition Disease

Monoclonal immunoglobulin deposition disease is a consequence of an uncontrolled production of abnormal light or heavy immunoglobulin chains. Recurrence in renal transplants heavily depends on the progression of the underlying condition. If the production of monoclonal immunoglobulins cannot be stopped, disease will recur in the allograft. In one recent series, recurrence was observed in five of seven patients between 2 and 45 months after transplantation (median 33 months) and all five cases resulted in either death or graft failure (1249). Interestingly, monoclonal kappa light chain deposits were not only found in the five patients with histologic signs of recurrence (including mesangial expansion and thickening of tubular basement membranes) but also in the two patients without apparent morphologic changes, one of them alive and well 13 years post transplantation. Thus, monoclonal immunoglobulin deposits may rarely occur without typical histologic signs of disease (1249).

## Fibrillary/Immunotactoid Glomerulopathy

Fibrillary/immunotactoid glomerulopathy is rare and our experience is limited (1250,1251). Although recurrent fibrillary deposits were noted in approximately 50% of grafts 2 to 9 years post transplantation (1252), functional deterioration progressed much slower than in native kidneys (1252,1253). Graft loss caused by disease recurrence is rare; it is only seen in approximately 20% of patients (1252).

## Diabetic Nephropathy

Diabetic nephropathy recurs in many patients over time. In a recent series disease recurrence was seen in 38% of patients 2 to 7 years post grafting (6 of 16 patients with biopsies among a total of 78 study subjects) (1254). Histologic evidence of diabetic nephropathy developed on average 8 years after surgery in another series of 14 patients, most commonly with signs of arteriolar hyalinosis (100%) and GBM thickening (64%); nodular glomerulosclerosis was uncommon and detected in only 14% (12 patients with recurrent and 2 with de novo disease) (1255). Nodular diabetic glomerulosclerosis (type Kimmelstiel-Wilson) has been reported as a late phenomenon, 5 to 15 years post grafting (1255–1258); this finding is similar to observations made in native kidneys in which the development of Kimmelstiel-Wilson nodules usually takes 10 years or more. The histologic diagnosis of recurrent diabetic nephropathy can be challenging, particularly if clinical data are incomplete and proteinuria levels are low. The most important differential diagnoses include arteriolar hyalinosis owing to hypertension (either pre-existing donor or de novo disease) and arteriolar hyalinosis owing to calcineurin inhibitors. A diagnosis of recurrent diabetic nephropathy is favored if hyalinosis is found in both afferent and efferent arterioles, if linear IgG and albumin deposits are observed along the GBM and TBM by immunofluorescence microscopy, and if thickening of the GBM is seen by elec-

tron microscopy. Five-year graft survival of patients with recurrent diabetic nephropathy was 71% to 92% and 10-year graft survival 34% to 58% (1254,1255); outcome was worse than that of a non-diabetic control group (1254). However, not all studies documented inferior graft survival in patients suffering from diabetes (at least in the short run [1259]).

The study of transplanted kidneys has delineated the sequence of changes in the development of diabetic nephropathy. The first change is an increase in allograft glomerular volume at 6 months (1260), followed by increases in mesangial volume (1261). Thickening of the GBM appears later, with a progressive increase that is first evident after 2 to 3 years (1261,1262). Increased linear staining of the GBM and TBM for IgG and albumin appears after about 2 years (1256,1257). Arteriolar hyalinosis follows in a similar time frame and is present in 83% of allografts in diabetics 2 to 5 years posttransplant (1257).

Pancreatic transplantation has also shown that some features of early diabetic glomerulopathy in the native kidney are reversible (1263). Renal biopsies were taken from 13 patients prior to and 5 years after pancreatic transplantation. These showed a reduction in glomerular size compared with the pretransplant biopsy and prevention of the progressive increase in mesangial volume that occurred over 5 years in 10 control patients without pancreas transplants. Reversal of diabetic glomerulosclerosis in a donor kidney transplanted into a non-diabetic recipient was documented by loss of proteinuria and mesangial hypercellularity at 7 months; thus, cadaver kidneys with mild diabetic lesions are potentially suitable donor organs (1264).

## Other Recurrent Diseases

Metabolic diseases owing to genetic abnormalities that cause renal disease in the recipient typically recur unless the metabolic lesion is ameliorated or the kidney serves as an important source of the defective molecule.

## Primary Hyperoxaluria Type I

Primary hyperoxaluria type I had a dismal rate of renal graft loss (92%) (13/14) owing to recurrent oxalate deposition in the kidney (1143). The mortality from oxalosis after transplantation was 37% in eight infants (1265). Probably the best results with kidney transplants alone have been reported from Minnesota. With a strict medical protocol (including extra hemodialysis, diuresis, pyridoxine, and avoidance of graft ischemia), graft survival of 70% was achieved in ten living related allografts. Renal function was good up to 7 years post transplant, and 60% of patients did not show any evidence of oxalate deposits in their graft biopsies (1267). Combined liver and kidney transplants offer a cure for the enzyme deficiency

(1268,1270–1274) and reversal of oxalosis cardiomyopathy (1275). Liver transplantation can delay or prevent the renal damage and may obviate the need for renal transplantation (1272).

In cases of oxalosis, transplant biopsies show characteristic birefringent sheaves of oxalate crystals in the tubules, sometimes with tubular cell endocytosis and cell proliferation (1269). Most specific are oxalate deposits in the interstitium and in arterial walls. We have seen a case in consultation in which the diagnosis was initially missed until the transplant nephrectomy was examined, which showed the pathognomonic deposition of oxalate in vascular walls.

## Miscellaneous Metabolic Diseases

In Fabry's disease, globoceramide deposits recur in the graft in minor amounts (often detected only by electron microscopy) and usually do not cause renal disease (1276,1277). Kidney transplant biopsies show the characteristic laminated osmophilic cytoplasmic inclusions in small vessel endothelium years after grafting (8 to 11 years) (1276,1278). It is likely that these lipids accumulate owing to uptake of circulating lipids rather than replacement of the endothelium by recipient cells, as once suggested (1278). On two occasions, a heterozygote was inadvertently used as a donor (1279,1280). Podocyte deposits were detected on a graft biopsy 11 days after transplantation, but these did not progress in a repeat biopsy 8 years later (1280). In the other case, renal failure developed 5 years after transplantation and a biopsy showed widespread globoceramide deposits in endothelial cells, podocytes, and mesangial cells, which probably caused the late dysfunction (1279). Patients who have received allografts often succumb to the cardiac manifestations of their disease, although several have long-term (more than 10 year) graft survival (1282). Recently the patient survival has improved and renal transplantation is viewed more favorably (1160), particularly with the advent of enzyme replacement therapy able to clear deposits from the tissue (1283).

Deficiency of adenine phosphoribosyltransferase (present in erythrocytes) usually causes urolithiasis (confused with gout) and can rarely cause renal failure by accumulation of crystals of the purine metabolite 2,8-dihydroxyadenine in tubules eliciting a chronic interstitial nephritis. One case recurred in an allograft 6 years posttransplant, leading to the correct diagnosis of the original disease (the crystals in the native kidney had been confused with oxalosis or radiocontrast material) (1284). The deposits are insoluble in water and xylene (as oxalate but not uric acid) and form sheaves of needle-shaped crystals, which have a brownish color, and an annular appearance with radial striations in polarized light. Definitive identification can be made by infrared microscopy analysis of crystal deposits in thick biopsy sections (1284).

Cystinosis is an autosomal recessive genetic disorder that affects lysosomal cystine efflux, causing cystine accumulation in cells and renal failure (1285). The diagnosis is made pathologically by the electron microscopic demonstration of intracellular hexagonal or rectangular crystals and extremely electron-dense (osmophilic) cytoplasm. The cytoplasmic changes indelibly mark recipient cells, which retain the metabolic defect. Macrophages with crystals and dense cytoplasm reappear in grafts in patients with cystinosis, whereas the parenchymal cells show no abnormality (1286). Cystine crystals (or cytoplasmic crystalline spaces compatible with cystine) occurred in inflammatory cells in 96% of biopsies (23/24) and in the glomerulus in 25% (1287). Macrophages with crystals and a dark cytoplasm can occasionally be found in the graft mesangium, elegant evidence in the human for a bone marrow origin of some mesangial cells (1287). Fortunately, patients with cystinosis generally do well with renal transplantation (1285).

## POST TRANSPLANT LYMPHOPROLIFERATIVE DISORDERS (PTLD) AND OTHER NEOPLASMS

The risk of certain neoplasms is substantially increased in renal allograft recipients compared with the general population and with patients maintained on hemodialysis (1293,1294). It has been extrapolated that with continued imunosuppression by the 20th year after transplantation, 70% of patients have one or more malignancies (1293). Most frequently allograft recipients suffer from carcinomas (squamous and basal cell) of the skin, lip, vulva, and cervix (occurring many years postgrafting), Kaposi's sarcoma, and B-cell lymphoproliferative disorders (commonly seen in the first years after transplantation) (1293,1295). These tumors have in common ultraviolet (UV)-induced mutations or viral causes, in both instances providing neoantigens that potentially provoke immune surveillance in immunocompetent hosts. This substantiated the hypothesis originally proposed by Sir Malcom Burnet that some human tumors may be antigenic to the host. The frequencies of the more common adenocarcinomas (breast, lung, prostate, colon) and melanomas are little affected. Renal transplant recipients also have an increased risk for renal cell carcinoma arising in their end-stage native kidneys (1296). Here we will limit our discussion to PTLD and the features confronting the renal pathologist.

According to the most recent 2001 World Health Organization (WHO) definition, "post transplant lymphoproliferative disorder is a lymphoid proliferation or lymphoma that develops as a consequence of immunosuppression in a recipient of a solid organ or bone marrow allograft. PTLDs

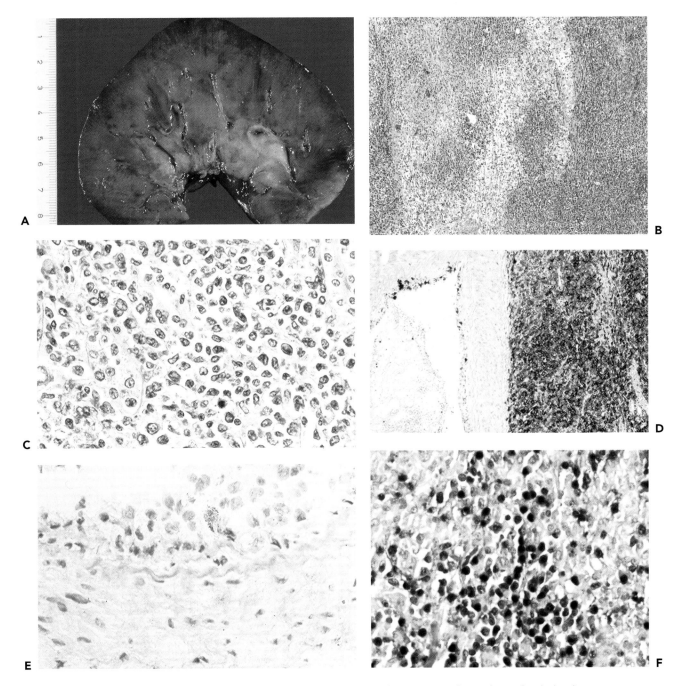

**Figure 28.91** Posttransplant lymphoproliferative disorder (PTLD)—polymorphic and polyclonal variant **(A–F)**. A failed allograft owing to PTLD shows marked swelling, an ill-defined corticomedullary junction, and minute irregular foci of hemorrhage **(A)**. Histologically, PTLD often presents with a nodular, destructive-appearing mononuclear cell infiltrate **(B)** that demonstrates on higher power examination **(C)** activated lymphoid cells and scattered blasts. Most PTLDs are B-cell dominant **(D** shows an immunohistochemical incubation for CD20). The lymphoproliferative disorder can also involve arterial intimal layers **(D** and **E)** and mimic an acute rejection episode with transplant endarteritis. Most PTLDs are promoted by Epstein-Barr virus (EBV) infections that can be detected either by immuno-histochemistry **(D** shows in the inflamed intima of an artery a single-cell staining for EBV-LMP [latent membrane protein] in the cytoplasm) or more easily by in situ hybridization detecting EBV-encoded RNA (EBER) **(F** shows EBER staining in many mononuclear cell nuclei). **(B** and **C:** H&E, ×40 and ×300; **D:** immunohistochemistry to detect CD20, ×150; **E:** immunohistochemistry to detect EBV-LMP, ×400; **F:** in situ hybridization to detect EBER, ×400.)

comprise a spectrum ranging from early, Epstein-Barr virus (EBV) driven polyclonal proliferations resembling infectious mononucleosis to EBV positive or EBV negative lymphomas of predominately B-cell or less often T-cell type" (1297). Overall PTLD developed in 1.4% of 25,127 renal allograft recipients transplanted in the United States between 1996 and 2000 (1298); patients on tacrolimus based immunosuppression showed PTLDs in one study (1299). PTLDs can involve the allograft (e.g. kidney, heart), can arise anywhere in the body, and can be widely disseminated. In the following paragraphs we will discuss changes seen in the kidney (340,1301–1312).

PTLDs involve the renal allograft in more than 30% of affected patients (340,1313); they were restricted to the kidney transplant in 12% of cases in one series (340). PTLDs restricted to the kidney transplant often occur early (on average 5 months) postsurgery, are more frequently of donor cell origin, and fare favorably (1314). Patients with kidney transplant involvement typically present with graft dysfunction (differential diagnosis: acute rejection) and may sometimes show a mass lesion in imaging studies. The kidney is more often involved in kidney transplant patients (14%) than in heart transplant patients (0.7%) (conversely, the heart is involved more often in heart than kidney transplant patients, 18% versus 7%), suggesting that the immunologic reaction in the allograft is a pathogenetic factor (1315).

When the allograft is involved diffusely, the kidneys are swollen with an ill-defined cortico-medullary junction and can show petechiae; the changes resemble those seen in severe acute rejection (Fig. 28.91). In our experience and according to literature reports, most cases of PTLD involving the kidneys are of the polymorphic variant (340,1313). The interstitial compartment typically shows vaguely nodular, expansile aggregates of mononuclear cell elements containing plasma cells and varying numbers of activated lymphocytes admixed with cell elements containing large nuclei and prominent nucleoli (i.e., blasts). Mitotic figures can usually be found and sometimes foci of serpiginous necrosis. The neoplastic mononuclear cells often invade tubules (i.e., tubulitis); they can also penetrate into arterial intimal layers (i.e., transplant endarteritis). Transplant glomerulitis is uncommon; viral inclusion bodies are not seen (Table 28.16).

It is not easy to establish a diagnosis of PTLD, especially in unsuspected cases limited to the donor organ (340,1301–1312) and the histologic changes can be confused with acute rejection (1303,1316). Both in rejection and PTLD, the mononuclear cells have enlarged nuclei with nucleoli and they can show mitotic activity (although 'blasts' and mitoses are typically more prominent in PTLD). In addition, tubulitis and endarteritis may be features of PTLD. To make things worse, it has been suggested that rejection can coexist with PTLD (340). Several features should raise the suspicion of PTLD. The most helpful clue in our experience is the presence of dense, vaguely nodular, expansile sheets of activated lymphoid cell elements without an admixture of granulocytes or macrophages. The presence of serpiginous necrosis is also a sign of PTLD (340), although its absence is not helpful, nor is hemorrhagic necrosis that can be seen in severe rejection episodes.

Diagnostic confirmation can usually be achieved by immunohistochemistry and in situ hybridization. Most cases of PTLD involving renal allografts are of B-cell lineage and express CD20 (approximately 85% to 90%) (in contrast to cases of cellular rejection that are CD3 and CD68 dominant; Fig. 28.91D). CD20-positive cells can also be found in foci of tubulitis and vessels with endothelialitis, thereby identifying these changes as PTLD induced. In situ hybridization for EBV-encoded RNA (EBER) usually shows widespread staining in mononuclear cell elements (typically in high copy numbers per cell). Immunohistochemical stains for LMP-1 and usually EBNA-2 are expected to be positive in PTLD, however, the staining signals can be weak and scattered and seem to be less reliable for diagnostic workup (Figs. 28.91E and F). In a systematic study of 14 cases of PTLD (1307), EBER was detected in all cases by in situ hybridization; 11 were positive for LMP-1 (CS1–4, Dako) and 9 for EBNA-2 (EBNA2/R3) by immunohistochemistry. The number of positive cells was highly variable, even within the same tumor; positivity was increased around areas of necrosis. Tests to detect clonality (e.g., immunoglobulin gene rearrangement) help to confirm the presence of a monomorphic PTLD; polyclonality, however, does not exclude early and polymorphic PTLD variants.

Therapy has typically included reduced immunosuppression, sometimes with added radiation, chemotherapy, and antiviral drugs (acyclovir, ganciclovir, alpha interferon) (1299,1317). Polymorphic PTLDs respond to antiviral therapy and a reduction in immunosuppression. Surgical resection has been performed for localized disease (limited to the allograft or ureters) with good success (1306,1318,1319). The monomorphic, monoclonal PTLDs that show mutations of the Bcl 6 gene require more aggressive therapy and have a poor long-term prognosis (1314). Anti-CD20 (rituximab) has shown promise in patients with monomorphic or polymorphic PTLDs, resulting in complete remission (mean duration 18 months) in 53% of patients (1320).

## ACKNOWLEDGMENTS

The authors thank Robert T. McCluskey for many detailed and thoughtful suggestions for this chapter and the many colleagues, fellows, and investigators who have collaborated on transplantation research over the years.

## REFERENCES

1. Evans RW, Kitzmann DJ. An economic analysis of kidney transplantation. Surg Clin North Am 1998;78:149.
2. Cecka JM. The OPTN/UNOS Renal Transplant Registry 2003. Clin Transplant 2003;17:1.
3. Hamilton DN. Kidney transplantation: A history. In: Morris PJ, ed. Kidney Transplantation: Principles and Practice, 5th ed. Philadelphia: WB Saunders, 2001:1.
4. Ullmann E. Experimentelle Nierentransplantation. Wein Klin Wochenschr 1902;15:281.
5. Druml W. The beginning of organ transplantation: Emerich Ullmann (1861–1937). Wien Klin Wochenschr 2002;114:128.
6. Carrel A. La technique operatoire des anastomoses vasculaires et al transplantation des visceres. Lyon Med 1902;98:859.
7. Jaboulay M. Greffe de reins au pli du coude par soudure arte. Bull Lyon Med 1906;107:575.
8. Unger E. Nierentransplantation. Berl Klin Wochenschr 1909;1:1057.
9. Hamilton DN, Reid WA. Yu Yu Voronoy and the first human kidney allograft. Surg Gynecol Obstet 1984;159:289.
10. Murray JE. The Nobel Lectures in Immunology. The Nobel Prize for Physiology or Medicine, 1990. The first successful organ transplants in man. Scand J Immunol 1994;39:1.
11. Hamilton DN. Kidney transplantation: A history. In: Morris PJ, ed. Kidney Transplantation: Principles and Practice. Philadelphia: WB Saunders, 1994:1.
12. Hume DM, Magee JH, Kauffman HM, et al. Experiences with renal homotransplantation in the human: Report of nine cases. J Clin Invest 1955;34:327.
13. Murray JE, Merrill JP, Harrison JH. Prolonged survival of human kidney homografts by immunosuppressive drug therapy. N Engl J Med 1963;268:1315.
14. Billingham RE, Brent L, Medawar PB. Actively acquired tolerance of foreign cells. Nature 1953;172:603.
15. Schwartz R, Dameshek W. Drug induced immunological tolerance. Nature 1959;183:1682.
16. Calne RY, Alexandre GP, Murray JE. A study of the effects of drugs in prolonging the survival of homologous renal transplantants in dogs. Ann N.Y Acad Sci 1962;99:743.
17. Starzl TE, Marchioro TL, Waddell WR. The reversal of rejection in human renal homografts with subsequent development of homograft tolerance. Surg Gynecol Obstet 1963;117:385.
18. Fudaba Y, Spitzer TR, Shaffer JM, et al. Evidence for "split" tolerance in multiple myeloma patients receiving combined HLA-identical related donor kidney and non-myeloablative bone marrow transplantation. Transplantation 2006, in press.
19. Williamson CS. Further studies on the transplantation of the kidney. J Urol 1926;16:231.
20. Dempster WJ. Kidney homotransplantation. Br J Surg 1953;40:447.
21. Simonsen M, Buemann J, Gammeltoft A, et al. Biological incompatibility in kidney transplantation in dogs. I. Experimental and morphological investigations. Acta Pathol Microbiol Scand 1953;32:1.
22. Simonsen M. Biological incompatibility in kidney transplantation in dogs. II. Serological investigations. Acta Pathol Microbiol Scand 1953;32:36.
23. Porter KA, Calne RY. The origin of the infiltrating cells in skin and kidney homografts. Transplant Bull 1960;26:458.
24. Dammin G. The kidney as a homograft and its host. U Mich Med Bull 1960;26:278.
25. Porter KA, Owen K, Mowbray JF, et al. Obliterative vascular changes in four human kidney homotransplants. Br Med J 1963;2:639.
26. Porter KA, Dossetor JB, Marchioro TL, et al. Human renal transplants. I. Glomerular changes. Lab Invest 1967;16:153.
27. Porter KA, Andres GA, Calder MW, et al. Human renal transplants. II. Immunofluorescence and immunoferritin studies. Lab Invest 1968;18:159.
28. Jeannet M, Pinn VW, Flax MH, et al. Humoral antibodies in renal allotransplantation in man. N Engl J Med 1970;282:111.
29. Kissmeyer-Nielsen F, Olsen S, Petersen VP, Fjeldborg O. Hyperacute rejection of kidney allografts, associated with pre-existing humoral antibodies against donor cells. Lancet 1966;2:662.
30. Glassock RJ, Feldman D, Reynolds ES, et al. Human renal isografts: A clinical and pathologic analysis. Medicine 1968;47:411.
31. Kincaid-Smith P. Histological diagnosis of rejection of renal homografts in man. Lancet 1967;1:849.
32. Lee HM. Surgical techniques of renal transplantation. In: Morris PJ, ed. Kidney Transplantation: Principles and Practice. Philadelphia: WB Saunders, 1994:127.
33. Leadbetter GW, Monaco AP, Russell PS. A technique for reconstruction of the urinary tract in renal transplantation. Surg Gynecol Obstet 1966;123:349.
34. Andres A, Morales JM, Herrero JC, et al. Double versus single renal allografts from aged donors. Transplantation 2000;69:2060.
35. Jerius JT, Taylor RJ, Murillo D, Leone JP. Double renal transplants from marginal donors: 2-year results. J Urol 2000;163:423.
36. Shimizu T, Tanabe K, Ishida H, et al. Histopathological evaluation of 0-h biopsy specimens of donor kidney procured by laparoscopic donor nephrectomy. Clin Transplant 2004;18(Suppl 11):24.
37. Troppmann C, Ormond DB, Perez RV. Laparoscopic (vs open) live donor nephrectomy: A UNOS database analysis of early graft function and survival. Am J Transplant 2003;3:1295.
38. Danovitch GM, ed. Handbook of Kidney Transplantation, 4th ed. Philadelphia: Lippincott Williams & Wilkins, 2005.
39. Danovitch GM, Cohen DJ, Weir MR, et al. Current status of kidney and pancreas transplantation in the United States, 1994–2003. Am J Transplant 2005;5:904.
40. Hariharan S, Johnson CP, Bresnahan BA, et al. Improved graft survival after renal transplantation in the United States, 1988 to 1996. N Engl J Med 2000;342:605.
41. Meier-Kriesche HU, Schold JD, Kaplan B. Long-term renal allograft survival: Have we made significant progress or is it time to rethink our analytic and therapeutic strategies? Am J Transplant 2004;4:1289.
42. Tilney NL. Transplantation between identical twins: A review. World J Surg 1986;10:381.
43. de Mattos AM, Bennett WM, Barry JM, Norman DJ. HLA-identical sibling renal transplantation: A 21-yr single-center experience. Clin Transplant 1999;13:158.
44. Krieger NR, Becker BN, Heisey DM, et al. Chronic allograft nephropathy uniformly affects recipients of cadaveric, non-identical living-related, and living-unrelated grafts. Transplantation 2003;75:1677.
45. Legendre C, Thervet E, Skhiri H, et al. Histologic features of chronic allograft nephropathy revealed by protocol biopsies in kidney transplant recipients. Transplantation 1998;65:1506.
46. Baltzan MA, Shoker AS, Baltzan RB, George D. HLA-identity—long-term renal graft survival, acute vascular, chronic vascular, and acute interstitial rejection. Transplantation 1996;61:881.
47. Danovitch GM, Cecka JM. Allocation of deceased donor kidneys: Past, present, and future. Am J Kidney Dis 2003;42:882.
48. Gjertson DW, Terasaki PI, Takemoto S, Mickey MR. National allocation of cadaveric kidneys by HLA matching. Projected effect on outcome and costs. N Engl J Med 1991;324:1032.
49. Remuzzi G, Cravedi P, Perna A, et al. Long-term outcome of renal transplantation from older donors. N Engl J Med 2006;354:343.
50. Brook NR, White SA, Waller JR, et al. Non-heart beating donor kidneys with delayed graft function have superior graft survival compared with conventional heart-beating donor kidneys that develop delayed graft function. Am J Transplant 2003;3:614.

51. Bains JC, Sandford RM, Brook NR, et al. Comparison of renal allograft fibrosis after transplantation from heart-beating and non-heart-beating donors. Br J Surg 2005;92:113.

52. Cecka JM, Terasaki PI. The UNOS scientific renal transplant registry. In: Cecka JM, Terasaki PI, eds. Clinical Transplants 1995. Los Angeles: UCLA Tissue Typing Laboratory, 1996:1.

53. Troppmann C, Gillingham KJ, Gruessner RW, et al. Delayed graft function in the absence of rejection has no long-term impact: A study of cadaver kidney recipients with good graft function at 1 year after transplantation. Transplantation 1996;61:1331.

54. Taylor RM, Ting A, Briggs J. Renal transplantation in the United Kingdom and Ireland-the centre effect. Lancet 1985;1:715.

55. Brenner BM, Cohen RA, Milford EL. In renal transplantation, one size may not fit all. J Am Soc Nephrol 1992;3:162.

56. Waltzer WC, Miller F, Arnold A, et al. Value of percutaneous core needle biopsy in the differential diagnosis of renal transplant dysfunction. J Urol 1987;137:1117.

57. Matas AJ, Tellis VA, Sablay L, et al. The value of needle renal allograft biopsy. III. A prospective study. Surgery 1985;98:922.

58. Parfrey PS, Kuo YL, Hanley JA, et al. The diagnostic and prognostic value of kidney transplant biopsy. Transplantation 1984;38:586.

59. Kiss D, Landman J, Mihatsch M, et al. Risks and benefits of graft biopsy in renal transplantation under cyclosporin-A. Clin Nephrol 1992;38:132.

60. Manfro RC, Lee JY, Lewgoy J, et al. The role of percutaneous renal biopsy in kidney transplant. Rev Assoc Med Brasil 1994;40:108.

61. Kon SP, Templar J, Dodd SM, et al. Diagnostic contribution of renal allograft biopsies at various intervals after transplantation. Transplantation 1997;63:547.

62. Pascual M, Vallhonrat H, Cosimi AB, et al. The clinical usefulness of the renal allograft biopsy in the cyclosporine era: A prospective study. Transplantation 1999;67:737.

63. Al-Awwa IA, Hariharan S, First MR. Importance of allograft biopsy in renal transplant recipients: Correlation between clinical and histological diagnosis. Am J Kidney Dis 1998;31:S15.

64. Colvin RB, Cohen AH, Saiontz C, et al. Evaluation of pathologic criteria for acute renal allograft rejection: Reproducibility, sensitivity, and clinical correlation. J Am Soc Nephrol 1997;8:1930.

65. Sorof JM, Vartanian RK, Olson JL, et al. Histopathological concordance of paired renal allograft biopsy cores. Effect on the diagnosis and management of acute rejection. Transplantation 1995;60:1215.

66. Gray DW, Richardson A, Hughes D, et al. A prospective, randomized, blind comparison of three biopsy techniques in the management of patients after renal transplantation. Transplantation 1992;53:1226.

67. Nast CC, Blifeld C, Danovitch GM, et al. Needle biopsy of renal allografts: Comparison of two techniques. Radiology 1990;174:273.

68. Mahoney MC, Racadio JM, Merhar GL, First MR. Safety and efficacy of kidney transplant biopsy: Tru-Cut needle vs sonographically guided Biopty gun. AJR Am J Roentgenol 1993;160:325.

69. Hanas E, Larsson E, Fellström B, et al. Safety aspects and diagnostic findings of serial renal allograft biopsies, obtained by an automatic technique with a midsize needle. Scand J Urol Nephrol 1992;26:413.

70. Wilczek H. Percutaneous needle biopsy of the renal allograft: A clinical safety evaluation of 1129 biopsies. Transplantation 1990;50:790.

71. Furness PN, Philpott CM, Chorbadjian MT, et al. Protocol biopsy of the stable renal transplant: A multicenter study of methods and complication rates. Transplantation 2003;76:969.

72. Beckingham IJ, Nicholson ML, Kirk G, et al. Comparison of three methods to obtain percutaneous needle core biopsies of a renal allograft. Br J Surg 1994;81:898.

73. Schwarz A, Gwinner W, Hiss M, et al. Safety and adequacy of renal transplant protocol biopsies. Am J Transplant 2005;5:1992.

74. Nicholson ML, Wheatley TJ, Doughman TM, et al. A prospective randomized trial of three different sizes of core-cutting needle for renal transplant biopsy. Kidney Int 2000;58:390.

75. Vidhun J, Masciandro J, Varich L, et al. Safety and risk stratification of percutaneous biopsies of adult-sized renal allografts in infant and older pediatric recipients. Transplantation 2003;76:552.

76. Benfield MR, Herrin J, Feld L, et al. Safety of kidney biopsy in pediatric transplantation: A report of the Controlled Clinical Trials in Pediatric Transplantation Trial of Induction Therapy Study Group. Transplantation 1999;67:544.

77. Merkus JW, Zeebregts CJ, Hoitsma AJ, et al. High incidence of arteriovenous fistula after biopsy of kidney allografts. Br J Surg 1993;80:310.

78. Cohen AH, Gonzalez S, Nast CC, et al. Frozen-section analysis of allograft renal biopsy specimens. Reliable histopathologic data for rapid decision making. Arch Pathol Lab Med 1991;115:386.

79. Solez K, Axelsen RA, Benediktsson H, et al. International standardization of criteria for the histologic diagnosis of renal allograft rejection: The Banff working classification of kidney transplant pathology. Kidney Int 1993;44:411.

80. Wilczek HE, Groth CG, Bohman SO. Effect of reduced cyclosporin dosage on long-term renal allograft histology. Transplant Int 1992;5:65.

81. Wang H, Nanra RS, Carney SL, et al. The renal medulla in acute renal allograft rejection: Comparison with renal cortex. Nephrol Dialysis Transplant 1995;10:1428.

82. Hamburger J. A reappraisal of the concept of organ "rejection," based on the study of homotransplanted kidneys. Transplantation 1967;37:564.

83. Nyberg G, Hedman L, Blohme I, Svalander C. Morphologic findings in baseline kidney biopsies from living related donors. Transplant Proc 1992;24:355.

84. Cahen R, Dijoud F, Couchoud C, et al. Evaluation of renal grafts by pretransplant biopsy. Transplant Proc 1995;27:2470.

85. Edwards EB, Posner MP, Maluf DG, Kauffman HM. Reasons for non-use of recovered kidneys: The effect of donor glomerulosclerosis and creatinine clearance on graft survival. Transplantation 2004;77:1411.

86. Wang HJ, Kjellstrand CM, Cockfield SM, Solez K. On the influence of sample size on the prognostic accuracy and reproducibility of renal transplant biopsy. Nephrol Dial Transplant 1998;13:165.

87. Sund S, Reisaeter AV, Fauchald P, et al. Living donor kidney transplants: A biopsy study 1 year after transplantation, compared with baseline changes and correlation to kidney function at 1 and 3 years. Nephrol Dial Transplant 1999;14:2445.

88. Furness PN, Taub N, Assmann KJ, et al. International variation in histologic grading is large, and persistent feedback does not improve reproducibility. Am J Surg Pathol 2003;27:805.

89. Fromer DL, Birkhoff JD, Hardy MA, et al. Bilateral intrarenal adrenal glands in cadaveric donor kidneys resembling renal cell carcinoma on intraoperative frozen section. J Urol 2001;166:1820.

90. Randhawa P. Role of donor kidney biopsies in renal transplantation. Transplantation 2001;71:1361.

91. Gaber LW, Moore LW, Alloway RR, et al. Glomerulosclerosis as a determinant of posttransplant function of older donor renal allografts. Transplantation 1995;60:334.

92. Seron D, Carrera M, Grino JM, et al. Relationship between donor renal interstitial surface and post-transplant function. Nephrol Dial Transplant 1993;8:539.

93. Taub HC, Greenstein SM, Lerner SE, et al. Reassessment of the value of post-vascularization biopsy performed at renal transplantation: The effects of arteriosclerosis. J Urol 1994;151:575.

94. Randhawa PS, Minervini MI, Lombardero M, et al. Biopsy of marginal donor kidneys: Correlation of histologic findings with graft dysfunction. Transplantation 2000;69:1352.

95. Kaplan C, Pasternack B, Shah H, Gallo G. Age-related incidence of sclerotic glomeruli in human kidneys. Am J Pathol 1975;80:227.

96. Escofet X, Osman H, Griffiths DF, et al. The presence of glomerular sclerosis at time zero has a significant impact on function after cadaveric renal transplantation. Transplantation 2003;75:344.

97. Pokorna E, Vitko S, Chadimova M, et al. Proportion of glomerulosclerosis in procurement wedge renal biopsy cannot alone discriminate for acceptance of marginal donors. Transplantation 2000;69:36.

98. Mizuiri S, Shigetomi Y, Sugiyama K, et al. Successful transplantation of a cadaveric kidney with post-infectious glomerulonephritis. Pediatr Transplant 2000;4:56.

99. Oda A, Morozumi K, Uchida K. Histological factors of 1-h biopsy influencing the delayed renal function and outcome in cadaveric renal allografts. Clin Transplant 1999;13(Suppl 1):6.

100. Bosmans JL, Woestenburg A, Ysebaert DK, et al. Fibrous intimal thickening at implantation as a risk factor for the outcome of cadaveric renal allografts. Transplantation 2000;69:2388.

101. Karpinski J, Lajoie G, Cattran D, et al. Outcome of kidney transplantation from high-risk donors is determined by both structure and function. Transplantation 1999;67:1162.

102. Howie AJ, Ferreira MA, Lipkin GW, Adu D. Measurement of chronic damage in the donor kidney and graft survival. Transplantation 2004;77:1058.

103. Badid C, Desmouliere A, Babici D, et al. Interstitial expression of alpha-SMA: An early marker of chronic renal allograft dysfunction. Nephrol Dial Transplant 2002;17:1993.

104. Abdi R, Slakey D, Kittur D, et al. Baseline glomerular size as a predictor of function in human renal transplantation. Transplantation 1998;66:329.

105. Li M, Nicholls KM, Becker GJ. Risk factors for late renal allograft dysfunction: Effects of baseline glomerular size. J Nephrol 2002;15:620.

106. Curschellas E, Landmann J, Durig M, et al. Morphologic findings in "zero-hour" biopsies of renal transplants. Clin Nephrol 1991;36:215.

107. McCall SJ, Tuttle-Newhall JE, Howell DN, Fields TA. Prognostic significance of microvascular thrombosis in donor kidney allograft biopsies. Transplantation 2003;75:1847.

108. Gaber LW, Gaber AO, Tolley EA, Hathaway DK. Prediction by postrevascularization biopsies of cadaveric kidney allografts of rejection, graft loss, and preservation nephropathy. Transplantation 1992;53:1219.

109. Rosenberg HG, Martinez PS, Vaccarezza AS, Martinez LV. Morphological findings in 70 kidneys of living donors for renal transplant. Pathol Res Pract 1990;186:619.

110. Cosyns JP, Malaise J, Hanique G, et al. Lesions in donor kidneys: Nature, incidence, and influence on graft function. Transpl Int 1998;11:22.

111. Ji S, Liu M, Chen J, et al. The fate of glomerular mesangial IgA deposition in the donated kidney after allograft transplantation. Clin Transplant 2004;18:536.

112. Silva FG, Chandler P, Pirani CL, Hardy MA. Disappearance of glomerular mesangial IgA deposits after renal allograft transplantation. Transplantation 1982;33:214.

113. Tolkoff-Rubin NE, Cosimi AB, Fuller T, et al. IgA nephropathy in HLA-identical siblings. Transplantation 1978;26:430.

114. Sanfilippo F, Croker BP, Bollinger RR. Fate of four cadaveric donor renal allografts with mesangial IgA deposits. Transplantation 1982;33:370.

115. Parker SM, Pullman JM, Khauli RB. Successful transplantation of a kidney with early membranous nephropathy. Urology 1995;46:870.

116. Nakazawa K, Shimojo H, Komiyama Y, et al. Preexisting membranous nephropathy in allograft kidney. Nephron 1999;81:76.

117. Lipkowitz GS, Madden RL, Kurbanov A, et al. Transplantation and 2-year follow-up of kidneys procured from a cadaver donor with a history of lupus nephritis. Transplantation 2000;69:1221.

118. Brunt EM, Kissane JM, Cole BR, Hanto DW. Transmission and resolution of type I membranoproliferative glomerulonephritis in recipients of cadaveric renal allografts. Transplantation 1988;46:595.

119. Koppel MH, Coburn JW, Mims MM, et al. Transplantation of cadaveric kidneys from patients with hepatorenal syndrome. Evidence for the functional nature of renal failure in advanced liver disease. N Engl J Med 1969;280:1367.

120. Benson SR, Ready AR, Savage CO. Donor platelet and leukocyte load identify renal allografts at an increased risk of acute rejection. Transplantation 2002;73:93.

121. Parmar MS, Kjellstrand CM, Solez K, Halloran PF. Glomerular endothelial cell detachment in paired cadaver kidney transplants: Evidence that some cadaver donors have pre-existing endothelial injury. Clin Transplant 1994;8:120.

122. Haas M, Ratner LE, Montgomery RA. C4d staining of perioperative renal transplant biopsies. Transplantation 2002;74:711.

123. Schwarz C, Hauser P, Steininger R, et al. Failure of BCL-2 up-regulation in proximal tubular epithelial cells of donor kidney biopsy specimens is associated with apoptosis and delayed graft function. Lab Invest 2002;82:941.

124. Oberbauer R, Rohrmoser M, Regele H, et al. Apoptosis of tubular epithelial cells in donor kidney biopsies predicts early renal allograft function. J Am Soc Nephrol 1999;10:2006.

125. Schwarz C, Regele H, Steininger R, et al. The contribution of adhesion molecule expression in donor kidney biopsies to early allograft dysfunction. Transplantation 2001;71:1666.

126. Mitterbauer C, Schwarz C, Hauser P, et al. Impaired tubulointerstitial expression of endothelin-1 and nitric oxide isoforms in donor biopsies with postischemic acute renal failure. Transplantation 2003;76:715.

127. Carver BS, Zibari GB, Venable DD, Eastham JA. Renal cell carcinoma detected in a cadaveric donor after orthotopic liver and contralateral renal transplantation in two recipients: Four-year follow-up. Transplantation 2001;71:1348.

128. Penn I. Primary kidney tumors before and after renal transplantation. Transplantation 1995;59:480.

129. Morris-Stiff G, Steel A, Savage P, et al. Transmission of donor melanoma to multiple organ transplant recipients. Am J Transplant 2004;4:444.

130. Rao KV, Kasiske BL, Bloom PM. Acute graft rejection in the late survivors of renal transplantation. Clinical and histological observations in the second decade. Transplantation 1989;47:290.

131. Reinke P, Fietze E, Docke WD, et al. Late acute rejection in long-term renal allograft recipients. Diagnostic and predictive value of circulating activated T-cells. Transplantation 1994;58:35.

132. Ahmad I, Abul-Ezz SR, Walker PD, et al. Acute rejection presenting as nephrotic syndrome. Transplantation 2000;69:2663.

133. Kasiske B, Gaston RS, Gourishankar S, et al. Long-term deterioration of kidney allograft function. Am J Transplant 2005;5:1405.

134. Cecka JM. The OPTN/UNOS Renal Transplant Registry. In: Clinical Transplants 2003, Los Angeles: UCLA Immunogenetics Center, 2004:1.

135. Porter KA, Marchioro TL, Starzl TE. Pathological changes in 37 human renal homotransplants treated with immunosuppressive drugs. Br J Urol 1965;37:250.

136. Trpkov K, Campbell P, Pazderka F, et al. Pathologic features of acute renal allograft rejection associated with donor-specific antibody: Analysis using the Banff grading schema. Transplantation 1996;61:1586.

137. Bishop GA, Hall BM, Duggin GG, et al. Immunopathology of renal allograft rejection analyzed with monoclonal antibodies to mononuclear cell markers. Kidney Int 1986;29:708.

138. Harry TR, Coles GA, Davies M, et al. The significance of monocytes in glomeruli of human renal transplants. Transplantation 1984;37:70.

139. Tuazon TV, Schneeberger EE, Bhan AK, et al. Mononuclear cells in acute allograft glomerulopathy. Am J Pathol 1987;129:119.

140. Olsen S, Spencer E, Cockfield S, et al. Endocapillary glomerulitis in the renal allograft. Transplantation 1995;59:1421.

141. Axelsen RA, Seymour AE, Mathew TH, et al. Glomerular transplant rejection: A distinctive pattern of early graft damage. Clin Nephrol 1985;23:1.

142. Herrera GA, Alexander RW, Cooley CF, et al. Cytomegalovirus glomerulopathy: A controversial lesion. Kidney Int 1986;29:725.

143. Maryniak R, First RM, Weiss MA. Transplant glomerulopathy: Evolution of morphologically distinct changes. Kidney Int 1985;27:799.

144. Richardson WP, Colvin RB, Cheeseman SH, et al. Glomerulopathy associated with cytomegalovirus viremia in renal allografts. New Engl J Med 1981;305:57.

145. Katafuchi R, Masutani K, Mizumasa T, et al. A case of persistent acute allograft glomerulopathy with long-standing stable renal function. Clin Transplant 2001;15:2.

146. Colvin RB, Cosimi AB, Burton RC, et al. Circulating T-cell subsets in human renal allograft recipients: The OKT4+/OKT8+ cell ratio correlates with reversibility of graft injury and glomerulopathy. Transplant Proc 1983;15:1166.

147. Messias NC, Eustace JA, Zachary AA, et al. Cohort study of the prognostic significance of acute transplant glomerulitis in acutely rejecting renal allografts. Transplantation 2001;72:655.

148. Resch L, Yu W, Fraser RB, et al. T-cell/periodic acid-Schiff stain: A useful tool in the evaluation of tubulointerstitial infiltrates as a component of renal allograft rejection. Ann Diagn Pathol 2002;6:122.

149. Nádasdy T, Ormos J, Stiller D, et al. Tubular ultrastructure in rejected human renal allografts. Ultrastruct Pathol 1988;12:195.

150. Marcussen N, Lai R, Olsen TS, Solez K. Morphometric and immunohistochemical investigation of renal biopsies from patients with transplant ATN, native ATN, or acute graft rejection. Transplant Proc 1996;28:470.

151. Iványi B, Hansen HE, Olsen S. Segmental localization and quantitative characteristics of tubulitis in kidney biopsies from patients undergoing acute rejection. Transplantation 1993;56:581.

152. Fonseca LE Jr, Shapiro R, Randhawa PS. Occurrence of urinary tract infection in patients with renal allograft biopsies showing neutrophilic tubulitis. Mod Pathol 2003;16:281.

153. Mauiyyedi S, Crespo M, Collins AB, et al. Acute humoral rejection in kidney transplantation. II. Morphology, immunopathology, and pathologic classification. J Am Soc Nephrol 2002;13:779.

154. Cohen AH, Border WA, Rajfer J, et al. Interstitial Tamm-Horsfall protein in rejecting renal allografts. Identification and morphologic pattern of injury. Lab Invest 1984;50:519.

155. Hancock WW, Atkins RC. Immunohistological analysis of sequential renal biopsies from patients with acute renal rejection. J Immunol 1985;136:2416.

156. Kirk AD, Mannon RB, Kleiner DE, et al. Results from a human renal allograft tolerance trial evaluating T-cell depletion with alemtuzumab combined with deoxyspergualin. Transplantation 2005;80:1051.

157. Leskinen R, Häyry P. Topographical distribution of inflammatory leukocyte subsets in acute cellular rejection of a kidney allograft. Acta Pathol Microbiol Immunol Scand 1986;94:69.

158. Andersen CB, Ladefoged SD, Larsen S. Acute kidney graft rejection: A morphological and immunohistological study on "zero-hour" and follow-up biopsies with special emphasis on cellular infiltrates and adhesion molecules. APMIS 1994;102:23.

159. Meehan S, McCluskey R, Pascual M, et al. Cytotoxicity and apoptosis in human renal allografts: Identification, distribution, and quantitation of cells with a cytotoxic granule protein GMP-17 (TIA-1) and cells with fragmented nuclear DNA. Lab Invest 1997;76:639.

160. Sako H, Nakane Y, Okino K, et al. Immunohistochemical study of the cells infiltrating human renal allografts by the ABC and the IGSS method using monoclonal antibodies. Transplantation 1987;44:43.

161. Sarwal M, Chua MS, Kambham N, et al. Molecular heterogeneity in acute renal allograft rejection identified by DNA microarray profiling. N Engl J Med 2003;349:125.

162. Charney DA, Nadasdy T, Lo AW, Racusen LC. Plasma cell-rich acute renal allograft rejection. Transplantation 1999;68:791.

163. Desvaux D, Le Gouvello S, Pastural M, et al. Acute renal allograft rejections with major interstitial oedema and plasma cell-rich infiltrates: High gamma-interferon expression and poor clinical outcome. Nephrol Dial Transplant 2004;19:933.

164. Aiello FB, Calabrese F, Rigotti P, et al. Acute rejection and graft survival in renal transplanted patients with viral diseases. Mod Pathol 2004;17:189.

165. David-Neto E, Ribeiro DS, Ianhez LE, et al. Acute interstitial nephritis of plasma cells: A new cause for renal allograft loss. Transplant Proc 1993;25:897.

166. Meehan SM, Domer P, Josephson M, et al. The clinical and pathologic implications of plasmacytic infiltrates in percutaneous renal allograft biopsies. Human Pathology 2001;32:205.

167. Danilewicz M, Wagrowska-Danilewicz M. Immunohistochemical analysis of the interstitial mast cells in acute rejection of human renal allografts. Med Sci Monit 2004;10:BR151.

168. Weir MR, Hall-Craggs M, Shen SY, et al. The prognostic value of the eosinophil in acute renal allograft rejection. Transplantation 1986;41:709.

169. Kormendi F, Amend W. The importance of eosinophil cells in kidney allograft rejection. Transplantation 1988;45:537.

170. Nickeleit V, Vamvakas EC, Pascual M, et al. The prognostic significance of specific arterial lesions in acute renal allograft rejection. J Am Soc Nephrol 1998;9:1301.

171. Hongwei W, Nanra RS, Stein A, et al. Eosinophils in acute renal allograft rejection. Transplant Immunology 1994;2:41.

172. Almirall J, Campistol JM, Sole M, et al. Blood and graft eosinophilia as a rejection index in kidney transplant. Nephron 1993;65:304.

173. Meleg-Smith S, Gauthier PM. Abundance of interstitial eosinophils in renal allografts is associated with vascular rejection. Transplantation 2005;79:444.

174. Ten RM, Gleich GJ, Holley KE, et al. Eosinophil granule major basic protein in acute renal allograft rejection. Transplantation 1989;47:959.

175. Colvin RB, Dvorak HF. Basophils and mast cells in renal allograft rejection. Lancet 1974;1:212.

176. McKenzie I, Colvin RB, Russell PS. Clinical immunopathology of transplantation. In: Miescher PA, Mueller-Eberhard HJ, eds. Textbook of Immunopathology, 2nd ed. New York: Grune and Stratton, 1976:1043.

177. Racusen LC, Solez K, Colvin RB, et al. The Banff 97 working classification of renal allograft pathology. Kidney Int 1999;55:713.

178. Sibley RK, Rynasiewicz J, Ferguson RM, et al. Morphology of cyclosporine nephrotoxicity and acute rejection in patients immunosuppressed with cyclosporine and prednisone. Surgery 1983;94:225.

179. Schroeder TJ, Weiss MA, Smith RD, et al. The efficacy of OKT3 in vascular rejection. Transplantation 1991;51:312.

180. Kooijmans-Coutinho MF, Hermans J, Schrama E, et al. Interstitial rejection, vascular rejection, and diffuse thrombosis of renal allografts. Predisposing factors, histology, immunohistochemistry, and relation to outcome. Transplantation 1996;61:1338.

181. Bates WD, Davies DR, Welsh K, et al. An evaluation of the Banff classification of early renal allograft biopsies and correlation with outcome. Nephrol Dial Transplant 1999;14:2364.

182. Bellamy CO, Randhawa PS. Arteriolitis in renal transplant biopsies is associated with poor graft outcome. Histopathology 2000;36:488.

183. Alpers CE, Gordon D, Gown AM. Immunophenotype of vascular rejection in renal transplants. Mod Pathol 1990;3:198.

184. Aita K, Yamaguchi Y, Horita S, et al. Peritubular capillaritis in early renal allograft is associated with the development

of chronic rejection and chronic allograft nephropathy. Clin Transplant 2005;19(Suppl 14):20.

185. Racusen LC, Colvin RB, Solez K, et al. Antibody-mediated rejection criteria—an addition to the Banff 97 classification of renal allograft rejection. Am J Transplant 2003;3:708.

186. Torbenson M, Randhawa P. Arcuate and interlobular phlebitis in renal allografts. Hum Pathol 2001;32:1388.

187. Katz JP, Hakki A, Katz SM, Simonian S. Rejection of the ureter: A new component of renal allograft rejection. Transplant Proc 1987;19:2200.

188. Paccione F, Enein AA, Shikata T, Dempster WJ. Changes in the transplanted ureter. Brit J Exp Pathol 1965;46:519.

189. Fusaro F, Murer L, Busolo F, et al. CMV and BKV ureteritis: Which prognosis for the renal graft? J Nephrol 2003;16:591.

190. Haber MH, Putong PB. Ureteral vascular rejection in human renal transplants. JAMA 1965;192:417.

191. Andrews PA, Finn JE, Lloyd CM, et al. Expression and tissue localization of donor-specific complement C3 synthesized in human renal allografts. Eur J Immunol 1995;25:1087.

192. Brooimans RA, Stegmann AP, van Dorp WT, et al. Interleukin 2 mediates stimulation of complement C3 biosynthesis in human proximal tubular epithelial cells. J Clin Invest 1991;88:379.

193. Endo T, Nakao S, Koizumi K, et al. Successful treatment with rituximab for autoimmune hemolytic anemia concomitant with proliferation of Epstein-Barr virus and monoclonal gammopathy in a post-nonmyeloablative stem cell transplant patient. Ann Hematol 2004;83:114.

194. Busch GJ, Galvanek EG, Reynolds ES. Human renal allografts. Analysis of lesions in long-term survivors. Human Pathol 1971;2:253.

195. Busch GJ, Reynolds ES, Galvanek EG, et al. Human renal allografts. The role of vascular injury in early graft failure. Medicine 1971;50:29.

196. McKenzie I, Whittingham S. Deposits of immunoglobulin and fibrin in human renal allografted kidneys. Lancet 1968;2:1313.

197. Colvin RB, Mosesson MW, Dvorak HF. Delayed-type hypersensitivity skin reactions in congenital afibrinogenemia lack fibrin deposition and induration. J Clin Invest 1979;63:1302.

198. Schwager I, Jungi TW. Effect of human recombinant cytokines on the induction of macrophage procoagulant activity. Blood 1994;83:152.

199. Mauiyyedi S, Colvin RB. Humoral rejection in kidney transplantation: New concepts in diagnosis and treatment. Curr Opin Nephrol Hypertens 2002;11:609.

200. Kuypers DR, Lerut E, Evenepoel P, et al. C3d deposition in peritubular capillaries indicates a variant of acute renal allograft rejection characterized by a worse clinical outcome. Transplantation 2003;76:102.

201. Shimamura T, Gyorkey F, Morgen RO, DeBakey ME. Fine structural observations in human kidney homografts. Invest Urol 1966;3:590.

202. Iványi B, Hamilton-Dutoit SJ, Hansen HE, Olsen S. Acute tubulointerstitial nephritis: Phenotype of infiltrating cells and prognostic impact of tubulitis. Virchows Archiv 1996;428:5.

203. Iványi B, Hansen HE, Olsen TS. Postcapillary venule-like transformation of peritubular capillaries in acute renal allograft rejection. An ultrastructural study. Arch Pathol Lab Med 1992;116:1062.

204. Oikawa T, Morozumi K, Koyama K, et al. Electron microscopic peritubular capillary lesions: A new criterion for chronic rejection. Clin Transplant 13 Suppl 1999;1:24.

205. Dvorak HF, Mihm MC Jr, Dvorak AM, et al. Rejection of first-set skin allografts in man. J Exp Med 1979;150:322.

206. Rosenberg AS, Mizuochi T, Singer A. Analysis of T-cell subsets in rejection of $K^b$ mutant skin allografts differing at class I MHC. Nature 1986;322:829.

207. Hansen TH, Carreno BM, Sachs DH. The major histocompatibility complex. In: Paul WE, ed. Fundamental Immunology. 3rd ed. New York: Raven Press; 1993:577.

208. Shiina T, Inoko H, Kulski JK. An update of the HLA genomic region, locus information and disease associations: 2004. Tissue Antigens 2004;64:631.

209. Daar AS, Fuggle SV, Fabre JW, et al. The detailed distribution of MHC Class II antigens in normal human organs. Transplantation 1984;38:293.

210. Fuggle SV, McWhinnie DL, Chapman JR, et al. Sequential analysis of HLA class II antigen expression in human renal allografts: Induction of tubular class II antigens and correlation with clinical parameters. Transplantation 1985;42:144.

211. Hancock WW, Kraft N, Atkins RC. The immunohistochemical demonstration of major histocompatibility antigens in the human kidney using monoclonal antibodies. Transplantation 1982;39:430.

212. Pober JS. Immunobiology of human vascular endothelium. Immunol Res 1999;19:225.

213. Maguire JE, Gresser I, Williams AH, et al. Modulation of expression of MHC antigens in the kidneys of mice by murine interferon-a/b. Transplantation 1990;49:130.

214. Skoskiewicz MJ, Colvin RB, Schneeberger EE, Russell PS. Widespread and selective induction of major histocompatibility complex-determined antigens in vivo by gamma interferon. J Exp Med 1985;162:1645.

215. Matas AJ, Sibley R, Mauer M, et al. The value of needle renal allograft biopsy. I. A retrospective study of biopsies performed during putative rejection episodes. Annals of Surgery 1983;197:226.

216. Halloran PF, Afrouzian M, Ramassar V, et al. Interferon-gamma acts directly on rejecting renal allografts to prevent graft necrosis. Am J Pathol 2001;158:215.

217. Grusby M, Auchincloss H, Lee R, et al. Mice lacking major histocompatibility complex class I and class II molecules. Proc Nat Acad Sci 1993;90:3913.

218. Lee RS, Grusby MJ, Laufer TM, et al. CD8$^+$ effector cells responding to residual class I antigens, with help from CD4$^+$ cells stimulated indirectly, cause rejection of "major histocompatibility complex-deficient" skin grafts. Transplantation 1997;63:1123.

219. Benacerraf B. Antigen processing and presentation. The biologic role of MHC molecules in determinant selection. J Immunol 1988;141:s17.

220. Moreau JF, Bonneville M, Peyrat MA, et al. T lymphocyte cloning from rejected human kidney allografts. Growth frequency and functional/phenotypic analysis. J Clin Invest 1986;78:874.

221. Shinohara N, Bluestone JA, Sachs DH. Cloned cytotoxic T lymphocytes that recognize an I-A region product in the context of a class I antigen. J Exp Med 1986;163:972.

222. Graff RJ, Brown DH. Estimates of histocompatibility differences between inbred mouse strains. Immunogenetics 1978;7:367.

223. Poindexter NJ, Steward NS, Shenoy S, et al. Cytolytic T lymphocytes from human renal allograft biopsies are tissue specific. Human Immunology 1995;44:43.

224. Moraes JR, Luo Y, Moraes ME, Stastny P. Clinical relevance of antibodies to non-HLA antigens in organ transplantation. Clin Lab Med 1991;11:621.

225. Krieger NR, Yin DP, Fathman CG. CD4+ but not CD8+ cells are essential for allorejection. J Exp Med 1996;184:2013.

226. Mosmann TR, Cherwinski H, Bond MW, et al. Two types of murine helper T-cell clone. I. Definition according to profiles of lymphokine activities and secreted proteins. J Immunol 1986;136:2348.

227. Yamane H, Zhu J, Paul WE. Independent roles for IL-2 and GATA-3 in stimulating naive CD4+ T-cells to generate a Th2-inducing cytokine environment. J Exp Med 2005;202:793.

228. Garcia-Zepeda EA, Rothenberg ME, Ownbey RT, et al. Human eotaxin is a specific chemoattractant for eosinophil cells and provides a new mechanism to explain tissue eosinophilia. Nat Med 1996;2:449.

229. Honjo K, Xu XY, Bucy RP. Heterogeneity of T-cell clones specific for a single indirect alloantigenic epitope (I-Ab/H-2Kd54–68) that mediate transplant rejection. Transplantation 2000;70:1516.

230. Hidalgo LG, Urmson J, Halloran PF. IFN-gamma decreases CTL generation by limiting IL-2 production: A feedback loop controlling effector cell production. Am J Transplant 2005; 5:651.

231. Catalfamo M, Henkart PA. Perforin and the granule exocytosis cytotoxicity pathway. Curr Opin Immunol 2003;15:522.

232. Pinkoski MJ, Waterhouse NJ, Heibein JA, et al. Granzyme B-mediated apoptosis proceeds predominantly through a Bcl-2-inhibitable mitochondrial pathway. J Biol Chem 2001;276: 12060.

233. Schulz M, Schuurman HJ, Joergensen J, et al. Acute rejection of vascular heart allografts by perforin-deficient mice. Eur J Immunol 1995;25:474.

234. Halloran PF, Urmson J, Ramassar V, et al. Lesions of T-cell-mediated kidney allograft rejection in mice do not require perforin or granzymes A and B. Am J Transplant 2004;4: 705.

235. Dai Z, Li Q, Wang Y, et al. CD4+CD25+ regulatory T-cells suppress allograft rejection mediated by memory CD8+ T-cells via a CD30-dependent mechanism. J Clin Invest 2004;113:310.

236. Walker LS. CD4+ CD25+ Treg: Divide and rule? Immunology 2004;111:129.

237. Fahlen L, Read S, Gorelik L, et al. T cells that cannot respond to TGF-beta escape control by CD4(+)CD25(+) regulatory T-cells. J Exp Med 2005;201:737.

238. Nelson PJ, Krensky AM. Chemokines, chemokine receptors, and allograft rejection. Immunity 2001;14:377.

239. Segerer S, Bohmig GA, Exner M, et al. Role of CXCR3 in cellular but not humoral renal allograft rejection. Transpl Int 2005;18:676.

240. Segerer S, Cui Y, Eitner F, et al. Expression of chemokines and chemokine receptors during human renal transplant rejection. Am J Kidney Dis 2001;37:518.

241. Ruster M, Sperschneider H, Funfstuck R, et al. Differential expression of beta-chemokines MCP-1 and RANTES and their receptors CCR1, CCR2, CCR5 in acute rejection and chronic allograft nephropathy of human renal allografts. Clin Nephrol 2004;61:30.

242. Grandaliano G, Gesualdo L, Ranieri E, et al. Monocyte chemotactic peptide-1 expression and monocyte infiltration in acute renal transplant rejection. Transplantation 1997;63:414.

243. Segerer S, Mac KM, Regele H, et al. Expression of the C-C chemokine receptor 5 in human kidney diseases. Kidney Int 1999;56:52.

244. Eitner F, Cui Y, Hudkins KL, et al. Chemokine receptor (CCR5) expression in human kidneys and in the HIV infected macaque. Kidney Int 1998;54:1945.

245. Cockwell P, Chakravorty SJ, Girdlestone J, Savage CO. Fractalkine expression in human renal inflammation. J Pathol 2002;196:85.

246. Pattison J, Nelson PJ, Huie P, et al. RANTES chemokine expression in cell-mediated transplant rejection of the kidney. Lancet 1994;343:209.

247. Schmouder RL, Streiter RM, Wiggins RC, et al. In vitro and in vivo production of interleukin-8 (IL-8) in renal cortical epithelium. Kidney Int 1992;41:191.

248. Vandenbroecke C, Caillat-Zucman S, Legendre C, et al. Differential in situ expression of cytokines in renal allograft rejection. Transplantation 1991;51:602.

249. Van Kooten C, Boonstra JG, Paape ME, et al. Interleukin-17 activates human renal epithelial cells in vitro and is expressed during renal allograft rejection. J Am Soc Nephrol 1998;9:1526.

250. Robertson H, Morley AR, Talbot D, et al. Renal allograft rejection: Beta-chemokine involvement in the development of tubulitis. Transplantation 2000;69:684.

251. Ali S, Malik G, Burns A, et al. Renal transplantation: Examination of the regulation of chemokine binding during acute rejection. Transplantation 2005;79:672.

252. Burdick JF, Beschorner WE, Smith WJ, et al. Characteristics of early routine renal allograft biopsies. Transplantation 1984; 38:679.

253. Preffer FI, Colvin RB, Leary CP, et al. Two-color flow cytometry and functional analysis of lymphocytes cultured from human renal allografts: Identification of a Leu-2+3+ subpopulation. J Immunol 1986;137:2823.

254. Sanfilippo F, Kolbeck PC, Vaughn WK, Bollinger RR. Renal allograft cell infiltrates associated with irreversible rejection. Transplantation 1985;40:679.

255. Ibrahim S, Dawson DV, Sanfilippo F. Predominant infiltration of rejecting human renal allografts with T-cells expressing CD8 and CD45RO. Transplantation 1995;59:724.

256. Raasveld MH, Bloemena E, Surachno S, ten Berge RJ. T gamma/delta lymphocytes in renal transplant recipients. Nephrol Dial Transplant 1992;7:530.

257. Kirk AD, Ibrahim S, Dawson DV, et al. Characterization of T-cells expressing the g/d antigen receptor in human renal allografts. Human Immunology 1993;36:11.

258. Frisman DM, Hurwitz AA, Bennett WT, et al. Clonal analysis of graft-infiltrating lymphocytes from renal and cardiac biopsies. Dominant rearrangements of TcR beta genes and persistence of dominant rearrangements in serial biopsies. Human Immunology 1990;28:208.

259. Obata F, Yoshida K, Ikeda Y, et al. Clonality analysis of T-cells mediating acute and chronic rejection in kidney allografts. Transpl Immunol 2004;13:233.

260. Obata F, Kumano K, Endo T, et al. T-cell receptor variable gene analysis of renal allograft-infiltrating cells in biopsy specimens using a nonradioisotopic micromethod. Transplantation 1998;66:1389.

261. Douillard P, Cuturi MC, Brouard S, et al. T-cell receptor repertoire usage in allotransplantation: An overview. Transplantation 1999;68:913.

262. Hu M, Zhang GY, Walters G, et al. Matching T-cell receptors identified in renal biopsies and urine at the time of acute rejection in pediatric renal transplant patients. Am J Transplant 2004;4:1859.

263. Kataoka K, Naomoto Y, Shiozaki S, et al. Infiltration of perforin-positive mononuclear cells into the rejected kidney allograft. Transplantation 1992;53:240.

264. Pascoe MD, Marshall SE, Welsh KI, et al. Increased accuracy of renal allograft rejection diagnosis using combined perforin, granzyme B, and Fas ligand fine-needle aspiration immunocytology. Transplantation 2000;69:2547.

265. Akasaka Y, Ishikawa Y, Kato S, et al. Induction of Fas-mediated apoptosis in a human renal epithelial cell line by interferon-gamma: Involvement of Fas-mediated apoptosis in acute renal rejection. Mod Pathol 1998;11:1107.

266. Kummer J, Wever P, Kamp A, et al. Expression of granzyme A and B proteins by cytotoxic lymphocytes involved in acute renal allograft rejection. Kidney Int 1995;47:70.

267. Rowshani AT, Florquin S, Bemelman F, et al. Hyperexpression of the granzyme B inhibitor PI-9 in human renal allografts: A potential mechanism for stable renal function in patients with subclinical rejection. Kidney Int 2004;66:1417.

268. Mengel M, Mueller I, Behrend M, et al. Prognostic value of cytotoxic T-lymphocytes and CD40 in biopsies with early renal allograft rejection. Transpl Int 2004;17:293.

269. Kurnick JT, Preffer FI, Colvin RB, et al. Functional analysis of lymphocyte subsets and clones infiltrating renal allografts. J Immunol 1987;141:4187.

270. Noronha IL, Hartley B, Cameron JS, Waldherr R. Detection of IL-1 beta and TNF-alpha message and protein in renal allograft biopsies. Transplantation 1993;56:1026.

271. Veronese F, Rotman S, Smith RN, et al. Foxp3 T regulatory cells (Tregs) in human kidney allograft biopsies: phenotype and relation to rejection type, tubulitis and outcome. Transplant Proc, in press.

272. Lee I, Wang L, Wells AD, et al. Recruitment of Foxp3+ T regulatory cells mediating allograft tolerance depends on the CCR4 chemokine receptor. J Exp Med 2005;201:1037.

273. Noronha IL, Eberlein-Gonska M, Hartley B, et al. In situ expression of tumor necrosis factor-alpha, interferon-gamma, and interleukin-2 receptors in renal allograft biopsies. Transplantation 1992;54:1017.

274. Biancone L, Segoloni G, Turello E, et al. Expression of inducible lymphocyte costimulatory molecules in human renal allograft. Nephrol Dial Transplant 1998;13:716.

275. Grimm PC, McKenna RM, Gospodarek EM, et al. Low frequency of infiltrating cells intensely expressing T-cell cytokine mRNA in human renal allograft rejection. Transplantation 1995;59:579.

276. Dugre FJ, Gaudreau S, Belles-Isles M, et al. Cytokine and cytotoxic molecule gene expression determined in peripheral blood mononuclear cells in the diagnosis of acute renal rejection. Transplantation 2000;70:1074.

277. Serinsoz E, Bock O, Gwinner W, et al. Local complement C3 expression is upregulated in humoral and cellular rejection of renal allografts. Am J Transplant 2005;5:1490.

278. Waltzer WC, Miller F, Arnold A, et al. Immunohistologic analysis of human renal allograft dysfunction. Transplantation 1987;43:100.

279. Copin MC, Noel C, Hazzan M, et al. Diagnostic and predictive value of an immunohistochemical profile in asymptomatic acute rejection of renal allografts. Transplant Immunology 1995;3:229.

280. Ito H, Kasagi N, Shomori K, et al. Apoptosis in the human allografted kidney. Analysis by terminal deoxynucleotidyl transferase-mediated DUTP-botin nick end labeling. Transplantation 1995;60:794.

281. Noronha IL, Oliveira SG, Tavares TS, et al. Apoptosis in kidney and pancreas allograft biopsies. Transplantation 2005; 79:1231.

282. August C, Schmid KW, Dietl KH, Heidenreich S. Prognostic value of lymphocyte apoptosis in acute rejection of renal allografts. Transplantation 1999;67:581.

283. Briscoe DM, Pober JSS, Harmon WE, Cotran RS. Expression of vascular cell adhesion molecule-1 in human renal allografts. J Am Soc Nephrol 1992;3:1180.

284. Wyburn KR, Jose MD, Wu H, et al. The role of macrophages in allograft rejection. Transplantation 2005;80:1641.

285. Dooper IM, Hoitsma AJ, Maass CN, et al. The extent of peritubular CD14 staining in renal allografts as an independent immunohistological marker for acute rejection. Transplantation 1994;58:820.

286. Hancock WW, Rickles FR, Ewan VA, Atkins RC. Immunohistological studies with A1-3, a monoclonal antibody to activated human monocytes and macrophages. J Immunol 1986; 136:2416.

287. Wang T, Dong C, Stevenson SC, et al. Overexpression of soluble fas attenuates transplant arteriosclerosis in rat aortic allografts. Circulation 2002;106:1536.

288. Watschinger B, Sayegh MH. Endothelin in organ transplantation. Am J Kidney Dis 1996;27:151.

289. Ozdemir BH, Ozdemir FN, Haberal N, et al. Vascular endothelial growth factor expression and cyclosporine toxicity in renal allograft rejection. Am J Transplant 2005;5:766.

290. Morel D, Normand E, Lemoine C, et al. Tumor necrosis factor alpha in human kidney transplant rejection–analysis by in situ hybridization. Transplantation 1993;55:773.

291. Wang Y, Thompson EM, Whawell SA, Fleming KA. Expression and localization of plasminogen activator inhibitor 1 mRNA in transplant kidneys. J Pathol 1993;169:445.

292. Roelofs JJ, Rowshani AT, van den Berg JG, et al. Expression of urokinase plasminogen activator and its receptor during acute renal allograft rejection. Kidney Int 2003;64:1845.

293. Grau V, Stehling O, Garn H, Steiniger B. Accumulating monocytes in the vasculature of rat renal allografts: Phenotype, cytokine, inducible no synthase, and tissue factor mRNA expression. Transplantation 2001;71:37.

294. Steinmetz OM, Panzer U, Kneissler U, et al. BCA-1/CXCL13 expression is associated with CXCR5-positive B-cell cluster formation in acute renal transplant rejection. Kidney Int 2005;67:1616.

295. Robertson H, Wheeler J, Kirby JA, Morley AR. Renal allograft rejection—in situ demonstration of cytotoxic intratubular cells. Transplantation 1996;61:1546.

296. Robertson H, Kirby JA. Post-transplant renal tubulitis: The

297. Wong WK, Robertson H, Carroll HP, et al. Tubulitis in renal allograft rejection: Role of transforming growth factor-beta and interleukin-15 in development and maintenance of CD103+ intraepithelial T-cells. Transplantation 2003;75:505.

298. Robertson H, Wong WK, Talbot D, et al. Tubulitis after renal transplantation: Demonstration of an association between CD103+ T-cells, transforming growth factor beta1 expression and rejection grade. Transplantation 2001;71:306.

299. Yuan R, El-Asady R, Liu K, et al. Critical role for CD103+CD8+ effectors in promoting tubular injury following allogeneic renal transplantation. J Immunol 2005;175:2868.

300. Robertson H, Wheeler J, Thompson V, et al. In situ lymphoproliferation in renal transplant biopsies. Histochem Cell Biol 1995;104:331.

301. Wever PC, Aten J, Rentenaar RJ, et al. Apoptotic tubular cell death during acute renal allograft rejection. Clin Nephrol 1998;49:28.

302. Du C, Guan Q, Yin Z, et al. IL-2-mediated apoptosis of kidney tubular epithelial cells is regulated by the caspase-8 inhibitor c-FLIP. Kidney Int 2005;67:1397.

303. Hagerty DT, Allen PM. Processing and presentation of self- and non-self foreign antigens by the renal proximal tubule. J Immunol 1992;126:2324.

304. Niemann-Masanek U, Mueller A, Yard BA, et al. B7–1 (CD80) and B7–2 (CD 86) expression in human tubular epithelial cells in vivo and in vitro. Nephron 2002;92:542.

305. Fuggle SV, McWhinnie DL, Morris PJ. Precise specificity of induced tubular HLA-class II antigens in renal allografts. Transplantation 1987;44:214.

306. Barrett M, Milton AD, Barrett J, et al. Needle biopsy evaluation of class II major histocompatibility complex antigen expression for the differential diagnosis of cyclosporine nephrotoxicity from kidney graft rejection. Transplantation 1987;44:223.

307. Ozdemir BH, Aksoy PK, Haberal AN, et al. Relationship of HLA-DR expression to rejection and mononuclear cell infiltration in renal allograft biopsies. Ren Fail 2004;26:247.

308. Nickeleit V, Hirsch HH, Zeiler M, et al. BK-virus nephropathy in renal transplants-tubular necrosis MHC-class II expression and rejection in a puzzling game. Nephrol Dial Transplant 2000;15:324.

309. Nickeleit V, Zeiler M, Gudat F, et al. Histological characteristics of interstitial renal allograft rejection. Kidney Blood Press Res 1998;21:230.

310. Alchi B, Nishi S, Kondo D, et al. Osteopontin expression in acute renal allograft rejection. Kidney Int 2005;67:886.

311. Faull RJ, Russ GR. Tubular expression of intercellular adhesion molecule-1 during renal allograft rejection. Transplantation 1989;48:226.

312. Fuggle SV, Sanderson JB, Gray DW, et al. Variation in expression of endothelial adhesion molecules in pretransplant and transplanted kidneys–correlation with intragraft events. Transplantation 1993;55:117.

313. Brockmeyer C, Ulbrecht M, Schendel DJ, et al. Distribution of cell adhesion molecules (ICAM-1, VCAM-1, ELAM-1) in renal tissue during allograft rejection. Transplantation 1993;55:610.

314. Bukovsky A, Labarrere CA, Carter C, et al. Novel immunohistochemical markers of human renal allograft dysfunction–antithrombin III, Thy-1, urokinase, and alpha-smooth muscle actin. Transplantation 1992;54:1064.

315. Robertson H, Ali S, McDonnell BJ, et al. Chronic renal allograft dysfunction: The role of T-cell-mediated tubular epithelial to mesenchymal cell transition. J Am Soc Nephrol 2004;15: 390.

316. Dvergsten J, Manivel JC, Correa-Rotter R, Rosenberg ME. Expression of clusterin in human renal diseases. Kidney Int 1994;45:828.

317. Murphy BF, Davies DJ, Morrow W, D'ApiceAJF. Localization of terminal complement components S-protein and SP-40,40 in renal biopsies. Pathology 1989;21:275.

318. Luo X, Yang H, Kim IS, et al. Systemic transforming growth

factor-beta1 gene therapy induces Foxp3+ regulatory cells, restores self-tolerance, and facilitates regeneration of beta cell function in overtly diabetic nonobese diabetic mice. Transplantation 2005;79:1091.

319. Russell PS, Chase CM, Colvin RB. Alloantibody- and T-cell-mediated immunity in the pathogenesis of transplant arteriosclerosis: Lack of progression to sclerotic lesions in B-cell-deficient mice. Transplantation 1997;64:1531.

320. Visscher D, Carey J, Oh H, et al. Histologic and immunophenotypic evaluation of pretreatment renal biopsies in OKT3-treated allograft rejections. Transplantation 1991;51:1023.

321. Cosimi AB, Burton RC, Colvin RB, et al. Treatment of acute renal allograft rejection with OKT3 monoclonal antibody. Transplantation 1981;32:535.

322. Woywodt A, Schroeder M, Gwinner W, et al. Elevated numbers of circulating endothelial cells in renal transplant recipients. Transplantation 2003;76:1.

323. Park SY, Kim HW, Moon KC, et al. mRNA expression of intercellular adhesion molecule-1 and vascular cell adhesion molecule-1 in acute renal allograft rejection. Transplantation 2000;69:2554.

324. Kirveskari J, Paavonen T, Hayry P, Renkonen R. De novo induction of endothelial L-selectin ligands during kidney allograft rejection. J Am Soc Nephrol 2000;11:2358.

325. Alpers CE, Davis CL, Barr D, et al. Identification of platelet-derived growth factor A and B chains in human renal vascular rejection. Am J Pathol 1996;148:439.

326. Bishop GA, Waugh JA, Landers DV, et al. Microvascular destruction in renal transplant rejection. Transplantation 1989;48:408.

327. Watschinger B, Vychytil A, Attar M, et al. Pattern of endothelin immunostaining during rejection episodes after kidney transplantation. Clin Nephrol 1994;41:86.

328. Segerer S, Bohmig GA, Exner M, et al. When renal allografts turn DARC. Transplantation 2003;75:1030.

329. Segerer S, Regele H, Mac KM, et al. The Duffy antigen receptor for chemokines is up-regulated during acute renal transplant rejection and crescentic glomerulonephritis. Kidney Int 2000;58:1546.

330. Hiki Y, Leong AY, Mathew TH, et al. Typing of intraglomerular mononuclear cells associated with transplant glomerular rejection. Clin Nephrol 1986;26:244.

331. Ko YJ, Sugar L, Zaltzman J, Paul LC: A-smooth muscle actin and collagen deposition in dysfunctional renal transplants. Transplantation 1997;63:156.

332. Ramos EL, Barri YM, Croker BP, et al. Thromboxane synthase expression in renal transplant patients with rejection. Transplantation 1995;59:490.

333. Zollinger HU, Mihatsch MJ. Renal Pathology in Biopsy. Berlin: Springer-Verlag, 1978.

334. Rubin RH, Colvin RB. Impact of cytomegalovirus infection on renal transplantation. In: Racusen LC, Solez K, Burdick JF, eds. Kidney Transplant Rejection: Diagnosis and Treatment, 3rd ed. New York: Marcel Dekker, 1998:605.

335. Cosio FG, Roche Z, Agarwal A, et al. Prevalence of hepatitis C in patients with idiopathic glomerulonephritis in native and transplant kidneys. Am J Kidney Dis 1996;28:752.

336. Browne G, Whitworth C, Bellamy C, Ogilvie MM. Acute allograft glomerulopathy associated with CMV viraemia. Nephrol Dial Transplant 2001;16:861.

337. Cosio FG, Sedmak DD, Henry ML, et al. The high prevalence of severe early posttransplant renal allograft pathology in hepatitis C positive recipients. Transplantation 1996;62:1054.

338. Gallay BJ, Alpers CE, Davis CL, et al. Glomerulonephritis in renal allografts associated with hepatitis C infection: A possible relationship with transplant glomerulopathy in two cases. Am J Kidney Dis 1995;26:662.

339. Meehan SM, Josephson MA, Haas M. Granulomatous tubulointerstitial nephritis in the renal allograft. Am J Kidney Dis 2000;36:E27.

340. Randhawa PS, Magnone M, Jordan M, et al. Renal allograft involvement by Epstein-Barr virus associated post-transplant lymphoproliferative disease. Am J Surg Pathology 1996;20:563.

341. Gonzalez-Posada JM, Garcia-Castro MC, Tamajon LP, et al. HLA-DR class II and ICAM-1 expression on tubular cells taken by fine-needle aspiration biopsy in renal allograft dysfunction. Nephrol Dial Transplant 1996;11:148.

342. Randhawa PS, Saad RS, Jordan M, et al. Clinical significance of renal biopsies showing concurrent acute rejection and tacrolimus-associated tubular vacuolization. Transplantation 1999;67:85.

343. Poduval RD, Kadambi PV, Josephson MA, et al. Implications of immunohistochemical detection of C4d along peritubular capillaries in late acute renal allograft rejection. Transplantation 2005;79:228.

344. Curtis JJ, Julian BA, Sanders CE, et al. Dilemmas in renal transplantation: When the clinical course and histological findings differ. Am J Kidney Dis 1996;27:435.

345. Meehan SM, Siegel CT, Aronson AJ, et al. The relationship of untreated borderline infiltrates by the Banff criteria to acute rejection in renal allograft biopsies. J Am Soc Nephrol 1999;10:1806.

346. McCarthy GP, Roberts IS. Diagnosis of acute renal allograft rejection: Evaluation of the Banff 97 Guidelines for Slide Preparation. Transplantation 2002;73:1518.

347. Regele H, Exner M, Watschinger B, et al. Endothelial C4d deposition is associated with inferior kidney allograft outcome independently of cellular rejection. Nephrol Dial Transplant 2001;16:2058.

348. Nickeleit V, Zeiler M, Gudat F, et al. Detection of the complement degradation product C4d in renal allografts: Diagnostic and therapeutic implications. J Am Soc Nephrol 2002;13:242.

349. Magil AB, Tinckam K. Monocytes and peritubular capillary C4d deposition in acute renal allograft rejection. Kidney Int 2003;63:1888.

350. Magil AB. Infiltrating cell types in transplant glomerulitis: Relationship to peritubular capillary C4d deposition. Am J Kidney Dis 2005;45:1084.

351. Fortin MC, Schurch W, Cardinal H, Hebert MJ. Complement factor H deficiency in acute allograft glomerulopathy and post-transplant hemolytic uremic syndrome. Am J Transplant 2004;4:270.

352. Ades L, Akposso K, Costa de Beauregard MA, et al. Bacterial endocarditis associated with crescentic glomerulonephritis in a kidney transplant patient: First case report. Transplantation 1998;66:653.

353. Banfi G, Imbasciati E, Tarantino A, Ponticelli C. Prognostic value of renal biopsy in acute rejection of kidney transplantation. Nephron 1981;28:222.

354. Herzenberg AM, Gill JS, Djurdjev O, Magil AB. C4d deposition in acute rejection: An independent long-term prognostic factor. J Am Soc Nephrol 2002;13:234.

355. Saad R, Gritsch HA, Shapiro R, et al. Clinical significance of renal allograft biopsies with "borderline changes," as defined in the Banff Schema. Transplantation 1997;64:992.

356. Schweitzer EJ, Drachenberg CB, Anderson L. Significance of the Banff borderline biopsy. Am J Kid Dis 1996;28:585.

357. Marcussen N, Olsen TS, Benediktsson H, et al. Reproducibility of the Banff classification of renal allograft pathology. Inter- and intraobserver variation. Transplantation 1995;60:1083.

358. Gough J, Rush D, Jeffery J, et al. Reproducibility of the Banff schema in reporting protocol biopsies of stable renal allografts. Nephrol Dial Transplant 2002;17:1081.

359. Veronese FV, Manfro RC, Roman FR, et al. Reproducibility of the Banff classification in subclinical kidney transplant rejection. Clin Transplant 2005;19:518.

360. Kazi JI, Furness PN, Nicholson M. Diagnosis of early acute renal allograft rejection by evaluation of multiple histological features using a Bayesian belief network. J Clin Pathol 1998;51:108.

361. Kirk A. CAMPATH path. Transplantatation, 2003.

362. Hibberd AD, Nanra RS, White KH, Trevillian PR. Reversal of acute glomerular renal allograft rejection: A possible effect of OKT3. Transpl Int 1991;4:246.

363. Caillat-Zucman S, Blumenfeld N, Legendre C, et al. The OKT3 immunosuppressive effect. In situ antigenic modulation of human graft-infiltrating T-cells. Transplantation 1990;49: 156.

364. Kerr PG, Atkins RC. The effects of OKT3 therapy on infiltrating lymphocytes in rejecting renal allografts. Transplantation 1989;48:33.

365. Mueller A, Schnuelle P, Waldherr R, van der Woude FJ. Impact of the Banff '97 classification for histological diagnosis of rejection on clinical outcome and renal function parameters after kidney transplantation. Transplantation 2000;69:1123.

366. Macdonald FI, Ashraf S, Picton M, et al. Banff criteria as predictors of outcome following acute renal allograft rejection. Nephrol Dial Transplant 1999;14:1692.

367. Gaber LW, Moore LW, Alloway RR, et al. Correlation between Banff classification, acute renal rejection scores and reversal of rejection. Kidney Int 1996;49:481.

368. Palomar R, Ruiz JC, Zubimendi JA, et al. Is there any correlation between pathologic changes for acute rejection in kidney transplantation (Banff 97) and graft function? Transplant Proc 2002;34:349.

369. Haas M, Kraus ES, Samaniego-Picota M, et al. Acute renal allograft rejection with intimal arteritis: Histologic predictors of response to therapy and graft survival. Kidney Int 2002;61:1516.

370. Kuypers DR, Chapman JR, O'Connell PJ, et al. Predictors of renal transplant histology at three months. Transplantation 1999;67:1222.

371. Herbertson BM, Evans DB, Calne RY, Banerjee AK. Percutaneous needle biopsies of renal allografts: The relationship between morphological changes present in the biopsies and subsequent allograft function. Histopathol 1977;1:161.

372. Kiaer H, Hansen HE, Olsen S. The predictive value of percutaneous biopsies from human renal allografts with early impaired function. Clin Nephrol 1980;13:58.

373. Cosio FG, Pesavento TE, Sedmak DD, et al. Clinical implications of the diagnosis of renal allograft infarction by percutaneous biopsy. Transplantation 1998;66:467.

374. Solez K, McGraw DJ, Beschorner WE, et al. Reflections on use of the renal biopsy as the "gold standard" in distinguishing transplant rejection from cyclosporine nephrotoxicity. Transplantation Proc. 1985;4(Suppl 1):123.

375. Kasiske BL, Kalil RS, Lee HS, Rao KV. Histopathologic findings associated with a chronic, progressive decline in renal allograft function. Kidney Int 1991;40:514.

376. Hsu AC, Arbus GS, Noriega E, Huber J. Renal allograft biopsy: A satisfactory adjunct for predicting renal function after graft rejection. Clin Nephrol 1976;5:260.

377. McWhinnie DL, Thompson JF, Taylor HM, et al. Morphometric analysis of cellular infiltration assessed by monoclonal antibody labeling in sequential human renal allograft biopsies. Transplantation 1986;2:352.

378. MacDonald AS; RAPAMUNE Global Study Group. A worldwide, phase III, randomized, controlled, safety and efficacy study of a sirolimus/cyclosporine regimen for prevention of acute rejection in recipients of primary mismatched renal allografts. Transplantation 2001;71:271.

379. Raftery MJ, Seron D, Koffman G, et al. The relevance of induced class II HLA antigens and macrophage infiltration in early renal allograft biopsies. Transplantation 1989;48:238.

380. Minervini MI, Torbenson M, Scantlebury V, et al. Acute renal allograft rejection with severe tubulitis (Banff 1997 grade IB). Am J Surg Pathol 2000;24:553.

381. Bonsib SM, Abul-Ezz SR, Ahmad I, et al. Acute rejection-associated tubular basement membrane defects and chronic allograft nephropathy. Kidney Int 2000;58:2206.

382. Verani RR, Bergman D, Kerman RH. Glomerulopathy in acute and chronic rejection: Relationship of ultrastructure to graft survival. Am J Nephrol 1983;3:253.

383. Nickeleit V, Mihatsch MJ. Kidney transplants, antibodies and rejection: Is C4d a magic marker? Nephrol Dial Transplant 2003;18:2232.

384. Feucht HE, Felber E, Gokel MJ, et al. Vascular deposition

385. Terasaki PI, Ozawa M. Predicting kidney graft failure by HLA antibodies: A prospective trial. Am J Transplant 2004;4:438.

386. Halloran PF, Schlaut J, Solez K, Srinivasa NS. The significance of the anti-class I antibody response. II. Clinical and pathologic features of renal transplants with anti-class I-like antibody. Transplantation 1992;53:550.

387. Halloran PF, Wadgymar A, Ritchie S, et al. The significance of the anti-class I antibody response. I. Clinical and pathologic features of anti-class I-mediated rejection. Transplantation 1990;49:85.

388. Rotman S, Collins AB, Colvin RB. C4d deposition in allografts: Current concepts and interpretation. Transplant Rev 2005;19:65.

389. Feucht HE, Schneeberger H, Hillebrand G, et al. Capillary deposition of C4d complement fragment and early renal graft loss. Kidney Int 1993;43:1333.

390. Collins AB, Schneeberger EE, Pascual MA, et al. Complement activation in acute humoral renal allograft rejection: Diagnostic significance of C4d deposits in peritubular capillaries. J Am Soc Nephrol 1999;10:2208.

391. Crespo M, Pascual M, Tolkoff-Rubin N, et al. Acute humoral rejection in renal allograft recipients. I. Incidence, serology and clinical characteristics. Transplantation 2001;71:652.

392. Takemoto SK, Zeevi A, Feng S, et al. National conference to assess antibody-mediated rejection in solid organ transplantation. Am J Transplant 2004;4:1033.

393. Lorenz M, Regele H, Schillinger M, et al. Risk factors for capillary C4d deposition in kidney allografts: Evaluation of a large study cohort. Transplantation 2004;78:447.

394. Kawai T, Sachs DH, Spitzer TR, et al. Combined kidney and bone marrow transplantation for induction of mixed chimerism and renal allograft tolerance in HLA mismatched transplantation. Am J Transplant 2004;4(Suppl 8):491.

395. Knechtle SJ, Pirsch JD, H. Fechner JJ, et al. Campath-1H induction plus rapamycin monotherapy for renal transplantation: Results of a pilot study. Am J Transplant 2003;3:722.

396. Baid S, Cosimi AB, Tolkoff-Rubin N, et al. Renal disease associated with hepatitis C infection after kidney and liver transplantation. Transplantation 2000;70:255.

397. Kato M, Morozumi K, Takeuchi O, et al. Complement fragment C4d deposition in peritubular capillaries in acute humoral rejection after ABO blood group-incompatible human kidney transplantation. Transplantation 2003;75:663.

398. Fidler ME, Gloor JM, Lager DJ, et al. Histologic findings of antibody-mediated rejection in ABO blood-group-incompatible living-donor kidney transplantation. Am J Transplant 2004;4:101.

399. Sund S, Reisaeter AV, Scott H, et al. Glomerular monocyte/macrophage influx correlates strongly with complement activation in 1-week protocol kidney allograft biopsies. Clin Nephrol 2004;62:121.

400. Herman J, Lerut E, Van Damme-Lombaerts R, et al. Capillary deposition of complement C4d and C3d in pediatric renal allograft biopsies. Transplantation 2005;79:1435.

401. Lobo PI, Spencer CE, Stevenson WC, Pruett TL. Evidence demonstrating poor kidney graft survival when acute rejections are associated with IgG donor-specific lymphocytotoxin. Transplantation 1995;59:357.

402. Hallgren R, Bohman SO, Fredens K. Activated eosinophil infiltration and deposits of eosinophil cationic protein in renal allograft rejection. Nephron 1991;59:266.

403. Eggertsen G, Nyberg G, Nilsson B, et al. Complement deposition in renal allografts with early malfunction. Apmis 2001;109:825.

404. Jabs WJ, Logering BA, Gerke P, et al. The kidney as a second site of human C-reactive protein formation in vivo. Eur J Immunol 2003;33:152.

405. Kanetsuna Y, Yamaguchi Y, Horita S, et al. C4d and/or immunoglobulins deposition in peritubular capillaries in perioperative graft biopsies in ABO-incompatible renal transplantation. Clin Transplant 2004;18(Suppl 11):13.

406. Meehan SM, Limsrichamrern S, Manaligod JR, et al. Platelets and capillary injury in acute humoral rejection of renal allografts. Hum Pathol 2003;34:533.

407. Liptak P, Kemeny E, Morvay Z, et al. Peritubular capillary damage in acute humoral rejection: An ultrastructural study on human renal allografts. Am J Transplant 2005;5: 2870.

408. Lajoie G. Antibody-mediated rejection of human renal allografts: An electron microscopic study of peritubular capillaries. Ultrastructural Pathology 1997;21:235.

409. Regele H, Bohmig GA, Habicht A, et al. Capillary deposition of complement split product C4d in renal allografts is associated with basement membrane injury in peritubular and glomerular capillaries: A contribution of humoral immunity to chronic allograft rejection. J Am Soc Nephrol 2002;13:2371.

410. Colvin RB, Smith RN. Antibody-mediated organ-allograft rejection. Nat Rev Immunol 2005;5:807.

411. Scornik JC, LeFor WM, Cicciarelli JC, et al. Hyperacute and acute kidney graft rejection due to antibodies against B-cells. Transplantation 1992;54:61.

412. Race RR, Sanger R. Blood Groups in Man. Oxford, UK: Blackwell Science, 1958.

413. Sumitran-Holgersson S, Wilczek HE, Holgersson J, Soderstrom K. Identification of the nonclassical HLA molecules MICA, as targets for humoral immunity associated with irreversible rejection of kidney allografts. Transplantation 2002;74:268.

414. Mizutani K, Terasaki P, Rosen A, et al. Serial ten-year follow-up of HLA and MICA antibody production prior to kidney graft failure. Am J Transplant 2005;5:1.

415. Cerilli J, Brasile L, Galouzis T, et al. The vascular endothelial cell antigen system. Transplantation 1985;39:286.

416. Kalil J, Guilherme L, Neumann J, et al. Humoral rejection in two HLA identical living related donor kidney transplants. Transplant Proc 1989;21:711.

417. Seigler HF, Ward FE, McCoy RE, et al. Long-term results with forty-five living related renal allograft recipients genotypically identical for HLA. Surgery 1977;81:274.

418. Mathew JM, Joyce S, Lawrence W, Mohanakumar T. Evidence that antibodies eluted from rejected kidneys of HLA-identical transplants define a non-MHC alloantigen expressed on human kidneys. Transplantation 1991;52:559.

419. Evans PR, Trickett LP, Gosney AR, et al. Detection of kidney reactive antibodies at crossmatch in renal transplant recipients. Transplantation 1988;46:844.

420. Sun Q, Liu Z, Yin G, et al. Detectable circulating antiendothelial cell antibodies in renal allograft recipients with C4d-positive acute rejection: A report of three cases. Transplantation 2005;79:1759.

421. Dragun D, Muller DN, Brasen JH, et al. Angiotensin II type 1-receptor activating antibodies in renal-allograft rejection. N Engl J Med 2005;352:558.

422. Austen WG Jr, Zhang M, Chan R, et al. Murine hindlimb reperfusion injury can be initiated by a self-reactive monoclonal IgM. Surgery 2004;136:401.

423. Mitchison NA. T-cell-B-cell cooperation. Nat Rev Immunol 2004;4:308.

424. Steele DJ, Laufer TM, Smiley ST, et al. Two levels of help for B-cell alloantibody production. J Exp Med 1996;183:699.

425. Edwards JC, Szczepanski L, Szechinski J, et al. Efficacy of B-cell-targeted therapy with rituximab in patients with rheumatoid arthritis. N Engl J Med 2004;350:2572.

426. Shapiro-Shelef M, Calame K. Regulation of plasma-cell development. Nat Rev Immunol 2005;5:230.

427. Baldwin WM, Ota H, Rodriguez ER. Complement in transplant rejection: Diagnostic and mechanistic considerations. Springer Semin Immunopathol 2003;25:181.

428. Auchincloss H Jr, Sachs DH. Xenogeneic transplantation. Annu Rev Immunol 1998;16:433.

429. Wasowska BA, Qian Z, Cangello DL, et al. Passive transfer of alloantibodies restores acute cardiac rejection in IgKO mice. Transplantation 2001;71:727.

430. Rahimi S, Qian Z, Layton J, et al. Non-complement- and

431. Menoret S, Plat M, Blancho G, et al. Characterization of human CD55 and CD59 transgenic pigs and kidney xenotransplantation in the pig-to-baboon combination. Transplantation 2004;77:1468.

432. Azimzadeh A, Zorn GL 3rd, Blair KS, et al. Hyperacute lung rejection in the pig-to-human model. 2. Synergy between soluble and membrane complement inhibition. Xenotransplantation 2003;10:120.

433. Gao ZH, McAlister VC, Wright JR Jr, et al. Immunoglobulin-G subclass antidonor reactivity in transplant recipients. Liver Transpl 2004;10:1055.

434. Albrecht EA, Chinnaiyan AM, Varambally S, et al. C5a-induced gene expression in human umbilical vein endothelial cells. Am J Pathol 2004;164:849.

435. Monsinjon T, Gasque P, Chan P, et al. Regulation by complement C3a and C5a anaphylatoxins of cytokine production in human umbilical vein endothelial cells. Faseb J 2003;17: 1003.

436. Nakashima S, Qian Z, Rahimi S, et al. Membrane attack complex contributes to destruction of vascular integrity in acute lung allograft rejection. J Immunol 2002;169:4620.

437. Hughes J, Nangaku M, Alpers CE, et al. C5b-9 membrane attack complex mediates endothelial cell apoptosis in experimental glomerulonephritis. Am J Physiol Renal Physiol 2000;278:F747.

438. Kilgore KS, Schmid E, Shanley TP, et al. Sublytic concentrations of the membrane attack complex of complement induce endothelial interleukin-8 and monocyte chemoattractant protein-1 through nuclear factor-kappa B activation. Am J Pathol 1997;150:2019.

439. Saadi S, Holzknecht RA, Patte CP, Platt JL. Endothelial cell activation by pore-forming structures: Pivotal role for interleukin-1alpha. Circulation 2000;101:1867.

440. Ikeda K, Nagasawa K, Horiuchi T, et al. C5a induces tissue factor activity on endothelial cells. Thromb Haemost 1997;77: 394.

441. Saadi S, Holzknecht RA, Patte CP, et al. Complement-mediated regulation of tissue factor activity in endothelium. J Exp Med 1995;182:1807.

442. van den Elsen JM, Martin A, Wong V, et al. X-ray crystal structure of the C4d fragment of human complement component C4. J Mol Biol 2002;322:1103.

443. Baldwin WM 3rd, Kasper EK, Zachary AA, et al. Beyond C4d: Other complement-related diagnostic approaches to antibody-mediated rejection. Am J Transplant 2004;4:311.

444. Sund S, Hovig T, Reisaeter AV, et al. Complement activation in early protocol kidney graft biopsies after living-donor transplantation. Transplantation 2003;75:1204.

445. Ichida S, Yuzawa Y, Okada H, et al. Localization of the complement regulatory proteins in the normal human kidney. Kidney Int 1994;46:89.

446. Nakanishi I, Moutabarrik A, Hara T, et al. Identification and characterization of membrane cofactor protein (CD46) in the human kidneys. Eur J Immunol 1994;24:1529.

447. Cosio FG, Sedmak DD, Mahan JD, Nahman NS Jr. Localization of decay accelerating factor in normal and diseased kidneys. Kidney Int 1989;36:100.

448. Campbell RD, Gagnon J, Porter RR. Amino acid sequence around the thiol and reactive acyl groups of human complement component C4. Biochem J 1981;199:359.

449. Meri S, Waldmann H, Lachmann PJ. Distribution of protectin (CD59), a complement membrane attack inhibitor, in normal human tissues. Lab Invest 1991;65:532.

450. Tamai H, Matsuo S, Fukatsu A, et al. Localization of 20-kD homologous restriction factor (HRF20) in diseased human glomeruli. An immunofluorescence study. Clin Exp Immunol 1991;84:256.

451. Hirschberg H, Thorsby E, Rolstad B. Antibody-induced cell-mediated damage to human endothelial cells in vitro. Nature 1975;255:62.

452. Yuan FF, Watson N, Sullivan JS, et al. Association of Fc gamma

receptor IIA polymorphisms with acute renal-allograft rejection. Transplantation 2004;78:766.

453. Gollackner B, Goh SK, Qawi I, et al. Acute vascular rejection of xenografts: Roles of natural and elicited xenoreactive antibodies in activation of vascular endothelial cells and induction of procoagulant activity. Transplantation 2004;77:1735.

454. Racusen L, Colvin RB, Solez K, Group IC. Standardization of scoring of C4d staining in renal allograft biopsies: Consensus from the Seventh Banff Conference on Allograft Pathology. J Am Soc Nephrol 2003;14:146A.

455. Magil AB, Tinckam KJ. Focal peritubular capillary C4d deposition in acute rejection. Nephrol Dial Transplant, 2006;5:1382.

456. Mengel M, Bogers J, Bosmans JL, et al. Incidence of C4d stain in protocol biopsies from renal allografts: Results from a multicenter trial. Am J Transplant 2005;5:1050.

457. Dickenmann M, Steiger J, Mihatsch M, Nickeleit V. The fate of C4d positive kidney allografts lacking histological signs of acute rejection. Clin Nephrol 2006;65:173.

458. Koo DD, Roberts IS, Quiroga I, et al. C4d deposition in early renal allograft protocol biopsies. Transplantation 2004;78:398.

459. Artz MA, Steenbergen EJ, Hoitsma AJ, et al. Renal transplantation in patients with hemolytic uremic syndrome: High rate of recurrence and increased incidence of acute rejections. Transplantation 2003;76:821.

460. Thurman JM, Lucia MS, Ljubanovic D, Holers VM. Acute tubular necrosis is characterized by activation of the alternative pathway of complement. Kidney Int 2005;67:524.

461. Lerut E, Kuypers D, Van Damme B. C4d deposition in the peritubular capillaries of native renal biopsies. Histopathology 2005;47:430.

462. Lederer SR, Kluth-Pepper B, Schneeberger H, et al. Impact of humoral alloreactivity early after transplantation on the long-term survival of renal allografts. Kidney Int 2001;59:334.

463. Bohmig GA, Exner M, Habicht A, et al. Capillary C4d deposition in kidney allografts: A specific marker of alloantibody-dependent graft injury. J Am Soc Nephrol 2002;13:1091.

464. Troxell ML, Sibley RK, Higgins JP, Kambham N. Comparison of immunofluorescence and immunohistochemical methods for C4d staining in renal allograft biopsies [Abstract]. Mod Pathol 2005;18:270A.

465. Nadasdy GM, Bott C, Cowden D, et al. Comparative study for the detection of peritubular capillary C4d deposition in human renal allografts using different methodologies. Hum Pathol 2005;36:1178.

466. Zwirner J, Felber E, Burger R, et al. Classical pathway of complement activation in mammalian kidneys. Immunology 1993;80:162.

467. Bhakdi S, Torzewski M, Paprotka K, et al. Possible protective role for C-reactive protein in atherogenesis: Complement activation by modified lipoproteins halts before detrimental terminal sequence. Circulation 2004;109:1870.

468. Kuraya M, Ming Z, Liu X, et al. Specific binding of L-ficolin and H-ficolin to apoptotic cells leads to complement activation. Immunobiology 2005;209:689.

469. Martin L, Guignier F, Mousson C, et al. Detection of donor-specific anti-HLA antibodies with flow cytometry in eluates and sera from renal transplant recipients with chronic allograft nephropathy. Transplantation 2003;76:395.

470. de Vries B, Walter SJ, Peutz-Kootstra CJ, et al. The mannose-binding lectin-pathway is involved in complement activation in the course of renal ischemia-reperfusion injury. Am J Pathol 2004;165:1677.

471. Sund S, Hovig T, Reisaeter AV, et al. Complement activation in early protocol kidney graft biopsies after living-donor transplantation. Transplantation 2003;75:1204.

472. Lederer SR, Kluth-Pepper B, Schneeberger H, et al. Impact of humoral alloreactivity early after transplantation on the long-term survival of renal allografts. Kidney Int 2001;59:334.

473. Fiebeler A, Mengel M, Merkel S, et al. Diffuse C4d deposition and morphology of acute humoral rejection in a stable renal allograft. Transplantation 2003;76:1132.

474. Shah A, Nadasdy T, Arend L, et al. Treatment of C4d-positive acute humoral rejection with plasmapheresis and rabbit polyclonal antithymocyte globulin. Transplantation 2004;77:1399.

475. White NB, Greenstein SM, Cantafio AW, et al. Successful rescue therapy with plasmapheresis and intravenous immunoglobulin for acute humoral renal transplant rejection. Transplantation 2004;78:772.

476. Rocha PN, Butterly DW, Greenberg A, et al. Beneficial effect of plasmapheresis and intravenous immunoglobulin on renal allograft survival of patients with acute humoral rejection. Transplantation 2003;75:1490.

477. Pascual M, Saidman S, Tolkoff-Rubin N, et al. Plasma exchange and tacrolimus-mycophenolate rescue for acute humoral rejection in kidney transplantation. Transplantation 1998;66:1460.

478. Toyoda M, Petrosyan A, Pao A, Jordan SC. Immunomodulatory effects of combination of pooled human gammaglobulin and rapamycin on cell proliferation and apoptosis in the mixed lymphocyte reaction. Transplantation 2004;78:1134.

479. Jordan SC, Vo A, Bunnapradist S, et al. Intravenous immune globulin treatment inhibits crossmatch positivity and allows for successful transplantation of incompatible organs in living-donor and cadaver recipients. Transplantation 2003;76:631.

480. Frank MM, Miletic VD, Jiang H. Immunoglobulin in the control of complement action. Immunol Res 2000;22:137.

481. Pfeiffer S, Zorn GL 3rd, Blair KS, et al. Hyperacute lung rejection in the pig-to-human model 4: Evidence for complement and antibody independent mechanisms. Transplantation 2005;79:662.

482. Pratt JR, Jones ME, Dong J, et al. Nontransgenic hyperexpression of a complement regulator in donor kidney modulates transplant ischemia/reperfusion damage, acute rejection, and chronic nephropathy. Am J Pathol 2003;163:1457.

483. Wang H, Rollins SA, Gao Z, et al. Complement inhibition with an anti-C5 monoclonal antibody prevents hyperacute rejection in a xenograft heart transplantation model. Transplantation 1999;68:1643.

484. Bohmig GA, Regele H, Exner M, et al. C4d-positive acute humoral renal allograft rejection: Effective treatment by immunoadsorption. J Am Soc Nephrol 2001;12:2482.

485. Lorenz M, Regele H, Schillinger M, et al. Peritransplant immunoadsorption: A strategy enabling transplantation in highly sensitized crossmatch-positive cadaveric kidney allograft recipients. Transplantation 2005;79:696.

486. Vieira CA, Agarwal A, Book BK, et al. Rituximab for reduction of anti-HLA antibodies in patients awaiting renal transplantation. 1. Safety, pharmacodynamics, and pharmacokinetics. Transplantation 2004;77:542.

487. Gloor JM, DeGoey SR, Pineda AA, et al. Overcoming a positive crossmatch in living-donor kidney transplantation. Am J Transplant 2003;3:1017.

488. Mohiuddin MM, Ogawa H, Yin DP, et al. Antibody-mediated accommodation of heart grafts expressing an incompatible carbohydrate antigen. Transplantation 2003;75:258.

489. Tyden G, Kumlien G, Fehrman I. Successful ABO-incompatible kidney transplantations without splenectomy using antigen-specific immunoadsorption and rituximab. Transplantation 2003;76:730.

490. Bariety J, Oriol R, Hinglais N, et al. Distribution of blood group antigen A in normal and pathologic human kidneys. Kidney Int 1980;17:820.

491. Alexandre GPJ, Squifflet JP, De Bruyère M, et al. Present experience in a series of 26 ABO-incompatible living donor renal allografts. Transplant Proc 1987;19:4538.

492. Segev DL, Simpkins CE, Warren DS, et al. ABO incompatible high-titer renal transplantation without splenectomy or anti-CD20 treatment. Am J Transplant 2005;5:2570.

493. Sonnenday CJ, Warren DS, Cooper M, et al. Plasmapheresis, CMV hyperimmune globulin, and anti-CD20 allow ABO-incompatible renal transplantation without splenectomy. Am J Transplant 2004;4:1315.

494. Montgomery RA, Zachary AA, Ratner LE, et al. Clinical results from transplanting incompatible live kidney donor/recipient pairs using kidney paired donation. JAMA 2005;294:1655.

495. Tanabe K, Takahashi K, Sonda K, et al. Long-term results of ABO-incompatible living kidney transplantation: A single-center experience. Transplantation 1998;65:224.

496. Gloor JM, Lager DJ, Moore SB, et al. ABO-incompatible kidney transplantation using both A2 and non-A2 living donors. Transplantation 2003;75:971.

497. Abe M, Sawada T, Horita S, et al. C4d deposition in peritubular capillary and alloantibody in the allografted kidney suffering severe acute rejection. Clin Transplant 17 Suppl 2003;(Suppl 10):14.

498. Gaber LW, Gaber AO, Vera SR, et al. Successful reversal of hyperacute renal allograft rejection with the anti-CD3 monoclonal OKT3. Transplantation 1992;54:930.

499. Williams GM, Hume DM, Huson RP Jr, et al. "Hyperacute" renal-homograft rejection in man. N Eng J Med 1968;279:611.

500. Starzl TE, Boehmig HJ, Amemiya H, et al. Clotting changes, including disseminated intravascular coagulation, during rapid renal-homograft rejection. N Engl J Med 1970;283:383.

501. Kohler TR, Tilney NL. Microangiopathic hemolytic anemia associated with hyperacute rejection of a kidney allograft. Transplant Proc 1982;14:444.

502. Iwaki Y, Terasaki PI. Primary nonfunction in human cadaver kidney transplantation: Evidence for hidden hyperacute rejection. Clin Transplant 1987;1:125.

503. Myburgh JA, Cohen I, Gecelter L, et al. Hyperacute rejection in human-kidney allografts Shwartzman or Arthus reaction? N Engl J Med 1969;281:131.

504. Starzl TE, Lerner RA, Dixon FJ, Groth CG. Shwartzman reaction after human renal homotransplantation. N Engl J Med 1968;278:642.

505. Sibley RK, Payne W. Morphologic findings in the renal allograft biopsy. Seminars in Nephrology 1985;5:294.

506. Lucas ZJ, Coplon N, Kempson R, Cohn RB. Early renal transplant failure associated with subliminal sensitization. Transplantation 1970;10:522.

507. Metzgar RS, Seigler HF, Ward FE, Rowlands DTJ. Immunological studies on elutes from human renal allografts. Transplantation 1972;13:131.

508. Matas AJ, Scheinman JI, Rattazzi LC, et al. Immunopathological studies of the ruptured human renal allograft. Transplantation 1976;22:420.

509. Ahern AT, Artruc SB, DellaPelle P, et al. Hyperacute rejection of HLA-AB-identical renal allografts associated with B lymphocyte and endothelial reactive antibodies. Transplantation 1982;33:103.

510. Paul L, Class F, van Es L, et al. Accelerated rejection of a renal allograft associated with pretransplantation antibodies directed against donor antigens on endothelium and monocytes. N Engl J Med 1979;300:1258.

511. Paul LC, van Es LA, de la Rivière GB, et al. Blood group B antigen on renal endothelium as the target for rejection in an ABO-incompatible recipient. Transplantation 1989;26:268.

512. Chapman JR, Taylor C, Ting A, Morris PJ. Hyperacute rejection of a renal allograft in the presence of anti-HLA-Cw5 antibody. Transplantation 1986;42:91.

513. Montoliu J, Cheigh JS, Mouradian JA, et al. Delayed hyperacute rejection in recipients of kidney transplants from HLA identical sibling donors. Am J Med 1979;67:590.

514. Jordan SC, Yap HK, Sakai RS, et al. Hyperacute allograft rejection mediated by antivascular endothelial antibodies with a negative monocyte crossmatch. Transplantation 1988;46:585.

515. Claas FHJ, Paul LC, van Es LA, van Rood JJ. Antibodies against donor antigens on endothelial cells and monocytes in eluates of rejected kidney allografts. Tissue Antigens 1980;15:19.

516. Brasile L, Rodman E, Shield CF, et al. The association of anti-vascular endothelial cell antibody with hyperacute rejection: A case report. Surgery 1986;99:637.

517. Lobo PI, Sturgill BC, Bolton WK. Cold-reactive alloantibodies and allograft malfunction occurring immediately posttransplant. Transplantation 1984;37:76.

518. Sturgill BC, Lobo PI, Bolton WK. Cold-reacting IgM antibody-induced renal allograft failure: Similarity to hyperacute rejection. Nephron 1984;36:125.

519. Schweitzer RT, Bartus SA, Perkins HA, Belzer FO. Renal allograft failure and cold red blood cell autoagglutinins. Transplantation 1982;33:77.

520. Busch GJ, Martins AC, Hollenberg NK, et al. A primate model of hyperacute renal allograft rejection. Am J Pathol 1975;79:31.

521. Ito S, Camussi G, Tetta C, et al. Hyperacute renal allograft rejection in the rabbit. Lab Invest 1984;51:148.

522. Sedmak DD, Orosz CG. The role of vascular endothelial cells in transplantation. Arch Pathol Lab Med 1991;115:260.

523. Shimizu A, Meehan SM, Kozlowski T, et al. Acute humoral xenograft rejection: Destruction of the microvascular capillary endothelium in pig-to-nonhuman primate renal grafts. Lab Invest 2000;80:815.

524. Shimizu A, Yamada K, Yamamoto S, et al. Thrombotic microangiopathic glomerulopathy in human decay accelerating factor-transgenic swine-to-baboon kidney xenografts. J Am Soc Nephrol 2005;16:2732.

525. Dalmasso AP, Vercellotti GM, Fischel RJ, et al. Mechanism of complement activation in the hyperacute rejection of porcine organs transplanted into primate recipients. Am J Pathol 1992;140:1157.

526. Patel R, Terasaki PI. Significance of the positive crossmatch test in kidney transplantation. N Engl J Med 1969;280:735.

527. Kirkman RL, Colvin RB, Flye MW, et al. Transplantation in miniature swine. VII. Evidence for cellular immune mechanisms in hyperacute rejection of renal alografts. Transplantation 1979;28:24.

528. Eichwald EJ, Shelby J. Serum and cell-mediated responses in tolerance and hyperacute rejection transplanted mouse hearts. Transplantation 1987;43:520.

529. Baid S, Pascual M, Williams WW Jr, et al. Renal thrombotic microangiopathy associated with anticardiolipin antibodies in hepatitis C-positive renal allograft recipients. J Am Soc Nephrol 1999;10:146.

530. Colovai AI, Vasilescu ER, Foca-Rodi A, et al. Acute and hyperacute humoral rejection in kidney allograft recipients treated with anti-human thymocyte antibodies. Hum Immunol 2005;66:501.

531. Cross DE, Whittier FC, Cuppage FE, et al. Hyperacute rejeciton of renal allografts following pulsatile perfusion with a perfusate containing specific antibody. Transplant 1974;17:626.

532. Light JA, Annable C, Perloff L, et al. Immune injury from organ preservation: A potential cause of hyepracute rejection in human cadaveric kidney transplantation. Transplantation 1975;19:511.

533. Gloor JM, DeGoey S, Ploeger N, et al. Persistence of low levels of alloantibody after desensitization in crossmatch-positive living-donor kidney transplantation. Transplantation 2004;78:221.

534. Warren DS, Zachary AA, Sonnenday CJ, et al. Successful renal transplantation across simultaneous ABO incompatible and positive crossmatch barriers. Am J Transplant 2004;4:561.

535. Palmer A, Taube DJ, Welsh K, et al. Successful removal of anti-HLA antibodies by extrcorporeal immunoadsorption allowing renal transplantation. Lancet 1989;1:10.

536. Bannett AD, Bensinger WI, Raja R, et al. Immunoabsorption and renal transplantation in two patients with a major ABO incompatibility. Transplantation 1987;43:909.

537. Fuller TC, Forbes JB, Delmonico FL. Renal transplantation with a positive historical donor crossmatch. Transplantation 1985;42:144.

538. Habib R, Zurowska A, Hinglais N, et al. A specific glomerular lesion of the graft: Allograft glomerulopathy. Kidney Int Suppl 1993;42:S104.

539. Cornell LD, Colvin RB. Chronic allograft nephropathy. Curr Opin Nephrol Hypertens 2005;14:229.

540. Colvin RB. Chronic allograft nephropathy. N Engl J Med 2003; 349:2288.

541. Joosten SA, van Kooten C, Sijpkens YW, et al. The pathobiology of chronic allograft nephropathy: Immune-mediated damage and accelerated aging. Kidney Int 2004;65:1556.

542. Briganti EM, Russ GR, McNeil JJ, et al. Risk of renal allograft loss from recurrent glomerulonephritis. N Engl J Med 2002;347:103.

543. Dickenmann MJ, Nickeleit V, Tsinalis D, et al. Why do kidney grafts fail?A long-term single-center experience. Transpl Int 2002;15:508.

544. Mihatsch MJ, Nickeleit V, Gudat F. Morphologic criteria of chronic renal allograft rejection. Transplant Proc 1999;31: 1295.

545. Ivanyi B, Kemeny E, Szederkenyi E, et al. The value of electron microscopy in the diagnosis of chronic renal allograft rejection. Mod Pathol 2001;14:1200.

546. Freese PM, Svalander CT, Molne J, Nyberg G. Renal allograft glomerulopathy and the value of immunohistochemistry. Clin Nephrol 2004;62:279.

547. Hara S, Matsushita H, Yamaguchi Y, et al. Allograft glomerulitis: Histologic characteristics to detect chronic humoral rejection. Transplant Proc 2005;37:714.

548. Lee SJ, Howie AJ. Changes at the glomerulo-tubular junction in renal transplants. J Pathol 1988;156:311.

549. Porter KA, Rendall JM, Stolinski C, et al. Light and electron microscopic study of biopsies from 33 human renal allografts and an isograft 1 3/4 to 2 1/2 years after transplantation. Ann N Y Acad Sci 1966;129:615.

550. Varkarakia MM, Murphy GP. Role of the juxtaglomerular apparatus in renal allograft rejection. N Y State J Med 1975;75: 531.

551. Pagtalunan ME, Oberbauer R, Haas M, et al. Atubular glomeruli in patients with chronic allograft rejection. Transplantation 1996;61:1166.

552. Gibson IW, Downie TT, More IA, Lindop GB. Atubular glomeruli and glomerular cysts—a possible pathway for nephron loss in the human kidney? J Pathol 1996;179:421.

553. Colvin RB, Dvorak AM, Dvorak HF. Mast cells in the cortical tubular epithelium and interstitium in human renal disease. Hum Pathol 1974;5:315.

554. Roberts IS, Brenchley PE. Mast cells: The forgotten cells of renal fibrosis. J Clin Pathol 2000;53:858.

555. Kerjaschki D, Regele HM, Moosberger I, et al. Lymphatic neoangiogenesis in human kidney transplants is associated with immunologically active lymphocytic infiltrates. J Am Soc Nephrol 2004;15:603.

556. Pardo J, Diaz L, Errasti P, et al. Mast cells in chronic rejection of human renal allografts. Virchows Archiv 2000;437:167.

557. Ishii Y, Sawada T, Kubota K, et al. Injury and progressive loss of peritubular capillaries in the development of chronic allograft nephropathy. Kidney Int 2005;67:321.

558. Burke BA, Chavers BM, Gillingham KJ, et al. Chronic renal allograft rejection in the first 6 months posttransplant. Transplantation 1995;60:1413.

559. Wells AF, Larsson E, Tengblad A, et al. The location of hyaluronan in normal and rejected human kidneys. Transplantation 1990;50:240.

560. Howie AJ, Bryan RL, Gunson BK. Arteries and veins formed within renal vessels: A previously neglected observation. Virchows Arch A Pathol Anat Histopathol 1992;420:301.

561. Sacchi G, Bertalot G, Cancarini C, et al. Atheromatosis and double media: Uncommon vascular lesions of renal allografts. Pathologica 1993;85:183.

562. Salomon RN, Hughes CC, Schoen FJ, et al. Human coronary transplantation-associated arteriosclerosis. Evidence for a chronic immune reaction to activated graft endothelial cells. Am J Pathol 1991;138:791.

563. Wieczorek G, Bigaud M, Menninger K, et al. Acute and chronic vascular rejection in non-human primate kidney tranplantation. Am J Transplant 2006;6(6):1285.

564. Smith RN, Kawai T, Boskovic S, et al. Chronic humoral rejection: Sequential development of alloantibody C4d deposition, allograft glomerulopathy and graft dysfunction. Am J Transplant, in press.

565. Rigg KM, Proud G, Taylor RM. Urological complications following renal transplantation. A study of 1016 consecutive transplants from a single centre. Transpl Int 1994;7:120.

566. Gough J, Yilmaz A, Yilmaz S, Benediktsson H. Recurrent and de novo glomerular immune-complex deposits in renal transplant biopsies. Arch Pathol Lab Med 2005;129:231.

567. Sijpkens YW, Joosten SA, Wong MC, et al. Immunologic risk factors and glomerular C4d deposits in chronic transplant glomerulopathy. Kidney Int 2004;65:2409.

568. Olsen S, Bohman SO, Petersen VP. Ultrastructure of the glomerular basement membrane in long term renal allografts with transplant glomerular disease. Lab Invest 1974;30: 176.

569. Rotellar C, Noel LH, Droz D, et al. Role of antibodies directed against tubular basement membranes in human renal transplantation. Am J Kidney Dis 1986;7:157.

570. Orfila C, Durand D, Vega VC, Suc JM. Immunofluorescent deposits on the tubular basement membrane in human renal transplant. Nephron 1991;57:149.

571. Bracamonte ER, Furmanczyk PS, Smith KD, et al. Tubular basement membrane immune deposits associated with polyoma virus nephropathy in renal allografts. Lab Invest 2006;86(Suppl 1):259A.

572. Mauiyyedi S, Pelle PD, Saidman S, et al. Chronic humoral rejection: Identification of antibody-mediated chronic renal allograft rejection by C4d deposits in peritubular capillaries. J Am Soc Nephrol 2001;12:574.

573. Mroz A, Durlik M, Cieciura T, et al. C4d complement split product expression in chronic rejection of renal allograft. Transplant Proc 2003;35:2190.

574. Vongwiwatana A, Gourishankar S, Campbell PM, et al. Peritubular capillary changes and C4d deposits are associated with transplant glomerulopathy but not IgA nephropathy. Am J Transplant 2004;4:124.

575. Andres GA, Accinni L, Hsu KC, et al. Human renal transplants. III. Immunopathologic studies. Lab Invest 1970;22:588.

576. Hsu HC, Suzuki Y, Churg J, Grishman E. Ultrastructure of transplant glomerulopathy. Histopathology 1980;4:351.

577. Zollinger HU, Moppert J, Thiel G, Rohr HP. Morphology and pathogenesis of glomerulopathy in cadaver kidney allografts treated with antilymphocyte globulin. Curr Top Pathol 1973;57:1.

578. Chicano SL, Cornell LD, Selig MK, et al. Distinctive ultrastructural features of chronic allograft glomerulopathy: new formation of circumferential glomerular basement membrane. Lab Invest. 2006;86(Suppl. 1).

579. Ivanyi B, Fahmy H, Brown H, et al. Peritubular capillaries in chronic renal allograft rejection: A quantitative ultrastructural study. Hum Pathol 2000;31:1129.

580. Porter KA. Renal transplantation. In: Heptinstall RH, ed. The Pathology of the Kidney, 4th ed. Boston: Little Brown and Company; 1990:1799.

581. Truong LD, Yoshikawa Y, Mawad J, Lederer E. Electron microscopic study of an unusual posttransplant glomerular lesion. Arch Pathol Lab Med 1991;115:382.

582. Nadasdy T, Abdi R, Pitha J, et al. Diffuse glomerular basement membrane lamellation in renal allografts from pediatric donors to adult recipients. Am J Surg Pathol 1999;23:437.

583. Petersen VP, Olsen TS, Kissmeyer NF, et al. Late failure of human renal transplants. An analysis of transplant disease and graft failure among 125 recipients surviving for one to eight years. Medicine 1975;54:45.

584. Reinholt FP, Bohman SO, Wilczek H, et al. Ultrastructural changes of tubular basement membranes in immunologic renal tubular lesions in humans. Ultrastruct Pathol 1990;14:121.

585. Monga G, Mazzucco G, Messina M, et al. Intertubular capillary changes in kidney allografts: A morphologic investigation on 61 renal specimens. Mod Pathol 1992;5:125.

586. Mazzucco G, Motta M, Segoloni G, Monga G. Intertubular capillary changes in the cortex and medulla of transplanted

kidneys and their relationship with transplant glomerulopathy: An ultrastructural study of 12 transplantectomies. Ultrastruct Pathol 1994;18:533.

587. Young-Ramsaran JO, Hruban RH, Hutchins GM, et al. Ultrastructural evidence of cell-mediated endothelial cell injury in cardiac transplant-related accelerated arteriosclerosis. Ultrastruct Pathol 1993;17:125.

588. Factor SM, Biempica L, Goldfischer S. Intralysosomal lipid in long-term maintenance transplant atherosclerosis. Arch Pathol Lab Med 1977;101:474.

589. Geraghty JG, Stoltenberg RL, Sollinger HW, Hullet DA. Vascular smooth muscle cells and neointimal hyperplasia in chronic transplant rejection. Transplantation 1996;62:502.

590. Kuwahara M, Jacobsson J, Kuwahara M, et al. Coronary artery ultrastructural changes in cardiac transplant atherosclerosis in the rabbit. Transplantation 1991;52:759.

591. McPhaul JJ Jr, Dixon FJ, Brettschneider L, Starzl, TE. Immunofluorescent examination of biopsies from long-term renal allografts. N Engl J Med 1970;282:412.

592. Rowlands DT Jr, Burkholder PM, Bossen EH, Lin HH. Renal allografts in HL-A matched recipients: Light, immunofluorescence and electron microscopic studies. Am J Pathol 1970; 61:177.

593. Cheigh JS, Chami J, Stenzel KH, et al. Renal transplantation between HLA identical siblings: Comparison with transplants from HLA semi-identical related donors. N Engl J Med 1977;296:1030.

594. Mannon RB, Griffiths R, Ruiz P, et al. Absence of donor MHC antigen expression ameliorates chronic kidney allograft rejection. Kidney Int 2002;62:290.

595. Basadonna GP, Matas AJ, Gillingham KJ, et al. Early versus late acute renal allograft rejection: Impact on chronic rejection. Transplantation 1993;55:993.

596. Almond PS, Matas A, Gillingham K, et al. Risk factors for chronic rejection in renal allograft recipients. Transplantation 1993;55:752.

597. Hostetter TH. Chronic transplant rejection. Kidney Int 1994; 46:266.

598. Isoniemi H, Nurminen M, Tikkanen MJ, et al. Risk factors predicting chronic rejection of renal allografts. Transplantation 1994;57:68.

599. Terasaki PI. Humoral theory of rejection. Amer J Transplantation 2003;3:1.

600. Worthington JE, Martin S, Al-Husseini DM, et al. Posttransplantation production of donor HLA-specific antibodies as a predictor of renal transplant outcome. Transplantation 2003;75:1034.

601. Hourmant M, Cesbron-Gautier A, Terasaki PI, et al. Frequency and clinical implications of development of donor-specific and non-donor-specific HLA antibodies after kidney transplantation. J Am Soc Nephrol 2005;16:2804.

602. Lee PC, Terasaki PI, Takemoto SK, et al. All chronic rejection failures of kidney transplants were preceded by the development of HLA antibodies. Transplantation 2002;74:1192.

603. Terasaki PI, Ozawa M. Predictive value of HLA antibodies and serum creatinine in chronic rejection: Results of a 2-year prospective trial. Transplantation 2005;80:1194.

604. Poggio ED, Clemente M, Riley J, et al. Alloreactivity in renal transplant recipients with and without chronic allograft nephropathy. J Am Soc Nephrol 2004;15:1952.

605. Opelz G. Non-HLA transplantation immunity revealed by lymphocytotoxic antibodies. Lancet 2005;365:1570.

606. Martin L, Guignier F, Bocrie O, et al. Detection of anti-HLA antibodies with flow cytometry in needle core biopsies of renal transplants recipients with chronic allograft nephropathy. Transplantation 2005;79:1459.

607. Nankivell BJ, Borrows RJ, Fung CL, et al. The natural history of chronic allograft nephropathy. N Engl J Med 2003;349: 2326.

608. Rush D, Nickerson P, Gough J, et al. Beneficial effects of treatment of early subclinical rejection: A randomized study. J Am Soc Nephrol 1998;9:2129.

609. Shishido S, Asanuma H, Nakai H, et al. The impact of repeated subclinical acute rejection on the progression of chronic allograft nephropathy. J Am Soc Nephrol 2003;14:1046.

610. Baboolal K, Jones GA, Janezic A, et al. Molecular and structural consequences of early renal allograft injury. Kidney Int 2002;61:686.

611. Nankivell BJ, Borrows RJ, Fung CL, et al. Delta analysis of posttransplantation tubulointerstitial damage. Transplantation 2004;78:434.

612. Cosio FG, Grande JP, Wadei H, et al. Predicting subsequent decline in kidney allograft function from early surveillance biopsies. Am J Transplant 2005;5:2464.

613. Tsamandas AC, Shapiro R, Jordan M, et al. Significance of tubulitis in chronic allograft nephropathy: A clinicopathologic study. Clin Transplant 1997;11:139.

614. Baker RJ, Hernandez-Fuentes MP, Brookes PA, et al. Loss of direct and maintenance of indirect alloresponses in renal allograft recipients: Implications for the pathogenesis of chronic allograft nephropathy. J Immunol 2001;167:7199.

615. Horita S, Nitta K, Kawashima M, et al. C4d deposition in the glomeruli and peritubular capillaries associated with transplant glomerulopathy. Clin Transplant 2003;17:325.

616. Aly ZA, Yalamanchili P, Cortese C, et al. C4d peritubular capillary staining in chronic allograft nephropathy and transplant glomerulopathy: An uncommon finding. Transpl Int 2005;18:800.

617. Kerby JD, Verran DJ, Luo KL, et al. Immunolocalization of FGF-1 and receptors in glomerular lesions associated with chronic human renal allograft rejection. Transplantation 1996;62:190.

618. Akalin E, Dikman S, Murphy B, et al. Glomerular infiltration by CXCR3+ ICOS+ activated T-cells in chronic allograft nephropathy with transplant glomerulopathy. Am J Transplant 2003;3:1116.

619. Harris PE, Bian H, Reed EF. Induction of high affinity fibroblast growth factor receptor expression and proliferation in human endothelial cells by anti-HLA antibodies: A possible mechanism for transplant atherosclerosis. J Immunol 1997;159:5697.

620. Alpers CE, Hudkins KL, Gown AM, Johnson RJ. Enhanced expression of "muscle-specific" actin in glomerulonephritis. Kidney Int 1992;41:1134.

621. Fellström B, Klareskog L, Heldin CH, et al. Platelet-derived growth factor receptors in the kidney—upregulated expression in inflammation. Kidney Int 1989;36:1099.

622. Nicholson ML, Bicknell GR, Barker G, et al. Intragraft expression of transforming growth factor *beta*1 gene in isolated glomeruli from human renal transplants. Br J Surg 1999; 86:1144.

623. Joosten SA, Sijpkens YW, van Ham V, et al. Antibody response against the glomerular basement membrane protein agrin in patients with transplant glomerulopathy. Am J Transplant 2005;5:383.

624. Gould VE, Martinez LV, Virtanen I, et al. Differential distribution of tenascin and cellular fibronectins in acute and chronic renal allograft rejection. Lab Invest 1992;67:71.

625. Jeong HJ, Sung SH, Hong SW, et al. Alterations in extracellular matrix components in transplant glomerulopathy. Virchows Archiv 2000;437:69.

626. Fukuda M, Morozumi K, Uchida K, et al. Glomerular capillary tenascin staining in renal allografts and its correlation with capillary loop 'double contours', proteinuria and graft outcome. Nephron Clin Pract 2004;96:c115.

627. Johnson TS, Abo-Zenah H, Skill JN, et al. Tissue transglutaminase: A mediator and predictor of chronic allograft nephropathy? Transplantation 2004;77:1667.

628. Eikmans M, Sijpkens YW, Baelde HJ, et al. High transforming growth factor-beta and extracellular matrix mRNA response in renal allografts during early acute rejection is associated with absence of chronic rejection. Transplantation 2002;73: 573.

629. Eremina V, Sood M, Haigh J, et al. Glomerular-specific alterations of VEGF-A expression lead to distinct congenital and acquired renal diseases. J Clin Invest 2003;111:707.

630. Ballermann BJ. Glomerular endothelial cell differentiation. Kidney Int 2005;67:1668.

631. Mui KW, van Son WJ, Tiebosch AT, et al. Clinical relevance of immunohistochemical staining for ecto-AMPase and ecto-ATPase in chronic allograft nephropathy (CAN). Nephrol Dial Transplant 2003;18:158.

632. Hayes JM, Steinmuller DR, Streem SB, Novick AC. The development of proteinuria and focal-segmental glomerulosclerosis recipients of pediatric donor kidneys. Transplantation 1991;52:813.

633. Woolley AC, Rosenberg ME, Burke BA, Nath KA. De novo focal glomerulosclerosis after kidney transplantation. Am J Med 1988;84:310.

634. Azuma H, Nadeau K, Mackenzie HS, et al. Nephron mass modulates the hemodynamic, cellular, and molecular response of the rat renal allograft. Transplantation 1997;63:519.

635. Uehara S, Chase CM, Kitchens WH, et al. NK cells can trigger allograft vasculopathy: The role of hybrid resistance in solid organ allografts. J Immunol 2005;175:3424.

636. Tellides G, Tereb DA, Kirkiles-Smith NC, et al. Interferon-gamma elicits arteriosclerosis in the absence of leukocytes. Nature 2000;403:207.

637. Tullius SG, Hancock WW, Heemann U, et al. Reversibility of chronic renal allograft rejection. Critical effect of time after transplantation suggests both host immune dependent and independent phases of progressive injury. Transplantation 1994;58:93.

638. Russell PS, Chase CM, Winn HJ, Colvin RB. Coronary atherosclerosis in transplanted mouse hearts. II. Importance of humoral immunity. J Immunol 1994;152:5135.

639. He C, Schenk S, Zhang Q, et al. Effects of T-cell frequency and graft size on transplant outcome in mice. J Immunol 2004;172:240.

640. Davenport A, Younie ME, Parsons JE, Klouda PT. Development of cytotoxic antibodies following renal allograft transplantation is associated with reduced graft survival due to chronic vascular rejection. Nephrol Dial Transplant 1994;9:1315.

641. Moreso F, Lopez M, Vallejos A, et al. Serial protocol biopsies to quantify the progression of chronic transplant nephropathy in stable renal allografts. Am J Transplant 2001;1:82.

642. Benzaquen LR, Nicholson-Weller A, Halperin JA. Terminal complement proteins C5b-9 release basic fibroblast growth factor and platelet-derived growth factor from endothelial cells. J Exp Med 1994;179:985.

643. Smith JD, Lawson C, Yacoub MH, Rose ML. Activation of NF-kappa B in human endothelial cells induced by monoclonal and allospecific HLA antibodies. Int Immunol 2000;12:563.

644. Jin YP, Singh RP, Du ZY, et al. Ligation of HLA class I molecules on endothelial cells induces phosphorylation of Src, paxillin, and focal adhesion kinase in an actin-dependent manner. J Immunol 2002;168:5415.

645. Coupel S, Leboeuf F, Boulday G, et al. RhoA activation mediates phosphatidylinositol 3-kinase-dependent proliferation of human vascular endothelial cells: An alloimmune mechanism of chronic allograft nephropathy. J Am Soc Nephrol 2004;15:2429.

646. Yamada K, Hatakeyama E, Sakamaki T, et al. Involvement of platelet-derived growth factor and histocompatibility of DRB 1 in chronic renal allograft nephropathy. Transplantation 2001;71:936.

647. Gouldesbrough DR, Axelsen RA. Arterial endothelialitis in chronic renal allograft rejection: A histopathological and immunocytochemical study. Nephrol Dial Transplant 1994;9:35.

648. Denton MD, Davis SF, Baum MA, et al. The role of the graft endothelium in transplant rejection: Evidence that endothelial activation may serve as a clinical marker for the development of chronic rejection. Pediatr Transplant 2000;4:252.

649. Fox WM, Hameed A, Hutchins GM, et al. Perforin expression localizing cytotoxic lymphocytes in the intimas of coronary arteries with transplant-related accelerated arteriosclerosis. Hum Pathol 1993;24:477.

650. Eitner F, Cui Y, Hudkins KL, Alpers CE. Chemokine receptor (CXCR4) mRNA-expressing leukocytes are increased in human renal allograft rejection. Transplantation 1998;66:1551.

651. Hall AV, Jevnikar AM. Significance of endothelial cell survival programs for renal transplantation. Am J Kidney Dis 2003;41:1140.

652. Shimizu A, Yamada K, Sachs DH, Colvin RB. Intragraft events preceding chronic renal allograft rejection in a modified tolerance protocol. Kidney Int 2000;58:2546.

653. Cailhier J-F, Laplante P, Hebert M-J. Endothelial apoptosis and chronic transplant vasculopathy: Recent results, novel mechanisms. Am J Transplant 2006;6:247.

654. Choy JC, Cruz RP, Kerjner A, et al. Granzyme B induces endothelial cell apoptosis and contributes to the development of transplant vascular disease. Am J Transplant 2005;5:494.

655. Choy JC, Kerjner A, Wong BW, et al. Perforin mediates endothelial cell death and resultant transplant vascular disease in cardiac allografts. Am J Pathol 2004;165:127.

656. Russell PS, Chase CM, Winn HJ, Colvin RB. Coronary atherosclerosis in transplanted mouse hearts. I. Time course and immunogenetic and immunopathological considerations. Am J Pathol 1994;144:260.

657. Cramer DV, Qian SQ, Harnaha J, et al. Cardiac transplantation in the rat. I. The effect of histocompatibility differences on graft arteriosclerosis. Transplantation 1989;47:414.

658. Adams DH, Tilney NL, Collins JJ, Karnovsky MJ. Experimental graft arteriosclerosis. I. The Lewis-to-F-344 allograft model. Transplantation 1992;53:1115.

659. Nadeau KC, Azuma H, Tilney NL. Sequential cytokine dynamics in chronic rejection of rat renal allografts: Roles for cytokines RANTES and MCP-1. Proc Nat Acad Sci U S A 1995;92:8729.

660. Russell PS, Chase CM, Colvin RB. Accelerated atheromatous lesions in mouse hearts transplanted to apolipoprotein E-deficient recipients. Am J Pathol 1996;149:91.

661. Adams DH, Wyner LR, Karnovsky MJ. Experimental graft arteriosclerosis. II. Immunocytochemical analysis of lesion development. Transplantation 1993;56:794.

662. Beranek JT, Cavarocchi NC. Smooth muscle cells and macrophages in rabbit cardiac allograft atherosclerosis. Arch Pathol Lab Med 1991;115:266.

663. Kennedy LJ, Weissman IL. Dual origin of intimal cells in cardiac allograft arteriosclerosis. N Engl J Med 1971;285:884.

664. Oguma S, Banner B, Zerbe T, et al. Participation of dendritic cells in vascular lesions of chronic rejection of human allografts. Lancet 1988;2:933.

665. Grimm PC, Nickerson P, Jeffery J, et al. Neointimal and tubulointerstitial infiltration by recipient mesenchymal cells in chronic renal-allograft rejection. New Engl J Med 2001;345:93.

666. Pollman MJ, Hall JL, Mann MJ, et al. Inhibition of neointimal cell bcl-x expression induces apoptosis and regression of vascular disease. Nat Med 1998;4:222.

667. Suzuki J, Isobe M, Morishita R, et al. Antisense Bcl-x oligonucleotide induces apoptosis and prevents arterial neointimal formation in murine cardiac allografts. Cardiovasc Res 2000;45:783.

668. Romagnani P, Pupilli C, Lasagni L, et al. Inducible nitric oxide synthase expression in vascular and glomerular structures of human chronic allograft nephropathy. J Pathol 1999;187:345.

669. McManus BM, Malcom G, Kendall TJ, et al. Prominence of coronary arterial wall lipids in human heart allografts. Implications for pathogenesis of allograft arteriopathy. Am J Pathol 1995;147:293.

670. Raymond MA, Desormeaux A, Laplante P, et al. Apoptosis of endothelial cells triggers a caspase-dependent anti-apoptotic paracrine loop active on VSMC. FASEB J 2004;18:705.

671. Grandaliano G, Di Paolo S, Monno R, et al. Protease-activated receptor 1 and plasminogen activator inhibitor 1 expression in chronic allograft nephropathy: The role of coagulation and fibrinolysis in renal graft fibrosis. Transplantation 2001;72:1437.

672. Alpers CE, Hudkins KL, Segerer S, et al. Localization of SPARC

in developing, mature, and chronically injured human allograft kidneys. Kidney Int 2002;62:2073.

673. Viklicky O, Matl I, Voska L, et al. TGF-beta1 expression and chronic allograft nephropathy in protocol kidney graft biopsy. Physiol Res 2003;52:353.

674. Russell PS, Chase CM, Winn HJ, Colvin RB. Coronary atherosclerosis in transplanted mouse hearts. III. Effects of recipient treatment with a monoclonal antibody to interferon-gamma. Transplantation 1994;57:1367.

675. Russell PS, Chase CM, Colvin RB. Coronary atherosclerosis in transplanted mouse hearts. IV. Effects of treatment with monoclonal antibodies to intercellular adhesion molecule-1 and leukocyte function-associated antigen-1. Transplantation 1995;60:724.

676. Molossi EM, Arrhenius T, Diaz R, et al. Blockage of VLA-4 integrin binding to fibronectin with CS1 peptide reduces accelerated coronary arteriopathy in rabbit cardiac allografts. J Clin Invest 1995;95:2601.

677. Vollmer E, Bosse A, Bogeholz J, et al. Apolipoproteins and immunohistological differentiation of cells in the arterial wall of kidneys in transplant arteriopathy. Morphological parallels with atherosclerosis. Patholy Res Pract 1991;187:957.

678. Faulk WP, Labarrere CA. Vascular immunopathology and atheroma development in human allografted organs. Arch Pathol Lab Med 1992;116:1337.

679. Yilmaz S, Paavonen T, Häyry P. Chronic rejection of rat renal allografts. II. The impact of prolonged ischemia time on transplant histology. Transplantation 1992;53:823.

680. Sijpkens YW, Doxiadis II, van Kemenade FJ, et al. Chronic rejection with or without transplant vasculopathy. Clin Transplant 2003;17:163.

681. Cosio FG, Pelletier RP, Sedmak DD, et al. Pathologic classification of chronic allograft nephropathy: Pathogenic and prognostic implications. Transplantation 1999;67:690.

682. Laine J, Etelamaki P, Holmberg C, Dunkel L. Apoptotic cell death in human chronic renal allograft rejection. Transplantation 1997;63:101.

683. Solez K, Vincenti F, Filo RS. Histopathologic findings from 2-year protocol biopsies from a U.S. multicenter kidney transplant trial comparing tarolimus versus cyclosporine: A report of the FK506 Kidney Transplant Study Group. Transplantation1998;66:1736.

684. Pilmore HL, Eris JM, Painter DM, et al. Vascular endothelial growth factor expression in human chronic renal allograft rejection. Transplantation 1999;67:929.

685. Boukhalfa G, Desmouliere A, Rondeau E, et al. Relationship between alpha-smooth muscle actin expression and fibrotic changes in human kidney. Exp Nephrol 1996;4:241.

686. Mas V, Alvarellos T, Giraudo C, et al. Intragraft messenger RNA expression of angiotensinogen: Relationship with transforming growth factor beta-1 and chronic allograft nephropathy in kidney transplant patients. Transplantation 2002;74:718.

687. Sharma VK, Bologa RM, Xu GP, et al. Intragraft TGF-beta 1 mRNA: A correlate of interstitial fibrosis and chronic allograft nephropathy. Kidney Int 1996;49:1297.

688. Nicholson ML, Waller JR, Bicknell GR. Renal transplant fibrosis correlates with intragraft expression of tissue inhibitor of metalloproteinase messenger RNA. Br J Surg 2002;89:933.

689. Ishimura T, Fujisawa M, Isotani S, et al. Transforming factor-beta1 expression in early biopsy specimen predicts long-term graft function following pediatric renal transplantation. Clin Transplant 2001;15:185.

690. Bakker RC, Koop K, Sijpkens YW, et al. Early interstitial accumulation of collagen type I discriminates chronic rejection from chronic cyclosporine nephrotoxicity. J Am Soc Nephrol 2003;14:2142.

691. Abrass CK, Berfield AK, Stehman-Breen C, et al. Unique changes in interstitial extracellular matrix composition are associated with rejection and cyclosporine toxicity in human renal allograft biopsies. Am J Kidney Dis 1999;33:11.

692. Roos-van Groningen MC, Scholten EM, Lelieveld PM, et al. Molecular comparison of calcineurin inhibitor-induced fibro-

693. Becker BN, Jacobson LM, Hullett DA, et al. Type 2 angiotensin II receptor expression in human renal allografts: An association with chronic allograft nephropathy. Clin Nephrol 2002;57:19.

694. Inigo P, Campistol JM, Lario S, et al. Effects of losartan and amlodipine on intrarenal hemodynamics and TGF-beta(1) plasma levels in a crossover trial in renal transplant recipients. J Am Soc Nephrol 2001;12:822.

695. De Heer E, Sijpkens YW, Verkade M, et al. Morphometry of interstitial fibrosis. Nephrol Dial Transplant 2000;15(Suppl 6):72.

696. Ho KM, Li AZ, Yiu MK, et al. Altered expression of aquaporin-2 in human explants with chronic renal allograft dysfunction. BJU Int 2005;95:1104.

697. Kalluri R, Neilson EG. Epithelial-mesenchymal transition and its implications for fibrosis. J Clin Invest 2003;112:1776.

698. Djamali A, Reese S, Yracheta J, et al. Epithelial-to-mesenchymal transition and oxidative stress in chronic allograft nephropathy. Am J Transplant 2005;5:500.

699. Slattery C, Campbell E, McMorrow T, Ryan MP. Cyclosporine A-induced renal fibrosis: A role for epithelial-mesenchymal transition. Am J Pathol 2005;167:395.

700. Halloran PF, Melk A, Barth C. Rethinking chronic allograft nephropathy: The concept of accelerated senescence. J Am Soc Nephrol 1999;10:167.

701. Chkhotua AB, Altimari A, Gabusi E, et al. Increased expression of p21 (WAF1/CIP1) cyclin-dependent kinase (CDK) inhibitor gene in chronic allograft nephropathy correlates with the number of acute rejection episodes. Transpl Int 2003;16:502.

702. Ferlicot S, Durrbach A, Ba N, et al. The role of replicative senescence in chronic allograft nephropathy. Hum Pathol 2003;34:924.

703. Melk A, Schmidt BM, Vongwiwatana A, et al. Increased expression of senescence-associated cell cycle inhibitor p16INK4a in deteriorating renal transplants and diseased native kidney. Am J Transplant 2005;5:1375.

704. Chkhotua AB, Gabusi E, Altimari A, et al. Increased expression of p16 and p27 cyclin-dependent kinase inhibitor genes in aging human kidney and chronic allograft nephropathy. Am J Kidney Dis 2003;41:1303.

705. Kerjaschki D, Huttary N, Raab I, et al. Lymphatic endothelial progenitor cells contribute to de novo lymphangiogenesis in human renal transplants. Nat Med 2006;12:230.

706. Cornell LD, Della Pelle P, Brousiadies N, et al. Endothelial response to rejection: Enhanced expression of complement regulatory proteins decay accelerating factor (DAF, CD55) and protectin (CD59) in human renal allografts. Mod. Pathol. 2004;17:285A.

707. Cardarelli F, Pascual M, Tolkoff-Rubin N, et al. Prevalence and significance of anti-HLA and donor-specific antibodies long-term after renal transplantation. Transpl Int 2005;18:532.

708. Seron D, Moreso F, Fulladosa X, et al. Reliability of chronic allograft nephropathy diagnosis in sequential protocol biopsies. Kidney Int 2002;61:727.

709. Nicholson ML, McCulloch TA, Harper SJ, et al. Early measurement of interstitial fibrosis predicts long-term renal function and graft survival in renal transplantation. Br J Surg 1996;83:1082.

710. Young EW, Ellis CN, Messana JM, et al. A prospective study of renal structure and function in psoriasis patients treated with cyclosporin. Kidney Int 1994;46:1216.

711. Grimm PC, Nickerson P, Gough J, et al. Computerized image analysis of Sirius Red-stained renal allograft biopsies as a surrogate marker to predict long-term allograft function. J Am Soc Nephrol 2003;14:1662.

712. Pape L, Henne T, Offner G, et al. Computer-assisted quantification of fibrosis in chronic allograft nephropaty by picosirius red-staining: A new tool for predicting long-term graft function. Transplantation 2003;76:955.

713. Masseroli M, O'Valle F, Andujar M, et al. Design and validation

of a new image analysis method for automatic quantification of interstitial fibrosis and glomerular morphometry. Lab Invest 1998;78:511.

714. Murphy GJ, Waller JR, Sandford RS, et al. Randomized clinical trial of the effect of microemulsion cyclosporin and tacrolimus on renal allograft fibrosis. Br J Surg 2003;90:680.

715. Diaz Encarnacion MM, Griffin MD, Slezak JM, et al. Correlation of quantitative digital image analysis with the glomerular filtration rate in chronic allograft nephropathy. Am J Transplant 2004;4:248.

716. Ellingsen AR, Nyengaard JR, Osterby R, et al. Measurements of cortical interstitium in biopsies from human kidney grafts: How representative and how reproducible? Nephrol Dial Transplant 2002;17:788.

717. Sund S, Grimm P, Reisaeter AV, Hovig T. Computerized image analysis vs semiquantitative scoring in evaluation of kidney allograft fibrosis and prognosis. Nephrol Dial Transplant 2004;19:2838.

718. Yilmaz S, Tomlanovich S, Mathew T, et al. Protocol core needle biopsy and histologic chronic allograft damage index (CADI) as surrogate end point for long-term graft survival in multicenter studies. J Am Soc Nephrol 2003;14:773.

719. Dimeny E, Wahlberg J, Larsson E, Fellström B. Can histopathological findings in early renal allograft biopsies identify patients at risk for chronic vascular rejection? Clin Transplant 1995;9:79.

720. Lachenbruch PA, Rosenberg AS, Bonvini E, et al. Biomarkers and surrogate endpoints in renal transplantation: Present status and considerations for clinical trial design. Am J Transplant 2004;4:451.

721. Andresdottir MB, Assmann KJ, Koene RA, Wetzels JF. Immunohistological and ultrastructural differences between recurrent type I membranoproliferative glomerulonephritis and chronic transplant glomerulopathy. Am J Kidney Dis 1998;32:582.

722. Morozumi K, Takeda A, Uchida K, Mihatsch MJ. Cyclosporine nephrotoxicity: How does it affect renal allograft function and transplant morphology? Transplant Proc 2004;36:251S.

723. Meehan SM, Pascual M, Williams WW, et al. De novo collapsing glomerulopathy in renal allografts. Transplantation 1998;65:1192.

724. Stokes MB, Davis CL, Alpers CE. Collapsing glomerulopathy in renal allografts: A morphological pattern with diverse clinicopathologic associations. Am J Kidney Dis 1999;33:658.

725. Nadasdy T, Allen C, Zand MS. Zonal distribution of glomerular collapse in renal allografts: Possible role of vascular changes. Hum Pathol 2002;33:437.

726. Sibley RK. Morphologic features of chronic rejection in kidney and less commonly transplanted organs. Clin Transplant 1994;8(Pt 2):293.

727. Nadasdy T, Krenacs T, Kalmar KN, et al. Importance of plasma cells in the infiltrate of renal allografts. An immunohistochemical study. Pathol Res Pract 1991;187:178.

728. Dell'Antonio G, Randhawa PS. "Striped" pattern of medullary ray fibrosis in allograft biopsies from kidney transplant recipients maintained on tacrolimus. Transplantation 1999;67:484.

729. Nickeleit V, Hirsch HH, Binet IF, et al. Polyomavirus infection of renal allograft recipients: From latent infection to manifest disease. J Am Soc Nephrol 1999;10:1080.

730. Randhawa PS, Vats A, Zygmunt D, et al. Quantitation of viral DNA in renal allograft tissue from patients with BK virus nephropathy. Transplantation 2002;74:485.

731. Celik B, Shapiro R, Vats A, Randhawa PS. Polyomavirus allograft nephropathy: Sequential assessment of histologic viral load, tubulitis, and graft function following changes in immunosuppression. Am J Transplant 2003;3:1378.

732. Mylonakis E, Goes N, Rubin RH, et al. BK virus in solid organ transplant recipients: An emerging syndrome. Transplantation 2001;72:1587.

733. Modena FM, Hostetter TH, Salahudeen AK, et al. Progression of kidney disease in chronic renal transplant rejection. Transplantation 1991;52:239.

734. Habib R, Malheiros D, Charbit M, Gagnadoux MF. Long term results in 70 pediatric renal transplants after more than 10 years. Histological study. Ann Pediatr (Paris) 1991;38:419.

735. Vathsala A, Verani R, Schoenberg L, et al. Proteinuria in cyclosporine-treated renal transplant recipients. Transplantation 1990;49:35.

736. Choi BS, Shin MJ, Shin SJ, et al. Clinical significance of an early protocol biopsy in living-donor renal transplantation: Ten-year experience at a single center. Am J Transplant 2005;5:1354.

737. Nankivell BJ, Borrows RJ, Fung CL, et al. Evolution and pathophysiology of renal-transplant glomerulosclerosis. Transplantation 2004;78:461.

738. Yakupoglu U, Baranowska-Daca E, Rosen D, et al. Posttransplant nephrotic syndrome: A comprehensive clinicopathologic study. Kidney Int 2004;65:2360.

739. Fernandez-Fresnedo G, Plaza JJ, Sanchez-Plumed J, et al. Proteinuria: A new marker of long-term graft and patient survival in kidney transplantation. Nephrol Dial Transplant 2004;19(Suppl 3):iii47.

740. Ramanathan V, Suki WN, Rosen D, Truong LD. Chronic allograft nephropathy and nephrotic range proteinuria. Clin Transplant 2005;19:413.

741. Isoniemi HM, Krogerus L, von Willebrand E, et al. Histopathological findings in well-functioning, long-term renal allografts. Kidney Int 1992;41:155.

742. Seron D, Moreso F, Ramon JM, et al. Protocol renal allograft biopsies and the design of clinical trials aimed to prevent or treat chronic allograft nephropathy. Transplantation 2000;69:1849.

743. Merville P, Berge F, Deminiere C, et al. Lower incidence of chronic allograft nephropathy at 1 year post-transplantation in patients treated with mycophenolate mofetil. Am J Transplant 2004;4:1769.

744. Ruiz JC, Campistol JM, Mota A, et al. Early elimination of cyclosporine in kidney transplant recipients receiving sirolimus prevents progression of chronic pathologic allograft lesions. Transplant Proc 2003;35:1669.

745. Bakker RC, Hollander AA, Mallat MJ, et al. Conversion from cyclosporine to azathioprine at three months reduces the incidence of chronic allograft nephropathy. Kidney Int 2003;64:1027.

746. Wilkinson A. Protocol transplant biopsies: Are they really needed? Clinical J Am Soc Nephrol 2006;1:130.

747. Rush D. Protocol transplant biopsies: An underutilized tool in kidney transplantation. Clinical J Am Soc Nephrol 2006;1:138.

748. Racusen L. Protocol transplant biopsies in kidney allografts: Why and when are they indicated? Clinical J Am Soc Nephrol 2006;1:144.

749. Rush DN, Jeffery JR, Gough J. Sequential protocol biopsies in renal transplant patients. Clinico-pathological correlations using the Banff schema. Transplantation 1995;59:511.

750. Shapiro R, Randhawa P, Jordan ML, et al. An analysis of early renal transplant protocol biopsies—the high incidence of subclinical tubulitis. Am J Transplant 2001;1:47.

751. Jain S, Curwood V, White SA, et al. Sub-clinical acute rejection detected using protocol biopsies in patients with delayed graft function. Transpl Int 2000;13(Suppl 1):S52.

752. Roberts IS, Reddy S, Russell C, et al. Subclinical rejection and borderline changes in early protocol biopsy specimens after renal transplantation. Transplantation 2004;77:1194.

753. Schwarz A, Mengel M, Gwinner W, et al. Risk factors for chronic allograft nephropathy after renal transplantation: A protocol biopsy study. Kidney Int 2005;67:341.

754. Jain S, Curwood V, Kazi J, et al. Acute rejection in protocol renal transplant biopsies-institutional variations. Transplant Proc 2000;32:616.

755. Nankivell BJ, Fenton-Lee CA, Kuypers DR, et al. Effect of histological damage on long-term kidney transplant outcome. Transplantation 2001;71:515.

756. Serón D, Moreso F, Bover J, et al. Early protocol renal allograft biopsies and graft outcome. Kidney Int 1997;51:310.

757. Kooijmans-Coutinho MF, Bruijn JA, Hermans J, et al. Evaluation by histology, immunohistology and PCR of proto-collized renal biopsies 1 week post-transplant in relation to subsequent rejection episodes. Nephrol Dial Transplant 1995;10:847.

758. Rush DN, Henry SF, Jeffery JR, et al. Histological findings in early routine biopsies of stable renal allograft recipients. Transplantation 1994;57:208.

759. Buehrig CK, Lager DJ, Stegall MD, et al. Influence of surveillance renal allograft biopsy on diagnosis and prognosis of polyomavirus-associated nephropathy. Kidney Int 2003;64:665.

760. Nankivell BJ, Borrows RJ, Fung CL, et al. Calcineurin inhibitor nephrotoxicity: Longitudinal assessment by protocol histology. Transplantation 2004;78:557.

761. Laftavi MR, Stephan R, Stefanick B, et al. Randomized prospective trial of early steroid withdrawal compared with low-dose steroids in renal transplant recipients using serial protocol biopsies to assess efficacy and safety. Surgery 2005;137:364.

762. Gwinner W, Suppa S, Mengel M, et al. Early calcification of renal allografts detected by protocol biopsies: Causes and clinical implications. Am J Transplant 2005;5:1934.

763. Pinheiro HS, Camara NO, Osaki KS, et al. Early presence of calcium oxalate deposition in kidney graft biopsies is associated with poor long-term graft survival. Am J Transplant 2005;5:323.

764. Alperovich G, Maldonado R, Moreso F, et al. Glomerular enlargement assessed by paired donor and early protocol renal allograft biopsies. Am J Transplant 2004;4:650.

765. Lachenbruch PA, Rosenberg AS, Bonvini E, et al. Biomarkers and surrogate endpoints in renal transplantation: Present status and considerations for clinical trial design. Am J Transplant 2004;4:51.

766. Nicholson ML, Bailey E, Williams S, et al. Computerized histomorphometric assessment of protocol renal transplant biopsy specimens for surrogate markers of chronic rejection. Transplantation 1999;68:236.

767. Kirk AD, Jacobson LM, Heisey DM, et al. Clinically stable human renal allografts contain histological and RNA-based findings that correlate with deteriorating graft function. Transplantation 1999;68:1578.

768. Scherer A, Krause A, Walker JR, et al. Early prognosis of the development of renal chronic allograft rejection by gene expression profiling of human protocol biopsies. Transplantation 2003;75:1323.

769. Midtvedt K, Hartmann A, Sund S. Can a diagnosis of renal allograft rejection be based on histology alone? Clin Transplant 1998;12:300.

770. Shimizu A, Yamada K, Meehan SM, et al. Acceptance reaction: Intragraft events associated with tolerance to renal allografts in miniature swine. J Am Soc Nephrol 2000;11:2371.

771. Russell PS, Chase CM, Colvin RB, Plate JM. Kidney transplants in mice. An analysis of the immune status of mice bearing long-term H-2 incompatible transplants. J. Exp. Med. 1978;147:1449.

772. Blancho G, Gianello PR, Lorf T, et al. Molecular and cellular events implicated in local tolerance to kidney allografts in miniature swine. Transplantation 1997;63:26.

773. Bugeon L, Cuturi MC, Paineau J, et al. Similar levels of granzyme A and perforin mRNA expression in rejected and tolerated heart allografts in donor-specific tolerance in rats. Transplantation 1993;56:405.

774. Kirby JA, Rajasekar MR, Lin Y, et al. Interaction between T lymphocytes and kidney epithelial cells during renal allograft rejection. Kidney Int 1993;39:S124.

775. Koch CA, Khalpey ZI, Platt JL. Accommodation: Preventing injury in transplantation and disease. J Immunol 2004;172:5143.

776. Delikouras A, Hayes M, Malde P, et al. Nitric oxide-mediated expression of Bcl-2 and Bcl-xl and protection from tumor necrosis factor-alpha-mediated apoptosis in porcine endothelial cells after exposure to low concentrations of xenoreactive natural antibody. Transplantation 2001;71:599.

777. Magee JC, Collins BH, Harland RC, et al. Immunoglobulin prevents complement-mediated hyperacute rejection in swine-to-primate xenotransplantation. J Clin Invest 1995; 96:2404.

778. Williams JM, Holzknecht ZE, Plummer TB, et al. Acute vascular rejection and accommodation: Divergent outcomes of the humoral response to organ transplantation. Transplantation 2004;78:1471.

779. Park WD, Grande JP, Ninova D, et al. Accommodation in ABO-incompatible kidney allografts, a novel mechanism of self-protection against antibody-mediated injury. Am J Transplant 2003;3:952.

780. Sinclair R. Origin of endothelium in human renal allografts. Br Med J 1972;4:15.

781. Sedmak D, Sharma H, Czajka C, Ferguson R. Recipient endothelialization of renal allografts. An immunohistochemical study utilitizing blood group antigens. Transplantation 1988;46:907.

782. Randhawa PS, Starzl T, Ramos HC, et al. Allografts surviving for 26 to 29 years following living-related kidney transplantation: Analysis by light microscopy, in situ hybridization for the Y chromosome, and anti-HLA antibodies. Am J Kidney Dis 1994;24:72.

783. Lagaaij EL, Cramer-Knijnenburg GF, van Kemenade FJ, et al. Endothelial cell chimerism after renal transplantation and vascular rejection. Lancet 2001;357:33.

784. Mengel M, Jonigk D, Marwedel M, et al. Tubular chimerism occurs regularly in renal allografts and is not correlated to outcome. J Am Soc Nephrol 2004;15:978.

785. Mestre M, Massip E, Bas J, et al. Longitudinal study of the frequency of cytotoxic T-cell precursors in kidney allograft recipients. Clin Exp Immunol 1996;104:108.

786. Steinmann J, Kaden J, May G, et al. Failure of in vitro T-cell assays to predict clinical outcome after human kidney transplantation. J Clin Lab Anal 1994;8:157.

787. Gao Z, Zhong R, Jiang J, et al. Adoptively transferable tolerance induced by CD45RB monoclonal antibody. J Am Soc Nephrol 1999;10:374.

788. Starzl TE, Demetris AJ, Murase N, et al. Cell migration, chimerism, and graft acceptance. Lancet 1992;339:1579.

789. Reinsmoen NL, Jackson A, McSherry C, et al. Organ-specific patterns of donor antigen-specific hyporeactivity and peripheral blood allogeneic microchimerism in lung, kidney, and liver transplant recipients. Transplantation 1995;60:1546.

790. Wood K, Sachs DH. Chimerism and transplantation tolerance: Cause and effect. Immunol Today 1996;17:584.

791. Starzl TE, Demetris AJ, Murase N, et al. The lost chord: Microchimerism and allograft survival. Immunol Today 1996; 17:577.

792. Sharabi Y, Sachs DH. Mixed chimerism and permanent specific transplantation tolerance induced by a nonlethal preparative regimen. J Exp Med 1989;169:493.

793. Strober S, Benike C, Krishnaswamy S, et al. Clinical transplantation tolerance twelve years after prospective withdrawal of immunosuppressive drugs: Studies of chimerism and anti-donor reactivity. Transplantation 2000;69:1549.

794. Gajewski JL, Ippoliti C, Ma Y, Champlin R. Discontinuation of immunosuppression for prevention of kidney graft rejection after receiving a bone marrow transplant from the same HLA identical sibling donor. Am J Hematol 2002;71:311.

795. Buhler LH, Spitzer TR, Sykes M, et al. Induction of kidney allograft tolerance after transient lymphohematopoietic chimerism in patients with multiple myeloma and end-stage renal disease. Transplantation 2002;74:1405.

796. Domenig C, Sanchez-Fueyo A, Kurtz J, et al. Roles of deletion and regulation in creating mixed chimerism and allograft tolerance using a nonlymphoablative irradiation-free protocol. J Immunol 2005;175:51.

797. Sykes M, Shimizu I, Kawahara T. Mixed hematopoietic chimerism for the simultaneous induction of T- and B-cell tolerance. Transplantation 2005;79:S28.

798. Sellers MT, Deierhoi MH, Curtis JJ, et al. Tolerance in renal

transplantation after allogeneic bone marrow transplantation-6-year follow-up. Transplantation 2001;71:1681.

799. Kawai T, Sogawa H, Boskovic S, et al. CD154 blockade for induction of mixed chimerism and prolonged renal allograft survival in nonhuman primates. Am J Transplant 2004;4:1391.

800. Strehlau J, Pavlakis M, Lipman M, et al. Quantitative detection of immune activation transcripts as a diagnostic tool in kidney transplantation. Proc Nat Acad Sci U S A 1997;94:695.

801. Sharma VK, Bologa RM, Li B, et al. Molecular executors of cell death—differential intrarenal expression of Fas ligand Fas, granzyme B, and perforin during acute and/or chronic rejection of human renal allografts. Transplantation 1996;62:1860.

802. Lipman ML, Stevens AC, Strom TB. Heightened intragraft CTL gene expression in acutely rejecting renal allografts. J Immunol 1994;152:5120.

803. Strehlau J, Pavlakis M, Lipman M, et al. The intragraft gene activation of markers reflecting T-cell-activation and -cytotoxicity analyzed by quantitative RT-PCR in renal transplantation. Clin Nephrol 1996;46:30.

804. Hoffmann SC, Hale DA, Kleiner DE, et al. Functionally significant renal allograft rejection is defined by transcriptional criteria. Am J Transplant 2005;5:573.

805. Suthanthiran M. Molecular analyses of human renal allografts: Differential intragraft gene expression during rejection. Kidney Int Suppl 1997;58:S15.

806. Desvaux D, Schwarzinger M, Pastural M, et al. Molecular diagnosis of renal-allograft rejection: Correlation with histopathologic evaluation and antirejection-therapy resistance. Transplantation 2004;78:647.

807. Nickel P, Lacha J, Ode-Hakim S, et al. Cytotoxic effector molecule gene expression in acute renal allograft rejection: Correlation with clinical outcome; histopathology and function of the allograft. Transplantation 2001;72:1158.

808. Einecke G, Melk A, Ramassar V, et al. Expression of CTL associated transcripts precedes the development of tubulitis in T-cell nediated kidney graft rejection. Am J Transplant 2005;5:1827.

809. Nast CC, Zuo XJ, Prehn J, et al. Gamma-interferon gene expression in human renal allograft fine-needle aspirates. Transplantation 1994;57:498.

810. Kirk AD, Bollinger RR, Finn OJ. Rapid, comprehensive analysis of human cytokine mRNA and its the study of acute renal allograft rejection. Hum Immunol 1995;43:113.

811. Xu GP, Sharma VK, Li B, et al. Intragraft expression of IL-10 messenger RNA: A novel correlate of renal allograft rejection. Kidney Int 1995;48:1504.

812. Akalin E, Hendrix RC, Polavarapu RG, et al. Gene expression analysis in human renal allograft biopsy samples using high-density oligoarray technology. Transplantation 2001;72:948.

813. Flechner SM, Kurian SM, Head SR, et al. Kidney transplant rejection and tissue injury by gene profiling of biopsies and peripheral blood lymphocytes. Am J Transplant 2004;4:1475.

814. Lipman ML, Shen Y, Jeffery JR, et al. Immune-activation gene expression in clinically stable renal allograft biopsies: Molecular evidence for subclinical rejection. Transplantation 1998;66:1673.

815. Aquino Dias EC, Veronese FJ, Santos Goncalves LF, Manfro RC. Molecular markers in subclinical acute rejection of renal transplants. Clin Transplant 2004;18:281.

816. Ode-Hakim S, Docke WD, Kern F, et al. Delayed-type hypersensitivity-like mechanisms dominate late acute rejection episodes in renal allograft recipients. Transplantation 1996;61:1233.

817. Alevy YG, Brennan D, Durriya S, et al. Increased expression of the HDJ-2 heat shock protein in biopsies of human rejected kidney. Transplantation 1996;61:963.

818. Becker BN, Jacobson LM, Becker YT, et al. Renin-angiotensin system gene expression in post-transplant hypertension predicts allograft function. Transplantation 2000;69:1485.

819. Sebekova K, Feber J, Carpenter B, et al. Tissue viral DNA is associated with chronic allograft nephropathy. Pediatr Transplant 2005;9:598.

820. Muthukumar T, Ding R, Dadhania D, et al. Serine proteinase inhibitor-9, an endogenous blocker of granzyme B/perforin lytic pathway, is hyperexpressed during acute rejection of renal allografts. Transplantation 2003;75:1565.

821. Tatapudi RR, Muthukumar T, Dadhania D, et al. Noninvasive detection of renal allograft inflammation by measurements of mRNA for IP-10 and CXCR3 in urine. Kidney Int 2004;65:2390.

822. Ding R, Li B, Muthukumar T, et al. CD103 mRNA levels in urinary cells predict acute rejection of renal allografts. Transplantation 2003;75:1307.

823. Dadhania D, Muthukumar T, Ding R, et al. Molecular signatures of urinary cells distinguish acute rejection of renal allografts from urinary tract infection. Transplantation 2003;75:1752.

824. Kotsch K, Mashreghi MF, Bold G, et al. Enhanced granulysin mRNA expression in urinary sediment in early and delayed acute renal allograft rejection. Transplantation 2004;77:1866.

825. Muthukumar T, Dadhania D, Ding R, et al. Messenger RNA for FOXP3 in the urine of renal-allograft recipients. N Engl J Med 2005;353:2342.

826. Simon T, Opelz G, Wiesel M, et al. Serial peripheral blood perforin and granzyme B gene expression measurements for prediction of acute rejection in kidney graft recipients. Am J Transplant 2003;3:1121.

827. Sabek O, Dorak MT, Kotb M, et al. Quantitative detection of T-cell activation markers by real-time PCR in renal transplant rejection and correlation with histopathologic evaluation. Transplantation 2002;74:701.

828. Vasconcellos LM, Schachter AD, Zheng XX, et al. Cytotoxic lymphocyte gene expression in peripheral blood leukocytes correlates with rejecting renal allografts. Transplantation 1998;66:562.

829. Simon T, Opelz G, Wiesel M, et al. Serial peripheral blood interleukin-18 and perforin gene expression measurements for prediction of acute kidney graft rejection. Transplantation 2004;77:1589.

830. Tan L, Howell WM, Smith JL, Sadek SA. Sequential monitoring of peripheral T-lymphocyte cytokine gene expression in the early post renal allograft period. Transplantation 2001;71:751.

831. Shoker A, George D, Yang H, Baltzan M. Heightened CD40 ligand gene expression in peripheral CD4+ T-cells from patients with kidney allograft rejection. Transplantation 2000;70:497.

832. Kasprzycka M, Klodos K, Nowaczyk M, et al. Expression of FasL gene in T-cells of renal allograft recipients. Immunol Lett 2002;80:9.

833. Hoffmann S, Park J, Jacobson LM, et al. Donor genomics influence graft events: The effect of donor polymorphisms on acute rejection and chronic allograft nephropathy. Kidney Int 2004;66:1686.

834. Tinckam K, Rush D, Hutchinson I, et al. The relative importance of cytokine gene polymorphisms in the development of early and late acute rejection and six-month renal allograft pathology. Transplantation 2005;79:836.

835. Melk A, Henne T, Kollmar T, et al. Cytokine single nucleotide polymorphisms and intrarenal gene expression in chronic allograft nephropathy in children. Kidney Int 2003;64:314.

836. Perico N, Cattaneo D, Sayegh MH, Remuzzi G. Delayed graft function in kidney transplantation. Lancet 2004;364:1814.

837. Renkens JJ, Rouflart MM, Christiaans MH, et al. Outcome of nonheart-beating donor kidneys with prolonged delayed graft function after transplantation. Am J Transplant 2005;5:2704.

838. Rudich SM, Kaplan B, Magee JC, et al. Renal transplantations performed using non-heart-beating organ donors: Going back to the future? Transplantation 2002;74:1715.

839. Sanchez-Fructuoso A, Prats Sanchez D, Marques Vidas M, et al. Non-heart beating donors. Nephrol Dial Transplant 2004;19(Suppl 3):iii26.

840. Nicholson ML, Metcalfe MS, White SA, et al. A comparison

of the results of renal transplantation from non-heart-beating, conventional cadaveric, and living donors. Kidney Int 2000;58:2585.

841. Smith KD, Wrenshall LE, Nicosia RF, et al. Delayed graft function and cast nephropathy associated with tacrolimus plus rapamycin use. J Am Soc Nephrol 2003;14:1037.

842. Solez K, Morel-Maroger L, Sraer JD. The morphology of "acute tubular necrosis" in man: Analysis of 57 renal biopsies and a comparison with the glycerol model. Medicine 1979;58:362.

843. Friedewald JJ, Rabb H. Inflammatory cells in ischemic acute renal failure. Kidney Int 2004;66:486.

844. Nádasdy T, Laszik Z, Blick KE, et al. Human acute tubular necrosis: A lectin and immunohistochemical study. Human Pathology 1995;26:230.

845. Olsen S, Burdick JF, Keown PA, et al. Primary acute renal failure ("acute tubular necrosis") in the transplanted kidney: Morphology and pathogenesis. Medicine 1989;68:173.

846. Rohr MS. Renal allograft acute tubular necrosis. II. A light and electron microscopic study of biopsies taken at procurement and after revascularization. Ann Surg 1983;197:663.

847. Burne-Taney MJ, Yokota N, Rabb H. Persistent renal and extrarenal immune changes after severe ischemic injury. Kidney Int 2005;67:1002.

848. Basile DP. Rarefaction of peritubular capillaries following ischemic acute renal failure: A potential factor predisposing to progressive nephropathy. Curr Opin Nephrol Hypertens 2004;13:1.

849. Keizer KM, de Fijter JW, Haase-Kromwijk BJ, Weimar W. Non-heart-beating donor kidneys in the Netherlands: Allocation and outcome of transplantation. Transplantation 2005;79:1195.

850. Matas AJ, Tellis VA, Quinn TA, et al. Timing of cyclosporine administration in patients with delayed graft function. J Surg Res 1987;43:489.

851. Howard RJ, Pfaff WW, Brunson ME, et al. Increased incidence of rejection in patients with delayed graft function. Clin Transplant 1994;8:527.

852. Merion RM, White DJ, Thiru S, et al. Cyclosporine: Five years' experience in cadaveric renal transplantation. N Engl J Med 1984;310:148.

853. Borel JF, Kis ZL. The discovery and development of cyclosporine (Sandimmune). Transplant Proc 1991;23:1867.

854. Borel JF, Feurer C, Gubler HU, Stahelin H. Biological effects of cyclosporine A. A new antilymphocytic agent. Agents Actions 1976;6:468.

855. Calne RY, White DJ, Thiru S, et al. Cyclosporin A in patients receiving renal allografts from cadaver donors. Lancet 1978;2:1323.

856. Powles RL, Barrett AJ, Clink H, et al. Cyclosporin A for the treatment of graft versus host disease in man. Lancet 1978;2:1327.

857. Pascual J, Marcen R, Burgos FJ, et al. Spanish experience with cyclosporine. Transplant Proc 2004;36:117S.

858. Wong W, Venetz JP, Tolkoff-Rubin N, Pascual M. 2005 immunosuppressive strategies in kidney transplantation: Which role for the calcineurin inhibitors? Transplantation 2005;80:289.

859. Halloran PF. Immunosuppressive drugs for kidney transplantation. N Engl J Med 2004;351:2715.

860. First MR. Tacrolimus based immunosuppression. J Nephrol 2004;17(Suppl 8):S25.

861. Webster AC, Woodroffe RC, Taylor RS, et al. Tacrolimus versus ciclosporin as primary immunosuppression for kidney transplant recipients: Meta-analysis and meta-regression of randomised trial data. BMJ 2005;331:810.

862. Kramer BK, Montagnino G, Del Castillo D, et al. Efficacy and safety of tacrolimus compared with cyclosporin A microemulsion in renal transplantation: 2 year follow-up results. Nephrol Dial Transplant 2005;20:968.

863. Mihatsch MJ, Kyo M, Morozumi K, et al. The side-effects of ciclosporine-A and tacrolimus. Clin Nephrol 1998;49:356.

864. Kaplan B, Schold JD, Meier-Kriesche HU. Long-term graft survival with neoral and tacrolimus: A paired kidney analysis. J Am Soc Nephrol 2003;14:2980.

865. Meier-Kriesche HU, Kaplan B. Cyclosporine microemulsion and tacrolimus are associated with decreased chronic allograft failure and improved long-term graft survival as compared with Sandimmune. Am J Transplant 2002;2:100.

866. Randhawa PS, Tsamandas AC, Magnone M, et al. Microvascular changes in renal allografts associated with FK506 (tacrolimus) therapy. Am J Surg Pathol 1996;20:306.

867. Stratta P, Canavese C, Quaglia M, et al. Posttransplantation chronic renal damage in nonrenal transplant recipients. Kidney Int 2005;68:1453.

868. Shulman H, Striker G, Deeg HJ, et al. Nephrotoxicity of cyclosporin A after allogeneic marrow transplantation. Glomerular thromboses and tubular injury. N Eng J Med 1981;305:1392.

869. Neild GH, Reuben R, Hartley RB, Cameron JS. Glomerular thrombi in renal allografts associated with cyclosporin treatment. J Clin Pathol 1985;38:253.

870. Van Buren D, Van Buren CT, Flechner SM, et al. De novo hemolytic uremic syndrome in renal transplant recipients immunosuppressed with cyclosporine. Surgery 1985;98:54.

871. Sommer BG, Innes JT, Whitehurst RM, et al. Cyclosporine-associated renal arteriopathy resulting in loss of allograft function. Am J Surg 1985;149:756.

872. Schwimmer J, Nadasdy TA, Spitalnik PF, et al. De novo thrombotic microangiopathy in renal transplant recipients: A comparison of hemolytic uremic syndrome with localized renal thrombotic microangiopathy. Am J Kidney Dis 2003;41:471.

873. Reynolds JC, Agodoa LY, Yuan CM, Abbott KC. Thrombotic microangiopathy after renal transplantation in the United States. Am J Kidney Dis 2003;42:1058.

874. Myers BD, Ross J, Newton L, et al. Cyclosporine-associated chronic nephropathy. N Eng J Med 1984;311:699.

875. Mihatsch MJ, Thiel G, Spichtin HP, et al. Morphological findings in kidney transplants after treatment with cyclosporine. Transplant Proc 1983;15(Suppl 1):2821.

876. Mihatsch MJ, Ryffel B, Gudat F. The differential diagnosis between rejection and cyclosporine toxicity. Kidney Int Supplement 1995;52:S63.

877. Mihatsch MJ, Morozumi K, Strom EH, et al. Renal transplant morphology after long-term therapy with cyclosporine. Transplant Proc 1995;27:39.

878. Mihatsch MJ, Gudat F, Ryffel B, Thiel G. Cyclosporine nephropathy. In: Tisher CC, Brenner BM, eds. Renal Pathology With Clinical and Functional Correlations, 2nd ed. Philadelphia: Lippincott Williams & Wilkins, 1994:1641.

879. Katari SR, Magnone M, Shapiro R, et al. Tacrolimus nephrotoxicity after renal transplantation. Transplant Proc 1997;29:311.

880. Mihatsch MJ, Gudat F, Ryffel B, Thiel G. Cyclosporine nephropathy. In: Tisher CC, Brenner BM, eds. Renal Pathology With Clinical and Functional Correlations. 2nd ed. Philadelphia: Lippincott Williams & Wilkins, 1994:1641.

881. Mihatsch M, Thiel G, Ryffel B. Cyclosporine nephrotoxicity. Adv Nephrol 1988;17:303.

882. Simpson MA, Madras PN, Cornaby AJ, et al. Sequential determinations of urinary cytology and plasma and urinary lymphokines in the management of renal allograft recipients. Transplantation 1989;47:218.

883. Kyo M, Gudat F, Dalquen P, et al. Differential diagnosis of kidney transplant rejection and cyclosporine nephrotoxicity by urine cytology. Transplant Proc 1992;24:1388.

884. Kyo M, Toki K, Nishimura K, et al. Differential diagnosis of kidney transplant rejection and cyclosporin/tacrolimus nephropathy using urine cytology. Clin Transplant 2002;16(Suppl 8):40.

885. Winkelmann M, Burrig KF, Koldovsky U, et al. Cyclosporin A-altered renal tubular cells in urinary cytology. Lancet 1985;2:667.

886. Wenzel-Seifert K, Harwig S, Keller F. Fulminant calcinosis in two patients after kidney transplantation. Am J Nephrol 1991;11:497.

887. Solez K, Racusen LC, Marcussen N, et al. Morphology of

ischemic acute renal failure, normal function, and cyclosporine toxicity in cyclosporine-treated renal allograft recipients. Kidney Int 1993;43:1058.

888. Bergstrand A, Bohman SO, Farnsworth A, et al. Renal histopathology in kidney transplant recipients immunosuppressed with cyclosporin A: Results of an international workshop. Clin Nephrol 1985;24:107.

889. Yamaguchi Y, Teraoka S, Yagisawa T, et al. Ultrastructural study of cyclosporine-associated arteriolopathy in renal allografts. Transplant Proc 1989;21:1517.

890. Strom EH, Epper R, Mihatsch MJ. Ciclosporin-associated arteriolopathy: The renin producing vascular smooth muscle cells are more sensitive to ciclosporin toxicity. Clin Nephrol 1995;43:226.

891. Strom EH, Thiel G, Mihatsch MJ. Prevalence of cyclosporine-associated arteriolopathy in renal transplant biopsies from 1981 to 1992. Transplant Proc 1994;26:2585.

892. Pei Y, Scholey JW, Katz A, et al. Chronic nephrotoxicity in psoriatic patients treated with low-dose cyclosporine. Am J Kidney Dis 1994;23:528.

893. Rossmann P, Jirka J, Chadimova M, et al. Arteriolosclerosis of the human renal allograft: Morphology, origin, life history and relationship to cyclosporine therapy. Virchows Archiv A Pathol Anat Histopathol 1991;418:129.

894. Antonovych TT, Sabnis SG, Austin HA, et al. Cyclosporine A-induced arteriolopathy. Transplant Proc 1988;20:951.

895. Savoldi S, Scolari F, Sandrini S, et al. Cyclosporine chronic nephrotoxicity: Histologic follow up at 6 and 18 months after renal transplant. Transplant Proc 1988;20:777.

896. Bren A, Pajek J, Grego K, et al. Follow-up of kidney graft recipients with cyclosporine-associated hemolytic-uremic syndrome and thrombotic microangiopathy. Transplant Proc 2005;37:1889.

896a. Sis B, Dadras F, Khoshjou F, et al. Reproducibility studies on arteriolar hyaline thickening scoring in calcineurin inhibitor-treated renal allograft recipients. Am J Transplant 2006;6:1444.

897. Takeda A, Morozumi K, Uchida K, et al. Is cyclosporine-associated glomerulopathy a new glomerular lesion in renal allografts using CyA? Transplant Proc 1993;25:515.

898. Goes N, Colvin RB. Renal failure nine years after a heart-lung transplant. New Engl J Med 2006, in press.

899. Mihatsch MJ, Thiel G, Basler V, et al. Morphological patterns in cyclosporine-treated renal transplant recipients. Transplant Proc 1985;17:101.

900. Ryffel B, Siegel H, Thiel G, Mihatsch MJ. Experimental cyclosporine nephrotoxicity. In: Burdick JF, Racusen LC, Williams GM, Solez K, eds. Kidney Transplant Rejection: Diagnosis and Treatment, 2nd ed. New York: Marcel Dekker, 1992:601.

901. Messana JM, Johnson KJ, Mihatsch MJ. Renal structure and function effects after low dose cyclosporine in psoriasis patients: A preliminary report. Clin Nephrol 1995;43:150.

902. Lewis RM, Verani RR, Vo C, et al. Evaluation of chronic renal disease in heart transplant recipients: Importance of pretransplantation native kidney histologic evaluation. J Heart Lung Transplant1994;13:376.

903. Fischer G, Wittmann-Liebold B, Lang K, et al. Cyclophilin and peptidyl-prolyl cis-trans isomerase are probably identical proteins. Nature 1989;337:476.

904. Takahashi N, Hayano T, Suzuki M. Peptidyl-prolyl cis-trans isomerase is the cyclosporin A-binding protein cyclophilin. Nature 1989;337:473.

905. Borel JF, Baumann G, Chapman I, et al. In vivo pharmacological effects of ciclosporin and some analogues. Adv Pharmacol 1996;35:115.

906. Kapturczak MH, Meier-Kriesche HU, Kaplan B. Pharmacology of calcineurin antagonists. Transplant Proc 2004;36:25S.

907. Wiederrecht G, Hung S, Chan HK, et al. Characterization of high molecular weight FK-506 binding activities reveals a novel FK-506-binding protein as well as a protein complex. J Biol Chem 1992;267:21753.

908. Maki N, Sekiguchi F, Nishimaki J, et al. Complementary DNA encoding the human T-cell FK506-binding protein, a peptidyl-prolyl cis-trans isomerase distinct from cyclophilin. Proc Nat Acad Sci U S A 1990;87:5440.

909. Sigal NH, Dumont F, Durette P, et al. Is cyclophilin involved in the immunosuppressive and nephrotoxic mechanism of action of cyclosporin A? J Exp Med 1991;173:619.

910. Nankivell BJ, Hibbins M, Chapman JR. Diagnostic utility of whole blood cyclosporine measurements in renal transplantation using triple therapy. Transplantation 1994;58:989.

911. Lo A, Burckart GJ. P-glycoprotein and drug therapy in organ transplantation. J Clin Pharmacol 1999;39:995.

912. Min DI. Cyclosporine. In: Schumacher D, ed. Therapeutic Drug Monitoring: Appleton Lange, 1995:449.

913. Lemahieu W, Maes B, Verbeke K, et al. Cytochrome P450 3A4 and P-glycoprotein activity and assimilation of tacrolimus in transplant patients with persistent diarrhea. Am J Transplant 2005;5:1383.

914. Remuzzi G, Perico N. Cyclosporine-induced renal dysfunction in experimental animals and humans. Kidney Int Suppl 1995;52:S70.

915. Reidy MA. Effect of cyclosporin on vascular smooth muscle cells. Lab Invest 1991;65:1.

916. Xue H, Bukoski RD, McCarron DA, Bennett WM. Induction of contraction in isolated rat aorta by cyclosporine. Transplantation 1987;43:715.

917. Bokemeyer D, Friedrichs U, Backer A, et al. Atrial natriuretic peptide inhibits cyclosporin A-induced endothelin production and calcium accumulation in rat vascular smooth muscle cells. Clin Sci 1994;87:383.

918. Bunchman TE, Brookshire CA. Cyclosporine-induced synthesis of endothelin by cultured human endothelial cells. J Clin Invest 1991;88:310.

919. Leszczynski D, Zhao Y, Yeagley TJ, Foegh ML. Direct and endothelial cell-mediated effect of cyclosporin A on the proliferation of rat smooth muscle cells in vitro. Am J Pathol 1993;142:149.

920. Abassi ZA, Pieruzzi F, Nakhoul F, Keiser HR. Effects of cyclosporin A on the synthesis, excretion and metabolism of endothelin in the rat. Hypertension 1996;27:1140.

921. Lanese DM, Conger JD. Effects of endothelin receptor antagonist on cyclosporine-induced vasoconstriction in isolated rat renal arterioles. J Clin Invest 1993;91:2144.

922. Lanese DM, Falk SA, Conger JD. Sequential agonist activation and site-specific mediation of acute cyclosporine constriction in rat renal arterioles. Transplantation 1994;58:1371.

923. Fogo A, Hellings EE, Inagami T, Kon V. Endothelin receptor antagonism is protective in in vivo acute cyclosporine toxicity. Kidney Int 1990;42:770.

924. Fasel J, Kaissling B, Ludwig KS, et al. Light and electron microscopic changes in the kidney of Wistar rats following treatment with cyclosporine A. Ultrastruct Pathol 1987;11:435.

925. Young BA, Burdmann EA, Johnson RJ, et al. Cyclosporine A induced arteriolopathy in a rat model of chronic cyclosporine nephropathy. Kidney Int 1995;48:431.

926. Franceschini N, Alpers CE, Bennett WM, Andoh TF. Cyclosporine arteriolopathy: Effects of drug withdrawal. Am J Kidney Dis 1998;32:247.

927. Pichler RH, Franceschini N, Young BA, et al. Pathogenesis of cyclosporine nephropathy: Roles of angiotensin II and osteopontin. J Am Soc Nephrol 1995;6:1186.

928. Neild GH, Rocchi G, Imberti L, et al. Effect of cyclosporin A on prostacyclin synthesis by vascular tissue. Thromb Res 1983;32:373.

929. Zoja C, Furci L, Ghilardi F, et al. Cyclosporin-induced endothelial cell injury. Lab Invest 1986;55:455.

930. Cohen H, Bull HA, Seddon A, et al. Vascular endothelial cell function and ultrastructure in thrombotic microangiopathy following allogeneic bone marrow transplantation. Eur J Haematol 1989;43:207.

931. Charba D, Moake JL, Harris MA, Hester JP. Abnormalities of von Willebrand factor multimers in drug-associated thrombotic microangiopathies. Am J Hematol 1993;42:268.

932. Seeber C, Hiller E, Holler E, Kolb HJ. Increased levels of tissue plasminogen activator (t-PA) and tissue plasminogen activator inhibitor (PAI) correlate with tumor necrosis factor alpha (TNF alpha)-release in patients suffering from microangiopathy following allogeneic bone marrow transplantation (BMT). Thromb Res 1992;66:373.

933. Carlsen E, Flatmark A, Prydz H. Cytokine-induced procoagulant activity in monocytes and endothelial cells. Further enhancement by cyclosporine. Transplantation 1988;46:575.

934. Brown Z, Neild GH, Willoughby JJ, et al. Increased factor VIII as an index of vascular injury in cyclosporine nephrotoxicity. Transplantation 1986;42:150.

935. Tsinalis D, Dickenmann M, Brunner F, et al. Acute renal failure in a renal allograft recipient treated with intravenous immunoglobulin. Am J Kidney Dis 2002;40:667.

936. Haas M, Sonnenday CJ, Cicone JS, et al. Isometric tubular epithelial vacuolization in renal allograft biopsy specimens of patients receiving low-dose intravenous immunoglobulin for a positive crossmatch. Transplantation 2004;78:549.

937. Moreau JF, Droz D, Sabto J, et al. Osmotic nephrosis induced by water-soluble triiodinated contrast media in man. A retrospective study of 47 cases. Radiology 1975;115:329.

938. Markowitz GS, Stokes MB, Radhakrishnan J, D'Agati VD. Acute phosphate nephropathy following oral sodium phosphate bowel purgative: An underrecognized cause of chronic renal failure. J Am Soc Nephrol 2005;16:3389.

939. Gonlusen G, Akgun H, Ertan A, et al. Renal failure and nephrocalcinosis associated with oral sodium phosphate bowel cleansing: Clinical patterns and renal biopsy findings. Arch Pathol Lab Med 2006;130:101.

940. Koop K, Bakker RC, Eikmans M, et al. Differentiation between chronic rejection and chronic cyclosporine toxicity by analysis of renal cortical mRNA. Kidney Int 2004;66:2038.

941. Hall BM, Tiller DJ, Duggin GG, et al. Post-transplant acute renal failure in cadaver renal recipients treated with cyclosporine. Kidney Int 1985;28:178.

942. Versluis DJ, Ten KFJ, Wenting GJ, et al. Histological lesions associated with cyclosporin: Incidence and reversibility in one year old kidney transplants. J Clin Pathol 1988;41:498.

943. Ojo AO, Held PJ, Port FK, et al. Chronic renal failure after transplantation of a nonrenal organ. N Engl J Med 2003;349:931.

944. English RF, Pophal SA, Bacanu SA, et al. Long-term comparison of tacrolimus- and cyclosporine-induced nephrotoxicity in pediatric heart-transplant recipients. Am J Transplant 2002;2:769.

945. Collins BS, Davis CL, Marsh CL, et al. Reversible cyclosporine arteriolopathy. Transplantation 1992;54:732.

946. Morozumi K, Thiel G, Albert FW, et al. Studies on morphological outcome of cyclosporine-associated arteriolopathy after discontinuation of cyclosporine in renal allografts. Clin Nephrol 1992;38:1.

947. Karthikeyan V, Parasuraman R, Shah V, et al. Outcome of plasma exchange therapy in thrombotic microangiopathy after renal transplantation. Am J Transplant 2003;3:1289.

948. Hochstetler LA, Flanigan MJ, Lager DJ. Transplant-associated thrombotic microangiopathy: The role of IgG administration as initial therapy. Am J Kidney Dis 1994;23:444.

949. Trimarchi HM, Truong LD, Brennan S, et al. FK506-associated thrombotic microangiopathy: Report of two cases and review of the literature. Transplantation 1999;67:539.

950. Katafuchi R, Saito S, Ikeda K, et al. A case of late onset cyclosporine-induced hemolytic uremic syndrome resulting in renal graft loss. Clin Transplant 1999;13(Suppl 1):54.

951. Galli FC, Damon LE, Tomlanovich SJ, et al. Cyclosporine-induced hemolytic uremic syndrome in a heart transplant recipient. J Heart Lung Transplant 1993;12:440.

952. Rabinowe SN, Soiffer RJ, Tarbell NJ, et al. Hemolytic-uremic syndrome following bone marrow transplantation in adults for hematologic malignancies. Blood 1991;77:1837.

953. Zarifian A, Meleg-Smith S, O'Donovan R, et al. Cyclosporine-associated thrombotic microangiopathy in renal allografts. Kidney Int 1999;55:2457.

954. Noel C, Saunier P, Hazzan M, et al. Incidence and clinical profile of microvascular complications in renal allografted patients treated with cyclosporine. Ann Med Interne (Paris) 1992;1:33.

955. Candinas D, Keusch G, Schlumpf R, et al. Hemolytic-uremic syndrome following kidney transplantation: Prognostic factors. Schweizer Med Wochenschr 1994;124:1789.

956. Dominguez J, Kompatzki A, Norambuena R, et al. Benefits of early biopsy on the outcome of kidney transplantation. Transplant Proc 2005;37:3361.

957. Langer RM, Van Buren CT, Katz SM, Kahan BD. De novo hemolytic uremic syndrome after kidney transplantation in patients treated with cyclosporine-sirolimus combination. Transplantation 2002;73:756.

958. Franco A, Hernandez D, Capdevilla L, et al. De novo hemolytic-uremic syndrome/thrombotic microangiopathy in renal transplant patients receiving calcineurin inhibitors: Role of sirolimus. Transplant Proc 2003;35:1764.

959. Tamura S, Sugawara Y, Matsui Y, et al. Thrombotic microangiopathy in living-donor liver transplantation. Transplantation 2005;80:169.

960. Wiener Y, Nakhleh RE, Lee MW, et al. Prognostic factors and early resumption of cyclosporin A in renal allograft recipients with thrombotic microangiopathy and hemolytic uremic syndrome. Clin Transplant 1997;11:157.

961. Young BA, Marsh CL, Alpers CE, Davis CL. Cyclosporine-associated thrombotic microangiopathy/hemolytic uremic syndrome following kidney and kidney-pancreas transplantation. Am J Kidney Dis 1996;28:561.

962. Bolin P Jr, Jennette JC, Mandel SR. Cyclosporin-associated thrombotic microangiopathy: Successful retreatment with cyclosporin. Ren Fail 1991;13:275.

963. Epstein M, Landsberg D. Cyclosporine-induced thrombotic microangiopathy resulting in renal allograft loss and its successful reuse: A report of two cases. Am J Kidney Dis 1991;17:346.

964. Franz M, Regele H, Schmaldienst S, et al. Posttransplant hemolytic uremic syndrome in adult retransplanted kidney graft recipients: Advantage of FK506 therapy? Transplantation 1998;66:1258.

965. Josephson MA, Chiu MY, Woodle ES, et al. Drug-induced acute interstitial nephritis in renal allografts: Histopathologic features and clinical course in six patients. Am J Kidney Dis 1999;34:540.

966. Abramowicz D, Pradier O, Marchant A, et al. Induction of thromboses within renal grafts by high-dose prophylactic OKT3. Lancet 1992;339:777.

967. Charpentier B, Hiesse C, Lantz O, et al. Evidence that antihuman tumor necrosis factor monoclonal antibody prevents OKT3-induced acute syndrome. Transplantation 1992;54:997.

968. Zlabinger GJ, Stuhlmeier KM, Eher R, et al. Cytokine release and dynamics of leukocyte populations after CD3/TCR monoclonal antibody treatment. J Clin Immunol 1992;12:170.

969. Durez P, Abramowicz D, Gérard C, et al. In vivo induction of interleukin 10 by anti-CD3 monoclonal antibody or bacterial lipopolysaccharide: Differential modulation by cyclosporin A. J Exp Med 1993;177:551.

970. Iitaka M, Iwatani Y, Row VV, Volpe R. Induction of monocyte procoagulant activity with OKT3 antibody. J Immunol 1987;139:1617.

971. Pradier O, Surquin M, Stordeur P, et al. Monocyte procoagulant activity induced by in vivo administration of the OKT3 monoclonal antibody. Blood 1996;87:3768.

972. Chatenoud L, Legendre C, Ferran C, et al. Corticosteroid inhibition of the OKT3-induced cytokine-related syndrome–dosage and kinetics prerequisites. Transplantation 1991;51:334.

973. Ferran C, Dy M, Sheehan K, et al. Cascade modulation by anti-tumor necrosis factor monoclonal antibody of interferon-gamma, interleukin 3 and interleukin 6 release after triggering of the CD3/T-cell receptor activation pathway. Eur J Immunol 1991;21:2349.

974. Kahan BD. Sirolimus. In: Morris PJ, ed. Kidney Transplantation: Principles and Practice, 5th ed. Philadelphia: WB Saunders, 2001:279.

975. Fellstrom B. Cyclosporine nephrotoxicity. Transplant Proc 2004;36:220S.

976. Stallone G, Infante B, Schena A, et al. Rapamycin for treatment of chronic allograft nephropathy in renal transplant patients. J Am Soc Nephrol 2005;16:3755.

977. Kirken RA, Wang YL. Molecular actions of sirolimus: Sirolimus and mTor. Transplant Proc 2003;35:227S.

978. Bruns CJ, Koehl GE, Guba M, et al. Rapamycin-induced endothelial cell death and tumor vessel thrombosis potentiate cytotoxic therapy against pancreatic cancer. Clin Cancer Res 2004;10:2109.

979. Guba M, Yezhelyev M, Eichhorn ME, et al. Rapamycin induces tumor-specific thrombosis via tissue factor in the presence of VEGF. Blood 2005;105:4463.

980. Guba M, von Breitenbuch P, Steinbauer M, et al. Rapamycin inhibits primary and metastatic tumor growth by antiangiogenesis: Involvement of vascular endothelial growth factor. Nat Med 2002;8:128.

981. Letavernier E, Pe'raldi MN, Pariente A, et al. Proteinuria following a switch from calcineurin inhibitors to sirolimus. Transplantation 2005;80:1198.

982. Sennesael JJ, Bosmans JL, Bogers JP, et al. Conversion from cyclosporine to sirolimus in stable renal transplant recipients. Transplantation 2005;80:1578.

983. Straathof-Galema L, Wetzels JF, Dijkman HB, et al. Sirolimus-associated heavy proteinuria in a renal transplant recipient: Evidence for a tubular mechanism. Am J Transplant 2006;6:429.

984. Coombes JD, Mreich E, Liddle C, Rangan GK. Rapamycin worsens renal function and intratubular cast formation in protein overload nephropathy. Kidney Int 2005;68:2599.

985. Dittrich E, Schmaldienst S, Soleiman A, et al. Rapamycin-associated post-transplantation glomerulonephritis and its remission after reintroduction of calcineurin-inhibitor therapy. Transpl Int 2004;17:215.

986. Sartelet H, Toupance O, Lorenzato M, et al. Sirolimus-induced thrombotic microangiopathy is associated with decreased expression of vascular endothelial growth factor in kidneys. Am J Transplant 2005;5:2441.

987. Oyen O, Strom EH, Midtvedt K, et al. Calcineurin inhibitor-free immunosuppression in renal allograft recipients with thrombotic microangiopathy/hemolytic uremic syndrome. Am J Transplant 2006;6:412.

988. Morelon E, Kreis H. Sirolimus therapy without calcineurin inhibitors: Necker Hospital 8-year experience. Transplant Proc 2003;35:52S.

989. Dean PG, Lund WJ, Larson TS, et al. Wound-healing complications after kidney transplantation: A prospective, randomized comparison of sirolimus and tacrolimus. Transplantation 2004;77:1555.

990. Gardner SD, Field AM, Coleman DV, Hulme B. New human papovavirus (B.K.) isolated from urine after renal transplantation. Lancet 1971;1:1253.

991. Mackenzie EF, Poulding JM, Harrison PR, Amer B. Human polyoma virus (HPV)–a significant pathogen in renal transplantation. Proc Eur Dial Transplant Assoc 1978;15:352.

992. Binet I, Nickeleit V, Hirsch HH, et al. Polyomavirus disease under new immunosuppressive drugs: A cause of renal graft dysfunction and graft loss. Transplantation 1999;67:918.

993. Drachenberg CB, Beskow CO, Cangro CB, et al. Human polyoma virus in renal allograft biopsies: Morphological findings and correlation with urine cytology. Hum Pathol 1999;30:970.

994. Howell DN, Smith SR, Butterly DW, et al. Diagnosis and management of BK polyomavirus interstitial nephritis in renal transplant recipients. Transplantation 1999;68:1279.

995. Pappo O, Demetris AJ, Raikow RB, Randhawa PS. Human polyoma virus infection of renal allografts: Histopathologic diagnosis, clinical significance, and literature review. Mod Pathol 1996;9:105.

996. Randhawa PS, Finkelstein S, Scantlebury V, et al. Human polyoma virus-associated interstitial nephritis in the allograft kidney. Transplantation 1999;67:103.

997. Nickeleit V, Steiger J, Mihatsch MJ. BK virus infection after kidney transplantation. Graft 2002;5(Suppl):S46.

998. Celik B, Randhawa PS. Glomerular changes in BK virus nephropathy. Hum Pathol 2004;35:367.

999. Drachenberg CB, Papadimitriou JC, Hirsch HH, et al. Histological patterns of polyomavirus nephropathy: Correlation with graft outcome and viral load. Am J Transplant 2004;4:2082.

1000. Drachenberg CB, Hirsch HH, Ramos E, Papadimitriou JC. Polyomavirus disease in renal transplantation: Review of pathological findings and diagnostic methods. Hum Pathol 2005;36:1245.

1001. Hirsch HH, Brennan DC, Drachenberg CB, et al. Polyomavirus-associated nephropathy in renal transplantation: Interdisciplinary analyses and recommendations. Transplantation 2005;79:1277.

1002. Nickeleit V, Mihatsch MJ. Polyomavirus nephropathy: Pathogenesis, morphological and clinical aspects. In: Kreipe HH, ed. Verhandlungen der Deutschen Gesellschaft fuer Pathologie, 88. Tagung. Muenchen Jena: Urban & Fischer, 2004:69.

1003. Nickeleit V, Mihatsch MJ. Polyomavirus nephropathy in native kidneys and renal allografts: An update on an escalating threat. Transpl Int. 2006, in press.

1004. Coleman DV, Mackenzie EF, Gardner SD, et al. Human polyomavirus (BK) infection and ureteric stenosis in renal allograft recipients. J Clin Pathol 1978;31:338.

1004a. Baksh FK, Finkelstein SD, Swalsky PA, et al. Molecular genotyping of BK and JC viruses in human polyomavirus-associated interstitial nephritis after renal transplantation. Am J Kidney Dis 2001;38:354.

1004b. Trofe J, Cavallo J, First MR, et al. Polyomavirus in kidney and kidney-pancreas transplantation: a defined protocol for immunosuppression reduction and histologic monitoring. Transplant Proc 2002;34:1788.

1004c. Kazory A, Ducloux D, Chalopin JM, et al. The first case of JC virus allograft nephropathy. Transplantation 2003;76:1653.

1004d. Milstone A, Vilchez RA, Geiger X, et al. Polymavirus simian virus 40 infection associated with nephropathy in a lung-transplant recipient. Transplantation 2004;77:1019.

1005. Drachenberg CB, Papadimitriou JC, Wali R, et al. BK polyoma virus allograft nephropathy: Ultrastructural features from viral cell entry to lysis. Am J Transplant 2003;3:1383.

1006. Haririan A, Ramos ER, Drachenberg CB, et al. Polyomavirus nephropathy in native kidneys of a solitary pancreas transplant recipient. Transplantation 2002;73:1350.

1007. Boldorini R, Veggiani C, Barco D, Monga G. Kidney and urinary tract polyomavirus infection and distribution: Molecular biology investigation of 10 consecutive autopsies. Arch Pathol Lab Med 2005;129:69.

1008. Chesters PM, Heritage J, McCance DJ. Persistence of DNA sequences of BK virus and JC virus in normal human tissues and in diseased tissues. J Infect Dis 1983;147:676.

1009. Heritage J, Chesters PM, McCane DJ. The persistence of papovavirus BK DNA sequences in normal human renal tissue. J Med Virol 1981;8:143.

1010. Nickeleit V, Singh HK, Gilliland MGF, et al. Latent polyomavirus type BK loads in native kidneys analyzed by TaqMan PCR: What can be learned to better understand BK virus nephropathy. J Am Soc Nephrol 2003;14:424A.

1011. Nickeleit V, Singh HK, Mihatsch MJ. Polyomavirus nephropathy: Morphology, pathophysiology, and clinical management. Curr Opin Nephrol Hypertens 2003;12:599.

1012. Bohl DL, Storch GA, Ryschkewitsch C, et al. Donor origin of BK virus in renal transplantation and role of HLA C7 in susceptibility to sustained BK viremia. Am J Transplant 2005;5:2213.

1013. Shah KV. Human polyomavirus BKV and renal disease. Nephrol Dial Transplant 2000;15:754.

1014. Mengel M, Marwedel M, Radermacher J, et al. Incidence of polyomavirus-nephropathy in renal allografts: Influence of modern immunosuppressive drugs. Nephrol Dial Transplant 2003;18:1190.

1015. Rocha PN, Plumb TJ, Miller SE, et al. Risk factors for BK polyomavirus nephritis in renal allograft recipients. Clin Transplant 2004;18:456.

1016. van Gorder MA, Della Pelle P, Henson JW, et al. Cynomolgus polyoma virus infection: A new member of the polyoma virus family causes interstitial nephritis, ureteritis, and enteritis in immunosuppressed cynomolgus monkeys. Am J Pathol 1999;154:1273.

1017. Dugan AS, Eash S, Atwood WJ. An N-linked glycoprotein with alpha(2,3)-linked sialic acid is a receptor for BK virus. J Virol 2005;79:14442.

1018. Eash S, Querbes W, Atwood WJ. Infection of vero cells by BK virus is dependent on caveolae. J Virol 2004;78:11583.

1019. Eash S, Atwood WJ. Involvement of cytoskeletal components in BK virus infectious entry. J Virol 2005;79:11734.

1020. Schmid H, Burg M, Kretzler M, et al. BK virus associated nephropathy in native kidneys of a heart allograft recipient. Am J Transplant 2005;5:1562.

1021. Schmid H, Nitschko H, Gerth J, et al. Polyomavirus DNA and RNA detection in renal allograft biopsies: Results from a European multicenter study. Transplantation 2005;80:600.

1022. Randhawa P, Shapiro R, Vats A. Quantitation of DNA of polyomaviruses BK and JC in human kidneys. J Infect Dis 2005;192:504.

1023. Bruno B, Zager RA, Boeckh MJ, et al. Adenovirus nephritis in hematopoietic stem-cell transplantation. Transplantation 2004;77:1049.

1024. Nada R, Sachdeva MU, Sud K, et al. Co-infection by cytomegalovirus and BK polyoma virus in renal allograft, mimicking acute rejection. Nephrol Dial Transplant 2005;20:994.

1025. Hirsch HH, Knowles W, Dickenmann M, et al. Prospective study of polyomavirus type BK replication and nephropathy in renal-transplant recipients. N Engl J Med 2002;347:488.

1026. Mayr M, Nickeleit V, Hirsch HH, et al. Polyomavirus BK nephropathy in a kidney transplant recipient: Critical issues of diagnosis and management. Am J Kidney Dis 2001;38:E13.

1027. Nickeleit V, Mihatsch MJ. Polyomavirus allograft nephropathy and concurrent acute rejection: A diagnostic and therapeutic challenge. Am J Transplant 2004;4:838.

1028. Mannon RB, Hoffmann SC, Kampen RL, et al. Molecular evaluation of BK polyomavirus nephropathy. Am J Transplant 2005;5:2883.

1029. Ahuja M, Cohen EP, Dayer AM, et al. Polyoma virus infection after renal transplantation. Use of immunostaining as a guide to diagnosis. Transplantation 2001;71:896.

1030. Jeong HJ, Hong SW, Sung SH, et al. Polyomavirus nephropathy in renal transplantation: A clinico-pathological study. Transpl Int 2003;16:671.

1031. Sachdeva MS, Nada R, Jha V, et al. The high incidence of BK polyoma virus infection among renal transplant recipients in India. Transplantation 2004;77:429.

1032. Vasudev B, Hariharan S, Hussain SA, et al. BK virus nephritis: Risk factors, timing, and outcome in renal transplant recipients. Kidney Int 2005;68:1834.

1033. Petrogiannis-Haliotis T, Sakoulas G, Kirby J, et al. BK-related polyomavirus vasculopathy in a renal-transplant recipient. N Engl J Med 2001;345:1250.

1034. Drachenberg CB, Papadimitriou JC, Wali R, et al. Improved outcome of polyoma virus allograft nephropathy with early biopsy. Transplant Proc 2004;36:758.

1035. Ramos E, Vincenti F, Lu WX, et al. Retransplantation in patients with graft loss caused by polyoma virus nephropathy. Transplantation 2004;77:131.

1036. Hirsch HH, Ramos E. Retransplantation after polyomavirus-associated nephropathy: Just do it? Am J Transplant 2006;6:7.

1037. Womer K, Meier-Krieschke HU, Patton P, et al. Preemptive retransplantation for BK virus nephropathy: Successful outcome despite active viremia. Am J Transplant 2006;6:209.

1038. Williams JW, Javaid B, Kadambi PV, et al. Leflunomide for polyomavirus type BK nephropathy. N Engl J Med 2005;352:1157.

1039. Kuypers DR, Vandooren AK, Lerut E, et al. Adjuvant low-dose cidofovir therapy for BK polyomavirus interstitial nephritis in renal transplant recipients. Am J Transplant 2005;5:1997.

1040. Vats A, Shapiro R, Singh Randhawa P, et al. Quantitative viral load monitoring and cidofovir therapy for the management of BK virus-associated nephropathy in children and adults. Transplantation 2003;75:105.

1041. Farasati NA, Shapiro R, Vats A, Randhawa P. Effect of leflunomide and cidofovir on replication of BK virus in an in vitro culture system. Transplantation 2005;79:116.

1042. Trofe J, Gaber LW, Stratta RJ, et al. Polyomavirus in kidney and kidney-pancreas transplant recipients. Transpl Infect Dis 2003;5:21.

1043. Kang YN, Han SM, Park KK, et al. BK virus infection in renal allograft recipients. Transplant Proc 2003;35:275.

1044. Drachenberg RC, Drachenberg CB, Papadimitriou JC, et al. Morphological spectrum of polyoma virus disease in renal allografts: Diagnostic accuracy of urine cytology. Am J Transplant 2001;1:373.

1045. Nickeleit V, Klimkait T, Binet IF, et al. Testing for polyomavirus type BK DNA in plasma to identify renal-allograft recipients with viral nephropathy. New Engl J Med 2000;342:1309.

1046. Hirsch HH, Drachenberg CB, Steiger J, Ramos E. Polyomavirus associated nephropathy in renal transplantation: Critical issues of screening and management. In: Ahsan N, ed. Polyomaviruses and Human Diseases. New York: Springer Science + Business Media, 2006:160.

1047. Drachenberg RC, Drachenberg CB, Papadimitriou JC, et al. Morphological spectrum of polyoma virus disease in renal allografts: Diagnostic accuracy of urine cytology. Am J Transplant 2001;1:373.

1048. Nickeleit V, Steiger J, Mihatsch MJ. Re: Noninvasive diagnosis of BK virus nephritis by measurement of messenger RNA for BK virus VP1. Transplantation 2003;75:2160.

1049. Singh HK, Bubendorf L, Mihatsch MJ, et al. Urine cytology findings of polyomavirus infections. In: Ahsan N, ed. Polyomaviruses and Human Diseases. New York: Springer Science+Business Media Landes Bioscience, 2006:201.

1050. Singh HK, Madden V, Shen YJ, et al. Negative staining electron microscopy of urine for the detection of polyomavirus infections. Ultrastruct Pathol 2006, in press.

1051. Tong CY, Hilton R, MacMahon EM, et al. Monitoring the progress of BK virus associated nephropathy in renal transplant recipients. Nephrol Dial Transplant 2004;19:2598.

1052. Randhawa P, Ho A, Shapiro R, et al. Correlates of quantitative measurement of BK polyomavirus (BKV) DNA with clinical course of BKV infection in renal transplant patients. J Clin Microbiol 2004;42:1176.

1053. Smith JM, McDonald RA, Finn LS, et al. Polyomavirus nephropathy in pediatric kidney transplant recipients. Am J Transplant 2004;4:2109.

1054. Battegay EJ, Mihatsch MJ, Mazzucchelli L, et al. Cytomegalovirus and kidney. Clin Nephrol 1988;30:239.

1055. Joshi K, Nada R, Radotra BD, et al. Pathological spectrum of cytomegalovirus infection of renal allograft recipients-an autopsy study from north India. Indian J Pathol Microbiol 2004;47:327.

1056. Cozzutto C, Felici N. Unusual glomerular change in cytomegalic inclusion disease. Virchows Arch A Pathol Anat Histol 1974;364:365.

1057. Beneck D, Greco MA, Feiner HD. Glomerulonephritis in congenital cytomegalic inclusion disease. Human Pathol 1986;17:1054.

1058. Onuigbo M, Haririan A, Ramos E, et al. Cytomegalovirus-induced glomerular vasculopathy in renal allografts: A report of two cases. Am J Transplant 2002;2:684.

1059. Detwiler RK, Singh HK, Bolin P Jr, Jennette JC. Cytomegalovirus-induced necrotizing and crescentic glomerulonephritis in a renal transplant patient. Am J Kidney Dis 1998;32:820.

1060. Ulrich W, Schlederer MP, Buxbaum P, et al. The histopathologic identification of CMV infected cells in biopsies of human renal allografts. An evaluation of 100 transplant biopsies by in situ hybridization. Pathol Res Pract 1986;181:739.

1061. Kadereit S, Michelson S, Mougenot B, et al. Polymerase chain reaction detection of cytomegalovirus genome in renal biopsies. Kidney Int 1992;42:1012.

1062. Liapis H, Storch GA, Hill DA, et al. CMV infection of the renal allograft is much more common than the pathology indicates: A retrospective analysis of qualitative and quantitative buffy coat CMV-PCR, renal biopsy pathology and tissue CMV-PCR. Nephrol Dial Transplant 2003;18:397.

1063. Reinke P, Fietze E, Ode-Hakim S, et al. Late-acute renal allograft rejection and symptomless cytomegalovirus infection. Lancet 1994;344:1737.

1064. Emovon OE, Chavin J, Rogers K, Self S. Adenovirus in kidney transplantation: An emerging pathogen? Transplantation 2004;77:1474.

1065. Ito M, Hirabayashi N, Uno Y, et al. Necrotizing tubulointerstitial nephritis associated with adenovirus infection. Hum Pathol 1991;22:1225.

1066. Lim AK, Parsons S, Ierino F. Adenovirus tubulointerstitial nephritis presenting as a renal allograft space occupying lesion. Am J Transplant 2005;5:2062.

1067. Asim M, Chong-Lopez A, Nickeleit V. Adenovirus infection of a renal allograft. Am J Kidney Dis 2003;41:696.

1068. Mathur SC, Squiers EC, Tatum AH, et al. Adenovirus infection of the renal allograft with sparing of pancreas graft function in the recipient of a combined kidney-pancreas transplant. Transplantation 1998;65:138.

1069. Bilic M, Nickeleit V, Howell DN, Self S. Necrotizing granulomatous tubulointerstitial nephritis due to adenovirus infection in the renal allograft: A characteristic morphologic pattern with major clinical implications. Lab Invest 2006;86(Suppl 1):259A.

1070. Nickeleit V. Critical commentary to: Acute adenoviral infection of a graft by serotype 35 following renal transplantation. Pathol Res Pract 2003;199:701.

1071. Singh HK, Nickeleit V. Kidney Disease caused by viral infections. Curr Diag Pathol 2004;10:11.

1072. Emovon OE, Lin A, Howell DN, et al. Refractory adenovirus infection after simultaneous kidney-pancreas transplantation: Successful treatment with intravenous ribavirin and pooled human intravenous immunoglobulin. Nephrol Dial Transplant 2003;18:2436.

1073. Friedrichs N, Eis-Hubinger AM, Heim A, et al. Acute adenoviral infection of a graft by serotype 35 following renal transplantation. Pathol Res Pract 2003;199:565.

1074. Pearson JC, Amend WJ Jr, Vincenti FG, et al. Post-transplantation pyelonephritis: Factors producing low patient and transplant morbidity. J Urology 1980;123:153.

1075. Dunn SP, Vinocur CD, Hanevold C, et al. Pyelonephritis following pediatric renal transplant: Increased incidence with vesicoureteral reflux. J Pediatr Surg 1987;22:1095.

1076. Yang CW, Kim YS, Yang KH, et al. Acute focal bacterial nephritis presented as acute renal failure and hepatic dysfunction in a renal transplant recipient. Am J Nephrol 1994;14:72.

1077. Gillum DM, Kelleher SP. Acute pyelonephritis as a cause of late transplant dysfunction. Am J of Med 1985;78:156.

1078. Hansen BL, Rohr N, Svendsen V, et al. Bacterial urinary tract infection in cyclosporine-A immunosuppressed renal transplant recipients. Scand J Infect Dis 1988;20:425.

1079. Kalra OP, Malik N, Minz M, et al. Emphysematous pyelonephritis and cystitis in a renal transplant recipient—computed tomographic appearance. Int J of Artif Organs 1993;16:41.

1080. Brook I. The role of anaerobic bacteria in perinephric and renal abscesses in children. Pediatrics 1994;93:261.

1081. Aguado JM, Morales JM, Salto E, et al. Encrusted pyelitis and cystitis by *Corynebacterium urealyticum* (CDC group D2): A new and threatening complication following renal transplant. Transplantation 1993;56:617.

1082. Thomalla JV, Gleason P, Leapman SB, Filo RS. Acute lobar nephronia of renal transplant allograft. Urology 1993;41:283.

1083. Hellman RN, Hinrichs J, Sicard G, et al. Cryptococcal pyelonephritis and disseminated cryptococcosis in a renal transplant recipient. Arch Intern Med 1981;141:128.

1084. Gibbs P, Berkley LM, Bolton EM, et al. Adhesion molecule expression (ICAM-1, VCAM-1, E-selectin and PECAM) in human kidney allografts. Transpl Immunol 1993;1:109.

1085. Hakim NS, Benedetti E, Pirenne J, et al. Complications of ureterovesical anastomosis in kidney transplant patients: The Minnesota experience. Clin Transplant 1994;8:504.

1086. Karam G, Maillet F, Parant S, et al. Ureteral necrosis after kidney transplantation: Risk factors and impact on graft and patient survival. Transplantation 2004;78:725.

1087. Jefferson RH, Burns JR. Urological evaluation of adult renal transplant recipients. J Urol 1995;153:615.

1088. Pollak R, Veremis SA, Maddux MS, Mozes MF. The natural history of and therapy for perirenal fluid collections following renal transplantation. J Urol 1988;140:716.

1089. Goel M, Flechner SM, Zhou L, et al. The influence of various maintenance immunosuppressive drugs on lymphocele formation and treatment after kidney transplantation. J Urol 2004;171:1788.

1090. Merion RM, Calne RY. Allograft renal vein thrombosis. Transplant Proc 1985;17:1746.

1091. Arruda JAL, Gutierrez LF, Jonasson O, et al. Renal-vein thrombosis in kidney allografts. Lancet 1973;2:585.

1092. Bakir N, Sluiter WJ, Ploeg RJ, et al. Primary renal graft thrombosis. Nephrol Dial Transplant 1996;11:140.

1093. Osman Y, Shokeir A, Ali-el-Dein B, et al. Vascular complications after live donor renal transplantation: Study of risk factors and effects on graft and patient survival. J Urol 2003;169:859.

1094. Benedetti E, Troppmann C, Gillingham K, et al. Short- and long-term outcomes of kidney transplants with multiple renal arteries. Ann Surg 1995;221:406.

1095. D'Cruz DP. Renal manifestations of the antiphospholipid syndrome. Lupus 2005;14:45.

1096. Simmons RL, Tallent MB, Kjellstrand CM, Najarian JS. Renal allograft rejection simulated by arterial stenosis. Surgery 1970;68:800.

1097. Bruno S, Remuzzi G, Ruggenenti P. Transplant renal artery stenosis. J Am Soc Nephrol 2004;15:134.

1098. Wong W, Fynn SP, Higgins RM, et al. Transplant renal artery stenosis in 77 patients—does it have an immunological cause? Transplantation 1996;61:215.

1099. Said R, Duarte R, Chaballout A, et al. Spontaneous rupture of renal allograft. Urology 1994;43:554.

1100. Heimbach D, Miersch WD, Buszello H, et al. Is the transplant-preserving management of renal allograft rupture justified? Br J Urol 1995;75:729.

1101. Shahrokh H, Rasouli H, Zargar MA, et al. Spontaneous kidney allograft rupture. Transplant Proc 2005;37:3079.

1102. Soler R, Perez-Fontan FJ, Lago M, et al. Renal allograft rupture: Diagnostic role of ultrasound. Nephrol Dial Transplant 1992;7:871.

1103. Chan YH, Wong KM, Lee KC, Li CS. Spontaneous renal allograft rupture attributed to acute tubular necrosis. Am J Kidney Dis 1999;34:355.

1104. Couser W. Recurrent glomerulonephritis in the renal allograft: An update of selected areas. Exp Clin Transplant 2005;3:283.

1105. Charpentier B, Lévy M. Étude coopérative des glomérulonephrites extra-membraneuses de novo sur allogreffe rénale humaine: Rapport de 19 nouveaux cas sur 1550 transplantés rénaux du groupe de transplantation de l'Île de France. Nephrol 1982;3:158.

1106. Berger BE, Vincenti F, Biava C, et al. De novo and recurrent membranous glomerulopathy following kidney transplantation. Transplantation 1983;35:315.

1107. Schwarz A, Krause PH, Offermann G, Keller F. Impact of de novo membranous glomerulonephritis on the clinical course after kidney transplantation. Transplantation 1994;58:650.

1108. Schwarz A, Krause PH, Offermann G, Keller F. Recurrent and de novo renal disease after kidney transplantation with or without cyclosporine A. Am J Kidney Dis 1991;17:524.

1109. Antignac C, Hinglais N, Gubler MC, et al. De novo membranous glomerulonephritis in renal allografts in children. Clin Nephrol 1988;30:1.

1110. Habib R, Antignac C, Hinglais N, et al. Glomerular lesions in the transplanted kidney in children. Am J Kidney Dis 1987;10:198.

1111. Honkanen E, Tornroth T, Pettersson E, Kuhlback B. Glomerulonephritis in renal allografts: Results of 18 years of transplantations. Clin Nephrol 1984;21:210.

1112. Truong L, Gelfand J, D'Agati V, et al. De novo membranous glomerulonephropathy in renal allografts: A report of ten cases and review of the literature. Am J Kidney Dis 1989;14:131.

1113. Cosyns JP, Kazatchkine MD, Bhakdi S, et al. Immunohistochemical analysis of C3 cleavage fragments, factor H, and the C5b-9 terminal complex of complement in de novo membranous glomerulonephritis occurring in patients with renal transplant. Clin Nephrol 1986;26:203.

1114. Monga G, Mazzucco G, Basolo B, et al. Membranous glomerulonephritis (MGN) in transplanted kidneys: Investigation on 256 renal allografts. Mod Pathol 1993;6:249.

1115. Josephson MA, Spargo B, Hollandsworth D, Thistlethwaite JR. The recurrence of recurrent membranous glomerulopathy in a renal transplant recipient: Case report and literature review. Am J Kidney Dis 1994;24:873.

1116. Marcen R, Mampaso F, Teruel JL, et al. Membranous nephropathy: Recurrence after kidney transplantation. Nephrol Dial Transplant 1996;11:1129.

1117. Hariharan S, Adams MB, Brennan DC, et al. Recurrent and de novo glomerular disease after renal transplantation: A report from Renal Allograft Disease Registry (RADR). Transplantation 1999;68:635.

1118. Heidet L, Gagnadoux ME, Beziau A, et al. Recurrence of de novo membranous glomerulonephritis on renal grafts. Clin Nephrol 1994;41:314.

1119. Morales JM, Pascual-Capdevila J, Campistol JM, et al. Membranous glomerulonephritis associated with hepatitis C virus infection in renal transplant patients. Transplantation 1997;63:1634.

1120. Cruzado JM, Carrera M, Torras J, Grinyo JM. Hepatitis C virus infection and de novo glomerular lesions in renal allografts. Am J Transplant 2001;1:171.

1121. Thoenes GH, Pielsticker K, Schubert G. Transplantation-induced immune complex kidney disease in rats with unilateral manifestations in the allografted kidney. Lab Invest 1979;41:321.

1122. Otani M, Shimojo H, Shiozawa S, Shigematsu H. Renal involvement in bone marrow transplantation. Nephrology (Carlton) 2005;10:530.

1123. Stevenson WS, Nankivell BJ, Hertzberg MS. Nephrotic syndrome after stem cell transplantation. Clin Transplant 2005;19:141.

1124. McCoy RC, Johnson HK, Stone WJ, Wilson CB. Absence of nephritogenic GBM antigen(s) in some patients with hereditary nephritis. Kidney Int 1982;21:642.

1125. Kashtan C, Fish AJ, Kleppel M, et al. Nephritogenic antigen determinants in epidermal and renal basement membranes of kindreds with Alport type familial nephritis. J Clin Invest 1986;78:1035.

1126. Fleming SJ, Savage CO, McWilliam LJ, et al. Anti-glomerular basement membrane antibody-mediated nephritis complicating transplantation in a patient with Alport's syndrome. Transplantation 1988;46:857.

1127. Kalluri R, Torre A, Shield CF III, et al. Identification of alpha3, alpha4, and alpha5 chains of type IV collagen as alloantigens for Alport posttransplant anti-glomerular basement membrane antibodies. Transplantation 2000;69:679.

1128. Gobel J, Olbricht CJ, Offner G, et al. Kidney transplantation in Alport's syndrome: Long-term outcome and allograft anti-GBM nephritis. Clin Nephrol 1992;38:299.

1129. Querin S, Noel LH, Grunfeld JP, et al. Linear glomerular IgG fixation in renal allografts: Incidence and significance in Alport's syndrome. Clin Nephrol 1986;25:134.

1130. Nyberg G, Friman S, Svalander C, Norden G. Spectrum of hereditary renal disease in a kidney transplant population. Nephrol Dial Transplant 1995;10:859.

1131. Kashtan CE. Alport syndrome and thin glomerular basement membrane disease. J Am Soc Nephrol 1998;9:1736.

1132. Kashtan CE. Alport syndrome: Renal transplantation and donor selection. Ren Fail 2000;22:765.

1133. Milliner DS, Pierdes AM, Holley KE. Renal transplantation in Alport's syndrome: Anti-glomerular basement membrane glomerulonephritis in the allograft. Mayo Clin. Proc 1982; 57:35.

1134. Vangelista A, Frasca GM, Martella D, Bonomini V. Glomerulonephritis in renal transplantation. Nephrol Dial Transplant 1990;1:42.

1135. Diaz JI, Valenzuela R, Gephardt G, et al. Anti-glomerular and anti-tubular basement membrane nephritis in a renal allograft recipient with Alport's syndrome. Arch Pathol Lab Med 1994;118:728.

1136. Goldman M, Depierreux M, De Pauw L, et al. Failure of two subsequent renal grafts by anti-GBM glomerulonephritis in Alport's syndrome: Case report and review of the literature. Transplant Int 1990;3:82.

1137. Mahan JD, Maver SM, Sibley RK, Vernier RL. Congenital nephrotic syndrome: Evolution of medical management and results of transplantation. J. Pediatr 1984;105:549.

1138. Patrakka J, Ruotsalainen V, Reponen P, et al. Recurrence of nephrotic syndrome in kidney grafts of patients with congenital nephrotic syndrome of the Finnish type: Role of nephrin. Transplantation 2002;73:394.

1139. Lane PH, Schnaper HW, Vernier RL, Bunchman TE. Steroid-dependent nephrotic syndrome following renal transplantation for congenital nephrotic syndrome. Pediatr Nephrol 1991;5:300.

1140. Flynn JT, Schulman SL, deChadarevian JP, et al. Treatment of steroid-resistant post-transplant nephrotic syndrome with cyclophosphamide in a child with congenital nephrotic syndrome. Pediatr Nephrol 1992;6:553.

1141. Bhathena DB. Glomerular size and the association of focal glomerulosclerosis in long-surviving human renal allografts. J Am Soc Nephrol 1993;4:1316.

1142. Neumayer HH, Huls S, Schreiber M, et al. Kidneys from pediatric donors: Risk versus benefit. Clin Nephrol 1994;41:94.

1143. Cameron JS. Recurrent primary disease and de novo nephritis following renal transplantation. Pediatr Nephrol 1991;5:412.

1144. Ramos EL, Tisher CC. Recurrent diseases in the kidney transplant. Am J Kidney Dis 1994;24:142.

1145. Floege J. Recurrent glomerulonephritis following renal transplantation: An update. Nephrol Dial Transplant 2003;18:1260.

1146. Leumann EP, Briner J, Donckerwolcke RA, et al. Recurrence of focal segmental glomerulosclerosis in the transplanted kidney. Acta Pathol Microbiol Immunol Scand 1980;94:69.

1147. Striegel JE, Sibley RK, Fryd DS, Mauer SM. Recurrence of focal segmental sclerosis in children following renal transplantation. Kidney Int Suppl 1986;19:S44.

1148. Zimmerman CE. Renal transplantation for focal segmental glomerulosclerosis. Transplantation 1980;29:172.

1149. O'Meara Y, Green A, Carmody M, et al. Recurrent glomerulonephritis in renal transplants: Fourteen years' experience. Nephrol Dial Transplant 1989;4:730.

1150. Tejani A, Stablein DH. Recurrence of focal segmental glomerulosclerosis posttransplantation: A special report of the North American Pediatric Renal Transplant Cooperative Study. J Am Soc Nephrol 1992;2:S258.

1151. Artero M, Biava C, Amend W, et al. Recurrent focal glomerulosclerosis: Natural history and response to therapy. Am J Med 1992;92:375.

1152. Weber S, Tonshoff B. Recurrence of focal segmental glomerulosclerosis in children after renal transplantation: Clinical and genetic aspects. Transplantation 2005;80(Suppl):S128.

1153. Hosenpud J, Piering WF, Garancis JC, Kauffman HM. Successful second kidney transplantation in a patient with focal glomerulosclerosis: A case report. Am J Nephrol 1985;5:299.

1154. Pinto J, Lacerda G, Cameron JS, et al. Recurrence of focal segmental glomerulosclerosis in renal allografts. Transplantation 1981;32:83.

1155. Broyer M, Gagnadoux MF, Guest G, et al. Kidney transplantation in children: Results of 383 grafts performed at Énfants Malades Hospital from 1973 to 1984. Adv Nephrol 1987;16:307.

1156. Maizel SE, Sibley RK, Horstman JP, et al. Incidence and significance of recurrent focal segmental glomerulosclerosis in renal allograft recipients. Nephron 1981;26:180.

1157. Senggutuvan P, Cameron JS, Hartley RB, et al. Recurrence of focal segmental glomerulosclerosis in transplanted kidneys: Analysis of incidence and risk factors in 59 allografts. Pediatr Nephrol 1990;4:21.

1158. Detwiler RK, Falk RJ, Hogan SL, Jennette JC. Collapsing glomerulopathy: A clinically and pathologically distinct variant of focal segmental glomerulosclerosis. Kidney Int 1994; 45:1416.

1159. Weber S, Tonshoff B. Recurrence of focal-segmental glomerulosclerosis in children after renal transplantation: Clinical and genetic aspects. Transplantation 2005;80:S128.

1160. Schwarz A, Krause PH, Offermann G, Keller F. Recurrent diseases in the renal allograft. J Am Soc Nephrol 1991;2:109.

1161. Schwimmer JA, Markowitz GS, Valeri A, Appel GB. Collapsing glomerulopathy. Semin Nephrol 2003;23:209.

1162. Toth CM, Pascual M, Williams WW Jr, et al. Recurrent collapsing glomerulopathy. Transplantation 1998;65:1009.

1163. Moudgil A, Shidban H, Nast CC, et al. Parvovirus B19 infection-related complications in renal transplant recipients: Treatment with intravenous immunoglobulin. Transplantation 1997;64:1847.

1164. Bhathena DB, Weiss JH, McMorrow RG, Curtis JJ. Focal and segmental glomerular sclerosis in reflux nephropathy. Am J Med 1980;68:886.

1165. Kiprov DD, Colvin RB, McCluskey RT. Focal and segmental glomerulosclerosis and porteinuria associated with unilateral renal agenesis. Lab Invest 1982;46:275.

1166. Axelsen RA, Seymour AE, Mathew TH, et al. Recurrent focal glomerulosclerosis in renal transplants. Clin Nephrol 1984;21:110.

1167. Conlon PJ, Butterly D, Albers F, et al. Clinical and pathologic features of familial focal segmental glomerulosclerosis. Am J Kidney Dis 1995;26:34.

1168. Goodman DJ, Clarke B, Hope RN, et al. Familial focal glomerulosclerosis: A genetic linkage to the HLA locus? Am J Nephrol 1995;15:442.

1169. Verani RR, Hawkins EP. Recurrent focal segmental glomerulosclerosis: A pathological study of the early lesion. Am J Nephrol 1986;6:263.

1170. Harrison DJ, Jenkins D, Dick J. An unusual interpodocyte cell junction and its appearance in a transplant graft kidney. J Clin Pathol 1988;41:155.

1171. Bariety J, Bruneval P, Hill G, et al. Posttransplantation relapse of FSGS is characterized by glomerular epithelial cell transdifferentiation. J Am Soc Nephrol 2001;12:261.

1172. Kemeny E, Mihatsch MJ, Durmuller U, Gudat F. Podocytes loose their adhesive phenotype in focal segmental glomerulosclerosis. Clin Nephrol 1995;43:71.

1173. Cochat P, Kassir A, Colon S, et al. Recurrent nephrotic syndrome after transplantation: Early treatment with plasmaphaeresis and cyclophosphamide. Pediatr Nephrol 1993;7:50.

1174. Torretta L, Perotti C, Costamagna L, et al. Usefulness of plasma exchange in recurrent nephrotic syndrome following renal transplant. Artif Organs 1995;19:96.

1175. Li PK, Lai FM, Leung CB, et al. Plasma exchange in the treatment of early recurrent focal glomerulosclerosis after renal transplantation: Report and review. Am J Nephrol 1993;13:289.

1176. Artero ML, Sharma R, Savin VJ, Vincenti F. Plasmapheresis reduces proteinuria and serum capacity to injure glomeruli in patients with recurrent focal glomerulosclerosis. Am J Kidney Dis 1994;23:574.

1177. Andresdottir MB, Assmann KJ, Hoitsma AJ, et al. Recurrence of type I membranoproliferative glomerulonephritis after renal transplantation: Analysis of the incidence, risk factors, and impact on graft survival. Transplantation 1997;63: 1628.

1178. Morzycka M, Croker BP Jr, Siegler HF, Tisher CC. Evaluation of recurrent glomerulonephritis in kidney allografts. Am J Med 1982;72:588.

1179. Little MA, Dupont P, Campbell E, et al. Severity of primary MPGN, rather than MPGN type, determines renal survival and post-transplantation recurrence risk. Kidney Int 2006;69:504.

1180. Dussol B, Tsimaratos M, Lerda D, et al. Viral hepatitis C and membranoproliferative glomerulonephritis in a renal transplant patient. Nephrologie 1995;16:223.

1181. Croker B, Ramos E. Pathology of the renal allograft. In: Tisher C, Brenner BM, eds. Renal Pathology With Clinical and Functional Correlations, 2nd ed. Philadelphia: JB Lippincott, 1989:1591.

1182. Curtis JJ, Wyatt RJ, Bhathena D, et al. Renal transplantation for patients with type I and type II membranoproliferative glomerulonephritis: Serial complement and nephritic factor measurements and the problem of recurrence of disease. Am J Med 1979;66:216.

1183. Andresdottir MB, Assmann KJ, Hoitsma AJ, et al. Renal transplantation in patients with dense deposit disease: Morphological characteristics of recurrent disease and clinical outcome. Nephrol Dial Transplant 1999;14:1723.

1184. Appel GB, Cook HT, Hageman G, et al. Membranoproliferative glomerulonephritis type II (dense deposit disease): An update. J Am Soc Nephrol 2005;16:1392.

1185. Braun MC, Stablein DM, Hamiwka LA, et al. Recurrence of membranoproliferative glomerulonephritis type II in renal allografts: The North American Pediatric Renal Transplant Cooperative Study experience. J Am Soc Nephrol 2005;16:2225.

1186. Beaufils H, Gubler MC, Karam J, et al. Dense deposit disease: Long term follow-up of three cases of recurrence after transplantation. Clin Nephrol 1977;7:31.

1187. Jansen JH, Hogasen K, Harboe M, Hovig T. In situ complement activation in porcine membranoproliferative glomerulonephritis type II. Kidney Int 1998;53:331.

1188. Droz D, Nabarra B, Noel LH, et al. Recurrence of dense deposits in transplanted kidneys. I. Sequential survey of the lesions. Kidney Int 1979;15:386.

1189. Muller T, Sikora P, Offner G, et al. Recurrence of renal disease after kidney transplantation in children: 24 years of experience in a single center. Clin Nephrol 1998;49:82.

1190. Hebert D, Kim EM, Sibley RK, Mauer MS. Post-transplantation outcome of patients with hemolytic-uremic syndrome: Update. Pediatr Nephrol 1991;5:162.

1191. Eijgenraam FJ, Donckerwolcke RA, Monnens LA, et al. Renal transplantation in 20 children with hemolytic-uremic syndrome. Clin Nephrol 1990;33:87.

1192. Van den Berg-Wolf MG, Kootte AM, Weening JJ, Paul LC. Recurrent hemolytic uremic syndrome in a renal transplant recipient and review of the Leiden experience. Transplantation 1988;45:248.

1193. Chiurchiu C, Ruggenenti P, Remuzzi G. Thrombotic microangiopathy in renal transplantation. Ann Transplant 2002;7:28.

1194. Pham PT, Pham PC, Danovitch GM, et al. Predictors and risk factors for recurrent scleroderma renal crisis in the kidney allograft: Case report and review of the literature. Am J Transplant 2005;5:2565.

1195. Bassani CE, Ferraris J, Gianantonio CA, et al. Renal transplantation in patients with classical haemolytic-uraemic syndrome. Pediatr Nephrol 1991;5:607.

1196. Grino JM, Caralps A, Carreras L, et al. Apparent recurrence of hemolytic uremic syndrome in azathioprine-allograft recipients. Nephron 1988;49:301.

1197. Folman R, Arbus GS, Churchill B, et al. Recurrence of the hemolytic uremic syndrome in a 3 1/2-year-old child, 4 months after second renal transplantation. Clin Nephrol 1978;10:121.

1198. Agarwal A, Mauer SM, Matas AJ, Nath KA. Recurrent hemolytic uremic syndrome in an adult renal allograft recipient: Current concepts and management. J Am Soc Nephrol 1995;6:1160.

1199. Berger J, Noel LH, Nabarra B. Recurrence of mesangial IgA nephropathy after renal transplantation. Contrib Nephrol 1984;40:195.

1200. Bachman U, Biava C, Amend W, et al. The clinical course of IgA-nephropathy and Henoch-Schönlein purpura following renal transplantation. Transplantation 1986;42:511.

1201. Odum J, Peh CA, Clarkson AR, et al. Recurrent mesangial IgA nephritis following renal transplantation. Nephrol Dial Transplant 1994;9:309.

1202. Ponticelli C, Traversi L, Feliciani A, et al. Kidney transplantation in patients with IgA mesangial glomerulonephritis. Kidney Int 2001;60:1948.

1203. Floege J. Recurrent IgA nephropathy after renal transplantation. Semin Nephrol 2004;24:287.

1204. Kessler M, Hiesse C, Hestin D, et al. Recurrence of immunoglobulin A nephropathy after renal transplantation in the cyclosporine era. Am J Kidney Dis 1996;28:99.

1205. Choy BY, Chan TM, Lo SK, et al. Renal transplantation in patients with primary immunoglobulin A nephropathy. Nephrol Dial Transplant 2003;18:2399.

1206. Obermiller LE, Hoy WE, Eversole M, Sterling WA. Recurrent membranous glomerulonephritis in two renal transplants. Transplantation 1985;40:100.

1207. Couchoud C, Pouteil-Noble C, Colon S, Touraine JL. Recurrence of membranous nephropathy after renal transplantation: Incidence and risk factors in 1614 patients. Transplantation 1995;59:1275.

1208. Cameron JS. Glomerulonephritis in renal transplants. Transplantation 1982;34:237.

1209. Lieberthal W, Bernard DB, Donohoe JF, et al. Rapid recurrence of membranous nephropathy in a related allograft. Clin Nephrol 1979;12:222.

1210. Crosson JT, Wathen RL, Raij L, et al. Recurrence of idiopathic membranous nephropathy in a renal allograft. Arch Internl Med 1975;135:1101.

1211. Cosyns JP, Couchoud C, Pouteil-Noble C, et al. Recurrence of membranous nephropathy after renal transplantation: Probability, outcome and risk factors. Clin Nephrol 1998;50:144.

1212. Briggs WA, Johnson JP, Teichman S, et al. Antiglomerular basement membrane antibody mediated glomerulonephritis and Goodpasture's syndrome. Medicine 1979;58:348.

1213. Collins AB, Colvin RB. Kidney and lung disease mediated by glomerular basement membrane antibodies: Detection by western blot analysis. In: Rose NR, de Macario EC, Folds JD, et al, eds. Manual of Clinical Laboratory Methods. Washington, DC: ASM Press, 1997:1008.

1214. Daly C, Conlon PJ, Medwar W, Walshe JJ. Characteristics and outcome of anti-glomerular basement membrane disease: A single-center experience. Ren Fail 1996;18:105.

1215. Deegens JK, Artz MA, Hoitsma AJ, Wetzels JF. Outcome of renal transplantation in patients with pauci-immune small vessel vasculitis or anti-GBM disease. Clin Nephrol 2003;59:1.

1216. Borza DB, Chedid MF, Colon S, et al. Recurrent Goodpasture's disease secondary to a monoclonal IgA1-kappa antibody autoreactive with the alpha1/alpha2 chains of type IV collagen. Am J Kidney Dis 2005;45:397.

1217. Trpkov K, Abdulkareem F, Jim K, Solez K. Recurrence of anti-GBM antibody disease twelve years after transplantation associated with de novo IgA nephropathy. Clin Nephrol 1998;49:124.

1218. Odorico JS, Knechtle SJ, Rayhill SC, et al. The influence of native nephrectomy on the incidence of recurrent disease following renal transplantation for primary glomerulonephritis. Transplantation 1996;61:228.

1219. Nachman PH, Segelmark M, Westman K, et al. Recurrent ANCA-associated small vessel vasculitis after transplantation: A pooled analysis. Kidney Int 1999;56:1544.

1220. Kuross S, Davin T, Kjellstrand CM. Wegener's granulomatosis with severe renal failure: Clinical course and results of dialysis and transplantation. Clin Nephrol 1981;16:172.

1221. Rostaing L, Modesto A, Oksman F, et al. Outcome of patients with antineutrophil cytoplasmic autoantibody-associated vasculitis following cadaveric kidney transplantation. Am J Kidney Dis 1997;29:96.

1222. Nyberg G, Åkesson P, Nordén G, Weislander J. Systemic vasculitis in a kidney transplant population. Transplantation 1997;63:1273.

1223. van der Woude FJ. Kidney transplantation and ANCA-associated vasculitis. Cleve Clin J Med 2002;69(Suppl 2):SII143.

1224. Reaich D, Cooper N, Main J. Rapid catastrophic onset of Wegener's granulomatosis in a renal transplant. Nephron 1994;67:354.

1225. Elmedhem A, Adu D, Savage CO. Relapse rate and outcome of ANCA-associated small vessel vasculitis after transplantation. Nephrol Dial Transplant 2003;18:1001.

1226. Boubenider SA, Akhtar M, Alfurayh O, et al. Late recurrence of Wegener's granulomatosis presenting as tracheal stenosis in a renal transplant patient. Clin Transplant 1994;8:5.

1227. Le Mao G, Rostaing L, Modesto A, et al. Recurrence of ANCA-associated microscopic polyangiitis after cadaveric renal transplant. Transplant Proc 1996;28:2803.

1228. Lobbedez T, Comoz F, Renaudineau E, et al. Recurrence of ANCA-positive glomerulonephritis immediately after renal transplantation. Am J Kidney Dis 2003;42:E2.

1229. Azevedo LS, Romao JE Jr, Malheiros D, et al. Renal transplantation in systemic lupus erythematosus: A case control study of 45 patients. Nephrol Dial Transplant 1998;13:2894.

1230. Mojcik CF, Klippel JH. End-stage renal disease and systemic lupus erythematosus. Am J Med 1996;101:100.

1231. Ramos EL. Recurrent diseases in the renal allograft. J Am Soc Nephrol 1991;2:109.

1232. Goral S, Ynares C, Shappell SB, et al. Recurrent lupus nephritis in renal transplant recipients revisited: It is not rare. Transplantation 2003;75:651.

1233. Moroni G, Tantardini F, Gallelli B, et al. The long-term prognosis of renal transplantation in patients with lupus nephritis. Am J Kidney Dis 2005;45:903.

1234. Mejia G, Zimmerman SW, Glass NR, et al. Renal transplantation in patients with systemic lupus erythematosus. Arch Intern Med 1983;143:2089.

1235. Rivera M, Marcen R, Pascual J, et al. Kidney transplantation in systemic lupus erythematosus nephritis: A one-center experience. Nephron 1990;56:148.

1236. Bumgardner GL, Mauer SM, Payne W, et al. Single-center 1-15-year results of renal transplantation in patients with systemic lupus erythematosus. Transplantation 1988;46:703.

1237. Ponticelli C, Moroni G. Renal transplantation in lupus nephritis. Lupus 2005;14:95.

1238. Ward MM. Outcomes of renal transplantation among patients with end-stage renal disease caused by lupus nephritis. Kidney Int 2000;57:2136.

1239. Jha V, Sakhuja V, Vaiphei K, et al. An unusual case of recurrence of AA amyloidosis in the renal allograft. Ren Fail 2004;26:89.

1240. Pasternack A, Ahonen J, Kuhlback B. Renal transplantation in 45 patients with amyloidosis. Transplantation 1986;42:598.

1241. Ozdemir BH, Ozdemir FN, Demirhan B, et al. Renal transplantation in amyloidosis: Effects of HLA matching and donor type on recurrence of primary disease. Transpl Int 2004;17:241.

1242. Hartmann A, Holdaas H, Fauchald P, et al. Fifteen years' experience with renal transplantation in systemic amyloidosis. Transpl Int 1992;5:15.

1243. Isoniemi H, Kyllonen L, Ahonen J, et al. Improved outcome of renal transplantation in amyloidosis. Transpl Int 1994;7(Suppl 1):S298.

1244. Heering P, Kutkuhn B, Frenzel H, et al. Renal transplantation in amyloid nephropathy. Int Urol Nephrol 1989;21:339.

1245. Nishikido M, Koga S, Kanetake H, et al. Renal transplantation in systemic amyloidosis. Clin Transplant 1999;13(Suppl 1):63.

1246. Giraud P, Adoue D, Durand D, et al. Kidney allograft in familial Mediterranean fever a case report and review of the literature [in French]. Annales de Medecine Interne 1981;132:507.

1247. Pras M, Gafni J, Jacob ET, et al. Recent advances in familial Mediterranean fever. Adv Nephrol 1984;13:261.

1248. Sherif AM, Refaie AF, Sobh MA, et al. Long-term outcome of live donor kidney transplantation for renal amyloidosis. Am J Kidney Dis 2003;42:370.

1249. Leung N, Lager DJ, Gertz MA, et al. Long-term outcome of renal transplantation in light-chain deposition disease. Am J Kidney Dis 2004;43:147.

1250. Carles X, Rostaing L, Modesto A, et al. Successful treatment of recurrence of immunotactoid glomerulopathy in a kidney allograft recipient. Nephrol Dial Transplant 2000;15:897.

1251. Pronovost PH, Brady HR, Gunning ME, et al. Clinical features, predictors of disease progression and results of renal transplantation in fibrillary/immunotactoid glomerulopathy. Nephrol Dial Transplant 1996;11:837.

1252. Samaniego M, Nadasdy GM, Laszik Z, Nadasdy T. Outcome of renal transplantation in fibrillary glomerulonephritis. Clin Nephrol 2001;55:159.

1253. Brady HR. Fibrillary glomerulopathy. Kidney Int 1998;53:1421.

1254. Kim H, Cheigh JS. Kidney transplantation in patients with type 1 diabetes mellitus: Long-term prognosis for patients and grafts. Korean J Intern Med 2001;16:98.

1255. Hariharan S, Smith RD, Viero R, First MR. Diabetic nephropathy after renal transplantation. Clinical and pathologic features. Transplantation 1996;62:632.

1256. Maryniak RK, Mendoza N, Clyne D, et al. Recurrence of diabetic nodular glomerulosclerosis in a renal transplant. Kidney Int 1985;27:799.

1257. Mauer SM, Barbosa J, Vernier RL, et al. Development of diabetic vascular lesions in normal kidneys transplanted into patients with diabetes mellitus. New Engl J Med 1976;295:916.

1258. Ianhez LE, Saldanha LB, Arap S, Sabbaga E. Renal biopsy in thirty-one kidney transplant recipients with more than ten years of follow-up. Transplant Proc 1989;21:2187.

1259. Shaffer D, Simpson MA, Madras PN, et al. Kidney transplantation in diabetic patients using cyclosporine. Five-year follow-up. Arch Surg 1995;130:283.

1260. Sterby R, Nyberg G, Karlberg I, Svalander C. Glomerular volume in kidneys transplanted into diabetic and non-diabetic patients. Diabet Med 1992;9:144.

1261. Wilczek HE, Jaremko G, Tyden G, Groth CG. Evolution of diabetic nephropathy in kidney grafts. Evidence that a simultaneously transplanted kidney exerts a protective effect. Transplantation 1995;59:51.

1262. Bohman SO, Tyden G, Wilczek H, et al. Prevention of kidney graft diabetic nephropathy by pancreas transplantation in man. Diabetes 1985;34:306.

1263. Fioretto P, Mauer SM, Bilous RW, et al. Effects of pancreas transplantation on glomerular structure in insulin-dependent diabetic patients with their own kidneys. Lancet 1993;342:1193.

1264. Abouna GM, Al Adnani MS, Kremer GD, et al. Reversal of diabetic nephropathy in human cadaveric kidneys after transplantation into non-diabetic recipients. Lancet 1983;2:1274.

1265. Najarian JS, Frey DJ, Matas AJ, et al. Renal transplantation in infants. Ann Surg 1990;212:353.

1266. Whelchel JD, Alison DV, Luke RG, et al. Successful renal transplantation in hyperoxaluria. A report of two cases. Transplantation 1983;35:161.

1267. Scheinman JI, Najarian JS, Mauer SM. Successful strategies for renal transplantation in primary oxalosis. Kidney Int 1984;25:804.

1268. Broyer M, Jouvet P, Niaudet P, et al. Management of oxalosis. Kidney Int 1886;53:S93.

1269. Lieske JC, Spargo BH, Toback FG. Endocytosis of calcium oxalate crystals and proliferation of renal tubular epithelial cells in a patient with type 1 primary hyperoxaluria. J Urol 1992;148:1517.

1270. Toussaint C, Vienne A, De Pauw L, et al. Combined liver-kidney transplantation in primary hyperoxaluria type 1: Histopathology and oxalate body content. Transplantation 1995;59:1700.

1271. Allen AR, Thompson EM, Williams G, et al. Selective renal transplantation in primary hyperoxaluria type 1. Am J Kidney Dis 1996;27:891.

1272. Latta A, Muller-Wiefel DE, Sturm E, et al. Transplantation procedures in primary hyperoxaluria type 1. Clin Nephrol 1996;46:21.

1273. Cibrik DM, Kaplan B, Arndorfer JA, Meier-Kriesche HU. Renal allograft survival in patients with oxalosis. Transplantation 2002;74:707.

1274. Millan MT, Berquist WE, So SK, et al. One hundred percent patient and kidney allograft survival with simultaneous liver and kidney transplantation in infants with primary hyperoxaluria: A single-center experience. Transplantation 2003;76:1458.

1275. Detry O, Honore P, DeRoover A, et al. Reversal of oxalosis cardiomyopathy after combined liver and kidney transplantation. Transpl Int 2002;15:50.

1276. Friedlander MM, Kopolovic J, Rubinger D, et al. Renal biopsy in Fabry's disease eight years after successful renal transplantation. Clin Nephrol 1987;27:206.

1277. Faraggiana T, Churg J, Grishman E, et al. Light- and electron-microscopic histochemistry of Fabry's disease. Am J Pathol 1981;103:247.

1278. Mosnier JF, Degott C, Bedrossian J, et al. Recurrence of Fabry's disease in a renal allograft eleven years after successful renal transplantation. Transplantation 1991;51:759.

1279. Popli S, Molnar ZV, Leehey DJ, et al. Involvement of renal allograft by Fabry's disease. Am J Nephrol 1987;7:316.

1280. Grünfeld JP, le Porrier M, Droz D, et al. La transplantation rénale chez le sujets atteints de maladie de Fabry: Transplantation du rein d'un suject hétérozygote à un sujet sain. Nouv Presse Med 1975;4:2081.

1281. Van Loo A, Vanholder R, Madsen K, et al. Novel frameshift mutation in a heterozygous woman with Fabry disease and end-stage renal failure. Am J Nephrol 1996;16:352.

1282. Bannwart F. Morbus Fabry: Licht und elektronenmikroskopischerherzbefund 12 Jahre nach erfolgreicher neirentransplantation. Schweiz Med Wochenschr 1982;112:1742.

1283. Thurberg BL, Rennke H, Colvin RB, et al. Globotriaosylceramide accumulation in the Fabry kidney is cleared from multiple cell types after enzyme replacement therapy. Kidney Int 2002;62:1933.

1284. Gagné ER, Deland E, Daudon M, et al. Chronic renal failure secondary to 2,8-dihydroxyadenine deposition: The first report of recurrence in a kidney transplant. Am J Kidney Dis 1994;24:104.

1285. Schneider JA. Therapy of cystinosis. N Engl J Med 1985;313:1472.

1286. Spear GS, Gubler MC, Habib R, Broyer M. Dark cells of cystinosis: Occurrence in renal allografts. Hum Pathol 1989;20:472.

1287. Bogan ML, Kopecky KK, Kraft JL, et al. Renal allografts in cystinosis and mesangial demography. Clin Nephrol 1989;32:256.

1288. Uranga VM, Simmons RL, Hoyer JR, et al. Renal transplantation for the nail patella syndrome. Am J Surg 1973;125:777.

1289. Chan PC, Chan KW, Cheng IK, Chan MK. Living-related renal transplantation in a patient with nail-patella syndrome. Nephron 1988;50:164.

1290. Djamali A, Cristol JP, Turc-Baron C, et al. Lipoprotein glomerulopathy: A new French case with recurrence on the transplant [in French]. Presse Med 1996;25:798.

1291. Miner DJ, Jorkasky DK, Perloff LJ, et al. Recurrent sickle cell nephropathy in a transplanted kidney. Am J Kidney Dis 1987;10:306.

1292. Barber WH, Deierhoi MH, Julian BA, et al. Renal transplantation in sickle cell anemia and sickle disease. Clin Transplantation 1987;1:169.

1293. Zeier M, Hartschuh W, Wiesel M, et al. Malignancy after renal transplantation. Am J Kidney Dis 2002;39:E5.

1294. Birkeland SA, Lokkegaard H, Storm HH. Cancer risk in patients on dialysis and after renal transplantation. Lancet 2000;355:1886.

1295. Penn I. The changing pattern of posttransplant malignancies. Transplant Proc 1991;23:1101.

1296. Neuzillet Y, Lay F, Luccioni A, et al. De novo renal cell carcinoma of native kidney in renal transplant recipients. Cancer 2005;103:251.

1297. Harris NL, Swerdlow SH, Frizzera G, Knowles DM. Posttransplant lymphoproliferative disorders. In: Jaffe ES, Harris NL, Stein H, Vardiman JW, eds. Pathology and Genetics of Tumours of Haematopoietic and Lymphoid Tissues. Lyon, France: IARC Press, 2001:264.

1298. Caillard S, Dharnidharka V, Agodoa L, et al. Posttransplant lymphoproliferative disorders after renal transplantation in the United States in era of modern immunosuppression. Transplantation 2005;80:1233.

1299. Shapiro R, Nalesnik M, McCauley J, et al. Posttransplant lymphoproliferative disorders in adult and pediatric renal transplant patients receiving tacrolimus-based immunosuppression. Transplantation 1999;68:1851.

1300. Doak PB, Montgomerie JZ, North JDK, Smith F. Reticulum cell sarcoma after renal homotransplantation and azathioprine and prednisone therapy. Br Med J 1968;4:746.

1301. Cockfield SM, Preiksaitis JK, Jewell LD, Parfrey NA. Posttransplant lymphoproliferative disorder in renal allograft recipients. Clinical experience and risk factor analysis in a single center. Transplantation 1993;56:88.

1302. Citterio F, Lauriola L, Nanni G, et al. Polyclonal lymphoma confined to renal allograft: Case report. Transplant Proc 1987;19:3732.

1303. Jones C, Bleau B, Buskard N, et al. Simultaneous development of diffuse immunoblastic lymphoma in recipients of renal transplants from a single cadaver donor: Transmission of Epstein-Barr virus and triggering by OKT3. Am J Kidney Dis 1994;23:130.

1304. Denning DW, Weiss LM, Martinez K, Flechner SM. Transmission of Epstein-Barr virus by a transplanted kidney, with activation by OKT3 antibody. Transplantation 1989;48:141.

1305. Nádasdy T, Park CS, Peiper SC, et al. Epstein-Barr virus infection-associated renal disease: Diagnostic use of molecular hybridization technology in patients with negative serology. J Am Soc Nephrol 1992;2:1734.

1306. Weissman DJ, Ferry JA, Harris NL, et al. Posttransplant lymphoproliferative disorders in solid organ recipients are predominately aggressive tumors of host origin. Am J Clin Pathol 1995;103:748.

1307. Delecluse H-J, Kremmer E, Rouault J-P, et al. The expression of Epstein-Barr virus latent proteins is related to the pathological features of post-transplant lymphoproliferative disorders. Am J Pathol 1995;146:1113.

1308. Thomas JA, Hotchin NA, Allday MJ, et al. Immunohistology of Epstein-Barr virus-associated antigens in B-cell disorders from immunocompromised individuals. Transplantation 1990;49:944.

1309. Renoult E, Aymard B, Gregoire MJ, et al. Epstein-Barr virus lymphoproliferative disease of donor origin after kidney transplantation: A case report. Am J Kidney Dis 1995;26: 84.

1310. Hjelle B, Evans HM, Yen TS, et al. A poorly differentiated lymphoma of donor origin in a renal allograft recipient. Transplantation 1989;47:945.

1311. Ulrich W, Chott A, Watschinger B, et al. Primary peripheral T-cell lymphoma in a kidney transplant under immunosuppression with cyclosporine A. Hum Pathol 1989;20:1027.

1312. Meduri G, Fromentin L, Vieillefond A, Fries D. Donor-related non-Hodgkin's lymphoma in a renal allograft recipient. Transplant Proc 1991;23:2649.

1313. Koike J, Yamaguchi Y, Hoshikawa M, et al. Post-transplant lymphoproliferative disorders in kidney transplantation: Histological and molecular genetic assessment. Clin Transplant 2002;16(Suppl 8):12.

1314. Mueller-Hermelink HK, Ott G, Kneitz B, Ruediger T. The spectrum of lymphoproliferations and malignant lymphoma after organ transplantation. In: Kreipe HH, ed. Verhandlungen der Deutschen Gesellschaft fuer Pathologie, 88. Tagung. Muenchen Jena: Urban & Fischer, 2004:63.

1315. Opelz G, Henderson R. Incidence of non-Hodgkins lymphoma in kidney and heart transplant recipients. Lancet 1993;342:1514.

1316. Lager DJ, Burgart LJ, Slagel DD. Epstein-Barr virus detection in sequential biopsies from patients with a posttransplant lymphoproliferative disorder. Mod Pathol 1993;6:42.

1317. O'Brien S, Bernert RA, Logan JL, Lien YH. Remission of post-transplant lymphoproliferative disorder after interferon alfa therapy. J Am Soc Nephrol 1997;8:1483.

1318. Senel MF, Van BCT, Riggs S, et al. Post-transplantation lymphoproliferative disorder in the renal transplant ureter. J Urol 1996;155:2025.

1319. Delbello MW, Dick WH, Carter CB, Butler FO. Polyclonal B-cell lymphoma of renal transplant ureter induced by cyclosporine: Case report. J Urol 1991;146:1613.

1320. Oertel SH, Verschuuren E, Reinke P, et al. Effect of anti-CD 20 antibody rituximab in patients with post-transplant lymphoproliferative disorder (PTLD). Am J Transplant 2005;5: 2901.

1321. Tinckam KJ, Djurdjev O, Magil AB. Glomerular monocytes predict worse outcomes after acute renal allograft rejection independent of C4d status. Kidney Int 2005;68:1866.

1322. Feucht HE, Schneeberger H, Hillebrand G, et al. Capillary deposition of C4d complement fragment and early renal graft loss. Kidney Int 1993;43:1333.

1323. Pins MR, Saidman S, Cosimi AB, et al. Accelerated acute rejection of an apparent $A_2$ renal allograft in an O recipient. Transplantation 1997;63:984.

1324. Mold C, Gewurz H, Du Clos TW. Regulation of complement activation by C-reactive protein. Immunopharmacology 1999;42:23.

# Renal Neoplasms

**29**

*David J. Grignon    John N. Eble*

A diverse array of tumors can arise in the human kidney. In this chapter, these will be covered using an approach that has become a standard one in dealing with this group of tumors. This is highlighted by the World Health Organization (WHO) classification of these tumors, as detailed in Table 29.1 (1). The first section will cover those tumors that characteristically are associated with the pediatric pop-ulation. This is a somewhat arbitrary designation, as most tumors can develop over a wide age range. This is followed by coverage of neoplasms in the more traditional categories of epithelial, mesenchymal, and other categories. Specific discussions of etiology and pathogenesis are dealt with in each of the sections on individual tumors, rather than as a freestanding section, as is used elsewhere in this text. The purpose of this chapter is to familiarize the reader with the tumor types encountered in the human rather than to provide a comprehensive diagnostic reference, which is better handled in more comprehensive textbooks and monographs.

## PEDIATRIC NEOPLASMS

### Wilms' Tumor

#### Clinical Findings and Epidemiology

More than 80% of renal tumors of childhood are Wilms' tumor (nephroblastoma) (1). Neonatal Wilms' tumor is rare (2). Most Wilms' tumor occurs in children between the ages of 2 and 4 years (3). It is uncommon in the first 6 months of life and after 6 years of age (4). It is slightly more common in girls than in boys (3). It is bilateral in about 5% of cases (5). Wilms' tumor may be associated with hemihypertrophy and aniridia, and with genital anomalies, such as cryptorchidism and hypospadias (6). Patients with Beckwith-Wiedemann syndrome and Drash syndrome have an increased risk of developing Wilms' tumor (7,8). Wilms' tumor is rare in adults (9,10). Wilms' tumor is believed to arise from embryonic tissues called *nephrogenic rests* that fail to undergo normal involution (11).

#### Pathology

##### Gross

Wilms' tumor often is greater than 5 cm in diameter, and more than 30% are larger than 10 cm (4). The cut surface is typically solid, soft, and gray or pink, with a texture and appearance resembling brain tissue. The tumor is usually circumscribed by a pseudocapsule formed of compressed renal and perirenal tissues. Cysts are common, as are foci of hemorrhage and necrosis (Fig. 29.1). Predominantly cystic Wilms' tumor that contains blastema and other Wilms' tumor tissues in its septa is called *cystic partially differentiated nephroblastoma* (12,13).

##### Microscopic

Although Wilms' tumor is typically composed of a mixture of blastema, epithelium, and stroma, sometimes one or two of these components are absent (Fig. 29.2) (14). Blastema consists of densely packed small cells randomly arranged in sheets. Blastemal cells have dense nuclei, frequent

## TABLE 29.1
### 2004 WHO CLASSIFICATION OF RENAL TUMORS

**Renal Cell Tumors**
Clear cell renal cell carcinoma
Multilocular clear cell renal cell carcinoma
Papillary renal cell carcinoma
Chromophobe renal cell carcinoma
Carcinoma of the collecting ducts of Bellini
Renal medullary carcinoma
Xp11 translocation carcinomas
Carcinoma associated with neuroblastoma
Mucinous tubular and spindle cell carcinoma
Renal cell carcinoma, unclassified
Papillary adenoma
Oncocytoma

**Metanephric tumors**
Metanephric adenoma
Metanephric adenofibroma
Metanephric stromal tumor

**Nephroblastic tumors**
Nephrogenic rests
Nephroblastoma
Cystic partially differentiated nephroblastoma

**Mesenchymal tumors**
Occurring mainly in children
Clear cell sarcoma
Rhabdoid tumor
Congenital mesoblastic nephroma
Ossifying renal tumor of infants
Occurring mainly in adults
Leiomyosarcoma (including renal vein)
Angiosarcoma
Rhabdomyosarcoma

Malignant fibrous histiocytoma
Hemangiopericytoma
Osteosarcoma
Angiomyolipoma
Epithelioid angiomyolipoma
Leiomyoma
Hemangioma
Lymphangioma
Juxtaglomerular cell tumor
Renomedullary interstitial cell tumor
Schwannoma
Solitary fibrous tumor

**Mixed mesenchymal and epithelial tumors**
Cystic nephroma
Mixed epithelial and stromal tumor
Synovial sarcoma

**Neuroendocrine tumors**
Carcinoid
Neuroendocrine carcinoma
Primitive neuroectodermal tumor
Neuroblastoma
Pheochromocytoma

**Hematopoietic and lymphoid tumors**
Lymphoma
Leukemia
Plasmacytoma

**Germ cell tumors**
Teratoma
Choriocarcinoma
**Metastatic tumors**

mitotic figures, and inconspicuous cytoplasm. Aggregates of blastema commonly form serpentine, nodular, and diffuse patterns that have sharp borders with the stromal component.

The epithelium of Wilms' tumor usually consists of small tubules or cysts lined by columnar or cuboidal cells. Occasionally, it forms structures resembling glomeruli or has mucinous, squamous, neural (15), or endocrine (16,17) differentiation (18).

The stroma of Wilms' tumor is variable and may differentiate toward almost any type of soft tissue. Nondescript myxoid and fibroblastic spindle cell stroma is most common, but smooth muscle, skeletal muscle, fat, cartilage, and bone are present in some tumors (18). When diffuse differentiation toward skeletal muscle occurs, the term *fetal rhabdomyomatous nephroblastoma* is applied (19,20). Complex combinations of differentiated epithelium and stroma are sometimes present. The term *teratoid Wilms' tumor* has been applied to these (21,22).

## Treatment and Outcome

The progress in the treatment of Wilms' tumor is one of the great success stories of oncology. Most cases are treated with surgery and dactinomycin and vinblastine chemotherapy with relatively low toxicity (23). Mortality declined approximately 10% per decade throughout the past century. This is owing in large part to the efforts of the National Wilms' Tumor Study (NWTS). From the results of the NWTS, Wilms' tumor has been classified as having either favorable or unfavorable histology, depending on whether or not anaplasia is present. In Wilms' tumor, anaplasia is defined as the combination of cells with enlarged hyperchromatic nuclei (at least three times as large as typical blastemal nuclei in both axes and having obvious hyperchromasia) and multipolar mitotic figures (Fig. 29.3). Recognition of anaplasia requires proper fixation, sectioning, and staining. The criteria for abnormal hyperdiploid mitotic figures are stringent; not only must there be structural abnormalities, but

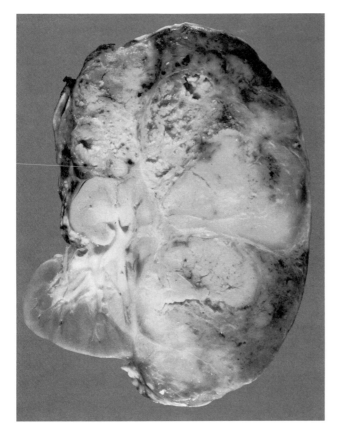

**Figure 29.1** Wilms' tumor. Typical gross appearance of Wilms' tumor with large, bulging variegated mass showing areas of necrosis and hemorrhage.

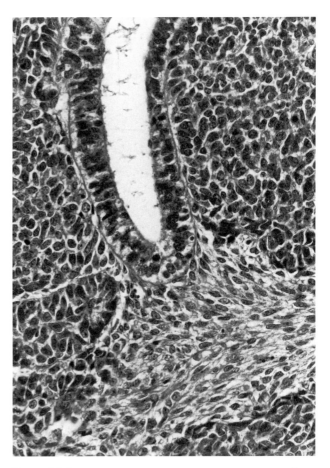

**Figure 29.2** Wilms' tumor. Typical triphasic histology with epithelial, blastemal, and mesenchymal elements. In this case, the mesenchymal component is primitive and undifferentiated.

the mitotic figure must also be enlarged as evidence of hyperploidy. Enlarged nuclei in skeletal muscle fibers in the stroma of Wilms' tumor are not evidence of anaplasia. Approximately 6% of Wilms' tumors contain anaplasia, mostly in patients older than 2 years (24). Anaplasia is not a marker of greater inherent aggressiveness; rather, it indicates a high likelihood of resistance to treatment with chemotherapy and radiation (25). The staging scheme for Wilms' tumor and other pediatric renal malignancies differs somewhat from that used for renal cell carcinoma (26).

## Congenital Mesoblastic Nephroma

### Clinical Findings and Epidemiology

Congenital mesoblastic nephroma makes up less than 3% of renal neoplasms in children; it is the predominant renal neoplasm in the first 3 months of life and is uncommon after 6 months (2,27). The births of patients with congenital mesoblastic nephroma often are complicated by polyhydramnios and prematurity (28,29). The presenting finding is almost always an abdominal mass. Congenital mesoblastic nephroma was first recognized in 1966 (30),

and subsequent studies (31) have shown it to be a morphologically distinct tumor with a good prognosis. Congenital mesoblastic nephroma has genetic similarities to infantile fibrosarcoma. (32–34).

## Pathology

### Gross

Congenital mesoblastic nephroma is usually large relative to the infant's kidney. The external surfaces of the tumor and kidney are smooth, and the renal capsule and renal pelvis and caliceal system are stretched over the tumor. Congenital mesoblastic nephroma may be spherical or bosselated. The cut surface resembles leiomyoma: firm, whorled or trabeculated, and pale (35). There is no true capsule. The tumor usually mingles with the surrounding kidney and may extend into perinephric soft tissue. Invasion of the renal vein occurs occasionally (35). Cysts, necrosis, and hemorrhage may be found occasionally, particularly in cases that are cellular on microscopic examination (35).

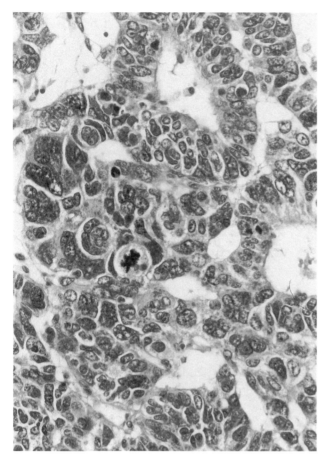

**Figure 29.3** Wilms' tumor. Focus of anaplasia in a Wilms' tumor with nucleomegaly, hyperchromasia, and multipolar mitotic figure.

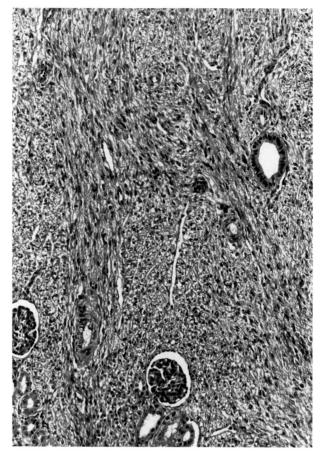

**Figure 29.4** Congenital mesoblastic nephroma. The tumor is composed of bland, spindle-shaped cells growing in an infiltrative manner; note the invasion between two glomeruli.

## Microscopic

Bolande (31) described the classic pattern of congenital mesoblastic nephroma: a moderately cellular neoplasm composed of interlacing bundles of spindle cells with elongate nuclei, usually infiltrating renal and perinephric tissues (Fig. 29.4). In the classic pattern, there is usually either none or one mitotic figure per 10 high-power fields (35). Some tumors contain small islands of cartilage or foci of extramedullary hematopoiesis.

Later, a second, more common, pattern was recognized. This pattern is densely cellular and composed of polygonal cells. Mitotic figures are present in the range of 8 to 30 per 10 high-power fields. Cysts are common in this pattern. Rather than being infiltrative, the borders usually are "pushing." This pattern is called *cellular congenital mesoblastic nephroma* (36). Often both the classic and cellular patterns are mixed in the same tumor.

Congenital mesoblastic nephroma is usually not difficult to diagnose when age and histology are considered. The major differential diagnostic consideration is Wilms' tumor with stromal predominance, especially if it has been treated preoperatively with chemother-

apy. Identification of blastema, which does not occur in mesoblastic nephroma, usually resolves the issue. Also, the sharply circumscribed borders of Wilms' tumor contrast with the infiltrative borders of mesoblastic nephroma.

## Treatment and Outcome

Almost all are cured by surgical resection (37–39). Recurrence and adverse outcome are rare and have mainly occurred in patients older than 3 months when the tumor was discovered (40,41). Congenital mesoblastic nephroma has infiltrative borders that the surgical pathologist must carefully study because recurrence may occur if resection is incomplete (42,43). Metastasis is exceptional (44). It has been suggested that the cellular pattern is prone to recur. Because it is the more common pattern and the great majority of patients are cured, any such tendency must be small, and age and completeness of resection are the prime risk factors.

## Clear Cell Sarcoma

### Clinical Findings and Epidemiology

Clear cell sarcoma occurs in the same age range as Wilms' tumor and makes up approximately 6% of renal neoplasms in children (45). Most patients are between 1 and 3 years old, and about two thirds are male. Clear cell sarcoma is invariably unilateral (1).

### Pathology

#### Gross
Clear cell sarcoma usually is large, well circumscribed, and often weighs more than 500 g (46). The cut surfaces of clear cell sarcoma have a variable appearance: Some are homogeneous, gray, and lobular; others are variegated and composed of firm gray whorled tissue with light pink soft areas (46). In some, an abundance of mucin imparts a glistening slimy appearance. Approximately 33% of tumors have cysts ranging from a few millimeters to centimeters in diameter (46).

#### Microscopic
The typical appearance of clear cell sarcoma at low magnification is of a monotonous sheet of cells with pale cytoplasm. At higher magnification, the cells are recognized to be organized in cords separated by branching septa composed of spindle cells with dark nuclei and of small blood vessels (47). The cells of the cords have pale cytoplasm with small vacuoles and indistinct cytoplasmic membranes (Fig. 29.5). Although the cytoplasm of clear cell sarcoma is pale, it usually is not clear in the same way as that of clear cell renal cell carcinoma, and clarity of cytoplasm is not key to making the diagnosis. Nuclear features are key to the diagnosis. The chromatin is finely dispersed and the nucleoli are small. This differs from the dark nuclei of blastema in Wilms' tumor and the prominent nucleoli typical of rhabdoid tumor. Another helpful feature is the infiltrative border in which renal tubules are frequently surrounded by sarcoma; this contrasts with the circumscribed border typical of Wilms' tumor (46). Confusing variations on the classic pattern occur—including spindle cell, cystic, hyaline sclerosis, and palisading (18). In such cases, generous sampling often reveals areas in which the pattern of cords and septa indicates the correct diagnosis. Other helpful points that distinguish clear cell sarcoma of kidney from Wilms' tumor include the following: blastema does not occur in clear cell sarcoma, heterologous elements such as cartilage or muscle do not occur in clear cell sarcoma, clear cell sarcoma is neither multicentric nor bilateral, and sclerotic stroma is uncommon in Wilms' tumor before therapy. Rarely, clear cell sarcoma contains foci in which the cells have prominent nucleoli, resembling those of rhabdoid tumor of kidney;

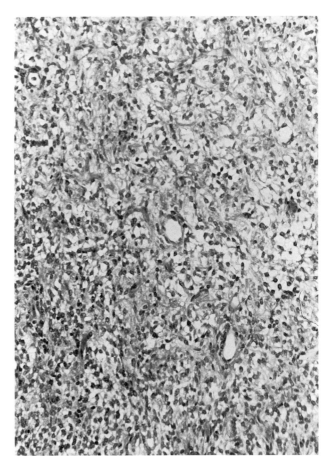

**Figure 29.5** Clear cell sarcoma. The tumor is composed of small, uniform spindle cells with scant clear cytoplasm growing in fascicles.

in other areas patterns typical of clear cell sarcoma often clarify the diagnosis.

### Treatment and Outcome

Clear cell sarcoma is highly malignant and at least 10 times as likely to metastasize to bone as any other pediatric renal cancer. It was originally called *bone-metastasizing renal tumor of childhood* by Marsden and Lawler (48). It is resistant to conventional therapy for Wilms' tumor, but survival under chemotherapy with doxorubicin is 60% to 70%, which makes the correct diagnosis clinically important (49).

## Rhabdoid Tumor of Kidney

### Clinical Findings and Epidemiology

Rhabdoid tumor is the most aggressive renal neoplasm of childhood and usually metastasizes widely to cause death within a year of the time of diagnosis (50). The NWTS median age at diagnosis is 11 months, and few rhabdoid tumors occur after 3 years. Boys predominate over girls in a ratio of 3:2 (51). Embryonal tumors of the central nervous system (52) and paraneoplastic hypercalcemia (53) occasionally are associated with rhabdoid tumor of the kidney.

## Pathology

### Gross

Rhabdoid tumor is less well circumscribed than Wilms' tumor or clear cell sarcoma. Most tumors are located in the center of the kidney (51), and it is usual for the renal sinus (the space formed by the medial concavity of the kidney) and pelvis to be infiltrated. The parenchyma of rhabdoid tumor is usually light tan or yellow-gray and friable with foci of necrosis and hemorrhage.

### Microscopic

Rhabdoid tumor consists of medium or large polygonal cells with abundant eosinophilic cytoplasm and round nuclei with thick nuclear membranes and large nucleoli. The cells are arranged in diffuse sheets (Fig. 29.6). The name

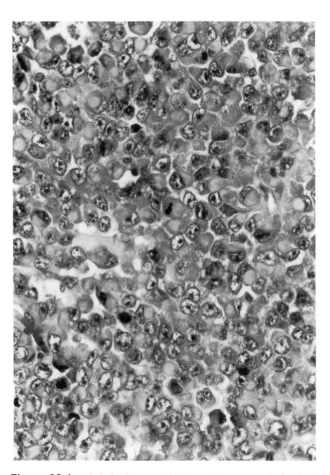

**Figure 29.6** Rhabdoid tumor. The tumor is composed of a sheet of loosely cohesive cells having vesicular nuclei and prominent nucleoli. Many of the cells have fibrillar eosinophilic cytoplasmic inclusions.

was given because the cytoplasm often bears a superficial resemblance to that of differentiating rhabdomyoblasts (49). The resemblance is spurious, and if there is definite differentiation toward skeletal muscle, the tumor is not a rhabdoid tumor. The cytoplasm commonly contains a large eosinophilic inclusion that forces the nucleus to one side. At the ultrastructural level, these are composed of whorled microfilaments (54). A variety of rare patterns have been recognized, including sclerosing, epithelioid, spindle cell, lymphomatoid, vascular, pseudopapillary, and cystic (51). These are usually mixed with the typical pattern and with each other and retain the characteristic nuclear features.

## Treatment and Outcome

Rhabdoid tumor of the kidney is not responsive to radiation or chemotherapy, so surgery is the principal treatment. Early and widespread metastasis is common, and approximately 75% of patients die from rhabdoid tumor within 12 months of diagnosis.

## Metanephric Adenoma

### Clinical Findings and Epidemiology

The rare tumor known as metanephric adenoma has only recently been described in detail (55–57). Epithelial neoplasms of the kidney are rare in children, but among them metanephric adenoma is the most common. It occurs at all ages but is most common in middle age, with a 2:1 female preponderance. Approximately 50% of metanephric adenomas are incidental findings, with others presenting with polycythemia, abdominal or flank pain, mass, or hematuria. The relationship, if any, of metanephric adenoma to other families of renal neoplasms has been debated. They do not have the chromosomal gains characteristic of papillary renal neoplasia (58), and some consider them to be related to Wilms' tumor (57). Metanephric adenoma is part of a family of neoplasms that includes the even more rare metanephric adenofibroma (59) and metanephric stromal tumor (60,61). The 2004 WHO classification places these tumors in a family by themselves (1).

## Pathology

### Gross

Metanephric adenoma is well circumscribed, gray or pale tan, solid or lobular, and its size ranges up to 15 cm. Small cysts and calcifications can be present (Fig. 29.7).

### Microscopic

Metanephric adenoma is composed of small, uniform, round tubules embedded in a loose stroma. At first glance, Wilms' tumor usually comes to mind. Nuclei are small

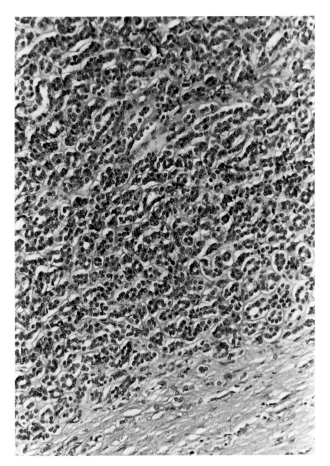

**Figure 29.7**  Metanephric adenoma. The tumor is composed of small uniform cells with scant cytoplasm and forms regular round tubules; note the thick capsule (*bottom*) that surrounds the mass.

and uniform with absent or inconspicuous nucleoli and scant cytoplasm (Fig. 29.7). Papillary or microcystic architectures are less common. Psammoma bodies are common, as are hemorrhage and necrosis. Wilms' tumor stroma and blastema are not found in metanephric adenoma.

### Special Studies
Metanephric adenoma cells usually react with antibody to WT1(62).

### Treatment and Outcome

Cases reported to date have not recurred or metastasized. Fewer than a handful of metanephric adenomas have been associated with psammoma bodies or even epithelial cells in lymph nodes draining the kidney with the metanephric adenoma; the nature of this process is unclear (63).

### Translocation Carcinomas

Over the last several years, a family of renal carcinomas that contain various translocations involving Xp11.2 has been identified (64). All of these translocations have resulted in gene fusions involving *TFE3*. This family of carcinomas

was classified as Xp11 translocation carcinomas in the 2004 WHO classification (1). Subsequently, carcinomas with a t(6;11) producing a fusion with *TFEB* have been identified. Since *TFE3* and *TFEB* are members of the MiTF/TFE family of transcription factor genes, it appears likely that further carcinomas may soon be discovered with fusions of other genes in the family and that the nomenclature will need to be revised (64).

### Clinical Findings and Epidemiology

Although carcinomas make up less than 5% of renal tumors in children, translocation carcinomas appear to make up at least 20% of pediatric renal carcinomas (65). However, translocation carcinomas also occur in adults although their frequency remains unclear. A number of cases have presented at a high stage and have undergone surprisingly indolent courses.

### Pathology

#### Gross
Translocation carcinomas are typically nondescript solid tan-yellow neoplasms, often with foci of hemorrhage and necrosis.

#### Microscopic
Xp11.2 translocation carcinomas often have large areas of papillary architecture in which the papillae are covered by cells with abundant clear or pale cytoplasm (Fig. 29.8). However, they also have an alveolar or nested architecture, and cells with eosinophilic cytoplasm are common. Psammoma bodies are common and may be quite numerous. There are subtle variations in morphology among carcinomas with the different Xp11 translocations.

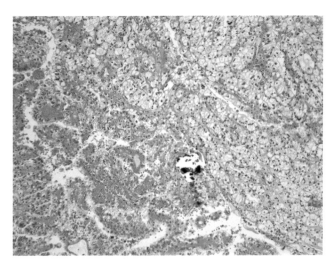

**Figure 29.8**  Xp11.2 translocation carcinoma. The tumor is composed of clear cells forming papillary and solid architectures.

The t(6;11) translocation carcinomas consist of nest and microscopic cysts composed of polygonal cells with pale or eosinophilic cytoplasm. Papillae are uncommon. A distinctive component consists of cells with small amounts of cytoplasm and denser chromatin arranged around nodules of hyaline material in large acini. At low magnification, these resemble rosettes.

### Special Studies

Translocation carcinomas with gene fusions involving *TFE3* typically show a positive intranuclear reaction with antibody to TFE3 (66). Carcinomas with gene fusions involving *TFEB* typically show positive intranuclear reactions with antibody to TFEB. Xp11 translocation carcinomas characteristically fail to mark or mark weakly with antibodies to epithelial markers, such as epithelial membrane antigen and cytokeratins. T(6;11) carcinomas are frequently positive for HMB45 and melanA.

### Treatment and Outcome

Because of the small number of cases studied so far, knowledge of the clinical aspects and outcome of these tumors is sketchy. Most have been found in children and young adults, but this may reflect a bias in the original populations studied. There may be more female than male patients, but that is not conclusive. Some patients have presented with metastases, yet have had prolonged survival. Some patients have had histories of chemotherapy for other conditions.

### Carcinoma Associated With Neuroblastoma

Roughly two dozen children and young adults have been diagnosed with renal cell carcinoma after surviving neuroblastoma in the first 2 years of life (67). In 1999, Medeiros et al (68) published an account of four survivors of neuroblastoma who had histologically distinctive renal tumors and suggested that they constituted a distinct clinicopathologic entity; subsequently, another series of similar tumors in neuroblastoma survivors was published (69). The participants in the World Health Organization consensus conference on the classification of renal neoplasms in December 2003 included the category of postneuroblastoma renal cell carcinoma in the classification to encompass this entity (1).

### Clinical Findings and Epidemiology

The patients had neuroblastoma at the usual age; two of them received neither radiation nor chemotherapy. They were diagnosed with renal cell carcinoma at ages ranging from 5 to 14 years. In one patient, the renal cell carcinoma metastasized to lymph nodes and liver.

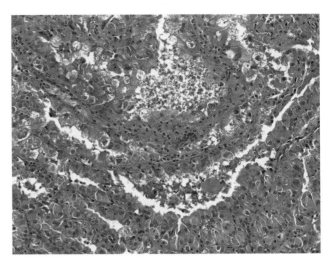

**Figure 29.9**  Postneuroblastoma carcinoma. The tumor is composed of cells with abundant eosinophilic cytoplasm.

## Pathology

### Gross

The major tumors have ranged in diameter from 35 to 80 mm; the 20 small tumors in the patient with multiple and bilateral tumors ranged from 1 mm to 24 mm. Two tumors were invasive of renal capsule, renal vascular system, or peripelvic lymphatics.

### Microscopic

The best-documented postneuroblastoma carcinomas of the kidney contain majority populations of cells with abundant eosinophilic cytoplasm that sometimes is reminiscent of the cytoplasm in oncocytomas (Fig. 29.9). The cells grow in both papillary and solid patterns. Psammoma bodies are infrequently present, as are small clusters of foamy histiocytes. The nuclei often are medium sized and have irregular contours. Nucleoli are easy to find, corresponding to nuclear grade 3. A few mitotic figures are usually present. All tumors studied have reacted with antibody to epithelial membrane antigen, vimentin, and cytokeratin Cam 5.2.

### Treatment and Outcome

Since so few patients have been reported, little is known of its responsiveness to radiation or chemotherapy, and the long-term outcome of these patients also is not clear.

## EPITHELIAL NEOPLASMS

### Renal Cortical Adenoma

### Clinical Findings and Epidemiology

All classifications of renal tumors include adenoma as an entity (1,23,70–72), although criteria for distinguishing adenoma from carcinoma in the kidney remain a significant and unresolved issue in surgical pathology. With increasing numbers of small tumors being detected with new imaging technology, resolution of this issue is important (73–75). Small cortical epithelial lesions have been found in 7% to 23% of kidneys in autopsy series (76,77). Eble and Warfel evaluated a series of 400 consecutive autopsies in which the kidneys were carefully sectioned and examined (78); in 83 instances (21%), epithelial cortical lesions were identified. The frequency increased with age (10% in 21- to 40-year-olds versus 40% in 70- to 90-year-olds). Similar tumors frequently develop in patients on long-term hemodialysis; papillary adenomas have been reported in up to one third of patients in association with acquired cystic disease (79,80). These are believed to be the precursors of carcinoma in this patient group. Papillary adenoma has similar cytogenetic changes to papillary carcinoma (81).

## Pathology

### Gross
Papillary adenoma is currently defined as being 5 mm or less in size (1,70). Tumors as small as 1 mm are identifiable with the naked eye. It is well circumscribed, yellow to gray, and located in the cortex.

### Microscopic
Adenoma is usually tubular, papillary, or tubulopapillary in architecture, corresponding to the chromophil–basophil cell type described by Thoenes et al (72). The cells have round to oval nuclei with stippled or clumped chromatin, and nucleoli are inconspicuous. Cytoplasm is usually scant and amphophilic to basophilic (Fig. 29.10). Although, in the past, small, low-grade clear cell lesions have been included in the adenoma category (72), this is not currently the case. The role of fine-needle aspiration biopsy in the diagnosis is limited; in general, examination of the entire tumor should be undertaken if a diagnosis of adenoma is considered.

## Treatment and Outcome

Reliable criteria for distinguishing adenoma from carcinoma remain elusive (11). In 1950, Bell (82) classified all tumors less than 3.0 cm in diameter as adenoma, despite the fact that metastases developed from 3 of 65 tumors (4.6%) in this size range. Small cortical tumors have repeatedly demonstrated malignant behavior, confirming that size alone is not a reliable diagnostic criterion. Thoenes et al (72) defined adenoma as any tumor up to 1.0 cm in size with grade 1 cytology (small uniform nuclei with delicate or condensed chromatin, inconspicuous nucleoli, absent mitotic figures) and included clear cell tumors in this definition. Murphy et al (23) consider one subset of cor-

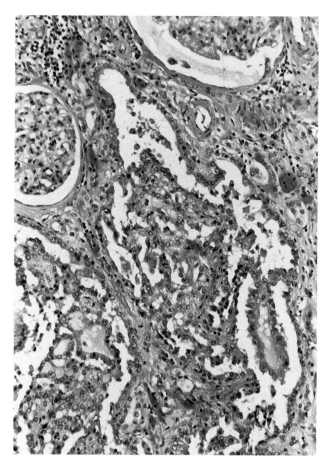

**Figure 29.10**  Cortical adenoma. Two small tubulopapillary lesions merge imperceptibly with adjacent normal tubules; the cells have small uniform nuclei without significant atypia.

tical epithelial lesions to be definable as adenoma: those with closely packed tubules with or without papillae and composed of "small, regular, cuboidal cells with rounded, uniform nuclei lacking any features of anaplasia." Mitotic figures are rare to absent. This description corresponds to the chromophil–basophil cell type (72). We agree that this is the most clearly identified benign tumor of cortical epithelium and consider all lesions composed of clear cells to be malignant regardless of size (70,83,84).

Treatment of small cortical epithelial tumors is determined on clinical grounds. A therapeutic decision should not be based on frozen section, which is associated with both false-positive and false-negative results (85). With the increasing popularity of partial nephrectomy for small tumors, the issue of frozen section is less pressing (86,87).

## Oncocytoma

### Clinical Findings and Epidemiology

In 1976, Klein and Valensi (88) described a subset of renal tumors in adults composed of oncocytes and having an apparently benign clinical course. This observation, subsequently, was confirmed by several other groups (89,90). Oncocytoma accounts for approximately 4% of renal tumors in adults. Most occur in adults older than age 50 years, with a male-to-female ratio of 2:1. They are most often detected as incidental findings, although oncocytoma may present with hematuria or a palpable mass (91). They are usually sporadic, but can develop as part of the Birt-Hogg-Dube syndrome (92).

Radiologic studies may suggest the diagnosis of oncocytoma, although they are not specific. Typical angiographic features include a sharp, smooth margin with the capsule, thereby creating a lucent rim; vasculature without marked disarray, with no pooling of contrast material or arteriovenous shunting; homogeneous capillary pattern, giving a density similar to normal renal parenchyma; and feeding arteries in a spoke-wheel pattern (93,94).

## Pathology

### Genetics
Cytogenetic studies have supported the view that oncocytoma is a distinct renal neoplasm. These tumors have a mosaic pattern of normal and aberrant karyotypes and consistently lack abnormalities in the 3p region (95–98). Evidence suggests that oncocytoma originates from the intercalated cell of the collecting duct (99,100).

### Gross
Oncocytoma is well circumscribed, homogeneous, and tan brown or mahogany brown (Fig. 29.11). It sometimes is bilateral or multifocal (101–103), and rarely, innumerable lesions are present, a process that has been termed *oncocytomatosis* or *oncocytosis* (102,104). There may be areas of hemorrhage, but necrosis is absent. A stellate central zone of edematous connective tissue is common in large tumors, but in smaller tumors it may be absent. Any tumor with a variegated appearance should be extensively sampled before making a diagnosis of oncocytoma; for this reason, the diagnosis of oncocytoma at frozen section or by fine-needle aspiration biopsy is discouraged.

### Microscopic
Renal oncocytoma is composed of cells with abundant intensely eosinophilic and coarsely granular cytoplasm (105). Focal cytoplasmic vacuolization and clearing can occur. The cells are cuboidal to columnar and are arranged in well-defined nests that are closely packed peripherally, but often are separated by a loose stroma near the center of the tumor (Fig. 29.12). Tubules (106) or small cysts (107) occur occasionally. Cysts may be associated with hemorrhage. Necrosis is absent. Nuclei are regular and round to oval, with granular chromatin and central nucleoli. The presence of cells with bizarre pleomorphic nuclei is well recognized and believed to be degenerative (Fig. 29.13). Mitotic figures are absent or rare, at most. Distinguishing

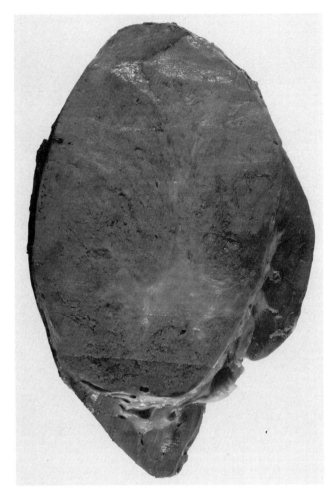

**Figure 29.11** Oncocytoma. The tumor is well circumscribed and solid with a dark brown color (compare the tumor with adjacent renal cortex) and an area of fibrous scarring (lower right part of mass).

oncocytoma from papillary carcinoma and chromophobe carcinoma is important because the latter two may show malignant behavior.

### Special Studies
Oncocytoma contains low–molecular-weight cytokeratin, but does not contain vimentin (108–111). Cytokeratin 7, typically, is expressed intensely by a few scattered single cells or small groups of cells (110,111). The tumor does not express the RCC antigen (112). Hale's colloidal iron stain is negative (positive in chromophobe carcinoma) (113) or shows luminal staining if tubules are present (114). Lectins show a pattern consistent with collecting duct origin (99,115). Ultrastructurally, the cells are filled with mitochondria (116).

### Treatment and Outcome
It now is generally accepted that renal oncocytoma is benign. Reports of oncocytoma with metastases (117,118) are believed by most authors to be examples of the eosinophilic

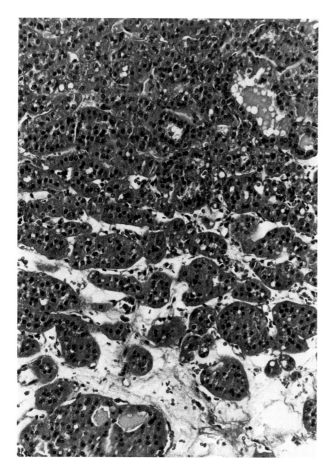

**Figure 29.12** Oncocytoma. Characteristic histology of oncocytoma, with uniform cells having abundant eosinophilic cytoplasm arranged in well-defined nests. Note the appearance of the nests in loose, fibrous connective tissue at the lower part of the photomicrograph; this pattern is almost pathognomonic for oncocytoma.

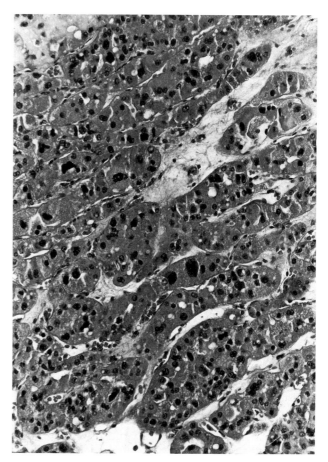

**Figure 29.13** Oncocytoma. Example of oncocytoma containing large pleomorphic hyperchromatic nuclei; this pattern is common in oncocytoma and is considered to represent a degenerative phenomenon.

variant of chromophobe renal cell carcinoma (23). Since oncocytoma is benign, there is no rationale for grading renal oncocytoma. Surgical resection, either by partial nephrectomy or by radical nephrectomy, is curative.

## Renal Cell Carcinoma

### Classification

Today the term *renal cell carcinoma* connotes a group of neoplasms having a common origin from the epithelium of the renal tubules but having distinct morphologic and genetic features (14). Until the mid-1980s, renal cell carcinoma was most often classified by its cytoplasmic appearance as clear cell or granular cell type. Tumors composed of mixtures of cells, with clear and granular cytoplasm, were recognized to be common. As detailed previously in the section on oncocytoma, in 1976, Klein and Valensi (88) extracted the benign renal oncocytoma from the granular cell end of this spectrum. In 1985, the Mainz group reported the first

cases of a subtype with distinctive morphologic features that they called the *chromophobe* type (119). Although the original chromophobe carcinomas emerged from what had previously been called clear cell carcinoma, an eosinophilic variant of chromophobe cell carcinoma soon developed from what had previously been called granular cell carcinoma. Around the same time, it was recognized that renal cell carcinoma may arise from segments distal to the proximal tubule and *collecting duct carcinoma* began to be recognized among tumors that previously would have been called granular cell carcinoma. In 1986, Thoenes et al (72) proposed a new classification of renal cell neoplasms that recognized these entities as well as clear cell renal cell carcinoma and *chromophil* renal cell carcinoma, also known as *papillary* renal cell carcinoma. The new entities make up 15% to 20% of renal cell neoplasms in surgical series, whereas clear cell renal cell carcinoma accounts for about 70%, with a few rarities and unclassified tumors making up the remainder. The recognition of so many new entities in the granular cell end of the spectrum, combined with the recognition that clear cell renal cell carcinoma may have areas in which the cells have eosinophilic cytoplasm, has made *granular cell renal cell carcinoma* useful only as a descriptive term and obsolete as a diagnosis. The new classification was developed from morphologic observations, but since 1985, genetic studies have validated it by discovering genetic abnormalities that are characteristic for each of the diagnostic groups (71). The most recent classifications have reaffirmed these changes and have added several newer entities (1,70). In the following sections, each of the currently recognized types of renal cell carcinoma is discussed.

## Clinical Findings and Epidemiology

The classic triad of presenting symptoms consists of hematuria, pain, and flank mass, a combination that is generally associated with advanced stage (120). However, approximately 40% of patients lack all of these and present with systemic symptoms. A common constellation is weight loss, abdominal pain, and anorexia, which may suggest carcinoma of the gastrointestinal tract (120). In approximately 18% of patients, there is fever without infection (121). The erythrocyte sedimentation rate is elevated in approximately 50% of cases (122). Although blood erythropoietin levels are elevated in almost two thirds of patients (123), erythrocytosis occurs in less than 4% (121). Hypochromic anemia unrelated to hematuria occurs in about one third of cases (121,124). Systemic amyloidosis occurs in about 3% of patients with renal cell carcinoma and is of the AA type (125).

Renal cell carcinoma occasionally causes paraneoplastic endocrine syndromes (126,127), which include pseudohyperparathyroidism, erythrocytosis, hypertension, and gynecomastia. Hypercalcemia occurs in the absence of bone metastases in approximately 10% of patients with renal cell carcinoma (128). Approximately 33% of patients are hypertensive (121,129); this is commonly associated with elevated renin concentrations (129). Typically, the blood pressure returns to normal after the tumor is resected. Gynecomastia may result from gonadotropin (130) or prolactin (131) production. Renal cell carcinoma also is notorious for presenting as metastatic carcinoma of unknown primary, sometimes in unusual sites (132,133).

Renal cell carcinoma occurs almost exclusively in adults, at rates of 5.6 and 4.1 per 100,000 among males and females, respectively (134). In the United States, approximately 36,160 new cases of cancer of the kidney and renal pelvis are diagnosed each year, and there are approximately 12,660 deaths attributed to these tumors (135). In the first two decades of life, renal cell carcinoma is rare (136). Few cases occur before age 40, but its incidence increases from that age to a peak in the sixth and seventh decades (134,135). Familial clusters of renal cell carcinoma are rare outside syndromes such as von Hippel–Lindau

disease (137). In recent years, a variety of hereditary renal cell carcinoma syndromes have been described; however, overall, these account for a small proportion of tumors (138–144).

As much as 30% of renal cell carcinoma is attributed to the carcinogenic effects of smoking (145,146). Obesity also is important, especially in women (146–148). Environmental risk factors include phenacetin and acetaminophen use for long periods (149), and exposure to cadmium (150), petroleum products (150,151), and industrial chemicals (150,152). In most cases, the carcinogenic influence is unknown.

Between one third and one half of patients with von Hippel–Lindau disease develop renal cell carcinoma (153,154); metastasis occurs in approximately 50% of these and causes death in about one third (155). Patients with tuberous sclerosis also have increased risk for renal cell carcinoma (156,157). Most have no recurrence, but a few cases with metastases have been documented (158,159). The association of autosomal dominant polycystic kidney disease with renal cell carcinoma is less well established (160). Acquired renal cystic disease in patients with chronic renal failure is also strongly associated with renal cell carcinoma (79,80,161,162).

## Staging

Since there is no effective treatment for metastases, the extent of spread of renal cell carcinoma dominates the prognosis. At present, the American Joint Commission on Cancer (AJCC) tumor, nodes, metastases (TNM) system is recommended for use (163) (Table 29.2). Tumors confined by the renal capsule are in the most favorable category. Within the most favorable group, the size of the tumor is used to subdivide these into three categories having different prognoses (164–166). Invasion of perinephric adipose tissue defines the pT3a category. Invasion of the renal sinus is included in this category (167,168). Direct invasion of the adrenal gland is also considered pT3a. The pT3b category is defined by grossly visible involvement of the renal vein and is not indicated by invasion of small veins inside the main tumor. Although the tumor thrombus may extend beyond the site of transection of the renal vein, this is not considered a positive margin unless the thrombus is adherent to the vein wall at the edge. In 10% to 15% of cases, there is metastasis to regional lymph nodes without distant metastasis (169,170). However, most regional lymphadenopathy is caused by inflammatory or hyperplastic changes (171). Although radical nephrectomy with regional lymph node dissection has long been the standard operation for renal cell carcinoma, the contribution of the lymph node dissection remains uncertain (172). The ipsilateral adrenal is involved by direct invasion or metastasis in about 5% of radical nephrectomy specimens (173–175).

**TABLE 29.2**

**AJCC-TNM STAGING OF RENAL CELL CARCINOMA (2002)**

**Primary tumor (T)**

| | |
|---|---|
| TX | Primary tumor cannot be assessed |
| T0 | No evidence of primary tumor |
| T1a | Confined to Kidney, $\leq$4.0 cm |
| T1b | Confined to kidney, >4.0 cm and $\leq$7.0 cm |
| T2 | Confined to kidney, >7.0 cm |
| T3a | Tumor invades the perinephric fat or the adrenal gland but not beyond Gerota's fascia |
| T3b | Tumor grossly extends into the renal vein(s) or vena cava below the diaphragm |
| T3c | Tumor grossly extends into the renal vein(s) or vena cava above the diaphragm |
| T4 | Tumor invades beyond Gerota's fascia |

**Regional lymph nodes (N)**

| | |
|---|---|
| NX | Regional lymph nodes cannot be assessed |
| N0 | No regional lymph node metastases |
| N1 | Metastases in a single regional lymph node |
| N2 | Metastasis in more than one regional lymph node |

**Distant metastases (M)**

| | |
|---|---|
| MX | Distant metastasis cannot be assessed |
| M0 | No distant metastasis |
| M1 | Distant metastasis |

### Grading

In 1971, Skinner et al (176) directed attention to the correlation between nuclear features and outcome. Currently, the Fuhrman et al (177) grading system is most widely used (Table 29.3). Grade 1 tumors are uncommon, making up less than 10% of cases. Approximately 20% are grade 4 (178). The middle grades each account for about 35% of cases (Fig. 29.14). Numerous reports have documented that this grading system correlates well with survival in a large series of patients with renal cell carcinoma (179–185). Actuarial, 5-year, disease-free survival ranges from 88% to 90% for patients with grade 1 tumors to 18% for patients with grade 4 tumors (182,184). The highest grade found is the grade assigned, regardless of extent (180,182). Mitotic figures are not included in this system, but more than one per 10 high-power fields has adverse significance (180). Störkel

et al (186) have proposed reducing the nuclear grades to three to improve the discriminatory power of the grades.

Areas resembling sarcoma are found in approximately 5% of renal cell carcinomas (187,188). Grossly, these areas are often dense and white and contrast with the rest of the carcinoma (Fig. 29.15). Sarcomatoid areas have been found in association with all the types of renal cell carcinoma. Usually, these resemble malignant fibrous histiocytoma, fibrosarcoma, or undifferentiated spindle cell sarcoma (Fig. 29.16) (189). Heterologous differentiation toward osteogenic sarcoma, chondrosarcoma, or rhabdomyosarcoma is uncommon (190,191). Patients with even small foci of sarcomatoid carcinoma have a much worse prognosis than those whose tumors do not have such foci (188,189,192,193), so thorough sampling of areas with differing gross appearances (especially firm, whitish areas) is important in evaluating renal cell carcinoma. The number of sections submitted is based on gross examination.

### Treatment and Outcome

Renal cell carcinoma is notorious for its unpredictable clinical course. There are documented cases of spontaneous regression of metastases (194–196) and of remarkably prolonged course (197). Recurrence, a decade or more after nephrectomy, is found in more than 10% of those who survive so long (198). The resistance of renal cell carcinoma to radiation and chemotherapy gives patients with remote metastases a poor prognosis (199,200). Treatment, in the last couple of decades, has focused on biologic therapies with limited success (201). Metastases to bone are frequent, and more than a third of these are to the scapula (202). In selected patients, resection of metastases may be beneficial (203).

### Clear Cell Renal Cell Carcinoma

### Clinical Findings and Epidemiology

The clinical and epidemiologic data presented in the previous section are largely based on clear cell renal cell carcinoma, as it composes most renal carcinomas, and will not be repeated here.

**TABLE 29.3**

**FUHRMAN NUCLEAR GRADING SYSTEM**

| Grade | Size (μm) | Shape | Chromatin | Nucleoli |
|---|---|---|---|---|
| 1 | <10 | Round | Dense | Inconspicuous |
| 2 | 15 | Round | Open | Small, not visible with 10× objective |
| 3 | 20 | Round/oval | Open | Prominent |
| 4 | >20 | Pleomorphic, multilobated | Open, hyperchromatic | Macro |

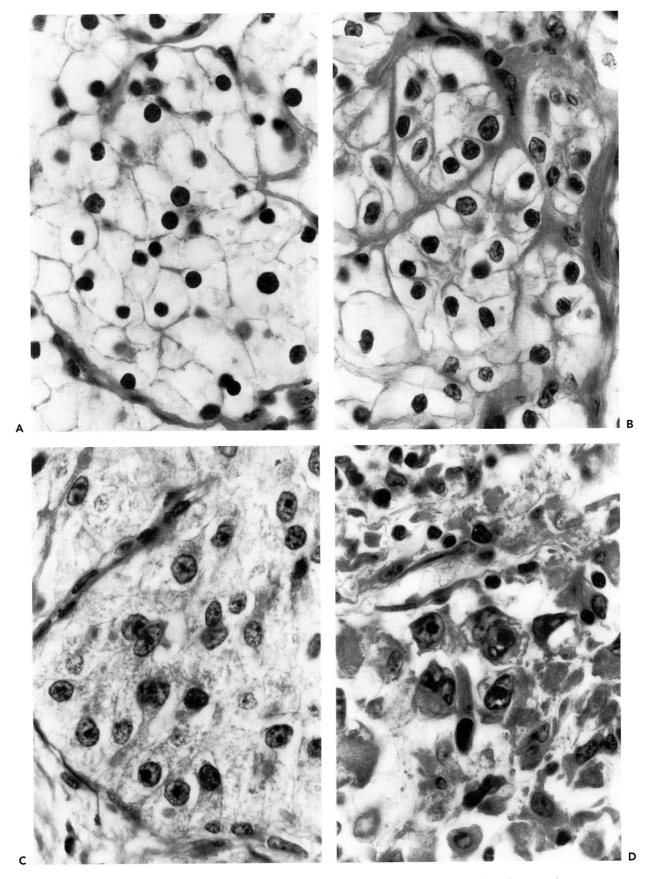

**Figure 29.14** Clear cell renal cell carcinoma. **A:** Nuclear grade 1 tumor with small, uniform round nuclei and dense chromatin. **B:** Nuclear grade 2 carcinoma with slightly larger nuclei having more open chromatin and inconspicuous (at intermediate magnification, ×10 objective) nucleoli. **C:** Nuclear grade 3 neoplasm has large, open nuclei with prominent nucleoli (readily visible at intermediate magnification). **D:** Nuclear grade 4 carcinoma with large bizarre nuclei, including binucleate cells.

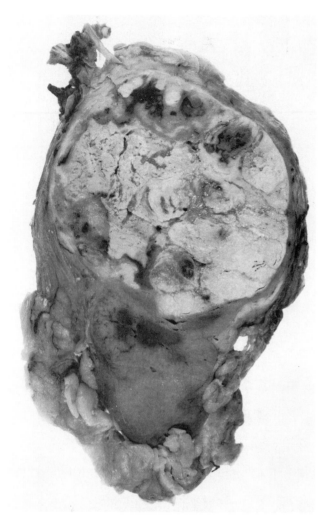

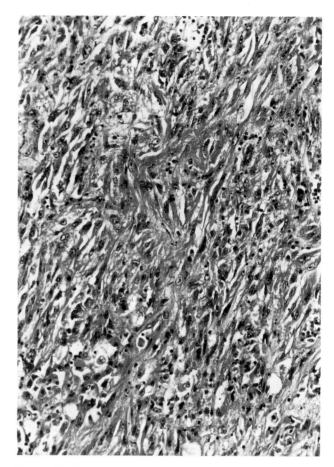

**Figure 29.16** Sarcomatoid renal cell carcinoma. The tumor is composed of pleomorphic spindle-shaped cells growing in a malignant fibrous histiocytomalike pattern.

**Figure 29.15** Sarcomatoid renal cell carcinoma. The tumor is well circumscribed with extensive necrosis; the sarcomatoid component is indicated by the fleshy gray-white areas (top and lower left parts of tumor).

## Pathology

### Genetics

Cytogenetic studies of clear cell renal cell carcinoma have consistently found losses in the short arm of chromosome 3 (3p) (204–209). Losses in 3p have been found in tumors as small as 11 mm (210). Renal cell carcinoma arising in patients with von Hippel–Lindau disease also, commonly, has deletion or partial deletion of chromosome 3p (211–213), with a breakpoint in the proximal short arm near the location (3p25) of the von Hippel–Lindau gene (214). A second commonly involved site is at 3p14, possibly, involving the *FHIT* gene (215). In one study, 96% of cases showed a continuous deletion from 3p14.2-p25, including both the *FHIT* and *VHL* genes (216). Although various other genetic abnormalities are common in clear cell renal cell carcinoma, loss in 3p appears to be required for it to develop.

### Gross

A bright yellow or light orange color is the most distinctive aspect of the gross appearance of clear cell renal cell carcinoma. Often its appearance is variegated, mottled by areas of hemorrhage and cream-colored foci of necrosis (Fig. 29.17). Tumors are now frequently discovered incidentally by radiologists and often are less than 3 cm in diameter (217). Clear cell renal cell carcinoma typically is solid and bulges above the cut surface. Most are roughly spherical and circumscribed by pseudocapsules, but diffuse infiltration and replacement of the kidney occur occasionally. Sometimes there are irregularly shaped areas of edematous gray connective tissue at the centers of large tumors. Cysts ranging from a few millimeters to 1 to 2 cm in diameter are common. Occasionally, clear cell renal cell carcinoma is almost completely cystic (218–221). The current classification recognizes multilocular cystic renal cell carcinoma as a specific subtype of clear cell carcinoma (1). Rarely, clear cell renal cell carcinoma arises in the wall of a simple cyst or becomes cystic through necrosis and degenerative changes. Gross features such as hemorrhage and granular eosinophilic cytoplasm and, sometimes, there are areas where most cells do not have clear cytoplasm. In some instances, the cells take on a rhabdoid morphology (225). Such areas may be associated with necrosis and should not be confusing if the other features typical of clear cell renal cell carcinoma are recognized. The nuclei usually are central and nearly spherical, ranging from small hyperchromatic ones lacking visible nucleoli, to large and pleomorphic ones with macronucleoli. The mitotic rate is highly variable.

The major architectural patterns are compact (alveolar), tubular, and cystic, occurring alone or in combinations. The vascular pattern, consisting of a conspicuous network of thin-walled blood vessels with little supporting fibrous tissue, is a diagnostically helpful feature of most clear cell renal cell carcinoma. The vascular pattern is most apparent in areas with alveolar architecture (Fig. 29.18). Tubular structures merge with the cystic pattern as they become dilated. The tubules are usually round or oval, but may occasionally elongate. Frequently, the small tubules are empty, but larger ones often contain eosinophilic fluid or blood. Rarely, clear cell renal cell carcinoma is grossly cystic and consists of

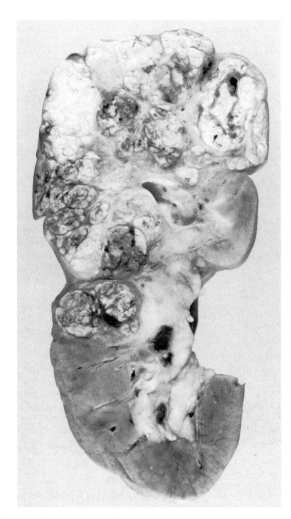

**Figure 29.17** Clear cell renal cell carcinoma. The tumor is multinodular and variegated with areas of necrosis and fibrosis.

necrosis, solid nodules, and a thick fibrotic capsule indicate a greater likelihood of a cystic lesion being neoplastic. Sampling should be directed to areas of the lesion with these features. Up to 13% of cases are multicentric within the same kidney (222), and renal cell carcinoma occurs bilaterally in approximately 1% of patients (223).

## Microscopic

Clear cell renal cell carcinoma is the most common carcinoma of the renal tubular epithelium. The cytoplasm of clear cell renal cell carcinoma is clear because it usually contains much lipid and glycogen, which dissolve during processing. The site of origin of clear cell renal cell carcinoma was controversial until 1960, when Oberling et al (224) demonstrated apical brush borders, which indicated origin from the proximal tubule. Although clear cytoplasm has given this carcinoma its name, it does not define it, and other morphologic features are diagnostically important. Clear cell renal cell carcinoma often contains cells with

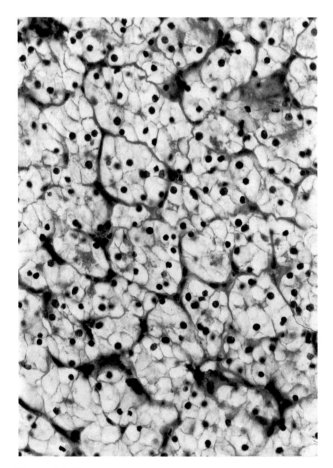

**Figure 29.18** Clear cell renal cell carcinoma. Characteristic alveolar pattern with nests of clear cells separated by a prominent sinusoidal vascular network.

fibrous septa with only a small population of carcinoma cells with clear cytoplasm and small, darkly staining nuclei that line the cysts and form small nodules within the septa (220,221,226–228). The term *multilocular cystic renal cell carcinoma* has been applied to these.

### Special Studies

Clear cell renal cell carcinoma frequently expresses both cytokeratins and vimentin; epithelial membrane antigen also, commonly, is present (111,229,230). Most also express the RCC (renal cell carcinoma) antigen and CD10 (112,231). These findings are especially helpful in evaluating metastases from unknown primaries. Abundant glycogen and lipid are seen in the cytoplasm by electron microscopy. Apical brush borders or microvilli are sometimes present, reflecting this tumor's origin from the epithelium of the proximal tubule.

### Papillary Renal Cell Carcinoma

#### Clinical Findings and Epidemiology

Approximately 10% to 15% of renal cell carcinoma, in surgical series, is papillary renal cell carcinoma (90,232–237). Males predominate in a ratio of approximately 2:1. Ages range from early adulthood to old age, with the mean between 50 and 55 years. These carcinomas have a mortality of up to 16% at 10 years (236) and sometimes present with metastases (238). Hereditary types of papillary renal cell carcinoma are well described (239). Papillary renal cell carcinoma has a significantly better prognosis than clear cell renal cell carcinoma (90,236).

#### Pathology

##### Genetics

Papillary renal cell carcinoma has a characteristic pattern of genetic abnormalities that differs from those of other renal cell neoplasms. The pattern of lesions is one of chromosomal gains, the most common of which are trisomy or tetrasomy of 17 and 7 (240,241). Most of these tumors in men lose the Y chromosome (241). These results are consistent and have been corroborated by several laboratories (98,242). Trisomy or tetrasomy of only chromosomes 7 and 17 appears to correlate with low grade and development of further trisomy correlates with progression (241).

##### Gross

Papillary renal cell carcinoma is usually a well-circumscribed, globular tumor with tan or brown parenchyma (Fig. 29.19). In about 66% of cases, hemorrhage and necrosis are prominent, which may cause the tumor to appear hypovascular radiographically (232,234). Many of these

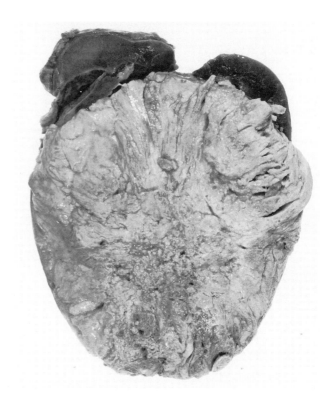

**Figure 29.19**  Papillary renal cell carcinoma. The tumor is well circumscribed, is pale tan, and has a soft, friable surface. The thick capsule is not apparent in this photograph as a result of bulging of the tumor.

tumors are large. Often the cut surface is friable or granular, a reflection of the papillae seen microscopically (Fig. 29.20). The larger tumors are often surrounded by a rim of dense fibrous tissue (243). In about one third of cases, there are calcifications (232,234).

##### Microscopic

In more than 90% of papillary renal cell carcinoma, the architecture is predominantly papillary or tubulopapillary (Fig. 29.21). The remaining tumors have a solid growth pattern that is the result of tight packing of papillae (244). The papillae usually have delicate fibrovascular cores covered by a single layer of carcinoma cells. The form of the papillae varies, ranging from complex branching to long parallel arrays (235). The cores are sometimes expanded by foamy macrophages. Psammoma bodies occasionally are present. Rarely, the papillary cores are wide and collagenous (235). The tubular architecture consists of small tubules lined by a single layer of cells identical to those covering papillae.

In papillary renal cell carcinoma, the cells range from small ones with inconspicuous cytoplasm to large ones with abundant eosinophilic cytoplasm. Tumors composed of small cells are more common. The small cells have high nuclear/cytoplasmic ratios because of their small volume

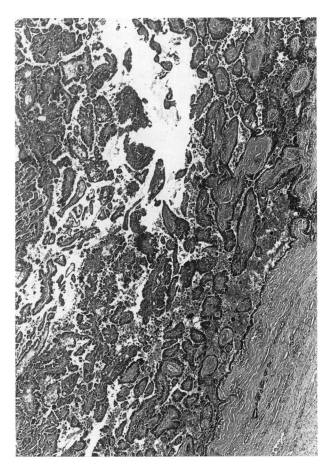

**Figure 29.20** Papillary renal cell carcinoma. The tumor has a thick, fibrous capsule and is composed of papillary structures. The dark staining of the tumor cells is due to abundant cytoplasmic hemosiderin, a feature often present in these tumors.

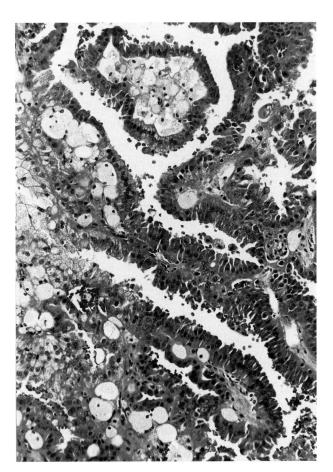

**Figure 29.21** Papillary renal cell carcinoma. In this eosinophilic variant, the cells are tall and columnar with abundant eosinophilic cytoplasm; note that some cells do have cytoplasmic clearing, particularly at the apical ends of the cytoplasm. The papillae often contain foamy histiocytes as in this example.

of cytoplasm. The cytoplasm of these cells typically is pale and nearly clear. The nuclei are nearly spherical and small, and nucleoli are small or invisible. In the larger cells with eosinophilic cytoplasm, the nuclei tend to be larger and to have prominent nucleoli (see Fig. 29.21). Delahunt and Eble (237) and others (245) have proposed subtyping papillary renal cell carcinoma into two groups, type 1 and type 2. There are data to support this distinction from both a clinicopathologic and molecular perspective (237,245–249). In several series, nuclear morphology correlated with stage and outcome (183,238); thus the nuclear grading system is recommended (177).

### Special Studies

Papillary renal cell carcinoma expresses cytokeratins, including cytokeratin 7, and frequently coexpresses vimentin (111,112,237). There is also consistent expression of the RCC marker and CD10 (231,250).

## Chromophobe Renal Cell Carcinoma

### Clinical Findings and Epidemiology

Thoenes et al (119) described the first cases of chromophobe renal cell carcinoma in 1985. The tumor makes up about 5% of all renal cell carcinomas (90,236,251–254). In contrast to clear cell renal cell carcinoma and papillary renal cell carcinoma, chromophobe renal cell carcinoma has no gender predilection. Patients range in age from 27 to 86 years, with a mean of approximately 55 years. Prognosis is significantly better than for clear cell and papillary renal cell carcinoma, with 5-year progression-free survival greater than 90% (90,236).

### Pathology

#### Genetics

Losses of multiple entire chromosomes—most often chromosomes 1, 2, 10, 13, 6, 21, and 17—occur in 90% of cases

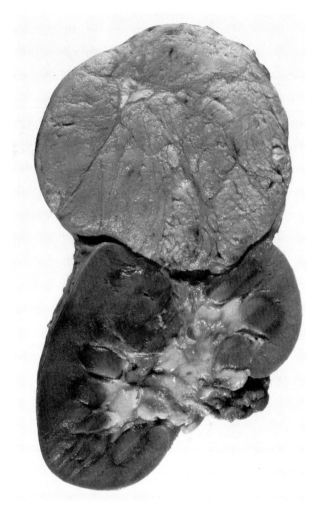

**Figure 29.22**  Chromophobe renal cell carcinoma. The tumor is well circumscribed, homogeneous, and pale tan.

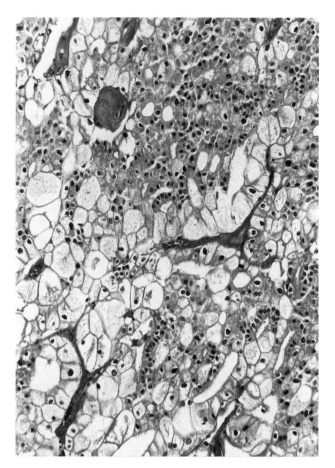

**Figure 29.23**  Chromophobe renal cell carcinoma. In this example of the classic type, there is a mixture of large cells with abundant flocculent cytoplasm and prominent cell borders and smaller cells with more dense eosinophilic cytoplasm.

of chromophobe renal cell carcinoma (255–258). The genetic lesions typical of clear cell renal cell carcinoma (loss of 3p) and of papillary renal cell carcinoma (trisomy and tetrasomy of chromosomes 17 and 7 with loss of Y) are not found.

## Gross

The typical chromophobe renal cell carcinoma is solid, beige or light brown, circumscribed, and nearly spherical (Fig. 29.22). Some have small foci of hemorrhage or necrosis. Occasionally, a few small cysts are present. Chromophobe renal cell carcinoma ranges in size from less than 2 cm to larger than 20 cm, and some tumors invade the renal vein (252).

## Microscopic

In sections stained with hematoxylin and eosin, chromophobe renal cell carcinoma has two variants: *typical* and *eosinophilic*. The former was recognized first (119). Its archi-

tecture usually is solid, but tubules and microscopic cysts sometimes are present. The cells vary in size and shape, tending to be large and polygonal. Their cytoplasm is abundant and pale staining, with a reticular or flocculent appearance. The cytoplasm is denser at the periphery, which makes the cytoplasmic membranes look thick (Fig. 29.23). Often some of the cells, particularly the smaller ones, have eosinophilic cytoplasm. The nuclei are of medium size and many have an irregular "raisinoid" shape. Many have small nucleoli; usually, there are few mitotic figures.

The eosinophilic variant of chromophobe cell renal cell carcinoma was recognized a few years later (253). Its cells have eosinophilic, finely granular cytoplasm. About the nucleus, the cytoplasm often is pale, creating a perinuclear halo (Fig. 29.24). On average, the cells are smaller than those of the typical variant. Tubular structures are more common. Tumors having features of both renal oncocytoma and chromophobe renal cell carcinoma have been described and the term *hybrid tumor* applied in such cases (104). How best to classify such tumors remains uncertain.

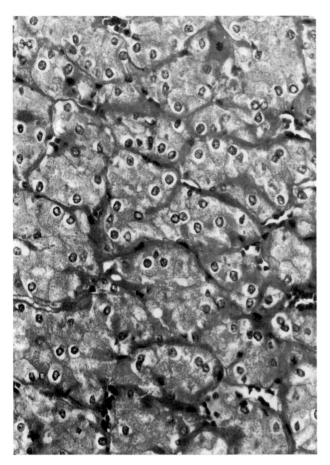

**Figure 29.24** Chromophobe renal cell carcinoma. The eosinophilic variant of chromophobe renal cell carcinoma has smaller cells than the classic type with granular eosinophilic cytoplasm and prominent perinuclear halos; the cells may be arranged in nests and mimic oncocytoma as in this example.

Although grading has not been validated for chromophobe renal cell carcinoma, most are nuclear grade 2 or 3 (251,252).

### Special Studies

For both variants, the Hale's colloidal iron stain is diagnostically helpful, staining the cytoplasm blue (113,114,119). Hale's colloidal iron stain reacts with acid mucosubstances from the characteristic cytoplasmic vesicles (259). The tumor expresses cytokeratins, including cytokeratin 7, but not vimentin (110–112). The RCC marker is expressed in about 50% of cases (112,250).

Electron microscopy also is valuable. In the typical variant, the cytoplasm is filled with 150- to 300-nm round-to-oval vesicles (116,253). Often, these are invaginated and resemble those of the intercalated cells of the collecting duct (260,261). In the eosinophilic variant, the cytoplasm contains numerous mitochondria interspersed among the vesicles.

## Collecting Duct Carcinoma

### Clinical Findings and Epidemiology

In a 1976 study of renal cell carcinoma with papillary architecture, Mancilla-Jimenez et al (234) described three cases with atypical hyperplastic changes in the collecting duct epithelium and postulated that these represented a distinct subset that probably originated from collecting ducts. Since then, several reports have further studied the clinical and pathologic features of this group of tumors (262–269). Collecting duct carcinoma often occurs at a younger age than other renal cell carcinomas and has an aggressive clinical course.

### Pathology

#### Genetics

Cytogenetic analysis of three examples of collecting duct carcinoma showed loss of chromosomes 1, 6, 14, 15, and 22 (270). Consistent involvement of chromosome 1 has been highlighted in other reports (271,272).

#### Gross

Collecting duct carcinoma has its epicenter in the renal medulla, although in larger tumors this may be impossible to define. It is white or gray-white and has an infiltrative growth pattern; variegation is common, with areas of necrosis frequent.

#### Microscopic

These tumors often have a mixed papillary and infiltrative tubular architecture (Fig. 29.25). The infiltrative component is associated with marked stromal desmoplasia. Foci of dysplasia, or carcinoma in situ, can be found in the adjacent collecting ducts in some cases. The tumors are of high nuclear grade, corresponding to Fuhrman grade 3 or 4. Some cases have been described with a urothelial carcinoma component (262,263). Sarcomatoid morphology has been described in collecting duct carcinoma (193,273).

#### Special Studies

Histochemical stains may help to separate collecting duct carcinoma from other types of renal cell carcinoma. This carcinoma contains relatively small amounts of glycogen and sometimes contains cytoplasmic mucin.

### Treatment and Outcome

Treatment has largely been surgical, with a poor overall survival. Of reported cases, 10 died of metastatic disease within 2 years (265–267). In the series from the M.D. Anderson Cancer Center, the median survival of 10 patients was only 22 months (264).

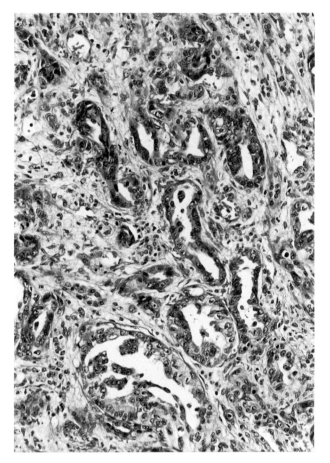

**Figure 29.25** Collecting duct carcinoma. The tumor is composed of infiltrating ductal structures in a desmoplastic stroma. Individual tumor cells are pleomorphic with irregular chromatin, prominent nucleoli, and frequent mitoses.

## Medullary Carcinoma

### Clinical Findings and Epidemiology

This tumor occurs most often in young African Americans with sickle cell trait or hemoglobin SC disease (234). The presentation is similar to other malignant kidney tumors.

### Pathology

#### Genetics

A *bcr/abl* gene rearrangement has been demonstrated in one case (276). Molecular profiling has demonstrated that medullary carcinoma clusters closer to urothelial carcinoma than renal cell carcinoma (277).

#### Gross

The tumors are located in the medullary region of the kidney. They are grey-white and infiltrative, usually involving the hilar fat. Satellite nodules are often present in the cortex.

#### Microscopic

The most characteristic histologic feature is a reticular or yolk saclike appearance combined with adenoid cysticlike areas. In other areas, tumor cells are in solid nests and sheets. An infiltrate of polymorphonuclear leukocytes is usually present. Individual cells have pleomorphic nuclei with frequent mitoses. In most cases, cells with a rhabdoid morphology are present. There is almost always a prominent desmoplastic stromal response. Sickled erythrocytes may be identified.

### Treatment and Outcome

The cases reported to date have been very aggressive with most patients dying within 1 year of diagnosis (274–276).

## Mucinous Tubular and Spindle Cell Carcinoma

### Clinical Findings and Epidemiology

A less common pattern of renal cell carcinoma that has been postulated to be of collecting duct and, possibly, loop of Henle origin (278–281) has now been included in current classifications as a distinct entity (1). The original description of low-grade collecting duct carcinoma of the kidney included tumors that now are included in this category (282). Most cases occur in females and are single although multifocality has been described.

### Pathology

#### Genetics

Cytogenetic studies have demonstrated consistent losses involving chromosomes 1, 4, 6, 8, 9, 13, 14, 15 and 22, supporting this lesion as being a distinctive entity (279,280).

#### Gross

Mucinous tubular and spindle cell tumors are solid, pale tan to yellow to gray-white lesions that may have slight focal areas of necrosis or hemorrhage.

#### Microscopic

Histologically, they manifest elongated branching tubules in a bubbly mucinous, myxoid stroma. The collapsed tubules result in a cordlike pattern, and spindle cell areas are also present. The tubules are striking with characteristic long profiles (Fig. 29.26). The basal lamina around the tubules is highlighted by PAS staining. The cells are cuboidal with scant clear to pale acidophilic cytoplasm and low-grade nuclear features.

#### Special Studies

Immunohistochemical studies have had widely varied results, but most tumors express CK18, CK19, and epithelial

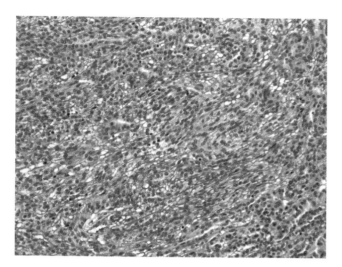

**Figure 29.26** Mucinous tubular and spindle cell carcinoma. This photomicrograph illustrates the well-formed elongated tubules in a solid spindle cell background.

membrane antigen (EMA) (279,280). Immunohistochemical and ultrastructural features of neuroendocrine differentiation have been reported in these tumors (283).

## Treatment and Outcome

The designation "carcinoma" appears warranted by the presence of documented lymph node metastases in some cases, although follow-up information is limited.

## Tubulocystic Carcinoma

### Clinical Findings and Epidemiology

In the third series AFIP fascicle, Murphy et al (23), illustrated an unusual tumor with a multicystic gross appearance and striking mixture of tubules and micro/macro cysts, histologically. Similar cases were subsequently included in the low-grade collecting duct carcinoma paper of MacLennan et al (282). Although this is not currently recognized in the classification as a distinct entity, it appears that it will be recognized as such in the future (1,70,284).

### Pathology

#### Gross

These tumors are well circumscribed with a complex, multicystic appearance.

#### Microscopic

The tubules and cysts are lined by cuboidal to columnar cells with eosinophilic cytoplasm. Nuclei are uniform and contain nucleoli. Whether these truly derive from the collecting system is uncertain.

## Treatment and Outcome

There is limited information on outcome in these tumors. Cases with regional and bone metastases are reported (282,284).

## Urothelial Carcinoma

### Clinical Findings and Epidemiology

Urothelial carcinoma of the renal pelvis accounts for 5% to 10% of renal tumors in adults (285). Risk factors include advanced age, smoking, exposure to various toxic industrial compounds, analgesic abuse, and Balkan nephropathy (285). Synchronous or asynchronous association with urothelial tumors elsewhere in the urinary tract occurs in up to 50% of cases. It is more common in males (3 to 4:1) and occurs in an older age group (peak in the seventh decade) (286–290). Presentation is typically with gross hematuria (80%); flank pain (20%) and palpable mass are less common (10%).

Staging is based on a modification of the system applied to bladder cancer: pTIS, carcinoma in situ; pTa, noninvasive papillary tumors; pT1, invasion of lamina propria; pT2, superficial muscularis propria; pT3, deep muscularis propria/pelvic fat; and pT4, adjacent structures (including kidney)(163). Fujimoto et al (291) suggested that if involvement of the kidney is restricted to intratubular growth without stromal invasion, the prognosis remains favorable.

### Pathology

#### Gross

Most tumors are papillary, producing an exophytic mass with a fine arborizing surface. In up to one third of cases, there are multiple lesions in the renal pelvis (287). Less often, the tumor forms a solid mass that sometimes extensively infiltrates the kidney or renal sinus soft tissue (Fig. 29.27). In a few cases, there is little if any growth within the renal pelvis, but the kidney is diffusely permeated (291). Tumors with a sarcomatoid component frequently have an exophytic, polypoid appearance (292).

#### Microscopic

More than 95% of renal pelvic tumors are urothelial, and adenocarcinoma (293), squamous cell carcinoma (294), and small cell carcinoma (295) are rare. Most tumors are composed of papillary fronds covered by urothelium having variable degrees of anaplasia. Most authorities apply the World Health Organization grading system used in bladder tumors to these lesions (1). High-grade tumors show the same diverse histology associated with urothelial carcinoma of the bladder (Fig. 29.28); squamous or glandular differentiation is found in up to 20% of such tumors

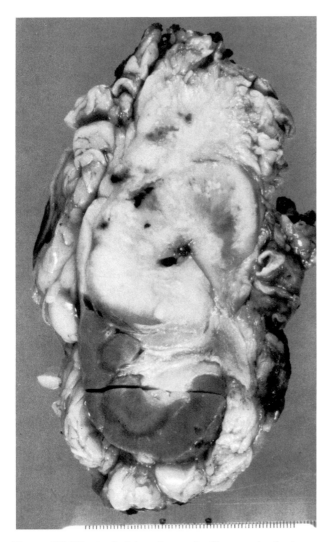

**Figure 29.27** Urothelial carcinoma. In this example, the tumor forms a large mass with extensive replacement of the upper pole of the kidney. Note the infiltrative margins and extension of the tumor into the perinephric fat.

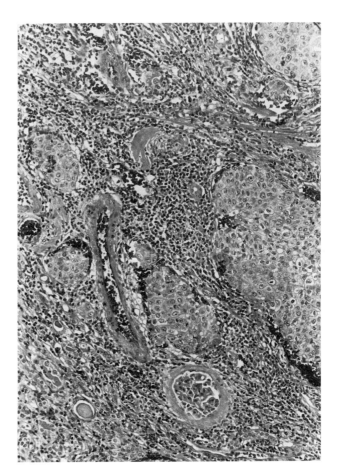

**Figure 29.28** Urothelial carcinoma (same case as Fig. 29.27). Histologically, this tumor is composed of well-circumscribed nests of cells diffusely permeating the renal parenchyma with a desmoplastic and inflammatory tissue response.

(288). These are diagnosed as urothelial carcinoma with squamous or glandular differentiation, and the diagnoses of squamous cell carcinoma and adenocarcinoma are reserved for tumors composed purely of those elements. Less often, areas of small cell or spindle cell differentiation are present (292,295). Rare examples with human chorionic gonadotropin production and syncytiotrophoblastic morphology have been described (296).

### Special Studies

Findings in urothelial carcinoma that help to distinguish it from renal cell carcinoma include mucin demonstrable with the mucicarmine stain (up to 50% of cases), or positive immunoreactivity for carcinoembryonic antigen (75%) or high–molecular-weight cytokeratin (50%) (297).

### Treatment and Outcome

The standard treatment is surgical resection by nephroureterectomy to prevent the development of additional tumors in the ureter. Overall, 5-year survival is in the range of 50%; however, this is strongly influenced by both stage and grade. Low-grade noninvasive tumors are associated with a greater than 90% 5-year survival, compared with less than 10% for advanced high-grade carcinomas (286–290).

### Unclassified Renal Cell Carcinoma

In approximately 5% to 7% of epithelial kidney tumors, classification into one of the categories defined above is extremely difficult (1,70,90,298). In most cases, the tumors are not undifferentiated, but have features that would fit into more than one category of classification. These include lesions with a well-defined differential diagnosis but for which a definitive conclusion cannot be reached. The most frequent problems in classification include the following: (a) separation of oncocytoma from chromophobe renal cell carcinoma; (b) the distinction of papillary renal cell carcinoma from clear cell renal cell carcinoma with pseudopapillary areas; and (c) the distinction of clear cell renal cell carcinoma from chromophobe renal cell carcinoma (298).

Another large group of these tumors are high-grade carcinomas or sarcomatoid carcinomas, in which the epithelial element cannot be recognized or classified. In sarcomatoid carcinomas, cases may have no identifiable epithelial element, with the diagnosis based on immunohistochemical or ultrastructural evidence of epithelial derivation. Tumors in these groups are associated with an aggressive clinical course (90,299). Additionally, carcinomas with mucin production, mixtures of epithelial and stromal elements, or unrecognizable cell types, not otherwise specified, are included here.

Unclassifiable renal tumors may not, necessarily, have an uncertain prognosis. The poorly differentiated and sarcomatoid carcinomas are predictably aggressive, whether or not they are included in a category of sarcomatoid renal cell carcinoma. Localized tumors lacking significant nuclear atypia are best considered to be low-grade malignancies. For other unusual tumors, pathologic features such as size, stage, and nuclear grade provide important clues to likely future events.

## Neuroendocrine Tumors

### Clinical Findings and Epidemiology

The full spectrum of neuroendocrine tumors—including carcinoid tumor (300–303), atypical carcinoid (304), and small cell carcinoma (305,306)—occurs in the kidney (307). Intrarenal pheochromocytoma (308,309) and neuroblastoma (310) have also been described. Several examples of primitive neuroectodermal tumor have been well documented (311,312). Small cell carcinoma is distinctly uncommon (295,306). Neuroendocrine tumors occur in older patients, show no gender predilection, present with hematuria and abdominal pain, and usually are advanced at diagnosis (295). Carcinoid syndrome and glucagon secretion have been reported (313,314).

### Pathology

#### Gross

Small cell carcinoma is large and bulky, with extensive necrosis and an infiltrative growth pattern. Some are located primarily within the renal parenchyma, whereas others have an epicenter in the renal pelvis. In most cases, it is impossible to be certain of the site of origin. Carcinoid tumors are well circumscribed, red-brown, and hemorrhagic.

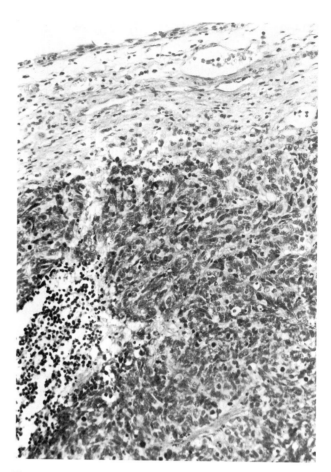

**Figure 29.29** Small cell carcinoma. The tumor is made up of loosely cohesive cells with hyperchromatic nuclei, inconspicuous nucleoli, nuclear molding, and scant cytoplasm. Attenuated urothelium of the renal pelvis is present at the top of the photomicrograph.

#### Microscopic

Histologically, these show similar features to neuroendocrine tumors elsewhere. Small cell carcinoma has small to large nuclei with finely distributed chromatin and inconspicuous or absent nucleoli. Cytoplasm is scant. There is prominent nuclear molding. Mitotic figures and individual cell necrosis are frequent (Fig. 29.29). A component of urothelial carcinoma may be present in cases arising in the renal pelvis, similar to small cell carcinoma elsewhere in the urothelial tract (315). Carcinoid tumors resemble such tumors elsewhere (316); in two such cases, the tumor was associated with teratoma (317,318).

#### Special Studies

Small cell carcinoma is usually cytokeratin-positive, with the characteristic cytoplasmic dotlike pattern of immunoreactivity associated with neuroendocrine carcinoma. Neuroendocrine markers such as neuron-specific enolase, chromogranin, and Leu-7 are demonstrable in about 50% of cases (306,316). Ultrastructural studies may show cytoplasmic processes and neurosecretory granules (306).

## Treatment and Outcome

To date, outcome has been poor, with 75% of reported patients dead of tumor, most within 5 years of diagnosis. Even carcinoid tumors have been associated with metastases (319,320). Primary treatment is surgical resection; the roles of radiation therapy and chemotherapy have not been defined.

# MESENCHYMAL NEOPLASMS

## Angiomyolipoma

### Clinical Findings and Epidemiology

Angiomyolipoma is a benign tumor of the kidney, typically composed of smooth muscle, fat, and thick-walled blood vessels. Previously, some have considered it to be a hamartoma, but genetic studies have shown it to be a clonal neoplastic proliferation (321). These tumors are believed to be derived from perivascular epithelioid cells (322). Approximately 50% are found as components of the tuberous sclerosis complex, and the remainder are sporadic (70,323–327). Between 50% and 80% of patients with tuberous sclerosis develop angiomyolipoma (328). In these patients, the tumors are diagnosed earlier (median 25 years), are smaller, and are less likely to be symptomatic, whereas sporadic cases present later (median, 45 years) with flank pain, mass, hematuria, or a combination of these. The most dangerous complication of angiomyolipoma is retroperitoneal hemorrhage (329).

Lymphangioleiomyomatosis of the lung occasionally occurs in association with angiomyolipoma (330–333). Imaging studies may be diagnostic, particularly computed tomography demonstrating fat within a renal tumor (334,335). Angiomyolipoma may also be present in regional lymph nodes or spleen and may extend into the renal vein. Patients with these findings have excellent outcomes, so these should not be misinterpreted as signs of malignancy (324,336,337). In contrast, the epithelioid variant has been shown to have malignant potential (338–340).

## Pathology

### Genetics

Angiomyolipoma is related to mutations in either the TSCI or *TSC2* genes (341).

### Gross

Angiomyolipoma is circumscribed but not encapsulated. Its cut surface has a variegated appearance (Fig. 29.30). Tumors composed predominantly of smooth muscle tend to have a fleshy, gray-white appearance, mimicking sarcoma or sarcomatoid carcinoma. Necrosis is uncommon, but hemorrhage may be extensive. In patients with tuberous sclerosis, the tumors are typically multiple, bilateral,

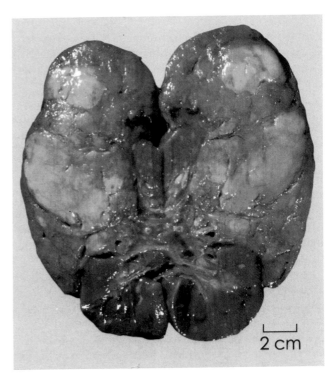

**Figure 29.30** Angiomyolipoma. Large, bulging tumor with a variegated appearance; note areas having a paler color corresponding to regions composed predominantly of fat.

and small, in contrast to sporadic cases that are single, unilateral, and large. Renal cell carcinoma occasionally occurs in the same kidney with angiomyolipoma (342,343).

### Microscopic

Angiomyolipoma has a tripartite composition of smooth muscle, fat, and thick-walled blood vessels in varying proportions (Fig. 29.31). When little fat is present, it may be difficult to decide whether the fat is an intrinsic part of the lesion or whether it represents invasion of perinephric fat by a spindle cell neoplasm. This is particularly problematic in lesions with predominance of smooth muscle when atypical features are present. Recognition of the thick-walled vessels is often the best clue to the true nature of the lesion. Atypical features such as nuclear pleomorphism, mitotic figures, and necrosis can be seen in angiomyolipoma (70,325). The smooth muscle can have an epithelioid appearance with abundant eosinophilic cytoplasm and eccentric large nuclei with prominent nucleoli (Fig. 29.32). Epithelioid angiomyolipoma is now recognized as a distinctive tumor that has malignant potential (338–340). Sarcomatous transformation, which is exceedingly rare, is indicated by the presence of unequivocal high-grade sarcoma (344).

### Special Studies

The smooth muscle component reacts with antibodies to vimentin, actin, and desmin; interestingly, it also reacts with antibodies to the melanoma-associated markers, including

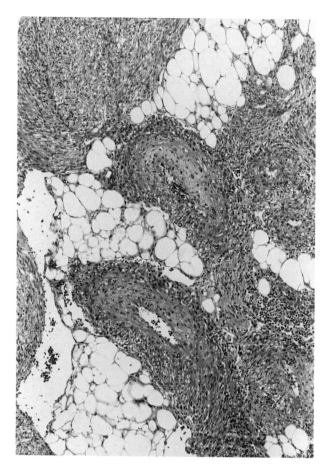

**Figure 29.31** Angiomyolipoma. Typical example with a mixture of smooth muscle, adipose tissue, and thick-walled blood vessels.

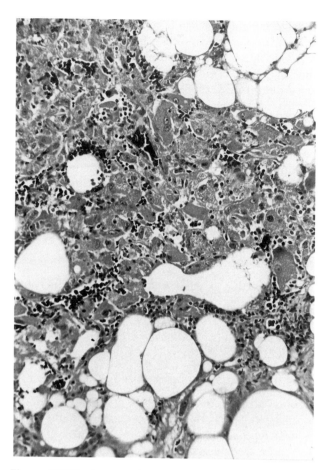

**Figure 29.32** Angiomyolipoma. In this angiomyolipoma, areas of the smooth muscle have a distinctly epithelioid morphology, with cells having abundant eosinophilic cytoplasm and large nuclei with prominent nucleoli.

HMB-45, MART1, and microphthalmia transcription factor (327,331,345–348), as do some of the other lesions of the tuberous sclerosis complex (349).

## Treatment and Outcome

Because angiomyolipoma is benign and can often be diagnosed radiographically because of its fat content, most are left in place unless they become symptomatic or exceed 4 cm in diameter (350). Leiomyosarcoma has arisen in angiomyolipoma only twice (344,351). Because of the potential for malignant behavior, epithelioid angiomyolipoma requires close clinical follow-up.

## Other Benign Mesenchymal Tumors

### Clinical Findings and Epidemiology

Mesenchymal tumors of almost every type have been reported as arising in the kidney (70,325), with leiomyoma and hemangioma being the most frequent (352–357). Other types include lymphangioma (358–361), lipoma (362), and the so-called capsuloma (363,364).

Smooth muscle neoplasms are the most common mesenchymal tumors of the adult kidney (352), but are rarely symptomatic (365). Hemangioma is rare, occurs mainly in adults, and has no gender predilection (353,355). It also occurs in association with the Klippel–Trenaunay and Sturge–Weber syndromes (366,367). Hematuria can be the presenting symptom, although most are asymptomatic.

## Pathology

### Gross

Leiomyoma is well circumscribed, gray-white, and has a bulging lobular cut surface. Necrosis and hemorrhage are absent. Hemangioma are single, small (less than 1 cm), and spongy red. The most frequent location of hemangioma is the renal medullary pyramids.

### Microscopic

Leiomyoma is composed of spindle-shaped cells with elongate nuclei and eosinophilic cytoplasm. The cells are arranged in intersecting fascicles. No established criteria reliably distinguish benign from malignant renal smooth muscle neoplasms. Most authors have stressed the absence of mitotic figures and nuclear pleomorphism (352,368). Grignon et al (325) indicated that the diagnosis of leiomyoma should be made cautiously; they considered large size, necrosis, nuclear pleomorphism, or one or more mitotic figures per 10 high-powered fields to be indicative of malignancy. In one series of primary renal sarcoma, a leiomyosarcoma with a mitotic rate of less than two per 10 high-power fields metastasized and caused the patient's death (369). The vascular spaces of hemangioma range from capillary to cavernous in size and are lined by benign endothelial cells.

## Treatment and Outcome

Surgical resection is curative for both leiomyoma and hemangioma.

## Primary Sarcoma

### Clinical Findings and Epidemiology

Sarcomas account for less than 1% of all kidney tumors in adults (325,369–372). Leiomyosarcoma is the most frequent type, making up approximately 50% of cases (369–372). Leiomyosarcoma develops in a younger age group than renal cell carcinoma, but occurs over a wide age range (369,372). The male-to-female ratio is roughly equal. There are no specific presenting symptoms. Abdominal or back pain, hematuria, and weight loss have been most frequent. Virtually all other types of sarcoma have been reported in the kidney (70,325). Among the more frequently described are liposarcoma (373,374), malignant fibrous histiocytoma (375–377), rhabdomyosarcoma (378), synovial sarcoma (379,380), and osteogenic sarcoma (381,382); vascular sarcomas also occur here (383).

## Pathology

### Gross

Most sarcomas are large, fleshy, and gray-white. Necrosis is often present. Leiomyosarcoma may be lobulated, bulging, and sharply circumscribed. Origin from the renal capsule or renal vein can be demonstrated in some cases.

### Microscopic

Leiomyosarcoma is characterized by intersecting fascicles of spindle cells with blunt-ended nuclei and eosinophilic cytoplasm. Nuclear pleomorphism and mitotic rate are variable (Fig. 29.33). Myxoid variants occur here. Grignon et al (369) recommended a diagnosis of leiomyosarcoma if there was necrosis, nuclear pleomorphism, or one or more

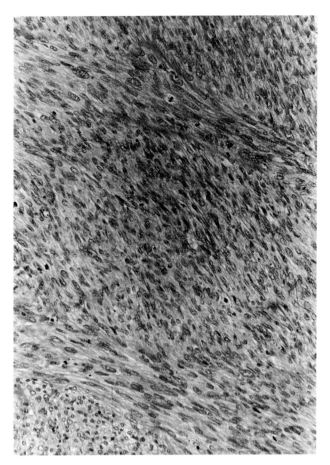

**Figure 29.33** Leiomyosarcoma. High-grade primary renal leiomyosarcoma composed of spindle-shaped cells in fascicles with frequent mitotic figures.

mitotic figures in 10 high-power fields of a smooth muscle tumor in the kidney.

### Special Studies

The results of immunohistochemical studies parallel those of sarcomas arising elsewhere. Vimentin, actin, and desmin should be positive in leiomyosarcoma. Nonreactivity for HMB-45 is useful in excluding angiomyolipoma (345,347,384). Although weak reactivity for cytokeratin can be present in smooth muscle tumors, it is usually negative. Primitive cell junctions, focal densities within groups of cytoplasmic microfilaments, pinocytotic vesicles along the cell membrane, and basal lamina are seen ultrastructurally.

### Treatment and Outcome

Treatment is primarily surgical, although given the poor prognosis, adjuvant chemotherapy may be appropriate (372). Outcome has been poor in the major reported series (369–372). The 3-year survival was 20% and the median survival was 18 months in the M.D. Anderson Cancer Center series (369).

## MISCELLANEOUS NEOPLASMS

### Cystic Nephroma

#### Clinical Findings and Epidemiology

Cystic nephroma is a tumor that occurs in adults and children (385). These cases are now considered to represent two distinct tumor types (1,70). Synonyms in common use are *multilocular cyst* (228) and *multilocular cystic nephroma* (386). In a review of 187 cases, Castillo et al (387) found a male predominance of nearly 2:1 in children younger than 2 years and a female predominance of more than 3:1 among adults.

#### Pathology

##### Gross

Cystic nephroma is a discrete globular mass that is contained by a fibrous capsule. Internally, it is composed of multiple locules with smooth linings and containing clear yellow fluid. The locules do not communicate with one another. The septa range from paper-thin to a few millimeters thick; solid areas are absent or scant.

##### Microscopic

The septa are composed of fibrous tissue of variable cellularity and may contain foci of calcification. Often the septa are densely collagenous. The septa may contain differentiated tubules (1,70). Usually the cysts are lined by flat or low cuboidal epithelium with little cytoplasm; sometimes the lining cells have a hobnail appearance (Fig. 29.34).

Most conditions that produce cysts in the kidneys are easily distinguished from cystic nephroma (388). Cystic Wilms' tumor and cystic renal cell carcinoma are the principal differential diagnostic considerations. Some authors have permitted foci of immature renal tissues, including blastema and tubules, in cystic nephroma, although some have considered these to be "cystic partially differentiated nephroblastoma." The predominance of females among adult patients, and the rarity of reports of blastema in the septa of tumors from adults, are evidence that cystic nephroma is a different entity from cystic partially differentiated nephroblastoma.

Multilocular cystic renal cell carcinoma differs from cystic nephroma in containing small populations of clear cells lining some of the locules and, occasionally, forming small collections in the septa (220). These cells are histologically identical to those of clear cell renal cell carcinoma.

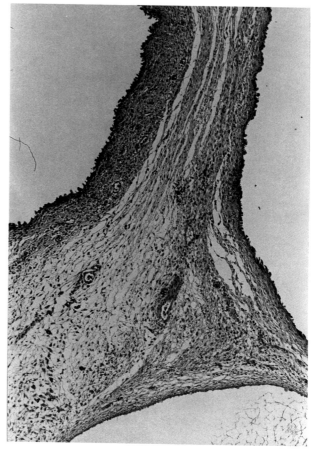

**Figure 29.34** Cystic nephroma. In this photomicrograph, the septae show variable cellularity with no normal renal elements being present. The cyst lining is a single cell layer, with some cells being flattened and others having a hobnail morphology.

### Treatment and Outcome

Cystic nephroma is benign and effectively treated by conservative surgery (387).

## Mixed Epithelial and Stromal Tumor

### Clinical Findings and Epidemiology

There have been reports of mixed epithelial and mesenchymal tumors in adults initially reported under the terms "cystic hamartoma of the renal pelvis" and "adult mesoblastic nephroma" (389–393). These have occurred more frequently in females (4 to 5:1) and over a broad age range. The descriptive term *mixed epithelial and stromal tumor* is now used in the current classification for this lesion (1,70). It is now believed that this lesion is unrelated to congenital mesoblastic nephroma (394). Because of the consistent expression of estrogen and progesterone receptors in the spindle cells, the possibility of a hormonal influence in the development of these neoplasms has been raised

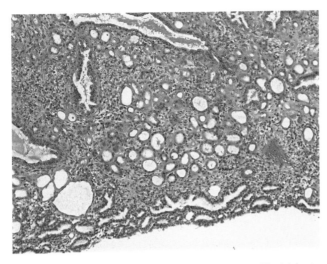

**Figure 29.35**  Mixed epithelial and stromal tumor. The biphasic nature of the tumor is illustrated. Note in particular the heterogeneous morphology of the epithelial element.

(392,393). Presentation has been similar to other renal neoplasms.

## Pathology

### Gross

Some tumors have been well circumscribed and others infiltrative; extensive growth into the renal pelvis, and even into the ureter, has been described. Most cases have a mixture of solid and cystic areas.

### Microscopic

The epithelial component in these tumors shows striking variability, from small tubules, to complex branching glandular formations, to microcyst and macrocyst formation (Fig 29.35). In some, there are leaflike arrangements resembling those seen in phyllodes tumors. Clear cells have also been noted in the tubular component of some cases. The mesenchymal component ranges from hypocellular and fibrotic to more cellular with fibroblastic and myofibroblastic foci to fairly cellular ovarianlike stroma. Smooth muscle differentiation, particular at the outer margin (capsule) can be prominent. A possibly related tumor, with predominantly smooth muscle stroma and a proliferative epithelial component, has been described under the name *benign angiomyoadenomatous tumor* (395).

### Special studies

The spindle cells are positive for vimentin, actin, and desmin. In most, the stromal cells express estrogen and progesterone receptors.

## Treatment and Outcome

To date, the reported cases have behaved in a benign fashion. There have been cases described that may represent a malignant counterpart with sarcomatous change in the mesenchymal component (396–398).

## Juxtaglomerular Cell Tumor

### Clinical Findings and Epidemiology

More than 50 cases of juxtaglomerular cell tumor have been reported since its discovery three decades ago (307,399–402). The tumor occurs in young adults and is more common in females; virtually all patients are hypertensive (307). Detection of elevated plasma renin levels by selective renal vein catheterization is diagnostic (403). No case of bilateral juxtaglomerular cell tumor has been reported.

### Pathology

#### Gross

Juxtaglomerular cell tumor is well circumscribed, small (less than 3 cm), and gray-white. Small cysts can be present.

#### Microscopic

The tumor is composed of small polygonal cells arranged in trabeculae in a myxoid stroma. The histology is, however, quite varied, and solid islands, tubules, cysts, and broad papillae (404) can all be seen (Fig. 29.36). Juxtaglomerular cell tumor is perhaps the most difficult renal tumor to diagnose in routine sections.

#### Special Studies

Renin can be demonstrated by immunohistochemistry, and characteristic rhomboid crystals are seen ultrastructurally (405). The tumors also express CD34 (401).

### Treatment and Outcome

Surgical resection results in cure of the hypertension. Juxtaglomerular cell tumor is benign, with no reported instance of recurrence or metastasis.

## Renomedullary Interstitial Cell Tumor

### Clinical Findings and Epidemiology

Renomedullary interstitial cell tumor is almost always an incidental finding (406). In one autopsy survey, it was identified in almost 50% of patients older than 20 years of age (407). It originates from the renomedullary interstitial cell, which is a specialized cell involved in blood pressure regulation.

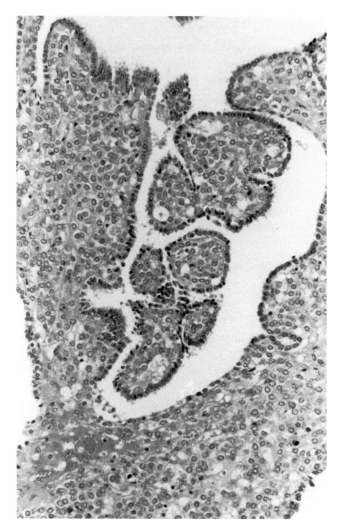

**Figure 29.36** Juxtaglomerular cell tumor. In this histologic variant, the tumor is composed of broad papillae filled with round to oval cells and covered by a columnar epithelium.

## Pathology

### Gross
The lesions are small and localized to the renal medulla, with most being less than 5 mm in diameter. They are well circumscribed, are gray-white, and do not bulge when cut.

### Microscopic
Renomedullary interstitial cell tumor is composed of stellate cells embedded in a loose fascicular stroma (Fig. 29.37). Amyloid may be present in the stroma (408).

## Treatment and Outcome

These are incidental benign lesions, and no specific treatment is required.

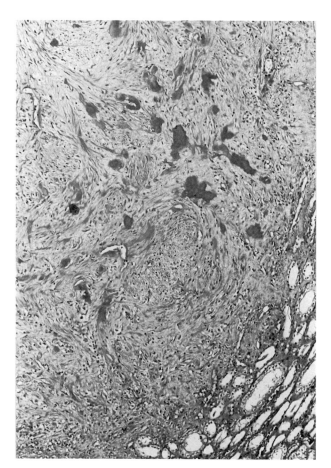

**Figure 29.37** Renomedullary interstitial cell tumor. The lesion is circumscribed but not encapsulated and is made up of spindle-shaped cells in a dense, collagenized stroma.

## Lymphoreticular and Hematopoietic Tumors

### Clinical Findings and Epidemiology

Malignant lymphoma infrequently presents as a renal mass, without detectable disease elsewhere (409–414). In most cases of renal involvement by lymphoma, however, systemic disease is discovered soon after the renal mass or the patient already is known to have lymphoma (415). In cases presenting as a renal mass, symptoms are similar to those of other kidney tumors.

### Pathology

#### Gross
Renal lymphoma appears relatively well circumscribed, but close inspection reveals infiltration at its edges. The tumor is soft, gray-white, and homogeneous. There may be a single mass or multiple nodules.

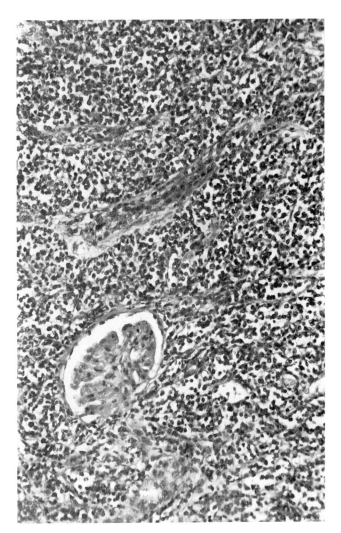

**Figure 29.38** Lymphoma. In this primary lymphoma of the kidney, the tumor is composed of sheets of small lymphocytes diffusely permeating the parenchyma and sparing some normal structures.

### Microscopic

Most characteristic is diffuse permeation of the renal interstitium by a monotonous population of lymphoid cells, with some degree of sparing of tubules and glomeruli (Fig. 29.38). Specific cytologic features depend on the type of lymphoma with large cell lymphoma of B-cell origin being most common (411). Rare examples of Hodgkin's disease (409) and plasmacytoma (416,417) have also been described.

### Special Studies

Immunohistochemistry reveals positive staining for leukocyte common antigen; in B-cell lymphoma, demonstration of clonality confirms the diagnosis. B- and T-cell gene rearrangement studies, as in lymphoma from any site, can be helpful.

## Treatment and Outcome

In most cases, the diagnosis is not made until after surgical resection. Additional treatment depends on the stage and histologic type.

## Metastases to the Kidney

### Clinical Findings and Epidemiology

In autopsy studies, the kidneys are involved by metastases in up to 7.2% of patients dying with cancer (418,419), with lung being the most common primary site. Much less frequently, tumors present with renal metastasis as the primary manifestation.

## Pathology

### Gross
Metastases can be single or multiple with no specific gross features.

### Microscopic
The histology of the tumor reflects its site of origin. In some cases, only microscopic involvement, limited to glomeruli, is present (420). In the latter instance, presentation with proteinuria or acute renal failure may result (178,421). Hyperplasia of Bowman's capsule, which rarely occurs in association with carcinoma elsewhere, should not be mistaken for metastasis (422).

## Treatment and Outcome

As indicated, metastatic involvement of the kidney most often occurs late in the course of the disease. However, in some cases, surgical resection of cancer metastatic to the kidney is indicated to treat intractable hematuria.

## REFERENCES

1. Eble JN, Sauter G, Epstein JI, Sesterhenn IA, eds. World Health Organization Classification of Tumours. Pathology and Genetics of Tumours of the Urinary System and Male Genital Organs. Lyon, France: IARC Press, 2004.
2. Hrabovsky EE, Othersen HB Jr, de Lorimier A, et al. Wilms' tumor in the neonate: A report from the National Wilms' Tumor Study. J Pediatr Surg 1986;21:385.
3. Breslow N, Beckwith JB, Ciol M, Sharples K. Age distribution of Wilms' tumor: Report from the National Wilms' Tumor Study. Cancer Res 1988;48:1653.
4. Lemerle J, Tournade M-F, Gerard-Marchant R, et al. Wilms' tumor: Natural history and prognostic factors. A retrospective study of 248 cases treated at the Institut Gustave-Roussy 1952–1967. Cancer 1976;37:2557.
5. Blute ML, Kelalis PP, Offord KP, et al. Bilateral Wilms' tumor. J Urol 1987;138:968.

6. Breslow NE, Beckwith JB. Epidemiological features of Wilms' tumor: Results of the National Wilms' Tumor Study. J Natl Cancer Inst 1982;68:429.

7. Heppe RK, Koyle MA, Beckwith JB. Nephrogenic rests in Wilms' tumor patients with the Drash syndrome. J Urol 1991;145:1225.

8. Sotelo-Avila C, Gonzalez-Crussi F, Fowler JW. Complete and incomplete forms of Beckwith-Wiedemann syndrome: Their oncogenic potential. J Pediatr 1980;96:47.

9. Arrigo S, Beckwith JB, Sharples K, et al. Better survival after combined modality care for adults with Wilms' tumor: A report from the National Wilms' Tumor Study. Cancer 1990;66:827.

10. Huser J, Grignon DJ, Ro JY, et al. Adult Wilms' tumor: A clinicopathologic study of 11 cases. Mod Pathol 1990;3:321.

11. Eble JN. Kidney. In: Henson DE, Albores-Saavedra J, eds. Pathology of Incipient Neoplasia. Philadelphia: WB Saunders, 1993:401.

12. Joshi VV. Cystic partially differentiated nephroblastoma: An entity in the spectrum of infantile renal neoplasia. Perspect Pediatr Pathol 1979;5:217.

13. Joshi VV, Banerjee AK, Yadav K, Pathak IC. Cystic partially differentiated nephroblastoma, a clinicopathologic entity in the spectrum of infantile renal neoplasia. Cancer 1977;40:789.

14. Eble JN. Neoplasms of the kidney. In: Bostwick DG, Eble JN, eds. Urologic Surgical Pathology. St Louis, MO: Mosby–Yearbook, 1996.

15. Grimes MM, Wolff M, Wolf JA, et al. Ganglion cells in metastatic Wilms' tumor: Review of a histogenetic controversy. Am J Surg Pathol 1982;6:565.

16. Cummins GE, Cohen D. Cushing's syndrome secondary to ACTH-secreting Wilms' tumor. J Pediatr Surg 1974;9:535.

17. Fetissof F, Dubois MP, Robert M, Jobard P. Néphroblastome avec cellules endocrines: Etude immunohistochimique. Ann Pathol 1985;5:279.

18. Beckwith JB. Wilms' tumor and other renal tumors of childhood: A selective review from the National Wilms' Tumor Study Pathology Center. Hum Pathol 1983;14:481.

19. Eble JN. Fetal rhabdomyomatous nephroblastoma. J Urol 1983;130:541.

20. Wigger HJ. Fetal rhabdomyomatous nephroblastoma. A variant of Wilms' tumor. Hum Pathol 1976;7:613.

21. Kotiloglu E, Kale G, Sevinir B, et al. Teratoid Wilms' tumor: A unilateral case. Tumori 1994;80:61.

22. Magee JF, Ansari S, McFadden DE, Dimmick J. Teratoid Wilms' tumour: A report of two cases. Histopathology 1992;20:427.

23. Murphy WM, Beckwith JB, Farrow GM. Atlas of Bladder, and Related Urinary Structures. Washington, DC: Armed Forces Institute of Pathology,1994.

24. Bonadio JF, Storer B, Norkool P, et al. Anaplastic Wilms' tumor: Clinical and pathologic studies. J Clin Oncol 1985;3:513.

25. Breslow NE, Palmer NF, Hill LR, et al. Wilms' tumor: Prognostic factors for patients without metastases at diagnosis: Results of the National Wilms' Tumor Study. Cancer 1978;41:1577.

26. Beckwith JB. Renal neoplasms of childhood. In: Sternberg SS, ed. Diagnostic Surgical Pathology. New York: Raven Press, 1994:1741.

27. Marsden HB, Lawler W. Primary renal tumours in the first year of life: A population based review. Virchows Arch 1983;399:1.

28. Blank E, Neerhout RC, Burry KA. Congenital mesoblastic nephroma and polyhydramnios. JAMA 1978;240:1504.

29. Favara BE, Johnson W, Ito J. Renal tumors in the neonatal period. Cancer 1968;22:845.

30. Kay S, Pratt CB, Salzberg AM. Hamartoma (leiomyomatous type) of the kidney. Cancer 1966;19:1825.

31. Bolande RP. Congenital mesoblastic nephroma of infancy. Perspect Pediatr Pathol 1973;1:227.

32. Rubin BP, Chen, C-J, Morgan TW, et al. Congenital mesoblastic nephroma t(12;15) is associated with ETV6-NTRK3 gene fusion; cytogenetic and molecular relationship to congenital (infantile) fibrosarcoma. Am J Pathol 1998;153:1451.

33. Argani P, Fritsch M, Kadkol SS, et al. Detection of the ETV6-NTRK3 chimeric RNA of infantile fibrosarcoma/cellular congenital mesoblastic nephroma in paraffin-embedded tissue: Application to challenging pediatric renal stromal tumors. Mod Pathol 2000;13:29.

34. Sandberg AA, Bridge JA. Updates on the cytogenetics and molecular genetics of bone and soft tissue tumors: Congenital (infantile) fibrosarcoma and mesoblastic nephroma. Cancer Genet Cytogenet 2002;132:1.

35. Pettinato G, Manivel JC, Wick MR, Dehner LP. Classical and cellular (atypical) congenital mesoblastic nephroma: A clinicopathologic, ultrastructural, immunohistochemical, and flow cytometric study. Hum Pathol 1989;20:682.

36. Beckwith JB. Mesenchymal renal neoplasms in infancy revisited. J Pediatr Surg 1974;9:803.

37. Chan HSL, Cheng M-Y, Mancer K, et al. Congenital mesoblastic nephroma: A clinicoradiologic study of 17 cases representing the pathologic spectrum of the disease. J Pediatr 1987;111:64.

38. Howell CG, Othersen HB, Kiviat NE, et al. Therapy and outcome in 51 children with mesoblastic nephroma: A report of the National Wilms' Tumor Study. J Pediatr Surg 1982;17:826.

39. Sandstedt B, Delemarre JFM, Krul EJ, Tournade MF. Mesoblastic nephromas: A study of 29 tumours from the SIOP nephroblastoma file. Histopathology 1985;9:741.

40. Gonzalez-Crussi F, Sotelo-Avila C, Kidd JM. Malignant mesenchymal nephroma of infancy: Report of a case with pulmonary metastases. Am J Surg Pathol 1980;4:185.

41. Joshi VV, Kasznica J, Walters TR. Atypical mesoblastic nephroma. Arch Pathol Lab Med 1986;110:100.

42. Beckwith JB, Weeks DA. Congenital mesoblastic nephroma. When should we worry? Arch Pathol Lab Med 1986;110:98.

43. Gormley TS, Skoog SJ, Jones RV, Maybee D. Cellular congenital mesoblastic nephroma: What are the options. J Urol 1989;142:479.

44. Heidelberger KP, Ritchey ML, Dauser RC, et al. Congenital mesoblastic nephroma metastatic to the brain. Cancer 1993;72:2499.

45. Argani P, Perlman EJ, Breslow NE, et al. Clear cell sarcoma of the kidney: A review of 351 cases from the National Wilms Tumor Study Group Pathology Center. Am J Surg Pathol 2000;24:4.

46. Sotelo-Avila C, Gonzalez-Crussi F, Sadowinski S, et al. Clear cell sarcoma of the kidney: A clinicopathologic study of 21 patients with long-term follow-up evaluation. Hum Pathol 1986;16:1219.

47. Marsden HB, Lawler W. Bone metastasizing renal tumour of childhood: Histopathological and clinical review of 38 cases. Virchows Archiv A Pathol Anat Histol 1980;387:341.

48. Marsden HB, Lawler W. Bone-metastasizing renal tumour of childhood. Br J Cancer 1978;38:437.

49. Beckwith JB, Palmer NF. Histopathology and prognosis of Wilms' tumor: Results from the First National Wilms' Tumor Study. Cancer 1978;41:1937.

50. Palmer NF, Sutow W. Clinical aspects of the rhabdoid tumor of the kidney: A report of the National Wilms' Tumor Study Group. Med Pediatr Oncol 1983;11:242.

51. Weeks DA, Beckwith JB, Mierau GW, Luckey DW. Rhabdoid tumor of kidney: A report of 111 cases from the National Wilms' Tumor Study Pathology Center. Am J Surg Pathol 1989;13:439.

52. Bonnin JM, Rubinstein LJ, Palmer, Beckwith JB. The association of embryonal tumors originating in the kidney and in the brain. A report of seven cases. Cancer 1984;54:2137.

53. Mayes LC, Kasselberg AG, Roloff JS, Lukens JN. Hypercalcemia associated with immunoreactive parathyroid hormone in a malignant rhabdoid tumor of the kidney (rhabdoid Wilms' tumor). Cancer 1984;54:882.

54. Haas JE, Palmer NF, Weinberg AG, Beckwith JB. Ultrastructure of malignant rhabdoid tumor of the kidney: A distinctive renal tumor of children. Hum Pathol 1981;12:646.

55. Davis CJ Jr, Barton JH, Sesterhenn IA, Mostofi FK. Metanephric adenoma. Clinicopathological study of fifty patients. Am J Surg Pathol 1995;19:1101.

56. Jones EC, Pins M, Dickersin GR, Young RH. Metanephric adenoma of the kidney. A clinicopathological, immunohistochemical, flow cytometric, cytogenetic, and electron microscopic study of seven cases. Am J Surg Pathol 1995;19:615.

57. Argani P. Metanephric neoplasms: The hyperdifferentiated, benign end of the Wilms tumor spectrum? Clin Lab Med 2005; 25:379.

58. Brunelli M, Eble JN, Zhang S, et al. Metanephric adenoma lacks the gains of chromosomes 7 and 17 and loss of Y that are typical of papillary renal cell carcinoma and papillary adenoma. Mod Pathol 2003;16:1060.

59. Arroyo MR, Green DM, Perlman EJ, et al. The spectrum of metanephric adenofibroma and related lesions: Clinicopathologic study of 25 cases from the National Wilms Tumors Study Group Pathology Center. Am J Surg Pathol 2001;25:433.

60. Argani P, Beckwith JB. Metanephric stromal tumor: Report of 31 cases of a distinctive pediatric renal neoplasm. Am J Surg Pathol 2000;24:917.

61. Palese MA, Ferrer F, Perlman E, Gearhart JP. Metanephric stromal tumor: A rare benign pediatric renal mass. Urol 2001;58:462.

62. Muir TE, Cheville JC, Lager DJ. Metanephric adenoma, nephrogenic rests, and Wilms' tumor: A histologic and immunophenotypic comparison. Am J Surg Pathol 2001;25:1290.

63. Paner GP, Turk TM, Clark JI, et al. Passive seeding in metanephric adenoma: A review of pseudometastatic lesions in perinephric lymph nodes. Arch Pathol Lab Med 2005;129:1317.

64. Argani P, Ladanyi M. Translocation carcinomas of the kidney. Clin Lab Med 2005;25:363.

65. Bruder E, Passera O, Harms D, et al. Morphologic and molecular characterization of renal cell carcinoma in children and young adults. Am J Surg Pathol 2004;28:1117.

66. Argani P, Lal P, Hutchinson B, et al. Aberrant nuclear immunoreactivity for TFE3 in neoplasm with TFE3 gene fusions: A sensitive and specific immunohistochemical assay. Am J Surg Pathol 2003;27:750.

67. Eble JN. Mucinous tubular and spindle cell carcinoma and postneuroblastoma carcinoma: Newly recognised entities in the renal cell carcinoma family. Pathology 2003;35:499.

68. Medeiros LJ, Palmedo G, Krigman HR, et al. Oncocytoid renal cell carcinoma after neuroblastoma: A report of four cases of a distinct clinicopathologic entity. Am J Surg Pathol 1999;23:772.

69. Koyle MA, Hatch DA, Furness PD 3rd, et al. Long-term urologic complications in survivors younger than 15 months of advanced stage abdominal neuroblastoma. J Urol 2001;166:1455.

70. Murphy WM, Grignon DJ, Perlman E. Tumors of the Kidney, Bladder, and Related Urinary Structures, 4th series fascicle. Washington, DC: Armed Forces Institute of Pathology, 2004.

71. Kovacs G. Molecular differential pathology of renal cell tumours. Histopathology 1993;22:1.

72. Thoenes W, Störkel S, Rumpelt H-J. Histopathology and classification of renal cell tumors (adenomas, oncocytomas and carcinomas). The basic cytological and histopathological elements and their use for diagnostics. Pathol Res Pract 1986;181:125.

73. Aso Y, Homma Y. A survey on incidental renal cell carcinoma in Japan. J Urol 1992;147:340.

74. Levine E, Huntrakoon M, Wetzel LH. Small renal neoplasms: Clinical, pathologic, and imaging features. AJR Am J Roentgenol 1989;153:69.

75. Thompson IM, Peek M. Improvement in survival of patients with renal cell carcinoma: The role of the serendipitously detected tumor. J Urol 1988;140:487.

76. Newcomb WD. The search for truth, with special reference to the frequency of gastric ulcer-cancer and the origin of Grawitz tumours of the kidney. Proc R Soc Med 1936;30:113.

77. Xipell JM. The incidence of benign renal nodules (a clinicopathologic study). J Urol 1971;106:503.

78. Eble JN, Warfel K. Early human renal cortical epithelial neoplasia [Abstract]. Mod Pathol 1991;4:45A.

79. Hughson MD, Buchwald D, Fox M. Renal neoplasia and acquired cystic kidney disease in patients receiving long-term dialysis. Arch Pathol Lab Med 1986;110:592.

80. Ishikawa I, Saito Y, Nakamura M, et al. Fifteen-year follow-up of acquired renal cystic disease—a gender difference. Nephron 1997;75:315.

81. Brunelli M, Eble JN, Zhang S, et al. Gains of chromosomes 7, 17, 12, 16, and 20 and loss of Y occur in the evolution of papillary

renal cell neoplasia: A fluorescent in situ hybridization study. Mod Pathol 2003;16:1053.

82. Bell ET. Renal Diseases, 2nd ed. Philadelphia: Lea & Febiger, 1950.

83. Murphy GP, Mostofi FK. Histologic assessment and clinical prognosis of renal adenoma. J Urol 1970;103:31.

84. Pfannkuch F, Leistenschneider W, Nagel R. Problems of assessment in the surgery of renal adenomas. J Urol 1981;125:95.

85. Dechet CR, Sebo T, Farrow G, et al. Prospective analysis of intraoperative frozen needle biopsy of solid renal masses in adults. J Urol 1999;162:1282.

86. Fergany A, Hafez KS, Novick AC. Long-term results of nephron sparing surgery for localized renal cell carcinoma: 10-year followup. J Urol 2000;163:442.

87. Lee C, Katz J, Shi W, et al. Surgical management of renal tumors 4 cm or less in a contemporary cohort. J Urol 2000;163:730.

88. Klein MJ, Valensi QJ. Proximal tubular adenomas of kidney with so-called oncocytic features. A clinicopathologic study of 13 cases of a rarely reported neoplasm. Cancer 1976;38:906.

89. Amin MB, Crotty TB, Tickoo SK, Farrow GM. Renal oncocytoma: A reappraisal of morphologic features with clinicopathologic findings in 80 cases. Am J Surg Pathol 1997;21:1.

90. Amin MB, Tamboli P, Javidan J, et al. Prognostic impact of histologic subtyping of adult renal epithelial neoplasms: An experience of 405 cases. Am J Surg Pathol 2002;26:281.

91. Davis CJ Jr, Mostofi FK, Sesterhenn IA, Ho CK. Renal oncocytoma; clinicopathological study of 166 patients. J Urogenital Pathol 1991;1:41.

92. Pavlovich CP, Walther MM, Eyler RA, et al. Renal tumors in the Birt-Hogg-Dube syndrome. Am J Surg Pathol 2002;26:1542.

93. Ambos MA, Bosniak MA, Valensi QJ, et al. Angiographic patterns in renal oncocytomas. Radiology 1978;129:615.

94. Weiner SN, Bernstein RG. Renal oncocytoma: Angiographic features of two cases. Radiology 1977;125:633.

95. Brauch H, Tory K, Linehan WM, et al.: Molecular analysis of the short arm of chromosome 3 in five renal oncocytomas. J Urol 1990;143:622.

96. Füzesi L, Gunawan B, Braun S, Boeckmann W. Renal oncocytoma with a translocation t (9;11) (p23;q13). J Urol 1994;152:471.

97. Morra MN, Das S. Renal oncocytoma: A review of histogenesis, histopathology, diagnosis, and treatment. J Urol 1993;150:295.

98. Presti JC Jr, Rao PH, Chen Q, et al. Histopathological, cytogenetic, and molecular characterization of renal cortical tumors. Cancer Res 1991;51:1544.

99. Lyzak JS, Farhood A, Verani R. Intracytoplasmic lumina in a case of bilaterally multifocal renal oncocytomas. Arch Pathol Lab Med 1994;118:275.

100. Störkel S, Pannen B, Thoenes W, et al. Intercalated cells as a probable source for the development of renal oncocytoma. Virchows Archiv B-Cell Pathol Incl Mol Pathol 1988;56:185.

101. Mead GO, Thomas LR Jr, Jackson JG. Renal oncocytoma: Report of a case with bilateral multifocal oncocytomas. Clin Imaging 1990;14:231.

102. Warfel KA, Eble JN. Renal oncocytomatosis. J Urol 1982;127:1179.

103. Shin LK, Badler RL, Bruno FM, et al. Radiology—Pathology conference: Bilateral renal oncocytoma. J Clin Imaging 2004;28:344.

104. Tickoo SK, Reuter VE, Amin MB, et al. Renal oncocytosis: A morphologic study of fourteen cases. Am J Surg Pathol 1999;23:1094.

105. Eble JN, Hull MT. Morphologic features of renal oncocytoma: A light and electron microscopic study. Hum Pathol 1984;15:1054.

106. Kragel PJ, Williams J, Emory TS, Merino MJ. Renal oncocytoma with cylindromatous changes: Pathologic features and histogenetic significance. Mod Pathol 1990;3:277.

107. Ogden BW, Beckman EN, Rodriguez FH Jr. Multicystic renal oncocytoma. Arch Pathol Lab Med 1987;111:485.

108. Holthöfer H. Renal oncocytoma: Immuno- and carbohydrate histochemical characterization. Virchows Archiv 1987;410:509.

109. Pitz S, Moll R, Störkel S, Thoenes W. Expression of intermediate filament proteins in subtypes of renal cell carcinomas and in renal oncocytomas. Distinction of two classes of renal cell tumors. Lab Invest 1987;56:642.

110. Wu SL, Kothari P, Wheeler TM, et al. Cytokeratins 7 and 20 immunoreactivity in chromophobe renal cell carcinomas and renal oncocytomas. Mod Pathol 2002;15:712.

111. Skinnider BF, Folpe AL, Hennigar RA, et al. Distribution of cytokeratins and vimentin in adult renal neoplasms and normal renal tissue: Potential utility of a cytokeratin antibody panel in the differential diagnosis of renal tumors. Am J Surg Pathol 2005;29:747.

112. Pan CC, Chen PC, Ho DM. The diagnostic utility of MOC31, BerEP4, RCC marker and CD10 in the classification of renal cell carcinoma and renal oncocytoma: An immunohistochemical analysis of 328 cases. Histopathology 2004;45:452.

113. DeLong WH, Sakr W, Grignon DJ. Chromophobe renal cell carcinoma: A comparative histochemical and immunohistochemical study. J Urol Pathol 1996;4:1.

114. Tickoo SK, Amin MB. Zarbo RJ. Colloidal iron staining in renal epithelial neoplasms including chromophobe renal cell carcinoma: Emphasis on technique and patterns of staining. Am J Surg Pathol 1998;22:419.

115. Eble JN, Hull MT. Glycoconjugate expression in human renal oncocytomas. Arch Pathol Lab Med 1988;112:805.

116. Tickoo SK, Lee MW, Eble JN, et al. Ultrastructural observations on mitochondria and microvesicles in renal oncocytoma, chromophobe renal cell carcinoma, and eosinophilic variant of conventional (clear cell) renal cell carcinoma. Am J Surg Pathol 2000;24:1247.

117. Jockle GA, Toker C, Shamsuddin AM. Metastatic renal oncocytic neoplasm with benign histologic appearance. Urology 1987;30:79.

118. Lewi HJE, Alexander CA, Fleming S. Renal oncocytoma. Br J Urol 1986;58:12.

119. Thoenes W, Storkel S, Rumpelt H-J. Human chromophobe cell renal carcinoma. Virchows Archiv B-Cell Pathol Incl Mol Pathol 1985;48:207.

120. Lee CT, Katz J, Fearn PA, Russo P. Mode of presentation of renal cell carcinoma provides prognostic information. Urol Oncol 2002;7:135.

121. Chisholm GD, Roy RR. The systemic effects of malignant renal tumours. Br J Urol 1971;43:687.

122. Dönmez T, Kale M, Özyürek Y, Atalay H. Erythrocyte sedimentation rates in patients with renal cell carcinoma. Eur Urol 1992;21(suppl):51.

123. Sufrin G, Mirand EA, Moore RH, et al. Hormones in renal cancer. J Urol 1977;117:433.

124. Cherukuri SV, Johenning PW, Ram MD. Systemic effects of hypernephroma. Urology 1977;10:93.

125. Vanatta PR, Silva FG, Taylor WE, Costa JC. Renal cell carcinoma and systemic amyloidosis: Demonstration of AA protein and review of the literature. Hum Pathol 1983;14:195.

126. Laski ME, Vugrin D. Paraneoplastic syndromes in hypernephroma. Semin Nephrol 1987;7:123.

127. Sufrin G, Chasan S, Golio A, Murphy GP. Paraneoplastic and serologic syndromes of renal adenocarcinoma. Semin Urol 1989; 7:158.

128. Fahn H-J, Lee Y-H, Chen M-T, et al. The incidence and prognostic significance of humoral hypercalcemia in renal cell carcinoma. J Urol 1991;145:248.

129. Steffens J, Bock R, Braedel HU, et al. Renin producing renal cell carcinomas—clinical and experimental investigations on a special form of renal hypertension. Urol Res 1992;20:111.

130. Golde DW, Schambelan M, Weintraub BD, Rosen SW. Gonadotropin-secreting renal carcinoma. Cancer 1974;33:1048.

131. Stanisic TH, Donovan J. Prolactin secreting renal cell carcinoma. J Urol 1986;136:85.

132. Melnick SJ, Amazon K, Dembrow V. Metastatic renal cell carcinoma presenting as a parotid tumor: A case report with immunohistochemical findings and review of the literature. Hum Pathol 1989;20:195.

133. Serretta V, Pavone C, Messina G, et al. Vaginal metastasis from renal cell carcinoma: The role of electron microscopy. Eur Urol 1989;16:78.

134. Kantor AF. Current concepts in the epidemiology and etiology of primary renal cell carcinoma. J Urol 1977;117:415.

135. Jemal A, Murray T, Ward E, et al. Cancer statistics, 2005. CA Cancer J Clin 2005;55:10.

136. Leuschner I, Harms D, Schmidt D. Renal cell carcinoma in children: Histology, immunohistochemistry, and follow-up of 10 cases. Med Pediatr Oncol 1991;19:33.

137. Levinson AK, Johnson DE, Strong LC, et al. Familial renal cell carcinoma: Hereditary or coincidental? J Urol 1990;144:849.

138. Gemmill RM, West JD, Boldog F, et al. The hereditary renal cell carcinoma 3;8 translocation fuses FHIT to a patched-related gene, TRC8. Proc Natl Acad Sci U S A 1998;95:9572.

139. Teh BT, Giraud S, Sari NF, et al. Familial non-VHL non-papillary clear-cell renal cancer. Lancet 1997;349:848.

140. Toro JR, Glenn G, Duray P, et al. Birt-Hogg-Dube syndrome: A novel marker of kidney neoplasia. Arch Dermatol 1999; 135:1195.

141. Kiuru M, Launonen V, Hietala M, et al. Familial cutaneous leiomyomatosis is a two-hit condition associated with renal cell cancer of characteristic histopathology. Am J Pathol 2001; 159:825.

142. Launonen V, Vierimaa O, Kiuru M, et al. Inherited susceptibility to uterine leiomyomas and renal cell cancer. Proc Natl Acad Sci U S A 2001;98:3387.

143. Haibach H, Burns TW, Carlson HE, et al. Multiple hamartoma syndrome (Cowden's disease) associated with renal cell carcinoma and primary neuroendocrine carcinoma of the skin (Merkel cell carcinoma). Am J Clin Pathol 1992;97:705.

144. Malchoff CD, Sarfarazi M, Tendler B, et al. Papillary thyroid carcinoma associated with papillary renal neoplasia: Genetic linkage analysis of a distinct heritable tumor syndrome. J Clin Endocrinol Metab 2000;85:1758.

145. La Vecchia C, Negri E, D'Avanzo B, Franceschi S. Smoking and renal cell carcinoma. Cancer Res 1990;50:5231.

146. Flaherty KT, Fuchs CS, Colditz GA, et al. A prospective study of body mass index, hypertension and smoking and the risk of renal cell carcinoma (United States). Cancer Causes Control 2005;16:1099.

147. Asal NR, Risser DR, Kadamani S, et al. Risk factors in renal cell carcinoma. I. Methodology, demographics, tobacco, beverage use, and obesity. Cancer Detect Prev 1988;11:359.

148. Wynder EL, Mabuchi K, Whitmore WF Jr. Epidemiology of adenocarcinoma of the kidney. J Natl Cancer Inst 1974;53:1619.

149. McLaughlin JK, Blot WJ, Mehl ES, Fraumeni JF Jr. Relation of analgesic use to renal cancer: Population-based findings. NCI Monogr 1985;69:217.

150. Pesch B, Haerting J, Ranft U, et al. Occupational risk factors for renal cell carcinoma: Agent-specific results from a case control study in Germany. Int J Epidemiol 2000;29:1014.

151. McLaughlin JK, Blot WJ, Mehl ES, et al. Petroleum-related employment and renal cell cancer. J Occup Med 1985;27:672.

152. Sharpe CR, Rochon JE, Adam JM, Suissa S. Case-control study of hydrocarbon exposures in patients with renal cell carcinoma. Can Med Assoc J 1989;140:1309.

153. Maher ER, Yates JRW, Harries R, et al. Clinical features and natural history of von Hippel-Lindau disease. Q J Med 1990;77:1151.

154. Solomon D, Schwartz A. Renal pathology in von Hippel-Lindau disease. Hum Pathol 1988;19:1072.

155. Horton WA, Wong V, Eldridge R. Von Hippel-Lindau disease: Clinical and pathological manifestations in nine families with 50 affected members. Arch Intern Med 1976;136:769.

156. Bernstein J, Robbins TO. Renal involvement in tuberous sclerosis. Ann N Y Acad Sci 1991;615:36.

157. Washecka R, Hanna M. Malignant renal tumors in tuberous sclerosis. Urology 1991;37:340.

158. Ahuja S, Loffler W, Wegener O-H, Ernst H. Tuberous sclerosis with angiomyolipoma and metastasized hypernephroma. Urology 1986;28:413.

159. Gutierrez OH, Burgener FA, Schwartz S. Coincidental renal cell carcinoma and renal angiomyolipoma in tuberous sclerosis. AJR Am J Roentgenol 1979;132:848.

160. Melicow MM, Gile HH. A hypernephroma in a polycystic kidney: Review of literature and report of a case. J Urol 1940;43:767.

161. Matson MA, Cohen EP. Acquired cystic kidney disease: Occurrence, prevalence and renal cancers. Medicine 1990;69:217.

162. Sule N, Yakupoglu U, Shen SS, et al. Calcium oxalate deposition in renal carcinoma associated with acquired cystic kidney disease: A comprehensive study. Am J Surg Pathol 2005;29:443.

163. American Joint Committee on Cancer. AJCC Cancer Staging Manual, 6th ed. Philadelphia: Lippincott-Raven, 2002.

164. Gettman MT, Blute ML, Spotts B, et al. Pathologic staging of renal cell carcinoma: Significance of tumor classification with the 1997 TNM staging system. Cancer 2001;91:354.

165. Ficarra V, Schips L, Guille F, et al. Multiinstitutional European validation of the 2002 TNM staging system in conventional and papillary localized renal cell carcinoma. Cancer 2005;104:968.

166. Frank I, Blute ML, Leibovich BC, et al. Independent validation of the 2002 American Joint Committee on Cancer primary tumor classification for renal cell carcinoma using a large single institution cohort. J Urol 2005;173:1889.

167. Bonsib SM, Gibson D, Mhoon M, Greene GF. Renal sinus involvement in renal cell carcinoma. Am J Surg Pathol 2000;24:451.

168. Bonsib SM. The renal sinus is the principal invasive pathway: A prospective study of 100 renal cell carcinomas. Am J Surg Pathol 2004;28:1594.

169. Giuliani L, Giberti C, Martorana G, Rovida S. Radical extensive surgery for renal cell carcinoma: Long-term results and prognostic factors. J Urol 1990;143:468.

170. Herrlinger A, Schrott KM, Sigel A, Giedl J. Results of 381 transabdominal radical nephrectomies for renal cell carcinoma with partial and complete en-bloc lymph-node dissection. World J Urol 1984;2:114.

171. Studer UE, Scherz S, Scheidegger J, et al. Enlargement of regional lymph nodes in renal cell carcinoma is often not due to metastases. J Urol 1990;144:243.

172. Ramon J, Goldwasser B, Raviv G, et al. Long-term results of simple and radical nephrectomy for renal cell carcinoma. Cancer 1991;67:2506.

173. Kobayashi T, Nakamura E. Ogura K, Ogawa O. Incidence of adrenal involvement and assessing adrenal function in patients with renal cell carcinoma: Is ipsilateral adrenalectomy indispensable during radical nephrectomy? BJU Int 2005;95:526.

174. O'Brien WM, Lynch JH. Adrenal metastases by renal cell carcinoma. Incidence at nephrectomy. Urology 1987;29:605.

175. Robey EL. The adrenal gland and renal cell carcinoma: Is ipsilateral adrenalectomy a necessary component of radical nephrectomy? J Urol 1986;135:453.

176. Skinner DG, Colvin RB, Vermillion CD, et al. Diagnosis and management of renal cell carcinoma. A clinical and pathological study of 309 cases. Cancer 1971;28:1165.

177. Fuhrman SA, Lasky LC, Limas C. Prognostic significance of morphologic parameters in renal cell carcinoma. Am J Surg Pathol 1982;6:655.

178. Gudbjartsson T, Hardarson S. Petursdottir V, et al. Histological subtyping and nuclear grading of renal cell carcinoma and their implications for survival: A retrospective, nationwide study of 629 patients. Eur Urol 2005;48:593.

179. Medeiros LJ, Gelb AB, Weiss LM. Renal cell carcinoma. Prognostic significance of morphologic parameters in 121 cases. Cancer 1988;61:1639.

180. Grignon DJ, Ayala AG, El-Naggar A, et al. Renal cell carcinoma: A clinicopathologic and DNA flow cytometric analysis of 103 cases. Cancer 1989;64:2133.

181. Green LK, Ayala AG, Ro JY, et al. Role of nuclear grading in stage I renal cell carcinoma. Urology 1989;34:310.

182. Cheville JC, Blute ML, Zincke H, et al. Stage pT1 conventional (clear cell) renal cell carcinoma: Pathological features associated with cancer specific survival. J Urol 2001;166:453.

183. Lohse CM, Blute ML, Zincke H, et al. Comparison of standardized and nonstandardized nuclear grade of renal cell carcinoma to predict outcome among 2042 patients. Am J Clin Pathol 2002;118:877.

184. Ficarra V, Righetti R, Martignoni G, et al. Prognostic value of renal cell carcinoma nuclear grading: Multivariate analysis of 333 cases. Urol Int 2001;67:130.

185. Zisman A, Pantuck AJ, Figlin RA, Belldegrun AS. Validation of the UCLA integrated staging system for patients with renal cell carcinoma. J Clin Oncol 2001;19:3792.

186. Störkel S, Thoenes W, Jacobi GH, Lippold R. Prognostic parameters in renal cell carcinoma: A new approach. Eur Urol 1989;16:416.

187. Bernoni F, Ferri C, Benati A, et al. Sarcomatoid carcinoma of the kidney. J Urol 1987;137:25.

188. Tomera KM, Farrow GM, Lieber MM. Sarcomatoid renal carcinoma. J Urol 1983;130:657.

189. Ro JY, Ayala AG, Sella A, et al. Sarcomatoid renal cell carcinoma: A clinicopathologic study of 42 cases. Cancer 1987;59:516.

190. Macke RA, Hussain MB, Imray TJ, et al. Osteogenic and sarcomatoid differentiation of a renal cell carcinoma. Cancer 1985;56:2452.

191. Menzies DW. Carcinoma and rhabdomyosarcoma in the same kidney; a study in the classification and histogenesis of mixed renal tumours. Aust N Z J Surg 1955;25:214.

192. Bonsib SM, Fischer J, Plattner S, Fallon B. Sarcomatoid renal tumors: Clinicopathologic correlation of three cases. Cancer 1987;59:527.

193. de Peralta-Venturina M, Moch H, Amin M, et al. Sarcomatoid differentiation in renal cell carcinoma: A study of 101 cases. Am J Surg Pathol 2001;25:275.

194. de Riese W, Goldenberg K, Allhoff E, et al. Metastatic renal cell carcinoma (RCC): Spontaneous regression, long-term survival and late recurrence. Int Urol Nephrol 1991;23:13.

195. Katz SE, Schapira HE. Spontaneous regression of genitourinary cancer: An update. J Urol 1982;128:1.

196. Kavoussi LR, Levine SR, Kadmon D, Fair WR. Regression of metastatic renal cell carcinoma: A case report and literature review. J Urol 1986;135:1005.

197. Takáts LJ, Csapó Z. Death from renal carcinoma 37 years after its original recognition. Cancer 1966;19:1172.

198. McNichols DW, Segura JW, DeWeerd JH. Renal cell carcinoma: Long-term survival and late recurrence. J Urol 1981;126:17.

199. Elson PJ, Witte RS, Trump DL. Prognostic factors for survival in patients with recurrent or metastatic renal cell carcinoma. Cancer Res 1988;48:7310.

200. Tobisu K-I, Kakizoe T, Takai K, Tanaka Y. Prognosis in renal cell carcinoma: Analysis of clinical course following nephrectomy. Jpn J Clin Oncol 1989;19:142.

201. Figlin RA. Renal cell carcinoma: Management of advanced disease. J Urol 1999;151:381.

202. Gurney H, Larcos G, McKay M, et al. Bone metastases in hypernephroma, frequency of scapular involvement. Cancer 1989;64:1429.

203. Pantuck AJ, Zisman A, Belldegrun AS. The changing natural history of renal cell carcinoma. J Urol 2001;166:1611.

204. Kovacs G, Erlandson R, Boldog F, et al. Consistent chromosome 3p deletion and loss of heterozygosity in renal cell carcinoma. Proc Natl Acad Sci U S A 1988;85:1571.

205. Kovacs G, Szücs S, De Riese W, Baumgärtel H. Specific chromosome aberration in human renal cell carcinoma. Int J Cancer 1987;40:171.

206. Nordenson I, Ljungberg B, Roos G. Chromosomes in renal carcinoma with reference to intratumor heterogeneity. Cancer Genet Cytogenet 1988;32:35.

207. Teyssier JR, Ferre D. Chromosomal changes in renal cell carcinoma. No evidence for correlation with clinical stage. Cancer Genet Cytogenet 1990;45:197.

208. Walter TA, Berger CS, Sandberg AA. The cytogenetics of renal tumors: Where do we stand, where do we go? Cancer Genet Cytogenet 1989;43:15.

209. Yoshida MA, Ohyashiki K, Ochi H, et al. Cytogenetic studies of tumor tissue from patients with nonfamilial renal cell carcinoma. Cancer Res 1986;46:2139.

210. Bergerheim USR, Frisk B, Stellan B, et al. Del (3p) (p13p21) in renal cell adenoma and del (4p) (p14) in bilateral renal cell carcinoma in two unrelated patients with von Hippel-Lindau disease. Cancer Genet Cytogenet 1990;49:125.

211. Goodman MD, Goodman BK, Lubin MB, et al. Cytogenetic characterization of renal cell carcinoma in von Hippel-Lindau syndrome. Cancer 1990;65:1150.

212. Jordan DK, Patil SR, Divelbiss JE, et al. Cytogenetic abnormalities in tumors of patients with von-Hippel-Lindau disease. Cancer Genet Cytogenet 1989;42:227.

213. King CR, Schimke RN, Arthur T, et al. Proximal 3p deletion in renal cell carcinoma cells from a patient with von Hippel-Lindau disease. Cancer Genet Cytogenet 1987;27:345.

214. Seizinger BR, Rouleau GA, Ozelius LJ, et al. Von Hippel-Lindau disease maps to the region of chromosome 3 associated with renal cell carcinoma. Nature 1988;332:268.

215. Takahashi M, Kahnoski R, Gross D, et al. Familial adult renal neoplasia. J Med Genet 2002;39:1.

216. Sukosd F, Kuroda N, Beothe T, et al. Deletion of chromosome 3p14.2-p25 involving the VHL and FHIT genes in conventional renal cell carcinoma. Cancer Res 2003;63:455.

217. Smith SJ, Bosniak MA, Megibow AJ, et al. Renal cell carcinoma: Earlier discovery and increased detection. Radiology 1989; 170:699.

218. Hartman DS, Davis CJ Jr, Johns T, Goldman SM. Cystic renal cell carcinoma. Urology 1986;28:145.

219. Madewell JE, Goldman SM, Davis CJ Jr, et al. Multilocular cystic nephroma: A radiographic-pathologic correlation of 58 patients. Radiology 1983;146:309.

220. Murad T, Komaiko W, Oyasu R, Bauer K. Multilocular cystic renal cell carcinoma. Am J Clin Pathol 1991;95:633.

221. Nassir A, Jollimore J, Gupta R, et al. Multilocular cystic renal cell carcinoma: A series of 12 cases and review of the literature. Urol 2002;60:421.

222. Cheng WS, Farrow GM, Zincke H. The incidence of multicentricity in renal cell carcinoma. J Urol 1991;146:1221.

223. Bennington JL, Beckwith JB. Atlas of Tumor Pathology: Tumors of the Kidney, Renal Pelvis, and Ureter, 2nd series, fascicle 12. Bethesda, MD: Armed Forces Institute of Pathology, 1975:1.

224. Oberling C, Rivière M, Hagueneau F. Ultrastructure of the clear cells in renal carcinomas and its importance for the demonstration of their renal origin. Nature 1960;186:402.

225. Gokden N, Nappi O, Swanson PE, et al. Renal cell carcinoma with rhabdoid features. Am J Surg Pathol 2000;24:1329.

226. Koga S, Yamasaki A, Nishikido M, et al. Multiloculated renal cell carcinoma. Int Urol Nephrol 1991;23:423.

227. Sherman ME, Silverman ML, Balogh K, Tan SS-G. Multilocular renal cyst. Arch Pathol Lab Med 1987;111:732.

228. Taxy JB, Marshall FF. Multilocular renal cysts in adults, possible relationship to renal adenocarcinoma. Arch Pathol Lab Med 1983;107:633.

229. Zhou M, Roma A, Magi-Galluzzi C. The usefulness of immunohistochemical markers in the differential diagnosis of renal neoplasms. Clin Lab Med 2005;25:247.

230. Ordonez NG. The diagnostic utility of immunohistochemistry in distinguishing between mesothelioma and renal cell carcinoma: A comparative study. Hum Pathol 2004;35:697.

231. Avery AK, Beckstead J, Renshaw AA. Use of antibodies to RCC and CD10 in the differential diagnosis of renal neoplasms. Am J Surg Pathol 2000;24:203.

232. Bard RH, Lord B, Fromowitz F. Papillary adenocarcinoma of kidney. II. Radiographic and biologic characteristics. Urology 1982;19:16.

233. Amin MB, Corless CL, Renshaw AA, et al. Papillary (chromophil) renal cell carcinoma: Histomorphologic characteristics and evaluation of conventional pathologic prognostic parameters in 62 cases. Am J Surg Pathol 1997;21:621.

234. Mancilla-Jimenez R, Stanley RJ, Blath RA. Papillary renal cell carcinoma: A clinical, radiologic, and pathologic study of 34 cases. Cancer 1976;38:2469.

235. Renshaw AA, Corless CL. Papillary renal cell carcinoma. Histology and immunohistochemistry. Am J Surg Pathol 1995;19: 842.

236. Cheville JC, Lohse CM, Zincke H, et al. Comparison of outcome and prognostic features among histologic subtypes of renal cell carcinoma. Am J Surg Pathol 2003;27:612.

237. Delahunt B, Eble JN. Papillary renal cell carcinoma: A clinicopathologic and immunohistochemical study of 105 tumors. Mod Pathol 1997;10:537.

238. Lager DJ, Huston BJ, Timmerman TG, Bonsib SM. Papillary re-

nal tumors, morphologic, cytochemical, and genotypic features. Cancer 1995;76:669.

239. Zbar B, Glenn G, Lubensky I, et al. Hereditary papillary renal cell carcinoma: Clinical studies in 10 families. J Urol 1995;153:907.

240. Kovacs G. Papillary renal cell carcinoma, a morphologic and cytogenetic study of 11 cases. Am J Pathol 1989;134:27.

241. Kovacs G, Fuzesi L, Emanuel A, Kung H-F. Cytogenetics of papillary renal cell tumors. Genes Chromosome Cancer 1991;3: 249.

242. Van den Berg E, van der Hout AH, Oosterhuis JW, et al. Cytogenetic analysis of epithelial renal-cell tumors: Relationship with a new histopathological classification. Int J Cancer 1993;55:223.

243. Reznicek SB, Narayana AS, Culp DA. Cystadenocarcinoma of the kidney: A profile of 13 cases. J Urol 1985;134:256.

244. Ngan KW, Chuang CK. Solid variant of papillary renal cell carcinoma. Chang Gung Med J 2001;24:582.

245. Delahunt B, Eble JN, McCredie MRE, et al. Morphologic typing of papillary renal cell carcinoma: Comparison of growth kinetics and patient survival in 66 cases. Hum Pathol 2001;32:590.

246. Leroy X, Zini L, Leteurtre E, et al. Morphologic subtyping of papillary renal cell carcinoma: Correlation with prognosis and differential expression of MUC1 between the two subtypes. Mod Pathol 2002;15:1126.

247. Mejean A, Hopirtean V, Bazin JP, et al. Prognostic factors for the survival of patients with papillary renal cell carcinoma: Meaning of histological typing and multifocality. J Urol 2003;170:767.

248. Sanders ME, Mick R, Tomaszewski JE, Barr FG. Unique pattern of allelic imbalance distinguish type 1 from type 2 sporadic papillary renal cell carcinoma. Am J Pathol 2002;161:997.

249. Yang XJ, Tan M-H, Kim HL. A molecular classification of papillary renal cell carcinoma. Cancer Res 2005;65:5628.

250. McGregor DK, Khurana KK, Cao C, et al. Diagnosing primary and metastatic renal cell carcinoma. The use of the monoclonal antibody "renal cell carcinoma marker." Am J Surg Pathol 2001;25:1485.

251. Bonsib SM, Lager DJ. Chromophobe cell carcinoma: Analysis of five cases. Am J Surg Pathol 1990;14:260.

252. Crotty TB, Farrow GM, Lieber MM. Chromophobe renal cell carcinoma: Clinicopathologic features of 50 cases. J Urol 1995;154:964.

253. Thoenes W, Störkel S, Rumpelt H-J, et al. Chromophobe cell renal carcinoma and its variants: A report on 32 cases. J Pathol 1988;155:277.

254. Peyromaure M, Misrai V, Thiounn N, et al. Chromophobe renal cell carcinoma: Analysis of 61 cases. Cancer 2004;100:1406.

255. Kovacs A, Kovacs G. Low chromosome number in chromophobe renal cell carcinomas. Genes Chromosome Cancer 1992;4: 267.

256. Speicher MR, Schoell B, du Manoir S, et al. Specific loss of chromosomes 1, 2, 6, 10, 13, 17, and 21 in chromophobe renal cell carcinomas revealed by comparative genomic hybridization. Am J Pathol 1994;145:356.

257. Mohamed AN, Koppitch FC, El-Naggar M, et al. Chromosome analysis of six chromophobe renal cell carcinomas. J Urologic Pathol 1998;9:223.

258. Brunelli M, Eble JN, Zhang S, et al. Eosinophilic and classic chromophobe renal cell carcinomas have similar frequent losses of multiple chromosomes from among chromosomes 1, 2, 6, 10, and 17, and this pattern of genetic abnormality is not present in renal oncocytoma. Mod Pathol 2005;18:161.

259. Bonsib SM. Renal chromophobe cell carcinoma: The relationship between cytoplasmic vesicles and colloidal iron stain. J Urol Pathol 1996;4:9.

260. Störkel S, Steart PV, Drenckhahn D, Thoenes W. The human chromophobe cell renal carcinoma: Its probable relation to intercalated cells of the collecting duct. Virchows Archiv B Cell Pathol Incl Mol Pathol 1989;56:237.

261. Thoenes W, Baum H-P, Störkel S, Müller M. Cytoplasmic microvesicles in chromophobe cell renal carcinoma demonstrated by freeze fracture. Virchows Archiv B-Cell Pathol Incl Mol Pathol 1987;54:127.

262. Aizawa S, Kikuchi Y, Suzuki M, Furusato M. Renal cell carcinoma of lower nephron origin. Acta Pathol Jpn 1987;37:567.

263. Balslev E, Fischer S. Transitional cell carcinoma of the renal collecting tubules ("renal urothelioma"). Acta Pathol Microbiol Scand 1983;1:419.

264. Dimopoulos MA, Logothetis CJ, Markowitz A, et al. Collecting duct carcinoma of the kidney. Br J Urol 1993;71:388.

265. Fleming S, Lewi HJE. Collecting duct carcinoma of the kidney. Histopathology 1986;10:1131.

266. Kennedy SM, Merino MJ, Linehan WM, et al. Collecting duct carcinoma of the kidney. Hum Pathol 1990;21:449.

267. Rumpelt HJ, Störkel S, Moll R, et al. Bellini duct carcinoma: Further evidence for this rare variant of renal cell carcinoma. Histopathology 1991;18:115.

268. Chao D, Zisman A, Pantuck AJ, et al. Collecting duct renal cell carcinoma: Clinical study of a rare tumor. J Urol 2002;167:71.

269. Peyromaure M. Thiounn N, Scott F, et al. Collecting duct carcinoma of the kidney: A clinicopathologic study of 9 cases. J Urol 2003;170:1138.

270. Füzesi L, Cober M, Mittermayer C. Collecting duct carcinoma: Cytogenetic characterization. Histopathology 1992;21:155.

271. Polascik TJ, Cairns P, Epstein JI, et al. Distal nephron renal tumors: Microsatellite allelotype. Cancer Res 1996;56:1892.

272. Steiner G, Cairns P, Polascik TJ, et al. High-density mapping of chromosomal arm 1q in renal collecting duct carcinoma: Region of minimal deletion at 1q32.1–32.2. Cancer Res 1996;56:5044.

273. Baer SC, Ro JY, Ordonez NG, et al. Sarcomatoid collecting duct carcinoma: A clinicopathologic and immunohistochemical study of five cases. Hum Pathol 1993;24:1017.

274. Davis CJ Jr, Mostofi FK, Sesterhenn IA. Renal medullary carcinoma: The seventh sickle cell nephropathy. Am J Surg Pathol 1995;19:1.

275. Swartz MA, Schneider DT, Rodriguez R, et al. Renal medullary carcinoma: Clinical, pathologic, immunohistochemical, and genetic analysis with pathogenetic implications. Urol 2002;60:1083.

276. Stahlschmidt J, Cullinane C, Roberts P, Picton SV. Renal medullary carcinoma: Prolonged remission with chemotherapy, immunohistochemical characterization and evidence of bcr/abl rearrangement. Med Pediatr Oncol 1999;33:551.

277. Yang XJ, Sugimura J, Tretiakova MS, et al. Gene expression profiling of renal medullary carcinoma: Potential clinical relevance. Cancer 2004;100:976.

278. Parwani AV, Husain AN, Epstein JI, et al. Low-grade myxoid renal epithelial neoplasms with distal nephron differentiation. Hum Pathol 2001;32:506.

279. Rakozy C, Schmahl GE, Bogner S, Störkel S. Low-grade tubular-mucinous renal neoplasms: Morphologic immunohistochemical, and genetic features. Mod Pathol 2002;15:1162.

280. Srigley JR, Kapusta L, Reuter V, et al. Phenotypic, molecular and ultrastructural studies of a novel low-grade epithelial neoplasm possibly related to the loop of Henle [abstract]. Mod Pathol 2002;15:182A.

281. Hes O, Hora M, Perez-Montiel DM, et al. Spindle and cuboidal renal cell carcinoma, a tumor having frequent association with nephrolithiasis: Report of 11 cases including a case with hybrid conventional renal cell carcinoma/spindle and cuboidal renal cell carcinoma components. Histopathology 2002;41:549.

282. MacLennan GT, Farrow GM, Bostwick DG. Low-grade collecting duct carcinoma of the kidney: Report of 13 cases of low-grade mucinous tubulocystic renal carcinoma of possible collecting duct origin. Urol 1997;50:679.

283. Kuroda N, Nakamura S, Miyazaki E, et al. Low-grade tubular-mucinous renal neoplasm with neuroendocrine differentiation: A histological, immunohistochemical and ultrastructural study. Pathol Int 2004;54:201.

284. Amin MB, MacLennan GT, Paraf F, et al. Tubulocystic carcinoma of the kidney: Clinicopathologic analysis of 29 cases of a distinctive rare subtype of renal cell carcinoma [abstract]. Mod Pathol 2004;17:137A.

285. Bonsib SM, Eble JN. Renal pelvis and ureters. In: Bostwick DG, Eble JN, eds. Urologic Surgical Pathology. Saint Louis, MO: Mosby–Yearbook, 1996.

286. Badalament RA, O'Toole RV, Kenworthy P, et al. Prognostic fac-tors in patients with primary transitional cell carcinoma of the upper urinary tract. J Urol 1990;144:859.

287. Charbit L, Gendreau M-C, Mee S, Cukier J. Tumors of the upper urinary tract: 10 years of experience. J Urol 1991;146:1243.

288. Davis BW, Hough AJ, Gardner WA. Renal pelvic carcinoma: Morphological correlates of metastatic behavior. J Urol 1987;137:857.

289. Mufti GR, Gove JRW, Badenoch DF. Transitional cell carcinoma of the renal pelvis and ureter. Br J Urol 1989;63:135.

290. Olgac S, Mazumdar M, Dalbagni G, Reuter VE. Urothelial carcinoma of the renal pelvis: A clinicopathologic study of 130 cases. Am J Surg Pathol 2004;28:1545.

291. Fujimoto H, Tobisu K-I, Sakamoto M-I, et al. Intraductal tumor involvement and renal parenchymal invasion of transitional cell carcinoma in the renal pelvis. J Urol 1995;153:57.

292. Suster S, Robinson MJ. Spindle cell carcinoma of the renal pelvis. Immunohistochemical and ultrastructural study of a case demonstrating coexpression of keratin and vimentin intermediate filaments. Arch Pathol Lab Med 1989;113:404.

293. Spires SE, Banks ER, Cibull ML, et al. Adenocarcinoma of renal pelvis. Arch Pathol Lab Med 1993;117:1156.

294. Nativ O, Reiman HM, Lieber MM, Zincke H. Treatment of primary squamous cell carcinoma of the upper urinary tract. Cancer 1991;68:2575.

295. Guillou L, Duvoisin B, Chobaz C, et al. Combined small-cell and transitional cell carcinoma of the renal pelvis: A light microscopic, immunohistochemical and ultrastructural study of a case with literature review. Arch Pathol Lab Med 1993;117:239.

296. Grammatico D, Grignon DJ, Eberwein P, et al. Transitional cell carcinoma of the renal pelvis with choriocarcinomatous differentiation: Immunohistochemical and immunoelectron microscopic assessment of human chorionic gonadotropin production by transitional cell carcinoma of the urinary bladder. Cancer 1993;71:1835.

297. Hart AP, Brown R, Lechago J, Truong LD. Collision of transitional cell carcinoma and renal cell carcinoma: An immunohistochemical study and review of the literature. Cancer 1994;73:154.

298. Reuter VE, Presti JC Jr. Contemporary approach to the classification of renal epithelial tumors. Semin Oncol 2000;27:124.

299. Zisman A, Chao DH, Pantuck AJ, et al. Unclassified renal cell carcinoma: Clinical features and prognostic impact of a new histological subtype. J Urol 2002;168:950.

300. Goldblum JR, Lloyd RV. Primary renal carcinoid: Case report and literature review. Arch Pathol Lab Med 1993;117:855.

301. Maera A, Ovak Z, Lamovec J, Pohar-Marinek Z. Primary carcinoid of the kidney. Int Urol Nephrol 1993;25:129.

302. Raslan WF, Ro JY, Ordonez NG, et al. Primary carcinoid of the kidney: Immunohistochemical and ultrastructural studies of five patients. Cancer 1993;72:2660.

303. Isobe H, Takashima H, Higoshi N, et al. Primary carcinoid tumor in a horseshoe kidney. Int J Urol 2000;7:184.

304. Fetissof F, Lanson Y, Dubois MP, Jobard P. Carcinome rénal avec cellules argyrophiles. Ann Pathol 1984;4:361.

305. Capella C, Eusebi V, Rosai J. Primary oat cell carcinoma of the kidney. Am J Surg Pathol 1984;8:855.

306. Tètu B, Ro JY, Ayala AG, et al. Small cell carcinoma of the kidney. A clinicopathologic, immunohistochemical, and ultrastructural study. Cancer 1987;60:1809.

307. Eble JN. Unusual renal tumors and tumor-like conditions. In: Eble JN, ed. Tumors and Tumor-like Conditions of the Kidneys and Ureters. New York: Churchill Livingstone, 1990:145.

308. Bezirdjian DR, Tegtmeyer CJ, Leef JL. Intrarenal pheochromocytoma and renal artery stenosis. Urol Radiol 1981;3:121.

309. Rothwell DL, Vorstman B, Patton I, Allan JS. Intrarenal pheochromocytoma. Urology 1983;21:175.

310. Gohji K, Nakanishi T, Hara I, et al. Two cases of primary neuroblastoma of the kidney in adults. J Urol 1987;137:966.

311. Marley EF, Liapis H, Humphrey PA, et al. Primitive neuroectodermal tumor of the kidney: Another enigma. A pathologic immunohistochemical and molecular diagnostic study. Am J Surg Pathol 1997;21:354.

312. Jiminez RE, Folpe AL, Lapham RL, et al. Primary Ewing's sarcoma/primitive neuroectodermal tumor of the kidney: A

clinicopathologic and immunohistochemical analysis of 11 cases. Am J Surg Pathol 2002;26:320.

313. Gleeson MH, Bloom SR, Polak JM, et al. Endocrine tumour in kidney affecting small bowel structure, motility, and absorptive function. Gut 1971;12:773.

314. Resnick ME, Unterberger H, McLoughlin PT. Renal carcinoid producing the carcinoid syndrome. Med Times 1966;94:895.

315. Grignon DJ, Ro JY, Ayala AG, et al. Small cell carcinoma of the urinary bladder: A clinicopathologic analysis of 22 cases. Cancer 1992;69:527.

316. Bégin LR, Jamison BM. Renal carcinoid: A tumor of probable hindgut neuroendocrine phenotype. Report of a case and literature review. J Urol Pathol 1993;1:269.

317. Fetissof F, Benatre A, Dubois MP, et al. Carcinoid tumor occurring in a teratoid malformation of the kidney: An immunohistochemical study. Cancer 1984;54:2305.

318. Kojiro M, Ohishi H, Isobe H. Carcinoid tumor occurring in cystic teratoma of the kidney: A case report. Cancer 1976;38:1636.

319. Ghazi MR, Brown JS, Warner RS. Carcinoid tumor of kidney. Urology 1979;14:610.

320. Stahl RE, Sidhu GS. Primary carcinoid of the kidney, light and electron microscopic study. Cancer 1979;44:1345.

321. Green AJ, Sepp T, Yates JRW. Clonality of tuberous sclerosis hamartomas shown by non-random X-chromosome inactivation. Hum Genet 1996;97:240.

322. Bonetti F, Pea M. The perivascular epithelioid cell and related lesions. Adv Anat Pathol 1997;4:343.

323. Blute ML, Malek RS, Segura JW. Angiomyolipoma: Clinical metamorphosis and concepts for management. J Urol 1988;139:20.

324. Farrow GM, Harrison EG Jr, Utz DC, Jones DR. Renal angiomyolipoma: A clinicopathologic study of 32 cases. Cancer 1968;22:564.

325. Grignon DJ, Ro JY, Ayala AG. Mesenchymal tumors of the kidney. In: Eble JN, ed. Tumors and Tumor-like Conditions of the Kidneys and Ureters. New York: Churchill Livingstone, 1990: 123.

326. Hajdu SI, Foote FW Jr. Angiomyolipoma of the kidney: Report of 27 cases and review of the literature. J Urol 1969;102:396.

327. L'Hostis H, Deminiere C, Ferriere J-M, Coindre J-M. Renal angiomyolipoma: A clinicopathologic, immunohistochemical, and follow-up study of 46 cases. Am J Surg Pathol 1999;23:1011.

328. Stillwell TJ, Gomez MR, Kelalis PP. Renal lesions in tuberous sclerosis. J Urol 1987;138:477.

329. Chan KW, Chan KL. Spontaneous rupture of renal tumours presenting as surgical emergency. Br J Urol 1993;71:253.

330. Kerr LA, Blute ML, Ryu JH, et al. Renal angiomyolipoma in association with pulmonary lymphangioleiomyomatosis: Forme fruste of tuberous sclerosis? Urology 1993;41:440.

331. Peccatori I, Pitingolo F, Battini G, et al. Pulmonary lymphangioleiomyomatosis and renal papillary cancer: Incomplete expression of tuberous sclerosis? Nephrol Dial Transplant 1977;12:2740.

332. Scully RE, Mark EJ, McNeely WF, McNeely BU. Case records of the Massachusetts General Hospital. Weekly clinicopathological exercises. Case 18-1994. A 37-year-old woman with interstitial lung disease, renal masses, and a previous spontaneous pneumothorax (clinical conference). N Engl J Med 1994;330:1300.

333. Uzzo RG, Libby DM, Vaughan ED Jr, Levey SH. Coexisting lymphangioleiomyomatosis and bilateral angiomyolipomas in a patient with tuberous sclerosis. J Urol 1994;151:1612.

334. Glenthj A, Partoft S. Ultrasound-guided percutaneous aspiration of renal angiomyolipoma: Report of two cases diagnosed by cytology. Acta Cytol 1984;28:265.

335. Kutcher R, Rosenblatt R, Mitsudo S, et al. Renal angiomyolipoma with sonographic demonstration of extension into the inferior vena cava. Radiology 1982;143:755.

336. Hulbert JC, Graf R. Involvement of the spleen by renal angiomyolipoma: Metastasis or multicentricity. J Urol 1983;130:328.

337. Ro JY, Ayala AG, El-Naggar A, et al. Angiomyolipoma of kidney with lymph node involvement. DNA flow cytometric analysis. Arch Pathol Lab Med 1990;114:65.

338. Eble JN, Amin MB, Young RH. Epithelioid angiomyolipoma of the kidney: A report of five cases with a prominent and diagnos-

tically confusing epithelioid smooth muscle component. Am J Surg Pathol 1997;21:1123.

339. Martignoni G, Pea M, Bonetti F, et al. Carcinomalike monotypic epithelioid angiomyolipoma in patients without evidence of tuberous sclerosis. A clinicopathologic and genetic study. Am J Surg Pathol 1998;22:663.

340. Cibas ES, Goss GA, Kulke MH, et al. Malignant epithelioid angiomyolipoma ('Sarcoma ex angiomyolipoma') of the kidney: A case report. Am J Surg Pathol 2001;25:121.

341. Martignoni G, Bonnetti F, Pea M, et al. Renal disease in adults with TSC2/PKD1 contiguous gene syndrome. Am J. Surg Pathol 2002;26:198.

342. Taylor RS, Joseph DB, Kohaut EC, et al. Renal angiomyolipoma associated with lymph node involvement and renal cell carcinoma in patients with tuberous sclerosis. J Urol 1989;141: 930.

343. Jimenez RE, Eble JN, Reuter VE, et al. Concurrent angiomyolipoma and renal cell neoplasia: A study of 36 cases. Mod Pathol 2001;14:157.

344. Ferry JA, Malt RA, Young RH. Renal angiomyolipoma with sarcomatous transformation and pulmonary metastases. Am J Surg Pathol 1991;15:1083.

345. Ashfaq R, Weinberg AG, Albores-Saavedra J. Renal angiomyolipoma and HMB-45 reactivity. Cancer 1993;71:3091.

346. Kaiserling E, Kröber S, Xiao J-C, Schaumberg-Lever G. Angiomyolipoma of the kidney: Immunoreactivity with HMB-45. Light- and electron-microscopic findings. Histopathology 1994;25:41.

347. Sturtz CL, Dabbs DJ. Angiomyolipomas: The nature and expression of the HMB45 antigen. Mod Pathol 1994;7:842.

348. Zavala-Pompa A, Folpe AL, Jimenez RE, et al. Immunohistochemical study of microphthalmia transcription factor and tyrosinase in angiomyolipoma of the kidney, renal cell carcinoma, and renal and retroperitoneal sarcomas. Comparative evaluation with traditional diagnostic markers. Am J Surg Pathol 2001;25:65.

349. Weeks DA, Chase DR, Malott RL, et al. HMB-45 staining in angiomyolipoma, cardiac rhabdomyoma, other mesenchymal processes, and tuberous sclerosis-associated brain lesions. Int J Surg Pathol 1994;1:191.

350. Oesterling JE, Fishman EK, Goldman SM, Marshall FF. The management of renal angiomyolipoma. J Urol 1986;135:1121.

351. Lowe BA, Brewer J, Houghton DC, et al. Malignant transformation of angiomyolipoma. J Urol 1992;147:1356.

352. Addison NV, Peach B. Smooth muscle tumours of the kidney (report on two cases). Br J Urol 1966;38:382.

353. Edward HG, DeWeerd JH, Woolner LB. Renal hemangiomas. Mayo Clin Proc 1962;37:545.

354. Imazu T, Nishimura K, Tsujimura A, et al. Leiomyoma of the Kidney. Hinyokika Kiyo 1994;40:519.

355. Peterson NE, Thompson HT. Renal hemangioma. J Urol 1971; 105:27.

356. Haas CA, Resnick MI, Abdul-Karim FW. Cavernous hemangioma presenting as a renal hilar mass. J Urol 1998;160:2139.

357. Hull GW 3rd, Genega EM, Sogani PC. Intravascular capillary hemangioma presenting as a solid renal mass. J Urol 1999;162:784.

358. Anderson C, Knibbs DR, Ludwig ME, Ely MG III. Lymphangioma of the kidney: A pathologic entity distinct from solitary multilocular cyst. Hum Pathol 1992;23:465.

359. Pickering SP, Fletcher BD, Bryan PJ, Abramowsky CR. Renal lymphangioma: A cause of neonatal nephromegaly. Pediatr Radiol 1984;14:445.

360. Singer DRJ, Miller JDB, Smith G. Lymphangioma of kidney. Scott Med J 1983;28:293.

361. Nakai Y, Namba Y, Sugao H. Renal lymphangioma. J Urol 1999; 162:484–485.

362. Dineen MK, Venable DD, Misra RP. Pure intrarenal lipoma: Report of a case and review of the literature. J Urol 1984;132:104.

363. Colvin SH Jr. Certain capsular and subcapsular mixed tumors of the kidney herein called "capsuloma." J Urol 1942;48:585.

364. Reese AJM, Winstanley DP. The small tumor-like lesions of the kidney. Br J Cancer 1958;12:507.

365. Di Palma S, Giardini R. Leiomyoma of the kidney. Tumori 1988; 74:489.

366. Fligelstone LJ, Campbell F, Ray DK, Ress RWM. The Klippel-Trenaunay syndrome: A rare cause of hematuria requiring nephrectomy. J Urol 1994;151:404.

367. Schofield D, Zaatari GS, Gay BB. Klippel-Trenaunay and Sturge-Weber syndromes with renal hemangioma and double inferior vena cava. J Urol 1986;136:442.

368. Palmer FJ, Tynan AP. Leiomyoma of the kidney. J Urol 1974;112:22.

369. Grignon DJ, Ayala AG, Ro JY, et al. Primary sarcomas of the kidney: A clinicopathologic and DNA flow cytometric study of 17 cases. Cancer 1990;65:1611.

370. Farrow GM, Harrison EG Jr, Utz DC, ReMine WH. Sarcomas and sarcomatoid and mixed malignant tumors of the kidney in adults. Part I. Cancer 1968;22:545.

371. Srinivas V, Sogani PC, Hajdu SI, Whitmore WF Jr. Sarcomas of the kidney. J Urol 1984;132:13.

372. Vogelzang NJ, Fremgen AM, Guinan PD, et al. Primary renal sarcoma in adults: A natural history and management study by the American Cancer Society, Illinois division. Cancer 1993;71:804.

373. Cano JY, D'Altorio RA. Renal liposarcoma: Case report. J Urol 1976;115:747.

374. Khan AN, Gould DA, Shah SM, Mouasher YK. Primary renal liposarcoma mimicking angiomyolipoma on ultrasonography and conventional radiology. J Clin Ultrasound 1985;13:58.

375. Joseph TJ, Becker DI, Turton AF. Renal malignant fibrous histiocytoma. Urology 1991;37:483.

376. Kollias G, Giannopoulos T. Primary malignant fibrous histiocytoma of the kidney: Report of a case. J Urol 1987;138:400.

377. Muretto P, Lemma E, Grianti C, et al. Inflammatory malignant fibrous histiocytoma of the kidney: An immunohistochemical and ultrastructural study. Tumori 1985;71:147.

378. Grignon DJ, McIsaac GP, Armstrong RF, Wyatt JK. Primary rhabdomyosarcoma of the kidney: A light microscopic, immunohistochemical, and electron microscopic study. Cancer 1988;62:2027.

379. Argani P, Faria P, Epstein JI, et al. Primary renal synovial sarcoma: Molecular and morphologic delineation of an entity previously included among embryonal sarcomas of the kidney. Am J Surg Pathol 2000;24:1087.

380. Kim DH, Sohn JH, Lee MC, et al. Primary synovial sarcoma of the kidney. Am J Surg Pathol 2000;24:1097.

381. Eble JN, Young RH, Störkel S, Thoenes W. Primary osteosarcoma of the kidney: A report of three cases. J Urogenital Pathol 1991;1:83.

382. O'Malley FP, Grignon DJ, Shepherd RR, Harker LA. Primary osteosarcoma of the kidney: Report of a case studied by immunohistochemistry, electron microscopy, and DNA flow cytometry. Arch Pathol Lab Med 1991;115:1262.

383. Manfredi RA, Govoni AF, Sassoon J. A 15-year-old black girl with a left abdominal mass. Clin Imaging 1991;15:62.

384. Chow LT-C, Chan S-K, Chow W-H. Fine needle aspiration cytodiagnosis of leiomyosarcoma of the renal pelvis: A case report with immunohistochemical study. Acta Cytol 1994;38:759.

385. Eble JN. Cystic nephroma and cystic partially differentiated nephroblastoma: Two entities or one? Adv Anat Pathol 1994;1:99.

386. Boggs LK, Kimmelstiel P. Benign multilocular cystic nephroma: Report of two cases of so-called multilocular cyst of the kidney. J Urol 1956;76:530.

387. Castillo OA, Boyle ET Jr, Kramer SA. Multilocular cysts of kidney: A study of 29 patients and review of literature. Urology 1991;37:156.

388. Bonsib SM. Non-neoplastic diseases of the kidney. In: Bostwick DG, Eble JN, eds. Urologic Surgical Pathology. Saint Louis, MO: Mosby–Yearbook, 1996:1.

389. Durham JR, Bostwick DG, Farrow GM, et al. Mesoblastic nephroma of adulthood: Report of three cases. Am J Clin Pathol 1993;17:1029.

390. Pawade J, Soosay GN, Delprado W, et al. Cystic hamartoma of the renal pelvis. Am J Clin Pathol 1993;17:1169.

391. Truong LD, Williams R, Ngo T, et al. Adult mesoblastic nephroma: Expansion of the morphologic spectrum and review of the literature. Am J Surg Pathol 1988;22:827.

392. Adsay NV, Eble JN, Srigley JR, et al. Mixed epithelial and stromal tumor of the kidney. Am J Surg Pathol 2000;24:958.

393. Michal M, Hes O, Bisceglia M, et al. Mixed epithelial and stromal tumors of the kidney. A report of 22 cases. Virchows Arch 2004;445:359.

394. Pierson CR, Schober MS, Wallis T, et al. Mixed epithelial and stromal tumor of the kidney lacks the genetic alterations of cellular congenital mesoblastic nephroma. Hum Pathol 2001;32:513.

395. Michal M, Hes O, Havlicek F. Benign renal angiomyoadenomatous tumor: A previously unreported renal tumor. Ann Diagn Pathol 2000;4:3111.

396. Svec A, Hes O, Michal M, Zachoval R. Malignant mixed epithelial and stromal tumor of the kidney. Virchows Archiv 2001;439:700.

397. Adsay NV, Che M, Basturk O, et al. Sarcomatous transformation in mixed epithelial and stomal tumors of the kidney (malignant MEST) [abstract]. Mod Pathol 2004;17:135A.

398. Nakagawa T, Kanai Y, Fujimoto H, et al. Malignant mixed epithelial and stromal tumours of the kidney: A report of the first two cases with a fatal outcome. Histopathology 2004;44:302.

399. Kihara I, Kitamura S, Hoshino T, et al. A hitherto unreported vascular tumor of the kidney: A proposal of "juxtaglomerular cell tumor." Acta Pathol Jpn 1968;18:197.

400. Robertson PW, Klidjian A, Harding LK, et al. Hypertension due to a renin-secreting renal tumour. Am J Med 1967;43:963.

401. Martin SA, Mynderse LA, Lager DJ, Cheville JC. Juxtaglomerular cell tumor. A clinicopathologic study of four cases and review of the literature. Am J Clin Pathol 2001;116:854.

402. Bonsib SM, Hansen KK. Juxtaglomerular cell tumors: A report of two cases with negative HMB 45 immunostaining. J Urol Pathol 1998;9:61.

403. Valdés G, Lopez JM, Martinez P, et al. Renin-secreting tumor: Case report. Hypertension 1980;2:714.

404. Tètu B, Vaillancourt L, Camilleri J-P, et al. Juxtaglomerular cell tumor of the kidney: Report of two cases with a papillary pattern. Hum Pathol 1993;24:1168.

405. Camilleri J-P, Hinglais N, Bruneval P, et al. Renin storage and cell differentiation in juxtaglomerular cell tumors: An immunohistochemical and ultrastructural study of three cases. Hum Pathol 1984;15:1069.

406. Mai KT. Giant renomedullary interstitial cell tumor. J Urol 1994;151:986.

407. Warfel KA, Eble JN. Renomedullary interstitial cell tumors. Am J Clin Pathol 1985;83:262.

408. Zimmermann A, Luscieti P, Flury B, et al. Amyloid-containing renal interstitial cell nodules (RICNs) associated with chronic arterial hypertension in older age groups. Am J Pathol 1981;105:288.

409. Farrow GM, Harrison EG Jr, Utz DC. Sarcomas and sarcomatoid and mixed malignant tumors of the kidney in adults. III. Cancer 1968;22:555.

410. Ferry JA, Harris NL, Papanicolaou N, Young RH. Lymphoma of the kidney: A report of 11 cases. Am J Surg Pathol 1995;19:134.

411. Osborne BM, Brenner M, Weitzner S, Butler JJ. Malignant lymphoma presenting as a renal mass: Four cases. Am J Surg Pathol 1987;11:375.

412. Silber SJ, Chang CY. Primary lymphoma of kidney. J Urol 1973;110:282.

413. Dimopoulos MA, Moulopoulos LA, Costantinides C, et al. Primary renal lymphoma: A clinical and radiological study. J Urol 1996;155:1865.

414. Da'as N, Polliack A, Cohen Y, et al. Kidney involvement and renal manifestations in non-Hodgkin's lymphoma and lymphocytic leukemia: A retrospective study in 700 patients. Eur J Haematol 2001;67:158.

415. Kandel LB, McCullough DL, Harrison LH, et al. Primary renal lymphoma. Does it exist? Cancer 1987;60:386.

416. Igel TC, Engen DE, Banks PM, Keeney GL. Renal plasmacytoma: Mayo Clinic experience and review of the literature. Urology 1991;37:385.

417. Jaspan T, Gregson R. Extra-medullary plasmacytoma of the kidney. Br J Radiol 1984;57:95.
418. Bracken RB, Chica G, Johnson DE, Luna M. Secondary renal neoplasms: An autopsy study. South Med J 1979;72:806.
419. Wagle DG, Moore RH, Murphy GP. Secondary carcinomas of the kidney. J Urol 1975;114:30.
420. Melato M, Laurino L, Bianchi P, Faccini L. Intraglomerular metastases: A possibly maldiagnosed entity. Zentralbl Allg Pathol 1991;137:90.
421. Naryshkin S, Tomaszewski JE. Acute renal failure secondary to carcinomatous lymphatic metastases to kidneys. J Urol 1991; 146:1610.
422. Grignon DJ, Eble JN. Adenomatoid metaplasia of the epithelium of Bowman's capsule. J Urol Pathol 1993;1:293.

# Index